Nursing Leadership & Management

SECOND EDITION

Nursing Leadership & Management

SECOND EDITION

Patricia Kelly, RN, MSN

Professor Emerita
Purdue University Calumet
School of Nursing
Hammond, Indiana

and

Faculty
Health Education Systems, Inc. (HESI)
Houston, Texas

DELMAR
CENGAGE Learning

Australia • Brazil • Japan • Korea • Mexico • Singapore • Spain • United Kingdom • United States

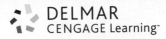

**Nursing Leadership & Management,
Second Edition**
Patricia Kelly

Vice President, Health Care Business Unit:
    William Brottmiller

Director of Learning Solutions: Matthew Kane

Acquisitions Editor: Tamara Caruso

Senior Product Manager: Elisabeth F. Williams

Editorial Assistant: Jennifer Waters

Director of Marketing: Jennifer McAvey

Marketing Channel Manager: Michele McTighe

Marketing Coordinator: Chelsey Iaquinta

Director of Technology: Laurie K. Davis

Director of Production: Carolyn Miller

Content Project Manager: Stacey Lamodi

Senior Art Director: Jack Pendleton

Library of Congress Control Number: 2007018346

ISBN-13: 978-1-4180-5026-9

ISBN-10: 1-4180-5026-1

Delmar
Executive Woods
5 Maxwell Drive
Clifton Park, NY 12065
USA

Cengage Learning is a leading provider of customized learning solutions with office locations around the globe, including Singapore, the United Kingdom, Australia, Mexico, Brazil, and Japan. Locate your local office at **international.cengage.com/region**

Cengage Learning products are represented in Canada by Nelson Education, Ltd.

For your course and learning solutions, visit **delmar.cengage.com**

Visit our corporate website at **www.cengage.com**

Notice to the Reader

Publisher does not warrant or guarantee any of the products described herein or perform any independent analysis in connection with any of the product information contained herein. Publisher does not assume, and expressly disclaims, any obligation to obtain and include information other than that provided to it by the manufacturer. The reader is expressly warned to consider and adopt all safety precautions that might be indicated by the activities described herein and to avoid all potential hazards. By following the instructions contained herein, the reader willingly assumes all risks in connection with such instructions. The publisher makes no representations or warranties of any kind, including but not limited to, the warranties of fitness for particular purpose or merchantability, nor are any such representations implied with respect to the material set forth herein, and the publisher takes no responsibility with respect to such material. The publisher shall not be liable for any special, consequential, or exemplary damages resulting, in whole or part, from the readers' use of, or reliance upon, this material.

Printed in the United States of America
2 3 4 5 6 7 11 10 09 08

CONTENTS

UNIT II
LEADERSHIP AND MANAGEMENT OF THE INTERDISCIPLINARY TEAM

CONTRIBUTORS

Rinda Alexander, PhD, RN, CS
Professor Emeritus, Nursing
Purdue University Calumet
Hammond, Indiana
and
Professor of Nursing
University of Florida
College of Nursing
Gainesville, Florida
and
Nursing Consultant
Health Care and Administration
Schererville, Indiana
Chapter 5: Evidence-Based Health Care

Margaret M. Anderson, EdD, RN, CNAA
Professor of Nursing and Chair
School of Nursing and Health Professions
Northern Kentucky University
Highland Heights, Kentucky
Chapter 13: Change, Innovation, and Conflict Management

Ida M. Androwich, PhD, RN, BC, FAAN
Professor and Director, Health Systems Management
Niehoff School of Nursing
Loyola University Chicago
Maywood, Illinois
Chapter 4: Basic Clinical Health Care Economics
Chapter 5: Evidence-Based Health Care
Chapter 10: Strategic Planning and Organizing Patient Care

Crisamar Javellana-Anunciado, MSN, APRN, BC
Inpatient Diabetes Nurse Practitioner
Sharp Chula Vista Medical Center
Chula Vista, California
Chapter 11: Effective Team Building

Anne Bernat, RN, MSN, CNAA
Vice President of Patient Care Services (Retired)
Arlington, Virginia
Chapter 15: Effective Staffing

Nancy Braaten, RN, MS
Adult Health Clinical Nurse Specialist
Clinical Analyst, Nursing Information Systems
Northeast Health Acute Care Division
Troy, New York
Chapter 19: Patient and Health Care Education

Sister Kathleen Cain, OSF, JD
Attorney
Franciscan Legal Services
Baton Rouge, Louisiana
Chapter 23: Legal Aspects of Health Care

Martha Desmond, RN, MS, Post Masters Certificate in Nursing Education
Clinical Nurse Specialist in Critical Care
Northeast Health Acute Care Division
Troy, New York
and
Adjunct Faculty
Excelsior College
Albany, New York
Chapter 19: Patient and Health Care Education

Joan Dorman, RN, MS, CEN
Clinical Assistant Professor
Purdue University Calumet
Hammond, Indiana
Chapter 24: Ethical Aspects of Health Care

Mary L. Fisher, PhD, RN, CNAA, BC
Professor and Department Chair
Environments for Health
Indiana University School of Nursing
Indianapolis, Indiana
Chapter 15: Effective Staffing

Corinne Haviley, RN, MS
Director of Medicine Nursing
Northwestern Memorial Hospital
Chicago, Illinois
Chapter 14: Budget Concepts for Patient Care

Paul Heidenthal, MS
Consultant
Accenture
Austin, Texas
Chapter 19: Patient and Health Care Education

Karen Houston RN, MS
Director of Quality and Continuum of Care
Albany Medical Center
Albany, New York
Chapter 20: Managing Outcomes Using an Organizational Quality Improvement Model

Ronda G. Hughes, PhD, MHS, RN
Senior Health Scientist Administrator
Senior Advisor on End-of-Life Care
Center for Primary Care, Prevention, and Clinical Partnerships
Agency for Healthcare Research and Quality
Rockville, Maryland
Chapter 2: The Health Care Environment

Mary Anne Jadlos, MS, APRN, BC, CWOCN
Coordinator—Wound, Skin and Ostomy Nursing Service
Northeast Health Acute Care Division
Samaritan Hospital
Troy, New York
and
Albany Memorial Hospital
Albany, New York
Chapter 21: Evidence-Based Strategies to Improve Patient Care Outcomes

Josette Jones, RN, PhD, BC
Assistant Professor
School of Nursing
School of Informatics
Indianapolis, Indiana
Chapter 6: Nursing and Health Care Informatics

Stephen Jones, MS, RNC, PNP, ET
Pediatric Clinical Nurse Specialist/Nurse Practitioner
The Children's Hospital at Albany Medical Center
Albany, New York
Founder, Pediatric Concepts
Averill Park, New York
Chapter 28: Emerging Opportunities

Patricia Kelly, RN, MSN
Professor Emerita
Purdue University Calumet
Hammond, Indiana
and
Faculty
Health Education Systems, Inc. (HESI)
Houston, Texas
Chapter 2: The Health Care Environment
Chapter 16: Delegation of Patient Care
Chapter 31: NCLEX Preparation and Professionalism

Glenda B. Kelman PhD, APRN, BC
Associate Professor and Chair
Nursing Department
The Sage Colleges
Troy, New York
and

Acute Care Nurse Practitioner
Wound, Skin, and Ostomy Nursing Service
Northeast Health Acute Care Division
Samaritan Hospital
Troy, New York
and
Albany Memorial Hospital
Albany, New York
Chapter 21: Evidence-Based Strategies to Improve Patient Care Outcomes

Mary Elaine Koren, RN, PhD
Assistant Professor of Nursing
Northern Illinois University School of Nursing
DeKalb, Illinois
Chapter 30: Healthy Living: Balancing Personal and Professional Needs

Lyn LaBarre, MS, RN
Patient Care Service Director
Critical Care, Specialty and Emergency Services
Albany Medical Center
Albany, New York
Chapter 29: Your First Job

Linda Searle Leach, PhD, RN, CNAA
Assistant Professor
UCLA School of Nursing
Los Angeles, California
Nurse Scientist
Kaiser Permanente
Southern California Nursing Research Program
Pasadena, California
Chapter 1: Nursing Leadership and Management

Camille B. Little, MS, RN, BSN
Instructional Assistant Professor (Retired)
Mennonite College of Nursing
Illinois State University
Normal, Illinois
Chapter 24: Ethical Aspects of Health Care

Sharon Little-Stoetzel, RN, MS
Associate Professor of Nursing
Graceland University
Independence, Missouri
Chapter 22: Decision Making and Critical Thinking

Dr. Miki Magnino-Rabig, PhD, RN
Assistant Professor
University of St. Francis
Joliet, Illinois
Chapter 29: Your First Job

Patsy Maloney, RN, BC, EdD, MSN, MA, CNAA
Associate Professor/Director Continuing Nursing Education
Pacific Lutheran University
Tacoma, Washington
Chapter 9: Politics and Consumer Partnerships
Chapter 12: Power
Chapter 18: Time Management and Setting Patient Care Priorities

Richard J. Maloney, BS, MA, MAHRM, EdD
Principal
Policy Governance Associates
Tacoma, Washington
Chapter 9: Politics and Consumer Partnerships
Chapter 12: Power

Maureen T. Marthaler RN, MS
Associate Professor
School of Nursing
Purdue University Calumet
Hammond, Indiana
Chapter 16: Delegation of Patient Care

Judith W. Martin, RN, JD
Attorney
Franciscan Legal Services
Baton Rouge, Louisiana
Chapter 23: Legal Aspects of Health Care

Edna Harder Mattson, RN, BN, BA(CRS), MDE, CTSN, CAE
President
Canadian Nursing Tutorial Services
Winnipeg, Manitoba, Canada
Chapter 27: Career Planning

Mary McLaughlin, RN, MBA
Assistant Director for Case Management and Social Work
Albany Medical Center
Albany New York
Chapter 20: Managing Outcomes Using an Organizational Quality Improvement Model

Terry W. Miller, PhD, RN
Dean and Professor
Pacific Lutheran University
School of Nursing
Tacoma, Washington
Chapter 9: Politics and Consumer Partnerships
Chapter 12: Power

Leslie H. Nicoll, PhD, MBA, RN, BC
President and Owner
Maine Desk, LLC
Portland, Maine
Chapter 6: Nursing and Health Care Informatics

Laura J. Nosek, PhD, RN
Doctor of Nursing Practice Faculty
The Bolton School of Nursing
Case Western Reserve University
Cleveland, Ohio
and
Adjunct Associate Professor of Nursing
Marcella Niehoff School of Nursing
Loyola University Chicago
Chicago, Illinois
and
Course Facilitator
Excelsior College
Albany, New York
Chapter 4: Basic Clinical Health Care Economics

Amy Androwich O'Malley MSN, RN
Education and Program Manager
Medela, Inc.
McHenry, Illinois
Chapter 5: Evidence-Based Health Care
Chapter 10: Strategic Planning and Organizing Patient Care

Kristine E. Pfendt, RN, MSN
Assistant Professor of Nursing
Northern Kentucky University
Highland Heights, Kentucky
Chapter 13: Change, Innovation, and Conflict Management

Chad S. Priest, RN, BSN, JD
Attorney
Baker and Daniels, LLP
Adjunct Lecturer
Indiana University School of Nursing
Indianapolis, Indiana
Chapter 23: Legal Aspects of Health Care

Jacklyn Ludwig Ruthman, PhD, RN
Associate Professor
Bradley University
Peoria, Illinois
Chapter 8: Personal and Interdisciplinary Communication

Patricia M. Schoon, MPH, RN
Associate Professor
Department of Nursing
Coordinator
Center of Excellence for Women and Health
College of St. Catherine
St. Paul, Minnesota
Chapter 7: Population-Based Health Care Practice

Kathleen F. Sellers PhD, RN
Associate Professor
School of Nursing and Health Systems
SUNY Institute of Technology
Utica, New York
Chapter 17: Organization of Patient Care

Susan Abaffy Shah, RN, MS, Post Masters Certificate in Nursing Education
Adult Health Clinical Nurse Specialist
Northeast Health Acute Care Division
Albany, New York
Chapter 19: Patient and Health Care Education

Maria R. Shirey, MS, MBA, RN, CNAA, BC, FACHE
Principal
Shirey and Associates
Evansville, Indiana
and
Adjunct Associate Professor
University of Southern Indiana
College of Nursing and Health Professions
Evansville, Indiana
Chapter 3: Organizational Behavior and Magnet Hospitals

Janice Tazbir RN, MS, CCRN
Associate Professor of Nursing
Purdue University Calumet
School of Nursing
Hammond, Indiana
Chapter 26: Collective Bargaining

Karen Luther Wikoff, RN, PhD
Assistant Professor
California State University, Stanislaus
Turlock, California
Chapter 25: Culture, Generational Differences, and Spirituality

REVIEWERS

Deborah Berkey, RN, MS
Professor
College of Nursing
Kent State University
Kent, Ohio

Sara L. Clutter, RN, MSN
Assistant Professor
Department of Nursing
Waynesburg College
Waynesburg, Pennsylvania

Deborah Kumer Coltrane, RN, MSN, MBA
Director of Marketing and Education
Pocket Nurse
Pittsburgh, Pennsylvania
and
Faculty
MBA/MSN and RN/BSN Programs
Waynesburg College
Waynesburg, Virginia

Karen Daley, RN, PhD
Assistant Professor
Department of Nursing
Western Connecticut State University
Stamford, Connecticut

Margaret S. Hamilton, RN, DNS
Clinical Associate Professor
School of Nursing
Florida International University
Miami, Florida

Karen Hartman, RN, PhD
Associate Professor
Murray State University
Murray, Kentucky

Marlene Huff, RN, PhD
Associate Professor
College of Nursing
The University of Akron
Akron, Ohio

Phyllis King, RN, C, MSN
Associate Professor of Nursing
Milligan College
Milligan College, Tennessee

Camille Little, MS, RN, BSN
Instructional Assistant Professor (Retired)
Mennonite College of Nursing
Illinois State University
Pleasant Hill, Missouri

James A. Metcalf, PhD
Professor
College of Health and Human Services
George Mason University
Fairfax, Virginia

Larry Purnell, RN, PhD, FAAN
Professor
College of Nursing
University of Delaware
Newark, Delaware

Rosemary Ricks-Saulsby, RN, MS, MA, PhD
Assistant Professor
Deparment of Nursing
Chicago State University
Chicago, Illinois

Stacey Sherwin, RN, PhD
Faculty
Nursing Department
Salish Kootenai College
Pablo, Montana

Barbara Warner, RN, CAN, DNSc
Chairperson
Nursing and Allied Health
Atlantic Cape Community College
Mays Landing, New Jersey

Mary A. Wcisel, RN, MSN
Assistant Professor, Nursing
Saint Mary's College
Notre Dame, Indiana

Antoinette Willsea, RN, MSN
Assistant Professor
R. H. Daniel School of Nursing
Piedmont College
Demorest, Georgia

Kelly Witter, RN, MSN
Program Director
Great Oaks School of Nursing
Bath, Indiana

PREFACE

Nurses play a crucial role in protecting patient safety and providing quality health care. A National Academy of Sciences, Institute of Medicine (IOM) report found that "how we are cared for by nurses affects our health, and sometimes can be a matter of life and death . . . nurses are indispensable to our safety" (Institute of Medicine, 2004). This finding was confirmed by an emerging body of research showing that nurses are much more likely than any other health professional to recognize, interrupt, and correct errors that are often life threatening (Rothschild et al., 2006), that higher levels of baccalaureate-prepared nurses in hospital settings reduce mortality and failure to rescue rates (Aiken et al., 2003), and that inadequate nurse staffing levels may lead to a higher incidence of complications and inadequate care (Aiken, Clarke, Cheung, Sloane, & Silber, 2002; Joint Commission, 2002; Needleman, Buerhaus, Mattke, Stewart, & Zelevinsky, 2002).

Another IOM report, *Health Professions Education: A Bridge to Quality* (2003), noted that nurses and other health professionals are currently not prepared to provide the highest quality and safest care possible. The IOM report concluded that education for the health professions is in need of a major overhaul and recommended that all programs that educate and train health professionals should adopt five core competencies. These core competencies are the ability to (1) provide patient-centered care, (2) work in interdisciplinary teams, (3) employ evidence-based practice, (4) apply quality improvement, and (5) utilize informatics (IOM, 2003).

The American Association of Colleges of Nursing (AACN) convened a task force to identify essential baccalaureate core competencies that should be achieved by professional nurses to assure high quality and safe patient care. These competencies include knowledge and skills related to critical thinking, including the application of evidence-based knowledge and quality improvement; health care systems and policies that contribute to safe and high-quality patient outcomes; communication, especially with the interdisciplinary team and shift handoff communication (JC, 2006); illness and disease management of individuals and communities; ethics; and information and health care technologies. These AACN competencies are essential for the nursing leader and manager of the future.

Nursing Leadership & Management, second edition, is designed to help beginning nurses address the IOM and AACN competencies. The text prepares beginning nurse leaders and managers for modern health care. It also reviews information from the Leapfrog Group, Thomson Medstat, the National Quality Forum, and the Institute for Healthcare Improvement (IHI), all focused on quality improvement of patient care.

The chapter contributors to this second edition include nurse educators, nursing faculty, clinical nurse specialists, nurse lawyers, nurse practitioners, wound and ostomy care nurses, nurse entrepreneurs, and others. These contributors are from the United States and Canada, thus allowing them to offer a broad view of nursing leadership and management. There are contributors from California, Florida, Illinois, Indiana, Kentucky, Maryland, Minnesota, Missouri, New York, Ohio, Texas, Washington, and Manitoba, Canada. Interviews with Loretta Ford, Tim Porter-O'Grady, and many other nurse experts are also included.

ORGANIZATION

Nursing Leadership & Management, second edition, consists of 31 chapters organized in a conceptual framework. This conceptual framework outlines the nurse's leadership and management responsibilities to the patient, to the health care team, to the institution, and to self. The five units of the framework provide beginning nurse leaders and managers with the knowledge needed in today's health care environment.

- Unit I introduces nursing leadership and management, including the health care environment, organizational behavior and magnet hospitals, basic clinical health care economics, evidence-based health care, nursing and health care informatics, and population-based health care practice.

- Unit II discusses leadership and management of the interdisciplinary team, including personal and interdisciplinary communication; politics and consumer partnerships; strategic planning and organizing patient care; effective team building; power; and change, innovation, and conflict management.

- Unit III discusses leadership and management of patient-centered care, including budget concepts for patient care, effective staffing, delegation of patient care, organization of patient care, time management and setting patient care priorities, and patient and health care education.

- Unit IV discusses quality improvement of patient outcomes, including managing outcomes utilizing an organizational quality improvement model; evidence-based strategies to improve patient care outcomes; decision making and critical thinking; legal aspects of health care; ethical aspects of health care; and culture, generational differences, and spirituality.

- Unit V discusses leadership and management of self and the future, including collective bargaining, career planning, emerging opportunities, your first job, healthy living: balancing personal and professional needs, and NCLEX preparation and professionalism.

Discussion of timely topics, such as the Joint Commission's National Patient Safety Goals, nurse-sensitive outcomes, evidence-based practice, information technology, Health Insurance Portability and Accountability Act (HIPAA), magnet hospitals, interdisciplinary teamwork, nurse entrepreneurs, quality and performance improvement, health care marketing, and population-based health care, is included throughout the chapters. Because many topics overlap and are intertwined, some topics appear in more than one chapter.

The second edition of *Nursing Leadership & Management* builds on the strengths of the first edition and embraces user feedback and the ever-changing health care landscape. Important changes include the following:

- A new conceptual framework to encourage reader understanding and development of key concepts of nursing leadership and management.

- A new chapter on NCLEX preparation and professionalism.

- A new chapter on organizational behavior and magnet hospitals.

- A new section on innovation included in the chapter on change and conflict management.

- A new section on generational differences appears in the chapter on culture and spirituality.

- All chapters are revised and strengthened, including those on evidence-based care, population-based health care, informatics, interdisciplinary teamwork, quality improvement, patient and health care education, balancing personal and professional needs, delegation, ethics, legal aspects, culture and spirituality, and change.

- The chapter on evidence-based strategies to improve patient care outcomes is enhanced with new Institute for Healthcare Improvement (IHI) guidelines.

- Detail has been added to legal charts on nursing malpractice to enhance learning.

- Enhanced content is included on patient safety, patient satisfaction, health care marketing, independent nursing practice, and nurse-sensitive outcomes.

- Stronger exercises and more Case Studies, Review Questions, and Activities are included for development of key concepts by the entry-level nurse.

CHAPTER FEATURES

Several standard chapter features are utilized throughout the text, which provide the reader with a consistent format for learning and an assortment of resources for understanding and applying the knowledge presented. Features include the following:

- Health care or nursing quote related to chapter content

- Photo that sets the scene for the chapter

- Objectives that state the chapter's learning goals

- Opening scenario, a mini entry-level nursing case study that relates to chapter, with two to three critical thinking questions

- Key Concepts, a listing of the primary understandings the reader is to take from the chapter

- Key Terms listing of important new terms presented in the chapter

- Review Questions, several NCLEX style questions at the end of chapter content

- Review Activities to apply chapter content to entry-level nursing situations

- Exploring the Web computer activities
- References
- Suggested Readings

Special elements are sprinkled throughout the chapters to enhance learning and encourage critical thinking and application:

- Evidence from the Literature with synopsis of key findings from nursing and health care literature
- Real World Interviews with nursing leaders and managers, including nursing staff, clinicians, administrators, risk managers, faculty, nursing and medical practitioners, patients, unlicensed assistive personnel (UAP), lawyers, and hospital administrators
- Critical Thinking exercises regarding an ethical, legal, cultural, spiritual, delegation, or quality improvement nursing or health care topic
- Case Studies to provide the entry-level nurse with a clinical nursing leadership/management situation calling for critical thinking to solve an open-ended problem

Additional materials can be found on the new **online companion** which accompanies this text, including the following:

- Discussion of opening scenario
- Discussion of Critical Thinking exercises
- Discussion of Case Studies
- Answers to Review Questions
- Discussion of Review Activities
- Web links
- Chapter Summaries

ELECTRONIC CLASSROOM MANAGER (ECM)

Order # 1-4180-5028-8

An *Electronic Classroom Manager* is available to adopters of the text. It is designed to assist faculty in presenting to nursing students the essential skills and information that are needed to help them secure a position as a beginning nursing manager and leader. The ECM will assist faculty in planning and developing their programs and classes for the most efficient use of time and resources. The ECM includes four elements:

1. An instructor manual offers practical resources for presenting material in the text and includes suggested answers to the Text Review Questions, Review Activities, and Case Studies.
2. PowerPoint templates serve as guides for presentation in the classroom.
3. A test bank offers approximately 750 questions in multiple-choice format.
4. Transition Guide to help you switch your notes from the first to the second edition of the text.

REFERENCES

Aiken, L. H., Clarke, S. P., Cheung, R. B., Sloane, D. M., Sochalski, J., & Silber, J. H. (2002, October 23). Hospital nurse staffing and patient mortality, nurse burnout, and job dissatisfaction. *Journal of the American Medical Association, 288,* 1987–1993.

Aiken, L. H., Clarke, S. P., Cheung, R. B., Sloane, D. M., & Silber, J. H. (2003, September 24). Educational levels of hospital nurses and surgical patient mortality. *Journal of the American Medical Association, 290,* 1617–1623.

American Association of Colleges of Nursing. (1998). *The essentials of baccalaureate education for professional nursing practice.* Washington, DC: Author.

American Association of Colleges of Nursing. (2006). *Hallmarks of quality and patient safety in baccalaureate nursing education.* Washington, DC: Author.

Institute of Medicine. (2003). *Health professions education: A bridge to quality.* Washington, DC: National Academies Press.

Institute of Medicine. (2004). *Keeping patients safe: Transforming the work environment of nurses.* Washington, DC: National Academies Press.

Joint Commission (JC). (2002). *Health care at the crossroads: Strategies for addressing the evolving nursing crisis.* Chicago: Author.

Joint Commission (JC). (2006). National Patient Safety Goals. Retrieved August 25, 2006, from http://www.jointcommission.org

Needleman, J., Buerhaus, P., Mattke, S., Stewart, M., & Zelevinsky, K. (2002, May 30). Nurse-staffing level and the quality of care in hospitals. *The New England Journal of Medicine, 346,* 1715–1722.

Rothschild, J. M., Hurley, A. C., Landrigan, C. P., Cronin, J. W., Martill-Waldrop, K., Foskitt, C. et al. (2006, February). Recovering from medical errors: The critical care nursing safety net. *Joint Commission Journal on Quality and Patient Safety, 32*(2), 63–72.

ACKNOWLEDGMENTS

A book such as this requires great effort and the coordination of many people with various areas of expertise. I would like to thank all of the contributors for their time and effort in sharing their knowledge gained through years of experience in both the clinical and academic setting. All of the contributing authors worked within tight time frames to accomplish their work. Special thanks go to Robyn Pozza, Attorney, Austin, Texas, for the legal charts and her contributions to the legal chapter. Thanks also to Dr. Patricia Padjen, Madison, Wisconsin; Dr. Susan Morrison, Houston, Texas; Steve Jones, Albany, New York; and Deborah Ennis, Etters, Pennsylvania, for their critical review and input into select chapters. I especially thank Jo Reidy and Corinne Haviley, Chicago, Illinois, for their help in arranging some of the photographs for the text.

I thank the reviewers for their time spent critically reviewing the manuscript and providing the valuable comments that have enhanced this text. Special thanks go to my Dad and Mom, Ed and Jean Kelly; my sisters, Tessie Dybel and Kathy Milch; my Aunt Pat and Uncle Bill Kelly (who convinced me to start writing); my Aunt Verna and Uncle Archie Payne; my nieces, Natalie Dybel Bevil, Melissa Milch Arredondo, and Stacey Milch; my nephew, John Milch; my grand nephew, Brock Bevil; my grand niece, Reese Bevil; and my dear friends, Patricia Wojcik, Florence Lebryk, Lee McGuan, and Dolores Wynen, who have supported me through this book and much of my life. Special thanks to my wonderful nursing friends, Zenaida Corpuz, Dr. Mary Elaine Koren, Dr. Barbara Mudloff, Dr. Patricia Padjen, Jane McKeon, Kerrie Ellingsen, and especially to Gerri Kane, Janice Klepitch, Sylvia Komyatte, and Julie Martini, as well as Anna Fizer, Judy Ilijanich, Trudy Keilman, Judy Rau, Lillian Rau, and Mary Kay Moredich, who have supported me throughout this book and during our forty-five years together as nurses. Special thanks to my faculty mentors, Dr. Imogene King, Dr. Joyce Ellis, and Nancy Weber.

I would like to acknowledge and sincerely thank the team at Delmar Cengage Learning who have worked to make this book a reality. Beth Williams, Senior Product Manager, is a great person who has worked tirelessly and brought knowledge, guidance, humor, and attention to help keep me motivated and on track throughout the project. Thanks also to Jane Woodruff for all the computer support.

ABOUT THE AUTHOR

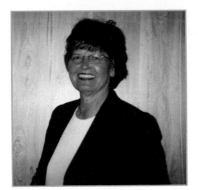

Patricia Kelly earned a Diploma in Nursing from St. Margaret Hospital School of Nursing, Hammond, Indiana; a Baccalaureate in Nursing from DePaul University in Chicago, Illinois; and a Master's Degree in Nursing from Loyola University in Chicago, Illinois. Pat is Professor Emerita, Purdue University Calumet, Hammond Indiana. She has worked as a staff nurse, school nurse, and nurse educator. Pat has traveled extensively in the United States, Canada, and Puerto Rico, teaching conferences for the Joint Commission, Resource Applications, Pediatric Concepts, and Kaplan, Inc. She currently teaches NCLEX-RN reviews for Health Education Systems, Inc. (HESI) and works part time as an emergency room staff nurse in Chicago, Illinois.

Pat was Director of Quality Improvement at the University of Chicago Hospitals and Clinics. She has taught at Wesley-Passavant School of Nursing, Chicago State University, and Purdue University Calumet, Hammond Indiana. She has taught Fundamentals of Nursing, Adult Nursing, Nursing Leadership and Management, Nursing Issues, Nursing Trends, Quality Improvement, and Legal Aspects of Nursing. Pat is a member of Sigma Theta Tau, the American Nurses Association, and the Emergency Nurses Association. She is listed in *Who's Who in American Nursing, 2000 Notable American Women,* and the *International Who's Who of Professional and Business Women.*

Pat has served on the Board of Directors of Tri City Mental Health Center, St. Anthony's Home, and the Quality Connection Journal. She is the author of *Nursing Leadership & Management,* Delmar Cengage Learning (2003), *Essentials of Nursing Leadership & Management,* Delmar Cengage Learning (2004), and *Delegation of Nursing Care,* Delmar Cengage Learning (2005). Pat contributed a chapter on "Preparing the Undergraduate Student and Faculty to Use Quality Improvement in Practice" to *Improving Quality,* Second Edition, by Claire Gavin Meisenheimer. She has written several articles, including "Chest X-Ray Interpretation" and many articles on quality improvement. Pat has served as a Disaster Volunteer for the American Red Cross and as a volunteer at several church food pantries in Austin, Texas, and Chicago, Illinois. Throughout most of her career, she has taught nursing at the university level. Pat has been licensed and has worked in many states over her career, including Indiana, Illinois, Wisconsin, Oklahoma, New York, and Pennsylvania. Pat may be contacted at patkh1@aol.com.

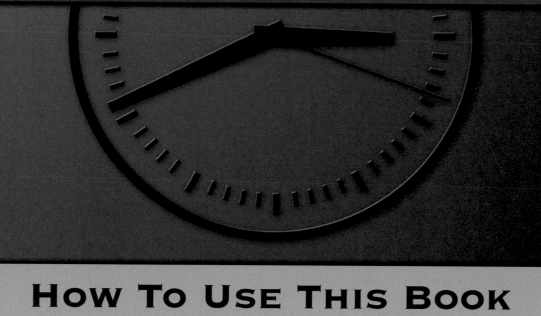

HOW TO USE THIS BOOK

Quote

A nursing or health care theorist quote gives a professional's perspective regarding the topic at hand; read this as you begin each new chapter and see whether your opinion matches or differs, or whether you are in need of further information.

Objectives

These goals indicate to you the performance-based, measurable objectives that are targeted for mastery upon completion of the chapter.

OBJECTIVES

Upon completion of this chapter, the reader should be able to:

1. Identify concepts of management.
2. Identify the management process.
3. Outline 10 roles that managers fulfill in an organization.
4. Relate management theories.
5. Summarize motivation theories.
6. Differentiate between leadership and management.
7. Distinguish characteristics of effective leaders.

Opening Scenario

Ed Harley was admitted to the cardiac observation unit earlier in the day. He had been diagnosed previously with heart disease and had experienced episodes of ventricular arrhythmias. His cardiologist had determined the need to change his antiarrhythmic medication to reduce the side effects Mr. Harley was experiencing. That evening, while Mr. Harley was talking to his wife on the phone, and as his nurse Maria, was walking to his bedside, he suddenly stopped talking and went into ventricular tachycardia and cardiac arrest. Maria reacted immediately and started cardiopulmonary resuscitation (CPR). Unable to use the

This mini case study with related critical thinking questions should be read prior to delving into the chapter; it sets the tone for the material to come and helps you identify your knowledge base and perspective.

Case Study

These short cases with related questions present a beginning clinical nursing management situation calling for judgment, decision making, or analysis in solving an open-ended problem. Familiarize yourself with the types of situations and settings you will later encounter in practice, and challenge yourself to devise solutions that will result in the best outcomes for all parties, within the boundaries of legal and ethical nursing practice.

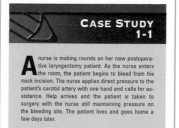

CASE STUDY 1-1

A nurse is making rounds on her new postoperative laryngectomy patient. As the nurse enters the room, the patient begins to bleed from his neck incision. The nurse applies direct pressure to the patient's carotid artery with one hand and calls for assistance. Help arrives and the patient is taken to surgery with the nurse still maintaining pressure on the bleeding site. The patient lives and goes home a few days later.

How does nursing leadership and management on a patient care unit ensure good patient care in an emergency?

How can you develop your leadership and management skills to improve your ability to care for a group of patients?

Evidence from the Literature

Study these key findings from nursing and health care research, theory, and literature, and ask yourself how they will influence your practice. Do you see ways in which your nursing could be affected by these literature findings and research results? Do you agree with the conclusions drawn by the author?

EVIDENCE FROM THE LITERATURE

Citation: Gordon, S. (2006). What do nurses really do? *Topics in Advanced Practice Nursing, 6*(1). Retrieved February 2, 2006 from http://www.medscape.com/viewarticle/520714.

Discussion: In this article by Suzanne Gordon, a journalist and author who writes about nursing, nurses are called upon to do a better job of accurately describing what nurses do and how they use expert knowledge acquired through scientific and technical mastery. She says, "What do nurses do? They save lives, prevent complications, prevent suffering, and save money." Her message to nurses is that there is a reason that the public has such little understanding of nursing and the importance of our work. The reason is twofold: traditional stereotypes about nursing cloud the reality of nursing as it is currently practiced, and nurses have been patterned to describe their contribution to health care in self-sacrificing and anonymous ways.

Implications for Practice: Nurses need to be clear about why it is important for the public to know what and how nurses contribute to health care. This article is an important vehicle from which nurses can begin to examine their own words and ways of discussing what nurses do and reflect upon the historical religious and societal practices that interfere with a clear, accurate, and realistic image of modern nursing. What nurses often think of as their ordinary work is really quite extraordinary. Nurses use scientific knowledge, expert judgment, and complex skills to make critical decisions that affect patient outcomes. Nurses need to be able to articulate how they do their work and the difference it makes.

CRITICAL THINKING

As we continue to learn more about what is involved in assuring quality, identifying patient safety errors, improving health care systems to avert subsequent errors, and applying evidence to daily practice, nurse managers and leaders are in critical positions to improve the quality of health care in their organizations. To realize this, many organizations will need to change the way they practice, train staff, reward high performance, and assess progress.

What can each staff member do to improve the quality of care, especially the safety of patient care?

How can we work toward a culture of continual improvement for those issues and situations that cause errors and almost lead to errors?

How much control do nurses have in identifying errors and reporting them?

What can you do to improve the quality of care afforded in your organization?

Critical Thinking

Ethical, cultural, spiritual, legal, delegation, and performance improvement considerations are highlighted in these boxes. Before beginning a new chapter, page through and read the Critical Thinking sections and jot down your comments or reactions, then see whether your perspective changes after you complete the chapter.

Real World Interviews

Interviews with well-known nursing leaders, such as Dr. Loretta Ford, Dr. Tim Porter O'Grady, and others are included as well as interviews with nursing and medical practitioners, hospital administrators, staff, patients, and family members. As you read these, ask yourself whether you had ever considered that individual's point of view on the given topic. How would knowing another person's perspective affect the care you deliver?

REAL WORLD INTERVIEW

It was a Monday. The Emergency Department was very busy as usual. A new patient, a sixty-nine year-old African-American female was admitted by ambulance following a motor vehicle accident. I went to assess this patient and noted that blood was dripping from a small laceration on her forehead. She was awake, alert, and oriented. She had no pain or nausea. She told me that she was feeling fine, but I noticed that her lips and mouth were pale. I told the charge nurse that I believed that the patient's hemoglobin level was below 5 and I asked her to please tell the physician to come to the room soon to assess the patient. As I believed this patient was not stable, I immediately took the lead and inserted a large-bore intravenous heplock in her vein and collected blood samples for a CBC, BMP, PT, PTT, INR, and type and cross match, just in case. I started a liter of 0.9% normal saline intravenous fluid and connected the patient to the cardiac monitor as well as to the blood pressure, pulse, and pulse oximeter monitors. The patient now began to complain of nausea. At this point, the doctor had not come to see the patient yet. I went and told the doctor to please come to the patient's room and assess her now. I told him that the patient was bleeding and that I believed that her hemoglobin would be reported as below 5. He then came to the room and assessed the patient. He removed the head laceration dressing which was now soaked in blood. He noted a 1-inch laceration on her forehead that was still bleeding. He sutured the wound and finally ordered the CBC. I asked him if he was sure he only wanted the CBC. He said, yes. When the CBC results came back, the patient's hemoglobin was 3.8. I felt good about my assessment and intervention with this patient. The physician then ordered a type and cross match for 4 units of blood and a CT of the head. After the patient received two units of blood, she was transferred to the ICU.

Nirmala Joseph, RN
Staff Nurse
Chicago, Illinois

KEY CONCEPTS

- Nurses are leaders and make a difference through their contributions of expert knowledge and leadership to health care organizations. Leadership development is a necessary component of preparation as a health care provider.

- All nurses are leaders because they have expert knowledge that they contribute to coordinate and provide patient care. Building expertise by gaining experience, setting goals to direct experiential learning, and gaining clinical skills and judgment are some of the ways that new nurses develop as leaders.

Key Concepts

This bulleted list serves as a review and study tool for you as you complete each chapter.

Key Terms

Study this list prior to reading the chapter, and then again as you complete a chapter to test your true understanding of the terms and concepts covered. Make a study list of terms you need to focus on to thoroughly appreciate the material of the chapter.

KEY TERMS

administrative principles
autocratic leadership
bureaucratic organization
consideration
contingency theory
democratic leadership
employee-centered
  leadership

formal leadership
Hawthorne effect
informal leader
initiating structure
job-centered leaders
knowledge workers
laissez-faire leadership
leader-member relations

REVIEW QUESTIONS

1. Management as a process that is used today by nurses or nurse managers in health care organizations is best described as
   A. scientific management.
   B. decision making.
   C. commanding and controlling others using hierarchical authority.
   D. planning, organizing, coordinating, and controlling.

2. According to Hersey and Blanchard and House, a participative leadership style is appropriate for employees who
   A. are not able to get the task done and are less mature.
   B. are able to contribute to decisions about getting the work done.
   C. are unable and unwilling to participate.
   D. need direction, structure, and authority.

Review Questions

These questions will challenge your comprehension of objectives and concepts presented in the chapter and will allow you to demonstrate content mastery, build critical thinking skills, and achieve integration of the concepts. Multiple choice, Multiple-Multiple, and all other types of NCLEX-RN questions are included.

Review Activities

These thought-provoking activities at the close of a chapter invite you to approach a problem or scenario critically and apply the knowledge you have gained.

REVIEW ACTIVITIES

1. Although it is difficult to modify the structure of health care, what could you do to implement a system to continually modify the process of health care delivery to improve health care quality in your organization?

2. What are strategies to ensure patient access to appropriate health care services in public and private health care agencies?

3. How can the five IOM health professions competencies for quality care be achieved in the current workplace?

EXPLORING THE WEB

Search the Web, checking the following sites.

- Emerging Leader: *www.emergingleader.com*

- Leadership Skills Development: *www.impactfactory.com* Search for leadership.

- LeaderValues: *www.leader-values.com*

- Don Clark's Big Dog Leadership: *http://management.about.com* Under topics, click Leadership.

- American Association of Critical Care Nurse's Standards for Establishing and Sustaining Healthy Work Environments: *www.aacn.org* Under Priority Issues, click Healthy Work Environments.

Exploring the Web

Internet activities encourage you to use your computer and reasoning skills to search the Web for additional information on quality and nursing leadership and management.

References

Evidence-based research, theory, and general literature, as well as nursing, medical, and health care sources, are included in these lists; refer to them as you read the chapter and verify your research.

REFERENCES

Aiken, L. H., Clarke, S. P., Sloane, D. M., Sochalski, J., & Silber, J. H. (2002). Hospital nurse staffing, patient mortality, nurse burnout, and job dissatisfaction. *Journal of American Medical Association, 288*(16), 1987–1993.

American Association of Critical Care Nurses. (2003). Written testimony to the IOM Committee on work environment of nurses and patient safety. Retrieved February 15, 2007, from http://www.aacn.org/

American Association of Critical Care Nurses. (2004). *AACN standards for establishing and sustaining healthy work environments: A journey of excellence.* Retrieved February 15, 2007, from http://www.aacn.org/aacn/hwe.nsf/vwdoc/HWEHomePage

Argyris, C. (1964). *Integrating the individual and the organization.* Hoboken, NJ: Wiley.

Barker, A. (1990). *Transformational nursing leadership: A vision for the future.* Baltimore: Williams & Wilkins.

Suggested Readings

These entries invite you to pursue additional topics, articles, and information in related resources.

SUGGESTED READINGS

Baggett, M. M., & Baggett, F. B. (2005, July). Move from management to high-level leadership. *Nursing Management, 36*(7), 12.

Bass, B. (1998). *Transformational leadership: Industrial, military, and educational impact.* Mahwah, NJ: Erlbaum.

Bass, B. M., & Riggo, R. (2006). *Transformational leadership* (2nd ed.). Mahwah, NJ: Erlbaum.

Buckingham, M., & Coffman, C. (2001). *First Break All the Rules.* New York: Simon & Schuster.

Calpin-Davies, P. J. (2003, Jan.). Management and leadership: A dual role in nursing education. *Nursing Education Today, 23*(1), 3–10.

Photos, Tables, and Figures

These items illustrate key concepts.

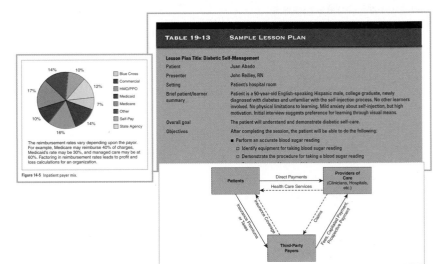

The reimbursement rates vary depending upon the payor. For example, Medicare may reimburse 40% of charges. Medicaid's rate may be 30%, and managed care may be at 60%. Factoring in reimbursement rates leads to profit and loss calculations for an organization.

Figure 14-5 Inpatient payer mix.

TABLE 19-13   SAMPLE LESSON PLAN

Lesson Plan Title: Diabetic Self-Management

Patient	Juan Abado
Presenter	John Reilley, RN
Setting	Patient's hospital room
Brief patient/learner summary	Patient is a 50-year-old English-speaking Hispanic male, college graduate, newly diagnosed with diabetes and unfamiliar with the self-injection process. No other learners involved. No physical limitations to learning. Mild anxiety about self-injection, but high motivation. Initial interview suggests preference for learning through visual means.
Overall goal	The patient will understand and demonstrate diabetic self-care.
Objectives	After completing the session, the patient will be able to do the following:

■ Perform an accurate blood sugar reading
  □ Identify equipment for taking blood sugar reading
  □ Demonstrate the procedure for taking a blood sugar reading

Figure 2-2 Economic Relationships in the Health Care Delivery System. (Adapted by Reinhardt, U. E. (1989). What can Americans learn from Europeans? *Health Care Financing Review* (Supplement), 97–103.)

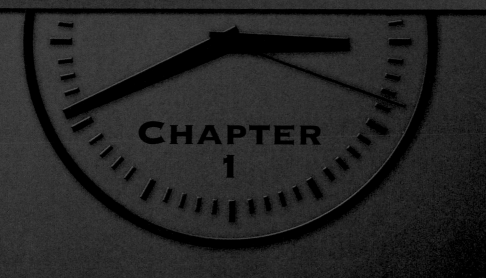

CHAPTER 1

Nursing Leadership and Management

Linda Searle Leach, PhD, RN, CNAA

Leadership is the essence of professionalism and should be considered an essential component of all nurse and other professional roles (Joyce Clifford, PhD, RN, FAAN).

OBJECTIVES

Upon completion of this chapter, the reader should be able to:

1. Identify concepts of management.
2. Identify the management process.
3. Outline 10 roles that managers fulfill in an organization.
4. Relate management theories.
5. Summarize motivation theories.
6. Differentiate between leadership and management.
7. Distinguish characteristics of effective leaders.
8. Identify leadership theories.
9. Apply knowledge of leadership theory in carrying out the nurse's role as a leader.

these leaders are highly visible and hold high-profile positions. We need leaders though at all levels of the organization. Leadership is a basic competency needed by all health professionals. Leadership development is a necessary part of the preparation of health care providers.

Nurses make a critical difference every day in the lives of their patients and patients' families, yet nurses believe those accomplishments are part of their ordinary work. Nurses are leaders, and by using their expert knowledge they manage and meet patient care needs.

Leadership and management are different. Leadership influences or inspires the actions and goals of others. One does not have to be in a position of authority to demonstrate leadership. Not all leaders are managers. Bennis and Nanus (1985) popularized the phrase, "leaders are people who do the right thing; managers are people who do things right." Both roles are crucial but different. Bennis stated that he often observes people in top positions doing the wrong things well. It is important to avoid thinking that leadership is important and management is insignificant. People need to be managed as well as inspired and led. Leadership is part of management, not a substitute for it. We need both.

This chapter lays the groundwork for the development of knowledge about nursing leadership and management. Many concepts touched on in this chapter will be developed in depth in other chapters of the book. The chapter introduces the process of management and explains management theories and functions. Management is defined, and current trends are discussed. This chapter also discusses motivation and leadership and provides a framework to differentiate leadership and management. Leadership characteristics, styles of leadership, and leadership theories are described.

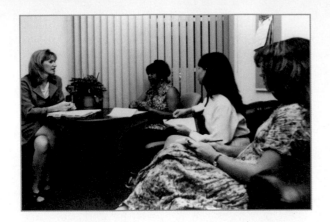

Ed Harley was admitted to the cardiac observation unit earlier in the day. He had been diagnosed previously with heart disease and had experienced episodes of ventricular arrhythmias. His cardiologist had determined the need to change his antiarrhythmic medication to reduce the side effects Mr. Harley was experiencing. That evening, while Mr. Harley was talking to his wife on the phone, and as his nurse Maria, was walking to his bedside, he suddenly stopped talking and went into ventricular tachycardia and cardiac arrest. Maria reacted immediately and started cardiopulmonary resuscitation (CPR). Unable to use the phone to call for help, she gave a precordial thump to his chest. Normal sinus rhythm appeared on the monitor before anyone else could respond to the code. Mr. Harley was then transferred to the coronary care unit (CCU).

Maria had been a registered nurse (RN) less than one year at the time, and although she had participated in code arrests a few times, she had never witnessed one occur right before her eyes. Her knowledgeable action saved this patient's life. In nursing, CPR is a mandatory skill and considered part of a nurse's ordinary work. Yet it is quite extraordinary work.

Everything had happened so quickly that evening that Maria did not have a chance to talk to the patient before he was transferred. She entered his room the next morning in CCU, as the sun was just rising. As he awoke, Maria spent that quiet time with him. While he embraced the start of a new day, his thoughts were intense. What he chose to share was this acknowledgment: "You saved my life. Thank you." This precious moment was a celebration of both of their lives.

What leadership characteristics did Maria demonstrate in preventing a nurse-sensitive outcome of cardiac arrest?

Why is Maria considered a leader, even though she is not in a leadership or management position?

Why is leadership important at all levels throughout a health care organization?

Professionals use their expertise and specialized knowledge to perform leadership roles. Many people think leaders are only top corporate executives and administrators, political representatives, military generals, or those who head organizations. This is because

DEFINITION OF MANAGEMENT

Management is defined as a process of coordinating actions and allocating resources to achieve organizational goals. Descriptive research (Mintzberg, 1973; McCall, Morrison, & Hanman, 1978; Hales, 1986) about what managers do has been a helpful way to expand our understanding of management. Managers often seem to work at a hectic pace and sustain that effort through long hours, frequently working without breaks. Yukl (1998) says that this reflects a preference by people in management positions who become adept at continuously seeking information and are constantly engaged in interactions with others who need information, help, guidance, or approval. Nurses at the bedside are continually helping patients, other practitioners, and staff meet their needs for such information, help, guidance, or approval. The typical manager is on the go. Research by McCall, Morrison, and

REAL WORLD INTERVIEW

The University of California at Los Angeles (UCLA) Medical Center was designated as a Magnet hospital by the American Nurses Credentialing Center (ANCC). I believe we earned this honor because of the quality of nurses and the quality of care these nurses have always provided to our patients and families. Some hospitals are faced with a vacancy rate of 20% and at times even higher. At UCLA's Medical Center, the nursing vacancy rate is very low, ranging from 2 to 5%. This is a satisfying place for nurses to work because it's a place with participatory leadership where there is a high degree of respect among colleagues. We don't seem to have issues between physicians and nurses. Perhaps being an academic institution helps. We share knowledge and experience, and we're surrounded by experts. If there's a problem, it's easy to reach out and ask, 'What do you think?' Education is a priority that we support, and the value of this is reflected in knowledgeable and competent nurses. Magnet status is nursing's top honor. It is accepted as the national gold standard in nursing excellence. This reflects the UCLA staff's compassion and commitment to creating an extraordinary environment of healing.

Heidi Crooks, RN, MA
Chief Nursing Executive
Senior Associate Director of Operations and Patient Care Services
Los Angeles, California

Hanman (1978) showed that the daily activities of managers are diverse and fast paced with regular interruptions. Priority activities are integrated among inconsequential ones. In the scope of one morning, a nurse manager may engage in serious decisions about a critically ill patient, a staff or patient complaint, a shortage of nurse staffing, and so forth. A nurse manager's work is driven by problems that emerge in random order and that have a range of importance and urgency. These circumstances create an image of the nurse manager as a "firefighter" involved in immediate and operational concerns. A significant proportion of a manager's time is spent in interaction with others, and more of the work is concerned with handling information than in making decisions (McCall et al., 1978). Nurse managers constantly interact with other members of a health care administrative team. This administrative team can include nurses, various health care practitioners, unit staff, and staff from other departments who share information and assure that quality patient outcomes are achieved.

MANAGERIAL ROLES

One of the most frequently referenced taxonomies of managerial roles is from an in-depth, month-long study of five chief executives by Henry Mintzberg. A **taxonomy** is a system that orders principles into a grouping or classification. Mintzberg's observations led to the identification of three categories of managerial roles: (1) information-processing role, (2) interpersonal role, and (3) decision-making role (Mintzberg, 1973).

A role includes behaviors, expectations, and recurrent activities within a pattern that is part of the organization's structure (Katz & Kahn, 1978). Specific or distinct roles are part of each of the three categories of managerial roles. The information processing roles are monitor, disseminator, and spokesperson, each of which is used to manage the information needs that people have. The interpersonal roles are figurehead, leader, and liaison, and each of these is used to manage relationships with people. The decisional roles are the entrepreneur, disturbance handler, allocator of resources, and negotiator roles that managers use to take action when making a decision.

THE MANAGEMENT PROCESS

In the early 1900s, an emphasis on management as a discipline emerged with a focus on the science of management and a view that management is an art of accomplishing things through people (Follet, 1924). Henri Fayol, a

CRITICAL THINKING 1-1

Note an administrative team during your clinical rotation. Who is part of the team? Does it include nurse managers, nursing staff, nurse clinicians, nurse practitioners, other health care practitioners, and staff from pharmacy, physical therapy, dietary, and so on? Does the team change depending on the problem it is working on?

manager, wrote a book in 1916 called *General and Industrial Management.* He described the functions of planning, organizing, coordinating, and controlling as the **management process** (Fayol, 1916/1949). His work has become a classic in the way that we define the process of managing. Two other individuals, Gulick and Urwick, in some part as a result of their esteemed status as informal advisers to President Franklin D. Roosevelt, served to define the management process according to seven principles (Henry, 1992). Their principles form the acronym POSDCORB, which stands for planning, organizing, staffing, directing, coordinating (CO), reporting, and budgeting (Gulick & Urwick, 1937; Henry, 1992). Their work is also considered to be a classic description of management functions and is still a relevant description of how the management process is carried out today.

More recently, Yukl (1998) and colleagues (Kim & Yukl, 1995; Yukl, Wall, & Lepsinger, 1990) described 13 management functions that address two broad aspects of the management process: managing the work and managing relationships. The management functions for managing the work are planning and organizing, problem solving, clarifying roles and objectives, informing, monitoring, consulting, and delegating. The management functions for managing relationships are networking,

supporting, developing and mentoring, managing conflict and team building, motivating and inspiring, and recognizing and rewarding.

The amount of time managers spend on particular roles or functions varies by the level of their position in an organization, ranging from the first-level positions, to the middle-level positions, to the executive-level positions. A first-level managerial role or function in health care organizations is the nurse manager at the clinical bedside. First-level nurse managers spend the majority of time directly managing patient care and supervising others as they deliver care. The next highest percentage of their time is spent in planning. The rest of first-level nurse managers' assignments take 10% or less of their time.

In contrast, middle-level nurse managers, often called nursing unit managers or nursing directors, spend less time in direct supervision and more time in the other managerial roles or functions, particularly, planning and coordinating. At the highest level of the organization, usually described as the executive level, planning and being a generalist are greatly expanded role functions. Direct supervision is not a major job assignment as it is in the other two levels. Nurses in executive-level roles in health care organizations usually have the title Chief Nurse Executive or, in acute care hospitals, their title may be Vice President of Patient Care Services.

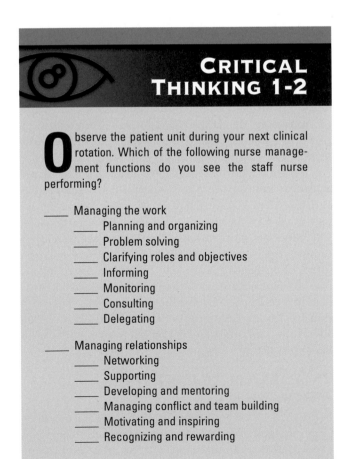

CRITICAL THINKING 1-2

Observe the patient unit during your next clinical rotation. Which of the following nurse management functions do you see the staff nurse performing?

_____ Managing the work
    _____ Planning and organizing
    _____ Problem solving
    _____ Clarifying roles and objectives
    _____ Informing
    _____ Monitoring
    _____ Consulting
    _____ Delegating

_____ Managing relationships
    _____ Networking
    _____ Supporting
    _____ Developing and mentoring
    _____ Managing conflict and team building
    _____ Motivating and inspiring
    _____ Recognizing and rewarding

MANAGEMENT THEORIES

The current management practices have evolved from earlier theories. Management practices were actually a part of the governance in ancient Samaria and Egypt as far back as 3000 B.C. (Daft & Marcic, 2001). Most of our current understanding of management, however, is based on the classical theories of management that were introduced in the 1800s during the industrial age as factories developed. Classical theory is based on the need to address efficiency in organizations. Classical theory is the oldest theory and is sometimes referred to as traditional management theory. The classical perspective includes three subfields of management: scientific management, bureaucratic management, and administrative management (Wren, 1979; Daft & Marcic, 2001) (Table 1-1).

SCIENTIFIC MANAGEMENT

While practicing managers, such as Fayol, who was mentioned earlier, were describing the functions of managers, a man named Frederick Taylor was focusing his attention on the operations within an organization by exploring production at the worker level. Taylor is acknowledged as the father of scientific management for his use

TABLE 1-1	MANAGEMENT THEORIES

Management Theory	Key Aspects
Scientific Management *Gulick & Urwick (1937),* *Mooney (1939), Taylor (1911)*	Focus is on goals and productivity. The organization is viewed as a machine to be run efficiently to increase production. Managers must closely supervise the work to assure maximum efficiency. Workers must have proper tools and equipment. There is a focus on training the worker to work most efficiently, and performance incentives are used. Time and motion studies are the vehicle for determining how to do and organize the work in the most efficient manner.
Bureaucratic Management *Weber (1864, reported in* *Mommsen, W. J. 1992)*	Focus is on superior-subordinate communication transmitted from the top down via a clear chain of command, a hierarchy of authority, and a division of labor chain. Uses rational, impersonal management process. Uses explicit rules and regulations for governing activities; focuses on exacting work processes and technical competence. Uses merit and skill as basis for promotion/reward. Emphasizes lifetime career service and salaried managers.
Administrative Management *Shortell & Kaluzny (2006)*	Focus is on the science of management and principles of an organization applicable in any setting. Identifies need for Planning, Organizing, Supervising, Directing, Controlling, Organizing, Reviewing and Budgeting (POSDCORB). Commonly referred to as the management process that involves planning, organizing, coordinating, and controlling. Concerned with the optimal approach for administrators to achieve economic efficiency.
Human Relations *Argyris (1964), Barnard (1938),* *Likert (1967), McGregor (1960),* *Roethlisberger & Dickson* *(1939)*	Focuses on empowerment of the individual worker as the source of control, motivation, and productivity in organizations. Hawthorne studies at Western Electric plant in Chicago led to belief that human relations between workers and managers and among workers were the main determinants of efficiency. The Hawthorne effect refers to the phenomena of how being observed or studied results in a change of behavior. Emphasizes that participatory decision making increases worker autonomy. Provides training to improve work.

of the scientific method and as the author of *Principles of Scientific Management* (1911). Productivity was the area of focus in scientific management. Taylor, an engineer, introduced precise procedures based on systematic investigation of specific situations. The underlying point of view is that the organization is a machine to be run efficiently to increase production.

Working independently of Taylor, Frank and Lillian Gilbreth also contributed significantly to scientific management. They pioneered studies of time and motion that emphasized efficiency and culminated in "one best way" of carrying out work. Frank Gilbreth (1912) revolutionized surgical efficiency in the operating room, resulting in operations of shorter duration that substantially reduced risks from surgery for patients at that time.

BUREAUCRATIC MANAGEMENT

Max Weber is the German theorist recognized for the organizational theory of bureaucracy. Weber's beliefs were in stark contrast to the typical European organization that was based on a family-type structure in which employees

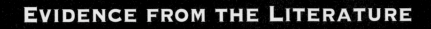

EVIDENCE FROM THE LITERATURE

Citation: Manojlovich, M. (2006). The effect of nursing leadership on hospital nurses' professional practice behaviors. *Journal of Nursing Administration, 35*(7/8), 366–374.

Discussion: This research study was conducted to evaluate the influence of nursing leadership on factors related to empowerment within a patient care unit and belief by nurses about their ability to express caring with patients, called self-efficacy. This reflects the idea that a nurse's perception of nursing leadership can have an impact on the nurse's behavior, particularly unit-level leadership, such as nurse manager leadership. This study was also based on the theory of empowerment where access to information, support, resources, and opportunities within the work environment can have the positive result of employee satisfaction as well as effectiveness. The results showed that nursing leadership is significantly related to empowerment and self-efficacy among acute care nurses in this study. In other words, the study results supported the idea that a nurse's self-efficacy is influenced by the self-efficacy of the unit-level nurse leader, both of which contribute to work effectiveness. Additionally, these results suggest that empowerment factors influence nurses' perceptions of their ability to care for patients; this is especially true when nursing leadership is strong.

Implications for Practice: One of the implications of this study is that leadership by nurses is important to all nurses and contributes to nurses being able to do their work better. The relationship between strong nursing leadership and professional practice behaviors, such as control over their practice environment and collaboration with practitioner colleagues, is also an important finding, indicating that strong and effective nurse leaders can support work environments that are conducive for other nurses. Therefore, when health care organizational leaders invest time and money for leadership development among nurses, the benefits are two-fold: unit-level nurse managers have more support and tools to carry out their role effectively, and all nurses feel they are more able to care for their patients and thus more effective at work. At a time when administrators are being called upon to base their management decisions on evidence, it is strategic to have empirical data that supports leadership development among unit-level nurse leaders.

were loyal to an individual, not to the organization—resources were used to benefit individuals rather than to advance the organization. Weber, however, believed efficiency is achieved through impersonal relations within a formal structure, competence should be the basis for hiring and promoting an employee, and decisions should be made in an orderly and rational way based on rules and regulations. The **bureaucratic organization** was a hierarchy with clear superior-subordinate communication and relations, based on positional authority, in which orders from the top were transmitted down through the organization via a clear chain of command.

ADMINISTRATIVE PRINCIPLES

Administrative principles are general principles of management that are relevant to any organization. In addition to some of the principles described as the management process (e.g., planning, organizing, directing, coordinating, and controlling), principles such as unity of command and direction were identified. Unity of command and direction means that a worker would get orders from only one supervisor, and related work would be grouped under one manager. These are examples of general principles generated during the early 1900s that were useful and relevant to all organizations (Fayol, 1916/1949).

Another key aspect of this perspective is attributed to Chester Barnard. Barnard (1938) is associated with the concept of the informal organization. The informal organization consists of naturally forming social groups that can become strong and powerful contributors to an organization. Barnard understood that these informal forces can be valuable in accomplishing the organization's goals and should be managed properly. He is also credited with the acceptance theory of authority. This theory identified people as having free will and that they actually choose to comply with orders they are given (Daft & Marcic, 2001). This view of people as making a difference in organizations was a precursor to the human relations movement that emerged from experiments at the Hawthorne plant of a Chicago electric company in the 1930s.

HUMAN RELATIONS

After the classical perspective, the next focus in the development of management is the human relations movement which started with the Hawthorne experiments. In contrast to the science of exact procedures, rules and regulations, and formal authority that characterized scientific management, the theories from the human relations school of thought espoused the individual worker as the source of control, motivation, and productivity in organizations. During the 1930s, labor unions became stronger and were instrumental in advocating for the human needs of employees. During this time, experiments were conducted at the Hawthorne plant of the Western Electric Company in Chicago that led to a greater understanding of the influence of human relations in organizations.

Electricity had become the preferred power source over gas; the Hawthorne plant experiments were run to show people that more light was necessary for greater productivity. This approach was designed to increase the use of electricity. Researchers Mayo (1933) and Roethlisberger and Dickson (1939) measured the effects on production of altering the intensity of lighting. They found that with more and brighter light, production increased as expected. However, production also increased each time they reduced the light, even when the light was extremely dim. Their research findings led to the conclusion that something else besides the light was motivating these workers.

The notion of social facilitation or the idea that people increase their work output in the presence of others was a result of the Hawthorne experiments. They also concluded that the effect of being watched and receiving special attention could alter a person's behavior. The phenomena of being observed or studied, resulting in changes in behavior, is now called the **Hawthorne effect**. Emerging from this study was the concept that people benefit and are more productive and satisfied when they participate in decisions about their work environment. This was the next phase in the evolution of management, called human relations management. In addition, social groupings, people's feelings, and their motivations became a focus of interest for future studies.

MOTIVATION THEORIES

The human relations perspective in management theory grew from the conclusion that worker output was greater when the worker was treated humanistically. This spawned a human resources point of view and a focus on the individual as a source of motivation. Motivation is not explicitly demonstrated by people but rather is interpreted from their behavior. **Motivation** is whatever influences our choices and creates direction, intensity, and persistence in our behavior (Hughes, Ginnett, & Curphy, 1999; Kanfer, 1990). Motivation is a process that occurs internally to influence and direct our behavior in order to satisfy needs (Lussier, 1999). Motivation theories are

not management theories per se; however, they are frequently considered along with management theories.

There are content motivation theories and process motivation theories (Lussier, 1999). The process motivation theories are expectancy theory and equity theory. The content motivation theories include Maslow's needs hierarchy; Aldefer's expectancy-relatedness-growth (ERG) theory and model of growth needs, relatedness needs, and existence needs; Herzberg's two-factor theory; and McClelland's manifest needs theory and model of achievement, power, and affiliation. Maslow's hierarchy of needs and Herzberg's two-factor theory are presented here along with Theory X, Theory Y, and Theory Z (Table 1-2 and Figure 1-1).

Motivation theories are useful because they help explain why people act the way they do and how a manager can relate to individuals as human beings and workers. When you are interested in creating change, influencing others, and managing patient care outcomes, it is helpful to understand the motivation that is reflected in a person's behavior. Motivation is a critical part of leadership because we need to understand each other in order to lead effectively. See Table 1-3 for common motivation problems and potential solutions.

MASLOW'S HIERARCHY OF NEEDS

One of the most well-known theories of motivation is Maslow's hierarchy of needs. Maslow (1970) developed a hierarchy of needs that shows how an individual is motivated. Motivation, according to Maslow, begins when a need is not met. For example, when a person has a physiological need, such as thirst, this unmet need has to be satisfied before a person is motivated to pursue higher-level needs. Certain needs have to be satisfied first, beginning with physiological needs, then safety and security needs, next social needs, followed by esteem needs, before an individual is motivated by the needs at the next level. The need for self-actualization drives people to the pinnacle of performance and achievement (Figure 1-2).

TWO-FACTOR THEORY

Frederick Herzberg (1968) contributed to research on motivation and developed the two-factor theory of motivation. He analyzed the responses of accountants and engineers and concluded that there were two sets of factors associated with motivation. One set of motivation factors must be maintained to avoid job dissatisfaction. These factors include such items as salary, working conditions, status, quality of supervision, relationships with others and so on. These factors have been labeled **maintenance or hygiene factors**. Factors such as achievement, recognition, responsibility, advancement, and so on, also contribute to job satisfaction. These factors are intrinsic and serve to satisfy or motivate people. Herzberg proposed

TABLE 1-2	**SELECTED MOTIVATION THEORIES**
Main Contributors	**Key Aspects**
Abraham Maslow (1908–1970) Hierarchy of needs	Motivation occurs when needs are not met. Certain needs have to be satisfied first, beginning with physiological needs, then safety and security needs, then social needs, followed by self-esteem needs, and then self-actualization needs. Needs at one level must be satisfied before one is motivated by needs at the next higher level of needs.
Frederick Herzberg (1964) Two-factor theory: Hygiene-Maintenance factors and Motivator factors	Hygiene-maintenance factors include adequate salary status, job security, quality of supervision, safe and tolerable working conditions, and relationships with others. When these factors are absent, they can be sources of job dissatisfaction. When they are present, job dissatisfaction can be avoided. However, these factors alone will not lead to job satisfaction. Motivator factors include satisfying and meaningful work, development and advancement opportunities, and responsibility and recognition. When these factors are present, people are motivated and satisfied with the job. When they are absent, people have a neutral attitude about their job/organization.
Douglas McGregor (1906–1964) Theory X	Leaders must direct and control because motivation results from reward and punishment. Employees prefer security, direction, and minimal responsibility, and they need coercion and threats to get the job done.
Theory Y	Leaders must remove work obstacles as under the right work conditions, workers have self-control and self-discipline. The workers' reward is their involvement in work and in the opportunity to be creative.
William Ouchi (1981) Theory Z	Uses collective decision making, long-term employment, mentoring, holistic concern, and use of quality circles to manage service and quality. This is a humanistic style of motivation based on the study of Japanese organizations.

that when these **motivation factors** are present, people are very motivated and satisfied with their jobs. When these factors are absent from a work setting, people have a neutral attitude about their organization. In contrast, when the maintenance factors are absent, people are dissatisfied. Herzberg believed that by providing the maintenance factors, job dissatisfaction could be avoided, but that these factors will not motivate people.

New graduate nurses can use Herzberg's theory by evaluating the maintenance factors present in a health care organization when they apply for a job. The pay, working conditions, and the beginning relationship that has been established with the supervisor are aspects of the job that the nurse should consider. If these maintenance factors are not adequate to begin with, then the nurse may become easily dissatisfied with the job. The higher-level needs that Herzberg describes as motivation factors should also be evaluated by the nurse before joining an organization. Are there opportunities for the nurse to achieve professional growth, to take on new responsibilities, to advance and be recognized for the contribution he has made?

It is important to recognize that not all employees respond to the same motivation factors. For example, a manager might be surprised to learn that some personnel will not respond to opportunities for autonomy and personal growth on the job. Rather, they may view their jobs as a means of providing income and seek various forms of personal fulfillment off-the-job through their families and leisure activities (Shortell & Kaluzny, 2006).

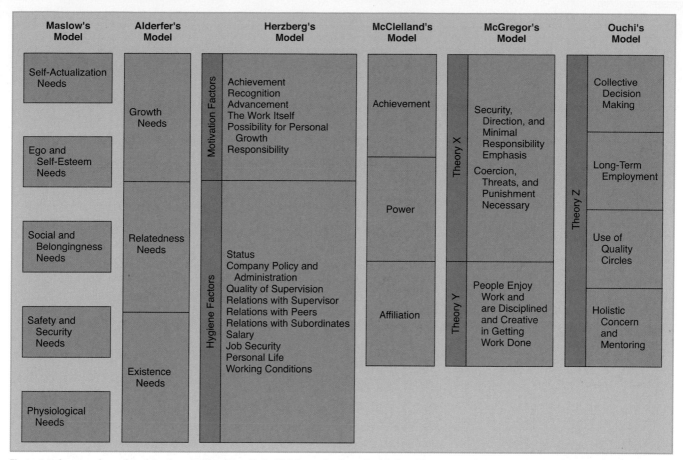

Maslow's Model	Alderfer's Model	Herzberg's Model	McClelland's Model	McGregor's Model	Ouchi's Model

Figure 1-1 A comparison of models of motivation. (Compiled with information from *Health Care Management* (5th ed.) by S. M. Shortell and A. D. Kaluzny, 2006, Clifton Park, NY: Thomson Delmar Learning; and Leadership and Management by L. S. Leach, from *Nursing Leadership & Management* by P. Kelly-Heidenthal, 2003, Clifton Park, NY: Thomson Delmar Learning.)

THEORY X AND THEORY Y

Continuing the emphasis on factors that stimulate job satisfaction and what motivates people to be involved and contribute productively at work, McGregor capitalized on his experience as a psychologist and university president to develop Theory X and Theory Y (McGregor, 1960). Theory X and Theory Y are about two different ways to motivate or influence others based on underlying attitudes about human nature. Each view reflects different attitudes about the nature of humans. The **Theory X** view is that in bureaucratic organizations, employees prefer security, direction, and minimal responsibility. Coercion, threats, or punishment are necessary because people do not like their work to be done. These employees are not able to offer creative solutions to help the organizations advance. McGregor's beliefs about Theory X were related to the classical perspective of organizations that included scientific management, bureaucracy theory, and administrative principles.

The assumptions of **Theory Y** are that in the context of the right conditions, people enjoy their work; can show self-control and discipline; are able to contribute creatively; and are motivated by ties to the group, the organization, and the work itself. In essence, this view espouses the belief that people are intrinsically motivated by their work. Theory Y was a guide for managers to take advantage of the potential of each person, which McGregor thought was being only partially utilized, and to provide support and encouragement to employees to do good work (McGregor, 1960).

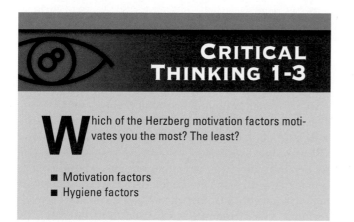

CRITICAL THINKING 1-3

Which of the Herzberg motivation factors motivates you the most? The least?

- Motivation factors
- Hygiene factors

TABLE 1-3	COMMON EMPLOYEE MOTIVATION PROBLEMS AND POTENTIAL SOLUTIONS

Motivational Problems

1. Inadequate performance definition, i.e., lack of goals, inadequate job descriptions, inadequate performance standards, inadequate performance assessment

2. Impediments to performance, i.e., bureaucratic or environmental obstacles, inadequate support or resources, poor employee-job matching, inadequate job information

3. Inadequate performance-reward linkages, i.e., inappropriate or inadequate job rewards, poor timing of rewards, low probability of receiving rewards, inequity in distribution of rewards

Potential Solutions

– Well-defined job descriptions

– Well-defined performance standards

– Goal setting

– Feedback on performance

– Improved employee selection

– Job redesign or enrichment

– Enhanced hygiene factors, i.e., safe and clean environment, good salary and fringe benefits, job security, good staffing, time off job, good equipment

– Behavior modification or positive reinforcement (individual or group)

– Pay for performance

– Enhanced job achievement or growth rewards, i.e., increased employee involvement and participation, job redesign or enrichment, career planning, professional development opportunities

– Enhanced job esteem or power factors, i.e., job autonomy or personal control, self-management, modified work schedule, recognition, praise or awards, opportunity to display skills or talents, opportunity to mentor or train others, promotions in rank or position, improved information concerning organization or department, preferred work activities or projects, letters of recommendation, preferred work space

– Enhanced affiliation or relatedness factors, i.e., recognized work teams and task groups; opportunities to attend conference, social activities, and professional and community group

Source: Compiled with information from Shortell, S. M., and Kaluzny, A. D. (2006). *Health Care Management* (5th ed.). Clifton Park, NY: Thomson Delmar Learning.

THEORY Z

Theory Z was developed by William Ouchi (1981) based on his years of study of organizations in Japan. He identified that Japanese organizations had better productivity than organizations in the United States and that they were managed differently with their use of quality circles to pursue better productivity and quality. Theory Z focuses on a better way of motivating people through their involvement. Collective decision making is a hallmark of

Theory Z as is a focus on long-term employment that involves slower promotions and less direct supervision. The organization and the worker are viewed more holistically. Through progressive development, the organization will be productive and quality goals will be achieved. The organization invests in its employees and addresses both home and work issues creating a path for career development. Democratic leaders, who are skilled in interpersonal relations, foster employee involvement (Ouchi, 1981).

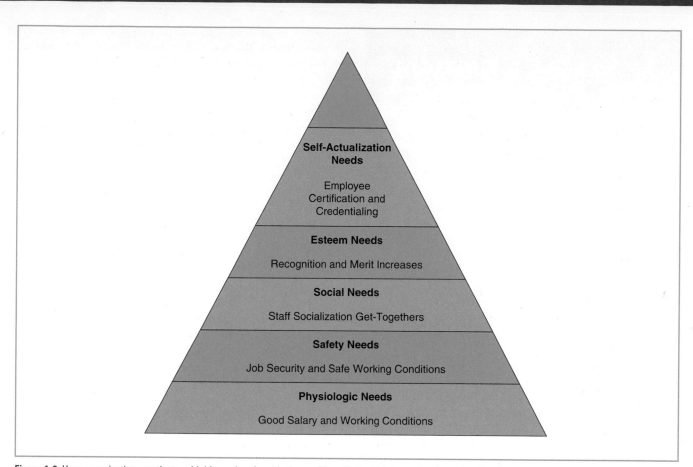

Figure 1-2 How organizations motivate with hierarchy of needs theory. (Compiled with information from How Organizations Motivate, Hierarchy of Needs Theory, figure in *Leadership: Theory, Application, Skill Building* by R. N. Lussier and C. F. Achua, 2000, Cincinnati, OH: South-Western College.)

THE CHANGING NATURE OF MANAGERIAL WORK

Current trends indicate that the numbers of managers in an organization, particularly at the middle level, are being reduced and that downsizing of staff has been a common phenomenon in most health care institutions. Those left in higher management positions after reorganizations are fewer in number and have taken on more responsibility over more areas. As individual nurses become more involved in managing consumer relations and consumer care, managers will become managers of systems rather than managers of nurses per se. The systems they will manage include clinical systems, cost information systems, and data systems on consumer satisfaction and feedback.

FEEDBACK

Because of their professional socialization and strong achievement needs, nurses want to deliver high-quality, excellent care to their patients. However, in order for them to know how well they are doing in this regard, they need to be able to assess how well they are doing with respect to their peers and their own past performance, and to benchmark quality performance goals. One way of accomplishing this is to develop high-quality information systems that provide feedback on a frequent basis. Such a system can allow health care professionals to know not only how well they are doing but also to enhance their confidence that they are doing things right (Kongstvedt, 2002).

Feedback can be a powerful tool to assist managers in motivating behavior; however, there are several factors that should be considered to maximize feedback effectiveness. First, for feedback to have value, nurses must truly see that their behavior needs to change. Second, feedback needs to be frequent, timely, and given at precise time intervals to sustain new behaviors. Third, feedback must be usable, consistent, correct, and of sufficient diversity. It should contain various important utilization, financial, and quality-related data that are valid representations of what is being measured. Otherwise, behavior problems can intensify as rewards flow to improvements based on flawed feedback data (Charns & Smith Tewksbury, 1993). Last, managers should not portray the feedback as "good" or "bad." Professionals, such as nurses, know when they

CRITICAL THINKING 1-4

Look for opportunities to gather data about your clinical performance. What other quality measures can you monitor in the following areas?

- *Patient Access:* Number of patients who are triaged within five minutes of arrival in the Emergency Department.
- *Utilization:* Number of patients who achieve quality outcomes under normal staffing ratios.
- *Financial:* Number of patients who meet patient care standards.
- *Quality:* Number of patients who state they are pleased with their nursing care.

have missed the goal (Shortell & Kaluzny, 2006). In the future, leadership responsibilities will be integrated among all organizational participants who function as **knowledge workers** and provide their professional expertise. Knowledge workers are those involved in serving others through their specialized knowledge. Among nurses, specialized knowledge is the practice and science of nursing used to serve patients and families. So leadership responsibilities are dispersed among all nurses, who are knowledge workers by virtue of their professional nursing expertise.

DEFINITION OF LEADERSHIP

Leadership is commonly defined as a process of influence in which the leader influences others toward goal achievement (Yukl, 1998). Influence is an instrumental part of leadership and means that leader's affect others, often by inspiring, enlivening, and engaging others to participate. The process of leadership involves the leader and the follower in interaction. This implies that leadership is a reciprocal relationship. Leadership can occur between the leader and another individual; between the leader and a group; or between a leader and an organization, a community, or a society. Defining leadership as a process helps us understand more about leadership than the traditional view of a leader being in a position of authority, exerting command, control, and power over subordinates. There are many more leaders in organizations than those who are in positions of authority. Each person has the potential to serve as a leader. What this means for

nurses as professionals is that they function as leaders when they influence others toward goal achievement. Nurses are leaders.

Leadership can be **formal leadership**, as when a person is in a position of authority or in a sanctioned, assigned role within an organization that connotes influence, such as a clinical nurse specialist (Northouse, 2001). An **informal leader** is an individual who demonstrates leadership outside the scope of a formal leadership role or as a member of a group rather than as the head or leader of the group. The informal leader is considered to have emerged as a leader when she is accepted by others and is perceived to have influence.

LEADERS VERSUS MANAGERS

Kotter (1990a) describes the differences between leadership and management in the following way: Leadership is about creating change and management is about controlling complexity in an effort to bring order and consistency. He says that leading change involves establishing a direction, aligning people through empowerment, and motivating and inspiring them toward producing useful change and achieving the vision, whereas management is defined as planning and budgeting, organizing and staffing, problem solving, and controlling complexity to produce predictability and order (Kotter, 1990b).

Nurses are leaders. Nurses function as leaders when they influence others toward goal achievement. RNs in staff nurse positions lead nursing practice by setting a direction, aligning people, and motivating and inspiring others toward a vision. Nurses lead other nurses and a community to achieve a collective vision of quality health care. See Table 1-4 for examples of nurses carrying out leadership role activities.

LEADERSHIP CHARACTERISTICS

According to Bennis and Nanus (1985), there are three fundamental qualities that effective leaders share. The first quality is a guiding vision. Leaders focus on a professional

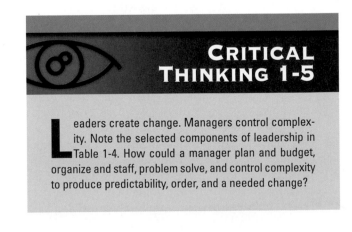

CRITICAL THINKING 1-5

Leaders create change. Managers control complexity. Note the selected components of leadership in Table 1-4. How could a manager plan and budget, organize and staff, problem solve, and control complexity to produce predictability, order, and a needed change?

TABLE 1-4   EXAMPLES OF NURSE LEADERSHIP ROLE ACTIVITIES

Leadership is about creating change through:	RN in a Staff Nurse Position	RNs Leading Other RNs	RNs Leading Communities/Society
Establishing direction and expressing a vision.	The RN read a current nursing journal and learned about a best-practice intervention that could reduce patient infection related to ventilator-associated pneumonia and reduce mortality (Pruitt & Jacobs, 2006). She uses this evidence to direct her nursing practice and reach the vision of quality patient outcomes (reduced pneumonia rate among hospitalized patients on her unit).	The American Association of Critical-Care Nurses (AACN) adopted the strategic initiative that identified the need for a healthy work environment, that is, work and patient care environments must be safe, healthy, humane, and respectful of the rights, responsibilities, needs, and contributions of patients, their families, nurses, and all health professionals (AACN, 2004).	Nurses take action toward the goal of a health care system where there is an adequate number of nurses with the appropriate education to carry out professional nursing practice in a variety of health settings and contribute optimally to the health care needs of all.
Aligning people.	The RN shared the article on reducing ventilator-related pneumonia with unit colleagues, the nurse manager, other practitioners, and respiratory therapists who are engaged in caring for ventilator patients. Together they identify the infection rate among these patients in their unit. They discuss the evidence and best practice interventions called, "ventilator bundle," which includes elevating the patient's head of the bed 30 degrees, sedation breaks, waking and weaning the patient, and prevention of deep vein thrombosis.	AACN provides testimony to the Institute of Medicine (IOM) Committee on Work Environment for Nurses and Patient Safety (AACN, 2003). "Ensuring patient safety and quality outcomes requires nurse leaders to prioritize strategic initiatives to cultivate a work environment of health." (Heath, Johanson, & Blake, 2004, p. 525)	The American Nurses Association (ANA) forms the American Nurses Credentialing Center to recognize excellence in the quality of professional nursing practice through the Magnet Recognition Program. The Scope and Standards for Nursing Administrators provides the framework for the Nursing Administration role to lead the creation and sustaining of professional nursing practice.

(Continues)

TABLE 1-4	**EXAMPLES OF NURSE LEADERSHIP ROLE ACTIVITIES (CONTINUED)**		

Leadership is about creating change through:	RN in a Staff Nurse Position	RNs Leading Other RNs	RNs Leading Communities/Society
Motivating and inspiring people.	The RN volunteers to contribute to a pilot project that introduces the "ventilator bundle" best practice interventions. The RN involves others to form a work group of colleagues interested in evaluating this innovation. They meet regularly to guide this project according to the hospital's and unit's policies and to share information with others as the project progresses.	AACN establishes the following standards for establishing and sustaining healthy work environments: Skilled Communication—Nurses must be as proficient in communication skills as they are in clinical skills. True Collaboration—Nurses must be relentless in pursuing and fostering true collaboration with the other nurses and health care staff. Effective Decision Making—Nurses must be valued and committed partners in making policy, directing and evaluating clinical care, and leading organizational operations. Appropriate Staffing—Staffing must ensure the effective match between patient needs and nurse competencies. Meaningful Recognition—Nurses must be recognized and must recognize others for the value each brings to the work of the organization. Authentic Leadership—Nurse leaders must fully embrace the imperative of a healthy work environment, authentically live it, and engage others in its achievement.	Research findings show that higher numbers of RN staff are associated with lower mortality (Aiken, 2002). Nurses in magnet hospitals report greater involvement in clinical decision making, more leadership support, and better quality of care than nonmagnet hospitals (Kramer & Schmalenberg, 2005; McClure & Hinshaw, 2002). These magnet professional nursing practice environments empower nurses and have a positive impact on nurse satisfaction and retention (Scott, Sochalski, & Aiken, 1999; Laschinger, Almost, & Tuer-Hodes, 2003; Upenieks, 2003).
Producing useful change and achieving the vision.	Based on the results of the ventilator bundle project, the RN helps to change the unit's policies and procedures in order to permanently adopt this change in practice. The RN has been a role model for others on how to engage and use evidence to improve practice. The RN has contributed to improved quality of care practices and improved health care outcomes for patients.	AACN publishes a call to action for nurses and all health professionals to embrace the personal obligation to participate in creating healthy work environments; for health care organizations to adopt and implement these standards; and for the community of nursing to bring urgent attention to the importance of establishing and sustaining a healthy work environment (AACN, 2004).	Nurses in magnet hospitals are leaders in attracting and retaining quality nurses and leaders and advancing nursing and health care in their communities.

Source: Compiled with information from Kotter, J. P. (1990). *A force for change: How leadership differs from management.* Glencoe, IL: Free Press.

and purposeful vision that provides direction toward the preferred future. The second quality is passion. Passion expressed by the leader involves the ability to inspire and align people toward the promises of life. The third quality is integrity that is based on knowledge of self, honesty, and maturity that is developed through experience and growth. McCall (1998) describes how self-awareness—knowing our strengths and weaknesses—can allow us to use feedback and learn from our mistakes. Daring and curiosity are also basic ingredients of leadership that leaders draw on to take risks, learning from what works as much as from what does not (Bennis & Nanus, 1985).

The American Association of Critical-Care Nurses in their landmark work, *AACN Standards for Establishing Healthy Work Environments: A Journey to Excellence,* cite authentic leadership as one of the key standards and assert that authentic leadership requires skill in the core competencies of self-knowledge, strategic vision, risk-taking and creativity, interpersonal and communication effectiveness, and inspiration (AACN, 2004).

Certain characteristics are commonly attributed to leaders. These traits are considered desirable and seem to contribute to the perception of being a leader. They include intelligence, self-confidence, determination, integrity, and sociability (Stodgill, 1948, 1974). Research among 46 hospitals designated as magnet hospitals for their success in attracting and retaining registered nurses emphasized the value of leaders who are visionary and enthusiastic, are supportive and knowledgeable, have high standards and expectations, value education and professional development, demonstrate power and status in the organization, are visible and responsive, communicate openly, and are active in professional associations (McClure & Hinshaw, 2002; Scott et al., 1999; Kramer, 1990; McClure, Poulin, Sovie, & Wandelt, 1983; Kramer & Schmalenberg, 2005). Research findings from studies on nurses revealed that caring, respectability, trustworthiness, and flexibility were the leadership characteristics most valued. In one study, nurse leaders identified managing the dream, mastering change, designing organization structure, learning, and taking initiative as leadership characteristics (Murphy & DeBack, 1991). Research by Kirkpatrick and Locke (1991) concluded that leaders are different from nonleaders across six traits: drive, the desire to lead, honesty and integrity, self-confidence, cognitive ability, and knowledge of the business. Although no set of traits is definitive and reliable in determining who is a leader or who is effective as a leader, many people still rely on personality traits to describe and define leadership characteristics.

LEADERSHIP THEORIES

Many believe that the critical factor needed to maximize human resources is leadership (Bennis & Nanus, 1985). A more in-depth understanding of leadership can be

REAL WORLD INTERVIEW

You're stepping forward to lead. It is important for you to know that leadership is different. It brings some very new responsibilities. Let me just put it this way—the stakes just went up a lot for all of you. How well you perform now really matters, not just in your career professionally, but to the people who are working with you and for you in your new leadership capacity.

Porter Goss
CIA Director, Washington, D.C.

gleaned from a review of leadership theories. The major leadership theories can be classified according to the following approaches: behavioral, contingency, and contemporary.

BEHAVIORAL APPROACH

Leadership studies from the 1930s by Kurt Lewin and colleagues at Iowa State University conveyed information about three leadership styles that are still widely recognized today: autocratic, democratic, and laissez-faire leadership (Lewin, 1939; Lewin & Lippitt, 1938; Lewin, Lippitt, & White, 1939). **Autocratic leadership** involves centralized decision making, with the leader making decisions and using power to command and control others. **Democratic leadership** is participatory, with authority delegated to others. To be influential, the democratic leader uses expert power and the power base afforded by having close, personal relationships. The third style, **laissez-faire leadership**, is passive and permissive, and the leader defers decision making. Lewin (1939) contrasted these styles and concluded that autocratic leaders were associated with high-performing groups, but that close supervision was necessary, and feelings of hostility were often present. Democratic leaders engendered positive feelings in their groups, and performance was strong whether or not the leader was present. Low productivity and feelings of frustration were associated with laissez-faire leaders.

Behavioral leadership studies from the University of Michigan and from Ohio State University led to the identification of two basic leader behaviors: job-centered behaviors and employee-centered behaviors. Effective leadership was described as having a focus on the human needs of subordinates and was called **employee-centered leadership** (Moorhead & Griffin, 2001). **Job-centered leaders** were seen as less effective because of their focus on

EVIDENCE FROM THE LITERATURE

Citation: Gordon, S. (2006). What do nurses really do? *Topics in Advanced Practice Nursing, 6*(1). Retrieved February 2, 2006 from http://www.medscape.com/viewarticle/520714.

Discussion: In this article by Suzanne Gordon, a journalist and author who writes about nursing, nurses are called upon to do a better job of accurately describing what nurses do and how they use expert knowledge acquired through scientific and technical mastery. She says, "What do nurses do? They save lives, prevent complications, prevent suffering, and save money." Her message to nurses is that there is a reason that the public has such little understanding of nursing and the importance of our work. The reason is twofold: traditional stereotypes about nursing cloud the reality of nursing as it is currently practiced, and nurses have been patterned to describe their contribution to health care in self-sacrificing and anonymous ways.

Implications for Practice: Nurses need to be clear about why it is important for the public to know what and how nurses contribute to health care. This article is an important vehicle from which nurses can begin to examine their own words and ways of discussing what nurses do and reflect upon the historical religious and societal practices that interfere with a clear, accurate, and realistic image of modern nursing. What nurses often think of as their ordinary work is really quite extraordinary. Nurses use scientific knowledge, expert judgment, and complex skills to make critical decisions that affect patient outcomes. Nurses need to be able to articulate how they do their work and the difference it makes.

CRITICAL THINKING 1-6

Among the individuals commonly identified as leaders (shown below), can you identify a set of traits that they all possess or traits that are associated with them? Are they perceived as leaders because they are characterized as intelligent, self-confident, and determined, have integrity, and are sociable? What other traits do (did) they have? Do you have any of these traits?

LEADERS AMONG US: PAST AND PRESENT

Mother Teresa	Martin Luther King
Sally Sample	Sister Rosemary Donley
Fay Bower	Polly Bednash
Joyce Clifford	Pam Cipriano
Margaret Sovie	Florence Nightingale
Virginia Henderson	Gale Pollock
Linda Burnes Bolton	John Thompson
Ida Androwich	Maggie McClure
Billye Brown	Leah Curtin
Imogene King	Peter Buerhaus
Muriel Poulin	Linda Aiken
Luther Christman	May Wykle
Rhonda Anderson	

schedules, costs, and efficiency, resulting in a lack of attention to developing work groups and high-performance goals (Moorhead & Griffin, 2001).

The researchers at Ohio State focused their efforts on two dimensions of leader behavior: initiating structure and consideration. **Initiating structure** involves an emphasis on the work to be done, a focus on the task, and production. Leaders who focus on initiating structure are concerned with how work is organized and on the achievement of goals. Leader behavior includes planning, directing others, and establishing deadlines and details of how work is to be done. For example, a nurse demonstrating the leader behavior of initiating structure could be a charge nurse who, at the beginning of a shift, makes out a patient assignment.

The dimension of **consideration** involves activities that focus on the employee and emphasize relating and getting along with people. Leader behavior focuses on the well-being of others. The leader is involved in creating a relationship that fosters communication and trust as a basis for respecting other people and their potential contribution. A nurse demonstrating consideration behavior will take the time to talk with coworkers, be empathetic, and show an interest in them as people.

The leader behaviors of initiating structure and consideration define leadership style. The styles are as follows:

- Low initiating structure, low consideration
- High initiating structure, low consideration
- High initiating structure, high consideration
- Low initiating structure, high consideration

The Ohio State University studies associate the high initiating structure–high consideration leader behaviors with better performance and satisfaction outcomes than the other styles. This leadership style is considered effective, although it is not appropriate in every situation.

Another model based on these two dimensions is the managerial grid developed by Blake and Mouton (1985). Five styles identify the extent of structure, called concern for production, and consideration, called concern for

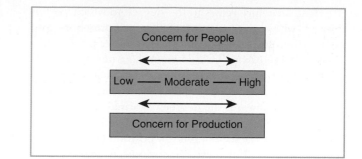

Figure 1-3 Key leadership dimensions. (Compiled with information from Blake, Mouton, and McCanse Leadership Grid from *Leadership: Theory, Application, Skill Building* by R. N. Lussier and C. F. Achua, 2000, Cincinnatti, OH: South-Western College.)

people, demonstrated by the leader. The five leader styles are impoverished leader for low production and people concern; authority compliance leader for high production concern and low people concern; country club leader for high people concern but low production concern; middle-of-the-road leader for moderate concern in both dimensions; and team leader for high production and people concern. Team management is usually a more effective leadership approach than an overemphasis on either concern for people or concern for production (Figure 1-3).

CONTINGENCY APPROACHES

Another approach to leadership is **contingency theory**. Contingency theory acknowledges that other factors in the environment influence outcomes as much as leadership style and that leader effectiveness is contingent upon or depends upon something other than the leader's behavior. The premise is that different leader behavior patterns will be effective in different situations. Contingency approaches include Fielder's contingency theory, the situational theory of Hersey and Blanchard, path-goal theory, and the idea of substitutes for leadership.

FIELDER'S CONTINGENCY THEORY. Fielder (1967) is credited with the development of the contingency model of leadership effectiveness. Fielder's theory of leadership effectiveness views the pattern of leader behavior as dependent upon the interaction of the personality of the leader and the needs of the situation. The needs of the situation or how favorable the situation is toward the leader involves leader-member relationships, the degree of task structure, and the leader's position of power (Fielder, 1967). **Leader-member relations** are the feelings and attitudes of followers regarding acceptance, trust, and credibility of the leader. Good leader-member relations exist when followers respect, trust, and have confidence in the leader. Poor leader-member relations reflect distrust, a lack of confidence and respect, and dissatisfaction with the leader by the followers.

CRITICAL THINKING 1-7

Identify the people who are leaders in your personal and professional life. In what way has their leadership affected you? As a person or as a nurse, identify the people that you lead. In what way has your interaction with those people influenced them? Influenced you?

Task structure refers to the degree to which work is defined, with specific procedures, explicit directions, and goals. High task structure involves routine, predictable, clearly defined work tasks. Low task structure involves work that is not routine, predictable, or clearly defined, such as creative, artistic, or qualitative research activities.

Position power is the degree of formal authority and influence associated with the leader. High position power is favorable for the leader and low position power is unfavorable. When all of these dimensions—leader-member relations, task structure, and position power—are high, the situation is favorable to the leader. When they are low, the situation is not favorable to the leader. In both of these circumstances, Fielder showed that a task-directed leader, concerned with task accomplishment, was effective. When the range of favorableness is intermediate or moderate, a human relations leader, concerned about people, was most effective. These situations need a leader with interpersonal and relationship skills to foster group achievement. Fielder's contingency theory is an approach that matches the organizational situation to the most favorable leadership style for that situation.

HERSEY AND BLANCHARD'S SITUATIONAL THEORY.

Situational leadership theory addresses follower characteristics in relation to effective leader behavior. Whereas Blake and Mouton focus on leader style and Fielder examines the situation, Hersey and Blanchard consider follower readiness as a factor in determining leadership style. Rather than using the words *initiating structure* and *contingency*, they use *task behavior* and *relationship behavior*.

High task behavior and low relationship behavior is called a telling leadership style. A high task, high relationship style is called a selling leadership style. A low task and high relationship style is called a participating leadership style. A low task and low relationship style is called a delegating leadership style.

Follower readiness, called maturity, is assessed in order to select one of the four leadership styles for a situation. For example, according to Hersey and Blanchard's situational leadership theory (2000), groups with low maturity, whose members are unable or unwilling to participate or are unsure, need a leader to use a telling leadership style to provide direction and close supervision. The selling leadership style is a match for groups with low to moderate maturity who are unable but willing and confident and need clear direction and supportive feedback to get the task done. Participating is the leadership style recommended for groups with moderate to high maturity who are able but unwilling or are unsure and who need support and encouragement. The leader should use a delegating style with groups of followers with high maturity who are able and ready to participate and can engage in the task without direction or support.

An additional aspect of this model is the idea that the leader not only changes leadership style according to followers' needs but also develops followers over time to increase their level of maturity (Lussier & Achua, 2000). Use of these four leadership styles helps a nurse manager assign work to others.

PATH-GOAL THEORY.

In this leadership approach, the leader works to motivate followers and influence goal accomplishment. The seminal author on path-goal theory is Robert House (1971). By using the appropriate style of leadership for the situation (i.e., directive, supportive, participative, or achievement oriented), the leader makes the path toward the goal easier for the follower. The directive style of leadership provides structure through direction and authority, with the leader focusing on the task and getting the job done. The supportive style of leadership is relationship oriented, with the leader providing encouragement, interest, and attention. Participative leadership means that the leader focuses on involving followers in the decision-making process. The achievement-oriented style provides high structure and direction as well as high support through consideration behavior. The leadership style is matched to the situational characteristics of the followers, such as the desire for authority, the extent to which the control of goal achievement is internal or external, and the ability of the follower to be involved. The leadership style is also matched to the situational factors in the environment, including the routine nature or complexity of the task, the power associated with the leader's position, and the work group relationship. This alignment of leadership style with the needs of followers is motivating and believed to enhance performance and satisfaction. The path-goal theory is based on expectancy theory, which holds that people are motivated when they believe they are able to carry out the work, they think their contribution will lead to the expected outcome, and they believe that the rewards for their efforts are valued and meaningful (Northouse, 2001).

SUBSTITUTES FOR LEADERSHIP.

Substitutes for leadership are variables that may influence followers to the same extent as the leader's behavior. Kerr and Jermier (1978) investigated situational variables and identified some aspects as substitutes that eliminate the need for leader behavior and other aspects as neutralizers that nullify the effects of the leader's behavior.

Some of these variables include follower characteristics, such as the presence of structured routine tasks, the amount of feedback provided by the task, and the presence of intrinsic satisfaction in the work; and organizational characteristics, such as the presence of a cohesive group, a formal organization, a rigid adherence to rules, and low position power. For example, an individual's experience substitutes for task-direction leader behavior

REAL WORLD INTERVIEW

It was a Monday. The Emergency Department was very busy as usual. A new patient, a 69 years-old African-American female was admitted by ambulance following a motor vehicle accident. I went to assess this patient and noted that blood was dripping from a small laceration on her forehead. She was awake, alert, and oriented. She had no pain or nausea. She told me that she was feeling fine, but I noticed that her lips and mouth were pale. I told the charge nurse that I believed that the patient's hemoglobin level was below 5 and I asked her to please tell the physician to come to the room soon to assess the patient. As I believed this patient was not stable, I immediately took the lead and inserted a large-bore intravenous heplock in her vein and collected blood samples for a CBC, BMP, PT, PTT, INR, and type and cross match, just in case. I started a liter of 0.9% normal saline intravenous fluid and connected the patient to the cardiac monitor as well as to the blood pressure, pulse, and pulse oximeter monitors. The patient now began to complain of nausea. At this point, the doctor had not come to see the patient yet. I went and told the doctor to please come to the patient's room and assess her now. I told him that the patient was bleeding and that I believed that her hemoglobin would be reported as below 5. He then came to the room and assessed the patient. He removed the head laceration dressing which was now soaked in blood. He noted a 1-inch laceration on her forehead that was still bleeding. He sutured the wound and finally ordered the CBC. I asked him if he was sure he only wanted the CBC. He said, yes. When the CBC results came back, the patient's hemoglobin was 3.8. I felt good about my assessment and intervention with this patient. The physician then ordered a type and cross match for 4 units of blood and a CT of the head. After the patient received two units of blood, she was transferred to the ICU.

Nirmala Joseph, RN
Staff Nurse
Chicago, Illinois

(Kerr & Jermier, 1978). Nurses and other professionals with a great deal of experience already have knowledge and judgment and do not need direction and supervision to perform their work. Thus, their experience serves as a leadership substitute. Another substitute for leader behavior is intrinsic satisfaction that emerges from just doing the work. Intrinsic satisfaction occurs frequently among nurses when they provide care to patients and families. Intrinsic satisfaction substitutes for the support and encouragement of relationship-oriented leader behavior.

CONTEMPORARY APPROACHES TO LEADERSHIP

Contemporary approaches to leadership address the leadership functions necessary to develop learning organizations. These approaches highlight charismatic

CRITICAL THINKING 1-8

Historical leadership traits attributed to leaders are the following:

- Intelligence
- Self-confidence
- Determination
- Integrity
- Sociability

- Caring
- Respectability
- Trustworthiness
- Flexibility

Review each of these traits attributed to leaders. Are these the characteristics you think are important for nurse leaders? To what extent do you portray each of these leadership traits?

CRITICAL THINKING 1-9

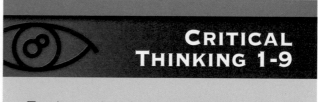

In what way do professional nursing standards, such as standards for nursing practice, standards for nursing performance, and the Code of Ethics for nurses serve as a substitute for leadership?

theory, transformational leadership theory, and knowledge workers.

CHARISMATIC THEORY

A charismatic leader has an inspirational quality that promotes an emotional connection from followers. House (1971) developed a theory of charismatic leadership that described how charismatic leaders behave as well as distinguishing characteristics and situations in which such leaders would be effective. Charismatic leaders display self-confidence, have strength in their convictions, and communicate high expectations and their confidence in others. They have been described as emerging during a crisis, communicating vision, and using personal power and unconventional strategies (Conger & Kanungo, 1987). One consequence of this type of leadership is a belief in the charismatic leader that is so strong that it takes on an almost supernatural purpose, and the leader is worshipped as if superhuman. Examples of charismatic leaders include Florence Nightingale and Martin Luther King.

Charismatic leaders can have a positive and powerful effect on people and organizations. Lee Iacocca, former chief executive officer (CEO) of Chrysler Corporation, and Herb Kelleher CEO of Southwest Airlines, are

REAL WORLD INTERVIEW

Saint Margaret Mercy Healthcare Centers, the largest hospital in Northwest Indiana with two campuses in Hammond and Dyer, Indiana, gives leadership and neighborhood watch a whole new meaning. We follow our Franciscan values every day, both inside the hospital and within our community. At Saint Margaret Mercy, we believe that everyone deserves a chance for good health and happiness. That's why we spent over $51 million in 2005 reaching out to our neighbors, including $39.8 million for the unpaid costs of Medicare and Medicaid, $8.2 million in uncompensated care, and $3.7 million in community support and services.

Saint Margaret Mercy's Hammond Campus 2006 payor mix includes 55% Medicare, 17% Medicaid, and 4% Self-Pay and Health Care for the Indigent (HCI). The Dyer Campus payor mix is 50% Medicare, 9% Medicaid, and 2% self-pay and HCI. Our Social Accountability investment in the communities that we serve is considerable based on these numbers. Managed care and commercial insurance make up about 24% of the payor mix at the Hammond Campus and 39% at the Dyer Campus. The hospital's bottom line is largely dependent on our ability to negotiate reasonable reimbursements from these managed care companies and to remain efficient with our expenses so that we can continue to meet our mission of serving all of those who come to us for health care services.

Whether it's offering free health screenings in the communities we serve, providing much-needed primary health care services for the working uninsured at our Catherine McAuley Clinic, helping teenage unwed mothers and babies who live at our St. Monica Home through counseling and parenting education, or helping troubled adolescents through the highly structured residential environment at our St. Francis Center, Saint Margaret Mercy does what it takes to give care and respect to those in need. We also provide free education for teens on sexual abstinence, and we founded the Volunteer Advocates for Seniors program. This program is dedicated to serving and safeguarding the health care, social service, and legal protection needs of incapacitated seniors who are inpatients in the Lake County, Indiana, health care system.

Saint Margaret Mercy has an ongoing commitment to excellent patient care. Our hospital is accredited by the Healthcare Facilities Accreditation Program and many of our patient service lines earn accreditation from various accrediting bodies and professional societies through our commitment to providing quality, evidence-based care.

In keeping with this philosophy, a multidisciplinary team is currently working to improve standards designed to increase the consistency and quality of care provided to patients with chest pain. Our efforts focus on developing policies and procedures to meet the Society of Chest Pain Centers' accreditation standards, thereby providing excellent care to our patients. This commitment to our beliefs might make us a little different. But we wouldn't have it any other way.

Thomas J. Gryzbek
President
Saint Margaret Mercy Healthcare Centers
Hammond and Dyer, Indiana

described as effective charismatic leaders. This type of leader can contribute significantly to an organization, even though all the leaders in an organization are not charismatic leaders. There are effective leaders who do not exhibit all the qualities associated with charismatic leadership. Charisma seems to be a special and valuable quality that some people have and some people do not.

TRANSFORMATIONAL LEADERSHIP THEORY

Burns defined transformational leadership as a process in which "leaders and followers raise one another to higher levels of motivation and morality" (Burns, 1978, p. 21). Transformational leadership theory is based on the idea of empowering others to engage in pursuing a collective purpose by working together to achieve a vision of a preferred future. This kind of leadership can influence both the leader and the follower to a higher level of conduct and achievement that transforms them both (Burns, 1978). Burns maintained that there are two types of leaders: the traditional manager concerned with day-to-day operations, called the **transactional leader**, and the leader who is committed to a vision that empowers others, called the **transformational leader**.

Transformational leaders motivate others by behaving in accordance with values, providing a vision that reflects mutual values, and empowering others to contribute. Bennis and Nanus (1985) describe this new leader as a leader who "commits people to action, who converts followers into leaders, and who converts leaders into agents of change" (p. 3). According to research by Tichy and Devanna (1986), effective transformational leaders identify themselves as change agents; are courageous; believe in people; are value driven; are lifelong learners; have the ability to deal with complexity, ambiguity, and uncertainty; and are visionaries. Yet transformational leadership may be demonstrated by anyone in an organization regardless of his position (Burns, 1978). The interaction that occurs between individuals can be transformational and motivate both to a higher level of performance (Bass, 1985).

Transformational leadership at the organizational level is about innovation and change. The transformational leader uses vision based on shared values to align people and inspire growth and advancement. It is both the inspiration and the empowerment aspects of transformational leadership that lead to commitment beyond self-interest, commitment to a vision, and commitment to action that creates change. Transformational leadership theory suggests that the relationship between the leader and the follower inspires and empowers an individual toward commitment to the organization.

Nurse researchers have described nurse executives according to transformational leadership theory and have used this theory to measure leadership behavior

---

CASE STUDY 1-1

A nurse is making rounds on her new postoperative laryngectomy patient. As the nurse enters the room, the patient begins to bleed from his neck incision. The nurse applies direct pressure to the patient's carotid artery with one hand and calls for assistance. Help arrives and the patient is taken to surgery with the nurse still maintaining pressure on the bleeding site. The patient lives and goes home a few days later.

How does nursing leadership and management on a patient care unit ensure good patient care in an emergency?

How can you develop your leadership and management skills to improve your ability to care for a group of patients?

---

among nurse executives and nurse managers (Leach, 2005; Dunham-Taylor, 2000; Wolf, Boland, & Aukerman, 1994; McDaniel & Wolf, 1992; Young, 1992). Additionally, transformational leadership theory has been the basis for nursing administration curriculum (Searle, 1996) and for investigation of relationships such as between a nurse's commitment to an organization and productivity in a hospital setting (Leach, 2005; McNeese-Smith, 1997). Cassidy and Koroll (1998) explored the ethical aspects of transformational leadership, and Barker (1990) comprehensively discussed nursing in terms of transformational leadership theory. Of the contemporary theories of leadership, transformational leadership has been a popular approach in nursing.

Most recently, the Institute of Medicine identified transformational leadership theory as a precursor to any change initiative and stated that transformational leadership can be a crucial approach toward achieving work environments that optimize patient safety (IOM, 2003).

KNOWLEDGE WORKERS

As mentioned earlier, the organizations that nurses are a part of are changing. They reflect the advance and the promise of the technology that enables us to perform our work. Peter Drucker (1994) identifies the organization of the future as a knowledge organization composed of knowledge workers. Knowledge workers are those who bring specialized, expert knowledge to an organization. They are valued for what they know. The knowledge organization shares, provides, and grows the information necessary to work efficiently and effectively. Drucker says that knowledge organizations, in which the knowledge worker is at the front lines with the expertise and the information to act, will be the dominant organizational type (Drucker, 1994; Helgesen, 1995). In organizations such as these, the ideas of leadership at the top and leadership equated with the power of a position are obsolete notions. Knowledge workers with the expertise and information to act are the organization's leaders. They provide the service, interact with the customer, represent the organization, and accomplish its goals.

Knowledge workers work in the information age, where the rapid, instant access to information makes information the medium of exchange. Knowledge workers are valued for what they know. Knowledge workers with the expertise and information to act are valued for their human capital (Lawler, 2001).

In the information age, it is the development of new knowledge and innovation and its meaningful interpretation and application that becomes the source for transactions with patients and staff. Nursing's transition to the information age is occurring within the context of rapidly advancing technology and nanotechnology and is influenced by three key trends. These trends have been termed mobility, virtuality, and user-driven practices (Porter O'Grady, 2001).

Mobility refers to the ability to change skill sets as well as having the work dispersed among a variety of work locations, rather than work occurring at fixed sites (Bennis, Spreitzer, & Cummings, 2001). Nurses are working in many new settings today and are constantly adding to their knowledge as new technologies emerge.

Virtuality means working through virtual means using digital networks, where the worker may be far from the patient but present in a digital reality. Nurses are working in outpatient settings today where they carry a computer and are in instant communication with other practitioners and patients.

User-driven practices mean that the individual, at a time when digital mediums have given us more access to information and therefore more choices, acts more independently and is increasingly accountable for those choices and actions. Nurses are constantly assessing patients using traditional assessment methods as well as newer digital methods, for example, computerized vital sign monitors, and taking action to safeguard their patients and improve their care.

Nursing leadership practices are evolving to match nurses' work within this mobile, changing, environment with nurses who act without much supervision or guidance. This is facilitated by the growth and sophistication of nursing research, the application of nursing science, and the translation of available evidence into evidence-based nursing practice. The journey to the information age is continually fulfilling for nurses as they are able to display the rich and valuable contribution that knowledgeable nurses make to the quality of patient care and to quality health care outcomes.

USING KNOWLEDGE

Good nursing leadership and management of patients includes getting to know the patient; spending time assessing normal behavior, physiological and psychological responses to illness and hospitalization; and using knowledge to recognize even subtle changes in the patient condition and further evaluate them. Another key aspect of using knowledge is developing the ability to anticipate patient care problems. When a nurse intervenes with a postoperative patient who is bleeding from his incision by applying pressure at the site, the nurse minimizes the amount of bleeding. What assists a nurse to intervene correctly is using knowledge and anticipating such complications, thinking in advance of what should be done if a particular complication occurs, and then monitoring the patient to assess and identify complications early or, when possible, to prevent them. Another aspect of using knowledge for good leadership and management on the patient care unit is to have the right type of personnel and the right amount of personnel; in other words, having patient care unit staffing with enough registered nurses, licensed practical nurses, or nursing assistants on the unit, so that they all can fulfill their roles appropriately and with enough people to adequately care for the patients.

Nurses can develop their leadership and management skills with continuing education and by increasing their knowledge and expertise in caring for a group of patients by taking care of those patients regularly. The more experience a nurse gains in caring for particular patients, the more opportunity for learning to recognize patterns that occur with these patients. Patterns can include the type of symptoms that are common, possible complications or emergencies, actions that can help prevent complications or negative outcomes. Good planning on how to spend their time and determining what actions are a nursing priority and what can be delegated to others will also help a nurse manage a group of patients.

Knowledgeable nursing leadership and management on a nursing unit fosters good patient care by providing a supportive environment for nurses to deliver care. A supportive leadership and management environment does such things as providing a clear chain of command, clear job descriptions, patient care standards, good staffing ratios, good Internet and library resources, continuing education support, and so on. This allows the nurse to set goals, seek a mentor, and continue employment in a setting that is supportive of quality nursing care.

THE NEW LEADERSHIP

Margaret Wheatley, in *Leadership and the New Science* (1999), says, "There is a simpler way to lead organizations, one that requires less effort and produces less stress than the current practices." She presents a new view of leadership, one encompassing connectedness and self-organizing systems that follow a natural order of both chaos and uncertainty, which is different from a linear order in a hierarchy. The leader's function is to guide an organization using vision, to make choices based on mutual values, and to engage in the culture to provide meaning and coherence. This type of leadership fosters growth within each of us as individuals and as members of a group. The notion of connection within a self-organizing system optimizes autonomy at all levels because the relationships among the individual and the whole are strong. For nursing, such systems might be the infrastructure that will foster interdisciplinary decision making and strengthen the connection with nonprofessional workers.

In Wheatley's subsequent book, *Finding Our Way: Leadership for an Uncertain Time* (2005) she discusses how humans learn best when they are engaged in relationships with others and can exchange knowledge and expertise through informal, self-organized communities. Wheatley refers to these as communities of practice and encourages us to develop new leaders using communities of practice. Her notion of a community of practice represents several elements nurses are familiar with, that is, forming informal groups, using a group process of organizing, using principles of learning, and sharing information. What is unique in her description of these communities of practice is that they form via self-organization. They come together naturally. What makes these communities

different from informal groups is Wheatley's characterization of a community built from relationships and participation in a way that connects nurses and allows the creation of meaning from information or the exchange of knowledge. In work done for the Center of Creative Leadership, communities of practice are described as being different from the ideas or experiences we have had with groups, teams, and collective forming because

CRITICAL THINKING 1-10

Becky is an Emergency Department (ED) nurse working with patients. Becky assesses her patients regularly and monitors their progress. She is certified in Advanced Cardiac Life Support and Trauma Nursing. One day, when she assesses her new patient, she notes that his pulse and respiration are increased and his blood pressure is decreased. She calls for the ED practitioner to see the patient immediately and simultaneously starts a large bore intravenous (IV) line and connects her patient to a cardiac monitor and the vital sign monitor. How has Becky demonstrated leadership? Do nurses regularly act to safeguard their patients in this way and prevent a negative nurse-patient outcome? Can the presence of safe staffing ratios affect a nurse's ability to deliver safe patient care and prevent negative nurse-sensitive patient care outcomes? Is Becky a knowledge worker?

REAL WORLD INTERVIEW

Leadership in nursing is probably one of the more personal forms of leadership. Nursing is one of the most intimate leadership relationships because of the vulnerability the patient brings to the relationship. With patients who are dying or in terrible situations, the nurse provides them with two vital leadership characteristics: optimism and courage. With patients who have lost their courage, it is the nurse who shows courage and strength that supports a patient and their family. Optimism and courage are the trademarks of great leaders. Nurses lead the patient, the patient's family, their nurse colleagues, and other health care providers. They have the courage to care in the face of fear and uncertainty, and in the face of disability or in death. Caring, hope, and support are a source of optimism that nurses provide. There are very few professions where you touch an individual's life so profoundly.

Jay Conger, PhD
Author, *Learning to Lead*
Los Angeles, California

communities of practice emerge from shared activity, shared knowledge, and ways of knowing that creates meaning and thus a culture of engagement, participation, and relationships (Drath & Palus, 1994). Wheatley directs nurses to name these communities of practice that bring people together, support these connections, nourish the community, and illuminate their work. These exciting notions hold great promise for health professionals as we learn how to collaborate within and across disciplines and countries to advance health care practices.

KEY CONCEPTS

- Nurses are leaders and make a difference through their contributions of expert knowledge and leadership to health care organizations. Leadership development is a necessary component of preparation as a health care provider.

- All nurses are leaders because they have expert knowledge that they contribute to coordinate and provide patient care. Building expertise by gaining experience, setting goals to direct experiential learning, and gaining clinical skills and judgment are some of the ways that new nurses develop as leaders.

- Management is a process used to achieve organizational goals. Management roles are classified as the information processing role, the interpersonal role, and the decision-making role. Managers use these roles to manage the work and to manage relationships with people to accomplish the work.

- The management process involves planning, coordinating, organizing, and controlling. The RN uses this process to manage patient care.

- Scientific management, based on the work of Taylor and others, viewed industrial organizations as machines where work was to be carried out in the most scientifically exact and efficient way to increase production.

- Weber is the theorist associated with bureaucratic theory. The idea of organizations as bureaucracies involves a formal organizational structure, impersonal relations, a hierarchy based on positional authority, and a clear chain of command.

- Human relations management is also known as organizational behavior and led to participative management. The human needs of employees and the motivation and satisfaction of the individual and groups were the focus of efforts to increase production.

- Motivation is an internal process that contributes to behavior in an effort to satisfy needs. Maslow's hierarchy of needs reflects the belief that the needs that motivate individuals have a priority order. Lower-level needs have to be satisfied first or individuals will not be motivated to address higher-level needs.

- Herzberg's two-factor theory of motivation identifies maintenance factors, such as security and salary, that are needed to prevent job dissatisfaction, and motivator factors, such as job development and opportunities to advance, that contribute to job satisfaction.

- Leadership is a process of influence that involves the leader, the follower, and their interaction. Followers can be individuals, groups of people, communities, and members of society in general.

- Leadership can be formal or informal. It can occur by being in a position of leadership and authority in an organization, such as a manager. Leadership can also occur outside the scope of a formal role, such as when an individual or member of a group moves to assume leadership.

- Leadership and management are different. Management is viewed as actions employed to cope with changes, whereas leadership is the effort to envision and inspire in order to create change.

- Nurses are leaders. They lead nursing practice. Nurses lead other nurses, and they lead patients and communities toward improved health.

- Leadership styles are described as autocratic, democratic, and laissez-faire and have been studied by examining job-centered or task-oriented approaches versus employee-centered or relationship-oriented approaches.

- Blake and Mouton's leadership model has five styles to address high- or low people concerns and high- or low production concerns.

- Contingency theories of leadership acknowledge that other factors in the environment, in addition to the leader's behavior, affect the effectiveness of the leader. Fielder's contingency theory describes the leader's behavior/style as being dependent upon the nature of the task, leader-member relations, and the power associated with the leader's position. Hersey and Blanchard's situational theory matches task and relationship needs with maturity or readiness of the followers to participate by using leadership styles called telling, selling, participating, or delegating. House's path-goal theory involves the leader using a directive style, a supportive style, a participative style, or an achievement-oriented leadership style to match the task.

- Substitutes for leadership are variables that eliminate the need for leadership or nullify the effect of the leader's behavior. These include work experience, professionalism, indifference to rewards, presence of routine tasks, feedback provided by the task, intrinsic satisfaction, cohesive groups, formal organizational structures, rigid adherence to rules, role distance, and low position power of the leader.

- Charismatic leadership theory describes leader behavior that displays self-confidence, passion, and communication of high expectations and confidence in others. These types of leaders often emerge in a crisis with a vision, have an appeal based on their personal power, and often use unconventional strategies and their emotional connections to succeed.

- Transformational leadership theory involves two styles of leadership: the transformational leader and the transactional leader. Transactional leaders focus on organizational operations and short-term goals. They use exchange and making trades as a way of accomplishing work. Transformational leaders inspire and motivate others to excel and participate in a vision that goes beyond self interests. Transformational leadership is believed to empower followers and contribute to their commitment to action and change.

- Organizations need to be viewed as self-organizing systems where what initially looks like chaos and uncertainty is indeed part of a larger coherence and a natural order. Such a living, self-organizing system, when understood better by participants, will be a less stressful and more holistic environment in which to carry out work.

- Future directions for nurses in organizations will continue to be influenced by technology and by the notions of mobility, virtuality, and user-driven practices. Knowledge workers, with specialized knowledge and expertise, are more self-directed. Future leadership practices need to adapt to them and to the changing work environments and circumstances.

- Nursing is in transition to the knowledge age where nursing research advances nursing science, and nursing science is translated into evidence-based nursing practice.

KEY TERMS

administrative principles
autocratic leadership
bureaucratic organization
consideration
contingency theory
democratic leadership
employee-centered
  leadership
formal leadership
Hawthorne effect
informal leader
initiating structure
job-centered leaders
knowledge workers
laissez-faire leadership
leader-member relations
leadership
maintenance or
  hygiene factors
management
management process
motivation
motivation factors
position power
substitutes for leadership
task structure
taxonomy
Theory X
Theory Y
Theory Z
transactional leader
transformational leader

REVIEW QUESTIONS

1. Management as a process that is used today by nurses or nurse managers in health care organizations is best described as
   A. scientific management.
   B. decision making.
   C. commanding and controlling others using hierarchical authority.
   D. planning, organizing, coordinating, and controlling.

2. According to Hersey and Blanchard and House, a participative leadership style is appropriate for employees who
   A. are not able to get the task done and are less mature.
   B. are able to contribute to decisions about getting the work done.
   C. are unable and unwilling to participate.
   D. need direction, structure, and authority.

3. If you applied the concepts of Theory Y to describe nurses, which of the following statements would be the best description?
   A. Nurses prefer to be directed and want job security more than other things.
   B. Nurses use self-direction and self-control to achieve work objectives in which they believe.
   C. Nurses have a hard time accepting responsibility, but they learn to do this over time.
   D. Nurses don't really want to work and would quit if they could.

4. Nurse retention is an important focus for health care organizations as we face a growing shortage of health care professionals in the future. According to Herzberg's motivation factors, which of the following would most likely contribute to increased job satisfaction?
   A. The organization recognizes and rewards those nurses who advance their education and achieve certification, such as the CCRN certification for critical care RNs.
   B. Hiring bonuses of up to $5,000 are given to nurses to reduce the vacant positions and prevent short-staffing.
   C. Nurse managers place an emphasis on establishing effective relationships with the nurses who work for them.
   D. Salary is increased.

5. Consider your role as a staff nurse in a patient care unit of a hospital. What factors are present that may serve as a substitute for your need for leadership from your nurse manager?
   A. Your desire for a promotion and an increase in pay.
   B. Professional nursing standards, code of ethics, and the intrinsic reward you get from this important work.
   C. Your manager spends time telling you exactly what to do and how to do it.
   D. Your nurse manager is inspiring and highly motivating to work for.

6. Leadership is defined as
   A. being in a leadership position with authority to exert control and power over subordinates.
   B. a process of interaction in which the leader influences others toward goal achievement.
   C. managing complexity.
   D. being self-confident and democratic.

7. Why is leadership development important for nurses if they are not in a management position?
   A. It is not really important for nurses.
   B. Leadership is important at all levels in an organization because nurses have expert knowledge and are interacting with and influencing the patient.
   C. Nurse leaders leave their jobs sooner for other positions.
   D. Nurses who lead are less satisfied in their jobs.

8. How does the human relations theory of management differ from earlier approaches?
   A. It focuses on precision to maximize efficiency.
   B. It emphasizes planning, organizing, coordinating, and controlling.
   C. It improves performance through participative management.
   D. It emphasizes long-term employment and job security.

REVIEW ACTIVITIES

1. Take the opportunity to learn about yourself by reflecting on five predominant factors identified as being influential in a nurse's leadership development: self-confidence, innate leader qualities/tendencies, progression of experiences and success, influence of significant others, and personal life factors. Consider what reinforces your confidence in yourself. What innate qualities or tendencies do you have that contribute to your development as a leader? Consider what professional experiences, mentors, and personal experiences or events can help you influence and change nursing practice.

2. Describe the type of leader you want to be as a nurse in a health care organization. Identify specific behaviors you plan to use as a leader. In what way are the transformational leadership and the charismatic leadership theories useful to your development as a leader?

3. Rate each of these twelve job factors that contribute to job satisfaction by placing a number from 1 to 5 on the line before each factor.

Very important 5	Somewhat important 4	3	2	Not important 1

_____ 1. An interesting job I enjoy doing
_____ 2. A good manager who treats people fairly
_____ 3. Getting praise and other recognition and appreciation for the work I do
_____ 4. A satisfying personal life at the job
_____ 5. The opportunity for advancement
_____ 6. A prestigious or status job
_____ 7. Job responsibility that gives me freedom to do things my way
_____ 8. Good working conditions (safe environment, nice office, cafeteria)
_____ 9. The opportunity to learn new things
_____ 10. Sensible company rules, regulations, procedures, and policies
_____ 11. A job I can do well and succeed at
_____ 12. Job security and benefits

Write the number from 1 to 5 that you selected for each factor. Total each column for a score between 6 and 30 points. The closer to 30 your score is, the more important these factors (motivating or maintenance) are to you.

Motivating factors		Maintenance factors	
1. _____		2. _____	
3. _____		4. _____	
5. _____		6. _____	
7. _____		8. _____	
9. _____		10. _____	
11. _____		12. _____	
Totals _____		_____	

From *Leadership: Theory, Application, Skill Development* (pp. 15–16), by R. N. Lussier and C. F. Achua, 2000, Cincinnati, OH: South-Western College Publishing.

4. What would a health care organization be like if it more closely resembled a self-organizing system and more holistic environment? How different would it be from a bureaucratic and more structured organization?

5. If nurses become more self-directed in the future, what kind of leadership practices will be the most effective?

6. What quality improvement projects are nurses in your work setting involved in? How is evidence being used to improve nursing practice? What sources of evidence from nursing science are you exploring through journals, attending educational conferences, the Internet, and participating in professional nursing associations?

EXPLORING THE WEB

Search the Web, checking the following sites:

- Emerging Leader: *www.emergingleader.com*

- Leadership Skills Development:
  www.impactfactory.com
  Search for leadership.

- LeaderValues: *www.leader-values.com*

- Don Clark's Big Dog Leadership:
  www.nwlink.com

- American Association of Critical Care Nurse's
  Standards for Establishing and Sustaining Healthy
  Work Environments: *www.aacn.org*
  Under Priority Issues, click Healthy Work Environments.

- American Organization of Nurse Executives
  Competencies: *www.aone.org*
  Click Resource Center and then click AONE Nurse
  Exec Competencies.

- Analyze My Career: *http://analyzemycareer.com*

- American Nurses Association Magnet Status Hospitals:
  www.nursingworld.org
  Search for ANCC.

- This site on classic management functions can keep you
  busy all week: *www.1000ventures.com*
  Review your character and personality, and click on
  other areas of interest.

REFERENCES

Aiken, L. H., Clarke, S. P., Sloane, D. M., Sochalski, J., & Silber, J. H. (2002). Hospital nurse staffing, patient mortality, nurse burnout, and job dissatisfaction. *Journal of American Medical Association, 288*(16), 1987–1993.

American Association of Critical Care Nurses. (2003). Written testimony to the IOM Committee on work environment of nurses and patient safety. Retrieved February 15, 2007, from http://www.aacn.org

American Association of Critical Care Nurses. (2004). *AACN standards for establishing and sustaining healthy work environments: A journey to excellence.* Retrieved February 15, 2007, from http://www.aacn.org/aacn/hwe.nsf/vwdoc/HWEHomePage

Argyris, C. (1964). *Integrating the individual and the organization.* Hoboken, NJ: Wiley.

Barker, A. (1990). *Transformational nursing leadership: A vision for the future.* Baltimore: Williams & Wilkins.

Barnard, C. (1938). *The functions of the executive.* Boston: Harvard University Press.

Bass, B. (1985). *Leadership and performance beyond expectations.* New York: Free Press.

Bennis, W., & Nanus, B. (1985). *Leaders: The strategies for taking charge.* New York: Harper & Row.

Bennis, W., Spreitzer, G. M., & Cummings, T. G. (2001). *The future of leadership.* San Francisco: Jossey-Bass.

Blake, R. R., & Mouton, J. S. (1985). *The managerial grid III.* Houston, TX: Gulf.

Burns, J. M. (1978). *Leadership.* New York: Harper & Row.

Cassidy, V., & Koroll, C. (1998). Ethical aspects of transformational leadership. In E. Hein (Ed.), *Contemporary leadership behavior: Selected readings* (5th ed., pp. 79–82). Philadelphia: Lippincott.

Charns, M., & Smith Tewksbury, L. (1993). *Collaborative management in health care.* San Francisco: Jossey-Bass.

Conger, J., & Kanungo, R. (1987). Toward a behavioral theory of charismatic leadership in organizational settings. *Academy of Management Review, 12,* 637–647.

Daft, R. L., & Marcic, D. (2001). *Understanding management* (3rd ed.). Philadelphia: Harcourt College.

Drath, W. H., & Palus, C. J. (1994). *Making common sense: Leadership as meaning-making in a community of practice.* Retrieved 2004 from http://www.ebookmall.com

Drucker, P. F. (1994). *The post-capitalist society.* New York: Harper & Row.

Dunham-Taylor, J. (2000). Nurse executive transformational leadership found in participative organizations. *Journal of Nursing Administration, 30*(5), 241–250.

Fayol, H. (1916/1949). (C. Storrs, Trans.). *General and industrial management.* London: Pitman.

Fielder, F. (1967). *A theory of leadership effectiveness.* New York: McGraw-Hill.

Follet, M. (1924). *Creative experience.* London: Longmans, Green.

Gilbreth, F. (1912). *Primer of scientific management.* New York: Van Nostrand.

Gordon, S. (2006). What do nurses really do? *Topics in Advanced Practice Nursing, 6*(1). Retrieved February 2, 2006, from http://www.medscape.com/viewarticle/520714

Gulick, L., & Urwick, L. (Eds.). (1937). *Papers on the science of administration.* New York: Institute of Public Administration.

Hales, C. P. (1986). What managers do: A critical review of the evidence. *Journal of Management Studies, 23,* 88–115.

Heath, J., Johanson, W., & Blake, N. (2004). Healthy work environments: A validation of the literature. *Journal of Nursing Administration, 34*(11), 524–530.

Helgesen, S. (1995). *The web of inclusion: A new architecture for building organizations.* New York: Doubleday Currency.

Henry, N. (1992). *Public administration and public affairs* (5th ed.). Englewood Cliffs, NJ: Prentice Hall.

Hersey, P., & Blanchard, K. (2000). *Management of organizational behavior* (8th ed.). Englewood Cliffs, NJ: Prentice Hall.

Herzberg, F. (1968, January/February). One more time: How do you motivate employees? *Harvard Business Review, 46*(1), 53–62.

House, R. H. (1971). A path-goal theory of leader effectiveness. *Administrative Science Quarterly, 16,* 321–338.

Hughes, R. L., Ginnett, R. C., & Curphy, G. J. (1999). *Leadership: Enhancing the lessons of experience* (3rd ed.). San Francisco: Irwin McGraw-Hill.

Institute of Medicine (2003). *Health professions education: A bridge to quality.* Washington, DC: The National Academies Press.

Kanfer, R. (1990). Motivation theory in industrial and organizational psychology. In M. D. Dunnette & L. M. Hough (Eds.), *Handbook of industrial and organizational psychology: Vol. 1* (pp. 53–68). Palo Alto, CA: Consulting Psychologists Press.

Katz, D., & Kahn, R. L. (1978). *The social psychology of organizations* (2nd ed.). New York: John Wiley.

Kerr, S., & Jermier, J. (1978). Substitutes for leadership: Their meaning and measurement. *Organizational Behavior and Human Performance, 22,* 374–403.

Kim, H., & Yukl, G. (1995). Relationships of self-reported and subordinate-reported leadership behaviors to managerial effectiveness and advancement. *Leadership Quarterly, 6,* 361–377.

Kirkpatrick, S. A., & Locke, E. A. (1991). Leadership: Do traits matter? *The Executive, 5,* 48–60.

Kongstvedt, P. R. (2002). *Managed care: What it is and how it works.* Gaithersburg, MD: Aspen Publishers.

Kotter, J. (1990a). *A force for change: How leadership differs from management.* Glencoe, IL: Free Press.

Kotter, J. (1990b). What leaders really do. *Harvard Business Review, 68,* 104.

Kramer, M. (1990). The magnet hospitals: Excellence revisited. *Journal of Nursing Administration, 20*(9), 35–44.

Kramer, M., & Schmalenberg, C. E. (2005, July–Sep.). Best quality patient care: A historical perspective on Magnet hospitals. *Nursing Administration Quarterly, 29*(3), 275–287.

Laschinger, H. K. S., Almost, J., & Tuer-Hodes, D. (2003). Workplace empowerment and magnet hospital characteristics: Making the link. *Journal of Nursing Administration, 33*(7/8), 410–422.

Lawler, E. (2001). The era of human capital has finally arrived. In W. Bennis, G. Spreitzer, & T. Cummings (Eds.), *The future of leadership.* San Francisco: Jossey-Bass.

Leach, L. S. (2005). Nurse executive leadership and organizational commitment among nurses. *Journal of Nursing Administration, 35*(5), 228–237.

Lewin, K. (1939). Field theory and experiment in social psychology: Concepts and methods. *Journal of Sociology, 44,* 868–896.

Lewin, K., & Lippitt, R. (1938). An experimental approach to the study of autocracy and democracy: A preliminary note. *Sociometry, 1,* 292–300.

Lewin, K., Lippitt, R., & White, R. (1939). Patterns of aggressive behavior in experimentally created social climates. *Journal of Social Psychology, 10,* 271–299.

Likert, R. (1967). *The human organization: Its management and value.* New York: McGraw-Hill.

Lussier, R. N. (1999). *Human relations in organizations: Applications and skill building* (4th ed.). San Francisco: Irwin McGraw-Hill.

Lussier, R. N., & Achua, C. F. (2000). *Leadership: Theory, application, skill development.* Cincinnati, OH: South-Western College.

Manojlovich, M. (2006). The effect of nursing leadership on hospital nurses professional practice behaviors. *Journal of Nursing Administration, 35*(7/8), 366–374.

Maslow, A. (1970). *Motivation and personality* (2nd ed.). New York: Harper & Row.

Mayo, E. (1933). *The Human problems of an industrial civilization.* New York: Macmillan.

McCall, M. W., Jr. (1998). *High flyers: Developing the next generation of leaders.* Boston: Harvard Business School Press.

McCall, M. W., Jr., Morrison, A. M., & Hanman, R. L. (1978). *Studies of managerial work: Results and methods* (Tech. Rep.). Greensboro, NC: Center for Creative Leadership.

McClure, M., & Hinshaw, A. (Eds.). (2002). *Magnet hospitals revisited.* Washington, DC: American Nurses Publishing.

McClure, M., Poulin, M., Sovie, M., & Wandelt, M. (1983). *Magnet hospitals: Attraction and retention of professional nurses.* Kansas City, MO: American Nurses Association.

McDaniel, C., & Wolf, G. (1992). Transformational leadership in nursing service. *Journal of Nursing Administration,12*(4), 204–207.

McGregor, D. (1960). *The human side of enterprise.* New York: McGraw-Hill.

McNeese-Smith, D. (1997). The influences of manager behavior on nurses' job satisfaction, productivity, and commitment. *Journal of Nursing Administration, 27*(9), 47–55.

Mintzberg, H. (1973). *The nature of managerial work.* New York: Harper & Row.

Mooney, J. (1939). *Principles of Organization.* New York: Harper.

Moorhead, G., & Griffin, R. W. (2001). *Organizational behavior: Managing people in organizations* (6th ed.). Boston: Houghton Mifflin.

Murphy, M., & DeBack, V. (1991). Today's nursing leaders: Creating the vision. *Nursing Administration Quarterly, 16*(1), 71–80.

Northouse, P. (2001). *Leadership: Theory and practice* (2nd ed.). Thousand Oaks, CA: Sage.

Ouchi, W. (1981). *Theory Z: How American business can meet the Japanese challenge.* Reading, MA: Addison-Wesley.

Porter O'Grady, T. (2001). Profound change: 21st century nursing. *Nursing Outlook, 41*(1), 182–186.

Pruitt, B., & Jacobs, M. (2006). Best practice interventions: Learn how you can prevent ventilator-associated pneumonia. *Nursing, 36*(2), 36–42.

Roethlisberger, J. F., & Dickson, W. J. (1939). *Management and the worker.* Cambridge, MA: Harvard University Press.

Scott, J. G., Sochalski, J., & Aiken, L. (1999). Review of magnet hospital research: Findings and implications for professional nursing practice. *Journal of Nursing Administration, 29*(1), 9–19.

Searle, L. (1996, January). 21st century leadership for nurse administrators. *Aspen's advisor for nurse executives, 11*(4), 1, 4–6.

Shortell, S. M., & Kaluzny, A. D. (2006). *Health Care Management* (5th ed.). Clifton Park, NY: Thomson Delmar Learning.

Stodgill, R. M. (1948). Personal factors associated with leadership: A survey of the literature. *Journal of Psychology, 25,* 35–71.

Stodgill, R. M. (1974). *Handbook of leadership: A survey of theory and research.* New York: Free Press.

Taylor, F. (1911). *Principles of scientific management.* New York: Harper & Row.

Tichy, N., & Devanna, D. (1986). *Transformational leadership.* New York: Wiley.

Upenieks, V. (2003). Nurse leaders' perceptions of what comprises successful leadership in today's acute inpatient environment. *Nursing Administration Quarterly, 27*(2), 140–152.

Weber, M. (1864), as reported in Mommsen, W. J. (1992). *The political and social theory of Max Weber: Collected essays.* Chicago: University of Chicago Press.

Wheatley, M. J. (1999). *Leadership and the new science: Learning about organization from an orderly universe.* San Francisco: Berrett-Koehler.

Wheatley, M. J. (2005). *Finding our way: Leadership for an uncertain time.* San Francisco, CA: Berrett-Koehler Publishers.

Wolf, G., Boland, S., & Aukerman, M. (1994). A transformational model for the practice of professional nursing. Part 1. *Journal of Nursing Administration, 24*(4), 51–57.

Wren, D. (1979). *Evolution of management thought.* New York: Wiley.

Young, S. (1992). Educational experiences of transformational nurse leaders. *Nursing Administration Quarterly, 17*(1), 25–33.

Yukl, G. (1998). *Leadership in organizations* (4th ed.). Upper Saddle River, NJ: Prentice Hall.

Yukl, G., Wall, S., & Lepsinger, R. (1990). Preliminary report on validation of the managerial practices survey. In K. E. Clarke & M. B. Clark (Eds.), *Measures of leadership* (pp. 223–238). West Orange, NJ: Leadership Library of America.

SUGGESTED READINGS

Baggett, M. M., & Baggett, F. B. (2005, July). Move from management to high-level leadership. *Nursing Management, 36*(7), 12.

Barker, A. M., Sullivan, D. T., & Emery, M. J. (2006). *Leadership competencies for clinical managers: The renaissance of transformational leadership.* Sudbury, MA: Jones and Bartlett.

Bass, B. (1998). *Transformational leadership: Industrial, military, and educational impact.* Mahwah, NJ: Erlbaum.

Bass, B., & Riggio, R. (2005). *Transformational leadership* (2nd ed.). Mahwah, NJ: Erlbaum.

Buckingham, M., & Coffman, C. (2001). *First break all the rules.* New York: Simon & Schuster.

Calpin-Davies, P. J. (2003, Jan.). Management and leadership: A dual role in nursing education. *Nursing Education Today, 23*(1), 3–10.

Cashman, K., & Forem, J. (2003). *Awakening the leader within: A story of transformation.* Hoboken, NJ: Wiley.

Conger, J., & Spreitzer, G. (Ed.). (1992). *Learning to lead.* San Francisco: Jossey-Bass.

Coughlin, L., Wingard, E., & Holihan, K. (Eds.). (2005). *Enlightened power: How women are transforming the practice of leadership.* San Francisco: Jossey-Bass.

Davenport, T. H. (2005). *Thinking for a living: How to get better performances and results from knowledge workers.* Cambridge, MA: Harvard School Press.

Donley, R. (2005). *Reflecting on 30 years of nursing leadership: 1975–2005.* Indianapolis, IN: Sigma Theta Tau International.

Dossey, B. M. (2000). *Florence Nightengale: Mystic, visionary, healer.* Springhouse, PA: Springhouse Corporation.

Enriquez, J. (2001). *As the future catches you.* New York: Crown Business.

Evans, M. G. (1996). R. J. House's "A path-goal theory of leader effectiveness." *Leadership Quarterly, 7*(3), 305–309.

Festa, M. S. (2005, July). Clinical leadership in hospital care: Leadership and teamwork skills are as important as clinical management skills. *British Medical Journal, 16,* 331(7509), 161–162.

Foley, B. J., Minick, M. P., & Kee, C. C. (2002). How nurses learn advocacy. *Journal of Nursing Scholarship, 34*(2), 181–186.

Gladwell, M. (2002). *The tipping point: How little things can make a big difference.* Boston: Little, Brown and Company.

Gordon, S. (2005). *Nursing against the odds: How health care cost-cutting, media stereotypes, and medical hubris undermine nurses and patient care.* Ithaca, NY: Cornell University Press.

Hesselbein, F., Goldsmith, M., & Beckhard, R. (Eds.). (1996). *The leader of the future: New visions, strategies, and practices for a new era.* San Francisco: Jossey-Bass.

Houser, B., & Player, K. (2004). *Pivotal moments in nursing: Leaders who changed the path of a profession.* Indianapolis, IN: Sigma Theta Tau International.

Huber, D. L. (2004, May). Nursing leadership: New initiatives in case management. *Nursing Outlook, 52*(3), 159–160.

Institute of Medicine Committee on the Work Environment for Nurses and Patient Safety. (2004). *Keeping patients safe: Transforming the work environment of nurses.* Washington, DC: The National Academies Press.

Johnson, S., & Blanchard, K. H. (1998). *Who moved my cheese? An amazing way to deal with change in your work and in your life.* New York: Putnam Adult.

Jumaa, M. O. (2006, Nov.). Developing nursing management and leadership capability in the workplace: Does it work? (2005). *Journal of Nursing Management, 13*(6), 451–458.

Kelly, T. (2005). *Ten faces of innovation: IDEOs strategies for beating the devil's advocate and driving creativity throughout your organization.* New York: Doubleday.

Kerfoot, K. M. (2006, Oct.–Dec.). Nursing research in leadership/management and the workplace: Narrowing the divide. *Nursing Administration Quarterly, 30*(4), 373–374.

Leonard, M., Frankel, A., & Simmonds, T. (2004). *Achieving safe and reliable health care: Strategies and solutions.* Chicago: Health Administration Press.

Lombardi, D. N. (2005, Nov.–Dec.). Preparing for the future: Management and leadership strategies. *Healthcare Executive, 20*(6), 8–12.

Lundin, S. C., Paul, H., & Christensen, J. (2000). *Fish!: A remarkable way to boost morale and improve results.* New York: Hyperion.

O'Neil, E., & Coffman, J. (Eds.). (1998). *Strategies for the future of nursing: Changing roles, responsibilities, and employment patterns of registered nurses.* San Francisco: Jossey-Bass.

Porter-O'Grady, T., & Malloch, K. (2002). *Quantum leadership: A textbook of new leadership.* Gaithersburg, MD: Aspen.

Santos, S. R., & Cox, K. (2000). Workplace adjustment and intergenerational differences between matures, boomers, and Xers. *Nursing Economic$, 18*(1), 7–13.

Schaffner, J. W., & Ludwig-Beymer, P. (2003). *Rx for the nursing shortage: A guidebook.* Chicago: Health Administration Press.

Secretan, L. (2004). *Inspire!* Hoboken, NJ: John Wiley & Sons.

Sellgren, S., Ekvall, G., & Tomson, G. (2006, July). Leadership styles in nursing management: Preferred and perceived. *Journal of Nursing Management, 14*(5), 348–355.

Senge, P. (1990). *The fifth discipline: The art and practice of the learning organization.* New York: Doubleday.

Sullivan, E. (2004). *Becoming influential: A guide for nurses.* Upper Saddle River, NJ: Pearson Prentice Hall.

Tomey, A. M., Arvin, K., Brown, W., Eslinger, S., Hamilton, C., Lofton, S., et al. (2001, March–April). Review of leadership and management literature. *Nurse Educator, 26*(2), 53, 63.

Upenieks, V. V. (2003). What constitutes effective leadership? Perceptions of magnet and nonmagnet nurse leaders. *Journal of Nursing Administration, 33*(9), 456–467.

The Health Care Environment

Ronda G. Hughes, PhD, MHS, RN ⊕ Patricia Kelly, RN, MSN

Health care in the twenty-first century will require a new kind of health professional: someone who is equipped to transcend the traditional doctor-patient relationship to reach a new level of partnership with patients; someone who can lead, manage, and work effectively in a team and organizational environment; someone who can practice safe high quality care but also constantly see and create the opportunities for improvement (Donaldson, 2001).

OBJECTIVES

Upon completion of this chapter, the reader should be able to:

1. Identify how health care is organized and financed in the United States.
2. Identify the major issues facing health care described in major national reports.
3. Relate efforts for improving the quality of health care.

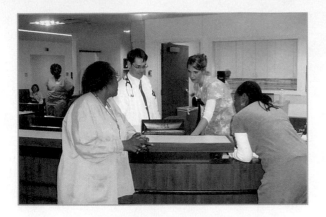

Your neighbor calls, asking you to come over and advise her as to what to do with her grandchild who is sick. Finding the three-year-old child with a runny nose, a slight fever, and a congested cough, you recommend that she take the child to her primary care clinician for an office visit, especially if the fever continues or rises. Your neighbor feels that there is no urgency because of the high cost of the office visit co-pay and her difficulty in getting the child to the clinician as the office hours coincide with her work schedule. Also, she is unable to get an appointment until two weeks later because her grandchild is covered by Medicaid. She opts to wait until after business hours on Friday and then take the child to the emergency department. By the time they arrive at the hospital five days later, the child is admitted to the pediatric intensive care unit with a temperature of 104°F (40°C) and is hospitalized for a week.

What do you think of the occurrence of this type of scenario in the United States?

How can access to health care be assured for all patients regardless of source of insurance?

Health care delivery in the United States is a combination of public and private initiatives organized to provide citizens with access to cost-effective quality health care. Most Americans are in good health, but many citizens are children, elderly, sick, disabled, or otherwise in need of access to quality health care services at a reasonable cost. The need for access, quality, and cost has driven various initiatives to improve health care in the past and present.

This chapter discusses a selected history of American health care. It discusses health care in various settings, disease management, and the influence of external forces on health care. The chapter reviews how health care is organized, funded, and accredited. It explores health care disparities and clinical variation, and reviews reports of the Institute of Medicine Committee on Health Care. Finally, the chapter discusses issues regarding quality health care and the education of health care professionals.

HISTORY OF HEALTH CARE

Advances in health care science and technology continually change what health care can accomplish. These advances are continuously improving patients' quality of life and saving the lives of other patients that would otherwise fail. Yet generations after the insights of Florence Nightingale were first set forth, some problems continue to challenge us, including preventing the spread of disease, structuring organizations to benefit both clinicians and patients, collecting and using data and information to encourage improvement, and understanding how external forces influence care delivery. An example of this is Nightingale's discovery of the link between adverse patient outcomes and cleanliness and hand-washing. Over 146 years after her discovery of this link, the simple task of hand-washing has failed to become habitual among clinicians. An estimated 2 million cases of health care-acquired infections, representing 5% of all hospitalizations, occur in acute care hospitalizations, causing additional health care expenditures in excess of $4.5 billion annually. The most prevalent and preventable infections are bloodstream infections, pneumonia, and surgical site and urinary tract infections (Gaynes et al., 2001). The highest rates of infection have been found to occur in Burn Intensive Care Units (ICUs), Neonatal ICUs, and Pediatric ICUs; areas where infections can easily be fatal (National Nosocomial Infections Surveillance [NNIS], 1998).

STRUCTURING HOSPITALS AROUND NURSING CARE

Nightingale also described the importance of structuring hospitals around nursing care. The initial design of hospitals followed that advice by building large wards where nurses could easily monitor and observe their patients. Later, hospital design evolved to placing patient rooms surrounding centrally located nursing stations. Then, as today, the physical environment of hospitals can create stress for patients, their families, and clinical staff. Research is finding links between the physical environment and patient outcomes, patient safety, and patient and staff satisfaction (Hamilton, 2003). Studies show that such elements of hospital design as exposure to natural light, private rooms, and facilities that are staff friendly and have less noise contribute to improved patient outcomes (Ulrich, Quan, Zimring, Joseph, & Choudhary, 2004).

Although little is known about how to best design the hospital environment to facilitate clinical advances and care delivery, an estimated $200 billion will be expended for new hospital construction across the United States during the next 10 years (Institute of Medicine [IOM], 2004a). The Robert Wood Johnson Foundation, the nation's largest philanthropy devoted exclusively to health and health care, has provided funding to the Center for Health Design, a nonprofit research organization, for the Designing the 21st Century Hospital Project, which is the most extensive review of the evidence-based approach to hospital design ever conducted. See www.healthdesign.org.

COLLECTING DATA

Nightingale also astutely recognized the importance of collecting and using data to assess the quality of health care. She employed coxcomb diagrams to present visual images of the number of preventable deaths during the Crimean war (Figure 2-1) and then later in London hospitals.

Today, data is collected through patient records, surveys, and administrative systems. From these, reports are developed, such as *To Err is Human* (IOM, 1999); the Centers for Disease Control and Prevention (CDC) National Vital Statistics Reports (Martin, Hamilton, Sutton, & Ventura, 2006); and The National Healthcare Disparities Report (NHDR) (Agency for Healthcare Research and Quality [AHRQ], 2005). These reports provide invaluable information, and data is displayed with charts and pictures to emphasize the successes and failure of health care throughout our nation. Evidence of significant disparities and low quality continue to demonstrate the need for significant healthcare improvement.

INFLUENCE OF EXTERNAL FORCES ON HEALTH CARE

Recognizing the influence of external forces on care delivery and scope of practice, Nightingale also kept informed of the activities of practitioners and government policy makers (Dossey, Selanders, & Beck, 2005). With health care being the largest sector of our economy, employers, clinicians, managers, and patients all have a vested interest in proposed changes to health care financing, organization, and the responsibilities and scope of practice for clinicians. Today, nursing leaders, managers, and staff need to be aware of and involved in the ongoing processes of making health policy.

ORGANIZATION OF HEALTH CARE

Health care systems have three simple components: structure, process, and outcome. The **structure** component of health care includes resources or structures needed to deliver quality health care, for example, human and physical resources, such as nurses and nurs-

ing and medical practitioners, hospital buildings, medical records, and pharmaceuticals. The **process** component of health care includes the quality activities, procedures, tasks, and processes performed within the health care structures, such as hospital admissions, surgical operations, and nursing and medical care delivery following standards and guidelines to achieve quality outcomes. The **outcome** component of health care refers to the results of good care delivery achieved by using quality structures and quality processes and includes the achievement of outcomes such as patient satisfaction, good health and functional ability, and the absence of health care-acquired infections and morbidity. See Table 2-1 for examples of structure, process, and outcome performance measures in clinical care, financial management, and human resources management.

It would be naïve to consider health care in the United States as it is currently being delivered as being an effective system of care. If that were true, it would imply that health care is based on shared values and goals; is organized around the patient; utilizes all pertinent information; ensures value-based and quality-based care; rewards quality care; is universally standardized and simplified; is available to everyone regardless of income, race, ethnicity, or education; is affordable; and reflects effective collaboration among clinicians and with patients (Davis, 2005; World Health Organization [WHO], 2000, p. 35). The World Health Organization (WHO) has put forth three primary goals for what good health care should do: (1) ensure that the health status of everyone is the best that is possible across the lifespan; (2) respond to patient's expectation of respectful treatment and include a focus on patients by health care clinicians; and (3) provide financial protection for everyone regardless of ability to pay (WHO, 2000).

REAL WORLD INTERVIEW

What can be said about the United States health care system is that it is not really a system, but rather a hodge-podge of systems, some great, some not so great, with a "sometimes" desire for universal service but with also the fierce energy of independent individuals seeking autonomy.

Ellyn Stecker, MD
Shipshewana, Indiana

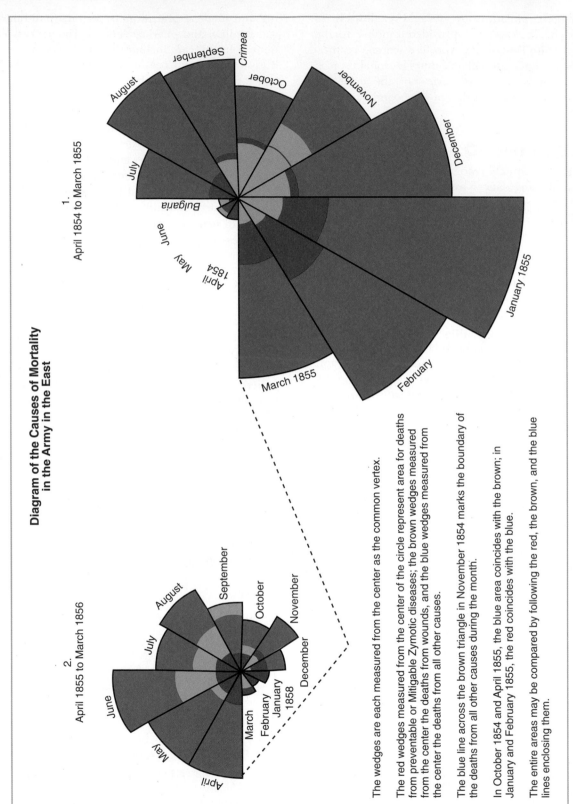

Diagram of the Causes of Mortality in the Army in the East

The wedges are each measured from the center of the circle as the common vertex.

The red wedges measured from the center of the circle represent area for deaths from preventable or Mitigable Zymotic diseases; the brown wedges measured from the center the deaths from wounds, and the blue wedges measured from the center the deaths from all other causes.

The blue line across the brown triangle in November 1854 marks the boundary of the deaths from all other causes during the month.

In October 1854 and April 1855, the blue area coincides with the brown; in January and February 1855, the red coincides with the blue.

The entire areas may be compared by following the red, the brown, and the blue lines enclosing them.

Figure 2-1 Florence nightingale's coxcomb diagram of the causes of mortality in the army in the east. (Reprinted with permission of the Houghton Library, Harvard University, Cambridge, MA.)

TABLE 2-1	**EXAMPLES OF PERFORMANCE MEASURES BY CATEGORY**

	Clinical Care	**Financial Management**	**Human Resources Management**
Structure	*Effectiveness* ■ Percent of nurses and physicians who are certified ■ JC (formerly JCAHO) accreditation ■ Presence of council for quality improvement planning ■ Presence of magnet recognition	*Effectiveness* ■ Qualifications of administrators in finance department ■ Use of preadmission criteria ■ Presence of an integrated financial and clinical information system and clinical decision-making technology	*Effectiveness* ■ Ability to attract desired nursing and medical practitioners, and other health professionals ■ Size or growth of nursing and medical staff ■ Salary and benefits competitive with competitors ■ Quality of in-house staff education
Process	*Effectiveness* ■ Ratio of medication errors ■ Ratio of nurse-sensitive complications ■ Ratio of health care-acquired infection ■ Ratio of postsurgical wound infection ■ Ratio of normal tissue removed during surgery	*Effectiveness* ■ Days in accounts receivable ■ Use of generic drugs and drug formulary ■ Market share ■ Size (or growth) of shared service arrangements	*Effectiveness* ■ Number and type of staff grievances ■ Number of promotions ■ Organizational climate
	Productivity ■ Ratio of total patient days to total full-time equivalent (FTE) nurses ■ Ratio of total admissions to total FTE staff ■ Ratio of patient visits to total FTE nursing and medical practitioners	*Productivity* ■ Ratio of collections to FTE financial staff ■ Ratio of total admissions to FTE in finance department ■ Ratio of new capital acquisitions to fund-raising staff	*Productivity* ■ Ratio of front-line staff to managers
	Efficiency ■ Average cost per admission ■ Average cost per surgery	*Efficiency* ■ Average cost per debt collection ■ Debt/equity ratio	*Efficiency* ■ Recruitment costs
Outcome	*Effectiveness* ■ Case-severity-adjusted mortality ■ Patient satisfaction ■ Patient functional health status ■ Number of deaths from medical errors	*Effectiveness* ■ Return on assets ■ Operating margins ■ Size and growth of federal, state, and local grants for teaching and research ■ Bond rating	*Effectiveness* ■ Staff turnover rate ■ Number of absenteeism days ■ Staff satisfaction

Source: Compiled with information from Shortell, S. M., & Kaluzny, A. D. (2006). *Health care management* (5th ed.). Clifton Park, NY: Thomson Delmar Learning.

ABSENCE OF A UNIVERSAL HEALTH CARE SYSTEM

The United States is one of only a few large countries in the world without a universal system of health care. Access to care in the United States is tied directly to having health insurance. As a result, serious gaps in health care payment coverage leave millions of people in the United States uninsured, thus leaving them sicker and dying younger than the insured (Muenning et al., 2005, p. 2–34). Compared to countries such as Great Britain, Canada, and Germany, health care services in the United States are far less organized and more expensive given the total health care expenditures as a percentage of the Gross Domestic Product (GDP) (Anell & Willis, 2000). As we go to press, several state governments have proposed state-run solutions for the problem. Several large consumer groups, for example, American Association for Retired People (AARP), and several business groups are also advocating for universal health care by the federal government.

EMPHASIS ON HOSPITAL CARE

In the United States, the emphasis on acute care health care services has successfully driven health care costs higher but has not necessarily improved the quality of care or patient outcomes (Werner & Bradlow, 2006; Jeffrey & Newacheck, 2006). Considering what health care services are needed by patients to improve their health status, only 8 out of 1,000 people will benefit from hospitalization, something that seems odd when considering where the research dollars are targeted and where the majority of health care dollars are devoted, that is, acute care settings in hospitals. When you look at a group of 1,000 people, it is estimated that 800 of them will experience symptoms of some disease or condition. Of this group of 800, 265 will be seen in a practitioner's office, hospital outpatient

CRITICAL THINKING 2-1

Think about how you could improve health care delivery in the United States. If only 8 out of 1,000 people need hospitalization, and 800 have symptoms, how could we best deliver this care? Health care that focuses on more delivery of prevention and primary care would increase health and decrease disease throughout the United States. How can you work individually and with your community to begin to accomplish this?

EVIDENCE FROM THE LITERATURE

Citation: States take on national health insurance crisis. *USA Today.* January 16, 2007, p 12A.

Discussion: The list of what is wrong with American health care is long. One in seven Americans lack insurance and either forego needed care or receive treatment that is inadequate and expensive at overcrowded emergency rooms. Most of this cost is passed on to others. Those lucky enough to have insurance have seen their premiums double in a decade, while they get less for their money. Co-pays are up, reimbursement rates are down, and some top doctors won't take insurance, making their services available only to wealthy patients. Nearly everyone squanders money and time fighting through payment hassles with their insurance companies, and anyone can abruptly be left without insurance at any time at enormous medical and financial peril.

California and Massachusetts have proposed similar reforms to cover nearly every resident. Roughly, these reforms look like this: Everybody is required to have insurance. Patients can pick a plan and an insurance carrier that suits them. Prices vary, as does what is provided, but everyone gets at least coverage for some preventive care plus major hospital bills. A national universal health care solution might be preferable but having states serve as laboratories for experiments will let us see which ideas work and which ones should be abandoned.

Implications for Practice: Nurses must participate in the health care delivery debate. Currently, half of U.S. bankruptcies are a result, in part, of medical illness or medical bills (McCanne, 2007). Money is not the problem. We are already spending enough on health care to provide high-quality, comprehensive services for everyone. But our inefficient, private-sector insurance bureaucracies have failed and need to be replaced with single-payer national health insurance, or something else that works. Every other developed nation has covered its citizens through some form of nonprofit health insurance (McCanne, 2007).

department or emergency department, or home health care. Only 8 will eventually be hospitalized. The majority doesn't need hospitalization and would benefit from primary health care delivery outside the hospital (Green, Gryer, Yawn, Lanier, & Dovery, 2000).

NEED FOR PRIMARY HEALTH CARE

Given that the majority of patient needs and patient care delivery occurs outside acute care settings, primary care "which provides integrated, accessible health care services by clinicians who are accountable for addressing a large majority of personal health care needs, developing a sustained partnership with patients, and practicing in the context of family and community (IOM 1996, p. 1), should be better understood and appreciated for the role it has in improving patient's health status and health outcomes. The key foundations of primary care (Starfield,

1998) can be applied across the health care continuum and across organizational settings because **primary care** emphasizes seven important features: care that is continuous, comprehensive, coordinated, community oriented, family centered, culturally competent, and begun at first contact with the patient. According to Starfield (1998), patients and clinicians need to work together to appropriately utilize services, based on the following four foundations of primary care:

- *First Contact:* Conduct the initial evaluation and define the health dysfunction, treatment options, and health goals.
- *Longitudinality:* Sustain a patient-clinician relationship continuously over time, throughout the patient's illness, acute need, and disease management.
- *Comprehensiveness:* Manage the wide range of health care needs, across health care settings and among different health care professionals.

CASE STUDY 2-1

You work in an Emergency Department (ED) that sees 6,000 patients a month. Patients are charged $200.00 per visit plus charges for tests and medications. Thus, these 6,000 patients can generate $1,200,000 in gross revenue for the hospital. Consider that there are 15 RNs making $30.00 per hour and 6 MDs, making $150.00 per hour working each shift. Salaries for the RNs total $324,000. Salaries for the MDs total $648,000. The total salary for these two groups is $972,000. Of these patients, 50% have Medicare/Medicaid, 45% are covered by managed care or insurance, and 5% have no insurance. Thus, just 95% of patients can pay their bills. The other 5% of patient's bills are written off by the hospital as bad debt.

Medicare/Medicaid/Managed Care/Insurance companies often only pay 55% of the bills for these patients. They may deny payment for 45% of the bills. Thus, for the $1,140,000 billed (95% of $1,200,000), the hospital will receive approximately $627,000 (55% of the $1,140,000 billed). Approximately $513,000 of the bill will not be paid by Medicare/Medicaid/Managed Care/Insurance. Consider the following:

What other expenses besides salary must the hospital pay out of the $627,000 that it receives? Consider hospital space, liability insurance, technology costs, and so on.

Notice the effect that increasing the volume of patients has on your budget figures. What happens to your budget if the patient volume goes to 8,000 patient ED visits per month and staffing stays the same?

Are patients receiving useful information about future illness prevention and healthy living practices in the ED?

Is this a cost-effective way to deliver health care?

How could we better serve the health care needs of Americans?

■ *Coordination:* Build upon longitudinality. Care received through referrals and other providers is followed and integrated, averting unnecessary services and duplication of services.

Primary care clinicians, which primarily include both medical and nursing practitioners, can be a patient's greatest asset in negotiating the health care system and improving patient outcomes. It is through understanding the patient's past and present, that future health care needs can be anticipated. Primary care interventions, such as health promotion and timely preventive care and medication administration, can reduce the need for hospitalizations, improve the health of patients, and avert adverse morbidity and mortality outcomes. Patients and their families can communicate with clinicians to understand their health care needs, how to achieve the best possible health, and how to partner with clinicians to improve decision making. This is what patient-centered care is based on, both primary care and patient decision making.

THE FEDERAL GOVERNMENT

The federal government is a major driver of health care organization and delivery. Distinct, major divisions of the U.S. Department of Health and Human Services (DHHS) include the following:

■ *Agency for Healthcare Research and Quality (AHRQ):* Funds health services research on the effectiveness of health care services and outcomes of care.

■ *Centers for Disease Control and Prevention (CDC):* Promotes health and quality of life by preventing and controlling disease, injury, and disability.

■ *Centers for Medicare and Medicaid Services (CMS):* Administers the Medicare program and regulates the Medicaid program.

■ *Food and Drug Administration (FDA):* Monitors the safety of food, the safety of cosmetic products, the safety and efficacy of drugs, and the safety and efficacy of medical devices.

■ *Health Resources and Services Administration (HRSA):* Administers training programs for health care clinicians, funding for pregnant women and children, programs for persons with HIV/AIDS, and programs serving low-income, underserved, and rural populations.

■ *Indian Health Service (IHS):* Maintains health services provided to American Indians and Alaska Natives.

■ *National Institutes of Health (NIH):* Funds biomedical research through 18 research institutes primarily organized according to specific diseases.

■ *Substance Abuse and Mental Health Services Administration (SAMHSA):* Provides leadership in services, policy, and information dissemination for mental health and substance abuse treatment and prevention.

STATE AND LOCAL LEVELS

Public health services at the state and local levels include boards of health and state and local health departments. Even with the 1988 IOM Report on public health, the ability of public health departments to engage in improving the health of the public has become limited (Tilson & Berkowitz, 2006). In addition, efforts for bioterrorism and disaster preparedness have brought the nation's infrastructure desolation to light, causing increased funding for this nation's disaster preparedness efforts, with little money focused on public health care funding and infrastructure redevelopment.

HOME HEALTH CARE

The location of care delivery is continually changing to adapt to technologies and patient needs. The fastest-growing segment of the health care delivery system has been the home health care business. In 1988, the Health Care Financing Administration expended approximately $2 billion for home health. By 1999, approximately $20 billion was expended. Almost as many persons receive health care in the home (an estimated 34,000,000 annually) as receive health care in acute-care settings (Kramarow, Lentzner, Rooks, Weeks, & Sayday, 1999).

HEALTH CARE DISPARITIES

Certain factors, known as enabling factors, affect a person's ability to have access to health care. Generally, these factors include income, type of insurance coverage, gender, race or ethnicity, geographic proximity, and system characteristics. Socioeconomic status is the number one predictor of poor health. The poor are more than three times as likely as the wealthy to die prematurely or have a disability from illness (Lantz et al., 1998), despite nearly two-thirds of the money for public health being directed to medical safety-net services. (Office of Management and Budget, 1999). Not enough health care delivery and attention is directed toward the top underlying causes of death in the United States (Table 2-2).

Analysis of large datasets illustrates that as one ages, more health care services are utilized; women use health care services more frequently then men; and whites have greater health care access, and therefore higher utilization rates, than do patients of color (National Healthcare Disparities Report [NHDR], 2005); (National Healthcare Quality Report [NHQR], 2005). Both financial and nonfinancial barriers to care delivery result in lack of attention to health care disparities and factors contributing to the underlying causes of death, which affects health outcomes. In-depth information on national health care disparities is reported in the annual National Health Disparities Report (NHDR, 2005), which now presents state variations (see www.ahrq.gov/qual/nhdr05/nhdr05.htm).

HEALTH CARE SPENDING

In the United States, health insurance is generally employment-based, so long as it is affordable for the employer to offer this health care coverage for employees. The higher one's income in this country, the greater the likelihood of having health insurance coverage. The opposite is true for those with low incomes, especially those with poverty-level incomes. Patients who are at poverty levels often cannot afford insurance premiums nor can they afford, in the majority of instances, out-of-pocket health care costs. Since the inception of private health insurance in the late 1920s following the development of hospitals as the "center" of health care and subsequent rising health care costs (Starr, 1983), private health insurance from third-party payers such as insurance companies has been generally voluntarily offered as a benefit to employees and sometimes their families. Patients may make payments to providers of health care and third-party payers. Providers of health care deliver service to patients and bill third-party payers. Third party-payers may make payment to providers as direct payment fees for individuals, capitated payment for services for a group of patients, or as prospective payments for future patients. Health insurance distributes health care funds from the healthy to the sick (Figure 2-2).

TABLE 2-2	TOP 10 UNDERLYING CAUSES OF DEATH IN THE UNITED STATES IN 1990		
1. Tobacco	4. Alcohol	7. Sexual behavior	9. Illicit drug use
2. Poor diet	5. Infectious agents	8. Motor vehicles	10. Pollutants/toxins
3. Lack of exercise	6. Firearms		

Source: © McGinnis, J. M., & Foege, W. H. (1993). Actual causes of death in the United States. *Journal of the American Medical Association, 270*(18), pp. 2207–2212.

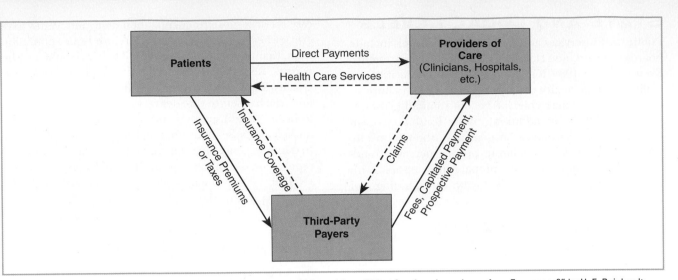

Figure 2-2 Economic relationships in the health care delivery system. (Adapted from "What Can Americans Learn from Europeans?" by U. E. Reinhardt, 1989, *Health Care Financing Review* [Supplement], p. 97–103.)

RISING HEALTH CARE COSTS

Over the years, by making health care more affordable, health insurance has contributed to rising health care costs. Even those with private health insurance can be faced with major expenses not covered by their insurance in the event of a serious illness or accident. Compounding this is the fact that health care costs grow faster than wages, due in large part to improvements in health care technology (Gilmer & Kronick, 2005). Health insurance premiums continue to increase, and employees are bearing more of the financial burden for their cost (Gabel et al., 2003). It is not uncommon for insurance plans to limit their maximum lifetime insurance coverage payout for a patient's health care expenses. Insurance companies also may include a limited catastrophic expenses exclusion clause and/or other insurance payment exclusions for pre-existing illnesses or services unless the beneficiary is willing to pay for higher premiums. It is common for insurance plans to feature patient cost-sharing items such as payment deductibles and copayments for services. Unfortunately, underinsurance and cost sharing items such as these reduce health service utilization for both appropriate and inappropriate medical services (Lohr et al., 1986; Lurie et al., 1987).

MEDICARE AND OTHER HEALTH CARE COSTS

One reason proposed for the steady incline in health care costs is that the elderly have virtually universal health care coverage through Medicare. This universal health care coverage indicates that the United States will likely experience very rapid growth in overall health expenditures in coming years, as the population continues to age. Other

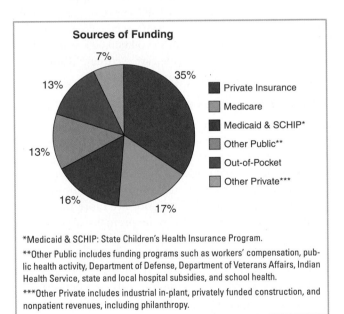

*Medicaid & SCHIP: State Children's Health Insurance Program.

**Other Public includes funding programs such as workers' compensation, public health activity, Department of Defense, Department of Veterans Affairs, Indian Health Service, state and local hospital subsidies, and school health.

***Other Private includes industrial in-plant, privately funded construction, and nonpatient revenues, including philanthropy.

Figure 2-3 The Nation's Health Services Dollars, 2005, Sources of Funding. (From "The Nation's Health Dollar, Calendar Year 2005: Where It Came From," 2006, Centers for Medicare & Medicaid Services, Office of the Actuary, National Health Statistics Group. Retrieved January 13, 2007, from http://www.cms.hhs.gov/NationalHealthExpendData/02_NationalHealthAccountsHistorical.asp#TopOfPage.)

sources of health care funding and where it went are shown in Figure 2-3 and Figure 2-4.

HEALTH CARE INSURANCE

Health care insurance is one of the most significant factors in facilitating access to health care services. Yet each year, those covered by insurance and the breadth and depth of health insurance coverage continues to deteriorate. All too often, people are not covered by private insurance because it is not affordable. As health care costs increase and

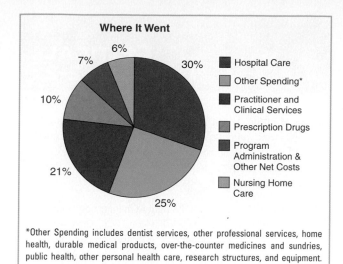

Where It Went

6%
7%
30%
10%
21%
25%

- Hospital Care
- Other Spending*
- Practitioner and Clinical Services
- Prescription Drugs
- Program Administration & Other Net Costs
- Nursing Home Care

*Other Spending includes dentist services, other professional services, home health, durable medical products, over-the-counter medicines and sundries, public health, other personal health care, research structures, and equipment.

Figure 2-4 The Nation's Health Services Dollars, 2005. (From "The Nation's Health Dollar, Calendar Year 2005: Where It Went," 2006, Centers for Medicare & Medicaid Services, Office of the Actuary, National Health Statistics Group. Retrieved January 13, 2007, from http://www.cms.hhs.gov/NationalHealthExpendData/ 02_NationalHealthAccountsHistorical.asp#TopOfPage.)

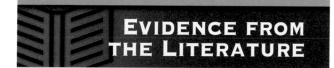

EVIDENCE FROM THE LITERATURE

Citation: Grose, T. (2007). How they do it better: Free health care for all. *U.S. News and World Report.* March 26, 2007, 65.

Discussion: Britain spends $2,546 annually per person for health care and offers all its citizens free care. The United States spends $6,102 annually per person for health care, and 47 million people are uninsured for health care. Britain's infant mortality rate is lower and its life expectancy rate is higher than the same rates in the United States. Patients in Britain wait for some elective surgeries, but they can buy private coverage for this, if desired. Appointments with general practitioners in Britain can be made quickly and Emergency Room treatment is good. Drugs are free to patients in Britain.

Implications for Practice: The United States would benefit from studies of other countries' health care systems. We can look to see what works well in other countries and what does not work so well and develop a system that is cost effective.

REAL WORLD INTERVIEW

I was admitted to the hospital in December for what was later diagnosed as angina. After being stabilized in the emergency room, I was admitted to the cardiac care unit. A series of tests were ordered by my cardiologist to determine enzyme levels in my blood. This would show if I had suffered a heart attack. Blood was drawn every eight hours for twenty-four hours. The news was good—no heart attack—until I received the bill. My insurance company said the enzyme tests for angina were frivolous and not necessary, and they would not pay. I had my cardiologist write a letter of explanation, saying the tests he ordered were routine for determining a diagnosis. After this second appeal, the insurance company rejected my payment claim again. After several more appeals, my insurance company ultimately paid the laboratory bill for these tests, but would not pay the pathologist for his interpretation of the blood tests. It has now been six months since I received my initial bill, and the hospital and pathologist's office have turned my case over to a collection agency. They did not take into consideration the fact that I was appealing the bill. They wanted me to pay upfront and then appeal. That was not going to happen.

Kathleen A. Milch
Patient
Whiting, Indiana

rising costs cut into business profits, employers are choosing to offer fewer insurance options, increase insurance premiums, or stop offering health insurance altogether. Between 2000 and 2004, the number of patients with employer-based insurance has been steadily dwindling from 63.6% to 59.8%. This was during a time of economic growth (Kaiser Family Foundation [KFF], 2004).

Decreases in the number of those with private insurance coverage increases the total number of uninsured. Other factors contributing to high numbers of uninsured can be attributed to patients being in between jobs or unemployed and not being eligible for public programs. These are all factors contributing to this nation's growing uninsured population. Together, the number of the uninsured increased from 38.8 million (14.2% of the U.S. population) in 2000 to over 46 million (15.3% of the U.S. population) in 2004. These numbers are expected to continue to increase in the years ahead (KFF & Health Research and Education Trust, 2006; KFF, 2006).

MEDICARE AND MEDICAID

Because we do not have national/universal health care insurance, public health care programs are intended to fill the gap, providing coverage for those without employer-based insurance. Beginning in 1965 under Titles XVIII (Medicare) and XIX (Medicaid) of the Social Security Act, eligibility for public insurance has been based on age (Medicare for those age 65 and older) or based on having a low income and/or having a disability (Medicaid). Medicare and Medicaid programs ensure access to many needed services for otherwise uninsured populations (Table 2-3).

OTHER PUBLIC PROGRAMS

Other large public insurance programs are associated with American Indian and Alaska Native heritage, and the Military Services, that is, veteran's health and insurance for active military personnel and their families. The Indian Health Service (IHS), under the U.S. Department of Health and Human Services, provides health services to American Indians and Alaska natives enrolled in more than 500 tribes, villages, and pueblos (IHS, 2006). The Indian Self-Determination Act of 1975 gave many tribal organizations the responsibility for the provision of health care services. IHS maintains some hospitals and clinics, yet recent legislation has severely cut funding for these sites of care.

The Department of Defense (DOD) finances and manages TRICARE, called the Civilian Health and Medical Program of the Uniformed Services (CHAMPUS) until 1993, for enlisted military personnel and their military dependents as well as for retirees and their dependents and survivors (Department of Defense, 2003). The Department of Veterans Affairs, established in 1921, finances and manages the Veterans Health Administration (VHA). This program is available for U.S. veterans if they need any medical, prescription, surgical, and rehabilitation care services.

STATE REGULATION OF HEALTH INSURANCE

Three key pieces of federal legislation set forth national standards that the individual states use to regulate health insurance. First, the Employee Retirement Income Security Act (ERISA) of 1974 provides a framework for states to regulate health insurers. Second, the Consolidated Omnibus Budget Reconciliation Act (COBRA) of 1985 ensures that employees who resigned, were laid off, were terminated, or lost their job due to family-related reasons can retain their health insurance coverage for up to 18 months and, in some cases, up to a maximum of 36 months if they are deemed qualified and pay the full premium. A third piece of legislation, the Health Insurance Portability and Accountability Act (HIPAA) of 1996 imposed restrictions on limitations and exclusions of insurance coverage for those with preexisting conditions and restricted other attempts to exclude employees from insurance coverage. It also provides protection of

insurance coverage as employees change employers, and it provides tax exclusions for medical savings accounts (Table 2-4).

THE RISING COST OF HEALTH CARE

U.S. national health care expenditures were $1.9 trillion in 2004 (KFF & Health Research and Education Trust, 2006). A staggering 16% of the GDP was spent on health care. From 1960 to 2000, the GDP for health care grew nearly 15-fold, from approximately $526 billion to the trillions of dollars spent today. It is projected that health care spending will rise to $4 trillion by 2015 (Borger et al., 2006). Health care spending continues to increase faster than the overall U.S. economy. This is 2.5 percentage points faster than the growth of the GDP (Centers for Medicare and Medicaid Services [CMS], 2006). In 2000, the percentage of GDP for health care was 15.3%, and analysts project this number to keep rising to 20% (Borger et al., 2006).

FACTORS CONTRIBUTING TO RISING HEALTH CARE COSTS

There are many factors contributing to the rising costs of health care. The key factors include the aging of the population with growth in the demand for health care, increased utilization of pharmaceuticals, expensive new technologies, rising hospital care costs, practitioner behavior, cost shifting, and administrative costs (Thorpe, Woodruff, & Ginsburg, 2005).

TABLE 2-3	OVERVIEW OF MEDICARE AND MEDICAID

	Medicare	**Medicaid**
Benefits	*Part A:* Coverage for hospitalization, skilled nursing facility (up to 100 days), hospice (up to 6 months for terminally ill), and some home health care. *Part B:* Coverage for ambulatory practitioner services; physical, occupational, and speech therapy; medical equipment; diagnostic tests; and some preventive care. *Part C:* Optional coverage for beneficiaries who can choose to receive all of their health care services through one of the provider organizations under Part C. (Medicare Advantage, formerly known as Medicare + Choice). These plans are available in many areas. *Part D:* Optional coverage for outpatient pharmaceuticals.	Comprehensive set of benefits, including coverage for the following: ■ Inpatient hospital, excluding inpatient services in institutions for mental disease. ■ Outpatient hospital, including Federally Qualified Health Centers, rural health clinics, and some other ambulatory services. ■ Other laboratory and x-ray services. ■ Services provided by medical practitioners, certified pediatric and family nurse practitioners, and nurse midwives. ■ Skilled nursing facility services for beneficiaries, age 21 and older. ■ Early and Periodic Screening, Diagnosis, and Treatment (EPSDT) for children under age 21. ■ Family planning services and supplies. ■ Medical and surgical services of a dentist. ■ Home health services for beneficiaries who are entitled to nursing facility services. ■ Home health agency services or services by an RN when there is no home health agency in the area. ■ Home health aides. ■ Medical supplies and appliances for use in the home. ■ Pregnancy-related services and services for other conditions that might complicate pregnancy, including 60 days postpartum pregnancy-related services.
Eligibility	*Medicare—Part A:* ■ 65 years of age and older and has worked 40 quarters—includes that person's spouse. ■ End-stage renal disease. ■ Totally and permanently disabled individuals (after receiving Social Security disability benefits for 2 years). *Medicare—Part B:* ■ If pay monthly premium (out-of-pocket or via Medicaid if patient qualifies).	■ Certain categories of low income people <65 (mainly women of child-bearing age and children). ■ People over age 65, the blind, and totally disabled who receive cash assistance under the federal Supplemental Security Income (SSI) program. ■ State Children's Health Insurance Program (SCHIP): Children, up to age 19, whose families earn up to $36,200 a year (for a family of four).

(Continues)

TABLE 2-3   OVERVIEW OF MEDICARE AND MEDICAID (CONTINUED)

	Medicare	**Medicaid**
Financing	*Source 1—Tax Dollars from Workforce:* 1.45% mandatory federal income tax on all covered wages matched by the employer, 2.9% mandatory federal income tax on self-employment income for self-employed persons, and individual enrollee premiums.	*Source 1—Federal Tax Dollars:* From general tax revenues, the federal government pays between 50% and 83% of total Medicaid costs in the state.
	Source 2—After Tax Dollars from Beneficiaries: Most people pay a monthly premium of $88.50 for Part B coverage.	*Source 2—State Tax Dollars:* From general state (and sometimes local) tax revenues.
	Source 3—Additional Insurance, Private: Prescription Drug Coverage is insurance provided by private companies.	*Source 3—Out-of-Pocket:* Beneficiaries either pay amount not covered by Medicaid or health care provider assumes cost.
	Source 4—Out-of-Pocket: For amounts not paid by Medicare, both Parts A and B. *Example:* Part B has an annual $124 deductible and, for most services, a 20% coinsurance.	
Administered by	Federal government's Department of Health and Human Services (DHHS) Centers for Medicaid & Medicare Services (CMS).	Individual state governments, with some federal oversight (CMS).

TABLE 2-4   HIPAA PRIVACY REGULATIONS

- Allows patient to review and request amendments to their medical records
- Gives consumers control over how their personal health information is used and limits the release of information without a patient's consent
- Restricts the amount of patient information shared between physicians and other caregivers to the "minimum necessary"
- Requires privacy-conscious business practices, such as hiring a privacy officer and training employees about patient confidentiality
- Requires that paper records and oral communications be protected from privacy breaches

AGING POPULATION

Because more baby-boomers are crossing the threshold age of 65, and the average life-expectancy is increasing, the elderly are becoming the largest group in the population. By 2035, the population of persons 65 years of age will exceed 80 million. In 1997, 1.6 million persons lived in long-term care facilities. By 2005, this figure will increase to an estimated 5 million. As this segment of the population increases, so does the utilization of health care. As more of the population ages, the number of nursing homes has increased from 16,091 in 1986 to 17,208 in 1996. The number of beds in these facilities increased from 1.298 million to 1.839 million (Kramarow et al., 1999). Given the increased utilization of pharmaceuticals and the need to manage and treat chronic illnesses and long-term care needs with increasing age, those patients aged 75 and older incur per capita health expenditures five times higher than those of people between 25 and 34 years of age (Boddenheimer, 2005a). On average, annual per capita expenditures on those patients aged 65 and older is $11,089, significantly higher than the annual expenditure of $3,352 for those aged 19 to 64 (Keehan, 2004). Despite the projected increases in demand from both growth in the elderly population and rising health care costs, estimates are that by the year 2018, federal funding will be able to cover only 80% of billings for inpatient care due to the projected nonsustainability of the long-run growth rate of Social Security or Medicare under current financing arrangements (CMS, 2006).

INCREASED UTILIZATION OF PHARMACEUTICALS

The increase in the cost of pharmaceuticals is attributed to increased utilization of medications, the cost of research and development, and increased insurance coverage (Scherer, 2004). Advertising directed to consumers has resulted in more prescriptions for the newer, costlier drugs, rather than prescriptions for the older drugs that are just as effective as the newer ones and have fewer side effects. The amount spent by consumers over the past decade on pharmaceuticals has steadily increased and shows no sign of slowing down.

TECHNOLOGICAL ADVANCES

Although technological advances have facilitated earlier diagnoses and better treatment of disease, factors such as the greater availability of new technology drive per capita expenditures higher (Boddenheimer, 2005b). Many health care procedures that were traditionally done on an inpatient basis have improved because of technological advances. For example, new techniques, equipment, and pharmaceuticals have resulted in 60–75% lower costs in outpatient settings (American Association for Accreditation of Ambulatory Surgery Facilities [AAAASF], 2001). In response to these lowered costs, the number of surgical procedures has rapidly increased. An estimated 400,000 surgeries were performed in 1984. This number grew to 8.3 million in 2000 (Lapetina & Armstrong, 2002), thus effectively increasing the amount of funding devoted to surgery.

RISING HOSPITAL COSTS

A large proportion of health care dollars are devoted to hospital care. The Hill-Burton Act of 1946, funded the development of the nation's infrastructure of hospitals. Today, there are almost 6,000 hospitals nationwide. As technology and scientific knowledge grow, and patients live longer, there has been a greater severity of illness in the hospitalized population. Hospital services contribute to the rise in health care costs due to the increased utilization of expensive technologies, high labor costs due to the shortage of nurses, rising malpractice premiums, and increased costs of hospitalization. Given the aging hospital infrastructure and increases in hospital reimbursements, future building of new hospital beds will also increase health care costs (Bazzoli, Gerland, & May, 2006).

PRACTITIONER BEHAVIOR

In response to the fear of malpractice lawsuits, greater numbers of patient diagnostic tests are ordered and patient procedures are done that may not be medically necessary. Practitioners have also expanded the number of patients deemed eligible for new procedures (Boddenheimer, 2005a).

COST SHIFTING

The popular practice of **cost shifting**, whereby health care providers raise prices for the privately insured to offset the lower health care payments from both Medicare and Medicaid as well as the often nonpayment of health care premiums from the uninsured, continues to raise the cost of health care. Medicare and Medicaid payments are less than 50% of what private insurers pay. Health care providers shift charges for health care costs to the private insurance sector. Some estimates of the cost shift are being valued at $6 billion annually. Cost shifting increases the cost of all health care. The health care facility or the health care professional shifts the cost of health care to other patients with health insurance or to those patients who can afford to pay. Costs to the public for these programs continue to increase. While the intent of the Medicaid program has been to ensure access to health care for mainly low-income pregnant women and children, over 72% of Medicaid's $295.9 billion dollars in expenditures in 2004 went toward care of the disabled and dual-eligibles. Dual-eligibles are the elderly who are eligible for both Medicaid and Medicare, and they are the fastest growing proportion enrolled in Medicaid (Holahan & Cohen, 2006).

ADMINISTRATIVE COSTS

According to Boddenheimer (2005a), the cost of administration of U.S. health care in 1999 was 24% of the nation's health care expenditures. In an attempt to reduce these costs, providers such as practitioner's offices, clinics, hospitals, and so on, have invested in Information Technology (IT). IT has played a role in improving quality through availability of the electronic medical record, aiding with HIPAA compliance and streamlining insurance coding and billing services. Because of the increased demand for such systems, the administrative cost of implementation has also gone up.

OTHER FACTORS CONTRIBUTING TO RISING HEALTH CARE COSTS

Because rising health care costs are based on utilization, it is important to understand other factors that can both increase and decrease utilization as listed in Table 2-5.

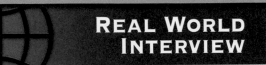

REAL WORLD INTERVIEW

Several years ago, I went to the hospital with excruciating pain. They admitted me to the hospital, and I had tests and x-rays for nine days before they found the cause. I had cancer in my left kidney, and I needed immediate surgery. I had the surgery and was discharged on my eighteenth hospital day. Thank heaven, I was now cancer free.

The hospital bill for this stay was $18,689.20. The radiologist and surgeon submitted additional bills. I was glad that I had Medicare and Blue Cross insurance, which paid it all. The only charge I had to pay was $25.00 per day for a private room. When I looked at the hospital bill, there were many charges for medications and treatments I never received. There were even charges for the day after I was discharged. I wonder how the hospital makes out the bill. I also wonder how people with no insurance pay these kinds of hospital bills.

Leona McGuan
Patient
Schererville, Indiana

COST CONTAINMENT STRATEGIES

Research has suggested the hazards and ethical problems in the overuse of services in fee-for-service settings (where payment is made based on service rendered to individuals for individual services) rather than service underuse in capitated care (where payment is made based on service rendered to a group of patients) (Berwick 1994; Leape et al., 1990). Over the years, cost containment strategies have targeted the financing and reimbursement sides of health care. Financing strategies have used health services regulation and limitation by means of taxes or insurance premiums and encouraged competition such as managed competition. Reimbursement containment strategies have used regulatory and competitive price controls and utilization controls, such as capitation, patient cost sharing, and utilization management. Capitation and prospective payment have had some of the most significant impact on cost containment.

CAPITATION

Even though legislation creating managed care was passed in 1973 (the Health Maintenance Organization Act), managed care did not become a major player or driving force in health care until the late 1980s. In an effort to reduce the number of hospitalizations and control profit incentives for health care providers, managed care plans offered hospitals and practitioners a capitated set fee for office visits and hospitalizations for a group of patients. Capitation is the payment of a fixed dollar amount, per person, for the provision of health services to a patient population for a specified period of time, for example, one year. Under capitation, health care organizations benefit from using their financial resources to

EVIDENCE FROM THE LITERATURE

Citation: Ginsburg, P. B. (2003). Can hospitals and physicians shift the effects of cuts in Medicare reimbursement to private payers? *Health Affairs, W3,* 472–479.

Discussion: Cost shifting occurs when employers lower the amount they pay for employee insurance by increasing the amount employees pay. The other cost shifting occurs when the cost of providing uncompensated health care services for the uninsured or lower Medicare reimbursement rates is covered by increasing the cost of health care from those with insurance. The ability to shift costs depends on the market power of hospitals and practitioners and can vary by geographic location. As attempts to control health care expenditures continue, cost shifting will continue to occur unless insurers and employers insist on fair prices and private and public reimbursement reflects the actual cost of care.

Implications for Practice: Nurses can help both patients and health care organizations avoid cost shifting by finding ways to use the most effective clinical practices to improve patient outcomes and lower preventable utilization of services.

| TABLE 2-5 | FORCES THAT AFFECT OVERALL HEALTH CARE UTILIZATION |

Force	Factors That May Decrease Health Services Utilization	Factors That May Increase Health Services Utilization
Financial incentives that reward practitioners and hospitals for performance (e.g., pay for performance [P4P] programs that reward quality practice)	■ Changes in clinician practice patterns (e.g., encouraging patient self-care and healthy lifestyles; reduced length of hospital stay)	■ Changes in clinician practice patterns (e.g., more aggressive treatment of the elderly)
Increased accountability for performance	■ Consensus documents or guidelines that recommend decreases in utilization	■ Consensus documents or guidelines that recommend increases in utilization
Technological advances in the biological and clinical sciences	■ Better understanding of the risk factors of diseases and prevention initiatives (e.g., smoking-prevention programs, cholesterol-lowering drugs)	■ New procedures and technologies (e.g., hip replacement, stent insertion, magnetic resonance imaging [MRI]) ■ New drugs, expanded use of existing drugs ■ Increased supply of services (e.g., ambulatory surgery centers, assisted living residences)
Increase in chronic illness	■ Aging of the population ■ Discovery/implementation of treatments that cure or eliminate diseases ■ Public health/sanitation advances (e.g., quality standards for food and water distribution)	■ Growing elderly population: – more functional limitations associated with aging – more illness associated with aging – more deaths among the increased number of elderly (elderly are correlated with high utilization of services)
Increased ethnic and cultural diversity of the population	■ Lack of insurance coverage ■ Low income	■ Growth in national population ■ Efforts to eliminate disparities in access and outcomes
Changes in the supply and education of health professionals	■ Decreased supply (e.g., hospital closures, large numbers of nursing and medical practitioners, and nurses retiring) ■ Shifts to other sites of care may cause declines in utilization of staff in the original sites: – as technology allows shifts (e.g., ambulatory surgery) – as alternative sites of care become available (e.g., assisted living)	■ Increase in chronic conditions ■ Growth in national population

(Continues)

	TABLE 2-5	FORCES THAT AFFECT OVERALL HEALTH CARE UTILIZATION (CONTINUED)

Force	Factors That May Decrease Health Services Utilization	Factors That May Increase Health Services Utilization
Social morbidity (e.g., increased AIDS, drugs, violence, disasters)	■ Disparities in access to health services and outcomes	■ New health problems (e.g., HIV/AIDS, bioterrorism)
Access to patient information	■ Changes in consumer preferences (e.g., home birthing, more self-care, alternative medicine)	■ Changes in consumer demand
Globalization and expansion of the world economy	■ Growth in uninsured population	■ Growth in national population
Cost control and competition for limited resources	■ Insurance payer pressures to reduce costs	■ Increased health insurance coverage ■ Consumer/employee pressures for more comprehensive insurance coverage ■ Changes in consumer preferences and demand (e.g., cosmetic surgery, hip and knee replacements, direct marketing of pharmaceuticals)

Source: Adapted from Bernstein, A. B., Hing, E., Moss, A. J., Allen, K. F., Siller, A. B., Tiggle, R. B. (2003). *Health care in America: Trends in utilization.* Hyattsville, MD: National Center for Health Statistics; and Shortell, S. M., & Kaluzny, A. D. (2006). *Health care management* (5th ed.). Clifton Park, NY: Thomson Delmar Learning.

keep people well. Otherwise, health care providers bear the financial loss. Then in the mid-1990s, the U.S. population had quality concerns with this system and "backlashed" against managed care organizations. Research has shown that resource use is lower for managed care beneficiaries, but it is not clear whether this lowered resource use is appropriate or causes adverse patient outcomes (Murry, Greenfield, Kaplan, & Yano, 1992; Hohlen et al., 1990).

PROSPECTIVE PAYMENT

Reacting to rapidly increasing costs to Medicare, the Tax Equity and Fiscal Responsibility Act (TEFRA) passed in 1982 mandated the Prospective Payment System (PPS) to control health care costs. For Medicare Part A services, PPS uses Medicare's administrative data to develop and continually refine PPS payments based on diagnosis-related groups (DRGs), that is, patients with similar diagnoses. The PPS is a method of reimbursement in which Medicare payment is made based on a predetermined, fixed amount for reimbursement to acute inpatient

hospitals, home health agencies, hospices, hospital outpatient and inpatient psychiatric facilities, inpatient rehabilitation facilities, long-term care hospitals, and skilled nursing facilities. For Medicare Part B services, the Resource-Based Relative Value Scale (RBRVS) is used to determine reimbursement amounts for practitioner services. The major problem that the CMS has encountered with funding prospective payment is DRG creep, where health care providers "up code" or over bill a patient to indicate a need for financial reimbursement for more expensive health care services to recoup what the health care provider believes is a more equitable payment.

HEALTH CARE QUALITY

The health care report, *To Err Is Human*, confronted health care clinicians and managers with concerns about the poor quality of health care attributable to misuse,

EVIDENCE FROM THE LITERATURE

Citation: Lankshear, A. J., Sheldon, T. A., & Maynard, A. (2005). Nurse staffing and healthcare outcomes: A systematic review of the international research evidence. *Advances in Nursing, 28*(2), 163–174.

Discussion: The relationship between quality of care and the cost of the nursing workforce is of concern to policymakers. This study assesses the evidence for a relationship between the nursing workforce and patient outcomes in the acute sector through a systematic review of international research produced since 1990 involving acute hospitals and adjusting for case mix. Twenty-two large studies of variable quality were included. They strongly suggest that higher nurse staffing and richer skill mix (especially of RNs) are associate with improved patient outcomes, such as failure to rescue and mortality, although the effect size cannot be estimated reliably.

Fundamental nursing care is often referred to as "basic," for much of what nurses do appears deceptively simple. However, it is during these "basic" tasks that a complex interaction occurs—nurses assess patients' physical and psychological status, and patients talk to and receive information from nurses. This can be important in detecting early signs of clinical deterioration or complications. If the nursing resource is stretched because of contextual factors (geographical disposition, decreased skill mix, increased patient dependence, and unit activity), then the ability to provide proactive care, cope with the unpredictable, and maintain flexibility can be adversely affected. Where RN ratios are lower, much of the frontline care may be given by less qualified and less empowered staff. In addition, noting deterioration does not of itself improve outcomes, and, having decided that an intervention is needed, a nurse may need to persuade medical staff to attend to the patient. This requires nurses to be able to present the case logically and confidently. Prompt attendance by medical staff is more likely if the doctor called has respect for the nurse.

In the United States, the California Department of Health Services has set absolute minimum ratios for licensed nurses (RNs and licensed vocational nurses) at 1:6 (4 Care Hours Per Patient Day [CHPPD]), day and night for medical and surgical areas, although the introduction of the 1:5 (4.8 CHPPD) ratio has recently been postponed to 2008. In Australia, the state of Victoria has recommended that RN ratios should be 1:4/5 (4.8-6 CHPPD) for day shifts in general medical and surgery units, depending on the type of hospital. However, the research evidence presented here does not support a precise recommendation on staffing levels, and evidence of diminishing returns implies that the cost-effectiveness of using nurse staffing as a quality improvement lever must fall as levels increase. More research is needed to investigate the resource implications alongside the impact on patient outcomes.

Implications for Practice: Overall, there is accumulating evidence of a relationship between nurse staffing, especially higher nursing skill mix, and patient outcomes. However, the estimates of the nurse staffing effects are likely to be unreliable. There is emerging evidence of a curvilinear relationship that suggests that the cost-effectiveness of using RN levels as a quality improvement tool will gradually become less cost-effective. The research is not yet clear.

overuse, and underuse of resources and procedures, which was responsible for thousands of deaths (IOM, 1999). The health care report, *Crossing the Quality Chasm* (IOM, 2001) and several large studies (McGlynn et al., 2003; Thomas et al., 2000) has shown that the quality of health care in the United States is at an unexpected low level and needs improvement in many dimensions given the amount of money the United States spends on health care (Table 2-6).

HEALTH CARE VARIATION

Groundbreaking research beginning in the 1970s and continuing in the 1990s demonstrated that there was significant variation in utilization of specific health care services associated with geographic location, provider preferences and training, type of health insurance, and patient-specific factors such as age and gender (Wennberg, & Gittelsohn, 1973; Leape, 1992; Adams, Fraser, & Abrams, 1973; Safran, Rogers, Tarlov, McHorney, & Ware, 1997; Greenfield et al., 1992). Associations between utilization rates of health care services have been found with availability of services and technologies, for example, MRIs, hospital beds, practitioners (Joines, Hertz-Picciotto, Carey, Gesler, & Suchindran, 2003), prevalence and severity of morbidities (Dunn, Lyman, & Marx, 2005; National Healthcare Quality Report, 2005), race/ethnicity (National Healthcare Quality Report, 2005), patient adherence, health-seeking behaviors of patients (Calvocoressi et al., 2004), and many other factors. Efforts to decrease variation and standardize care with quality-care guidelines are underway to improve health care outcomes.

TABLE 2-6	HEALTH CARE DIMENSIONS NEEDING IMPROVEMENT

Health care should be:

- Effective—providing services based on scientific knowledge to all who could benefit and refraining from providing services to those not likely to benefit (avoiding overuse and underuse).

- Patient-centered—providing care that is respectful of and responsive to individual patient preferences, needs, and values and ensuring that patient values guide all clinical decisions.

- Timely—reducing waits and sometimes harmful delays for both those who receive and those who give care.

- Efficient—avoiding waste, in particular waste of equipment, supplies, ideas, and energy.

- Safe—avoiding injuries to patients from care intended to help them.

- Equitable—providing care that does not vary in quality because of personal characteristics, such as gender, ethnicity, geographic location, and socioeconomic data.

Source: Compiled with information from the Institute of Medicine. (2001). *Crossing the quality chasm: A new health system for the 21st century.* Washington, DC: National Academy Press.

IMPROVEMENTS IN THE PROCESS OF CARE

Using the example of the management of hypertension, recent research findings illustrate the need for significant improvements in the process of health care delivery. Blood pressure control is strongly linked to the delivery of evidence-based quality care for those with hypertension (Goldstein, Lavori, Coleman, Advani, & Hoffman, 2005). Each year, uncontrolled blood pressure contributes to more than 68,000 deaths (Woolf, 1999). When 61% of patients with a myocardial infarction were appropriately given aspirin, which has been shown to reduce the risk of death by 15%, the risk of nonfatal myocardial infarction was reduced by 30%, and the risk of nonfatal stroke was reduced by 40% (Antman, Lau, Kupelnick, Mosteller, & Chalmers, 1992). When simple evidence-based changes of administering aspirin and beta-blockers is done, thus changing the processes of care for patients who have had a myocardial infarction, it can lower health care dollars and save lives associated with heart disease. This is true even if it is because aspirin use is being measured to assess provider performance (Williams, Schmaltz, Morton, Koss, & Loeb, 2005). Such change in the processes of care delivery could change this list of the top ten health care conditions, both in cost and mortality (Table 2-7).

PERFORMANCE AND QUALITY MEASUREMENT

Performance and quality measurement is an essential component of health care improvement efforts. Performance and quality are measured to determine resource allocation, organize care delivery, assess clinician competency, and improve health care delivery processes. Hospitals and practitioners have been given past and present financial incentives to score well on measures of quality from both public and private health care payers. When the quality of care is measured, it improves (Brook, Kamberg, & McGlynn, 1996; Chassin & Galvin, 1998) possibly largely due to the Hawthorne effect, which has illustrated that observed activity shows improvement. Unfortunately, those aspects of care not being measured may not improve. Nursing leaders have also recognized the need to establish classifications that can be used to measure nursing care. Selected classifications are listed in Table 2-8.

Note that setting standards for appropriate care and guideline development should have a basis in validated measures of quality, using reliable performance data, and making appropriate adjustments in care delivery. However, it is important to know that the majority of quality care is not measurable using current methods (Epstein, 1995; Smith, Atherly, Kane, & Pacala, 1997). Reliable methods and measures need to be developed and tested. Also, practitioners have been resistant to their care delivery being measured because they have believed that it would interfere with their professionalism and autonomy. If this belief persists, the majority of health care delivery will not be measured.

MALCOLM BALDRIDGE NATIONAL QUALITY AWARD

Health care organizations are eligible to consider another framework for health care quality and to apply for

TABLE 2-7   TOP 10 CONDITIONS—COST AND DEATH

Cost	Death
1. Heart Disease ($58B)	1. Heart Disease
2. Cancer ($46B)	2. Cancer
3. Trauma ($44B)	3. Cerebrovascular Disease
4. Mental Disorders ($30B)	4. Chronic Pulmonary Disease
5. Pulmonary Conditions ($29B)	5. Accidents (unintentional injures)
6. Diabetes ($20B)	6. Diabetes Mellitus
7. Hypertension ($18B)	7. Influenza and Pneumonia
8. Cerebrovascular Disease ($16B)	8. Alzheimer's Disease
9. Osteoarthritis ($16B)	9. Kidney Disease
10. Pneumonia ($16B)	10. Septicemia

Source: Compiled with information from National Vital Statistics Reports. (2005). Vol. 53, No. 15.

TABLE 2-8   SELECTED CLASSIFICATION SYSTEMS

North American Nursing Diagnosis Association (NANDA): www.nanda.org

Home Health Care Classification (HHCC): www.sabacare.com

PeriOperative Nursing Data Set: www.aorn.org

National Quality Forum-endorsed Nursing-sensitive Consensus Standards: www.qualityforum.org

Omaha System: www.omahasystem.org

ABC Codes: www.alternativelink.com

Logical Observation Identifiers Names and Codes: www.loinc.org

Patient Care Data Set: e-mail: judy.ozbolt@vanderbilt.edu

SNOMED CT: www.snomed.org

International Classification of Nursing Practice: www.icn.ch

the Malcolm Baldridge National Quality Award. The Baldridge Award highlights the importance of leadership; strategic planning; and a focus on patients, other customers, and markets in building a quality health care system. Baldridge also stresses the importance of measurement, analysis, and knowledge management; workforce focus; process management; and results (Baldridge National Quality Program, 2007).

OUTCOME MEASUREMENT

Outcome measurements can be done indicating an individual's clinical state, such as their severity of illness, course of illness, and the effect of interventions on their clinical state. Outcome measures involving a patient's functional status evaluate a patient's ability to perform activities of daily living (ADLs). These can include measures of physical health in terms of function, mental and social health, cost of care, health care access, and general health perceptions. The measures can distinguish the concepts of physical and mental health and identify the five indicator categories of clinical status, functioning, physical symptoms, emotional status, and patient/family evaluation and perceptions about quality of life. Selected quality-of-life measures include quality-adjusted life years (QALY), quality-adjusted life expectancy (QALE), and quality-adjusted healthy life years (QUALY) (Drummond, Stoddart, & Torrance, 1994).

The Medical Outcomes Study (MOS) "Short Form 36" Health Survey is one of the many health indices that have been developed since 1950. The SF-36, as it is commonly known (Ware & Sherbourne, 1992), measures physical functioning, role limitations due to physical health, bodily pain, social functioning, general mental health, role limitations due to emotional problems, vitality, and general health perceptions.

OTHER HEALTH ASSESSMENT TOOLS

Other health status assessment surveys in use today include the Quality of Life Index (Spitzer, 1998), developed to measure the general health and well-being of terminally ill individuals; the COOP Charts for primary care practice patients; the functional status questionnaire (Jette & Cleary, 1987), a self-administered general health and social well-being survey for ambulatory patients; the Duke Health Profile (Parkerson, Broadhead, & Tse, 1990), which evaluates health status in primary care patients; the Sickness Impact Profile (Bergner, Bobbit, Carter, & Gilson, 1981), which was developed to measure changes in an individual's behavior as a result of illness; and the Nottingham Health Profile (Hunt, McKenna, McEwen, Williams, & Papp, 1981), developed as a measure of perceived general health status for primary care patients and general population health surveys.

PUBLIC REPORTING OF PERFORMANCE

Public reporting of organizational performance and quality information is being driven by several forces. As more data about quality becomes available electronically, individuals reporting the data and those wanting to make comparisons among organizations want the data analyzed and the findings reported. This information can be used to determine where there are health care inefficiencies and poor quality of care. Public reporting of the information is also used to influence reimbursement policies where payment is linked to the ability to achieve standards and benchmarks, for example, pay-for-performance (P4P) (Dudley & Rosenthal, 2006). Performance reporting to demonstrate quality status on minimum reporting standards can also be used by major health care payers as a condition of doing business with an organization

(Lansky, 2002). Performance reporting is also used to influence clinician and patient utilization behavior. It also moves health care toward a population-based approach as opposed to focusing on individual patient care.

INSTITUTE OF MEDICINE HEALTH CARE REPORTS

In 1996, the Institute of Medicine (IOM) launched a concerted, ongoing effort focused on assessing and improving the nation's quality of care. This effort is now in its third phase. The first phase of this quality initiative documented the serious and pervasive nature of the nation's overall quality problem. This phase established that the nature of the problem was one of overuse, misuse, and underuse of health care services. More specifically, the *Ensuring Quality Cancer Care Report* (1999), documented the wide gulf that exists between ideal cancer care and the reality many Americans with cancer experience.

During the second phase, spanning 1999 to 2001, the Committee on Quality of Health Care in America laid out a vision for how the health care system and related policy environment must be radically transformed to close the chasm between what we know to be good quality care and what actually exists in practice. The reports released during this phase, *To Err is Human: Building a Safer Health System* (1999), and *Crossing the Quality Chasm: A New Health System for the 21st Century* (2001), stress that partial reform is inadequate to address system ills. The *To Err Is Human* report put the spotlight on how tens of thousands of Americans die each year from medical errors and raised the issue of patient safety and quality. The *Quality Chasm* report described broader quality issues, defined the six aims mentioned earlier in Table 2-6, and highlighted ten rules for care delivery redesign (IOM, 2001).

Phase three of the IOM quality initiative focuses on operationalizing the vision of a future health system described in the *Quality Chasm* report. This phase has generated several publications, including *Preventing Medication Errors* (2006), *Performance Measurement: Accelerating Improvement* (2005), *Patient Safety: Achieving a New Standard for Care* (2003), *Keeping Patients Safe: Transforming the Work Environment of Nurses* (2003), *Health Professions Education: A Bridge to Quality* (2003), and *Priority Areas for National Action: Transforming Health Care Quality* (2003).

OTHER NATIONAL PUBLIC QUALITY REPORTS

Several key national public quality sources of interest for health care and nursing leaders and managers for purposes of performance measurement and benchmarking or comparison are as follows:

■ *AHRQ National Healthcare Quality Report (2005):* Available at www.ahrq.gov/qual/nhqr05/ nhqr05.htm.

- *AHRQ National Healthcare Disparities Report (2005):* Available at www.ahrq.gov/qual/nhdr05/nhdr05.htm.
- *Healthy People 2010:* Accessible at www.healthypeople.gov.
- *Health Grades for Hospitals and Physicians:* Available at www.healthgrades.com.
- *Leapfrog:* Available at www.leapfroggroup.org.

Public reporting of quality performance has been shown to influence declines in cardiac surgery mortality (Peterson, DeLong, Jollis, Muhlbaier, & Mark, 1998); improvements in the processes of obstetrics care (Bost, 2001); and employee enrollment and desire to switch health care providers (Beaulieu, 2002). While providers and policymakers do seek out these public quality reports, the general public does not search them out, does not understand them, distrusts them, and fails to make use of them (Marshall, Hiscock, & Sibbald, 2002).

In many respects, hospitals are providing quality care. Data to assess clinical performance from the Joint Commission (JC), formerly known as the Joint Commission on Accreditation of Healthcare Organizations (JCAHO), core measures program, which uses standardized, evidence-based measures, and data from the Medicare program show improvements in the quality of care in hospitals (Williams et al., 2005; Jencks, Huff, & Cuerdon, 2003). Yet at hospitals that do not meet the sample-size requirement for national comparisons, quality performance remains mediocre (Jha, Li, Orav, & Epstein, 2005).

DISEASE MANAGEMENT

A key challenge for health care is the numerous deficiencies in the delivery of care to patients with chronic conditions (IOM, 2001). The amount and breadth of knowledge about the effectiveness of regular disease management for improving care across populations and disease states is building (Ofman et al., 2004). Disease management is a systematic population-based approach to identifying persons at risk, intervening with specific programs of care, and measuring clinical and other outcomes (Epstein & Sherwood, 1996). What makes caring for patients with chronic diseases problematic is that usually multiple chronic conditions are involved. In the elderly, nine out of ten patients with ischemic heart disease or congestive heart failure had three or more chronic conditions, including hypertension, diabetes, urinary incontinence, and chronic pain; the majority of these patients had an average of five chronic conditions (Bierman, 2004). Because of this, condition-specific disease management will not be successful given the likelihood of disease comorbidities, that is, other diseases. Documented widespread variation in disease management and treatment interventions have led health care payors to consider the option of paying-for-

performance (P4P). These types of financial incentives may be an effective way of changing professional behavior (Robinson, 2001; Chaix-Couturier, Durand-Zaleski, Jolly, & Durieux, 2000) and the quality of care delivered.

EVIDENCE-BASED PRACTICE

Evidence-based practice involves supplementing clinical expertise with the judicious and conscientious implementation of the most current and best evidence along with patient values and preferences to guide health care decision making (Jennings & Loan, 2001). The body of evidence supporting clinical practice is steadily growing. However, even when evidence-based quality care guidelines are available for numerous conditions, for example, diabetes, congestive heart failure, and asthma, they have not been fully implemented in actual patient care, and variation in clinical practice is abundant (Timmermans & Mauck, 2005; IOM, 2001; McGlynn et al., 2003). Health care knowledge continues to expand. This requires practice guidelines and the measures of quality on which they are based to be continually updated. It also requires attention to continuing to develop health care quality (Table 2-9).

IMPACT OF ACCREDITATION

Health care accreditation is a mechanism used to ensure that organizations meet certain national standards. Hospitals and other organizations seek accreditation by the Joint Commission (JC) to demonstrate their ability to meet national quality standards. Accreditation status is directly linked to a hospital's ability to serve Medicare beneficiaries. One of the greatest forces driving quality-improvement efforts in hospitals is the JC's patient safety requirements, in large part due to hospital's fears of possibly losing accreditation if the JC standards are not achieved and sustained (Devers, Pham, & Liu, 2004). The JC accreditation is also tied into hospital regulation, primarily by the CMS, which establishes regulations setting forth minimum standards of quality tied to reimbursement for patient care services. Currently there is no direct linkage between the JC accreditation and seeking accreditation for magnet status (Table 2-10).

MAGNET PROGRAM

The Magnet Recognition Program of the American Nurses Credentialing Center can potentially be a tool to establishing an environment that recognizes excellence in nursing services in a health care system (Magnet Recognition Program [MRP], 2005). Research continues to demonstrate positive implications of the magnet program, relating magnet characteristics to nurse job satisfaction and retention, prevention of job burnout, and improvement in perceived quality of care (Aiken, Havens, & Sloane, 2000; Friese, 2005; Lake & Friese, 2006).

TABLE 2-9	RULES OF EFFECTIVE HEALTH CARE TO IMPROVE HEALTH CARE QUALITY

Current Health Care Rule	Requirement to Improve Health Care Quality
Care requires a face-to-face visit with health care clinician.	Patients participate in shared decision making whenever they need care.
Professional practitioner autonomy drives variability in health care delivery.	Care that patient is offered is customized according to patient's needs and values.
Clinicians control health care utilization.	Care is patient-centered and driven by patients' preferences and shared decision making.
Information is recorded privately in the patient record.	Clinicians and patients communicate effectively and share information.
Clinical decision making is based on the training and experience of the clinician.	Decision making is based on evidence.
"Do no harm" is a professional responsibility.	Health care systems require that patients are safe from injury.
Secrecy is necessary.	Transparency is necessary.
The system is reactive.	The system is proactive and anticipates needs.
Cost reduction is sought.	Waste is continuously decreased.
Preference is given to some professional roles in the system.	Cooperation among clinicians to achieve high-quality care is a priority.

Source: Compiled with information from Berwick, D. M. (2002). A user's manual for the IOM's "Quality Chasm" report. *Health Affairs, 21*(3), 80–90.

TABLE 2-10	HOSPITAL ACCREDITATION STANDARDS OVERVIEW

Patient-focused functions

- Ethics, rights, and responsibilities
- Provision of care, treatment, and services
- Medication management
- Surveillance, prevention, and control of infection

Organization functions

- Improving organization performance
- Leadership

- Management of the environment of care
- Management of human resources
- Management of information

Structures with functions

- Medical staff
- Nursing

Source: © Joint Commission: *CAMH: 2006 Comprehensive Accreditation Manual for Hospitals.* Oakbrook Terrace, IL: Joint Commission, 2006.

IMPROVING QUALITY THROUGH HEALTH PROFESSIONS EDUCATION

While there is currently concern about the supply and distribution of health care clinicians, there is also a need to focus on retooling the health care workforce with new knowledge and requisite skills to function in better, re-designed health care systems. To begin to realize the quality agenda set forth by the IOM (IOM, 2001), a subsequent report, *Health Professions Education: A Bridge to Quality* (IOM, 2003), delineates a needed "overhaul" of the curriculum of health professionals' education to transform current skills and knowledge (IOM, 2003, p. 1). This curriculum includes training clinicians to effectively work in interdisciplinary teams; have an educational foundation in informatics; and deliver patient-centered care fully exploiting evidence-based practice, quality improvement approaches, and informatics. A set of five competencies are set forth:

1. *Ability to provide patient-centered care:* Patient-centered care requires a complex set of knowledge about the characteristics of shared responsibility between patients and clinicians and knowledge of effective communication approaches that allows patient access to information and achieves patient understanding. Patient-centered care respects patients' individuality, values, and needs, and uses related population-based strategies to improve appropriate utilization of health care services. Patient-centered care is important because research continues to

find that involving patients in decision making about their care results in higher functional status, better outcomes, and lower costs.

2. *Ability to effectively work in interdisciplinary teams:* Even though interdisciplinary teams have been shown to enhance quality and lower costs, training in effective interdisciplinary teamwork is challenged by differences in communication norms across disciplines and power and turf controversies among disciplines. This may only be achieved through collaborative interdisciplinary education and research.

3. *Understanding of evidence-based practices:* Actual evidence-based practice integrates available research evidence, clinical expertise, and patient values in making care decisions about individual patients. To actively provide evidence-based care (EBC), clinicians need the following knowledge and skills: how to locate the best sources of evidence, how to formulate clear clinically-based questions, and how to determine when and how to translate new knowledge into practice. Unfortunately for many clinical scenarios, the evidence base is often thin.

4. *Ability to measure the quality of care:* Clinicians need to be able to measure the quality of care; use comparison benchmarks to identify opportunities for improvement; design, test, and assess quality improvement interventions; identify current and potential errors in care; and implement safety design principles such as recognizing human factors and the need for standardization.

5. *Ability to use health information technology:* Health care informatics applications can enhance patient safety by driving standardization, as well as facilitating knowledge management, communication, and

decision making. As more technology becomes available, database systems are linked within and across health care settings. As our evidence-based measures and decision-making tools improve, clinicians will need to be able to fully utilize health information technology to improve the quality of health care delivery.

CRITICAL THINKING 2-4

Think about the five competencies needed to improve health care education:

1. Patient-centered care delivery
2. Interdisciplinary teamwork
3. Evidence-based practice
4. Measurement of the quality of care
5. Health information technology skill

How can you improve your education and experience in each of the competencies now and throughout your career?

CURRENT PRACTICES

The current education of health professionals and their subsequent practice can be limited by the use of external oversights of clinician credentialing, certification, and licensure to assure clinician competence and quality patient outcomes. These oversight processes currently have minimal expectations, and the review of the five competencies previously identified among individual clinicians at various times during their career is generally not part of the current oversight of individual clinicians (IOM, 2003).

KEEPING PATIENTS SAFE

The IOM's 2004 *Report on Patient Safety* was the first in a series of three reports published since the year 2000 to emphasize the connections among nursing, patient safety, and quality of care. *Keeping Patients Safe* sets forth the structures and processes health care workers use in the delivery of care and emphasizes the need to design the nurses' environment to promote the practice of safe nursing care (IOM, 2004b). The importance of organizational management practices, strong nursing leadership, and adequate nurse staffing for providing a safe care environment is critical (Laschinger & Leiter, 2006). Until recently, shortages of nurses have been cyclical. These nurse shortages are associated with increased demand for patient care services at a time of falling nursing school enrollment, salary compression, and nominal increases

---

EVIDENCE FROM THE LITERATURE

Citation: Soukup, Sr. M. (2000, June). Preface to section on Evidence-based Nursing Practice. *Nursing Clinics of North America, 35*(2), xvii–xviii.

Discussion: The author discusses a nurse's response to queries as to whether she has integrated evidence-based practice. The nurse responds, "Yes, I practice state-of-the-art nursing. My education and professional practice experiences have prepared me to care for more than 700 chronically ill patients annually, in the past five years. These patients have an average reported expected pain rating of 6.9 (using a scale of 1 to 10, with 10 being severe pain), and my pain management interventions have kept these patients, during my hours of care, at a reported actual pain rating of 4. Also, as a team member, these patients have not had any known pressure ulcers, skin tears, or catheter-related infections. On two occasions, for patients who were dying, I created a humanizing environment for the patients and their families when they were rapidly transferred from the critical care unit. My documentation has met organizational standards during monthly peer reviews; I have provided leadership for emergencies with positive outcomes; and physician and patient satisfaction ratings for clinical practice on our unit is 9.5 on a scale of 10, with 10 being the highest. Our unit-based team has not had a needle stick-related or back-related injury during the past two years. This has contributed to a significant cost avoidance and benefit to the organization."

Implications for Practice: Nurses practicing in the twenty-first century must embrace the principles of evidence-based practice, interdisciplinary teamwork, quality measurement, and use of health information technology as an approach to the provision of patient-centered clinical care and professional accountability.

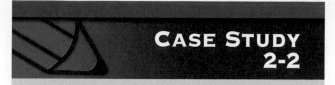

CASE STUDY 2-2

Review the ratings of hospitals in your area of the country at www.healthgrades.com, www. solucient.com, www.100tophospitals.com, www. leapfroggroup.org, and one of the weekly July issues of *US News and World Report,* published annually.

What kinds of ratings are given to hospitals in your area?

Review the criteria and evaluation system used to rate the hospitals. Is it valid and reliable?

Will you choose a hospital for your own family's care using a rating system like this?

in wages. With an aging nursing workforce (Norman et al., 2005), more nursing faculty is needed to train larger numbers of students, and wages will need to increase. Shortages are strongly associated with wages that are

lower than other occupations. The nursing shortage continues to push the current workforce to its limits. The challenges posed by current nurse recruitment and retention strategies may not address the anticipated long-term crisis (Buerhaus & Staiger, 1999). Without significant changes in educational institutions, shortages of nursing and medical clinicians will have a devastating effect on the quality of health care and lead to changes in scope of practice (Cooper, Getzen, McKee, & Laud, 2002) and patient outcomes.

DOCTORATE OF NURSING PRACTICE

Relatively new, the Doctorate of Nursing Practice (DNP) may in time supplant current masters-level nurse practitioner (NP) programs. These programs are designed to prepare nurse experts in specialized advanced nursing practice. They focus on practice that is innovative, evidence based, and reflective of the application of current research. A challenge is to clearly establish the scope of work and reimbursement for DNPs and avoid the confusion of patients and other clinicians as to exactly what a DNP is and how they differ from the current public understanding of nursing and medical practitioners. You can check for current updates at www.aacn.nche.edu (click on Doctor of Nursing Practice).

KEY CONCEPTS

- Health care reports provide invaluable information that emphasizes the successes and failures of health care throughout our nation.

- Evidence of significant disparities and low quality continue to demonstrate the need for significant health care improvement.

- Today, leaders, managers, and staff need to be aware of and involved in the ongoing processes of the making of health policy.

- Health care systems have three simple components: structure, process, and outcome.

- The United States is one of only a few large countries in the world without a universal system of health care.

- In the United States, the emphasis on acute care health care services has successfully driven health care costs higher but has not necessarily improved the quality of care or patient outcomes.

- Primary care provides integrated, accessible health care services by clinicians who are accountable for addressing a large majority of personal health care needs, developing a sustained partnership with

patients, and practicing in the context of family and community.

- Patients and clinicians need to work together to appropriately utilize services based on the following four foundations of primary care: First Contact, Longitudinality, Comprehensiveness, and Coordination.

- The federal government is a major driver of health care organization and delivery

- Today, almost as many persons receive health care in the home as receive health care in acute-care settings.

- Enabling factors such as income, type of insurance coverage, gender, race or ethnicity, geographic proximity, and system characteristics affect a person's ability to have access to health care.

- Private health insurance has been generally voluntarily offered as a benefit to employees and sometimes their families in the United States.

- The elderly have virtually universal health care coverage through Medicare.

- Because the United States does not have national/universal health care insurance, public health care programs are intended to fill the gap, providing coverage for those without employer-based insurance.

- Health care spending continues to increase faster than the overall U.S. economy, growing at an average annual rate of 9.9%.

- There are many contributing factors to the rising costs of health care. The key factors include the aging of the population with growth in the demand for health care, increased utilization of pharmaceuticals, expensive new technologies, rising hospital care costs, practitioner-behavior, cost shifting, and administrative costs.

- Because rising health care costs are based on utilization, it is important to understand other factors that can both increase and decrease utilization.

- Capitation and prospective payment have had some of the most significant impact on cost containment.

- The health care report, *To Err Is Human,* confronted health care clinicians and managers with concerns about the poor quality of health care attributable to misuse, overuse, and underuse of resources and procedures, which was responsible for thousands of deaths (IOM, 1999).

- The health care report, *Crossing the Quality Chasm* (IOM, 2001) and several large studies (McGlynn et al., 2003; Thomas et al., 2000) have shown that the quality of health care in the United States is at an unexpected low level and needs improvement in many dimensions given the amount of money the United States spends on health care.

- Groundbreaking research beginning in the mid-1980s and continuing in the 1990s demonstrated that there was significant variation in utilization of specific health care services associated with geographic location, provider preferences and training, type of health insurance, and patient-specific factors such as age and gender.

- Recent research findings illustrate the need for significant improvements in the process of health care delivery.

- Health care performance and quality are measured to determine resource allocation, organize care delivery, assess clinician competency, and improve health care delivery processes.

- Public reporting of organizational performance and quality information is being driven by several forces.

- Several key national public quality reports of interest for health care and nursing leaders and managers for purposes of performance measurement and benchmarking are available.

- A key challenge for health care is the numerous deficiencies in the delivery of care of patients with chronic conditions.

- Evidence-based practice involves supplementing clinical expertise with the judicious and conscientious implementation of the most current and best evidence along with patient values and preferences to guide health care decision making.

- Health care accreditation is a mechanism used to ensure that organizations meet certain national standards.

- The Magnet Recognition Program of the American Nurses Credentialing Center can potentially be a tool to establishing an environment that recognizes excellence in nursing services in a health care system.

- There is a need to focus on retooling the health care workforce with new knowledge and requisite skills to function in better, redesigned health care systems.

- Health professionals' education to transform current skills and knowledge includes training clinicians to effectively work in interdisciplinary teams; have an educational foundation in informatics; and deliver patient-centered care, fully exploiting evidence-based practice, quality improvement approaches, and informatics.

- The Institute of Medicine's 2004 *Report on Patient Safety* was the first in a series of reports published since the year 2000 to emphasize the connections among nursing, patient safety, and quality of care.

- The Doctorate of Nursing Practice (DNP) may in time supplant current masters-level nurse practitioner programs.

KEY TERMS

cost shifting	process
outcome	structure
primary care	

REVIEW QUESTIONS

1. The national organization that accredits health care organizations is known as which of the following?
   A. American Nurses Association
   B. Health Professions Commission
   C. Agency for Health Care Research and Quality
   D. Joint Commission

2. The largest purchaser of health care in America is which of the following?
   A. Private individuals
   B. Private insurance companies
   C. Health Maintenance Organizations
   D. Medicare, Medicaid, and other governmental programs

3. Who identified a structure, process, and outcome framework for quality?
   A. Nightingale
   B. Donabedian
   C. Starr
   D. Lohr

4. What is the top underlying cause of health care disparity in the United States?
   A. Socioeconomic status
   B. Race
   C. Ethnicity
   D. Gender

REVIEW ACTIVITIES

1. Although it is difficult to modify the structure of health care, what could you do to implement a system to continually modify the process of health care delivery to improve health care quality in your organization?

2. What are strategies to ensure patient access to appropriate health care services in public and private health care agencies?

3. How can the five IOM health professions competencies for quality care be achieved in the current workplace?

EXPLORING THE WEB

Federal Government:

- Agency for Healthcare Research and Quality (AHRQ): *www.ahrq.gov*

- Centers for Disease Control and Prevention (CDC): *www.cdc.gov*

- Centers for Medicare and Medicaid Services (CMS): *www.cms.gov*

- Department of Defense (DOD) TRICARE program: *www.tricare.mil*

- Food and Drug Administration (FDA): *www.fda.gov*

- Health Resources and Services Administration (HRSA): *www.hrsa.gov*

- Indian Health Service (IHS): *www.ihs.gov*

- National Center for Health Statistics: *www.cdc.gov*. Search for National Center for Health Statistics.

- National Guidelines Clearinghouse: *www.guidelines.gov*

- National Institutes of Health (NIH): *www.nih.gov*

- Substance Abuse and Mental Health Services Administration (SAMHSA): *www.samhsa.gov*

- Veterans Health Administration (VHA): *www.va.gov*

Private Foundations and Organizations:

- Commonwealth Fund: *www.cmwf.org*

- Henry J. Kaiser Family Foundation (KFF): *www.kff.org*

- Joint Commission (JC): *www.jointcommission.org*

- National Committee for Quality Assurance (NCQA): *www.ncqa.org*

- National Quality Forum (NQF): *www.qualityforum.org*

- Robert Wood Johnson Foundation (RWJF): *www.rwjf.org*

- Malcolm Baldridge Quality Award (MBQA): *www.quality.nist.gov*

REFERENCES

Adams, D. F., Fraser, D. B., & Abrams, H. L. (1973). The complications of coronary arteriography. *Circulation, 48*(3), 609–618.

Aiken, L. H., Havens, D. S., & Sloane, D. M. (2000). The Magnet Nursing Services Recognition Program. *American Journal of Nursing, 100*(3), 26–36.

American Association for Accreditation of Ambulatory Surgery Facilities (AAAASF). (2001). About AAAASF. Retrieved October 4, 2006 from www.aaaasf.org/aboutAAAASt/about.cfm

Anell, A., & Willis, M. (2000). International comparison of health care systems using resource profiles. *Bulletin of the World Health Organization, 78*(6), 770–778.

Antman, E. M., Lau, J., Kupelnick, B., Mosteller, F., & Chalmers, T. C. (1992). A comparison of results of meta-analyses of randomized control trials and recommendations of clinical experts: Treatments for myocardial infarction. *The Journal of the American Medical Association, 268*, 240–258.

Baldridge National Quality Program. (2007). *Health care criteria for performance excellence.* Gaithersburg, MD: Baldridge National Quality Program.

Bazzoli, G. J., Gerland, A., & May, J. (2006). Construction activity in U.S. hospitals. *Health Affairs, 25*(3), 783–791.

Beaulieu, N. D. (2002). Quality information and consumer health plan choices. *Journal of Health Economics, 21*(1), 43–63.

Bergner, M., Bobbit, R. A., Carter, W. B., & Gilson, B. S. (1981). The Sickness Impact Profile: Development and final revision of a health status measure. *Medical Care, 19*(8), 787–805.

Berwick, D. M. (1994). Eleven worthy aims for clinical leadership of health system reform. *Journal of the American Medical Association, 272*, 797–802.

Berwick, D. M. (2002). A user's manual for the IOM's "Quality Chasm" report. *Health Affairs, 21*(3), 80–90.

Bierman, A. S. (2004). Coexisting illness and heart disease among elderly Medicare managed care enrollees. *Health Care Financing Review, 25*(4), 485–488.

Boddenheimer, T. (2005a). High and rising health care costs. Part 1: Seeking an explanation. *Annals of Internal Medicine, 142*(10), 847–854.

Boddenheimer, T. (2005b). High and rising health care costs. Part 2: Technologic innovation. *Annals of Internal Medicine, 142*(11), 932–937.

Borger, C., Smith, S., Truffer, C., Keehan, S., Sisko, A., Poisal, J., et al. (2006). Health spending projections through 2015: Changes on the horizon. *Health Affairs, 25*(2), 61–73.

Bost, J. (2001). Managed care organization publicly reporting 3 years of HEDIS data. *Managed Care Interface, 14,* 50–54.

Brook, R. H., Kamberg, C. H., & McGlynn, E. A. (1996). Health system reform and quality. *The Journal of the American Medical Association, 276,* 476–480.

Buerhaus, P. I., & Staiger, D. O. (1999, Jan–Feb). Trouble in the nurse labor market? Recent trends and future outlook. *Health Affairs,* 214–222.

Calvocoressi, L., Kasl, S. V., Lee, C. H., Stolar, M., Claus, E. B., & Jones, B. A. (2004). A prospective study of perceived susceptibility to breast cancer and nonadherence to mammography screening guidelines in African American and white women ages 40 to 79 years. *Cancer Epidemiology Biomarkers Preview, 13*(12), 2096–2105.

Centers for Medicare and Medicaid Services (CMS). (2006). Historical National Health Expenditure Data. Retrieved June 4, 2006, from http://www.cms.hhs.gov/NationalHealthExpendData/02_NationalHealthAccountsHistorical.asp#TopOfPage

Chaix-Couturier, C., Durand-Zaleski, I., Jolly, D., & Durieux, P. (2000). Effects of financial incentives on medical practice: Results from a systematic review of the literature and methodological issues. *International Journal on Quality Health Care, 12,* 133–142.

Chassin, M. R., & Galvin, R. W. (1998). The urgent need to improve health care quality: Institute of Medicine National Roundtable on Health Care Quality. *The Journal of the American Medical Association, 280,* 1000–1005.

Cooper, R. A., Getzen, T. E., McKee, H. M., & Laud, P. (2002). Economic and demographic trends signal an impending physician shortage. *Health Affairs, 21*(1), 140–154.

Davis, K. (2005). Ten points for transforming the U.S. health care system. Retrieved October 4, 2006, from http://www.cmwf.org/aboutus/aboutus_show.htm?doc_id=259233

Department of Defense (DOD). (2003). TRICARE: The Basics. Retrieved October 4, 2006, from http://www.tricare.mil/Factsheets/viewfactsheet.cfm?id=127

Devers, K. J., Pham, H. H., & Liu, G. (2004). What is driving hospitals' patient-safety efforts? *Health Affairs, 23*(2), 103–115.

Donaldson, L. (2001). Safe high-quality health care: Investing in tomorrow's leaders. *Quality in Health Care, 10*(suppl II), ii8–ii12.

Dossey, B., Selanders, L., & Beck, D. (2005). *Florence Nightingale today: Healing, leadership, global action.* Washington, DC: American Nurses Publishing.

Drummond, M. F., Stoddart, F. L., & Torrance, G. W. (1994). *Methods for the economic evaluation of health care programmes.* Oxford, England: Oxford University Press.

Dudley, R. A., & Rosenthal, M. B. (2006). *Pay for performance: A decision guide for purchasers.* Rockville, MD: Agency for Healthcare Research and Quality. AHRQ Pub. No. 06-0047.

Dunn, W. R., Lyman, S., & Marx, R. G. (2005). Small area variation in orthopedics. *Journal of Knee Surgery, 18*(1), 51–56.

Epstein, A. M. (1995). Performance reports on quality—prototypes, problems, and prospects. *New England Journal of Medicine, 333,* 57–61.

Epstein, R. S., & Sherwood, L. M. (1996). From outcomes research to disease management: A guide for the perplexed. *Annuals of Internal Medicine, 124*(9), 832–837.

Friese, C. R. (2005). Nurse practice environments and outcomes: Implications for oncology nursing. *Oncology Nursing Forum, 32*(4), 765–772.

Gabel, J., Claxton, G., Holve, E., Pickreign, J., Whitmore, H., Dhont, K., et al. (2003). Health benefits in 2003: Premiums reach thirteen-year high as employers adopt new forms of cost sharing. *Health Affairs, 22*(5), 117–126.

Gaynes, R., Richards, C., Edwards, J., Emori, T. G., Horan, T., Alonso-Eschanove, J., et al. (2001, Mar.–Apr.). Feeding back surveillance data to prevent hospital acquired infections. *Emerging Infectious Diseases, 7*(2), 295–298.

Gilmer, T., & Kronick, R. (2005). It's the premiums stupid: Projections of the uninsured through 2013. *Health Affairs, 24,* w143–w151, (published online April 5, 2005).

Ginsburg, P. B. (2003). Can hospitals and physicians shift the effects of cuts in Medicare reimbursement to private payers? *Health Affairs, W3,* 472–479.

Goldstein, M. K., Lavori, P., Coleman, R., Advani, A., & Hoffman, B. B. (2005). Improving adherence to guidelines for hypertension drug prescribing: Cluster-randomized controlled trial of general verses patient-specific recommendation. *American Journal of Managed Care, 11*(11), 677–685.

Green, L. A., Gryer, G. E., Yawn, B. P., Lanier, D., & Dovery, S.M. (2000). The ecology of medical care revisited. *New England Journal of Medicine, 344,* 2021–2025.

Greenfield, S., Nelson, E. C., Zubkoff, M., Manning, W., Rogers, W., Kravitz, R. L., et al. (1992). Variations in resource utilization among medical specialties and systems of care. Results from the medical outcomes study. *Journal of the American Medical Association, 267*(12), 1624–1630.

Hamilton, K. (2003). The four levels of evidence based practice. *Healthcare Design, 3,* 18–26.

Hohlen, M. M., Manheim, L. M., Fleming, G. V., Davidson, S. M., Yadkowsky, B. K., Weiner, S. M., et al. (1990). Access to office-based physicians under capitation reimbursement and Medicaid case management: Findings from the Children's Medicaid Program. *Medical Care, 28,* 59–68.

Holahan, J., & Cohen, M. (2006). Understanding the recent changes in Medicaid spending and enrollment growth between 2000–2004. Issue Paper. Kaiser Commission on Medicaid and the Uninsured. Retrieved October 4, 2006, from http://www.kff.org/medicaid/upload/7499.pdf

Hunt, S. M., McKenna, P., McEwen, J., Williams, J., & Papp, E. (1981). The Nottingham Health Profile: Subjective health status and medical consultations. *Social Science and Medicine, 15*(3, Pt. 1), 221–229.

Indian Health Service (IHS). (2006). Indian Health Service Fact Sheet. Retrieved October 4, 2006, from http://info.ihs.gov/Files/IHSFacts-June2006.pdf

Institute of Medicine (IOM). (1996). *Primary care: America's health in a new era.* Washington, DC: National Academy Press.

Institute of Medicine (IOM). (1999). *To Err Is Human.* Washington, DC: National Academy Press.

Institute of Medicine. (2001). *Crossing the quality chasm: A new health system for the 21st century.* Washington, DC: National Academy Press.

Institute of Medicine (IOM). (2003). *Health Professions Education: A bridge to quality.* Washington, DC: National Academies Press.

Institute of Medicine (IOM). (2004a). *Evidence-based hospital design improves healthcare outcomes for patients, families, and staff.* Washington, DC: National Academy Press.

Institute of Medicine (IOM). (2004b). *Keeping patients safe: Transforming the work environment of nurses.* Washington, DC: National Academy Press.

Jeffrey, A. E., & Newacheck, P. W. (2006). Role of insurance for children with special health care needs: A synthesis of the evidence. *Pediatrics, 118*(4), e1027–1038.

Jencks, S. F., Huff, E. D., & Cuerdon, O. (2003). Change in the quality of care delivered to Medicare beneficiaries. *Journal of the American Medical Association, 289,* 305–312.

Jennings, B. M., & Loan, L. A. (2001). Misconceptions among nurses about evidence-based practice. *Journal of Nursing Scholarship, 33*(2), 121–127.

Jette, A. M., & Cleary, P. D. (1987). Functional disability assessment. *Physical Therapy, 67,* 1854–1859.

Jha, A. K., Li, Z., Orav, E. J., & Epstein, A. M. (2005). Care in U.S. hospitals—The Hospital Quality Alliance program. *New England Journal of Medicine, 353*(3), 265–274.

Joines, J. D., Hertz-Picciotto, I., Carey, T. S., Gesler, W., & Suchindran, C. (2003). A spatial analysis of count-level variation in hospitalization rates for low back problems in North Carolina. *Social Science and Medicine, 56*(12), 2541–2553.

Kaiser Family Foundation (KFF). (2004). Trends and Indicators in the Changing Health Care Marketplace. Publication number: 7031. Retrieved October 4, 2006, from http://www.kff.org/insurance/7031/ti2004-1-1.cfm

Kaiser Family Foundation (KFF). (2006). The uninsured: A primer. Key facts about americans without health insurance. Publication number 7451-02. Retrieved October, 2006, from http://www.kff.org/KCMU

Kaiser Family Foundation (KFF) and Health Research and Education Trust. (2006). Employer Health Benefits: 2006 Annual Survey. Publication number 7527. Retrieved October, 2006, from http://www.kff.org

Keehan, S. (2004). Health spending by age. *Health Affairs, 23*(6), 280–281.

Kramarow, E., Lentzner, H., Rooks, R., Weeks, J., & Sayday, S. (1999). *Health and aging chartbook: Health,* United States, 1999. Hyattsville, MD: National Center for Health Statistics, U.S. Department of Health and Human Services.

Lake, E. T., & Friese, C. R. (2006). Variations in nursing practice environments: Relation to staffing and hospital characteristics. *Nursing Research, 55*(1), 1–9.

Lankshear, A. J., Sheldon, T. A., & Maynard, A. (2005). Nurse staffing and healthcare outcomes: A systematic review of the international research evidence. *Advances in Nursing, 28*(2), 163–174.

Lansky, D. (2002, July–Aug.). Improving quality through public disclosure of performance information. *Health Affairs,* 52–62.

Lantz, P., House, J. S., Lepkroski, J. M., Williams, D. R., Mero, R. P., & Chen, J. (1998). Socioeconomic factors, health behaviors, and mortality. *Journal of the AMA, 279,* 1703.

Lapetina, E. M., & Armstrong, E. M. (2002, July–Aug.). Preventing errors in the outpatient setting: A tale of three states. *Health Affairs,* 26–39.

Laschinger, H. K. S., & Leiter, M. P. (2006). The impact of nursing work environments on patient safety outcomes: The mediating role of burnout/engagement. *Journal of Nursing Administration, 36*(5), 259–267.

Leape, L. L. (1992). Unnecessary surgery. *Annual Review Public Health, 13,* 363–383.

Leape, L .L., Park, R. E., Solomon, D. H., Chassin, M. R., Kisecoff, J., & Brook, R. H. (1990). Does inappropriate use explain small area variations in the use of health care services? *Journal of the American Medical Association, 263,* 669–672.

Lohr, K. N., Brook, R. H., Kamberg, C. J., Goldberg, G. A., Leibouitz, A., Keesey, J., et al. (1986). Use of medical care in the Rand Health Insurance Experiment. *Medical Care,* Supplement 24, S1.

Lurie, N., Manning, G. W., Peterson, C., Goldberg, G. A. Phelps, C. A., & Lillard, L. (1987). Preventive care: Do we practice what we preach? *New England Journal of Medicine, 329,* 478.

Magnet Recognition Program (MRP). (2005). *Force of magnetism statement of evidence* (pp. 32–45). Silver Spring, MD.

Marshall, M. N., Hiscock, J., & Sibbald, B. (2002). Attitudes to the public release of comparative information on the quality of general practice care: A qualitative study. *British Medical Journal, 325*(7375), 1278.

Martin, J. A., Hamilton, B. E., Sutton, P. D., & Ventura, S. J. (2006). Births: Final data for 2004. *National vital statistics reports* (Vol. 55, No. 1). Hyattsville, MD: National Center for Health Statistics.

McCanne, D. (2007, January). State plans miss the point. *USA Today,* 12A.

McGinnis, J. M., & Foege, W. H. (1993). Actual causes of death in the United States. *Journal of the American Medical Association, 270*(18), 2207–2212.

McGlynn, E. A., Asch, S. M., Adams, J., Keesey, J., Hicks, J., DeCristofaro, A., et al. (2003). The quality of health care delivered to adults in the United States. *New England Journal of Medicine, 348,* 2635–2645.

Muenning, P., Franks, P., Jia, H., Lubetkin, E., & Gold, M. R. (2005). The income-associated burden of disease in the United States. *Social Science Medicine, 61*(9), 2018–2026.

Murry, J. P., Greenfield, S., Kaplan, S. H., & Yano, E. M. (1992). Ambulatory testing for capitation and fee-for-service patients in the same practice setting: Relationship to outcomes. *Medical Care, 30,* 252–261.

National Healthcare Disparities Report. (2005). Agency for Healthcare Research and Quality, Rockville, MD. Retrieved November 4, 2006, from http://www.ahrq.gov/qual/nhdr05/nhdr05.htm

National Healthcare Quality Report (NHQR). (2005). Agency for Healthcare Research and Quality, Rockville, MD. http://www.ahrq.gov/qual/nhqr05/nhqr05.htm

National Nosocomial Infections Surveillance (NNIS) System Report. (1998, Oct.). Data summary from October 1986–April 1998, issued June 1998. *American Journal of Infectious Control, 26*(5), 522–533.

Norman, L. D., Donelan, K., Buerhaus, P. I., Willis, G., Williams, M., Ulrich, B., et al. (2005). The older nurse in the workplace: Does age matter? *Nursing Economics, 23*(6), 279, 282–289.

Ofman, J. J., Badamgarav, E., Henning, J. M., Knight, K., Gano, A. D., Jr., Levan, R. K., et al. (2004). Does disease management improve clinical and economic outcomes in patients with chronic diseases? A systematic review. *American Journal of Medicine, 117*(3), 182–192.

Parkerson, G. R., Jr., Broadhead, W. E., & Tse, C.-K. J. (1990). The Duke health profile: A 17 item measure of health and dysfunction. *Medical Care, 28,* 1056–1072.

Peterson, E. D., DeLong, E. R., Jollis, J. G., Muhlbaier, L. H., & Mark, D. B. (1998). The effects of New York's bypass surgery provider profiling on access to care and patient outcomes in the elderly. *Journal of the American College of Cardiology, 32*(4), 993–999.

Robinson, J. C. (2001). Theory and practice in the design of physician payment incentives. *Milbank Quarterly, 79,* 149–177.

Safran, D. G., Rogers, W. H., Tarlov, A. R., McHorney, C. A., & Ware, J. E., Jr. (1997). Gender differences in medical treatment: The case of physician-prescribed activitiy restrictions. *Social Science Medicine, 45*(5), 711–722.

Scherer, F. M. (2004). The pharmaceutical industry: Prices and progress. *New England Journal of Medicine, 351*(9), 927–932.

Shortell, S. M., & Kaluzny, A. D. (2006). Health Care Management (5th ed., p. 9). Clifton Park, NY: Thomson Delmar Learning.

Smith, M. A., Atherly, A. J., Kane, R. L., & Pacala, J. T. (1997). Peer review of the quality of care: Reliability and sources of variability for outcome and process assessment. *The Journal of the American Medical Association, 278,* 1573–1578.

Soukup, Sr. M. (2000, June). Preface to section on evidence-based nursing practice. *Nursing Clinics of North America, 35*(2), xvii–xviii.

Spitzer, W. O. (1998). Quality of life. In D. Burley & W. H. W. Inman (Eds.), *Therapeutic risk: Perception, measurement, and management.* New York: Wiley.

Starfield, B. (1998). *Primary care: Balancing health needs, services, and technology.* New York: Oxford University Press.

Starr, P. (1983). The social transformation of American medicine. Jackson, TN: Basic Books.

States take on national health insurance crisis, January 15, 2007, *USA Today,* 12A.

Thomas, E. J., Studdert, D. M., Burstin, H. R., Orav, E. J., Zeena, T., Williams, E. J., et al. (2000). Incidence and types of adverse events and negligent care in Utah and Colorado. *Medical Care, 38,* 261–271.

Thorpe, K., Woodruff, R., & Ginsburg, P. (2005). Factors driving cost increases. Retrieved on June 6, 2006, from http://www.ahrq.gov/news/ulp/costs/ulpcosts1.htm

Tilson, H., & Berkowitz, B. (2006). The public health enterprise: Examining our twenty-first century policy challenges. *Health Affairs, 25*(4), 900–910.

Timmermans, S., & Mauck, A. (2005). The promises and pitfalls of evidence-based medicine. *Health Affairs, 24*(1), 18–28.

Ulrich, R., Quan, X., Zimring, C., Joseph, A., & Choudhary, R. (2004). *The role of the physical environment in the hospital of the 21st century.* Concord, CA: Center for Health Design.

U.S. Office of Management and Budget. (1998). *The Budget for Fiscal Year 1999, Analytical Perspectives.*

Ware, J. E., & Sherbourne, C. D. (1992). The MOS 36-item short form health survey I: Conceptual framework and item selection. *Medical Care, 30,* 473–478.

Wennberg, J. E., & Gittelsohn, A. M. (1973). Small area variations in health care delivery. *Science, 182*(117), 1102–1108.

Werner, R. M., & Bradlow, E. T. (2006). Relationship between Medicare's hospital compare performance measures and mortality rates. *Journal of the American Medical Association, 296*(22), 2694–2702.

Williams, S. C., Schmaltz, S. P., Morton, D. J., Koss, R. G., & Loeb, J. M. (2005). Quality of care in U.S. hospitals as reflected by standard measures, 2003–2004. *New England Journal of Medicine, 353*(3), 255–264.

Woolf, S. H. (1999). The need for perspective in evidence-based medicine. *Journal of the American Medical Association, 282,* 2358–2365.

World Health Organization (WHO). (2000). The World Health Report 2000—Health systems: Improving performance (pp. 27–35). Geneva: World Health Organization.

SUGGESTED READINGS

Anderson, R. M., Rice, T. H., & Kominski, G. F. (2007). *Changing the U.S. health care system: Key issues in health services policy and management* (3rd ed.). San Francisco: Jossey-Bass.

Brown, M. A., Draye, M. A., Zimmer, P. A., Magyary, D., Woods, S. L., Whitney, J., et al. (2006, May–Jun.). Developing a practice doctorate in nursing: University of Washington perspectives and experience. *Nursing Outlook, 54*(3), 130–138.

Centers for Medicare and Medicaid Services (CMS). (2006). 2006 Annual Report of the Boards of Trustees of the Federal Hospital Insurance and Federal Supplementary Medical Insurance Trust Funds. Retrieved October 4, 2006, from http://www.cms.hhs.gov/ReportsTrustFunds/downloads/tr2006.pdf

Centers for Medicare & Medicaid Services, Office of the Actuary, National Health Statistics Group. (2006). Retrieved October 4, 2006, from http://www.cms.hhs.gov/NationalHealthExpendData/downloads/PieChartSourcesExpenditures2004.pdf

Centers for Medicare and Medicaid Services, Office of the Actuary, National Health Statistics Group. (2006). Retrieved October 4, 2006, from http://www.cms.hhs.gov/NationalHealthExpendData

Cohen, J., & Krauss, N. (2003, Mar.–Apr.). Spending and service use among people with the fifteen most costly medical conditions, 1997. *Health Affairs, 22*(2), 129–138.

Donabedian, A. (1966). Evaluating the quality of medical care. *Milbank Quarterly, 20*(1), 137–141.

Dracup, K., Cronenwett, L., Meleis, A. I., & Benner, P. E. (2005). Reflections on the doctorate of nursing practice. *Nursing Outlook, 53*(4), 177–182.

Draye, M. A., Acker, M., & Zimmer, P. A. (2006, May–Jun.). The practice doctorate in nursing: Approaches to transform nurse practitioner education and practice. *Nursing Outlook, 54*(3), 123–129.

Headrick, L. A. (2000). Learning to improve complex systems of care. In *Collaborative education to ensure patient safety* (pp. 75–88). Washington, DC: HRSA/Bureau of Health Professions.

Kahn, C. N., Ault, T., Isenstein, H., Potetz, L., & Van Gelder, S. (2006). Snapshot of hospital quality reporting and pay-for-performance under Medicare. *Health Affairs, 25*(1), 148–162.

Kaiser Family Foundation (KFF). (2005a). *Navigating Medicare and Medicaid, 2005: Medicaid.* Washington, DC: Kaiser Family Foundation. Accessible at http://www.kff.org/medicare/7240/medicaid.cfm

Kaiser Family Foundation (KFF). (2005b). *Navigating Medicare and Medicaid, 2005: Medicare.* Washington, DC: Kaiser Family Foundation. Accessible at http://www.kff.org/medicare/7240/medicare.cfm

Kaiser Family Foundation (KFF). (2006). *The uninsured: Key facts about Americans without health insurance.* Washington, DC: Kaiser Family Foundation. Accessible at http://www.kff.org/uninsured/upload/7451-021.pdf

Lee, J. S., Berenson, R. A., Mayes, R., & Gauthier, A. K. (2003). Medicare payment policy: Does cost shifting matter? *Health Affairs, W3,* 480–488.

Mundinger, M. O. (2005). Who's who in nursing: Bringing clarity to the doctor of nursing practice. *Nursing Outlook, 53,* 173–176.

National Bureau of Economic Research. (2006). Healthcare expenditures in the OECD. Retrieved June 4, 2006, from http://www.nber.org/aginghealth/winter06/w11833.html

Rosenthal, M. B., Fernandopulle, R., Song, H. R., & Landon, B. (2004). Paying for quality: Providers' incentives for quality improvement. *Health Affairs, 23*(2), 127–141.

U.S. Department of Health and Human Services. (2006). Annual Update of the HHS Poverty Guidelines. Accessible at http://aspe.hhs.gov/poverty/06fedreg.pdf

The viewpoints expressed in this chapter are the responsibility of the author and do not represent those of the federal government.

CHAPTER 3

Organizational Behavior and Magnet Hospitals

Maria R. Shirey, MS, MBA, RN, CNAA, BC, FACHE

Magnet hospitals are living evidence that creating professional nurse practice environments is the solution to the flight of nurses from hospital practice (Aiken, 2002).

OBJECTIVES

Upon completion of this chapter, the reader should be able to:

1. Relate organizational behavior.
2. Identify the evolution of organizational behavior and its impact on autocratic, custodial, supportive, and collegial organizational behavior.
3. Identify the characteristics of a high-performance organization.
4. Identify the organizational characteristics that define magnet nursing services.
5. Relate the historical evolution and significance of magnet hospitals.
6. Support the 14 Forces of Magnetism.

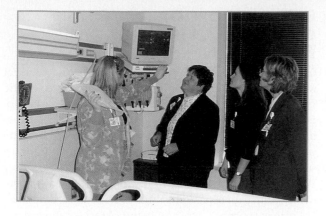

Anne and Maria are new nurses who went to nursing school together. Now, one year after both became registered nurses, they still maintain their commitment to having dinner together at their favorite restaurant at least once a month. Both nurses started their careers with a great deal of excitement and anticipation. Anne is now concerned that Maria's "flame" is starting to lose its vibrancy.

When Anne and Maria get together, they invariably talk about their relatively new positions as staff nurses in two different local hospitals. Anne works on a medical-surgical unit at Midwest Community Hospital (MCH) that has been magnet-designated for about five years. At MCH, Anne joyously reports working on a cohesive unit adequately staffed with capable nurses who are true team players and contribute to outstanding patient outcomes. Anne raves about her unit-based clinical nurse specialist (her mentor) and about her nurse manager who both seem very interested in Anne's personal and professional development. Maria, on the other hand, also works on a medical-surgical unit, but at a nonmagnet-designated facility. Maria reports that her nurse manager is not supportive of magnet designation. In fact, when Maria initiated a conversation to inquire about the possibility of her Good Spirit Hospital pursuing such a journey, her manager's response was "That magnet 'thing' is nothing more than a marketing ploy; it offers no real benefits." Fearing that her manager would see her as confrontational and not wanting to get on her manager's bad side, Maria dropped the conversation. Over the past few months, Maria has been working many mandatory overtime hours at her hospital. Every shift worked on her unit feels like an exercise in "survival of the fittest." With more nurses resigning from her unit and patient care outcomes not being what they should be, Maria still loves nursing, yet she is beginning to wonder if she made the right choice in going to work at Good Spirit Hospital.

Compare and contrast the characteristics of Anne's and Maria's professional nursing practice environments.

As a new nurse entering the workforce, what objective and subjective resources should you review to guide an assessment of the professional nursing practice environment at a potential place of employment?

From an organizational behavior standpoint, how can the practice environments at MCH and Good Spirit Hospital be explained?

The health care industry is in the midst of a workforce shortage that includes both nurses and other health care professionals. Facing an aging society and the rising need for health care services, the ability to attract and retain current and future health care professionals is of paramount concern. The literature suggests a link between desirable practice environments, such as those seen in magnet hospitals, and the ability to attract and retain health care professionals. A better appreciation of the links between employee attitudes and behaviors related to work environments, however, requires an understanding of organizational behavior.

This chapter introduces the concept of organizational behavior and explains how an understanding of organizational behavior may favorably shape the professional work environment to directly affect individuals, groups, and organizations. The chapter highlights **magnet hospitals** as high-quality health care organizations that have met the rigorous nursing excellence requirements of the American Nurses Credentialing Center (ANCC), a division of the American Nurses Association (ANA), and that are supportive and collegial practice settings that incorporate principles of organizational behavior to achieve positive individual, group, and organizational outcomes.

ORGANIZATIONAL BEHAVIOR

Organizational behavior can be defined as the study of human behavior in organizations (Schermerhorn, Hunt, & Osborn, 2005). Organizational behavior is specifically concerned with work-related behavior and addresses individuals and groups, interpersonal processes, and organizational dynamics and systems. Organizational behavior draws from many disciplines, including psychology, sociology, social psychology, anthropology, and political science (Robbins, 2005).

An **organization** is a coordinated and deliberately structured social entity that consists of two or more individuals, functioning on a relatively continuous basis to achieve a predetermined set of goals (Daft, 2006). Organizations are complex entities that exist as **open systems**, that must interact with the environment in order to survive (Daft, 2006). An organization's long-term effectiveness may be determined by its capability to anticipate, manage, and respond to changes in its environment. These changes may result from **external forces**, that is, influences originating outside the organization such as, the labor force and economy, or from **stakeholders**, that is, people or groups with an interest in the performance of the organization such as customers, competitors, suppliers, government, and regulatory agencies.

The field of organizational behavior emphasizes people skills in addition to technical skills and involves the systematic study of the actions and attitudes people exhibit within organizations (Robbins, 2005). Attitudes of interest in organizational behavior include **job satisfaction**, how organizational members feel about their job, and **organizational commitment**, how committed or loyal employees feel to the goals of the organization. Actions or behaviors of interest in organizational behavior also include three important determinants of employee performance. The determinants are **productivity**, which is the quantity and quality of output an employee generates for an organization; **absenteeism**, which is the rate of employee absences from work; and **turnover**, which is the number of employees who resigned divided by the total number of employees during the same time period. All of these determinants can be measured.

IMPORTANCE OF ORGANIZATIONAL BEHAVIOR

Learning about organizational behavior enables organizational members to better understand their own behaviors as well as those of peers, superiors, and/or subordinates within an organization. This understanding helps individuals become more effective employees, team members, and managers within organizations. Research suggests that employees who demonstrate high levels of organizational commitment are generally more satisfied in their jobs and more likely to stay employed within their organizations (Lynn & Redman, 2005). Employees who experience empowering structures in the workplace are generally more engaged (Laschinger & Finegan, 2005) and may have lower absenteeism and lower employee turnover. Because excessive employee turnover is costly and detrimental to quality outcomes, organizations need to proactively concern themselves with the important issues related to organizational behavior.

Organizational behavior allows individuals to increase organizational effectiveness to ultimately meet the needs of the organization, its members, and society. **Organizational effectiveness** refers to an organization's sustainable high performance in accomplishing its mission and objectives (Schermerhorn et al., 2005). In the long run, the primary criterion to evaluate organizational effectiveness is the organization's capability to survive and thrive under conditions of uncertainty. Important contributors to the effectiveness of any organization are the quality of its workforce and their commitment to the goals and success of the organization. Maintaining a satisfied and committed workforce, however, is a planned effort that requires the contributions of many members within an organization.

EVOLUTION OF ORGANIZATIONAL BEHAVIOR

Organizational behavior traces its roots to the original work of Frederick Taylor and to the advent of scientific management in the late 1800s and early 1900s. Proponents of scientific management emphasized the machine-like or assembly-line focus of work processes and the precise sets of instructions and time-motion studies assumed to enhance productivity (Wikipedia, 2006). After World War I and the identification of the **Hawthorne effect**, which demonstrated that a change in employee behavior occurs as a result of being observed, the organizational behavior focus shifted to how human relations and psychology affected organizations. This era was followed by the introduction of the human motivation theories by Abraham Maslow (hierarchy of needs theory), Douglas McGregor (Theory X and Theory Y), and William Ouchi (Theory Z). See Chapter 1 for more on these theories.

Over the past century, the U.S. economy has shifted from an industrial focus and an assembly line mentality in the 1900s to a knowledge economy in the 2000s. A knowledge economy requires highly educated employees for a more technologic information age and thus necessitates a new way of leading and developing future employees and organizations. Increasingly, today's health care professionals see themselves as **knowledge workers** who are well educated and technologically savvy and who see themselves as owning their intellectual capital. This **intellectual capital** includes an individual's knowledge, skills, and abilities that have value and portability in a knowledge economy. This shift to a knowledge economy means that health care professionals today possess well-developed abilities and require supportive and collegial organizations to cultivate their much in-demand talents or they will take their knowledge, skill, and ability to another organization. The supportive and collegial work environments that today's knowledge workers prefer are consistent with McGregor's Theory Y, that is, environments in which leaders remove obstacles for motivated and empowered individuals. These environments appear to be in sharp contrast with the autocratic and custodial organizational frameworks of earlier centuries. Table 3-1 summarizes and compares the common organizational models of autocratic, custodial, supportive, and collegial organizations (Clark, 2000).

In addition to supportive and collegial organizations, today's health care industry places great emphasis on global diversity, technological intensity, change as a constant, superior quality and safety outcomes, and continuous learning and process improvements. Organizational behavior today continues to be influenced by the human relations movement and by the human

TABLE 3-1		MODELS OF ORGANIZATIONAL BEHAVIOR			
Type of Model	**Basis of the Model**	**Managerial Orientation**	**Employee Orientation**	**Employee Need(s) Met**	**Performance Outcomes**
Autocratic	Power	Authority	Dependence on the boss	Subsistence	Minimal
Custodial	Economics	Money	Security Benefits Dependence on the organization	Security	Passive cooperation
Supportive	Leadership	Support	Good job performance Participation	Status Recognition	Awakened work drive and cooperation Passion
Collegial	Partnership	Teamwork	Responsible behavior Self-discipline	Self-actualization	Enthusiasm Engagement

motivation theories that capitalize on humanistic, motivational, team-based, and collaborative strategies. Business practice models emphasizing quality leadership and management (Drucker, 2006) and developing life-long learning organizations (Senge, 1990) further contribute to contemporary organizational development and effectiveness.

HIGH-PERFORMANCE ORGANIZATIONS

Health care organizations operate within a competitive environment of constant change and scarcity of human and financial resources. Given the rising shortages of qualified health care professionals and compounded by an aging population requiring greater access to health care services, many health care organizations have seen the need to reposition their organizations for the future. These changing forces have contributed to the reinvention of many health care institutions as high-performance organizations. A **high-performance organization** operates in a way that brings out the best in people and produces sustainable high-performance over time. High-performance organizations pay close attention to the dynamics of the workplace and are known for also having high quality-of-work-life environments (Schermerhorn et al., 2005).

High quality-of-work-life environments are those work environments in which the quality of the human experience in the workplace meets and surpasses employee expectations. Employees in high quality-of-work-life environments are respected and treated well at work, thus keeping employees motivated, engaged, continuously growing, and retained within their organizations.

Maintaining high quality-of-work-life environments requires the commitment of both leaders and employees in organizations. Leaders in high-performance organizations recognize that the single best predictor of an organization's success is its capability to attract, motivate, and retain talented people (Schermerhorn et al., 2005). So important is the quality of the work environment in health care that the Institute of Medicine (IOM), a major policy influencing organization, has specifically called for the transformation of the nurse's work environment in order to retain nurses in the profession and to keep patients safe (IOM, 2004). Table 3-2 summarizes the five characteristics of high-performance organizations that contribute to a high quality-of-work-life environment and to quality patient care. A magnet hospital represents an example of a supportive and collegial work environment for nurses that also may be classified as a high-performance organization and a high quality-of-work-life environment.

TABLE 3-2	FIVE CHARACTERISTICS OF HIGH-PERFORMANCE ORGANIZATIONS

High-Performance Organizations

- Value people as human assets, respect diversity, and empower individuals to use their talents to advance personal and organizational performance

- Mobilize teams that build synergy from the talents of its members and are empowered to use self-direction and personal initiative to maximize performance

- Successfully bring people and technology together in a performance context

- Thrive on learning, encourage knowledge sharing, and enable members to continuously grow and develop

- Are achievement-oriented, sensitive to the external environment, and focused on total quality management to deliver outstanding and sustainable results

MAGNET HOSPITALS

As mentioned earlier, a magnet hospital is a health care organization that has met the rigorous nursing excellence requirement of the American Nurses Credentialing Center (ANCC), a division of the American Nurses Association (ANA). Magnet designation involves a voluntary credentialing process. Achieving magnet designation represents the highest level of recognition the ANCC accords to health care organizations that provide the services of registered professional nurses (ANCC, 2004). As a testament to the increasing recognition given to magnet hospitals, *U.S. News and World Report* recently included magnet designation in its criteria for its annual "100 Best Hospitals of America" list (U.S. News & World Report, 2005).

Of 5,759 hospitals in the United States (AHA, 2006), 202 (or 3.5%) are magnet-designated facilities (ANCC, 2006a). This figure is rising daily. Community hospitals, teaching hospitals, and hospital systems, large (more than 1,000 beds) and small (less than 100 beds), in rural and urban settings, have achieved magnet recognition. Although pursuing magnet designation is an individual organizational decision, implementing the magnet standards in hospital settings can potentially benefit institutions independent of whether they achieve magnet designation or not.

HISTORICAL OVERVIEW OF MAGNET HOSPITALS

In 1983, the American Academy of Nursing (AAN), an organization affiliated with the ANA, appointed a Task Force on Nursing Practice in Hospitals. The purpose of the task force was to identify workplace characteristics that were successful in recruiting and retaining hospital nurses. The task force studied 163 hospitals in the United States based on their reputation for successfully attracting and retaining nurses and for delivering high-quality nursing care. Of the 163 hospitals studied, 41 (25%) were described as magnet hospitals (McClure, Poulin, Sovie, & Wandelt, 1983). A magnet designation was earned through demonstrated high nurse satisfaction, low nurse turnover, and low nurse vacancy rates. Interestingly, the 41 original magnet hospitals were able to recruit and retain nurses despite concurrent health care industry changes in the payment system; an unprecedented number of hospital mergers, acquisitions, and consolidations; and a major nursing shortage. The AAN's landmark study concluded that the 41 original magnet hospitals shared a set of core organizational attributes that were desirable. The study stimulated additional independent research that provided further evidence to highlight the achievement of superior outcomes in magnet hospitals.

By June 1990, the ANA established the ANCC as a separate, incorporated, nonprofit organization that was to serve as the credentialing arm for magnet hospitals. The initial proposal for the Magnet Hospital Recognition Program was approved by the ANA Board of Directors in December 1990. The Magnet Program proposal indicated that the program would be built upon the 1983 AAN magnet hospital study. Further, the Magnet Program would use as a baseline for program development, the 1999 *ANA Scope and Standards for Nurse Administrators*, now in its second revision (ANA, 2004).

THE ANCC MAGNET FACILITIES

The University of Washington Medical Center in Seattle became ANCC's first magnet facility in 1994. By 1998, 13 hospitals achieved magnet designation. By the 2000s,

REAL WORLD INTERVIEW

With magnet hospitals recognized for low RN turnover rates, higher nurse-patient staffing ratios, and greater autonomy and influence over practice decisions, it is anticipated that high nurse satisfaction will exist across nursing units. A professional nursing practice model, such as ours at Columbus Regional Hospital in Indiana, includes clinical practice development, positive nurse-physician relationships, supportive nurse-manager relationships, ongoing educational support, and adequate nurse staffing. It is the synergy of these factors within the Nursing Services Department that will create high nurse satisfaction.

Cherona Hajewski, RN, MSN, CNAA
Senior Vice-President, Patient Care Services
Columbus, Indiana

TABLE 3-3	NINE CHARACTERISTICS DEFINING MAGNET NURSING SERVICES

- High-quality patient care
- Clinical autonomy and responsibility
- Participatory decision making
- Strong nurse leaders
- Two-way communication with staff

- Community involvement
- Opportunity and encouragement of professional development
- Effective use of staff resources
- High levels of job satisfaction

the growth of magnet hospitals was exponential, resulting in more than 200 magnet-designated facilities by mid-2006. Hundreds of facilities are continuously in the pipeline seeking to become magnet hospitals. To date, the Magnet Recognition Program has been expanded to include both acute care hospitals and long-term facilities. The Magnet Recognition Program reviews applications from both U.S. and international health care organizations.

GOALS OF THE MAGNET RECOGNITION PROGRAM

The Magnet Recognition Program (ANCC, 2004) was created to achieve three major goals:

1. Promote quality in a milieu that supports professional nursing practice.
2. Identify excellence in the delivery of nursing services to patients.
3. Provide a mechanism for the dissemination of best practices in nursing services.

CRITICAL THINKING 3-1

To learn more about some of the most important questions that must be addressed at the beginning of the magnet application process, access and complete the document entitled, Staff Nurse Opinion Questionnaire (ANCC, 2007) at www.nursingworld.org. Click on American Nurses Credentialing Center. Click on Calling All Staff Nurses. Complete the Nurse Opinion Questionnaire that you find there.

Nine characteristics define magnet nursing services (Table 3-3). These characteristics form the assessment framework for the Magnet Recognition Program's appraisal process.

BENEFITS OF MAGNET RECOGNITION

Hospitals attaining magnet designation may achieve multiple benefits that include improved patient quality outcomes, enhanced organizational culture, improved nurse recruitment and retention, enhanced safety outcomes, and enhanced competitive advantage (Table 3-4). A major benefit of magnet designation is that it enhances the image of nursing within the health care organization and the community. Magnet recognition raises the bar for nursing services and contributes to upgrading the quality of nursing services delivered at the local, national, and international levels.

IMPROVEMENT IN QUALITY PATIENT OUTCOMES

Improved patient quality outcomes have been reported in magnet organizations. Much of the evidence documenting better patient outcomes in these hospitals supports the underlying assumption that work environments that are attractive to nurses yield better outcomes for patients (Aiken, 2002). Historical research by Aiken over the past two decades and more current studies conducted by her team and others continue to support the significant importance of the nurse's work environment (Lake & Friese, 2006).

In a study comparing patient quality outcomes between magnet and nonmagnet facilities, Aiken, Smith, & Lake (1994) demonstrated that magnet hospitals, after adjusting for differences in severity of patient illness, had a 4.6% lower Medicare mortality than comparison hospitals. In another study comparing AIDS mortality in magnet versus nonmagnet facilities, researchers documented better outcomes in the magnet facilities (Aiken, Sloane, Lake, Sochalski, & Weber, 1999). The higher nurse-to-patient ratio in the magnet hospitals was found to be the major factor explaining the lower patient mortality.

Increased levels of patient satisfaction have also been documented in magnet hospitals. In a study comparing patients on dedicated AIDS units in magnet hospitals versus patients on a medical unit in conventionally organized hospitals, patient satisfaction was highest in the AIDS units in the magnet hospitals (Aiken, Sloan, & Lake, 1997; Aiken et al., 1999). The researchers found that the single most important factor explaining differences in patient satisfaction was the superior nurse practice environment of the magnet hospitals and the dedicated AIDS units. Patients in the magnet hospitals and dedicated AIDS units reported better nurse accountability with their care, a factor presumed to enhance continuity of patient care. As outcomes in magnet hospitals continue to be disseminated in the lay literature, more patients are beginning to associate higher levels of perceived quality of care with magnet hospitals. Increasingly, patients are actively seeking magnet facilities to meet their health care needs.

TABLE 3-4   BENEFITS OF MAGNET DESIGNATION

Improved patient quality outcomes

- Lower patient morbidity and mortality
- Increased patient satisfaction

Enhanced organizational culture

- Greater nurse empowerment structures
- Improved nurse well-being
- Supportive, people-oriented, and visible nurse leaders and administrators
- Shared decision making
- Increased culture of respect for nurses

Improved nurse recruitment and retention

- Higher levels of nurse job satisfaction
- Increased perception by nurses of presence of a work environment that allows them to give quality patient care

- Higher levels of nurse autonomy and control over practice
- More positive nurse-physician relationships
- Greater support for ongoing professional development

Enhanced safety outcomes

- Lower incidence of needle stick injury rates among nurses
- Lower incidence of near-miss patient injuries

Enhanced competitive advantage

- More validation of excellence in nursing services
- Enhanced public confidence with the facility
- Enhanced public perception of overall facility quality
- Lower nurse turnover
- Higher nurse job satisfaction

REAL WORLD INTERVIEW

At Columbus Regional, Indiana's first magnet hospital, a primary strategy we use to emphasize the need for renewal in the workplace is to focus on reflective nursing practice. We have in place unit-based and hospital-based practice councils as part of our shared governance structure. We participate in storytelling grand rounds as well as in nursing leadership forums. These venues allow us to partner with others to examine any "fuel leaks" in our organization. By fuel leaks, I mean negative thinking or unnecessary depleting actions that detract us from pursuing our passion and purpose. We also do not lose sight of the need to engage in celebrations to summon our human spirit, reattach us to our human roots, and help us to soar toward new visions.

Mary Sitterding, RN, MSN, CNS
Magnet Recognition Progam Director
Columbus, Indiana

ENHANCED ORGANIZATIONAL CULTURE

Core values such as empowerment, pride, mentoring, nurturing, respect, integrity, and teamwork are reported in magnet facilities (ANCC, 2006a). There is evidence to suggest that nurses in magnet facilities work within greater empowerment structures that enhance the work environment, improve nurse well-being (Laschinger & Finegan, 2005), and make professional nursing practice more desirable in those settings (Laschinger, Almost, & Tuer-Hodes, 2003). Magnet workplace cultures report people-oriented, visible, and empowering nurse leaders (Upenieks, 2003; Steinbinder & Scherer, 2006) who contribute in a significant way toward building positive organizational cultures. Shared decision making is a hallmark of magnet cultures that allows nurses to practice in a workplace where professional autonomy is both valued and encouraged. Overall, magnet hospital nurses report a culture of respect for nurses. This culture of respect manifests itself in the form of more supportive hospital administrators and more value attributed to nurses (Havens & Aiken, 1999) and nurses' contributions to the organizational mission, quality patient care.

IMPROVED NURSE RECRUITMENT AND RETENTION

Magnet hospitals are considered to be good places to practice nursing (Scott, Sochalski, & Aiken, 1999). These facilities are named magnet hospitals due to their capability to attract and retain nurses and maintain high levels of job satisfaction (Brady-Schwartz, 2005). In fact, nurse turnover and vacancy rates are generally lower in magnet hospitals than they are in other facilities (Kramer, 1990; Kramer & Schmalenburg, 1991; Coile, 2001). It is not unusual to observe both new and experienced nurses

REAL WORLD INTERVIEW

I choose to drive the hour to Columbus Regional Hospital (CRH) in Indiana to work because of the respect the nursing profession receives at CRH. Nursing administration gives bedside nurses a voice. My ideas are encouraged, good and bad.

Sheri McDole, RN
Staff Nurse and Member, Nursing Practice Council
Columbus, Indiana

making hospital employment decisions based on whether or not a facility is magnet designated. Given today's ready electronic access, determination of an organization's magnet status requires a simple Web-based search (http://nursecredentialing.org/magnet). Click on Find a Facility. Interestingly, nonnursing health care professionals such as practitioners (ANCC, 2006a), pharmacists, physical therapists, social workers, and others (McClure & Hinshaw, 2002) also seem to benefit from magnet workplace cultures.

Additional research supports the essentials of magnetism and their role in nurse retention. For example, nurses in magnet facilities report higher levels of nurse autonomy and control over practice with more positive nurse-physician relationships (Aiken, Sloane, & Lake, 1997; Laschinger et al., 2003). These findings are significant given the important patient safety implications of

TABLE 3-5	EIGHT ESSENTIALS OF MAGNETISM

- Opportunities to work with other nurses who are clinically competent.
- Good nurse-physician relationships and communication.
- Nurse autonomy and accountability.
- Supportive nurse manager-supervisor.

- Control over nursing practice and practice environment.
- Support for education.
- Adequate nurse staffing.
- Concern for the patient is paramount.

cohesive interdisciplinary teams capable of initiating open communication and collaborative dialogue on behalf of patients. Nurses at magnet facilities also report strong organizational support for continuing professional development (Kramer & Schmalenberg, 2004). Support for ongoing professional development is an important retention strategy that benefits patients and helps nurses meet their lifelong learning requirements.

Two decades of research by Kramer and Schmalenberg (2002) suggests that nurses in magnet facilities indicate high levels of job satisfaction because they perceive that magnet practice environments allow nurses the ability to give quality patient care. The eight essentials to giving quality care reported by staff nurses in magnet hospitals are also known as the Essentials of Magnetism (Table 3-5).

ENHANCED SAFETY OUTCOMES

Magnet hospitals are known for better patient and staff safety outcomes. Specifically, magnet hospitals have been found to have fewer needle stick injury rates among nurses (Aiken, Sloane, & Klocinski, 1997). Better nurse-to-patient ratios in magnet hospitals are also known to result in reduced near-miss patient injury (Clarke, Rockett, Sloane, & Aiken, 2002). The Agency for Health Care Research and Quality (AHRQ) defines a near miss as a close call or an event or situation that did not produce patient injury but could have done so (AHRQ, 2006). The literature clearly supports the value of nurses in establishing and maintaining the vigilant surveillance systems that are crucial for patient safety (Aiken, 2002; Aiken, Clarke, Cheung, Sloane, & Silber, 2003; Clarke & Aiken, 2006).

ENHANCED COMPETITIVE ADVANTAGE

Magnet designation represents a gold seal of approval that validates excellence in nursing services. Achieving such distinction enhances the public's confidence with the facility and speaks to the organization's overall quality (ANCC, 2004). The low turnover and high job

CRITICAL THINKING 3-2

After reading the three interviews in this chapter, identify one common theme that emerges from all three of the interviews. Based on your assessment, describe the quality-of-work-life environment and the patient outcomes you would expect to see at a magnet-designated organization.

satisfaction of nurses in magnet facilities also provides competitive advantage by increasing staff continuity, maintaining patient care quality, and minimizing the costs associated with employee turnover. Achieving the prestigious magnet hospital designation can be used powerfully in hospital-wide promotional materials, thus adding to the hospital's capability to gain marketing advantage.

FORCES OF MAGNETISM

The 14 Forces of Magnetism represent the foundation of the Magnet Recognition Program (Urden & Monarch, 2002). These Forces incorporate the nine characteristics defining magnet nursing services and the eight essentials of magnetism discussed earlier in this chapter. The 14 Forces of Magnetism are the outcomes of innovative and dynamic implementation of the Scope and Standards for Nurse Administrators by visionary nurse leaders creating supportive and collegial environments for nursing practice (ANCC, 2004) (Table 3-6).

Magnet designation requires the full expression of the 14 Forces of Magnetism (ANCC, 2004, p. 5). This means that facilities seeking magnet designation must show evidence to support the existence of all the

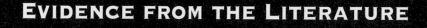

EVIDENCE FROM THE LITERATURE

Citation: Havens, D.S. & Johnston, M.A. (2004). Achieving magnet hospital recognition: Chief nurse executives and magnet coordinators tell their stories. *Journal of Nursing Administration, 34*(12), 579–588.

Discussion: This research was designed to add to the understanding of how hospitals successfully pursue magnet recognition. Although extensive literature exists to demonstrate the benefits of magnet hospitals, few studies have been conducted to explain how to get there. A convenience sample of twenty-four participants (six chief nurse executives and eighteen magnet program coordinators) attending the October 2003 National Magnet Hospital Conference in Houston, Texas, was selected. Three two-hour focus groups were conducted with questions guided by the literature on magnet hospitals. This article reports on the results of one question: How did you pursue ANCC magnet recognition?

Data analysis from the interviews revealed the nine following themes related to the research question. First, securing buy-in from key stakeholders is key. Having the support of hospital administrators, chief executive officers, the board of trustees, practitioners, nurses, and staff from other departments is important. The researchers found nurses to be the hardest sell, primarily because nurses were concerned with the perceived added workload that a magnet journey would entail. Second, the importance of celebrating throughout the process was highlighted. Because the magnet journey may be a long one, participants reported on the importance of celebrating along the way with large, themed, kick-off events and functions after achieving specified milestones and formal galas after the attainment of magnet designation. Third, the use of external consultants was found to be mostly beneficial. The consultants were seen as expert guides who could serve as validators and encouragers. Satisfaction with the use of consultants was mixed. Fourth, putting the structure for magnet in place required time. Some facilities reported needing a lead-time of about three years, whereas others appeared to have significant components of the magnet structure already in place earlier. The need to identify champions and cheerleaders early in the process was mentioned. Fifth, communicating frequently was crucial in helping to spread the magnet message. Newsletters, flyers, personal communications, and addressing an ongoing magnet agenda at multiple venues were strategies used to reach all levels of the organization. Sixth, educating nurses and others was identified as a key strategy for a successful magnet journey. Magnet education was included as part of an ongoing component of new employee orientation. Seventh, mentoring by ANCC magnet hospitals was reported to be most helpful early in the magnet journey. Mentoring took the form of on-site visits by teams at mentor hospitals, phone calls, and email exchanges. Eighth, telling the story while collecting the organization's magnet evidence was important. Although the hospitals reported a variety of methods to collecting magnet evidence, most agreed on the importance of gathering a variety of rich and robust examples from across the organization. Ninth, paying the costs of the magnet journey involved a significant time commitment with the magnet coordinator assuming a great deal of the responsibility. Most organizations undertaking a magnet journey underestimate the time commitment it requires. Interestingly, there was no consensus among participants as to the monetary costs associated with the journey. Sources of funding for the magnet journey ranged from internal budgets to grants from hospital foundations. The participants agreed that a significant value of the magnet journey was in the magnet appraisal process.

Implications for Practice: The process of pursuing magnet designation is as meaningful as attaining the actual magnet designation. Pursuing a magnet journey is consistent with implementing a change process and should be approached from an organizational change perspective. The effort requires frequent communication and the involvement and support of multiple disciplines. The success of the magnet journey rests with the understanding that nursing exists within a larger culture and thus must pursue the contributions of many within the organization. To this end, buy-in and support from multiple stakeholders is crucial to the success and sustainability of magnet hospitals.

Forces of Magnetism in the organization. An emerging body of literature exists to help navigate the magnet journey (Goode, et al, 2005; Ellis & Gates, 2005; Havens & Johnston, 2004; Shirey, 2004). Articles that describe the magnet application process (Bumgarner & Beard, 2003; Bliss-Holtz, Winter, & Scherer, 2004) provide guidance in meeting difficult standards (Messmer, Jones, & Rosillo, 2002; Turkel, Reidinger, Ferket, & Reno, 2005). Help to document the Forces of Magnetism (Shirey, 2005; Drenkard, 2005; Poduska, 2005) is also available.

MAGNET APPRAISAL PROCESS

The magnet appraisal process addresses specific requirements, processes, and activities necessary to achieve

| TABLE 3-6 | THE FOURTEEN FORCES OF MAGNETISM |

Forces of Magnetism	Definition
Quality nursing leadership	■ Nurse leaders are perceived as knowledgeable, strong risk-takers who follow an articulated philosophy of nursing. ■ Nurse leaders are strong staff advocates and supporters. ■ The outcomes of quality nursing leadership are evident in nursing practice at the patient's bedside.
Organizational structure	■ Organizational structures are flat with decentralized, unit-based decision making. ■ Strong nursing representation is evident in the organizational committee structure. ■ Chief nursing officer reports to the organization's chief executive officer and is a member of the executive team.
Management style	■ Nursing and hospital administrators share a participative management style that incorporates feedback from staff at all levels of the organization.
Personnel policies and programs	■ Organization offers competitive salaries and benefits. ■ Flexible staffing models are utilized. ■ Personnel policies reflect staff involvement and clinical promotional opportunities.
Professional models of care	■ Nurses have accountability for their nursing practice. ■ Practice model reflects nurses as coordinators of care.
Quality of care	■ Providing quality of care is seen as an organizational priority. ■ Nurse leaders develop the work environment so that quality of care can be delivered, and nurses perceive they are able to provide high-quality care.
Quality improvement	■ Staff nurses participate in quality improvement processes, and they perceive the process as educational and beneficial to quality patient care.
Consultation and resources	■ Knowledgeable experts, including advanced practice nurses, are available and utilized. ■ Adequate consultation with other health care human resources are available within the organization.
Autonomy	■ Nurses engage in autonomous practice consistent with professional standards. ■ Independent professional judgment is expected within the context of interdisciplinary collaboration in patient care.
Community and the hospital	■ The hospital maintains a strong community presence with the community perceiving the hospital as a productive and positive corporate citizen.
Nurses as teachers	■ Nurses are expected to incorporate teaching in all aspects of their professional practice.
Image of nursing	■ Nurses are seen as crucial to the hospital's capability to provide patient care services, a perception also held by other members of the health care team.
Interdisciplinary relationships	■ Positive interdisciplinary relationships are present with a sense of mutual respect exhibited among all disciplines.
Professional development	■ Significant emphasis is placed on the professional development of the staff, including orientation, inservice education, continuing education, formal education, and ongoing competency maintenance. ■ Value is given to personal and professional growth, including emphasis on employee career development.

magnet designation. Magnet-aspiring organizations generally begin the process by purchasing the most current issue of the *Magnet Recognition Program Application Manual* (ANCC, 2004). This manual guides the aspiring magnet organization's Chief Nursing Officer (CNO), Magnet Program Coordinator, and Magnet Steering Team members in pursuing the magnet journey. The magnet appraisal process requires collecting detailed demographic information from applicant organizations and reviewing comprehensive documents and magnet evidence reflecting how applicants meet all program requirements. Additionally, the process considers feedback acquired from public comment opportunities. Magnet appraisers conduct a variety of site visits to verify and expand upon the submitted application materials.

The magnet appraisal process consists of four sequential phases: application, evaluation, site visit, and award decision. The application phase involves review of the application manual and the decision to apply for magnet designation. Early in the magnet journey, organizations will need to establish a database to collect data on **nursing-sensitive indicators**, that is, measures that reflect the outcome of nursing actions. Joining the National Database of Nursing Quality Indicators (NDNQI, 2006) is a means to achieve this data-collection requirement. Membership in the NDNQI is beneficial because it provides organizations with the capability to benchmark data on nursing-sensitive indicators gathered at the unit level. Benchmarking is the process of comparing outcomes with similar organizations to identify and establish best practices.

Organizations will also conduct a gap analysis in the application process. A **gap analysis** is an assessment of the differences between the expected magnet requirements and the organization's current performance on those requirements. A **gap** is the space between where the organization is and where it wants to be. A gap analysis serves as a tool that provides direction in developing the necessary activities to bridge a gap.

The evaluation phase occurs following the written application and submission of the aspiring hospital's magnet evidence. These comprehensive documents and demographic data are reviewed by a team of ANCC magnet appraisers who independently score the evidence for each of the 14 Forces of Magnetism. Arrangements for a site visit will follow if the written documentation earns the necessary points to score at a level of excellence.

The site visit involves the magnet appraisal team making a planned site visit to the magnet-aspiring facility. While on site, the magnet appraisers visit the units of the organization where nurses work to verify the content of the written magnet evidence previously submitted and scored. Following the site visit, the appraisal team

CRITICAL THINKING 3-3

Review the 14 Forces of Magnetism in Table 3-6 at your clinical facility. How does your unit compare with a magnet facility?

prepares a Consensus Report summarizing the written documentation review and the site visit findings.

The award decision involves review of the Consensus Report by the Commission on Magnet Recognition of the ANCC. Magnet awards are made when the Commission on Magnet Recognition members agree that the evidence reflects magnet-defined excellence in an organization's nursing services (ANCC, 2004). After magnet designation is conferred, facilities must maintain compliance with the magnet standards to sustain the magnet workplace culture and to position the organization for magnet redesignation. Magnet hospitals submit annual reports for interim reporting and repeat the original application, evaluation, and site visit activities every four years for the redesignation process.

PROFESSIONAL NURSING PRACTICE

The quality of a professional nursing practice environment is crucial in attracting and retaining professional nurses. Nurse leaders play a key role in creating practice environments that are supportive of and conducive to professional nursing practice. Magnet hospitals represent one example of supportive and collegial work environments that are both high performance and high quality-of-work-life organizations for nurses and other health care professionals. These desired work environments do not happen overnight. They require significant investment of time, energy, and resources by individuals, groups, and organizations. Although the investment required to create magnet workplaces is significant, the rewards to individuals, groups, and organizations are even greater. Ultimately, the investment in building supportive and collegial work environments results in organizational effectiveness, a key desired outcome of organizational behavior.

CASE STUDY 3-1

A new nurse, Latisha, has just joined the staff of a busy cardiovascular unit. The nurse manager has assigned a clinical nurse specialist and a senior staff nurse mentor to assist with Latisha's orientation and integration into the unit. As part of this orientation, Latisha has been asked to develop a personal career plan that addresses measurable goals at three months, six months, one year, and three years. The nurse manager also gives Latisha a list of the unit-based and hospital-based committees and asks her to think about which committees she would like to join. Latisha should pick committees that maximize her gifts and talents to best contribute to her personal goals and to the hospital's goals. Involvement in committees and in quality improvement activities is very important. The organization is so committed to these activities that it not only regularly provides release time for employees to participate in these very important activities but also funds attendance at outside educational programs to build the nursing knowledge base in these areas.

What model of organizational behavior does this case study depict?

What is your preliminary assessment regarding the 14 Forces of Magnetism and their presence in this unit and organization?

How can Latisha, a new staff nurse joining the staff on this unit, further contribute toward building and sustaining the workplace culture?

KEY CONCEPTS

- Organizational behavior is the study of human behavior in organizations. Common organizational behavior models include autocratic, custodial, supportive, and collegial models.

- Creating desirable work environments is key to positively influencing employee attitudes, behaviors, and organizational performance. Failure to understand individual and group dynamics within organizations makes it difficult to create and sustain desirable work environments for professional practice.

- As organizations strive for sustainable high performance, they must consider material resources, such as technology, capital, quality improvement, and other information, yet they cannot lose sight of the human element, such as the people and teams who do the required work.

- Maintaining a satisfied and committed workforce requires a planned and dedicated effort by all members of the organization to create and sustain desirable work environments for practice.

- Health care professionals in a knowledge economy possess valuable knowledge, skills, and abilities that individuals and organizations need to cultivate to retain employees, generate quality outcomes, and gain competitive advantage.

- High performance organizations that bring out the best in people generally focus on creating high quality-of-work-life environments. Nurses practicing in such organizations benefit from these organizational cultures and enjoy high levels of job satisfaction.

- Magnet hospitals are known to have supportive and collegial work environments for nurses and may be classified as both high-performance and high quality-of-work-life environments. Nine characteristics define magnet nursing services.

- A strong body of evidence exists to support the achievement of quality outcomes for nurses, patients, and organizations by magnet hospitals.

- There are five major benefits of magnet designation.

- The magnet process and magnet designation both create organizational value and meaning for individuals and groups within those organizations. Magnet designation should be seen as not merely a destination but rather an ongoing commitment to excellence in nursing services.

- In the face of a highly competitive health care industry, health care leaders have a compelling obligation to create supportive and collegial work environments that are conducive to keeping patients safe and nurses retained within the profession.

- The eight Essentials of Magnetism help a health care organization move toward achieving the 14 Forces of Magnetism.

KEY TERMS

absenteeism
external forces
gap
gap analysis
Hawthorne effect
high quality-of-work-life
  environments
high-performance
  organizations
intellectual capital
job satisfaction

knowledge workers
magnet hospitals
nursing-sensitive indicators
open systems
organization
organizational behavior
organizational commitment
organizational effectiveness
productivity
stakeholders
turnover

REVIEW QUESTIONS

1. As a new nurse attending the hospital's employee orientation program, you are told the hospital recognizes its employees as its most valuable asset. Which of the following does not demonstrate congruence between this statement and what you observe in the workplace?
   A. Employees are treated with respect and fairness.
   B. The hospital supports employee attendance at continuing education programs.
   C. Employee suggestions are encouraged but are rarely acted upon.
   D. Employee job satisfaction is evaluated on a yearly basis.

2. Magnet hospitals foster the philosophy that nurse leaders are needed at all levels of the organization. As a staff nurse and clinical leader on your unit, which of the following activities would not be viewed as supportive of the hospital's philosophy in a magnet facility?
   A. Staff nurse serving as the chairperson of the nursing practice council
   B. Medical practitioner serving in the role of chairperson of the nursing practice council
   C. Staff nurses conducting breast cancer self-exam classes in the community
   D. Medical practitioners collaborating with nursing personnel on an interdisciplinary task force

3. A body of evidence spanning two decades of research exists to support the value of magnet hospitals. Which of the following statements offers the strongest support for the pursuit of magnet hospital designation?
   A. In a longitudinal, multisite study of more than 2,000 U.S. hospitals, researchers reported that 1-year and 3-years following implementation of a magnet workplace culture, employee turnover dropped by 50%.
   B. The nurses at Community Hospital stated that they liked working there because it was a magnet-designated hospital.

   C. The nurses at Harper Hospital state they should become a magnet hospital because others in the area also are becoming magnet designated.
   D. *People* magazine, one of the most popular and well read magazines in one community, recently had an article supporting the benefits of magnet hospitals.

4. A nurse evaluating an organization's potential for long-term success knows that high performance environments offer a competitive advantage. Which of the following examples does not exemplify a high-performance organization?
   A. The organization partners with a technology center that readily integrates new and emerging technologies into clinical practice.
   B. The organization demonstrates a commitment to continuous quality improvement.
   C. The organization controls information available to employees and follows the company policy that what employees don't know will not hurt them.
   D. The organization developed a succession strategy that identifies and plans for the education of future leaders within the organization.

5. As a nurse, you are increasingly reading about magnet hospitals and noticing that these hospitals are also known as high-performance organizations. Which of the following most accurately characterizes why magnet hospitals may be classified as high-performance organizations?
   A. High-performance organizations and magnet hospitals possess no similarities, and therefore this association in terminology is not well founded.
   B. High-performance organizations, like magnet hospitals, recognize the importance of attracting and retaining talented employees.
   C. High-performance organizations, like magnet hospitals, are known for high employee turnover.
   D. High-performance organizations, like magnet hospitals, focus on maintaining the status quo and benefit from the fact that they do not experience change or turmoil.

6. A nurse was visiting with a relative who is not a nurse. The relative had been reading about the benefits of magnet hospitals in a recent issue of *Reader's Digest*. She wanted to know more about these benefits. In responding to the relative's question, which of the following outcomes listed on a magnet hospital's Website would the nurse not use to illustrate the benefits of magnet hospitals?
   A. Patient satisfaction scores in the 99th percentile
   B. Nurse turnover rate of 2%
   C. Employee waiting lists for new hires in 50% of the hospital's departments
   D. Nurse-to-patient ratio of 1 nurse to 20 patients

7. Part of the role of the staff nurse champion for a hospital's magnet journey is to prepare and present an in-service on the historical evolution of the Magnet Recognition Program. As part of this program's discussion, which primary goal should be presented to describe the primary reason for creation of the Magnet Recognition Program?
   A. To start the re-engineering efforts in the health care industry
   B. To promote excellence in the delivery of nursing services to patients
   C. To increase the incidence of medication error reporting
   D. To promote staff and physician satisfaction

8. Demonstrating that all the Forces of Magnetism exist in an organization is crucial to meeting the magnet requirements. As a staff nurse working on a magnet committee, you have been asked to help evaluate the magnet evidence to be submitted with the hospital's magnet application. Which of the following pieces of evidence is not evidence to support professional development, the fourteenth Force of Magnetism?
   A. Documentation of annual certification preparation courses offered in all the nursing specialty areas within the hospital
   B. Access to Web-based educational programs for nurses working at the unit level or nurses working from their own homes
   C. A 12-month financial report that details on a unit-by-unit basis the economic support provided to all staff nurses on that unit attending educational programs outside the health care organization
   D. A statement describing how decision making is done by the medical staff

9. As a new nurse seeking a supportive and collegial work environment, which of the following workplace cultures would be most consistent with your aspirations?
   A. The unit manager is known to hold staff meetings only when they are needed to address hospital economic concerns.
   B. The unit scheduling system is not flexible, and staff nurses work when they are told to work.
   C. The unit has a staff retention committee that hosts a quarterly luncheon and an employee-of-the quarter recognition event.
   D. The nature of the nurse and practitioner relationship is paternalistic, and nurses seek practitioner orders for matters pertaining to independent nursing practice.

10. A staff nurse just finished taking a course entitled, "Becoming a Charge Nurse." Organizational behavior was part of the course content. Which of the following statements most readily explains the reason why such a course would be beneficial?
    A. The course may be beneficial to those interested in a true managerial role, but the course is not really beneficial for staff nurses.
    B. The course helps employees better understand themselves and others as a basis for good contributions toward achieving top organizational performance.
    C. The course is not based on sound theoretical evidence, therefore, its value is questionable for nurses.
    D. The course is helpful in assisting nurses to practice in static, noncomplex work environments.

REVIEW ACTIVITIES

1. To learn more about the magnet eligibility criteria, access and review the document entitled "Is Your Hospital Ready for the Magnet Status Recognition Challenge?" (ANCC, 2006b). To access the document, go to www.healthevolutions.com. Click on Resources, Articles. Enter the key word, Magnet. Click on ANCC Magnet Recognition Program. Download the ANCC Magnet Recognition Program. Complete the document entitled "Is Your Hospital Ready for the Magnet Status Recognition Challenge?" After you have found the document, use this eight-page article to familiarize yourself with the requirements that must be in place to achieve magnet designation. Reflect on the extent to which you see your current health care work environment meeting the specified requirements.

2. To identify your organization's behavioral model, access and review the document entitled "Organizational Behavior Survey" (Clark, 2002). To access the document, go to www.nwlink.com/~donclark/. Click on Content. Type *organizational behavior survey* in the Google Search section of the Table of Contents. Click on Leadership—Organizational Behavior. After you have found the Organizational Behavior Survey, identify the congruence between what the survey score says about your organization (autocratic, custodial, supportive, or collegial) and your own preferred model of organizational behavior. Reflect on your work environment selection and consider some of the strategies you will pursue to better align your organizational model with your preferred model of organizational behavior.

EXPLORING THE WEB

Search the Web, checking the following sites:

- Agency for Health Care Research and Quality: *www.ahrq.gov* Explore the various elements of the Website.

- Big Dog's Leadership Page—Organizational Behavior: *www.nwlink.com* Click on the following sites and review what you find there: Performance, Learning, Leadership, and Knowledge. Review some of the other sites you find there.

■ Institute of Medicine: *www.iom.edu*
Explore the various elements of the Website.

■ ANCC list of magnet facilities that is updated regularly can be found at *www.nursingworld.org*
Click on ANCC, and then click on Magnet Recognition. View the list of all the designated magnet facilities.

■ National Student Nurses' Association (NSNA) Career Center: *www.nsna.org*

REFERENCES

Agency for Health Care Research and Quality. (2006). *AHRQ patient safety network: Glossary.* Retrieved May 6, 2006, from http://psnet.ahrq.gov/glossary.aspx

Aiken, L. H. (2002). Superior outcomes for magnet hospitals: The evidence base. In M. L. McClure & A. S. Hinshaw (Eds.), *Magnet hospitals revisited: Attraction and retention of professional nurses* (pp. 61–81). Washington, DC: American Nurses Publishing.

Aiken, L. H., Clarke, S. P., Cheung, R. B., Sloane, D. M., & Silber, J. H. (2003). Educational levels of hospital nurses and surgical patient mortality. *Journal of the American Medical Association, 290*(12), 1617–1623.

Aiken, L. H., Sloane, D. M., & Klocinski, J. L. (1997). Hospital nurses' occupational exposure to blood: Prospective, retrospective, and institutional reports. *American Journal of Public Health, 87,* 103–107.

Aiken, L. H., Sloane, D. M., & Lake, E. T. (1997). Satisfaction with inpatient acquired immunodeficiency syndrome care: A national comparison of dedicated and scattered-bed units. *Medical Care, 36*(9), 948–962.

Aiken, L. H., Sloane, D. M., Lake, E. T., Sochalski, J., & Weber, A. L. (1999). Organization and outcomes of inpatient AIDS care. *Medical Care, 37*(8), 760–772.

Aiken, L. H., Smith, H., & Lake, E. (1994). Lower medicare mortality among a set of hospitals known for good nursing care. *Medical Care, 32*(8), 771–785.

American Hospital Association. (2006). *Statistics and studies: Fast facts on U.S. hospitals.* Retrieved May 6, 2006, from http://www.aha.org/aha/resource-center

American Nurses Association. (2004). *Scope and standards for nurse administrators.* Washington, DC: American Nurses Publishing.

American Nurses Credentialing Center. (2004). *Magnet recognition program: Application manual 2005.* Washington, DC: American Nurses Credentialing Center.

American Nurses Credentialing Center. (2006a). *Benefits of becoming a magnet-designated facility.* Retrieved May 6, 2006, from http://nursingworld.org/ancc/magnet/benes.html

American Nurses Credentialing Center. (2006b). *Is your hospital ready for the magnet status recognition challenge?* Retrieved May 6, 2006 from http://www.healthevolutions.com/resources/articles.aspx

American Nurses Credentialing Center. (2007). *Staff nurse self-assessment to determine readiness to pursue magnet recognition.* Retrieved May 15, 2006, from http://www.nursingworld.org/ancc/magnet/forms/selfassess.pdf

Bliss-Holtz, J., Winter, N., & Scherer, E. M. (2004). An invitation to magnet accreditation. *Nursing Management, 35*(9), 36–43.

Brady-Schwartz, D. C. (2005). Further evidence on the Magnet Recognition Program: Implications for nursing leaders. *Journal of Nursing Administration, 35*(9), 397–403.

Bumgarner, S. D., & Beard, E. L. (2003). The magnet application. *Journal of Nursing Administration, 33*(11), 603–606.

Clark, D. (2000). *Big dog's leadership page: Organizational behavior.* Retrieved May 6, 2006, from http://www.nwlink.com/~donclark/leader/leadob.html

Clark, D. (2002). *Organizational behavior survey.* Retrieved May 15, 2006, from http://nwlink.com/~donclark/leader/obsurvey.html

Clarke, S. P., & Aiken, L. H. (2006). More nursing, fewer deaths. *Quality & Safety in Health Care, 15*(1), 2–3.

Clarke, S. P., Rockett, J. L., Sloane, D. M., & Aiken, L. H. (2002). Organizational climate, staffing and safety equipment as predictors of needlestick injuries and near-misses in hospital nurses. *American Journal of Infection Control, 30*(4), 207–216.

Coile, R. C. (2001). Magnet hospitals use culture, not wages, to solve nursing shortage. *Journal of Health Care Management, 46*(4), 224–227.

Daft, R. L. (2006). *Organization theory and design* (9th ed.). Mason, OH: South-Western College Publishing.

Drenkard, K. N. (2005). Sustaining Magnet: Keeping the forces alive. *Nursing Administration Quarterly, 29*(3), 214–222.

Drucker, P. F. (2006). *Classic Drucker: Wisdom from Peter Drucker from the pages of Harvard Business Review.* Boston: Harvard Business School Press.

Ellis, B., & Gates, J. (2005). Achieving Magnet status. *Nursing Administration Quarterly, 29*(3), 241–244.

Goode, C. J., Krugman, M. E., Smith, K., Diaz, J., Edmonds, S., & Mulder, J. (2005). The pull of magnetism: A look at the standards and the experience of a western academic medical center hospital in achieving and sustaining magnet status. *Nursing Administration Quarterly, 29*(3), 202–213.

Havens, D. S., & Aiken, L. H. (1999). Shaping systems to promote desired outcomes: The magnet hospital model. *Journal of Nursing Administration, 29*(2), 14–20.

Havens, D. S., & Johnston, M. A. (2004). Achieving magnet hospital recognition: Chief nurse executives and magnet coordinators tell their stories. *Journal of Nursing Administration, 34*(12), 579–588.

Institute of Medicine. (2004). Keeping patients safe: Transforming the work environment of nurses. Washington, DC: The National Academies Press.

Kramer, M. (1990). The magnet hospitals: Excellence revisited. *Journal of Nursing Administration, 20*(9), 35–44.

Kramer, M., & Schmalenberg, C. (1991). Job satisfaction and retention insights for the 90's. *Nursing '91,* 50–55.

Kramer, M., & Schmalenberg, C. (2002). Staff nurses identify essentials of magnetism. In M. L. McClure, & A. S. Hinshaw (Eds.), *Magnet hospitals revisited: Attraction and retention of professional nurses* (pp. 25–59). Washington, DC: American Nurses Publishing.

Kramer, M., & Schmalenberg, C. (2004). Magnet hospitals: What makes nurses stay? *Nursing 2004, 34*(6), 50–54.

Lake, E. T., & Friese, C. R. (2006). Variations in nursing practice environments: Relation to staffing and hospital characteristics. *Nursing Research, 55*(1), 1–9.

Laschinger, H. K. S., & Finegan, J. (2005). Empowering nurses for work engagement and health in hospital settings. *Journal of Nursing Administration, 35*(10), 438–449.

Laschinger, H. K. S., Almost, J., & Tuer-Hodes, D. (2003). Workplace empowerment and magnet hospital characteristics. *Journal of Nursing Administration, 33*(7/8), 410–422.

Lynn, M. R., & Redman, R. W. (2005). Faces of the nursing shortage: Influences on staff nurses' intentions to leave their positions or nursing. *Journal of Nursing Administration, 35*(5), 264–270.

McClure, M. L., & Hinshaw, A. S. (2002). *Magnet hospitals revisited: Attraction and retention of professional nurses.* Washington, DC: American Nurses Publishing.

McClure, M., Poulin, M., Sovie, M., & Wandelt, M. (1983). *Magnet hospitals: Attraction and retention of professional nurses.* American Academy of Nursing Task Force on Nursing Practice in Hospitals. Kansas City, MO: American Academy of Nursing.

Messmer, P. R., Jones, S. G., & Rosillo, C. (2002). Using nursing research projects to meet magnet recognition program standards. *Journal of Nursing Administration, 32*(10), 538–543.

NDNQI. (2006). *National Database for Nursing Quality Indicators.* Retrieved May 6, 2006, from http://www.nursingquality.org

NSNA. National Student Nurses' Association Career Center. Retrieved February 15, 2007, from http://www.nsna.org

Poduska, D. D. (2005). Magnet designation in a community hospital. *Nursing Administration Quarterly, 29*(3), 223–227.

Robbins, S. P. (2005). Essentials of organizational behavior (8th ed.). Upper Saddle River, NJ: Pearson Prentice Hall.

Schermerhorn, J. R., Hunt, J. G., & Osborn, R. N. (2005). Organizational behavior (9th ed.). Hoboken, NJ: John Wiley & Sons.

Scott, J. G., Sochalski, J., & Aiken, L. H. (1999). Review of magnet hospital research: Findings and implications for professional nursing practice. *Journal of Nursing Administration, 29*(11), 1, 9–19.

Senge, P. (1990). *The fifth discipline: The art and practice of the learning organization.* New York: Doubleday.

Shirey, M. R. (2004). Preparing an organization for achieving magnet designation. (2004 Fellow project available from The American College of Health Care Executives, 1 N. Franklin Street, Suite 1700, Chicago, IL 60606).

Shirey, M. R. (2005). Celebrating certification in nursing: Forces of magnetism in action. *Nursing Administration Quarterly, 29*(3), 245–253.

Steinbinder, A., & Scherer, E. M. (2006). Creating nursing system excellence through the forces of magnetism. In K. Malloch & T. Porter O'Grady (Eds.), *Introduction to evidence-based practice in nursing and health care* (pp. 235–266). Boston: Jones & Bartlett Publishers.

Turkel, M. C., Reidinger, G., Ferket, K., & Reno, K. (2005). An essential component of the Magnet journey: Fostering an environment for evidence-based practice and nursing research. *Nursing Administration Quarterly, 29*(3), 254–262.

Upenieks, V. V. (2003). What constitutes effective leadership? Perceptions of magnet and nonmagnet nurse leaders. *Journal of Nursing Administration, 33*(9), 456–467.

Urden, L. D., & Monarch, K. (2002). The ANCC Magnet recognition program: Converting research into action. In M. L. McClure & A. S. Hinshaw (Eds.), *Magnet hospitals revisited: Attraction and retention of professional nurses* (pp. 103–115). Washington, DC: American Nurses Publishing.

U.S. News & World Report. (2005). *America's best hospitals: 2005 methodology.* Retrieved May 9, 2006, from http://www.usnews.com

Wikipedia. (2006). *Organizational studies.* Retrieved May 6, 2006, from http://en.wikipedia.org/wiki/Organizational_behavior

SUGGESTED READINGS

Aiken, L. H., Clarke, S., Sloane, D., Sochalski, J., & Silber, J. (2002). Hospital nurse staffing and patient mortality, nurse burnout, and job dissatisfaction. *Journal of the American Medical Association, 288*(16), 1987–1993.

Aiken, L. H., Havens, D. S., & Sloane, M. (2000). The magnet nursing services recognition program: A comparison of two groups of magnet hospitals. *American Journal of Nursing, 100*(3), 26–35.

American Nurses Credentialing Center. (2004). *Magnet: Best practices in today's challenging health care environment.* Washington, DC: American Nurses Credentialing Center.

Brooks, B. A., & Anderson, M. A. (2005). Defining quality of nursing work life. *Nursing Economics, 23*(6), 319–326, 279.

Havens, D. S. (2001). Comparison of nursing department infrastructure and outcomes: ANCC magnet and nonmagnet chief nurse executives report. *Nursing Economics, 19*(6), 258–266.

Laschinger, H. K. S., Shamian, J., & Thomason, D. (2001). Impact of magnet hospital characteristics on nurse's perception of trust, burnout, quality of care and work satisfaction. *Nursing Economics, 19*(5), 12, 51–52.

Laschinger, H. K. S., & Finegan, J. (2005). Using empowerment to build trust and respect in the workplace: A strategy for addressing the nursing shortage. *Nursing Economics, 23*(1), 6–13.

Maslow, A. (1970). Motivation and personality (2nd ed.). New York: Harper & Row.

McGregor, D. (1960). The human side of enterprise. New York: McGraw Hill.

McNeese-Smith, D. (1996). Increasing employee productivity, job satisfaction, and organizational commitment. *Hospital & Health Services Administration, 41*(2), 160–175.

Morey, D., Maybury, M., & Thuraisingham, B. (Eds.). (2002). Knowledge management: Classic and contemporary works. Cambridge, MA: The MIT Press.

Ouchi, W. (1981). *Theory Z: How American business can meet the Japanese challenge.* Reading, MA: Addison-Wesley.

SearchSMB.com. (2006). *SMB definitions: Gap analysis.* Retrieved May 11, 2006, from http://searchsmb.techtarget.com/sDefinition/0,290660,sid44_gci831294,00.html

Smith, H. L., Hood, J. N., Waldman, J. D., & Smith, V. L. (2005). Creating a favorable practice environment for nurses. *Journal of Nursing Administration, 35*(12), 525–532.

Stolzenberger, K. M. (2003). Beyond the magnet award: The ANCC Magnet program as the framework for culture change. *Journal of Nursing Administration, 33*(10), 522–531.

Taylor, F. (1911). *Principles of scientific management.* New York: Harper & Row.

Triolo, P. K., Scherer, E. M., & Floyd, J. M. (2006). Evaluation of the Magnet Recognition Program. *Journal of Nursing Administration, 36*(1), 42–48.

Upenieks, V. V. (2003). The interrelationship of organizational characteristics of magnet hospitals, nursing leadership, and nursing job satisfaction. *Health Care Manager, 22*(2), 83–98.

Urden, L. D. (2006). Transforming professional practice environments: The Magnet Recognition Program. In P. S. Yoder-Wise & K. E. Kowalski (Eds.), *Beyond leading and managing: Nursing administration for the future* (pp. 23–34). St. Louis, MO: Mosby Elsevier.

CHAPTER 4

Basic Clinical Health Care Economics

Laura J. Nosek, PhD, RN ✛ Ida M. Androwich, PhD, RN, BC, FAAN

The purpose of creating and analyzing records of what transpires in hospitals is to know how the money is being spent; whether it is, in fact, doing good, or whether it is doing mischief (Florence Nightingale, 1859).

OBJECTIVES

Upon completion of this chapter, the reader should be able to:

1. Analyze why health care must be managed as a business.
2. Apply the cost equation to the mission statement of a health care enterprise to discover why the enterprise may be thriving or struggling.
3. Analyze the impact of at least three contemporary economic or social pressures driving health care enterprises.
4. Apply the break-even formula to compute a break-even point for a piece of equipment your health care organization is planning to purchase.
5. Discover how a health care enterprise is balancing quality and profit by assigning its satisfaction rating and margin to an appropriate square on the Nosek-Androwich Profit: Quality (NAPQ) Matrix.

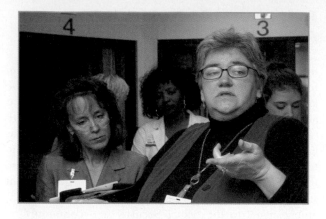

You and your spouse are vacationing in a foreign country. You rent small hand-held aqua scooters that pull you through the saltwater lagoon and you gleefully romp in the quiet water. As you make a turn near the island of dead coral in the center of the lagoon, you lose your balance and are dragged along the sharp coral, lacerating both thighs. A lifeguard hears your screams and dashes to your aid. Hotel personnel put you in a taxi, and send you to a nearby hospital emergency room. There, with your limited local language and the help of one person who speaks limited English, you discover that all health care is socialized and provided free to all citizens. You are told that you cannot be treated because there is no provision for accepting your American insurance and no provision for paying cash.

What do you think the hospital perceives the problem to be?

Do you perceive the problem to be the same as the hospital does?

When cost is removed from the equation, what drives the decision to provide or not provide health care?

Is that driver a universal need, or is it culturally dependent?

If cost were not a driving consideration in providing health care in the United States, what would the health care system be like?

Regardless of how expert, creative, collaborative, and altruistic a health care system may be, it cannot function without money. Over the ages, that money has flowed from varying sources, including philanthropy, volunteerism, fees for services, insurance, and government subsidies. Securing the bottom line is basic to achieving the mission of providing health care and is now viewed as the shared responsibility of humans around the world.

It was once thought that nurses need only be educated in the art and the science of providing clinical care to patients. Today, nurses must be much more broadly educated. In addition to clinical care expertise, they must demonstrate beginning competence in the humanities, management science, and computer science, as well as be skilled in evaluating and applying new knowledge suggested by scientific research.

The United States spends more per capita on health care than any other country in the world, yet morbidity and mortality statistics, in terms of improved health outcomes, lead us to question the value that we receive for our dollars. Nightingale's early search for the "good" versus "mischievous" outcomes of the money spent on health care may have initiated an unspoken commitment to financial stewardship among nurses. All nurses are required to participate knowledgeably in designing care systems that provide the best possible care at the lowest cost. Consequently, every nurse today needs to have a basic understanding of clinical health care **economics**—the study of how scarce resources are allocated among possible uses—in order to make appropriate choices among the increasingly scarce resources of the future.

The study of economics is based on three general premises: (1) scarcity—resources exist in finite quantities, and consumption demand is typically greater than resource supply; (2) choice—decisions are made about which resources to produce and consume among many options; and (3) preference—individual and societal values and preferences influence the decisions that are made. In a traditional market economy, the sellers sell to the buyers who buy, with each trying to maximize their gains from the transactions. Health care does not fit well in this model. For example, consider the concept of price elasticity, which is related to the price that an individual is willing to pay for a given item. Normally, as the price goes up, the demand goes down. When the purchase is health care, however, the price may be viewed as irrelevant to the decision to purchase. Think of a wristwatch that you might always purchase for $5, would likely not buy at $50, and would never consider at $500. Now, imagine that instead of a wristwatch, the item in question is a medication or therapy needed to save your sick child. Now the consideration of price in the decision-making process is likely quite different. Thus, health care is much less "elastic" with reference to price than many other consumer goods.

Another aspect of health care's difference from the traditional economic model relates to the knowledge of options and payment mechanisms available to the consumer. In a typical market, the buyer is also the payer. In health care, the health care provider (buyer) ordering a hospitalization or treatment is a doctor or nurse. The provider is not the payer, nor is the patient (buyer) using the hospital or treatment the payer. The actual **payer** is the third-party reimburser (insurance company or government). Consequently, the financial impact of the decision on the provider (buyer) and the patient user (buyer) is skewed. Neither of these buyers is the payer.

This chapter presents basic clinical health care economics concepts that are important to the novice nurse entering clinical practice. Included are perspectives on the role cost has played and will play in directing health care delivery, the methods for determining the cost of delivering nursing care, and the effect of health care policy on the delivery of nursing care. Recognized nurse experts provide comments on the future impact of economics on clinical nursing.

TRADITIONAL PERSPECTIVE ON THE COST OF HEALTH CARE: HEALTH CARE AS ALTRUISM

The long-standing tradition of health care is to help people achieve their optimal level of health so that they can enjoy their maximum quality of life. **Altruism**, the unselfish concern for the welfare of others, and **ethics**, the doctrine that the general welfare of society is the proper goal of an individual's actions as opposed to **egoism**, the tendency to be self-centered or to consider only oneself and one's own interests (Agnes, 2000), drove the way health care was viewed and provided. Several early nursing leaders, including Florence Nightingale and Isabel Adams Hampton Robb, were members of socially prominent families instilled with the value that altruistic service was the expected role of the privileged. Such feelings of dedication to the less fortunate stemmed from medieval infirmaries established by convents and monasteries to care for the aged, orphaned, poor, and disabled. The first hospitals to care for the sick and injured were also charitable institutions established around the 14th century to provide illness care to those who did not have a home or who could not afford home care. The people cared for in hospitals were called patients from the Latin *patiens*, meaning, to suffer.

NEED FOR HEALTH CARE DETERMINED BY PROVIDER

Prior to the 1980s, mainstream health care was delivered from a paternalistic model of governance and control. Health professionals, led by practitioners controlled a vast body of scientific knowledge and skill rendered awesome and mystical by complex scientific language. Command of that scientific knowledge and skill required extensive and expensive education and was not shared with "outsiders." The practitioner determined what health care was needed independent of the patient and even independent of professional colleagues. The practitioner also decided how much to charge for that care. Decision making about all aspects of health care was the exclusive domain of the professionals.

RIGHT TO HEALTH CARE AT ANY COST

The cost of health care was not considered, let alone questioned, until the early 1960s. The American belief system firmly held that every individual was entitled to all the knowledge, skill, and technology related to health care at any cost. It was claimed to be a "right"; it was the "American way." The spiraling cost of providing health care was noted, but it was antithetical to the American value system to consider rationing health care. In an attempt to ease the burden of health care costs, the U.S. government stepped up in 1965 and enacted Titles XVIII and XIX, amendments to the Social Security Act, commonly referred to as the Medicare and Medicaid programs, which provide health care coverage for the elderly and the indigent, respectively. These programs require documentation of the kind and amount of services provided. It was anticipated that by requiring health care providers to account for the cost of Medicare and Medicaid patients' care, spending would be curbed. Other insurers soon followed with their own requirements, launching the overall budgeting of health care.

COST PLUS

Despite the initiation of budgets in the late 1960s, the cost of health care continued to spiral upward as hospitals became the preferred site for provision of intermediate care and the high technology necessary for state-of-the-art illness care. That cost was determined by the actual cost the provider incurred for the care plus a profit incentive for being in the business. The method was known as "cost plus," and clearly the incentive was "the more you spend, the more you get," not "how can this be accomplished more economically?"

CONTEMPORARY PERSPECTIVE ON COST OF HEALTH CARE: HEALTH CARE AS A BUSINESS

Possibly the most common reason given for entering a health care profession is "to help people." Virginia Henderson, viewed by some as the contemporary Florence Nightingale, defined nursing as

> . . . *primarily helping people (sick or well) in the performance of those activities contributing to health, or its recovery (or to peaceful death) that they would perform unaided if they had the necessary strength, will, or knowledge. It is*

likewise the unique contribution of nursing to help people to be independent of such assistance as soon as possible (Henderson & Nite, 1978).

Nurses fervently believe and state that this definition applies irrespective of the site where nursing care is given. Yet, nurses also have begun to recognize that the cost of providing care in the traditional altruistic way was prohibitive and that achieving independence from nursing care as quickly as possible conserves scarce nursing resources.

Taxes to cover the ever-increasing costs of the government health care programs were climbing. In the late 1970s medicare insolvency was a threat. Again, the government, the major payer, stepped in. The Health Care Financing Administration (HCFA), the department responsible for the Medicare and Medicaid programs, was authorized to change the way it paid for health care. The Tax Equity and Fiscal Responsibility Act (TEFRA) of 1982 established new payment regulations. Instead of reimbursing the provider's cost, the government would henceforth pay a flat rate stated up front. The new system would therefore be called the prospective payment system.

The new payment system considerably changed institutions' incentives for spending. If the provider was able to provide the care for less than the prospective payment, the provider could make a profit. If the provider spent more than that payment, the provider lost money. Because length of hospital stay is a surrogate measure of hospital cost, reducing length of stay was seen as the easiest and most logical way to reduce the cost of care enough to ensure adequacy of the payment.

One of the first hospital lengths of stay to be shortened was that for obstetrical patients. It was an unforgettable October morning in 1983 when the headlines of the *Cleveland Plain Dealer* shocked the city with the news. Effective immediately, hospital care for those experiencing normal vaginal delivery would be three calendar days starting with the day of admission, the story read. At that time in that city, the usual stay for a normal vaginal delivery was five days; for a Cesarean delivery, it was seven days. If a woman were admitted shortly before midnight, that constituted day one. If she experienced a long labor, she could end up being discharged on her first postpartum day. Patients were crying in the halls. Nurses were outraged, trying to figure out how they could possibly teach breastfeeding when breast milk does not come in until postpartum day three. Practitioners were threatening a variety of actions, citing unsafe care.

Out with altruism. In with health care that clinicians had to recognize was truly a business. In with a whole new language, that of business and consumers and profit and margin and competition and cost, *cost*, COST. The bottom line (cost) became the focus, not only of managers and administrators but of all employees at all levels of all health care entities. Everyone needed to question what they did, how they did it, and how many it took to do it in order to determine whether it was required for safe care and quality outcomes and whether there was a less costly way of attaining a safe, quality outcome. In 1960, Abdellah had challenged health care providers to determine the care that was needed and to provide no more, no less (Abdellah, Beland, Martin, & Matheney, 1960). Nearly 50 years later, health care providers are still trying to come to grips with just that.

NEED FOR HEALTH CARE DETERMINED BY THE CONSUMER

Attention has shifted toward safety and quality and the need for measurable outcomes. Total quality improvement (TQI) and continuous quality improvement (CQI) programs were initiated to assure society that cost management was not compromising safety or quality. These programs required all stakeholders, including patients, to work together to evaluate and improve outcomes. The expertise of allied health care providers was recognized, and through the growing access to information technology, consumers were empowered to better understand their own health, the complex technologies available, their options for choosing to manage the decisions about their care, and the cost implications of those decisions. No longer was health care the exclusive realm of the practitioner and other professionals.

Serb (2006) points out that more than a decade ago, Harvard Business School Professor Regina Herzlinger predicted a revolution in health care toward a consumer-based model, with greater choice, i.e., focused factories of provider teams, flexible insurance products, and widely available information on quality and cost. Many dismissed her ideas, and Herzlinger herself delayed publication of her award-winning book, *Market-Driven Health Care*, until after the heyday of HMOs—whose gatekeepers, top-down managements, and tight networks seemed the antithesis of consumerism. Since Herzlinger's predictions, access to reliable, extensive health care information, as well as cost and quality data, have become ever more available on the Internet. In addition, the 2003 Medicare Modernization Act established Health Savings Accounts (HSAs), insurance policies that offer consumers a choice of tax-advantaged low premiums in exchange for higher deductibles and co-pays. It was hoped that the Act could potentially curb indiscriminate use of health care services by encouraging consumers to shop for cost-effective quality health care.

RIGHT TO HEALTH CARE AT A REASONABLE COST

The contemporary value system holds that individuals have the right to health care at a reasonable cost. Reasonable cost is currently determined by insurers. When it refers to fees charged for services, a *reasonable cost* is the usual and customary fee charged in the region. When referring to technology; complex and expensive procedures; or expensive, extensive pharmacologic therapies, there is no established standard for how much it should cost to provide someone enhanced quality of life over time. Clearly, the lack of consensus on what constitutes reasonable cost is at the heart of the controversies among insurers, patients, and their professional providers.

MANAGED CARE

The effort to control cost through the Medicare and Medicaid programs marked the beginning of health care reform. There was keen anticipation that if the care of the neediest—the elderly and the poor—was managed centrally, access, cost, and quality would be optimally controlled. When it became evident that the program costs had been woefully underestimated, health maintenance organizations (HMOs), or managed care, emerged as the answer to cost-efficient and quality care.

Managed care is not easily defined and categorized. It is the product of a series of efforts to establish an effective program for all **stakeholders** (providers, employers, customers, patients, and payers who may have an interest in, and seek to influence, the decisions and actions of an organization) and it has resulted in a complex, still-evolving array of structures and processes to deliver health care.

Managed care integrates the financial and the clinical care delivery functions of health care into a single organized system by contracting to be responsible for the clinical outcomes of an enrolled population for a capitated (fixed) fee. Managed care emphasizes delivery of a coordinated continuum of services across the care spectrum from wellness to death using financial incentives to achieve cost-efficiency. Managed care grew rapidly in the 1980s and 1990s and by 1993, the average annual growth in health care cost stabilized from year to year. Figure 4-1 shows the growth rate from the immediately preceding year, for example, the growth from 1992 to 1993 was 11.5%; the growth rate from 1997 to 1998 was way down in comparison, only 5.3%; by 2002, the growth rate from 2001 was back up to 7.9%. The growth rate has steadily declined a little each year since 2002 and it is projected to remain fairly stable through 2014.

It is important to note that managed care is the only health services delivery model generated from a market response rather than a formal federal government

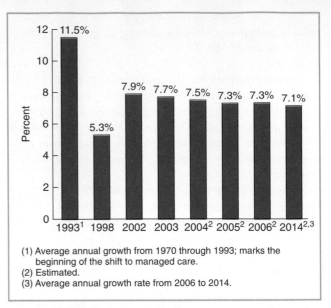

(1) Average annual growth from 1970 through 1993; marks the beginning of the shift to managed care.
(2) Estimated.
(3) Average annual growth rate from 2006 to 2014.

Figure 4-1 National health care expenditures, average annual percent growth from prior year, 1993–2014. (Centers for Medicare and Medicaid Services, Office of the Actuary: U.S. Department of Commerce, Bureau of Economic Analysis and Bureau of the Census. Retrieved March 31, 2006 from http://www.iii.org.)

legislative initiative (Liberman & Rotarius, 2001). The first recorded managed care program in the United States was established for maritime workers in 1798. The mission and vision of managed care was to provide wellness care at a minimal cost to keep people healthy and thus avoid providing illness care at a higher, even astronomical, cost. A secondary mission was to standardize diagnostic and treatment decisions across the nation.

Often, preapproval of care is required under managed care, and coverage is selective, effectively rationing care. Choice of practitioner or other provider and choice of site for care are restricted, which are additional methods of rationing care. An added incentive to rationing is a copayment for care that must be paid by the patient at the time that care is received. Despite industry assurances that care is not rationed, rationing is the undergirding concept of managed care. Managed care is not about providing health care; it is about being a for-profit brokerage business in which the managed care company acts as an agent who negotiates the contract about how the provision of health care will be accomplished.

There are a variety of models of managed care companies. Included are staff, group, network, **preferred provider organization (PPO)**, point of service (POS), mixed, each having its own unique structure and risk arrangements. The most common form is the PPO. A PPO generally consists of a hospital and a number of practitioner providers. The PPO contracts with health care providers (both practitioners and hospitals) and payers (self-insured employers, insurance companies, or managed care organizations) to provide health care services to a defined population for predetermined fixed fees. Discount rates may be negotiated with the providers in return for expedited claims payment and a somewhat predictable market share. In the PPO model, patients have a choice of using PPO or non-PPO providers; however, financial incentives are built in to encourage utilization of PPO providers.

Nongovernmental health insurance is predominantly accessed through employment. Employers provide coverage to employees as a benefit for working for their company. Therefore, the employer chooses the coverage with cost in mind and negotiates an acceptable package of benefits on behalf of the employees. If the employer offers a selection of benefit packages, the employee may choose the package that is most suitable. The range of available packages has narrowed to being nearly exclusively HMOs.

Examination of the percentage of the gross domestic product (gross national product statistics were used until 1999) spent on health care over the past few years shows that the *percentage* growth of costs was temporarily controlled in the 1990s (Figure 4-2), despite the continued *dollar* growth of costs, as shown in Figure 4-3. As

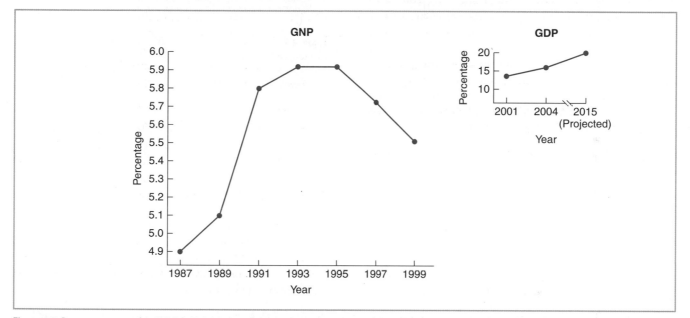

Figure 4-2 Percentage growth—U.S. health care costs as a percentage of gross national product, 1987–1999. (From "Industry Accounts Data. Gross National Product by Industry," 2000, Bureau of Economic Analysis. Retrieved June 16, 2001 from http://www.bea.doc.gov.)

NCHC health care cost as percentage of gross domestic product 2001–2004. (Retrieved June 20, 2006, from http://www.nchc.org.)

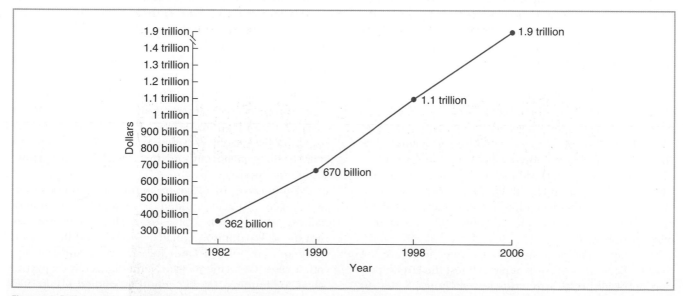

Figure 4-3 Dollar growth—Health care costs in dollars, 1982–2006.

shown in Figure 4-2, the percentages from 1987 through 1999 are expressed in terms of the gross *national* product and are incrementally small, all within a single percentage point. By 2001 a different analysis was adopted that expresses the percentages in terms of gross *domestic* product and shows much larger percentage increases. To view the trend over time, a double line near the top of the vertical percentage line in Figure 4-2 indicates the change in the vertical scale. If the scale were maintained at the original one tenth percentage, the figure would need to be extremely tall. The time intervals shown on the horizontal scale from 1987 through 2001 are every two years. The only available data following 2001 is for 2004, a three year interval. Health care costs are increasing yearly and are projected to increase to 20% of gross *domestic* product by 2015.

Managed care has become the focus for the anger of many health care providers and much of American society. Because care decisions are driven, in significant part, by the care options for which insurance coverage will pay, rather than by the free choice of the patient in consultation with a professional provider, feelings of distrust and anger about necessary compromises in care are often strongly held by both patients and providers. As the public becomes more knowledgeable, it also becomes more demanding.

To ease the pressure from practitioners, patients, consumer advocates, and employers, many HMO programs recently dropped the requirement for managed care preapproval prior to hospitalization or consultation with a specialist. In response to the demand for greater choice of provider, care plans were adapted to permit those who can afford to pay higher premiums and copayments to have broader choices. Efforts to salvage the reputation of managed care have spawned a new name—*coordinated care* is replacing the term *managed care* to better describe a system of mutual decision making among insurers, providers, and patients. In 2001, a patient's bill of rights was introduced into Congress to, among other things, allow patients to sue their coordinated care providers.

Such changes diminished the insurer's clout and with it the ability to contain costs. The news media reported that nationally renowned health care economist, Uwe Reinhardt of Princeton University, stated that "health plans can no longer bully and threaten the providers of care." Dr. David Lawrence, chief executive of the Kaiser Foundation Health Plan and Hospitals, noted, "When one uses financial tools to try to change the delivery of care, A, they are not very powerful, and B, they make people mad."

It may come as a surprise to note in Figure 4-4 that the Federal Government pays almost the largest proportion of all health care costs in the United States. In

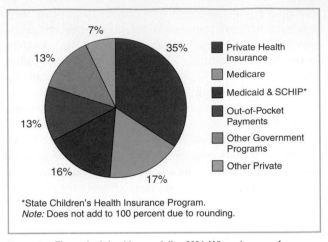

Figure 4-4 The nation's health care dollar, 2004: Where it comes from. (Centers for Medicare and Medicaid Services, Office of the Actuary, National Health Statistics Group. Retrieved March 21, 2006 from http://www.iii.org.)

addition to Medicare, State Children's Health Insurance Program (SCHIP), and Medicaid programs, government tax funds pay for the health care of members of the military, eligible veterans, Native Americans, federal prisoners, selected vulnerable or at-risk populations, and developmentally disabled and mentally ill patients who are institutionalized. Such government funding bears some resemblance to the socialized health care programs of other nations. This is a significant, but gradual, shift from 1960 when out-of-pocket payments were nearly three times as much as government payments.

SOCIALIZED HEALTH CARE

Socialized systems of providing health care (socialized medicine) are in place around the world. Philosophically, under such systems, complete health and hospital care is provided to all the citizens in a community, district, or nation (universal access). However, it is important to realize that the term, *socialized health care,* now refers to a variety of programs, each specific about what coverage is provided and how it is funded. Savage, Hoelscher, and Walker (1999) studied seven industrialized European countries and Canada for commonalities in coverage and funding. Their work reveals both centralized and decentralized compulsory single-payer systems with fee-for-service components, as well as some private insurance components.

Funding for the programs in the 1999 study also varied. In general, care is funded through public taxation of citizens, who are then eligible for care but who may or may not use it. Programs in Canada, Sweden, and the United Kingdom are funded from income taxes and selected other taxes. Germany and the Netherlands rely on payroll taxes for funding. Of the countries studied using 1999

TABLE 4-1	PROJECTED COMPARISON OF HEALTH CARE SPENDING, INFANT MORTALITY RATE, AND LIFE EXPECTANCY FOR 2006 ACROSS FOUR INDUSTRIALIZED COUNTRIES

Country	% GDP	Infant Mortality Rate	Male Life Expectancy (years)	Female Life Expectancy (years)
United States	16.0	6.50	72.95	79.67
Germany	10.7	4.16	74.01	80.50
Canada	9.7	4.75	76.12	82.79
United Kingdom	6.9	5.16	74.73	80.15

Source: Percent of GNP and Infant Mortality Rate retrieved June 20, 2006, from www.en.wikipedia.org. Life Expectancy retrieved March 31, 2006, from www.photius.com.

statistics (selected statistics for 2004 are shown in parentheses), Canada, the industrialized country most similar to the United States, spends 9.2% (9.7%) of its Gross National Product (GNP) on health care. Germany spends the most at 10.5% (10.7%), with the others spending as follows: Netherlands, 8.6%; Norway, 7.9%; Finland, 7.5%; Sweden, 7.2%; and Denmark, 6.4% in comparison to the 13.6% (16%) spent in the United States (Table 4-1).

The 1999 study also examined per capita health care spending and found that Canada spends $2,002; Germany, $2,222; and the United Kingdom, $1,304 per person. The 1999 study revealed life expectancy for males in Canada as 75.3 years (76.2 in 2004), in Germany as 73 years (74.1 in 2004), and in the United Kingdom as 74.3 years (74.7 in 2004). Life expectancy for females in Canada was reported as 81.3 years (82.8 in 2004), in Germany as 79.5 years (80.5 in 2004), and in the United Kingdom as 79.7 years (80.2 in 2004). The authors of the 1999 study pointed out that the countries studied face similar challenges of aging populations with chronic disease, the need to ration costly technology, severe budget shortages, managed competition, decentralization, and vertical integration. Compare the 1999 study findings to the 16% of gross domestic product ($6,280 per capita) spent in 2004 by the United States, more than any other country in the world and nearly twice that of many of the European countries studied, as shown in Table 4-1. Still, there are nearly 46 million people in the United States without health insurance, and the United States continues to experience a stubbornly high infant mortality rate.

With U.S. life expectancy for males at 72.95 years and for females at 79.67 years in 2004, the benefits reaped in the U.S. health care system seem to be those of enhanced quality of life rather than enhanced longevity. Quality of life must be defined within the specific cultures and value systems of each country. In the United States, qualities of life highly valued by Americans include prompt access to diagnostic and treatment services, even when health problems are not life threatening; ready availability of cutting-edge technology and pharmaceuticals; the ability to choose among health care practitioners and sites for care; and participation in health care decisions. All these contribute to the cost of health care. Is that enough to justify spending more than any other country in the world and nearly twice as much as European countries with similar health and financial circumstances? Perhaps.

THE INSTITUTE FOR HEALTHCARE IMPROVEMENT

The Institute for Healthcare Improvement (IHI) is a not-for-profit organization leading the improvement of health care throughout the world (www.ihi.org). IHI developed a campaign to reduce morbidity and mortality in the United States through the use of six health care interventions designed to save 100,000 Lives. These six IHI interventions include the following: deploy rapid response teams, improve care of patients with acute myocardial infarction, prevent adverse drug events through the use of medication reconciliation, and prevent central line infections, surgical site infections, and ventilator-associated pneumonia.

CENTRAL LINE BUNDLE

As part of the approaches to prevent central line infections mentioned above, several interventions have been developed (Institute for Healthcare Improvement, 2007). These interventions include the following:

1. Hand hygiene, including the following:
   ■ Before and after palpating catheter insertion site

- Before and after inserting, replacing, accessing, repairing, or dressing an intravascular catheter
- When hands are soiled
- Before and after invasive procedures
- Between patients
- Before donning and after removing gloves
- After using the bathroom

2. Maximal barrier precautions when inserting central lines, including the following:
   - Cap
   - Mask and sterile gown
   - Sterile gloves
   - Covering patient with large sterile drape
3. Chlorhexidine skin antisepsis
4. Optimal catheter site selection
   - Whenever possible and not contraindicated, the subclavian line site is preferred over the jugular and femoral sites for nonfunneled catheters in adult patients
5. Daily review of central line necessity, with prompt removal of unnecessary lines

RAPID-RESPONSE TEAM DEPLOYMENT TO PREVENT FAILURE TO RESCUE

Failure to Rescue describes the clinician's inability to save a patient's life when the patient experiences complications. Rapid-response teams have been developed to rescue the patient by mobilizing hospital resources quickly, including bringing nursing and medical practitioners and nurses to the bedside when a patient's condition deteriorates. Failure to rescue often stems from having a lack of sufficiently trained clinicians who have too little time to maintain close surveillance. Two examples of Failure to Rescue include the following:

- Nursing or medical surveillance systems fail to act on signs of a complication in a timely manner, resulting in a missed opportunity or seriously delayed rescue effort.
- Necessary supplies and equipment are not ready when a patient presents with a problem.

EVIDENCE-BASED PRACTICE

Clinicians have identified the need to use evidence-based practice (EBP) to improve the quality and cost-effectiveness of care delivery. Elements of EBP include the following:

- Identify an EBP question
- Assign responsibility for leadership
- Schedule a team conference with an interdisciplinary team
- Conduct a search for evidence, for example, www.pubmed.gov, www.cochrane.org, and so on

- Review and summarize evidence
- Rate strength of evidence
- Develop recommendations for change in care or guidelines on the basis of strength of evidence
- Create action plan
- Implement change
- Evaluate outcomes
- Communicate findings

EBP will be discussed in more detail in Chapter 5.

INSTITUTE OF MEDICINE (IOM) REPORTS

The Institute of Medicine (IOM), established in 1970 under the charter of the National Academy of Sciences, provides independent, objective, evidence-based advice to policymakers, health professionals, the private sector, and the public. IOM has released a series of reports on the quality of health care (www.iom.edu), for example, *Patient Safety: Achieving a New Standard for Care* (2003), *Crossing the Quality Chasm: A New Health System for the 21st Century* (2001), *Measuring the Quality of Health Care* (1999), *To Err is Human: Building A Safer Health System* (1999), *The Computer-Based Patient Record: An Essential Technology for Health Care, Revised Edition* (1997), and so on. These important Reports are profoundly affecting health care delivery today, and selected elements of these Reports are discussed in other chapters.

PAY-FOR-PERFORMANCE PROJECTS

An example of a Pay-for-Performance health care demonstration project is one that the Centers for Medicare and Medicaid Services (CMS) is doing in conjunction with Premier, Inc., a nationwide organization of not-for-profit hospitals. CMS will reward participating top-performing hospitals by increasing their payment for Medicare patients. Top-performing hospitals will receive bonuses based on their performance on evidence-based quality measures for inpatients with heart attack, heart failure, pneumonia, coronary artery bypass graft, and hip and knee replacements. This is a three-year demonstration project that's expected to cost roughly $7 million a year for each of the three years. CMS has indicated that financial awards will be paid as follows:

- Hospitals in the top decile of hospitals for a given diagnosis will be provided a 2% bonus of their Medicare payments for the measured condition
- Hospitals in the second decile will be paid a 1% bonus
- In year three, hospitals that don't achieve performance improvements above demonstration baseline will have adjusted payments

REAL WORLD INTERVIEW

During my many experiences over the past years with the Ontario, Canada, Health Care System and Ontario Health Insurance Program (OHIP), I have had annual visits to my General Practitioner (GP) with referrals to specialists for various tests, including x-rays, blood work, and hospital stays as needed. All my medical expenses while in these doctors' care is covered completely by the OHIP funds. Medications, glasses, and dental work are not covered unless one's gross annual income is a very minimal amount, in which case, some medications, dental, and hospitalizations are covered.

My husband was a diabetic, and he had a stroke 20 years ago at the age of 53. His GP met us at the hospital and assessed him through triage. My husband lost the use of his right arm and leg and his ability to comprehend language. The supreme care and compassion of his doctors and nurses helped my husband and family cope with the severity of this horrific disease. We paid for an upgrade to a semiprivate room. All other expenses while he was in the hospital were covered by OHIP. His rehabilitation began two weeks after his stroke, and he was transferred to the rehabilitation center, where he stayed for three months. All expenses while he was there were funded by OHIP.

After his acute illness, my husband saw a specialist every three months to monitor his blood sugar levels. He saw his GP every three months for his hypertension and saw his optometrist every year. He went for speech therapy once a week, physical therapy three times a week, and went to a nutritionist twice a year. This was all covered by OHIP.

He had several episodes of congestive heart failure through the years. Each time, I called 911, and the fire department came within minutes, administered oxygen, and inquired about his medical problems and medications while waiting for the ambulance medics to arrive. The medics took his vitals, gave him nitro, and called the admitting hospital.

We have four hospitals in Hamilton, Ontario, where I live. In the emergency department (ED), my husband was always processed immediately. When a heart specialist was called in, it took about an hour for him to arrive. Then the heart specialist would decide whether my husband was to be admitted to Intensive Care or a ward. There were times when a bed was not available until the next day, and we had to wait in the ED.

All emergencies in our ED are taken care of fairly promptly, the most severe first. Elective surgery such as knee or hip replacements, eye cataracts, etc., require a longer waiting period, sometimes up to six months. Hospital and emergency patients are on the priority list for magnetic resonance imaging (MRI) and CT scans. Other patients may have to wait for a couple of months for these tests. I also have the option, if I can afford it, of visiting the Buffalo, New York area clinics for MRIs, etc., if it is not an emergency, and I want to do it quicker. I would have to pay for these visits and tests out of pocket. All in all, I have been fairly pleased with our Canadian health system.

Flo Paradisi
Hamilton, Ontario, Canada

■ Hospitals will receive 1% lower DRG payment for clinical conditions that score below the ninth decile and 2% less if they score below the tenth decile (Centers for Medicare and Medicaid Services, 2006)

FUTURE PERSPECTIVE ON COST OF HEALTH CARE

Futurists are in demand to guide health care to organize for success. Health care providers have been thrashing in chaos for many years, reinventing their structures and processes, right-sizing their enterprises, outsourcing to better focus on their core business, and merging to share scarce or expensive resources. Although there have been some short-term cost savings, and the rise in health care spending has slowed, several evolving trends keep the overall cost growing.

Highly complex and expensive technology, including microsurgery, continues to develop. New diseases that require expensive or long-term treatment, such as AIDS and Ebola, continue to emerge. With the eradication or successful management of selected diseases, such as tuberculosis, populations are surviving longer. With that lengthened survival comes debilitating diseases of aging.

We look to futurists to help us make decisions about what business we ought to be prepared to provide. Will the Veterans Affairs hospitals go out of business when all the veterans with illness or injuries related to their military service or who are indigent die? Will a few strategically located hospitals provide only an intensive level of care, while acute care is managed on an ambulatory basis without invasive procedures? Will preventive, primary, and restorative care be the purview of advanced nurse practitioners practicing in community sites? Will altruism no longer be the basis for caring careers? Will nurses be "ordered to care" in a society that no longer values caring (Reverby, 1987)? Will the United States adopt a health care delivery system similar to those in European countries and Canada?

THE COST EQUATION: MONEY = MISSION = MONEY

The mission statement of any health care business describes the purpose for existence of the business and the rationale that justifies that existence. The statement directs decision making about what is or is not within the purview of the business. The vision statement is a logical extension of the mission into the future that establishes long-range goals for the business. After the vision is established and the business can articulate where it wants to go, a strategic plan for how to achieve the vision, or how to get to the goals, is developed. There must be cohesion and consistency across the mission, vision, and strategic plan for the business to successfully achieve its mission. There must also be money, for without it no mission can be accomplished.

COHESION AND CONSISTENCY OF THE BUSINESS

The question, then, is what is the cost of achieving the mission? Part of the cost may be in providing health care services that are not directly related to the mission, in the interest of political viability. Consider the Veterans Affairs (VA) health care system, established to provide intensive, acute, and rehabilitative care to military veterans (not active or reserve duty personnel or family members) who meet complex care-eligibility criteria for service-related illness and injury and/or indigency. Among the seventy-two VA medical centers in the United States and Puerto Rico are five Blind Centers, which provide unique mechanical aids, training for activities of daily living, and job training. When a center still has beds available after admitting all veteran applicants who meet the VA eligibility criteria, it may admit others using more lenient

standards. This practice may result in inconsistency with the core mission but can maintain the program at capacity and better assure its ongoing viability. A great deal of soul-searching regularly occurs about whether the political obligation to provide this unique and valued health care service justifies the cost of existence—and its occasional extension beyond the VA mission—in a cost-sensitive health care environment.

A more familiar example of providing a costly service that is inconsistent with the mission of the health care business may be the small maternity service of a remote region that claims few women of childbearing age as inhabitants. Without the service, the women would need to relocate to a distant facility miles away for the duration of the pregnancy. A sense of commitment to the well-being of the surrounding community is viewed as justification for keeping the service open. Similarly, a commitment to charity as a component of their mission drives religious organizations that are otherwise astute businesses to provide free care to the poor. However, modern health care organizations have limited tolerance for diversification from their core business.

Refer to Chapter 10 in this text for more in-depth discussion of mission-vision-strategic plan cohesion.

BUSINESS PROFIT

Revenue (income) minus cost (expense) equals profit. Profit is not restricted to for-profit businesses. Profit is not a dirty word. All businesses must realize a profit to remain in business. In for-profit businesses, a portion of the profit is distributed to stockholders in appreciation for their investing in the business, and the remainder is used to maintain and grow the organization. In nonprofit businesses, there are no stockholders to share the profit, so all of it is fed back into the business for maintenance and growth.

Not-for-profit organizations desiring a purer image than the term *profit* engenders refer to their profit as contribution to **margin**, with the rule of thumb being to secure 4% to 5% of the total budget as profit or margin. Mission and margin are strategically and operationally linked by the reality that resources are required to carry out the organization's strategic plan and achieve its mission. Without margin, or with limited margin, there would be a lack of money to replace worn-out equipment, to establish new services or enlarge existing services in response to changing community needs for health care, to purchase state-of-the-art technology, to maintain existing buildings or undertake new construction, and to replace heating and lighting systems. Failure to maintain such infrastructure can impair the organization's ability to be competitive, resulting in failure to meet its mission and eventual organizational failure. Profit is the elasticity that accommodates improvements in patient and staff education, recruitment and hiring of expert staff, and special

REAL WORLD INTERVIEW

The age of "volume" as a measure of anything is long past. In health care, for so many years, the notion of unlimited growth and expansion and providing anything for anyone was common. Subsequent introduction of broader concepts that reflect understanding of value and longevity now drive rational thinking about the availability and delivery of health services. In an era of unmatched cost that cannot continue to be supported, the issue of "value" now drives all elements of health service from access to delivery and, in the end, to making a difference in the individual's health status. Now we can more clearly identify the relationship between inputs and outcomes and between the process of delivering health care and the outcome of that care based on evidence-based practices. Health services must now be able to establish the connection between what is done and what is achieved. Health professions' addictions to what they do now gives way to tightening the connection between what is done and what difference it makes in the health status of individuals and of society. The "noise," or challenge, for nurses, physicians, and other health care providers is for everyone to more closely look at the "value" of their health care interventions in the light of the promise those interventions hold for improvement. The issue: either deliver improved health, or rethink why you're doing what you're doing. This critical examination and expectation will radically alter the economics and values of health care for the next two decades.

Tim Porter-O'Grady, EdD, ScD, APRN, FAAN
Prolific Nurse Author and Speaker on New-Edge Health Care
Otto, North Carolina

programming that yields personal professional growth. Profit is a critical requirement for doing business. A truism of business is, no margin, no mission.

Achieving and sustaining margin is a constant challenge for health care enterprises. New Jersey's governor recently proposed a "sick tax" on acute care enterprises in his state at the rate of $1,400 per patient bed per month to help bolster the state's 2007 budget. In his Letter to the Editor of the June, 2006 issue of *Hospitals and Health Networks,* Gary Carter, CEO and President of the New Jersey Hospital Association, walks through the ripple effect of such a heavy additional tax burden. Mr. Carter predicts that New Jersey's health care enterprises will be unable to maintain their buildings and infrastructure or to purchase the supplies, equipment, and personnel required to obtain expensive new technology required for exemplary care. He predicts that the organizations would probably look first to cutting personnel cost by adjusting their benefit packages, shifting more health care cost to employees and retirees. In addition, because hospitals in New Jersey are required by law to provide care to anyone who comes through their doors, some enterprises might not survive financially, depriving some populations of health care services (Carter, 2006).

FUNDAMENTAL COSTS

There are many ways to examine or classify the costs of care. One fundamental method is to view costs as direct

or indirect. A **direct cost** is directly related to patient care within a manager's unit, such as the cost of nurses' wages and the cost of patient care supplies. An **indirect cost** is not explicitly related to care within a manager's unit but is necessary to support care. The costs of electricity, heat, air conditioning, and maintenance of the facility are all considered indirect.

Those same costs may also be considered either fixed or variable. These distinctions are somewhat artificial and are related to the volume of services that are provided. A **fixed cost** is one that exists irrespective of the number of patients for whom care is provided, as shown in Figure 4-5. Examples of this are the cost of the rent or the monthly mortgage for the space in which the care is provided and the cost of salaried (but not hourly) wage earners such as the nurse manager or nurse administrator. These costs would be the same whether one patient was served or 1,000 patients were served. A **variable cost**, on the other hand, varies with volume and will increase or decrease depending on the number of patients, as shown in Figure 4-6. The costs of medical supplies, laundry for the linens used in patient care, or patient meals are variable costs that increase or decrease in proportion to the number of patients served.

Some costs are step variable; that is, they vary with volume, but not smoothly. The key to step costs is that they are fixed over volume intervals but vary within the relevant range. For instance, a fixed number of nurses

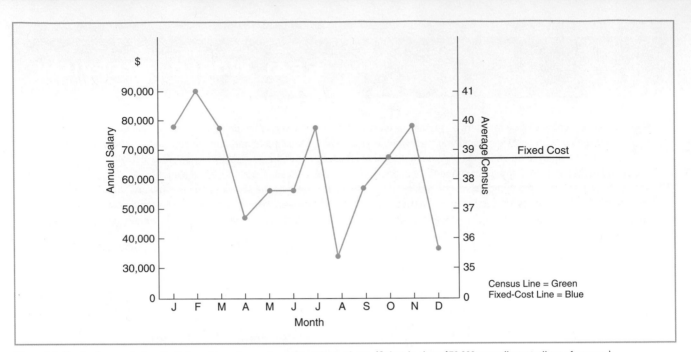

Figure 4-5 Fixed salary cost of a salaried employee does not vary by patient volume. (Salary is about $70,000 annually regardless of census.)

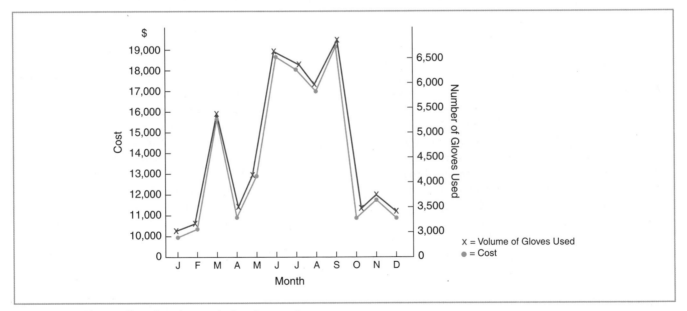

Figure 4-6 Variable cost of latex-free gloves varies by volume used.

may be able to care for eleven to twenty-one patients. However, as depicted in Figure 4-7, when even one additional patient beyond twenty-one requires care, additional nurses are required.

COST ANALYSIS

There is an old saying that numbers don't lie. There is also an old saying that statistics can be manipulated to show whatever is desired. Both sayings are true, and therein lies the challenge, the frustration, and occasionally the glory of clinical cost management. The health care industry

commonly embraces the position that the past is prologue for forecasting its future. The ability to predict the behavior of cost in the future based on its past behavior, then, is considered requisite to successful cost management and thereby the achievement of mission and vision. A **budget** is a plan that provides formal quantitative expression for acquiring and distributing funds over the ensuing time period (generally one year). This budget is based on what is known about how much was spent in the past and how that will inevitably change in the coming year. A cost prediction is simply a tool for developing a budget. The three most common methods of cost prediction are

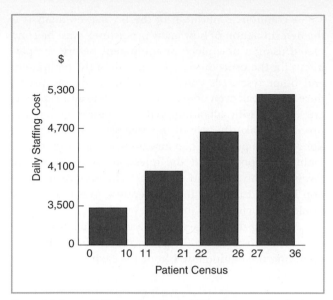

Figure 4-7 Step variable costs are fixed within a range and then increase when volume exceeds the upper end of the range.

high-low cost estimation, regression analysis, and break-even analysis.

HIGH-LOW COST ESTIMATION

This is not the tool to choose if a sophisticated, statistically rigorous prediction is needed, but it does surpass just guessing. Examining both fixed and variable cost information from the most recent five years for each category of expense provides a "good enough" cost projection for many items that remain relatively constant in volume of consumption and cost. Both fixed and variable dollars need to be adjusted upward to account for inflation, and the total projected cost needs to be adjusted upward to cover anticipated cost of living or other wage increases and to cover bad debt when services are rendered but payment does not occur.

The following is an example that clarifies the math:

Highest wage cost = $500,000
Lowest wage cost = $300,500
Difference = $199,500

Highest number of patient days = 9,000
Lowest number of patient days = 7,500
Difference = 1,500

Difference in cost ($199,500)/Difference in volume (1,500) = $133 per patient day variable cost

Variable cost ($133) × Lowest number of patient days (7,500) = $997,500 = Total annual variable cost

Total annual labor cost for the unit from this year's fiscal department records ($1,100,000) − Total annual variable cost ($997,500) = $102,500 Fixed cost

If 1,000 additional patient days are anticipated in the ensuing year, there would be an additional cost as follows:

$133 per patient day variable cost × 1,000 additional days	= $133,000
+ Fixed cost (regardless of the number of patient days)	= $102,500
Total additional cost	= $235,500

Thus, the total cost for this unit next year, using high-low cost estimation, will be this year's cost of $1,100,000 plus $235,500 in new costs, or $1,335,500.

REGRESSION ANALYSIS

A more precise prediction of cost can be realized using the statistical tool, regression analysis. Whereas the high-low method relies on only two data points—the highest and the lowest—for historical cost behavior, regression analysis examines all available past cost information over a specific time period. It assumes there is only one dependent variable—cost—with only one independent variable—volume—causing change in that dependent variable. It also assumes that mathematically, cost behavior can be shown in a linear fashion by drawing a straight line through a scatter diagram of all fixed and variable costs at all volumes of use. When all cost information is plotted on a vertical axis, and all volume information is plotted on the horizontal axis, a scatter diagram results. The straight line through the scatter diagram that best approximates all the points is used to predict cost at a specific volume of use. Selecting a volume on the horizontal axis and examining where a vertical line from that point intersects the straight regression line, then moving horizontally to the vertical cost axis, provides the cost prediction for that specific volume as shown by the dotted lines in the scatter diagram in Figure 4-8. The analysis is carried out for each item for which cost needs to be predicted.

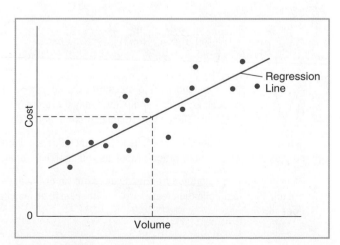

Figure 4-8 Regression analysis.

BREAK-EVEN ANALYSIS

Because accruing profit to enhance the quality of services provided and to achieve optimal competitive market position is the business goal of health care organizations, projecting whether and when profitability will be achieved is necessary for both proposed and well-established programs and services. The third basic cost analysis tool is break-even analysis. It assists the provider to predict the volume of services that must be provided (and for which payment must be received) for the cost of providing the services to be equally matched by the payment received, yielding neither a profit nor loss. The formula for computing a break-even analysis (Finkler & Kovner, 2000) is as follows:

Volume of procedures = Fixed cost/Payment − Variable cost

A common application of the break-even analysis is the determination of how many procedures must be completed using a new piece of equipment before the payments for the procedure cover the cost of the equipment and other resources consumed while doing the procedure (the **break-even point** at which income and expenses are equal), with all additional procedures generating profit. To make the use of the analysis more clear, consider that the purchase of a new piece of radiology equipment is proposed, and the question has been posed, "Would this be a good investment?" The underlying question is, would the purchase generate a profit, a loss, or would the organization just break even?

Applying the breakeven analysis formula, if the new procedure costs $50,000, the wages of the technician operating the equipment 1 hour for each use is $20 per

CRITICAL THINKING 4-1

Reducing costs and improving quality at the same time is a very realistic goal. Frequently, quality problems are very costly. Examples of this are found in Chassin and Galvin's (1998) article on improving health care quality. They cite underuse, overuse, and misuse of potentially effective interventions as a costly problem. Underuse—failing to use treatments that are known to be effective, such as thromboembolytics, beta blockers, aspirin, and angiotensin-converting enzyme inhibitors in myocardial infarctions—may account for as many as 18,000 preventable deaths each year. Overuse of drugs such as antibiotics is not only ineffective and expensive, but it is believed to lead to antibiotic resistance. Misuse is generally the failure to prevent complications of treatment and adds thousands of dollars to the costs of health care.

Identify some ways in which nurses can participate in reducing waste, influence best practices, and improve quality in these areas. Is keeping current with the literature in your specialty necessary to be effective in doing this?

CRITICAL THINKING 4-2

Nursing is a collaborative profession existing in a complex health care system. At one time it was influenced by three factors: cost, access, and quality. Today there are five influencing factors: cost, access, cost, quality, and cost (John M. Lantz, RN, PhD, Dean and Professor, School of Nursing, University of San Francisco).

Is this an accurate description of the things that influence contemporary nursing practice? What do these five influencing factors suggest may be an organization's focus as you interview for a staff nurse position?

You notice that a colleague frequently does not record patient charge items for elderly patients. When you inquire about it, you are told that your colleague feels sorry for those on fixed incomes and wants to save them money. Who pays when your colleague does this?

use, and the payment for each procedure is $50, it would take 1,667 procedures to pay for the equipment and technician wages before a profit would begin to accrue.

$$\text{Volume} = \$50,000 / (\$50 - \$20) = 1,667$$

If the payment for the procedure were $100, a profit would begin to accrue after only 625 procedures.

$$\text{Volume} = \$50,000 / (\$100 - \$20) = 625$$

Thus, a projection can be made about how long it will take before the new equipment would be a profitable venture, guided by the decision about how much cost the purchaser of the procedure is likely to tolerate.

DIAGNOSTIC, THERAPEUTIC, AND INFORMATION TECHNOLOGY COST

A common perception held by both society and the health care industry is that payroll costs constitute the largest expense item in organizational budgets and that the most expensive health care personnel are registered nurses (RNs). Therein lies the rush to downsize RNs when a determination is made that costs need to be cut and better managed. Close examination of the entire budget, however, is likely to reveal that although the nursing payroll is the most expensive payroll item and the most expensive operating budget item, the most expensive item on the total budget is diagnostic, therapeutic, and information technology. This technology is required to meet society's demand for state-of-the-art care; professionals' demand for quicker, keener ways to work; and the organization's need to maintain a competitive business edge. Such items characteristically appear on the capital budget because of their considerable cost. With cost management generally focused on the operating budget, the cost of diagnostic, therapeutic, and information technology is often conveniently overlooked because it is deemed "strategic" and therefore untouchable during cost-cutting initiatives. Moreover, despite a rise in nursing payroll costs over the past 20 years, proportionately that rise has been considerably more gradual than the rise in diagnostic, therapeutic, information technology, and total hospital costs, resulting in a widening gap in costs that suggests that nursing is a cost bargain. A hypothetical example of the proportional broadening of total hospital costs (including technology) and nursing payroll costs is shown in Figure 4-9.

Yet, the high cost of technology in particular has been recognized by regulatory agencies for many years. In pursuit of cost control in hospitals, the states independently established laws more than 30 years ago creating Certificate of Need (CON) agencies to oversee, regulate, and

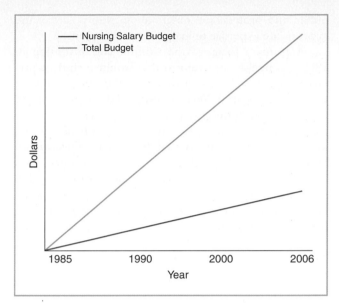

Figure 4-9 Comparison of nursing pay to total budget.

approve major technology and construction expenditures. A secondary goal was to ensure equitable distribution of and access to high-end technology across the states. The CON approach was not successful because it focused only on hospitals and provided no incentives to change either practitioner or patient behavior. Hospitals were given spending limits, but there was no incentive for practitioners to change their practice, so they didn't. Without incentives, patients' expectations and demands for care also remained unchanged.

More recently, managed care programs have exerted oversight of the use of complex, expensive technology by requiring justification and approval prior to its use for payment to occur. Only when less costly approaches had been exhausted would the possibility of using highly specialized technology be considered. Diagnostically, movement has been away from "fishing expeditions" such as ordering the comprehensive metabolic panel (CMP) and routine chest x-ray on all patients and toward completing only that which is minimally required to reach a reasonable diagnosis based on overt signs and symptoms. Exploration of subtle or subclinical signs or symptoms—the heart of the art of medical care—has, as a result, largely gone begging. The question that arises is whether assurance of correct diagnosis has been critically compromised or whether sharper clinical skill has resulted.

Therapeutically, there has been a movement toward rationing the most expensive technology to those with the ability and willingness to pay for it over and above their health insurance coverage. Underscoring public and professional concern about rationing was the best-selling book by John Kilner (1992), *Who Lives? Who Dies? Ethical Criteria in Patient Selection.* We have begun to see managed care programs become more lenient in response to a public and professional outcry about who possesses the appropriate expertise to make clinical decisions.

A primary focus of the Clinton administration in 1993 was health care reform that would include a prescription drug benefit provided by the government. It took Congress until 2005 to design and adopt Medicare Part D. Congress designed Medicare Part D not to cover all prescription drugs or even the total cost of selected drugs. Congress claimed that the federal government budget could only provide assistance to enrollees with low incomes and high drug costs. Rules for membership eligibility, rules for coverage eligibility, and a gap in coverage that has come to be called the "doughnut hole" have Americans confused, appalled, disappointed, and, in some cases, worse off than they were without the plan. The June 2006 American Association of Retired People (AARP) Bulletin provides the following explanation of the "doughnut hole" that is currently generating much high emotion:

> Medicare drug coverage is generally divided into three phases. Depending on your plan, in the first phase (initial coverage period), you may pay a deductible and about 25% of your drug costs. In the third phase (catastrophic coverage), you pay about 5%. In between these two periods, there is a gap in coverage (commonly called the doughnut hole), when most people must pay 100% of their drug costs out of their own pocket.

Another less-recognized aspect of the Medicare drug plan is that the initial coverage phase of the plan that pays up to a $2,250 limit in drug costs includes both the cost paid by the insured and the cost paid by the plan. These two significant pitfalls are illustrated in Table 4-2.

TABLE 4-2	IMPACT OF THE MEDICARE "DOUGHNUT HOLE" GAP ON A PATIENT'S DRUG COST		
	Total Drug Cost ($)	Drug Insurance Covers ($)	Patient Out of Pocket Pays ($)
Month 1	825.00	412.50	275.00 deductible 137.50 co-pay
Month 2	825.00	618.75	206.25
Month 3 pre Gap	600.00	450.00	150.00
Pre-Gap Total	2250.00	1481.25	768.75
Month 3 in Gap	225.00	0.00	225.00
Month 4	825.00	0.00	825.00
Month 5	825.00	0.00	825.00
Month 6	825.00	0.00	825.00
Month 7 in Gap	131.25	0.00	131.25
Gap Total	2831.25	0.00	2831.25
Month 7 post Gap Catastrophic	693.75	659.06	34.69
Month 8	825.00	783.75	41.25
Month 9	825.00	783.75	41.25
Month 10	825.00	783.75	41.25
Month 11	825.00	783.75	41.25
Month 12	825.00	783.75	41.25
Catastrophic Total	4818.75	4577.81	240.94
Year Total	9900.00	6059.06	3840.94

Note: The "Doughnut Hole" Gap is effective when drug costs reach $2250.00. While in the Gap the patient must pay the full cost of drugs. Catastrophic coverage becomes effective when the patient has paid $3600.00 out of pocket (in this example, $768.75 + $2831.25). Under catastrophic coverage the patient pays 5% of drug cost.

Source: Adapted from Barry, P. (2006, June). One trip through the coverage gap. *AARP Bulletin,* 16–18.

NURSING COST

Fiscally, most organizations view nursing as a cost center that does not independently generate revenue. Although some deviation from that fiscal philosophy may occur when selected nursing practitioners are permitted by law to bill directly for their unique professional services, the cost of providing nursing care (wages, benefits, selected supplies and equipment, overhead) is commonly bundled into a catchall, room, or per diem, cost that assumes that every patient consumes identical nursing resources each day. Such a view is not only antiquated, it is incorrect. Nursing care is not an identical product delivered in assembly-line fashion. It varies remarkably in intensity, in depth, and in breadth across patients, consistent with patients' unique, individual dependency needs.

Those unique needs have contributed to nursing care being more broadly available than ever before across a variety of sites. Access to a high degree of nursing care is still accepted as second only in importance to access to medical technology as a reason for hospitalization. When access to both nursing care and medical technology is needed, hospitalization is unquestionably appropriate. Consequently, the revenue generated from hospitalization is, in fact, payment, primarily, for consumption of medical technology and nursing services and should be recognized as such. The revenue generated from consumption of nursing resources also should be accurately quantified to each patient and charged at a rate consistent with the level and intensity of care consumed.

Ongoing efforts to measure and establish the cost of the diverse, yet related, components of nursing care are disappointing. That care includes direct hands-on care, teaching, and coordinating discharge, as well as indirect documentation, consultation, critical problem solving and decision making, and supervision of multiple levels of workers. These same components contribute to the long-established cost of other practitioner and therapist services, yet the value, and thus the cost, of nursing care eludes measurement and agreement. Perhaps reluctance to legitimize the independent professional practice of the largest unit of health care providers (more than 2.9 million RNs are employed in nursing in the United States) contributes to the inability to reach agreement about how to cost out nursing.

Consequently, nursing cost is narrowly associated with budgeted and actual nursing care hours per patient day, a measure of time rather than a measure of type or level of care. Guiding the budgeted hours are historical consumption and projected changes in future demand for nursing care in response to market competition and projected changes in community demographics or consumer demands. Volume, acuity, and complexity of required care comprise workload and drive the actual nursing hours consumed.

While volume and acuity are relatively straightforward concepts that lend themselves to measurement, measuring complexity is multifaceted. Various federal, state, and local laws regulate who can accomplish what work based on educational preparation and ability to

REAL WORLD INTERVIEW

The ongoing and escalating shortage of nurses and other health care professionals may be the major health care issue well into the twenty-first century and at least for the next 20 years. There must be valid and reliable mechanisms for calculating the requirement for nursing care time and intensity.

Models of care delivery that maximize the use of unlicensed assistive personnel (UAP) and provide for sufficient professional nursing expertise and time for both care delivery and supervision are a necessity. The number of nursing hours provided to each patient over a 24-hour period (nursing hours per patient day) that is commonly used to project staffing needs provides insufficient and inadequate information for planning and staffing decisions that can best assure quality clinical outcomes for patients. Mechanisms used to track or predict nursing workload must be able to differentiate between the care that requires professional nurses and the care that can safely and effectively be done by assistive personnel. Definitions and measurements of nursing workload must be standardized so that comparative data can be collected and analyzed.

Sheila Haas, PhD, RN
Dean and Professor
Loyola University, Chicago, Illinois

EVIDENCE FROM THE LITERATURE

Citation: Aiken, L. H., Clarke, S. P., Cheung, R. B., Sloane, D. M., & Silber, J. H. (2003, Sept.). Educational levels of hospital nurses and surgical patient mortality. *Journal of American Medical Association, 290*(12), 1617–1623.

Discussion: Article discusses results of study done to determine the association between the educational levels of hospital RNs and the mortality of surgical patients. The study examined 168 adult acute care hospitals in Pennsylvania reporting a total of 232,342 surgical discharges to the Pennsylvania Health Care Cost Containment Council in 1999. The researchers also surveyed a random sample of 50% of hospital nurses who live in Pennsylvania and were registered with the Pennsylvania Board of Nursing. In all, 10,184 nurses (52% of nurses surveyed) responded.

According to the survey results, the average age of respondents was between 40 and 41 years, and between 30% and 31% of respondents had earned a BSN or higher degree. Hospital nurses who participated in the study had 14.2 years' nursing experience with a mean patient load of 5.7 per day. The researchers examined how the education of hospital nurses affected the death rates of surgical patients within 30 days of admission and death rates within 30 days of admission among patients who experienced complications. The study also took into consideration whether a board-certified surgeon performed the surgery. The types of surgeries examined included general surgery, orthopedic, and vascular procedures.

The study found that years of nursing experience don't predict a patient's outcome and that patients cared for in hospitals with a higher proportion of nurses holding a BSN degree or higher have a better chance of postsurgical survival. Specifically, the study stated that "a 10% increase in the proportion of nurses holding a bachelor's degree (in hospitals) was associated with a 5% decrease in both the likelihood of patients dying within 30 days of admission and the odds of failure to rescue." Failure to rescue was defined as "deaths in patients with serious complications." The researchers recognized two limitations to their study:

- The low (52%) response rate of the nurses surveyed
- The examination of hospitals from only one state

The researchers concluded that although these preliminary findings raise concerns over nurse education as it relates to patient outcomes, further study of nurses and hospitals nationwide would be required to make these results irrefutable.

Implication for Practice: This study offers powerful insights into the need for higher nursing education levels. The study bears repeating for validation.

---

demonstrate command of a minimum body of knowledge on a standardized examination. These laws affect workload. The efficiency and effectiveness of work flow, the way work is accomplished, affect workload. This may involve something as simple as the nurse making multiple trips back and forth to access supplies in an awkward physical configuration of the work environment. It may also involve something as complex as making innovative adjustments to a familiar work pattern to accommodate physical, cognitive, behavioral, or sociocultural challenges presented by a "difficult" patient.

PATIENT CLASSIFICATION SYSTEM (PCS)

The tool most broadly used to identify nursing cost is the **patient classification system (PCS)**, a system for distinguishing among different patients based on their acuity (level of need or dependency of an individual patient),

functional ability, or resource needs. Originally developed to predict staffing, it is used across diverse settings as a moderately robust measure of cost, as well as to predict staffing. Patients with similar requirements for care are assigned to one of five progressively weighted categories of acuity from minimal to maximal. The weights are the average number of hours of nursing care deemed required by all of the patients in each respective category; some patients within the category will actually require more hours, while others will require fewer hours (Finkler & Kovner, 2000).

Most PCSs are designed commercially and tailored to the descriptive data and information provided by the actual workgroup that will be using the PCS. The users describe the acuity and complexity of their typical workload and the volume and mix of nursing resources typically needed to do the work. Changes to the profile of the work or to the profile of the workers are expensive, so it is important not to minimize or exaggerate either description when working with the vendor. To protect the business interest of the PCS vendor, the specific formula used to compute the nursing hours needed for each category is not revealed to the organization in which the PCS will be used.

Each work shift, on-site nurses, who are providing direct care and can therefore best judge the actual patient acuity, select the activity category of care each patient requires from a standard weighted menu of procedures. Patient acuity is often rated with a nursing-driven system yielding a number from 1 (low) to 5 (high) acuity. A formula (often institution specific) is used to determine staffing. Besides the usual aspects of acuity, the formula may include considerations of psychosocial, education, family, and bereavement issues that are not included in usual staffing formulas. Other factors to consider in determining staffing level are the number of admissions, deaths, and discharges. When lengths of stay are short, more staffing is needed to manage the admissions. If there are many patients discharged alive, the discharge planning and family teaching burden is high. If there are many deaths in a given time period, this increases the staffing required.

Most units develop their own system of determining acuity. Frequently, this means a conversion factor is developed. Based on the kinds of factors described, an acuity level is ascribed to each patient (for example, 1–5). Then, a conversion factor for each acuity level is applied to determine the amount of staffing required. For example:

- (# patients) × (Acuity 1 conversion factor) = x hours nursing
- (# patients) × (Acuity 2 conversion factor) = x hours nursing
- (# patients) × (Acuity 3 conversion factor) = x hours nursing
- (# patients) × (Acuity 4 conversion factor) = x hours nursing
- (# patients) × (Acuity 5 conversion factor) = x hours nursing

The hours are totalled, and the number of FTE nursing is determined.

Highest acuity usually means the patient requires 1:1 or 1:2 nursing care. Many patients today are acuity level 3 or 4. There are other types of patient acuity scales also. The higher the total weight of the required care, the higher the acuity. The higher the total acuity for all the patients assessed, the more nursing resources the PCS assigns. The more resources assigned, the higher the cost. Perfect logic? Not quite.

There are several shortcomings to a formula that measures only time. First, it cannot account for the presence, or absence, of knowledge, skill, or experience in

EVIDENCE FROM THE LITERATURE

Citation: Hall, L. M., Pink, L., Lalonde, M., Murphy, G. T., O'Brien-Pallas, L., Laschinger, H. K., et al. (2006). Decision making for nurse staffing. *Policy Politics in Nursing Practice, 7*(4), 261–269.

Discussion: The effectiveness of methods for determining nurse staffing is unknown. Despite a great deal of interest, efforts conducted to date indicate that there is a lack of consensus on nurse staffing decision-making processes. This study explored nurse staffing decision-making processes, supports in place for nurses, nursing workload being experienced, and perceptions of nursing care and outcomes. Substantial information was provided from participants about the nurse staffing decision-making methods currently employed, including frameworks for nurse staffing, nurse-to-patient ratios, workload measurement systems, and "gut" instinct. A number of key themes emerged from the study that can form the basis for policy and practice changes related to determining appropriate workload for nursing. These include the use of staffing principles and frameworks, nursing workload measurement systems, and nurse-to-patient ratios. There is a need for more evidence related to nurse staffing.

Implications for Practice: It appears there is no one method to determine patient acuity and staffing requirements. While research must continue in this area, current systems use combinations of the above to determine safe staffing.

the nurses providing the hours of care. Even the gross categories of RN and LPN cannot be taken into account. It cannot, therefore, account for the richness in clinical assessment and decision making that occurs when the same procedure or care is provided by an RN versus an LPN. Second, there is no ability to account for the atypical physical, cognitive, behavioral, or sociocultural challenges that consume above-average hours. Similarly, the way one patient manages pain, fear, or anxiety is seldom identical to the way another patient copes, and supporting one may require very different resources than supporting the other, identical acuity notwithstanding. In other words, a category 4 patient is not a category 4 patient is not a category 4 patient. Innumerable nursing hours are spent attempting to justify the actual nursing hours consumed when that number slides above the number of hours assigned by the PCS.

RELATIVE VALUE UNIT (RVU)

A **relative value unit (RVU)** is an index number assigned to various health care services based on the relative amount of resources (labor and capital) used to produce the service. The actual consumption of nursing resources is not linear; that is, caring for an acuity level 2 patient does not consume twice as many nursing resources as caring for an acuity level 1 patient. RVUs provide a proportional comparison between the resources required by level 1 acuity (always a value of 1) and any other level. For example, only 20% (1.2 RVUs) more resources may be consumed by a level 2 acuity patient than a level 1, but twice as many resources may be consumed by a level 3 acuity (2.0 RVUs), and more than three times as much by a level 4 acuity (3.33 RVUs), and so forth, as shown in Table 4-3.

The RVUs can be used to calculate the relative costs of nursing care using the following reasoning:

For the time period of interest, the total cost of nursing wages = $1,250,000.

For the time period of interest, the total RVUs by acuity level and patient days are as follows:

Acuity	Days		RVU weight		Total RVUs
1	125	×	1.00	=	125.00
2	200	×	1.20	=	240.00
3	500	×	2.00	=	1,000.00
4	550	×	3.33	=	1,831.50
5	400	×	5.00	=	2,000.00
Total	1775				5,196.50

Dividing the total nursing costs by the total RVUs yields the cost per RVU.

$1,250,000 / 5,196.50 = $240.55 per RVU

The cost for one level 5 acuity patient for one day, then, is $240.55 × 5 (the RVU weight for acuity level 5), or $1,202.75.

Patients acuity varies, even within the same day, as they experience invasive procedures, intensive treatments and medication, complications, or progress toward wellness. As acuity varies, consumption of nursing resources varies. It follows that the cost for direct nursing care would be consistent with nursing resource consumption and could be determined using RVU calculations.

This approach provides a reasonably accurate per-patient costing approach. It does not account for the difference in cost based on the category of worker providing the care. Indirect fixed costs that do not vary dependent on patient classification such as salaried wages, overhead, service contracts, and noncapital equipment purchases must be added to arrive at the full cost of nursing care. Both administrators and clinicians recognize the serious shortcomings of the current methods available to calculate the cost of nursing care and the critical need for something more accurate. But the current tools offer at least a rudimentary method for capturing nursing cost.

QUALITY MEASUREMENT

An evidence-based concept of quality is grounded on scientific evidence that a diagnostic or therapeutic approach improves patient outcomes. This concept exploded into the health care industry in the early 1990s with evidence-based clinical practices. The four core components are (1) a mechanism that establishes local or regional consensus about what constitutes the best practices based on scientific research findings, (2) strong feasible processes to accomplish such practices, (3) a deliberate program of outreach to the community on disease prevention and health promotion, and (4) a rigorous system to review actual performance and clinical outcomes, as well as identification and implementation of improvement

TABLE 4-3	COMPARATIVE VALUES OF ACUITY, CARE HOURS, AND RELATIVE VALUE UNITS	
Acuity	**Care Hours**	**Relative Value Weight**
1	3.00	1.00
2	3.60	1.20
3	6.00	2.00
4	9.99	3.33
5	15.00	5.00

CRITICAL THINKING 4-3

Securing a profit might suggest that high quality is also secured because it facilitates purchase of state-of-the-art equipment and expert practitioners. Quality and profit do not necessarily go together. The Nosek-Androwich Profit: Quality (NAPQ) Matrix shown here models four possible relationships between profit and quality that may exist in a health care organization. Any organization can fit into any quadrant, and a single organization may shift among quadrants from time to time in response to market forces. The challenge for the organization is to maintain existence in the high-profit, high-quality quadrant to be best positioned for clinical success and for business success, the mission of the organization. A common mission, consistent vision, collaboration, and constant vigilance to the elements of quality and profit by all employees and stakeholders together are keys to maintaining organizational positioning and achieving economic and quality success.

Access the annual report published by any health care enterprise. Based on the margin reported by the Finance Department, as compared to the rule of thumb of 3% to 5% margin required for business success, would you rate that organization as high profit or as low profit? Based on the overall satisfaction score reported for all services of that organization, would you rate it as high quality or as low quality? (Hint: If the satisfaction score is not published, it may be because that score is relatively low.) Which quadrant of the NAPQ Matrix does the health care enterprise fit?

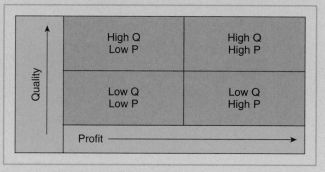

Nosek-Androwich Profit: Quality (NAPQ) matrix.

methodologies that achieve a dynamic balance between economy and quality. The essence of that dynamic balance may be the "value" Dr. Tim Porter-O'Grady projects as the future focus of health care (see Real World Interview within this chapter).

Regardless of its particular size or mission, every contemporary health care **enterprise** (an organization of any size established as a business venture) must commit to cost improvement and quality improvement as core goals for strategic business success and for strategic clinical success. Clearly, this is not a new notion, but the recent intensification of the focus on cost and quality improvement and its expansion from hospitals to diverse ambulatory and home care sites is startling and is being referred to as the Q-revolution (Carpenter, 2006). The more critical cost containment and cost management become, the more critical attention to quality management becomes. Quality and cost are inextricably linked.

Logic suggests that higher quality could lead to a higher volume of use of the organization by patients and providers who have the flexibility to make choices about where they seek health care. Higher volume generally leads to higher profits, which, in turn, may be directed toward improving programs and services, thus achieving higher quality, a very positive spiral that can result in the organization's thriving.

Increased quality > Increased volume >
Increased profit > Enhanced programs/services >
Increased quality

The obverse spiral is more likely when quality is shoddy, a very negative and potentially fatal spiral.

Decreased quality > Decreased volume >
Decreased profit > Cutting corners >
Decreased quality

REGULATORY OVERSIGHT

The quality industry measures and tracks organizational performance to ensure that organizations' structures and processes are designed, monitored, and constantly ratcheted toward improved performance and improved patient outcomes. The Joint Commission (JC), formerly known as the Joint Commission on Accreditation of Healthcare Organizations (JCAHO), is the preeminent regulatory body overseeing health care quality. Its review processes are extensive, and payments to an organization by government insurers of health care (Medicare and

Medicaid) are dependent on the organization's ability to meet JC standards with a high degree of compliance. In addition, other federal, state, local, and voluntary regulatory agencies oversee the quality of specific organizational components such as pharmacy, laboratory, long-term care, rehabilitative care, dietary, behavioral health, and fire safety. Accreditation, which signifies that the organization meets the standards for practice of these oversight agencies, influences market perception about the quality of health care that the organization provides and engenders trust and confidence in the organization. Accreditation also ensures payment from both governmental and nongovernmental insurers.

Sally Sample was the first nurse appointed by the JC to the at-large seat created on the board of commissioners. She was appointed to the board in 1992 and has witnessed firsthand the tumultuous changes in the perspective on health care quality and in the operations of the commission. She characterizes the mission and the work of the JC in the following Real World Interview.

CUSTOMER SATISFACTION

Regardless of how superior providers may perceive their own product or service to be, if customers fail to perceive it to be the needed or wanted service provided conveniently by skilled and knowledgeable people in a caring manner at a reasonable cost and consistent with their own culture and value system, the organization may fail. Perception, accurate or not, is the key. Therefore, organizations use a variety of indices to measure both internal and external customer satisfaction.

Commercial surveys such as Press-Ganey measure how satisfied the patients are with their care, food, physical environment, emotional ambiance, and their interactions with various health care workers, and then provide comparison rankings across similar organizations and populations nationally. The Veterans Affairs system of hospitals conducts its own unique survey after patient discharge. Many organizations use instruments developed internally to measure attributes of unique interest to that organization. Research protocols use a variety of statistical methods to test satisfaction. Results of such surveys are analyzed as part of the organization's quality-management program.

HEALTH CARE SITE ECONOMICS

The study of economics focuses on how choices are made to overcome a scarcity of resources. Christensen, Bohmer, and Kenagy (2000) rate health care as possibly the most entrenched, change-aversive industry in the United States. Their thesis is that the three Rs, redesigning, restructuring, and **reengineering** (despite the latter's

claim to turn organizations upside down and inside out through fundamental rethinking and radical redesign of processes to achieve dramatic improvements in critical performance), simply tweak the existing health care structure and processes. They believe that changes that offer cheaper, simpler, more convenient products or services aimed at the lower end of the market are key to the survival of the industry. They further believe that only a whole host of large and small changes—"disruptive innovations"—in technologies and business models that "sneak up from the bottom" can end the health care crisis. These disruptive innovations should come from workers in the trenches who know what would work better. Disruptive innovations in the usual setting for health care may already be underway as more care moves away from the hospital site.

HEALTH CARE PROVIDER ECONOMICS

Economic risk is borne by individuals, as well as by organizations. Both individuals and organizations may experience actual or perceived pressure to provide less health care service than is optimal in order to contain costs. Individual professionals risk what can be referred to as "dumbing down" of their respective professions. Dumbing down occurs when cost-saving strategies include using individuals with less knowledge to perform health care services usually performed by people with advanced knowledge. When this happens, the quality of the services delivered may decrease without actual harm occurring to patients and without patient recognition that the services are not optimal. If the enterprise is willing to provide less-than-optimal services to save money, those with the advanced knowledge may face loss of job security. Eventually, if care is judged to be inadequate or inappropriate, there may be risk of expensive litigation that can threaten both individuals and the organization with loss of licensure and livelihood.

Organizations' attempts to provide more economical care by changing the mix of caregivers is ultimately regulated by the respective state's practice acts (laws) with their accompanying rules. State nursing and medical practice acts define the scope of practitioner practice. Both types of acts regulate the practice components that can be delegated and the accountability that follows delegation of care. The law determines the extent to which an organization can stipulate that medical care or nursing care will be managed by delegation of that care in order to capture fiscal economies.

Individual providers such as practitioners and therapists receiving direct payment from insurers bear risk

REAL WORLD INTERVIEW

The Joint Commission (JC) is a nonprofit organization that is committed to continuously improve the safety and quality of health care provided to the public. The JC accomplishes this mission primarily through regular inspection and survey of health care organizations by a multidisciplinary professional team using extensive standardized measures of facility, clinical care, and material standards that support improvement in quality. A health care organization is assigned a numeric score that must meet a minimum level for the enterprise to be accredited. The JC currently accredits nearly 19,000 health care organizations in the United States, including burn hospitals and home care organizations, and more than 8,000 organizations that provide long-term care or behavioral health care, as well as laboratory and ambulatory services. Extensive education about the nature of quality and how to best achieve it is also provided to health care enterprises by the JC.

Health care organizations commit a great deal of time and energy to preparing for both prescheduled and "surprise" on-site surveys in order to successfully comply with the JC standards and receive a favorable accreditation status. The JC standards are developed through a definitive process of input from the field, expert consultation, and research to validate the standard as a measure of quality.

Sally A. Sample, RN, MN, ND, DSc, FAAN
Nurse at Large, Board of Governors, Joint Commission
Tucson, Arizona

REAL WORLD INTERVIEW

One generally does not associate nurse practice acts with nursing economics. However, a connection can be formulated. Nurse practice acts delineate scope of practice and define the educational preparation necessary to perform nursing acts. These laws restrict the health care agencies from unilaterally determining that an RN, practical nurse, or nursing assistant may work beyond their scope of practice. The agencies must conform to the law and employ qualified nurses, which invariably may impact health care costs.

Anita Ristau, RN, MS
Executive Director, Vermont State Board of Nursing
Montpelier, Vermont

when they must lower their usual fees to a flat rate in order to be included for payment by the HMO. A catch-22 exists for individual providers. If the provider agrees to participate in an HMO as a preferred provider, a lower payment rate may be part of the agreement. If the provider chooses not to participate in an HMO as a preferred provider, there is risk of attracting only the limited number of patients willing and able to pay out-of-pocket fee-for-service rates. To minimize their own expenses for providing services, individual providers regulate the amount and selection of services they provide, as well as the time spent with each patient. As a result, patients may be dissatisfied with the services and choose an alternate provider.

Patients bear the risk of being unable to access services they regard as optimal, or that they perceive as bearing the least risk of harm. Clearly, frivolous services are not available under the managed care philosophy, but patients may find themselves co-opted from their demands for health care services by incentives to accept less expensive levels of service. Their out-of-pocket expense, or co-payment, is usually considerably lower if they accept care from a member of the PPO than if they choose to obtain

EVIDENCE FROM THE LITERATURE

Citation: Nosek, L. (1986). Explanation of hospital stay by nursing diagnoses, medical diagnoses, and social position. (Doctoral dissertation, Case Western Reserve University, 1986). *Dissertation Abstracts International, 47*(07B), 00215. (University Microfilms No. AAG8622844).

Discussion: The importance of this research is becoming more evident as RNs continue to assume broader authority and responsibility for clinical decision making, for management of clinical systems, and for operational supervision of multiple and diverse personnel. The findings have significant economic implication at a time when health care enterprises are struggling to balance quality and cost through innovative use of human and material resources. The study describes the amount of variation in length of hospital stay explained by 127 nursing diagnoses, 288 diagnosis-related groups of medical diagnoses, and 8 demographic descriptors of social and economic status. These three elements explain a very high proportion of the total variation, 71.48%. Of that, 59.98% of the variation is attributed to nursing diagnoses; an additional 11.12% to medical diagnoses; and merely 0.38% is attributed to social position descriptors. The decision about when a patient is able to be discharged, then, is based on that patient's progress toward independence from nursing care, a concept consistent with Henderson's 1978 definition of nursing. The proposal that emerges from the findings is that while practitioners may be best able to determine the need for hospital admission, decisions about when hospital discharge could best occur and the appropriate sequential site for the patient's health care could best be managed by nurses.

Implications for Practice: Hospital length of stay (LOS) continues to be reduced. No longer is the discharge criterion independent from the need for skilled nursing care. Often, independence from skilled nursing care is not accomplished for several days, or even weeks, following acute care hospital discharge. Rather, hospital discharge involves transfer of the management and delivery of skilled nursing care from an acute care hospital to a less expensive site for provision of skilled care, such as a rehabilitation, home care, or hospice care organization. The findings of this study suggest that the most appropriate clinician to make the discharge decision is the RN responsible for the patient's discharge planning because that is the person most knowledgeable about the patient's needs for ongoing nursing care. The quality implications for such an innovation include transfer to the most appropriate level of nursing care to manage the nursing diagnoses, increased assurance of safe passage across the health care system, and reducing the risk of patient abandonment. Cost implications include facilitation of discharge through decreasing the wait time for discharge orders and thereby decreasing the consumption of multidisciplinary goods and services.

CASE STUDY 4-1

Y ou have just been hired as a nurse in a home care agency. One of the first things you noticed when you took a tour of the facility during your interview process was the disarray of the supply area. In fact, as you peered into the area, you overheard a staff member letting off frustration at once again not being able to find the supplies he needed for his day's assignments. Although she looked a bit sheepish, your tour guide quickly dismissed the incident, stating that a STAT delivery of the supplies could easily and promptly be arranged. Now that you are an employee, you, too, are having difficulty locating things in that supply area. Broken and outdated supplies take up significant space and new supplies sit unopened in stacks around the room. No one seems to have the time or interest to change the situation. You volunteer to lead a team effort to improve both the quality and the cost impact of the lack of organization in the supply area.

What method will you use to identify the issues?

What are some of the issues the staff might identify?

What are some of the options the staff might identify to address the issues?

How will you implement the options chosen?

care from a provider that is not a member of the PPO. Employers who provide health insurance as part of an employee's compensation package choose the insurance plan most economical for the employer, not necessarily the plan providing the best quality (Finkler, 2001).

Authors of the two seminal magnet hospital studies (McClure, Poulin, Sovie, & Wandelt, 1983; Kramer, 1990) eloquently concluded that a high level of performance by RNs is inseparable from high-quality patient care. Protagonists of disruptive innovation as the answer to the health care crisis believe that most ailments are relatively straightforward disorders whose diagnosis and treatment tap but a small fraction of what medical practitioners are educated to do and what nurse practitioners do so capably. They point out that most of the powerful innovations that disrupted other industries did so by enabling a larger population of less-skilled people to do, in a more convenient and less expensive way, things that historically were carried out only by a defined group of "experts." The findings of the cited studies are consistent with the magnet hospital findings and with disruptive innovation as an appropriate tool for change.

KEY CONCEPTS

- Health care economics is grounded in past values and culture. Nearly 150 years ago, Florence Nightingale recognized that the resources being used to care for sick people ought to be tracked and analyzed to improve clinical and business outcomes.

- Contemporary health care is characterized as a business struggling to balance cost and quality. Patients are fearful that health care is rapidly becoming unaffordable and are demanding care at a reasonable cost.

- In the United States, multiple programs exist to pay for health care. Managed care is the most common non-governmental structure for health care payment, with a variety of health maintenance organizations (HMOs) operating independently, and offering a variety of health insurance packages.

- Government programs for eligible individuals are tax supported. Other industrialized countries around the world offer tax-supported socialized health care to every citizen through centralized or decentralized programs at about half of the U.S. per capita cost.

- Futurists agree that significant change will occur in the health care industry. They predict that the mechanism of change will be tumultuous. Futurists believe the focus on value received for dollars spent, the inextricable link of cost and quality, will grow.

- The ability to track and manage both cost and quality is critical. To achieve the organization's economic and quality goals, administrators and clinicians at all levels and in diverse health care organizations must focus on a common mission and consistent vision.

- Accounting for the cost of nursing care must be simplified and standardized. Regression analysis, patient classification systems (PCS), and relative value units (RVU) computations are complex, time consuming, and lack the support of both administrators and clinicians.

- Quality measurement in organizations is supplemented by external regulatory bodies that oversee safety and quality on behalf of society. Satisfaction indices may be measured both internally and externally and then compared to the performance of similar organizations.

- Nurses at all levels of all health care organizations are responsible for basic economic processes.

- An economic break-even formula can be used to compute the cost of health care equipment.

- The Nosek-Androwich Profit: Quality Matrix identifies the balance between quality and profit.

KEY TERMS

altruism	margin
break-even point	patient classification
budget	system (PCS)
direct cost	payer
economics	preferred provider
egoism	organization (PPO)
enterprise	reengineering
ethics	relative value unit (RVU)
failure to rescue	stakeholder
fixed cost	variable cost
indirect cost	

REVIEW QUESTIONS

1. Identify the health care insurer that contributes the largest proportion of the health care dollar in the United States.
   A. U.S. Government
   B. Private health insurance
   C. Out-of-pocket payers
   D. Other private payers

2. Compare the life expectancy of women in Canada to the life expectancy of women in the United States.
   A. Canadian women have the same life expectancy as U.S. women.
   B. Canadian women have a shorter life expectancy than U.S. women.
   C. Canadian women can expect to die about three years after U.S. women.

D. Canadian women can expect to live six years longer than U.S. women born in 2006.

3. Select the most important reason for managing health care as a business.
   A. Patients need to know how the system works.
   B. Profit must be assured for the system to continue.
   C. Business ethics assure that patients are treated fairly.
   D. A competitive market keeps providers more responsive to patients.

4. Differentiate which of the following documents articulates the purpose for which a health care organization is in business?
   A. Strategic plan
   B. Mission statement
   C. Vision statement
   D. Corporate philosophy

5. Distinguish which of the following nurse leaders was not mentioned in this chapter as having a perspective on economics?
   A. Nightingale
   B. Sample
   C. Barton
   D. Henderson

6. Select the concept that is synonymous with profit.
   A. Dividends
   B. Billing privileges
   C. Contribution to margin
   D. Certificate of Need

REVIEW ACTIVITIES

1. Interview the chief financial officer of a health care organization to gain an understanding of how various costs are managed. Use the following questions to guide the interview:

   What method is used to measure nursing cost?
   What level of confidence does Fiscal Services have in its accuracy and why?
   How are contracts with various insurers such as Medicare, Medicaid, preferred provider organizations (PPOs), and Blue Cross discounted?
   What percentage of profit did the organization make last year and how was it allocated? How typical was this?
   Which therapists' services are billed directly?

2. Consult a seasoned member of the medical staff for a personal perspective on the adjustments in practice that person made, if any, related to cost and quality issues in practice as his or her career unfolded. Compare and contrast what you discover to the experiences of a second person you consult who has been in practice for only the past 10 years. What level of passion about the discussion was demonstrated by each interviewee? What did they view as their greatest challenge?

3. Explore with the chief nursing officer what the most challenging clinical economic issue currently is for nursing in the organization and how it is being addressed.

4. Using the formulas provided in this chapter, determine the cost of nursing care for the past 24 hours for your work unit or for any manageable unit to which you have access.

EXPLORING THE WEB

What sites could you recommend to a colleague interested in tracking health care cost trends over time?

- Centers for Medicare and Medicaid Services: *www.cms.hhs.gov*

- Search an alternate government bureau site. What does the Bureau of Labor Statistics offer at *www.stats.bls.gov*

  Is it relevant to cost or quality issues?

- Search the following Websites for information of interest to nurses:
  www.florence-nightingale.co.uk
  www.aahn.org
  www.onhealth.com
  www.medexplorer.com
  www.medicarerights.org

REFERENCES

Abdellah, F., Beland, I., Martin, A., & Matheney, R. (1960). *Patient centered approaches to nursing.* New York: Macmillan.

Agnes, M. (2000). (Ed.) *Webster's new world collegiate dictionary* (4th ed.). Foster City, CA: IDG Books Worldwide.

Aiken, L. H., Clarke, S. P., Cheung, R. B., Sloane, D. M., & Silber, J. H. (2003, Sept.) . Educational levels of hospital nurses and surgical patient mortality. *Journal of the American Medical Association, 290*(12), 1617–1623.

Barry, P. (2006, June). [AARP Bulletin]. (p. 16–18).

Carpenter, D. (2006, May). Attention, investors: The Q-revolution is spreading. *Hospitals & Health Networks,* 4–8.

Carter, G. (2006, June). "Sick tax" would hurt everyone. *Hospitals & Health Networks,* 6, 8.

Centers for Medicare and Medicaid Services. (2006). Changes in sources of funds for health care. Retrieved June 20, 2006, from http://www.cms.hhs.gov/statistics

Centers for Medicare and Medicaid Services Office of the Actuary, National Health Statistics Group. (2006). Retrieved March 31, 2006, from http://www.iii.org/media

Chassin, M. R., & Galvin, R. W. (1998). The urgent need to improve health care quality. Institute of Medicine National Roundtable on Health Care Quality. *Journal of the American Medical Association, 280*(11), 1000–1005.

Christensen, C., Bohmer, R., & Kenagy, J. (2000, September/October). Will disruptive innovations cure health care? *Harvard Business Review,* 102–112, 199.

Finkler, S. (2001). *Budgeting concepts for nurse managers* (3rd ed.). Philadelphia: Saunders.

Finkler, S., & Kovner, C. (2000). *Financial management for nurse managers and executives* (2nd ed.). Philadelphia: Saunders.

Hall, L. M., Pink, L., Lalonde, M., Murphy, G. T., O'Brien-Pallas, L., Laschinger, H. K., et al. (2006). Decision making for nurse staffing. *Policy Politics in Nursing Practice, 7*(4), 261–269.

Henderson, V., & Nite, G. (1978). *Principles and practice of nursing* (6th ed.). New York: Macmillan.

Infant mortality rate. (2006). Retrieved June 20, 2006, from http://www.en.Wikipedia.org

Institute for Healthcare Improvement (IHI). Getting started kit: Prevent central line infections. Retrieved March 20, 2007 from http://www.ihi.org/NR/rdonlyres/of4cc102-CS64-4436-AC3A-OC57B1202872/o/Ccentrallineshowtoguidefind720.pdf

Kilner, J. (1992). *Who lives? Who dies? Ethical criteria in patient selection.* New Haven, CT: Yale University Press.

Kramer, M. (1990, June). Trends to watch at the magnet hospitals. *Nursing90,* 67–74.

Liberman, A., & Rotarius, T. (2001). Managed care evolution—where did it come from and where is it going? In E. Hein (Ed.), *Nursing Issues in the 21st century: Perspectives from the literature.* Philadelphia: Lippincott.

Life expectancy. (2006). Retrieved June 20, 2006, from http://www.en.Wikipedia.org

Male and female life expectancy. (2006). Retrieved June 20, 2006, from http://www.photius.com

McClure, M., Poulin, M., Sovie, M., & Wandelt, M. (1983). *Magnet hospitals: Attraction and retention of professional nurses.* Kansas City, MO: American Academy of Nursing.

National Coalition on Health Care. (2006). Health care cost as percentage of gross domestic product. Retrieved June 20, 2006, from http://www.nchc.org

Nightingale, F. (1859). *Notes on hospitals;* being two papers read before the National Association for the Promotion of Social Science, at Liverpool in October, 1858. With evidence given to the Royal Commissioners on the State of the Army in 1857 (2nd ed.). London: Parker.

Nosek, L. J. (1986). Explanation of hospital stay by nursing diagnoses, medical diagnoses, and social position. (Doctoral dissertation, Case Western Reserve University, 1986). *Dissertation Abstracts International, 47*(07B), 00215. (University Microfilms No. AAG8622844).

Reverby, S. (1987). *Ordered to care: The dilemma of American nursing, 1850–1945.* New York: Cambridge.

Savage, G., Hoelscher, M., & Walker, E. (1999). International health care: A comparison of the United States, Canada, and Western Europe. In L. Wolper (Ed.), *Health care administration: Planning, implementing, and managing organized delivery systems* (3rd ed). Gaithersburg, MD: Aspen.

Serb, C. (2006, June). Financial fitness test: 10 Ways to get in shape for a new payment era. *Hospitals & Health Networks,* 34–36, 38, 40, 49.

SUGGESTED READINGS

(2006, May). Aging baby boomers will have less impact than other trends on inpatient needs. *Hospitals & Health Networks,* 73.

Borkowski, N. (Ed). (2005). *Organizational behavior in health care.* Sudbury, MA: Jones and Bartlett.

California Health Care Foundation. (2005, March). Health care costs 101. Retrieved March 19, 2007, from http://www.chcf.org

Cleverly, W. O., & Cameron, A. E. (2002). *Cost concepts and decision making. Essentials of health care finance.* Gaithersburg, MD: Aspen.

Dunham-Taylor, J., & Pinczuk, J. Z. (2006). *Health care financial management for nurse managers: Merging the heart with the dollar.* Sudbury, MA: Jones and Bartlett.

Fortin, L., & Douglas, K. (2006). Shift bidding technology: A substantial return on investment. *Nurse Leader, 4*(1), 26–28.

Gullatte, M. (2005). *Nursing management: Principles and practice.* Pittsburgh: Oncology Nursing Society.

Henry, J. Kaiser Family Foundation. (2005, Sept.). Employee health benefits: 2005. Annual Survey.

Herzlinger, R. (2006, May). Why innovation in healthcare is so hard. *Harvard Business Review, 84*(5), 58–66, 156.

Hospitals & Health Networks. (2006, May). U.S. ranks lowest of six affluent nations in patients' opinions, health care equity. *Author, 80*(5), 74.

Malloch, K., & Porter-O'Grady, T. (2005). *The quantum leader: Applications for the new world of work.* Sudbury, MA: Jones and Bartlett.

National League for Nursing Public Policy Action Center. (2006). Health Resources and Services Administration 2004 National Sample Survey of Registered Nurses, p. 2. Retrieved February 28, 2006, from http://capwiz.com/nln/home

Premier Hospital Quality Incentive Demonstration. (2006). Retrieved January 30, 2006 from http://www.cms.hhs.gov/Hospital-QualityInits/35_HospitalPremier.asp

Sandrick, K. (2006, Feb.). A tale of two turnarounds. *Hospitals & Health Networks,* 66–70.

U.S. Census Bureau. (2005). IDB Summary Demographic Data, Canada, Germany, United Kingdom, United States. Retrieved March 31, 2006, from http://www.census.gov

Watson Wyatt Worldwide. (2006). Health care costs: Up, down and around the world. Retrieved June 20, 2006, from http://www.WatsonWyattWorldwide.com

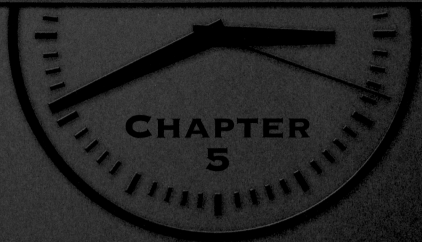

CHAPTER 5

Evidence-Based Health Care

Rinda Alexander, PhD, RN, CS ⊕ Amy Androwich O'Malley, MSN, RN ⊕
Ida M. Androwich, PhD, RN, BC, FAAN

Not all "literature" is "evidence" and not all evidence is valid or relevant to the patient at hand (Dr. Feldstein, Wisconsin Medical Journal, 2005).

OBJECTIVES

Upon completion of this chapter, the reader should be able to:

1. Discuss the history of evidence-based care (EBC) in nursing.

2. Develop an understanding of evidence and its use in decision making.

3. Assume responsibility for developing an evidence-based approach to patient care.

4. Understand the terminology used to describe types of evidence and evidence-based care processes.

5. Develop an informed view of the current state of evidence-based care and an understanding of the role of nursing in evidence-based decision making.

6. Apply the steps needed to incorporate evidence-based care in practice.

7. Conduct a search for evidence on a given topic.

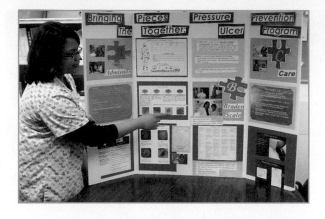

You are at the annual Nurses' Day luncheon, and the vice president for nursing has just announced that your institution is applying for magnet status. The nursing manager of your unit and three other units stop to chat. She said that she is concerned because she has noticed variability in the use of nursing interventions on the units and that this variability may be negatively affecting patient outcomes in the institution. In light of the plan to achieve magnet designation, she would like to see all units incorporate evidence in patient care processes, and she wants to appoint you to a task force to consider using evidence-based care (EBC) as a means of reducing variability and improving patient outcomes. This scenario is becoming more and more common in health care institutions as managers of care explore new ways to improve the quality of care.

What do you know about EBC?

What are some things you need to know before you can accept the appointment to the task force?

How will you prepare yourself for the task?

Many professionals and society in general accept the position that nurses are the coordinators of care within institutions. However, as the health care system continues to evolve, nurses and other health professionals must consider new ways to deliver more effective and efficient interventions. In fact, there is probably no greater challenge for nursing than to ensure that we have the competencies needed in the twenty-first century for evidence-based health care delivery. Nursing leaders and managers are particularly well placed to see that health care institutions have EBC and work processes in place that provide professional nurses with support to meet new challenges in the clinical delivery of care. **Evidence-based care (EBC)** is clinically competent care based on the best scientific evidence available. It incorporates clinical expertise and the patient's preferences. All nurses have responsibility for promoting patient care based on the best scientific evidence available.

The purpose of this chapter is to define what constitutes evidence for clinical practice, to discuss the

importance of EBC to patients and nursing, and to develop individual strategies to provide EBC. Future trends in health care will require the use of sophisticated evidence-based tools to deliver care and measure outcomes of care. This suggests that nursing must become more comfortable using a scientific process driven by evidence-based standards and practice guidelines while also emphasizing continuing quality improvement. Refer to Table 5-1 for an overview of research terminology useful in developing skill in EBC.

HISTORY OF EBC

The term evidence-based medicine (EBM) was coined at McMaster Medical School in Canada during the 1980s. D. L. Sackett, well known in the EBM and EBC movement, along with his Oxford colleagues, encouraged EBM as a way to integrate individual clinical medical experience with external clinical evidence using a systematic research approach. Sackett, Rosenberg, Gray, Haynes, and Richardson, in their classic 1996 definition, define **evidence-based medicine (EBM)** as ". . . the conscientious, explicit, and judicious use of current best evidence in making decisions about the care of individual patients. The practice of EBM means integrating individual clinical expertise with the best available external clinical evidence from systematic research."

REAL WORLD INTERVIEW

There are several key components of an effective strategy for the implementation of evidence-based practice. First, it is essential to find a source of evidence-based content that is developed using a strict and rigorous methodology that includes both review and classification of the sources of the evidence and routine updating. Second, the evidence-based content itself must be efficient for clinicians to use at the bedside. This efficiency factor can be accomplished through easy-to-read, succinct summaries of the evidence. And also, it can be achieved by integrating evidence-based content in order sets, plans of care, and documentation forms. This integration delivers evidence-based content and direction to the clinician at the bedside, at the point of decision making.

Patricia S. Button, EdD, RN, Director
Nursing Content, Zynx Health
Lyme, New Hampshire

TABLE 5-1   RESEARCH TERMINOLOGY

Absolute benefit increase (ABI)	The absolute arithmetic difference in rates of good outcomes between experimental and control groups, calculated as the rate of good outcomes in the experimental group minus the rate of good outcomes in the control group.
Best practice	In application, best practice includes the use of rigorous scientific evidence to support the effectiveness of specific clinical interventions for explicit patients, groups, or populations; implementation monitoring to assure accurate application; and outcome measurement to validate effectiveness.
Case-control study	A research study designed to determine the association between an exposure of interest and an outcome. Those cases with the outcome (study group) are compared to those cases without the outcome (control group) to identify the effect of exposure to the suspected harmful agent on the study group.
Clinical practice guidelines (or practice guidelines)	Systematically developed statements or recommendations to assist practitioner and patient decisions about appropriate health care for specific clinical circumstances. Practice guidelines present indications for performing a test, procedure, or intervention, or the proper management for specific clinical problems. Guidelines may be developed by government agencies, institutions, organizations such as professional societies or governing boards, or by expert panels.
Cohort study	When used to study potential causes of a disorder, it is a prospective investigation in which a group (cohort) of individuals who do not have evidence of an outcome of interest but who are exposed to the suspected cause are compared with a concurrent cohort who are also free of the outcome but were not exposed to the suspected cause. Both cohorts are then followed forward in time to compare the incidence of the outcome of interest.
Control group	Subjects in an experiment who do not receive the experimental treatment and whose performance provides a baseline against which the effects of the treatment can be measured.
Correlational research	Research that explores the interrelationships among variables of interest without any active intervention on the part of the researcher.
Dependent variable	The outcome variable of interest; the variable that is hypothesized or thought to depend on or be caused by another variable, called the independent variable.
Descriptive research	Research studies that have as their main objective the accurate portrayal of the characteristics of people, situations, or groups, and the frequency with which certain phenomena occur.
Evidence-based health care	The conscientious, explicit, and judicious use of current best evidence in making decisions about the care of individual patients. Evidence-based clinical practice requires integration of individual clinical expertise and patient preferences with the best available external clinical evidence from systematic research, and consideration of available resources.
Follow-up study	A study undertaken to determine the subsequent development of individuals with a specified condition or a study of people who have received a specified treatment.

TABLE 5-1 CONTINUED

Health outcomes	All possible changes in health status that may occur for a defined population or that may be associated with exposure to an intervention. These include changes in the length and quality of life as a result of detecting or treating disease when it is present, the false security associated with failing to detect disease when it is present, and the mislabeling associated with detecting disease when it is really absent.
Independent variable	The variable that is believed to cause or influence the dependent variable; in experimental research, the independent variable is the variable that is manipulated.
Integrative review	A type of evidence summary; concludes with implications from research for practice.
Longitudinal study	A study designed to collect data at more than one point in time, in contrast to a cross-sectional study.
Matching	A deliberate process to make a study group and comparison group comparable with respect to factors or confounders that are unrelated to the purpose of the investigation but that might interfere with the interpretation of the study's findings.
Meta-analysis	A procedure for quantitatively combining the results of many research studies that measure the same outcome into a single pooled or summary estimate of the results.
Nonexperimental research	A study in which the researcher collects data without introducing an intervention.
Number needed to treat (NNT)	The number of patients who need to be treated over a specific period of time to achieve one additional good outcome. When discussing NNT, it is important to specify the intervention, its duration, and the good outcome. If risk of an event is high, the NNT is low and vice versa; NNT aids in deciding if benefit of intervention is worth the potential risk.
Outcomes research	Research designed to document the effectiveness of health care services and the end results of patient care.
Prospective study	A study that begins with an examination of presumed causes (e.g., cigarette smoking) and then goes forward in time to observe presumed effects (e.g., lung cancer).
Qualitative analysis	The organization and interpretation of nonnumeric data for the purpose of discovering important underlying dimensions and patterns of relationships.
Quantitative analysis	The manipulation of numeric data through statistical procedures for the purpose of describing phenomena or assessing the magnitude and reliability of relationships among them.
Quasi-experiment	An intervention study in which subjects are not randomly assigned to treatment conditions, but the researcher exercises certain controls to enhance the internal validity of the research results .
Randomized clinical trial	A study in which individuals are randomly allocated to receive or not receive an experimental preventive, therapeutic, or diagnostic procedure. Individuals are then followed to determine the effect of the intervention.
Relative risk (or risk ratio)	Ratio of the risk of an event among an exposed population to the risk among the unexposed.

(Continues)

TABLE 5-1   RESEARCH TERMINOLOGY (CONTINUED)

Research utilization	The use of some aspect of a study in an application unrelated to the original research.
Retrospective design	A study design that begins with the manifestation of the dependent variable in the present (e.g., lung cancer) and then searches for the presumed cause occurring in the past (e.g., cigarette smoking).
Systematic review	Type of evidence summary that uses a rigorous scientific approach to combine results from a body of original research studies into a clinically meaningful whole.
Time series design	A quasi-experimental design that involves the collection of data over an extended period of time, with multiple data collection points both prior to and after the introduction of an intervention. The time series design monitors the occurrence of outcomes or end points over a number of cycles and determines if the pattern changes coincide with the intervention.
Translation	Translation is the process that transforms the evidence from a systematic review into clinical practice guidelines.
Treatment effect	The results of comparative clinical studies can be expressed using various intervention effect measures, for example, absolute risk reduction, relative risk reduction, odds ratio, number needed to treat, and effect size. The appropriateness of using these to express an intervention effect, and whether probabilities, means, or medians are used to calculate them depends upon the type of outcome variable used to measure health outcomes.
Variable	An attribute of a person or object that varies (i.e., takes on different values) within the population under study (e.g., body temperature, heart rate).

Source: Compiled with information from Polit, D., & Beck, C. (2004). *Nursing research: Principles and methods* (7th ed.). Philadelphia: Lippincott; and DiCenso, A., Guyatt, G., & Ciliska, D. (2005). *Evidence-based nursing: A guide to clinical practice.* St. Louis, MO: Elsevier Mosby.

EBC is a newer term and has broadened the EBM methods to include other clinical health care providers. Currently, there are a number of excellent sites for finding information about evidence-based nursing and evidence-based practice (EBP), which are listed at the end of this chapter. Since the early work of the McMaster's group, methods for review and summarization of evidence have undergone dramatic advances. A. Cochrane of the Cochrane Library group was a pioneer in the movement and preparation of high-quality reviews. In 1978, Cochrane suggested that only 15 to 20% of practitioner interventions were supported by objective evidence. This led to much variation in patient care delivery and patient care outcomes. Since then, with increasing technology, there have been major improvements in our ability to access information. Haase-Herrick (2004) calls this the "journey to evidence-based health care" and states that it "... requires a shift from knowing a static body of information to knowing how to access the evolving knowledge base to support the needs of those whose care is managed."

THE ACE STAR MODEL OF KNOWLEDGE TRANSFORMATION

Table 5-2 provides information on the ACE Star Model of Knowledge Transformation which is useful in assisting with the transformation of research evidence into practice.

TABLE 5-2   **ACE STAR MODEL OF KNOWLEDGE TRANSFORMATION**

The ACE Star Model provides a framework for systematically putting evidence-based practice (EBP) processes into operation. Configured as a simple five-point star, the model illustrates five major stages of knowledge transformation:

- Knowledge discovery
- Evidence summary
- Translation into practice recommendations
- Integration into practice
- Evaluation

Evidence-based processes and methods vary from one point on the Star Model to the next.

STAR POINT 1. Knowledge Discovery: In this knowledge-generating stage, new knowledge is discovered through traditional research methodologies and scientific inquiry. Research results are generated through the conduct of a single study.

STAR POINT 2. Evidence Summary: Evidence summary is the first unique step in EBP. The task is to synthesize the body of research knowledge into a single, meaningful statement of the state of the science.

STAR POINT 3. Translation into Practice Recommendations: The transformation of evidence summaries into actual practice requires two stages—translation of evidence into practice recommendations and integration into practice.

STAR POINT 4. Integration into Practice: This step involves changing both individual and organizational practices through formal and informal channels.

STAR POINT 5. Evaluation: The final state in knowledge transformation is evaluation of the impact of EBP on patient health outcomes, provider and patient satisfaction, efficacy, efficiency, economic analysis, and health status.

Source: Compiled with information from Stevens, K. R. (2004). ACE star model of EBP: Knowledge transformation. Academic Center for Evidence-based Practice. The University of Texas Health Science Center at San Antonio. Retrieved September 8, 2006, from http://www.acestar.uthscsa.edu

IMPORTANCE OF EBC

Why is EBC important? About 100 people die each day because the current paper-based health care system introduces error or delays in treatment or limits what health care professionals know (Hudak, 2004). Grol and Grimshaw (2003) found that only 10 to 20% of clinician actions are supported by scientific evidence as to the efficacy of the action or treatment; 20 to 25% of care provided is not needed or is potentially harmful, and 30 to 40% of patients do not receive care according to present scientific evidence. Consequently, there is nothing more important to patients and professional nursing than evidence-based clinical interventions that can be linked to clinical outcomes and used as a basis for care within the institution. However, there has been a lack of generally agreed-upon standards or processes that are based on evidence. This lack of standards has been addressed of late with the development of EBC.

Generally speaking, nursing, medicine, health care institutions and health policy makers recognize EBC as care based on state-of-the-art science reports. It is a process approach to collecting, reviewing, interpreting, critiquing, and evaluating research and other relevant literature for direct application to patient care. EBC uses evidence from research; performance data; quality improvement studies such as hospital or nursing report cards, program evaluations, and surveys; national and local consensus recommendations of experts; and clinical experience.

The EBC process further involves the integrating of both clinician-observed evidence and research-directed evidence. This then leads to state-of-the-art integration of available knowledge and evidence in a particular area of clinical concern that can be evaluated and measured through outcomes of care.

Applying the best available evidence does not guarantee good decisions, yet it is one of the keys to improving outcomes affecting health. EBC should be viewed as

REAL WORLD INTERVIEW

With over 20 years in nursing and hospice care, I have increasingly realized that a large part of the health care system, both doctors and nurses, do not understand the need for adequate pain control. One of my patients was a young man with cancer of the throat. He had received a radical laryngectomy and had had his tongue removed. He was left with a tracheotomy and was rendered speechless. His doctors at a top-rated university hospital seemed amazed that he was in as much pain as he was. It was not until he entered hospice care, where we emphasized an evidence-based holistic pain protocol, that he received some degree of comfort. This man was an exceptional person who never complained. He also had exceptionally strong support from his wife and family.

As nurses, please advocate for adequate pain relief for your patient. I have seen over and over that patients do not abuse the medications or the system. Our hospice saying is, "Meet the patients where they are, not where you think they should be!" When our patients are comfortable, there is peace for everyone.

Sylvia Komyatte, RN, MPS
Chaplain, Hospice
Munster, Indiana

REAL WORLD INTERVIEW

We believe that a patient admitted to a small rural hospital should expect the same level of safety as those in large urban facilities. To this end, Appalachian Regional Healthcare is striving to provide an evidence-based practice approach as the foundation for our bar-coded medication administration system. This has included a focused, evidence-based literature review of best practices, and we are building them into our care. We recognize that incorporating technology into the workflow of the front line staff is a major culture change. Therefore, we have studied the current practice and plan to work alongside of the staff encouraging them to take the journey with us as we use systems and technology to advance practice and improve patient safety. We are fortunate to have a bright and caring nursing staff, dedicated to incorporating current best evidence into their patient care.

Beatrice A. Miller, BSN, RN
Clinical Informatics Coordinator
Appalachian Regional Healthcare
Whitesburg, Kentucky

the highest standard of care so long as critical thinking and sound clinical judgment support it. Nurses and practitioners will always need to search for the best evidence available to support their clinical decisions. Sometimes, there is little research backing for clinical actions. In that case, nurse and practitioner clinicians should use their critical thinking skills and apply the consensus of experts. Institutions of care have a responsibility to provide nurses and others in health care with an environment supportive of EBC.

Demonstrating that outcomes of health care are effective, efficient, and safe is a major responsibility for nursing. It is evident as we consider the art and science of nursing that recognizing the importance of EBC and stimulating an environment within institutions in which evidence-based models of care can flourish will result in improved outcomes of clinical care. Table 5-3 summarizes trends driving the development of EBC in nursing.

A common misconception about EBC is that it ignores patient values and preferences. This is not the case; rather, the nurse works with the patient in deciding treatment options based on which tradeoffs the patient is willing to accept.

NURSING AND EBC

It was inevitable that nursing would move to EBC. One of the earlier proponents for EBC in nursing was the Joanna Briggs Institute for Evidence Based Nursing and Midwifery

TABLE 5-3	CURRENT ISSUES AND TRENDS DRIVING DEVELOPMENT OF EBC IN NURSING

- Significant contribution to the body of clinical research by nursing science
- Need for decreased variability in implementation of nursing practice
- Need for implementation of research in practice to improve effectiveness and efficiency
- Societal demands for evidence-based, clinically competent care (Institute of Medicine, 1999 and 2001)
- Growth of advanced practice roles with development of prescriptive power and evidence-based diagnostic decision making
- Increased experience in clinical pathways, standards, protocols, and algorithms
- Increase in integrated systematic reviews of research studies found in the nursing, medical, and health care literature
- Need for outcome data to guide patient care
- Explosion in information technology with better-organized, rapidly retrievable information in the literature and on the Internet
- Improved knowledge base facilitating research capable of supporting EBC models
- Need to collaborate in complex decision making with patients and other members of the health care team
- Requirement for evidence-based standards of care implemented by the Joint Commission (JC) and National Database on Nursing Quality Indicators (NDNQI) (www.nursingquality.org)

(JBIEBN), established in 1996. Significant work has been done worldwide to implement EBC into Australian, Canadian and U.K. institutions of care.

In the United States, the Agency for Healthcare Research and Quality (AHRQ) has provided stimulus for the EBC movement through recognition of a need for evidence to guide practice throughout the health care system. In 1997, the AHRQ launched its initiative establishing twelve evidence-based practice centers. This initiative partnered AHRQ with other private and public organizations in an effort to improve the quality, effectiveness, and appropriateness of care. The initiative is discussed later in this chapter.

ATTRIBUTES OF EBC

A new culture that can support EBC needs to evolve in institutions. There is a need to define the meaning of evidence in each agency, a need to begin to use the term *evidence* in daily practice, and a need to look for the best evidence when evaluating new goals and new programs. Where possible, the use of visible, formal supports for EBC should be encouraged as well as the development of systems in the health care agency that support EBC on an ongoing basis. According to Guyatt and Rennie (2002), EBC is an approach to patient care that involves two fundamental principles:

- Evidence alone is never sufficient to make a clinical decision
- EBC involves a hierarchy of evidence to guide decision making

In a landmark study completed as recently as 2005, Pravikoff, Tanner, and Pierce surveyed more than 2,000 nurses and found that while 64.5% of nurses report needing information weekly or several times a week, only 26.7% have received training in using tools to access evidence. Furthermore, only 11% of nurses state that they search for information from the evidence weekly or more often, and nearly half (48.5%) were not familiar with the term, *evidence-based practice*.

EVIDENCE: HOW IT IS DEVELOPED AND EVALUATED

The literature available to both nursing and medicine is immense, but only a small portion is immediately useful for answering clinical questions. To recognize that the available evidence in the literature for any clinical question exists at various levels can help nurses retrieve the highest level of evidence available for use in providing care. There are two major challenges that nurses face in

I have been a nurse for 39 years and have seen many changes in health care during that time. About five years ago, I had a ruptured brain aneurysm, which occurred after having an angiogram. I was airlifted to a nearby university hospital. The knowledge and competence of the air transport team was impeccable. I was glad to be in the hands of people who were up to date on the best way to care for me. They were definitely in control—a nice thing to have when you're not.

Before the surgery, I was unconscious, and my family was informed of the dangers and the necessity to either coil or clip the aneurysm. During the 14-hour operation, the neurosurgeon's nurse updated them periodically on my progress. During my entire hospital stay, she visited me daily and was available by pager if my husband had any questions, doubts, or fears. While I was in the ICU, I was the only patient cared for by one nurse for three days. Although I had short-term memory loss at the time, I do remember that I did not have any concerns about my needs not being met. In fact, I felt the nurses predicted the problems I had before I even vocalized them. I was given quality patient care, and as an RN, I am very proud to say that. I am back working as a nurse now, and my experience has given me a whole new level of understanding for patients. I am glad that the people who cared for me were up to date on the latest!

Janice Klepitch, RN
Office Nurse, Schererville, Indiana

using available evidence. The first is the rapidly growing body of scientific literature, that is, no unaided human being can read, recall, and act effectively on the volume of clinically relevant scientific literature (IOM, 2001). Each year, 10,000 new randomized clinical trials (RCTs) are introduced in the literature, and more than 350,000 studies have been identified by the Cochrane Collaboration alone (Grol & Grimshaw, 2003). Therefore, methods such as systematic reviews are required to synthesize all the research in one area into a meaningful, comprehensible summary.

The second challenge is that often the literature is not in a form that is suitable for application to practice but needs to be evaluated and transformed to be useful for clinical decision making. Table 5-4 provides a summary of recommended criteria for grading and leveling the scientific merit or strength of evidence.

The *Online Journal of Clinical Innovations* (OJCI), published by Cumulative Index to Nursing and Allied Health Literature (CINAHL), uses a slightly different method of evaluating and grading evidence, reflective of the types or sources of evidence and the strength of evidence that nurses may use (Tables 5-5 and 5-6).

CONDUCTING EVIDENCE REPORTS IN NURSING

For the new nurse, understanding how evidence is judged can seem to be a very complex task. However, experience in reviewing and critiquing research and using research in

Citation: Haller, K. (2006, Summer). Safe staffing saves lives. *John Hopkins Nursing, 4*(2), 16.

Discussion: Despite the recent focus on "safe" staffing nationally and internationally, there are few available policy statements that actually examine staffing in light of patient safety rather than workload. Much of what has been written or discussed on staffing really refers to nurse-patient ratios. We do not have good evidence to support our understanding of optimal levels of staffing or, conversely, minimal levels that are needed before patient safety is impacted. However, recent research demonstrates that institutions with higher levels of nurses have decreased nurse-sensitive complications in the areas of urinary tract infections and upper gastrointestinal bleeds, have fewer cases of hospital-acquired pneumonia, and have a decrease in the rate of shock and cardiac arrest.

Implications for Practice: There is evidence to support that the quality of care is increased with improved RN staffing. Although, we do not have evidence of optimal nurse patient ratios, we do know that improved staffing is associated with better patient outcomes.

TABLE 5-4   SCALE OF RESEARCH GRADES AND LEVELS

Grade of Research

A	Strongly recommend; good evidence
B	Recommend; at least fair evidence
C	No recommendation for or against; balance of benefits and harms too close to justify a recommendation
D	Recommend against; fair evidence is ineffective or harm outweighs the benefit
E	Evidence is insufficient to recommend for or against routinely; evidence is lacking or of poor quality; benefits and harms cannot be determined.

Level of Evidence

Level I	Meta-analysis of multiple studies
Level II	Experimental studies
Level III	Well-designed, quasi-experimental studies
Level IV	Well-designed, nonexperimental studies
Level V	Case reports and clinical examples

TABLE 5-5   TYPE OR SOURCE OF EVIDENCE

- Published research
- Published research utilization report
- Published quality improvement report
- Published meta-analysis
- Published systematic or integrative literature review
- Published review of the literature
- Policies, procedures, protocols
- Published guidelines
- Practice exemplars, stories, opinions
- General or background information/texts/reports
- Unpublished research, reviews, poster presentations, or other such materials
- Conference proceedings, abstracts, presentations

Source: CINAHL Information Systems. (2004). *The Online Journal of Clinical Innovations.* Reprinted with permission from CINAHL Information Systems, Glendale, California.

TABLE 5-6   **STRENGTH OF EVIDENCE**

- Supported by two or more clinical trials
- Supported by one clinical trial or two or more methodologically sound studies
- Supported by one methodologically sound study
- Supported by rigorous quality improvement study
- Supported by research utilization or clinical adoptions report using structured evaluation
- Supported by expert opinion
- Supported by strong consensus

Source: CINAHL Information Systems. (2004). *The Online Journal of Clinical Innovations.* Reprinted with permission from CINAHL Information Systems, Glendale, California.

TABLE 5-7   **METHOD FOR CONDUCTING EVIDENCE REPORTS IN NURSING**

Select a problem.	Risk Management has reported that falls in the evening on your unit seem excessive, and the plan is to try to reduce them using principles of EBC.
Review the evidence using a standard scheme for assigning strength and level to the evidence.	Using Tables 5-4 and 5-6, several well-designed, nonexperimental, methodologically sound, Level IV studies are found.
Summarize the evidence, including a statistical summary if appropriate.	The studies are summarized.
Report the results.	Report specific research results to the interdisciplinary team.
Make recommendations for potential clinical applications.	Discuss potential practice changes based on the evidence found in the evidence summary. Develop protocol for frequent assessment of patients who are weak or confused; insure that patients are reminded to ask for help to use the bathroom; place call lights within easy reach; use side rails to support, do not restrain patients, and so on, based on review of the evidence.
Implement agreed-upon practice changes.	Implement protocol and evaluate outcomes of practice changes.

---

clinical activities can be very rewarding. A framework to guide you in the process, such as that shown in Table 5-7, can be useful.

USING EBC REFERENCES

Several evidence-based sources are listed in Table 5-8.

EBC CENTERS IN THE UNITED STATES

As mentioned earlier, clinicians have coped with accusations for many years that only a small percentage of treatments provided have scientific foundations. Many within

TABLE 5-8   EVIDENCE-BASED RESOURCES

Resource	URL
National guideline clearinghouse, Agency for Health Care Quality and Research	www.guideline.gov
Evidence-Based Nursing	http://ebn.bmj.com
Sigma Theta Tau International	www.nursingsociety.org
Global evidence	www.globalevidence.com
Cochrane collaboration	www.cochrane.org
Joanna Briggs Institute for Evidence-Based Nursing and Midwifery	www.joannabriggs.edu.au
Sarah Cole Hirsh Institute for Best Nursing Practices Based on Evidence	http://fpb.case.edu
Evidence-Based Nursing Practice, Welch Library	www.welch.jhu.edu
Centre for Evidence-Based Nursing	www.york.ac.uk
Royal College of Nursing	www.rcn.org.uk
Registered Nurses' Association of Ontario	www.rnao.org
Gerontological Nursing Interventions Research Center (GNIRC)	www.nursing.uiowa.edu
Research Centre for Transcultural Studies in Health	www.mdx.ac.uk
Academic Center for Evidence-Based Nursing (ACE)	www.acestar.uthscsa.edu
Cumulative Index to Nursing and Allied Health (CINAHL)	www.cinahl.com
Evidence-Based Nursing Journal	www.evidencebasednursing.com
McGill University Health Centre, Clinical and Professional Staff Development, Research & Clinical Resources for Evidence-Based Nursing	www.muhc-ebn.mcgill.ca
MEDLINE via PubMed, free resource provided by the National Library of Medicine	www.ncbi.nlm.nih.gov
Netting the Evidence—A ScHARR Introduction to Evidence-based Practice on the Internet	www.shef.ac.uk
PubMed Tutorial (NLM), an in-depth tutorial from the National Library of Medicine	www.nlm.nih.gov
Search Strategies to Identify Reviews and Meta-analyses in MEDLINE and CINAHL	www.york.ac.uk
University of Minnesota Evidence-based nursing site	http://evidence.ahc.umn.edu

EVIDENCE FROM THE LITERATURE

Citation: Block, L. M., & LeGrazie, B. A. (2006). Research to practice: Don't get lost in translation: Successfully communicate evidence with fact and follow up. *Nursing Management, 37*(5), 37–40.

Discussion: A challenge in using evidence is translating the evidence found in the literature into the actual, real world environment. Virtua Health in their Translating Research into Practice (TRIP) program set out to accomplish just that. They established a nursing research committee and educated staff and managers about EBC and how to translate the current best evidence into daily practice.

They developed a five-step process:

1. Assess the current situation.
2. Research best practices in the field.
3. Develop a program that meets the organization's needs.
4. Implement the program.
5. Evaluate the program.

Examples of TRIP programs they developed included EBC of patients on a ventilator receiving IV sedation, patients having ambulatory surgery, and a program on the need for hand washing.

Implications for Practice: Nurses need to be on the alert for opportunities to improve practice. The use of evidence-based protocols can significantly improve patient care.

CRITICAL THINKING 5-1

You work on a unit delivering care to patients. You want to be sure your care delivery is state of the art.

How will you as a new nurse begin to provide EBC?

What contributions can you make to EBC?

How can we as nurses help overcome potential resistance to EBC?

the health care system have supported this accusation. In response to this ongoing lack of evidence to make clinical decisions, the AHRQ has undertaken the development and funding of twelve evidence-based centers to carry out development and dissemination of best practice models based on available scientific information and data. Development of these special centers has been a driving force for state-of-the-art evaluations of current knowledge used in EBC in the United States. An example of an evidence-based center for nursing is the ACE Center at the University of Texas health Science Center in San Antonio, discussed earlier (www.acestar.uthscsa.edu).

PROMOTING EVIDENCE-BASED BEST PRACTICES

The U.S. health care system is a $1 trillion industry, and yet it is difficult to get all clinical health care providers to carefully consider the findings of both nursing and medical research and then deliver quality outcomes. Clinicians, nursing leaders, and nursing managers must promote the use of EBC to develop best practices at all levels of care. Research can be facilitated within the institution and then the findings can be reviewed and implemented. A change in practice can be facilitated through the collaboration of nursing and medicine working closely with quality improvement teams to deliver quality outcomes.

REAL WORLD INTERVIEW

I entered the hospital last year for a complete knee replacement. I was confident that I had the best orthopedic surgeon. He had told me of the pain that would follow the surgery and accompany the therapy. He told me that the hospital followed a clinical protocol for pain management that had been developed from the best research possible, and so I approached surgery confidently. The anesthetist administered the epidural and enough anesthesia to keep me semiawake during surgery. I relaxed and slept until I was moved to my room. When I was awake, I experienced the most excruciating pain I had ever experienced. My family was in the room, and when I asked for the nurse, she came in and told me I was going to have pain. She also said I would be able to press the button and receive measured doses of the epidural and be relieved. Each time she checked on me, she asked what number between one and ten was my pain. I told her for seven hours that the pain was unbearable. My family pleaded for the nurse to get help. She said she had called the anesthetist, who finally appeared and checked the epidural. He said it was not working, but he would be happy to insert a new tube, and if he did it, it would work. That means for seven solid hours I had no working treatment to manage postsurgery bone pain. What's the use of having well-researched pain protocols if they are not used properly?

Instead of having another epidural inserted, I asked for the morphine, which I was not able to tolerate. The next day, they gave me Demerol, which made my therapy bearable. I did not fill out the patient satisfaction survey they sent following my dismissal because I was disgusted, and I did not feel they would ever take any action anyway. Something was definitely wrong with their pain-management system. So much for the best research possible! It only works if it is administered properly. I want to add that caring and compassion should be the most important qualities a health caregiver should be taught. I did have one nurse who was very considerate and informative. I wish she were working the day I went to surgery. Maybe she would have gotten help for my pain.

Patricia A. Murry Kelly
Patient
Munster, Indiana

KEY CONCEPTS

- The focus on EBC can be expected to remain a driving force in the health care arena in the foreseeable future.

- Nursing can make significant contributions to the advancement of EBC.

- Nursing leaders and managers can promote a culture receptive to the practice of EBC, and all nurses can support this.

- Ultimately, EBC is the gold standard in clinical care.

- By accepting the challenge to provide EBC, nursing can pursue its future, confident of its ability to contribute to an increasingly complex health care system.

KEY TERMS

evidence-based care (EBC)
evidence-based medicine (EBM)

REVIEW QUESTIONS

1. What is the major purpose of evidence-based care (EBC)?
   A. To increase variability of care
   B. To cause a link to be missing in clinical care
   C. To determine what medical models can be applied by nursing
   D. To provide EBC supporting clinical competency

2. Concerning EBC, which of the following is an accurate statement at this time?
   A. EBC takes the place of continuous quality improvement.
   B. Because we can already demonstrate effective and efficient care, EBC is redundant.
   C. Leaders and managers in nursing are not clinicians, generally speaking, and so do not have a part in EBC processes.
   D. Generally speaking, EBC is recognized by nursing, medicine, and health policy makers as state-of-the-art science reports.

3. Which of the following organizations develops clinical practice guidelines?
   A. American Heart Association
   B. Agency for Healthcare Research and Quality (AHRQ)
   C. Pew Health Professions Commission
   D. Joint Commission (JC)

4. Which of the following is a research design that always involves testing of a clinical treatment with assignments of research subjects to either experimental or control conditions?
   A. Lonitudinal study
   B. Randomized controlled trial
   C. Meta-analysis
   D. Time series design

5. The following is true about evidence for use in clinical practice:
   A. It is typically quickly adopted by clinicians.
   B. It always needs to be interpreted for appropriateness with a specific patient.
   C. It should never be challenged by nurses.
   D. It provides unarguable direction for patient care.

6. Which of the following is likely to provide the strongest evidence about a diabetic patient care?
   A. A study found in the literature about a patient with Type II diabetes
   B. An article about diabetes in a nursing research journal
   C. An article about diabetes in a medical research journal
   D. A systematic synthesized review of the literature on diabetes

Review Activities

1. Review Table 5-4. Are the evidence levels clear to you? Look at a patient's condition that you encounter in your clinical lab experience. Which level of evidence supports the care delivery approaches to this patient? Are any clinical pathways or standards in use in caring for this patient?

2. To understand some of the studies used in EBC, it is necessary to understand some of the research terminology. Review the research terminology in Table 5-1. Check the library and see whether you can find an example of one of the studies.

3. Using Table 5-7 on conducting evidence reports in nursing, study the treatment of depression.

Exploring the Web

Go to the following sites to develop your knowledge of evidence-based health care:

- American College of Physicians (ACP) ACP Journal Club. ACP Journal Club's general purpose is to select from the biomedical literature those articles reporting original studies and systematic reviews that warrant immediate attention by clinicians attempting to keep pace with important advances in internal medicine.
  www.acpjc.org

- Agency for Healthcare Research and Quality (AHRQ).
  www.ahrq.gov

- Center for Evidence-Based Medicine, University of Toronto. Note the evidence-based nursing syllabi and resources.
  www.cebm.utoronto.ca

- Cumulative Index to Nursing and Allied Health (CINAHL). The CINAHL database covers nursing, allied health, biomedical and consumer health journals, and publications of the American Nursing Association and the National League for Nursing. More than 350,000 records and 900 journals are included.
  www.cinahl.com

- Cochrane Library. The aim of the Cochrane Library is to prepare, maintain, and promote the accessibility of systematic reviews of the effects of health care interventions. It contains four databases: the Cochrane Database of Systematic Reviews (CDSR), the Database of Abstracts of Reviews of Effectiveness (DARE), the Cochrane Controlled Trials Register (CCTR), and the Cochrane Review Methodology Database (CRMD).

  View introductory information free.
  www.cochrane.org/index.htm

  Free access to Cochrane Reviewer's Handbook.
  www.cochrane.org/cochrane/hbook.htm

- EBM Education Center of Excellence, North Carolina.
  http://library.ncahec.net

- Evaluating the Literature: Quality Filtering and Evidence-based Medicine and Health. Available from the National Library of Medicine.
  www.nlm.nih.gov

- Evidence-based Medicine.
  www.acponline.org

- Evidence-based Medicine ToolKit.
  www.med.ualberta.ca

- Health Information Research Unit, McMaster University.
  http://hiru.mcmaster.ca

- Health Sciences Library, University of North Carolina, Chapel Hill. Evidence-based medicine tutorial.
  www.hsl.unc.edu

- Searching the Medical Literature for the Best Evidence, University of North Carolina at Chapel Hill Health Sciences Library.
  www.hsl.unc.edu

- Searching CINAHL Using the Ovid Web Gateway, Duke University Medical Center Library. *www.mclibrary.duke.edu*

- University of North Carolina Health Sciences Library. *www.hsl.unc.edu*

REFERENCES

Block, L. M., & LeGrazie, B. A. (2006). Research to practice: Don't get lost in translation: Successfully communicate evidence with fact and follow up. *Nursing Management, 37*(5), 37–40.

DiCenso, A., Guyatt, G., & Ciliska, D. (2005). *Evidence-based nursing: A guide to clinical practice* (Glossary, pp. 547–573). St. Louis, MO: Elsevier Mosby.

Grol, R., & Grimshaw, J. (2003). From best evidence to best practice: Effective implementation of change in patients' care. *Lancet, 362*(9391), 1225–1230.

Guyatt, G., & Rennie, D. (2002). *Users guide to the medical literature: A manual for evidence-based clinical practice* (p. 2). Chicago: AMA.

Haase-Herrick, K. (2004). The journey to evidence-based healthcare. *Modern Healthcare, 4*(19).

Haller, K. (2006, Summer). Safe staffing saves lives. *John Hopkins Nursing, 4*(2), 16.

Hudak, C. (2004, July–August). Using simulations to promote learning in higher education: An introduction. *Nursing Education Perspectives, 25*(4), 198.

Institute of Medicine. (1999). *To err is human.* Washington, DC: National Academies Press.

Institute of Medicine. (2001). *Crossing the quality chasm.* Washington, DC: National Academies Press.

Polit, D., & Beck, C. (2004). *Nursing research: Principles and methods* (7th ed.). (Glossary, p. 711–735). Philadelphia, PA: Lippincott.

Pravikoff, D. S., Tanner, A. B., & Pierce, S. T. (2005). Readiness of U.S. nurses for evidence-based practice. *American Journal of Nursing, 105*(9), 40–51.

Sackett, D. L., Rosenberg, W. M. C., Gray, J. A. M., Haynes, R. B, & Richardson, W. S. (1996). Evidence-based medicine: What it is and what it isn't. *British Medical Journal, 312*(7023), 71–72.

Stevens, K. R. (2004). ACE star model of EBP: Knowledge transformation. Academic Center for Evidence-based Practice. The University of Texas Health Science Center at San Antonio. Retrieved September 8, 2006, from http://www.acestar.uthscsa.edu

SUGGESTED READINGS

Allen, D. E., Bockenhauer, B., Egan, C., & Kinnaird, L. S. (2006). Relating outcomes to excellent nursing practice. *The Journal of Nursing Administration (JONA), 36*(3), 140–147.

Arnold, L., Campbell, A., Dubree, M., Fuchs, M. A., Davis, N., Hertzler, et al. (2006). Priorities and challenges of health system chief nursing executives: Insights for nursing educators. *Journal of Professional Nursing, 22*(4), 213–220.

Brewer, C. S. (2005). Health services research and the nursing workforce: Access and utilization issues. *Nursing Outlook, 53*(6), 281–290.

CINAHL Information Systems. (2004). Job satisfaction of hospital-based registered nurses. *Online Journal of Clinical Innovations, 7*(1), 1–48.

Clancy, C., Sharp, B. A., & Hubbard, H. B. (2005). Guest editorial: Intersections for mutual success in nursing and health services research. *Nursing Outlook, 53*(6), 263–265.

Cochrane Library at McMaster University. *Using Medline to search for evidence.* Retrieved March, 2000, from http://www.londonlinks.ac.uk/evidence_strategies/coch_search.htm

Engelke, M. K., & Marshburn, D. M. (2006). Collaborative strategies to enhance research and evidence-based practice. *The Journal of Nursing Administration (JONA), 36*(3), 131–135.

Ervin, N. E. (2006). Does patient satisfaction contribute to nursing care quality? *The Journal of Nursing Administration (JONA), 36*(3), 126–130.

Goode, C. J. (2000). What constitutes the "evidence" in evidence-based practice? *Applied Nursing Research, 13,* 222–225.

Guyatt, G. H., Haynes, R. B., Jaeschke, R. Z., Cook, D. J., Green, L., Naylor, C. D., et al. (2000). Users guides to the medical literature: XXV. Evidence-based medicine: Principles for applying the users guides to patient care. *Journal of American Medical Association, 284,* 1290–1296.

Healy, B. (2006). Who says what's best? *U.S. News & World Report, 141*(9), 75.

Hutchinson, A. M., & Johnston, L. (2006). Beyond the BARRIERS scale: Commonly reported barriers to research use. *The Journal of Nursing Administration (JONA), 36*(4), 189–199.

Jangold, K. L., Pearson, K. K., Schmitz, J. R., Scherb, C. A., Specht, J. P., & Loes, J. L. (2006). Perceptions and characteristics of registered nurses' involvement in decision making. *Nursing Administration Quarterly, 30*(3), 266–272.

Joanna Briggs Institute for Evidence Based Nursing & Midwifery. Retrieved March 9, 2007, from http://www.joannabriggs.edu.au/services/search.php

Jones, C. B., & Mark, B. A. (2005). The intersection of nursing and health services research: Overview of an agenda setting conference. *Nursing Outlook, 53*(6), 270–273.

Jones, C. B., & Mark, B. A. (2005). The intersection of nursing and health services research: An agenda to guide future research. *Nursing Outlook, 53*(6), 324–332.

Meyer, T. C. (2005). Following up on evidence-based medicine. *Wisconsin Medical Journal, 104*(3), 1.

Newhouse, R. P., Pettit, J. D., Poe, S., & Rocco, L. (2006). The slippery slope: Differentiating between quality improvement and research. *The Journal of Nursing Administration (JONA), 36*(4), 211–219.

Potylycki, M. J., Kimmel, S. R., Ritter, M., Capuano, T., Gross, L., Riegel-Gross, K. I., et al. (2006). Nonpunitive medication error reporting: 3-years findings from one hospital's primum nonnocere initiative. *The Journal of Nursing Administration (JONA), 36*(7/8), 370–376.

Pravikoff, D. S., Pierce, S., & Tanner A. (2003). Are nurses ready for evidence-based practice? *American Journal of Nursing. 103*(5), 95–96

Pravikoff, D. S., Pierce, S. T., & Tanner, A. (2005, Jan.–Feb.). Evidence-based practice readiness study supported by academy nursing informatics expert panel. *Nursing Outlook, 53*(1), 49–50.

Sackett, D. L., Rosenberg, W. M., Gray, J. A., Haynes, R. B., & Richardson, W. S. (2007). Evidence based medicine: What it is and What it isn't. *Clinical Orthopaedics and Related Research, 455,* 3–5.

Simpson, R. L. (2006). Evidence-based practice: How nursing administration makes it happen. *Nursing Administration Quarterly, 30*(3), 291–294.

Stevens, K. R., & Staley, J. M. (2006). The Quality Chasm reports, evidence-based practice, and nursing's response to improve healthcare. *Nursing Outlook, 54*(2), 94–101.

Tanner, A., Piece, S., & Pravikoff, D. (2004). Readiness for evidence-based practice: Information literacy needs of nurses in the United States. *Medinfo, 11*(2), 936–940.

CHAPTER 6

Nursing and Health Care Informatics

Leslie H. Nicoll, PhD, MBA, RN, BC ⊕ Josette Jones, RN, PhD, BC

Health Information Technology (IT) is not just about better treatments for the ailing and ill among us, nor just for all of us who want to prevent or limit illness in its early stages. It is ultimately about treating the industry itself so that we can have not only the best science, infrastructure, and professionals in the world, but also the best value, safety, and productivity (David Brailer, National Coordinator for Health Information Technology, HIMSS, 2005).

OBJECTIVES

Upon completion of this chapter, the reader should be able to:

1. List the components that define a nursing specialty and discuss how nursing informatics meets these requirements.

2. Relate educational opportunities for nurses interested in pursuing a career in nursing informatics.

3. Identify current challenges for health information technology applications.

4. Relate how ubiquitous computing and virtual reality have the potential to influence nursing education and practice.

5. Use established criteria to evaluate the content of health-related sites found on the Internet.

6. Identify the role of informatics in evidence-based practice (EBP) and patient safety.

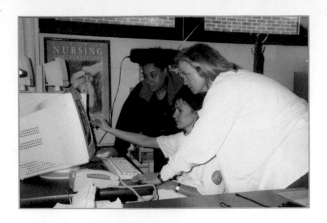

Consider the health care consumer of the year 2010:

Everyone could carry around their health care history on a Smart card with their Personal Health Record (PHR), a type of electronic Smart card that stores lots of individual health data accessible anytime and anywhere.

Patients could be diagnosed and treated with the aid of telemedicine at the point where they are living. Clinicians are no longer the only sources of health care advice for consumers. Electronic E-patients are placing themselves at the center of a network of electronic resources, including search engines, online support groups, and health care Websites. Providers can be contacted by e-mail 24/7. Self-diagnosis, self-care, and self-medication are in!

How will all of this affect the health care consumer and the health care provider?

Like it or not, computers and the Internet are here to stay. Computers and the Internet have changed the way we communicate, obtain information, work, entertain, and make important health decisions. As documented in the PEW Report from April 19, 2006 (Horrigan & Rainie, 2006), some 21 million Americans rely on the Internet in a crucial or important way for career training, 17 million rely on it when helping someone else with a major illness or health care condition, and another 17 million rely on it when choosing a school for themselves or for a child.

Computers and the Internet are changing health care delivery, too. For example, in an outpatient mental health clinic, computer reminders were shown to be superior to manual reminders in improving adherence to a clinical practice guideline for depression (Cannon & Allen, 2000). An integrated electronic reminder system also resulted in variable improvement in care for diabetes and coronary artery disease (Sequist et al., 2005). Another study showed that onscreen computer-generated reminders sent to practitioners of patients lacking a recent potassium test increased potassium testing by 9.8% (p < 0.001) (Hoch et al., 2003). On a regional and national level, health care communities are moving

forward with health information exchange to create Local or Regional Health Information Infrastructures (LHII) and are improving the efficiency, quality, and safety of care by interconnecting local as well as national health information resources (Overhage, Evans, & Marchibroda, 2005).

Nurses are not immune to the changes that computers are bringing to both everyday life and nursing practice. As professionals, information technology can help achieve the goals of quality patient-centered care and increased patient safety. Whether you are a nursing student learning a clinical procedure using a computer-based instruction program; a nurse on the floor using electronic devices such as ventilators, intravenous pumps, telemetry, and the electronic health record; a nursing administrator using a spreadsheet and database to plan a budget; or a nursing researcher or clinician keeping updated with the latest evidence-based nursing care, it is evident that information technology has become an essential part of professional nursing practice, both on the individual and institutional level.

In this day and age, most everyone is involved with computers to some degree. Some have chosen to specialize within the field of computer science, information, and technology. Just over a decade ago, the term *nursing informatics* might have induced puzzled looks. Since then, the burgeoning field of nursing informatics has become an essential element of health care delivery. In the past decade alone, there has been a significant increase in the demand for nurses whose knowledge of nursing and specialization in informatics contributes to nursing practice, leadership, education, and research throughout the United States, Canada, and other countries (Carroll, Bradford, Foster, Cato, & Jones, 2006).

This chapter will introduce you to both the world of nursing informatics and the world of computing. Although it may not be your career choice to become a nursing informaticist, the professional RN of the twenty-first century will not be effective in the role without a solid base of knowledge related to information technology and its impact on nursing practice, patient care, and patient outcomes.

NURSING INFORMATICS

The Special Interest Group of the International Medical Informatics Association—Nursing Informatics (IMIA-NI) definition, agreed upon at their General Assembly in Stockholm in 1997, and amended for clarity at the General Assembly in Seoul, 1998, defined **nursing informatics** as the integration of nursing, its information, and information management with information processing and communication technology to support the health of people worldwide. The focus of IMIA is to:

- Foster collaboration among nurses and others who are interested in nursing informatics
- Explore the scope of nursing informatics and its implication for information handling activities associated with nursing care delivery, nursing administration, nursing research and nursing education, and the various relationships with other health care information systems
- Support the development of nursing informatics in the member countries
- Provide appropriate informatics meetings, conferences and postconferences, and provide opportunities to share knowledge and research to facilitate communication of developments in the field
- Encourage the publication and dissemination of research and development materials in the field of nursing informatics
- Develop recommendations, guidelines and courses related to nursing informatics (www.imia.org)

The term, *informatics,* has its foundations with the French term, *informatique,* which concerns all the aspects of the computer as a tool for use in processing of information. The term, *medical informatics,* is also used. Medical informatics is the use of computers for the classification and retrieval of data and for the management of health care information, enabling us to explore and better understand the informational and cognitive foundations of medicine (Blois, 1986).

In 1985, Hannah defined nursing informatics as the use of information technology by nurses carrying out their duties in relation to any function in the purview of nursing (as cited in Ball, Hannah, Newbold, & Douglass, 2000). Graves and Corcoran (1989) state that nursing informatics is a combination of computer science, information science, and nursing that is designed to assist in the management and processing of nursing data, information, and knowledge to support the practice of nursing and the delivery of nursing care. Grobe, cited in Ball et al. (2000), adds a further dimension to this definition by asserting that nursing informatics is the application of the principles of information science and theory to the study, scientific analysis, and management of nursing information for the purposes of establishing a body of nursing knowledge. This added dimension suggests that the contribution of nursing informatics is not limited to clinical and administrative nursing practice, but it also contributes to the development of nursing knowledge.

Romano, as cited in Ball et al. (2000), departs from the view that nursing informatics is the integration of information science, computer science, and nursing by maintaining that the focus of nursing informatics is the nature of nursing and how nursing information is acquired,

manipulated, and used. Goossens (1996) adds that nursing informatics is the multidisciplinary scientific endeavor of analyzing, formalizing, and modeling how nurses collect and manage data, process data into information and knowledge, make knowledge-based decisions and inferences for patient care, and use this empirical and experiential knowledge to broaden the scope and enhance the quality of their professional practice. The scientific methods central to nursing informatics are focused on using a discourse about motives for computerized systems; analyzing, formalizing and modeling nursing information processing and nursing knowledge for all components of nursing practice, that is, clinical practice, management, education and research; investigating determinants, conditions, elements, models, and processes to design and implement as well as test the effectiveness and efficiency of computerized information, (tele)communication, and network systems for nursing practice; and studying the effects of these systems on nursing practice.

In sum, several definitions of nursing informatics have been proposed. The definitions can be categorized as:

- Technology-focused, for example, Ball and Hannah, Saba and McCormick
- Conceptually focused, for example, Graves and Corcoran, Grobe
- Role-oriented, for example, American Nurses Association, Henry, Turley

A 1997 Delphi study, incorporating these definitions, gained consensus about the framework and definition of nursing informatics. It was the foundation of the IMIA-NI definition given at the beginning of this section. Ball et al. (2000) provide a comprehensive description of nursing informatics as nurses' use of information technology for the substitution, innovation, and transformation of patient care, nursing administration, or educational preparation for nurses (Figure 6-1).

E-HEALTH AND TELEHEALTH

Related terms in the field of Informatics are *e-health* and *telehealth.* E-health is an emerging field in the intersection of medical informatics, public health, and business, referring to health services and information delivered or enhanced through the Internet and related technologies. In a broader sense, the term characterizes not only a technical development but also a state of mind, a way of thinking, an attitude, and a commitment for networked, global thinking to improve health care locally, regionally, and worldwide by using information and communication technology (Eysenbach, G., 2001).

Telehealth is the delivery of health-related services and information via telecommunications technologies. It may be as simple as two health professionals discussing a case over the telephone or as sophisticated as using

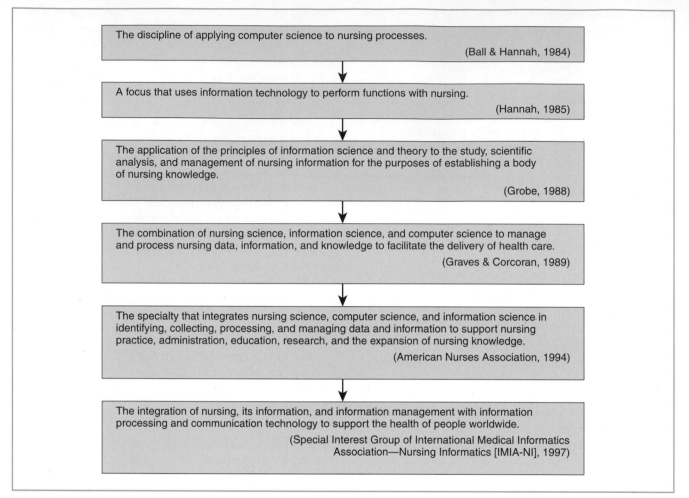

The discipline of applying computer science to nursing processes.

(Ball & Hannah, 1984)

A focus that uses information technology to perform functions with nursing.

(Hannah, 1985)

The application of the principles of information science and theory to the study, scientific analysis, and management of nursing information for the purposes of establishing a body of nursing knowledge.

(Grobe, 1988)

The combination of nursing science, information science, and computer science to manage and process nursing data, information, and knowledge to facilitate the delivery of health care.

(Graves & Corcoran, 1989)

The specialty that integrates nursing science, computer science, and information science in identifying, collecting, processing, and managing data and information to support nursing practice, administration, education, research, and the expansion of nursing knowledge.

(American Nurses Association, 1994)

The integration of nursing, its information, and information management with information processing and communication technology to support the health of people worldwide.

(Special Interest Group of International Medical Informatics Association—Nursing Informatics [IMIA-NI], 1997)

Figure 6-1 Evolution of a definition: Nursing informatics.

satellite technology to broadcast a consultation between providers at facilities in two countries, using videoconferencing equipment or robotic technology. It may include transmission of patient images or data for diagnosis or disease management; groups or individuals exchanging health services, education, health care advice, or research via live videoconference; or home monitoring of dialysis or cardiac patients.

ELEMENTS OF NURSING INFORMATICS

Some common elements of NI include clinical information systems such as the following:

- Computerized order entry
- Electronic Health Records
- Patient decision support tools, clinical and business related
- Laboratory and x-ray results reporting and viewing systems
- Electronic prescribing and order entry, including barcoding
- Community and population health management and information

- Communication, staffing, and administrative systems
- Evidence-based knowledge and information retrieval systems
- Quality improvement data collection/data summary systems
- Documentation and care planning
- Patient monitoring and problem alerts

NEED FOR NURSING INFORMATICS

As of 2006, less than 10% of American hospitals have implemented health information technology (Medical Records Institute, 2006), and a mere 16% of primary care practitioners use Electronic Health Records (EHR) (Johnston et al., 2003). The vast majority of health care transactions in the United States still take place on paper, a system that has remained unchanged since the 1950s. The health care industry spends only 2% of gross revenues on technology, which is meager compared to other information-intensive industries such as finance, which spend upwards of 10% (Raymond & Dold, 2001).

The development of standards for EHRs is at the forefront of the national health care agenda (MRI, 2006).

Without accessible, standardized EHRs, practicing clinicians, pharmacies, and hospitals cannot share patient information, which is necessary for timely, patient-centered, and portable care. There are currently multiple competing vendors of EHR systems, each selling a software suite that in many cases is not compatible with those of their competitors. Only counting the outpatient vendors, there are more than 25 major brands currently on the market. In 2004, President Bush created the Office of the National Coordinator for Health Information Technology (ONC) to address interoperability issues and to establish a National Health Information Network (NHIN). Under the ONC, Regional Health Information Organizations (RHIOs) have been established in many states to promote the sharing of health information. As of 2005, one of the largest projects for a national EHR is by the National Health Service (NHS) in the United Kingdom. The goal of the NHS is to have 60,000,000 patients with a centralized electronic medical record by 2010.

JOINT COMMISSION NATIONAL PATIENT SAFETY GOALS

Several other forces have highlighted the need for increased patient technology and nursing informatics. The Joint Commission (JC), formerly the Joint Commission on Accreditation of Healthcare Organizations (JCAHO), has set the following National Patient Safety Goals for 2006, many of which require the use of technology:

- Improve the accuracy of patient identification
- Improve the effectiveness of communication among caregivers
- Improve the safety of medication use
- Eliminate wrong site, wrong patient, wrong procedure surgery
- Improve the effectiveness of patient-specific clinical alarm systems that alert staff to patient emergencies
- Reduce the risk of health care-associated infections
- Accurately and completely reconcile medications across the continuum of care
- Reduce the risk of patient harm from falls
- Reduce the risk of influenza and pneumococcal disease in older adults
- Reduce the risk of surgical fires
- Encourage active involvement of patients and families in patient's own care as a patient safety strategy
- Prevent health care-associated pressure ulcers

In 2007, the changes and additions to these Goals are as follows:

- Provide a complete list of medications to the patient when discharged
- Encourage patient's active involvement in his own care as a patient safety strategy

- Tell patients and their families how they can report concerns about safety and encourage them to do so
- Offer influenza vaccine to all staff
- Identify safety risks in the patient population
- Psychiatric hospitals should identify patients at risk for suicide
- General hospitals should identify those patients being treated for emotional or behavioral disorders who are at risk for suicide (www.jointcommission.org/ PatientSafetyNationalPatientSafety)

Attainment of many of these Goals requires the judicious use of technology.

LEAPFROG GROUP

The Leapfrog Group is another force advocating for technology. Leapfrog is a voluntary program aimed at using employer purchasing power to alert America's health industry that big leaps in health care safety, quality, and customer value will be recognized and rewarded. Among other initiatives, Leapfrog works with its employer members to encourage transparency and easy access to health care information as well as rewards for hospitals that have a proven record of high quality care. Leapfrog measures how hospitals are doing on the following:

- Computerized practitioner order entry into computers linked to error-prevention software
- ICU's staffed by practitioner intensivists
- Evidence-based hospital performance on five high-risk procedures and care for two high-risk neonatal conditions
- Progress on 27 National Quality Forum Safe Practices (www.leapfroggroup.org). Data support services are offered to Leapfrog by Thomson medstat (see www.medstat.com)

THE NATIONAL QUALITY FORUM

The National Quality Forum (NQF) is a not-for-profit membership organization created to develop and implement a national strategy for health care quality measurement and reporting. (www.qualityforum.org). A shared sense of urgency about the impact of health care quality on patient outcomes, workforce productivity, and health care costs prompted leaders in the public and private sectors to create the NQF as a mechanism to bring about national change.

Established as a public-private partnership, the NQF has broad participation from all parts of the health care system, including national, state, regional, and local groups representing consumers, public and private purchasers, employers, health care professionals, provider organizations, health plans, accrediting bodies, labor

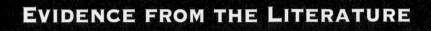

EVIDENCE FROM THE LITERATURE

Citation: Stevens, K. R., & Staley, J. M. (2004). The Quality Chasm Reports, evidence-based practice, and nursing response to improve healthcare. *Nursing Outlook, 54*(2), 94–101.

Discussion: In a growing set of landmark reports, the institute of Medicine (IOM) set in motion a sweeping quality initiative for reform of the health care system. Many of the IOM recommendations incorporate evidence-based practice and technology applications. New rules to redesign and improve care are highlighted in this article as follows. Patient care requires:

- *Care based on continuous healing relationships:* Patients should receive care whenever they need it and in many forms, not just face-to-face visits. This rule implies that the health care system should be responsive at all times (24 hours a day, every day) and that access to care should be provided over the Internet, by telephone, and by other means in addition to face-to-face visits.
- *Customization based on patient needs and values:* The system of care should be designed to meet the most common types of needs but have the capability to respond to individual patient choices and preferences.
- *The patient as the source of control:* Patients should be given the necessary information and the opportunity to exercise the degree of control they choose over health care decisions that affect them. The health care system should be able to accommodate differences in patient preferences and encourage shared decision making.
- *Shared knowledge and the free flow of information:* Patients should have unfettered access to their own medical information and to clinical knowledge. Clinicians and patients should communicate effectively and share information.
- *Evidence-based decision-making (EBD-M):* Patients should receive care based on the best available scientific knowledge. Care should not vary illogically from clinician to clinician or from place to place.
- *Safety as a system property:* Patients should be safe from injury caused by the care system. Reducing risk and ensuring safety require greater attention to systems that help prevent and mitigate errors.
- *The need for transparency:* The health care system should make information available to patients and their families that allows them to make informed decisions when selecting a health plan, hospital, or clinical practice, or when choosing among alternative treatments. This should include information describing the system's performance on safety, EBD-M, and patient satisfaction.
- *Anticipation of needs:* The health system should anticipate patient needs, rather than simply react to events.
- *Continuous decrease in waste:* The health system should not waste resources or patient time.
- *Cooperation among clinicians:* Clinicians and institutions should actively collaborate and communicate to ensure an appropriate exchange of information and coordination of care. (Institute of Medicine [IOM], 2001)

The IOM also offers analysis of the current health system and recommends changes in education of health professionals. These include several core competencies requiring the use of technology. Health professionals must:

- *Provide patient-centered care:* Identify, respect, and care about patients' differences, values, preferences, and expressed needs; relieve pain and suffering; coordinate continuous care; listen to, clearly inform, communicate with, and educate patients; share decision making and management; and continuously advocate disease prevention, wellness, and promotion of healthy lifestyles, including a focus on population health.
- *Work in interdisciplinary teams:* Cooperate, communicate, and integrate care in teams to ensure that care is continuous and reliable.
- *Employ evidence-based practice (EBP):* Integrate best research with clinical expertise and patient values for optimum care; participate in learning and research activities to the extent feasible.
- *Apply quality improvement:* Identify errors and hazards in care; understand and implement basic safety design principles, such as standardization and simplification; continually understand and measure quality of care in terms of structure, process, and outcome in relation to patient and community needs; and design and test interventions to change processes and systems of care, with the objective of improving quality.
- *Utilize informatics:* Communicate, manage knowledge, mitigate error, and support decision making using information technology. (IOM, 2003)

Implications for Practice: Health care professionals will be expected to be familiar with technology, EBP, and EBDM as they deliver care to patients in the future. Schools of Nursing must move to prepare students and faculty to meet this demand.

EVIDENCE FROM THE LITERATURE

Citation: Wickham, V., Miedema, F., Gamerdinger, K., & DeGooyer, J. (2006). Bar-coded patient ID: Review an organizational approach to vendor selection. *Nursing Management, 37*(12), 22–26.

Discussion: Article discusses implementation of various technologies, for example, bar-coded patient ID system, IV pumps, and so on, as well as technologies to improve care in the ER and neonatal units. The authors state that as important as it is to implement new technology to improve patient care, it's also important to measure the outcomes. They use the reports available from the systems and monitor the documentation of the care processes, for example, pain management, restraints, patient education, and ED turnaround time.

Implications for Practice: The use of technology in this agency is improving care. Nurses in other agencies will begin to see more use of technology to improve patient care.

---

unions, supporting industries, and organizations involved in health care research or quality improvement. Together, the organizational members of the NQF work to promote a common approach to measuring health care quality and fostering systemwide capacity for quality improvement.

In 2003, the NQF endorsed a set of 30 safe practices that should be universally utilized in applicable clinical care settings to reduce the risk of harm to patients. NQF has now formally launched the Safe Practices Consensus Standards Maintenance Committee to review the practices and recommend additions or changes for members to consider so that the set remains current and appropriate (see www.qualityforum.org).

THE SPECIALTY OF NURSING INFORMATICS

According to the American Nurses' Association (ANA, 2001), nursing informatics (NI) is a discipline-specific practice within the broader perspective of health informatics. NI was recognized as a specialty for RNs in 1992. NI includes, but is not limited to the following:

- Use of decision-making systems or artificial intelligence to support the nursing process
- Use of software application to support health care organization, for example, staffing, bed allocation, and so on
- Integration of information technology in patient education
- Use of computer-aided learning for nursing education
- Development and use of nursing databases and Nursing Information Systems (NIS)
- Use of research related to nurses' information management and communication

The focus of NI is on representation of nursing data, information, and knowledge and the management and communication of nursing information within the broader context of health informatics. Nursing informatics is a specialty in nursing due to the following:

- *Differentiated practice:* In addition to the four phenomena of interest to the discipline of nursing, NI focuses on the structure and algorithm of data, information, and knowledge used by nurses.
- *Defined research program:* Priorities for NI research are the development of nursing languages and terminologies, databases for clinical information, information for patients as users of information technology, telehealth, and maintenance of data privacy and confidentiality.
- *Organizational representation:* In International (for example IMIA), national (for example, American Medical Informatics Association [AMIA]), regional, and local level organizations, NI provides opportunities for networking and professional development.
- *Educational programs:* This is done through emerging NI graduate programs.
- *Credentialing:* This is done through the American Nurses Credentialing Center (ANCC).
- *Application of principles:* This is done using Human Computer Interaction (HCI) and ergonomics principles.

The Informatics Nurse Specialist has at least a master's degree in nursing informatics (system degree) and functions in the role of project manager, consultant, educator, researcher, development supporter, policy developer, or entrepreneur related to nursing information technology applications. Although NI is considered a specialty practice within the discipline of nursing, some

EVIDENCE FROM THE LITERATURE

Citation: McNeil, B. J., Elfrink, V. L., Pierce, S. T., Beyea, S. C., Bickford, C. J., & Averill, C. (2005, Dec.). Nursing informatics knowledge and competencies: A national survey of nursing education programs in the United States. *International Journal of Medical Informatics, 74*(11–12), 1021–1030.

Discussion: An online survey of deans/directors of 266 baccalaureate and higher nursing programs in the United States was developed by informatics expert nurses. Participants (1) identified nursing informatics (NI) competencies and knowledge of undergraduate and/or graduate students in their nursing programs, (2) determined faculty preparedness to teach NI and to use informatics tools, and (3) provided perceptions of NI requirements of local practicing nurses. Frequency data and qualitative responses were analyzed. Approximately half of undergraduate nursing programs were teaching information literacy skills and required students to enter with word-processing and e-mail skills. Least visible informatics content at all levels included the use of information system data standards, the Nursing Information and Data Set Evaluation Center criteria, the unified medical language system (UMLS), and the nurse's role in the life cycle of an information system. Almost 50% of respondents perceived faculty as "novice" and "advanced beginners" in teaching and using NI applications. Participants reported no future plans to offer NI training in their region.

Implications for Practice: Nursing faculty and students will want to consider this study's results. Findings have major implications for planning continuing education opportunities and designing nursing curricula that prepare nurses for use of the electronic health record and twenty-first century professional practice.

---

informatics competencies are required for all nurses. A beginning nurse may have fundamental computer literacy skills and information access skills related to patient care. Experienced nurses may have more proficiency in information management and communication in their areas of practice such as community health, patient education, and so on. The Informatics Nurse Specialist then would be probably expected to have all of the competencies outlined previously for the beginning and experienced nurse and demonstrate the competencies enumerated in the Standard of Practice for Nursing Informatics (ANA, 2001), collaborate with other informaticists, and function within interdisciplinary environments such as health care, Human Computer Interactions, information science, and computer science.

EDUCATION IN INFORMATICS

There are both formal and informal opportunities for education in nursing informatics. The first formal programs that offered specific degrees in nursing informatics were established within the past 20 years, and the number of programs has been increasing steadily. However, because educational options were limited, there are many nurses practicing in informatics that have been prepared for their role through on-the-job training or by receiving education outside of nursing. For example, a nurse may have a bachelor of science in nursing (BSN) plus a second degree in computer science or information technology. Nurses have been successful in educating themselves using formal and informal resources. Nurses considering a career in informatics need to carefully consider options that are available and plan their educational program accordingly.

FORMAL PROGRAMS

As the health care industry relies more on information technology for the delivery of care, it is imperative that basic computer skills and nursing informatics competencies are incorporated in all levels of professional nursing education programs.

It was as recent as 1989 that the first Masters program in Nursing Informatics was established at the University of Maryland, following by a doctoral program in 1992. Now, there are numerous universities nationwide offering master's degrees, doctoral degrees, and postgraduate certifications in Nursing Informatics. For a comprehensive list of programs for nursing, medical, and health informatics, refer to the AMIA site at www.amia.org/informatics/acad&training.

INFORMAL EDUCATION

For many nurses, graduate education is not an option or personal choice, but they still desire to become more knowledgeable about informatics. There are numerous venues for all nurses to stay abreast of emerging health information technologies and trends. A popular continuing education seminar is the Weekend Immersion in Nursing Informatics (WINI), which can be accessed at www.winiconference.net. Additionally, groups such as the American Medical Informatics Association (AMIA) and the Healthcare Information and Management Systems Society (HIMSS) have annual conferences that attract thousands of health information technology professionals and vendors, offering educational and networking opportunities for all informatics appetites. Many regions have formed nursing informatics groups that function at the local, national, and even international levels. These groups, such as the Capital Area Roundtable on Informatics in Nursing Group (CARING), offer vital networking and educational services to their members. In 2004, 18 of these regional nursing informatics groups, representing 2,000 nurses, formed the Alliance for Nursing Informatics (ANI) in collaboration with HIMSS, the American Nurses Association (ANA), and CARING. There are several nursing and health informatics scholarly journals, such as *Computers, Informatics, and Nursing* (www.cinjournal.com) and *Journal of Medical Informatics Association* (www.jamia.org), which provide essential elements of continuing industry trends and nursing informatics education.

CERTIFICATION

Whether a nurse has pursued a formal or informal educational path in nursing informatics, many practicing in the specialty choose to become certified. Certification in a specialty is a formal, systematic mechanism whereby nurses can voluntarily seek a credential that recognizes their quality and excellence in professional practice and continuing education (American Nurses Credentialing Center, 1993). For many nurses, becoming certified is a professional milestone and validation of their qualifications, knowledge, and skills in a defined area of nursing practice. The American Nurses Credentialing Center (ANCC) offers certification examinations for a variety of specialties in nursing, including informatics. The ANCC Website (www.nursingworld.org/ancc) details the nursing candidate's requirements for the Informatics Nurse Certification Exam, as such:

- A baccalaureate degree or higher
- An active RN license, with at least two years of professional practice
- Practice of at least 2,000 hours of nursing informatics within the past three years

OR

- Twelve hours of graduate work and 1,000 hours of nursing informatics practice

OR

- Completion of a graduate program in nursing informatics that included at least 200 hours of clinical practicum

- Completion of 30 continuing education contact hours in specialty area within the past three years for those who have not completed a graduate informatics program

Those RNs with a baccalaureate or higher degree in the field of nursing that successfully pass the informatics certification exam are recognized as Board Certified with the initials, RN, BC. For RNs with a baccalaureate or higher degree in a nonnursing field, their certification is recognized as Certified with the initials RN, C.

CAREER OPPORTUNITIES

Career opportunities in the fields of computer science and information technology are growing at an exponential rate, and nursing is no exception. Nurses working in informatics can look forward to multiple job opportunities, with new roles continuously being developed as technology changes and matures. Changes in health care delivery, particularly managed care, have caused shifts in computer systems to care management, clinical systems, clinical data repositories, care mapping, and outcomes measures (Hersher, 2000).

These shifts have resulted in the recognition of the need for computerization within the health care industry to collect, manage, analyze, and report data that come from a variety of sources and across the continuum of care. Rapid advances in technology have enabled the development of complex interfaces, communication, and networking of diverse systems. Workers are needed to define, develop, install, consult, and market these systems. Nurses in informatics have taken leadership roles in all these areas (Hersher, 2000).

In acute care and long-term care health care organizations, as well as industry or vendor companies, nursing informatics specialists hold roles that offer such diverse titles as Nursing Informatics Specialist, Clinical Analyst, Clinical Project Manager, and Nursing Informatics Manager. Some of these roles are integrated in the Information Technology (IT) department, whereas others report to the Chief Nursing Officer and have a close working

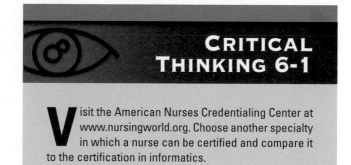

CRITICAL THINKING 6-1

Visit the American Nurses Credentialing Center at www.nursingworld.org. Choose another specialty in which a nurse can be certified and compare it to the certification in informatics.

How are they similar? How are they different?

relationship with the IT department and the education staff. Nursing informatics positions are also seen in practice in senior management positions holding such titles as Clinical IT Directors, Chief Information Officers (CIO), and Chief Nursing Officers. The Nursing Informatics Working Group of the AMIA maintains a repository of NI role descriptions at www.amia.org (Carroll et al., 2007).

CLINICAL INFORMATION SYSTEMS

As mentioned earlier, clinical information systems (CISs) are changing the way that health care is delivered, whether in the hospital, the clinic, the provider's office, or the patient's home. With capabilities ranging from advanced instrumentation to high-level decision support, CISs offer nurses and other clinicians information when, where, and how they need it. Increasingly, CIS applications function as the mechanisms to improve outcomes and reduce errors, as well as to control costs by realizing a host of efficiencies in clinical data entry and patient care and supporting the move toward the computer-based patient record (CPR) or Electronic Health Record (EHR).

What exactly is a CIS? Definitions vary, often from organization to organization. In general, a **clinical information system (CIS)** is a computer-based system used to inform clinicians about tests, procedures, and treatment in an effort to improve the quality of care through real-time assistance in decision making and to increase efficiency and effectiveness of care delivery.

A CIS can be patient-focused or departmental in focus. In patient-focused systems, automation supports patient care processes. Typical applications found in a patient-focused system include order entry, test results reporting, clinical documentation, care planning, and clinical pathways. As data are entered into the system, data repositories are established that can be accessed to look for trends in patient care.

Departmental systems evolved to meet the operational needs of particular departments, such as the laboratory, radiology, pharmacy, medical records, or billing. Early systems often were stand-alone systems designed for an individual department. A major challenge facing CIS developers is to integrate these stand-alone systems to work with each other and with the newer patient-focused systems.

COMPUTERIZED PATIENT RECORDS

A **computerized patient record (CPR)** or electronic patient record will include all information about an individual's lifetime health status and health care. The CPR is a replacement for the paper medical record as the primary source of information for health care, meeting all clinical, legal, and administrative requirements. However, the CPR is more than today's medical record. Information technology permits much more data to be captured, processed, and integrated, which results in information that is broader than that found in a linear paper record.

The CPR is not a record in the traditional sense of the term. *Record* connotes a repository with limitations of size, content, and location. The term traditionally has suggested that the sole purpose for maintaining health data is to document events. Although this is an important purpose, the CPR permits health information to be used to support the generation and communication of knowledge.

REAL WORLD INTERVIEW

To me, the greatest contribution of health care information technology and systems is its power to support clinician decision making. Far too often we focus on the technical aspects of hardware and software design while minimizing the real intent of this powerful technology, which is to support clinicians in their practice endeavors. We need to make clinicians' knowledge paramount as we transform our clinical practice environments through the design and implementation of new health care information technology and systems.

Rita Snyder-Halpern, PhD, RN, CNAA
Associate Professor
San Diego, California

The health care delivery system is dramatically changing, with a strong emphasis on improving outcomes of care and maintaining health. The CPR needs to be considered in a broader context and is not applicable only to patients, that is, individuals with the presence of an illness or disease. Rather, in the CPR, the focus is on the individuals' health, encompassing both wellness and illness.

As a result of this focus on the individual, the CPR is a virtual compilation of nonredundant health data about the person across her lifetime, including facts, observations, interpretations, plans, actions, and outcomes. Health data include information on allergies, history of illness and injury, functional status, diagnostic studies, assessments, orders, consultation reports, and treatment records. Health data also include wellness information such as immunization history, behavioral data, environmental information, demographics, health insurance, administrative data for care delivery processes, and legal data such as consents. The who, what, when, and where of data capture also are identified. The structure of the data includes text, numbers, sounds, images, and full–motion video. These are thoroughly integrated so that any given view of health data may incorporate one or more structural elements.

Within a CPR, an individual's health data are maintained and distributed over different systems in different locations, such as a hospital, clinic, practitioner's office, and pharmacy. Intelligent software agents with appropriate security measures are necessary to access data across these distributed systems. The nurse or other user who is retrieving these data must be able to assemble the data in such a way as to provide a chronology of health information about the individual.

The CPR is maintained in a system that captures, processes, communicates, secures, and presents the data about the patient. This system may include the CIS. Other components of the CPR system include clinical rules, literature for patient education, expert opinions, and payer rules related to reimbursement. When these elements work together in an integrated fashion, the CPR becomes much more than a patient record—it becomes a knowledge tool. The system is able to integrate information from multiple sources and provides decision support; thus, the CPR serves as the primary source of information for patient care.

A fully functional CPR is a complex system. Consider a single data element (datum), such as a person's weight. The system must be able to record the weight, store it, process it, communicate it to others, and present it in a different format, such as a bar graph or chart. It may also be necessary to convert a weight in pounds to kilograms or vice versa. All of this must be done in a secure environment that protects the patient's confidentiality and privacy. The complexity of these issues and the development of the necessary systems help to explain why few fully functional CPR systems are in place today.

DATA CAPTURE

Data capture refers to the collection and entry of data into a computer system. The origin of the data may be local or remote, with the data coming from patient-monitoring devices, from telemedicine applications, directly from the individual recipient of health care, and even from others who have information about the recipient's health or environment, such as relatives, friends, and public health agencies. Data may be captured by multiple means, including key entry, pattern recognition (voice, handwriting, or biological characteristics), and medical device transmission.

All data entered into a computer are not necessarily structured for subsequent processing. Document imaging systems, for example, provide for creation of electronically stored text but have limitations on the ability to process that text. Data capture includes the use of controlled vocabularies and code systems to ensure common meaning for terminology and the ability to process units of information. As noted earlier, great strides have been made in the development of standardized nursing languages. These languages provide structured data entry and text processing that result in common meaning and processing.

Data capture also encompasses authentication to identify the author of an entry and to ensure that the author has been granted permission to access the system and change the CPR.

STORAGE

Storage refers to the physical location of data. In CPR systems, health data are distributed across multiple systems at different sites. For this reason, there needs to be common access protocols, retention schedules, and universal identification.

Access protocols permit only authorized users to obtain data for legitimate uses. The systems must have backup and recovery mechanisms in the event of failure. Retention schedules address the maintenance of the data in active and inactive form and the permanence of the storage medium.

A person's identity can be determined by many types of data in addition to common identifiers such as name and number. Universal identifiers or other methods are required for integrating health data of an individual distributed across multiple systems at different sites.

INFORMATION PROCESSING

Computer processing functions provide for effective retrieval and processing of data into useful information. These include decision-support tools such as alerts and alarms for drug interactions, allergies, and abnormal laboratory results. Reminders can be provided for appointments, critical path actions, medication administration, and other activities. The systems also may provide access to consensus-driven and evidence-driven diagnostic and treatment guidelines and protocols (Weaver, Warren, & Delaney, 2005). The nurse could integrate a standard guideline, protocol, or critical path into a specific individual's CPR, modify it to meet unique circumstances, and use it as a basis for managing and documenting care. Outcome data communicated from various caregivers and health care recipients themselves also may be analyzed and used for continual improvement of the guidelines and protocols.

INFORMATION COMMUNICATION

Information communication refers to the interoperability of systems and linkages for the exchange of data across disparate systems. To integrate health data across multiple systems at different sites, identifier systems (unique numbers or other methodology) for health care recipients, caregivers, providers, payers, and sites are essential. Local, regional, and national health information infrastructures that tie all participants together using standard data communication protocols are key to the linkage function. Hundreds of types of transactions or messages must be defined and agreed to by the participating stakeholders. Vocabulary and code systems must permit the exchange and processing of data into meaningful information. CPR systems must provide access to point-of-care information databases and knowledge sources, such as pharmaceutical formularies, referral databases, and reference literature.

Electronic data sharing of any kind of data as described previously raises concerns of security and confidentiality. Existing challenges in protecting security while

EVIDENCE FROM THE LITERATURE

Citation: Levine, C. (2006). HIPAA and Talking with Family Caregivers. *American Journal of Nursing, 106*(8), 51–53.

Discussion: HIPAA has alarmed and confused many conscientious health care providers. Providers can share needed information with family and friends or with anyone a patient identifies as involved in his care as long as the patient does not object and/or the provider believes that doing so is in the best interests of the patient. The article shares the U.S. Department of Health & Human Services Website for a list of Frequently Asked Questions about HIPAA, available at www.hhs.gov/hipaafaq

Implications for Practice: Health care providers concerned with quality patient care will want to review HIPAA and ensure that they do not use HIPAA to avoid difficult conversations.

allowing for increased ease of data retrieval have been significantly complicated by the Health Insurance Portability and Accountability Act of 1996 (HIPAA). Specific legal and ethical issues vary from state to state, from specialty to specialty, and from caregiver to caregiver. Incorporating these variations into a cohesive, comprehensive CIS presents a considerable challenge.

SECURITY

Computer-based patient record systems provide better protection of confidential health information than paper-based systems because they support controls that ensure that only authorized users with legitimate uses have access to health information. Security functions address the confidentiality of private health information and the integrity of the data. Security functions must be designed to ensure compliance with applicable laws, regulations, and standards. Security systems must ensure that access to data is provided only to those who are authorized and have a legitimate purpose for using the data. Security functions also must provide a means to audit for inappropriate access.

Three important terms are used when discussing security: privacy, confidentiality, and security. It is important to understand the differences among these concepts.

- *Privacy* refers to the right of individuals to keep information about themselves from being disclosed to

CRITICAL THINKING 6-2

In your clinical practice, you have likely interacted with a clinical information system to both enter and access data for the patient you were caring for.

What security systems were in place to maintain the confidentiality of patient data, for example, passwords, identification cards, and so on? Do you believe the security system was effective? Was it updated on a regular basis? Did the security system present any barriers to your obtaining necessary information for providing quality patient care—for example, were the results of certain tests or past history restricted in any way?

anyone. If a patient had an abortion and chose not to tell a health care provider this fact, the patient would be keeping that information private.

- *Confidentiality* refers to the act of limiting disclosure of private matters. After a patient has disclosed private information to a health care provider, that provider has a responsibility to maintain the confidentiality of that information.
- *Security* refers to the means to control access and protect information from accidental or intentional disclosure to unauthorized persons and from alteration, destruction, or loss. When private information is placed in a confidential CPR, the system must have controls in place to maintain the security of the system and not allow unauthorized persons access to the data (CPRI Work Group on Confidentiality, Privacy & Security, 1995).

INFORMATION PRESENTATION

The wealth of information available through CPR systems must be managed to ensure that authorized caregivers, including nurses and others with legitimate uses, have the information they need in their preferred presentation form. A nurse, for example, may like to see data organized by source, caregiver, encounter, problem, or date. Data can be presented in detail or summary form. Tables, graphs, narrative, and other forms of information presentation must be accommodated. Some users may

need to know only of the presence or absence of certain data, not the nature of the data itself. For example, blood donation centers test blood for HIV, hepatitis, and other conditions. If a donor has a positive test result, the center may not be given the specific information regarding the test but just general information that a test result was abnormal and that the patient should be referred to an appropriate health care provider.

INTERFACE BETWEEN THE INFORMATICS NURSE AND THE CLINICAL INFORMATION SYSTEM

Information demands in health care systems are pushing the development of CISs and CPRs. The ongoing development of computer technology—smaller, faster machines with extensive storage capabilities and the ability for cross-platform communication—is making the goal of an integrated electronic system a realistic option, not just a long-term dream. As these systems evolve, informatics nurses will play an important role in their development, implementation, and evaluation.

Informatics nurses, because of their expertise, are in an ideal position to assist with the development, implementation, and evaluation of CISs. Their knowledge of policies, procedures, and clinical care is essential as work-flow systems are redesigned within a CIS. It is not unusual for nurses within an institution to have more hands-on interaction with and knowledge of different departments than any other group of employees in an institution. Jenkins (2000) suggests that the process model of nursing (assessment, planning, implementation, and evaluation) works well during a CIS implementation, thus nurses have a familiar framework from which to understand the complexity of a major system change.

TRENDS IN COMPUTING

As noted earlier, computers have moved from the realm of a "nice to know" luxury item to a "need to know" essential resource for professional practice. Nurses are knowledge workers who require accurate and up-to-date information for their professional work. The explosion in information—some estimate that all information is replaced every 9 to 12 months—requires nurses to be on the cutting edge of knowledge to practice ethically and safely. Trends in computing will also affect the work of professional nurses and not just through the development of CISs and CPRs. Research advances, new devices, monitoring equipment, sensors, and "smart body parts" will all change the way that health care is conceptualized, practiced, and delivered.

Within this context, not every nurse will need to be an informatics specialist, but every nurse must be computer literate. **Computer literacy** is defined as the knowledge and understanding of computers combined with the ability to use them effectively (Joos, Whitman, Smith, & Nelson, 1996). Computer literacy may be interpreted as different levels of expertise for different people in various roles. On the least specialized level, computer literacy may involve knowing how to turn on a computer, start and stop simple application programs, and save and print information. For health care professionals, computer literacy requires having an understanding of systems used in clinical practice, education, and research settings. In clinical practice, for example, electronic patient records and clinical information systems are being used more often. The computer literate nurse must be able to use these systems effectively and address issues discussed earlier, such as confidentiality, security, and privacy. At the same time, the more advanced nurse must be able to effectively use applications typically found on PCs, such as word processing software, spreadsheets, and power-point. The nurse will want to develop the ability to use statistics for research. Finally, the computer literate nurse must know how to access information from a variety of electronic sources and how to evaluate the appropriateness

of the information at both the professional and patient level. The computer literate nurse has information literacy. **Information literacy** is defined as the understanding of the architecture of information; the ability to navigate among a variety of print and electronic tools to effectively access, search, and critically evaluate appropriate resources and synthesize accumulated information into an existing body of knowledge and practice (Jacobs, Rosenfeld, & Haber, 2003). The remainder of this chapter is designed to help you gain a broader understanding of computer literacy and the computing environment of PCs and the online world, and includes a discussion of future trends.

DEVELOPMENT OF MODERN COMPUTING

Weiser and Brown (1996) have characterized the history and future of computing as having three phases. The first phase is known as the "mainframe era" in which many people share one computer. Computers were found behind closed doors and run by experts with specialized knowledge and skills. Although we have mostly moved beyond the mainframe era, it still exists in CISs (hence, some of the problems discussed previously) or other situations with large mainframe systems, such as banking, weather forecasting, and academic institutions.

The archetypal computer of the mainframe era must be the ENIAC, developed at the University of Pennsylvania in 1945. The Electronic Numerical Integrator and Computer (ENIAC) was conceived by John Mauchly, an American physicist, and built at the Moore School of Engineering by Mauchly and J. Presper Eckert, an engineer. It is regarded as the first successful digital computer. It weighed more than 60,000 pounds and contained more than 18,000 vacuum tubes. About 2,000 of the computer's vacuum tubes were replaced each month by a team of six technicians. Even though one vacuum tube blew approximately every 15 minutes, the functioning of the ENIAC was still considered to be reliable! Many of the ENIAC's first tasks were for military purposes, such as calculating ballistic firing tables and designing atomic weapons. Because the ENIAC was initially not a stored program machine, it had to be reprogrammed for each task.

Phase II in modern computing is the "PC era," which is characterized by one person to one computer. In this era, the computing relationship is personal and intimate. Similar to a car, the computer is seen as a special, relatively expensive item, which requires attention but provides a very valuable service in one's life.

The first harbinger of the PC era was in 1948 with the development of the transistor at Bell Telephone Laboratories. The transistor, which could act as an electric switch, replaced the costly, energy-inefficient, and unreliable vacuum tubes in computers and other devices, including televisions. By the late 1960s, integrated circuits, tiny transistors, and other electrical components arranged on a single chip of silicon replaced individual transistors in computers. Integrated circuits became miniaturized, enabling more components to be designed into a single computer circuit. In the 1970s, refinements in integrated circuit technology led to the development of the modern microprocessor, integrated circuits that contained thousands of transistors. Weiser and Brown (1996) date the true start of the second phase as 1984, when the number of people using PCs surpassed the number of people using shared computers.

Manufacturers used integrated circuit technology to build smaller and cheaper computers. The first PCs were sold by Instrumentation Telemetry Systems. The Altair 8800 appeared in 1975. Graphical user interfaces were first designed by the Xerox Corporation in a prototype computer, the Alto, developed in 1974. This prototype computer incorporated many of the features found on computers today, including a mouse, a graphical user interface, and a "user friendly" operating system. However, the Xerox Corporation made a corporate decision to not pursue commercial development of the PC, the rationale being that the core business strategy of Xerox was copiers, not computers. One only has to look at how PCs have proliferated throughout the world to realize that this may not have been the smartest business decision ever made. In fact, this whole episode has become a bit of a computer history legend (Hiltzik, 2000; Smith & Alexander, 1988). Continuing development of sophisticated operating systems and miniaturization of components (modern microprocessors contain as many as ten million transistors) have enabled computers to be developed that can run programs and manipulate data in ways that were unimaginable in the era of the ENIAC.

UBIQUITOUS COMPUTING

Phase III has been dubbed the era of ubiquitous computing (UC), in which computers are no longer distinct objects but are integrated in the environment, thus enabling people to interact with information-processing devices more naturally and casually. Weiser and Brown (1996) estimate that the crossover with the PC era will be between 2005 and 2020. In this phase, computers will be everywhere—in walls, chairs, clothing, light switches, cars, appliances, and so on. Computers will become so fundamental to our human experience that they will "disappear," and we will cease to be aware of them. The result will be "calm technology," in which computers do not cause stress and anxiety for the user but, rather, recede into the background of life. For those who are skeptical that this will come to pass, consider two other ubiquitous technologies: writing and electricity (Weiser, 1991). In Egyptian times, writing was a secret art, known and performed only by specially trained scribes who lived on a level close to royalty. Clay tablets and later papyrus were precious commodities. Many people died without ever having seen a piece of paper in their lives! Now, paper and writing are everywhere. Within the course of an average day, most people use and discard hundreds of pieces of paper, never giving them a second thought. Electricity has a similar history. When electricity was first invented in the nineteenth century, entire factories were designed to accommodate the presence of light bulbs and bulky motors. The placement of workers, machines, and parts was designed around the need of electricity and motors. Today, electricity is everywhere. It is hidden in the walls and stored in tiny batteries. The average car has more than 22 motors and 25 solenoids.

One only has to look around a typical house to see how UC is becoming part of our lives. Microprocessors exist in every room: appliances in the kitchen, remote controls for the TV and stereo in the den, and clock radios and cordless phones in the bedroom. And the bathroom? Matsushita of Japan has developed a prototype toilet (dubbed the "smart toilet") that includes an online, real-time health monitoring system. It measures the user's weight, fat content, and urine sugar level; plots the recorded data on a graph; and sends the data instantaneously to a health care provider for monitoring (Watts, 1999).

Another dimension of UC is the Internet. Each time you connect to the Internet, you are connecting with millions of information resources and hundreds of information delivery systems. A person truly does become one person to hundreds of computers. It is ironic that the interface to the UC world of the Internet is still through a PC. But this is changing. Wireless, infrared connections are eliminating wires; handheld devices are eliminating the bulky PC. Once we become wireless and mobile, UC will become a reality.

VIRTUAL REALITY

Virtual reality (VR) puts people inside a computer-generated world. Virtual reality, while still somewhat limited in its development, does have enormous potential in health care applications.

Virtual reality, despite recent popularization, is not new. Just like the Internet, it had its beginnings within the Department of Defense and innovations developed during the 1960s. A brief review of history: during the time of the Cold War, there was great fear of a nuclear attack. Military leaders sought to develop systems that would remain intact in the face of great destruction. The Internet, which is a worldwide network of computers (there is not one large "Internet computer"), was developed so that the electronic communication infrastructure could not be destroyed. Electronic mail (e-mail) was created to ensure rapid and secure communication in the event the wire-based telephone system was destroyed. Virtual reality

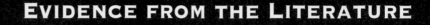

EVIDENCE FROM THE LITERATURE

Citation: Miller, J., Shaw-Kokot, J. R., Arnold, M. S., Boggin, T., Crowell, K. E., Allegri, F., et al. (2005). A study of personal digital assistants to enhance undergraduate clinical nursing. *Nursing Outlook, 44*(1), 19–24.

Discussion: This article reports on personal digital assistants (PDAs) as a means to prepare competent nurse professionals who value and seek current information. Through the incorporation of PDAs in undergraduate clinical courses, it is anticipated that the value and skill of seeking current information will become a routine that nursing students take into their professional practice. PDA software is available for such things as DrugGuides, Medical Laboratory Reference, Medical Abbreviations, Medical Spanish, and so on.

Implications for Practice: PDAs bring evidence-based care (EBC) to the bedside. The development of skill in using this technology is a basis for the development of ongoing technology skills and increased use of EBC.

CRITICAL THINKING 6-3

Many nurses are now using PDAs to deliver quality patient care. What are the benefits? What precautions need to be in place?

Do wireless applications in health care settings improve the efficiency of care delivery systems? Explain.

---

simulations were developed so that jet pilots could have training that would mimic a world turned upside down: flying through fire, mushroom clouds, and poisonous gases in planes that might lack air-to-ground control systems.

Current virtual reality systems have developed from these early applications. With VR, a person can see, move through, and react to computer-simulated items or environments. Using certain tools such as a head-mounted computer display and a handheld input device, the user feels immersed in and can interact with this world. The virtual world can represent the current world or a world that is difficult or impossible to experience firsthand—for example, the world of molecules, the interior of the human body, or the surface of Pluto. By putting the sensors on the person (head-mounted computer display, sensors in gloves, shoes, and glasses), the person can move and experience the world in a typical way—by walking, moving, and using the senses of touch, sight, smell, and hearing.

VR has allowed practitioners to develop minimally invasive surgical techniques. Traditionally, surgery is per-

formed by making incisions and directly interacting with the organs and tissues. Recent innovations in video technology allow direct viewing of internal body cavities through natural orifices or small incisions. The surgeon operates on a virtual image. The manipulation of instruments by the surgeon or assistants can be direct or via virtual environments. In the latter case, a robot reproduces the movements of humans using virtual instruments. The precision of the operation may be augmented by data or images superimposed on the virtual patient (Satava, 1995).

Applications in health care education also exist. Virtual reality allows information visualization through the display of enormous amounts of information contained in large databases. Through 3-D visualization, students can understand important physiological principles or basic anatomy. Students can go "inside" the body to visualize structures and see how they work. It is also possible to observe changes in physiologic functioning. For example, a student can visualize the vascular system of a patient going into shock (Satava, 1993, 1995).

A popular use in psychology has been in exposure therapy for patients with specific phobias. Hodges et al. (1995) used a VR simulation to treat patients with a fear of flying. Other researchers have found significant improvements in patients with agoraphobia using exposure therapy and VR (North, North, & Coble 1996).

At the University of Dayton Research Institute, Dayton, OH, researchers collaborated with the Miami Valley Transit Authority to assist disabled students to learn to ride the bus. Using a simulation of a public bus, students were able to learn how to get on, get off, and negotiate the interior, which gave them increased confidence and skills when faced with a real bus for the first time (Buckert-Donelson, 1995).

EVIDENCE FROM THE LITERATURE

Citation: Beyea, S. C., & Kobokovich, L. J. (2004, Oct.). Human patient simulation: A teaching strategy. *AORN Journal,* 719–724.

Discussion: Article discusses use of patient simulators for teaching purposes. A human patient simulator is a highly sophisticated, technologically advanced mannequin in adult, child, or infant size. These mannequins fully integrate with computer software that supports the development of preplanned scenarios that mimic a wide variety of clinical situations. Most human patient simulators produce lung, heart, and bowel sounds; have anatomically correct pulses; and respond to medical and pharmacological interventions with expected physiologic responses. Human patient simulators can be programmed to speak and, thus, interact with clinicians much like an actual patient. Simulators come equipped with a number of different features that support a variety of learning experiences. For example, one simulator model allows the insertion of a chest tube or application of a trauma or wound care kit. Such features support educators' abilities to create learning situations that address a variety of specific clinical problems or needs. Human patient simulation also can provide clinicians with an opportunity to care for a simulated patient with acute clinical problems, such as airway obstruction or cardiac arrest, hemorrhage, shock, or various other common emergencies.

Implications for Practice: Working with patient simulators allows students to solve problems, work as a team, and communicate effectively with their colleagues and other providers. Role play provides an opportunity to improve communication and enhance patient safety. By integrating concepts related to patient safety, such as human factors engineering, staff management, and situational awareness, participants learn approaches and concepts related to patient safety and develop clinical skills that reduce the potential for errors. Patient safety and avoidable medical errors are a concern in any institution. The Institute of Medicine report *To Err Is Human: Building a Safer Health System* recommends simulation training as one strategy to prevent errors in the clinical setting.

Applications in nursing are similar. For students learning clinical procedures, VR gives them the opportunity to practice invasive and less commonly occurring procedures in the lab so they have both the skill and confidence necessary when encountering a patient requiring the procedure for the first time. Likewise, VR enhances patient education materials. Diabetic patients needing to understand the physiologic processes of the pancreas may visualize the organ to more fully understand their disease and treatment. Patients requiring painful or unusual procedures may experience a VR simulation as a means of preparation. By providing an alternate environment, VR also has the potential to mitigate or minimize the side effects of certain procedures such as chemotherapy in patients with cancer.

THE INTERNET

The other major trend in modern computing—the Internet—is changing the way we communicate and obtain information. Many mistakenly believe that the Internet is a recent development. But, like VR, it has been around for more than three decades. The modern Internet started out in 1969 as a U.S. Defense Depart-

ment network called ARPAnet. Scientists built ARPAnet with the intention of creating a network that would still be able to function efficiently if part of the network were damaged. Since then, the Internet has grown, changed, matured, and mutated, but the essential structure of interconnected domains randomly distributed throughout the world has remained the same. ARPAnet no longer exists, but many of the standards established for that first network still govern the communication and structure of the modern Internet.

For many years, the Internet was more or less the private domain of scientists, researchers, and university professors who verdict to communicate and exchange files and software. A number of events transpired in the 1980s and early 1990s that resulted in the enormous growth of the Internet and its ensuing popularity.

In 1989, English computer scientist Timothy Berners-Lee introduced the World Wide Web (WWW). Berners-Lee initially designed the WWW to aid communication between physicists who were working in different parts of the world for the European Laboratory for Particle Physics (CERN). As it grew, however, the WWW revolutionized the use of the Internet. During the early 1990s, increasingly large numbers of users who were not part of the scientific or academic communities began to use the Internet, in large part because of the ability of the WWW

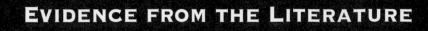

EVIDENCE FROM THE LITERATURE

Citation: Littlejohns, P., Wyatt, J. C., & Garvican, L. (2003). Information in practice, Evaluating computerized health information systems: hard lessons still to be learnt. *British Medical Journal, 326,* 860–863.

Discussion: The overall goal of the failed technology project discussed in this report was to improve the efficiency and effectiveness of health and welfare services through the creation and use of information for clinical, administrative, and monitoring purposes. Functions required to support these objectives in each hospital included the following:

- Master patient index
- Admission, discharges, and transfers
- Patient record tracking
- Appointments
- Order entry and reporting of results
- Departmental systems for laboratory, radiology, operating theater, other clinical services, dietary services, laundry
- Financial management

Some reasons for failure of the project included the following:

- Failure to take into account the social and professional cultures of health care organizations and to recognise that education of users and computer staff is an essential precursor of technology implementation
- Underestimation of the complexity of routine clinical and managerial processes
- Dissonance among the expectations of the administrators, the suppliers, and the users of the system
- Failure of developers to look for and learn lessons from past projects.

Implications for Practice: New technology systems are expensive. Implementation of new systems requires the ability to learn from past failures as well as the development of an interdisciplinary team of administrators, health care professionals, and technology representatives and users to assure successful implementation of new technology.

---

to easily handle multimedia documents. Other changes have also influenced the growth of the Internet, such as the High-Performance Computing Act of 1991; the decision to allow computers other than those used for research and military purposes to connect to the network; and the development of "user-friendly" software and tools that allowed less experienced computer users to obtain information quickly and easily.

The Internet is attractive. Information can be presented in different forms and in different languages. It also provides different organizational structures for information storage and access to accommodate the user's preference and need. Even though computer-stored and displayed information resources are potentially very useful in relation to patient education, their integration into nursing practice is rather inconsistent. Several problems, such as time requirements to filter the long and undifferentiated list of computer search results and the unknown quality and appropriateness of information, hamper the integration of electronic resources into clinical practice.

USING THE INTERNET FOR CLINICAL PRACTICE

A major use of the Internet is to obtain information. In clinical practice, this dimension of the Internet is becoming essential to ensure that you have accurate and up-to-date information for your nursing work. To use information that exists on the Internet, it is important to develop skills for searching quickly and efficiently. There are a variety of strategies you can use for searching, including quick and dirty searching, links, and brute force.

Keep in mind that you must be persistent. No one search strategy is going to work all the time, nor is any one search engine more effective than any other. Here are some strategies and tactics to render Internet searches more efficient and reduce search time (Jones, 2003):

- Use Websites published by governmental or professional organizations such as the American Heart Association (www.americanheart.org) or the National Heart, Lung & Blood Institute (www.nhlbi.nih.gov) for questions related to cardiovascular diseases; CancerNet (http://cancer-net.nci.nih.gov) for cancer information; and the National Institute of Diabetes and Digestive and Kidney Diseases (http://digestive.niddk.nih.gov) for information on diabetes and digestive disorders. The Center for Disease Control and Prevention (www.cdc.gov) is a primary resource for developing and applying disease prevention and control, environmental health, and health promotion activities; the National Institute on Aging (www.nia.nih.gov) focuses on well-being and health of older adults. Also helpful is the American Dietetic Association (www.eatright.org) offering information related to food and diet. The American Medical Association's consumer health information site (www.ama-assn.org) is a valuable resource for general health information.

■ Use reputable health care organizations' Websites such as www.mayoclinic.com from the Mayo Clinics and www.intelihealth.com from Harvard Medical School.

■ Use Consumer health sites organized by medical librarians. These offer a wealth of organized information on disease management. Examples are MEDLINE*plus* (www.medlineplus.gov) maintained by the National Library of Medicine and the New York Online Access to Health (NOAH) (www.noah-health.org), a multilingual Website organized and maintained by medical librarians in New York City.

■ Use precise terms, such as "Diabetes Type I" instead of just "Diabetes," to reduce the number of hits when searching for very specific information.

■ Draw on search engines, such as Mayo Clinic (www.mayoclinic.com); WebMD (www.webmd.com); and so forth, that collect information from reliable online health resources rather than relying on the "bots" or robots typically used by search engines to "crawl" the Web, such as Google.

■ Refine your Internet searches with filters. Filtering is mechanically blocking Internet content from being retrieved through the identification of key words and phrases. For example, you can narrow your search by the type of medical viewpoint (traditional or alternative), reading level (easy, moderate, or complex), and type of site (commercial, non-commercial, government, or nonprofit) that you use in your key words to filter your search.

The result of your searches after using these strategies will probably be a more focused and helpful list of links matching your specific request. You will then want to evaluate your search data using the method discussed in this chapter.

THE P-F-A ASSESSMENT

One strategy to develop your search is to conduct a "purpose-focus-approach" (P-F-A) assessment. To determine your purpose, ask yourself why you are doing the search and why you need the information. Consider questions such as the following:

■ Is it for personal interest?
■ Do you want to obtain information to share with coworkers or a client?
■ Are you verifying information given to you by someone else?
■ Are you preparing a report or writing a paper for a class or project?

Based on your purpose, your focus may be as follows:

■ Broad and general (basic information for yourself)
■ Lay oriented (to give information to a patient) or professionally oriented (for colleagues)
■ Narrow and technical with a research orientation

Purpose combined with focus determines your approach. For example, information that is broad and general can be found using brute force methods or quick and dirty searching. Lay information can be quickly accessed at a few key sites, including MEDLINE*plus* and consumer health organizations. Similarly, professional associations and societies are a good starting point for professionally oriented information. Scientific and research information usually requires literature resources that can be found in databases such as MEDLINE or CINAHL (Cumulative Index to Nursing and Allied Health Literature).

QUICK AND DIRTY SEARCHING

Quick and dirty searching is a very simple but surprisingly effective search strategy. First, start with a search engine, such as AltaVista (www.altavista.com). Next, type in the term of interest. At this point, do not worry about being overly broad or general. You will retrieve an enormous number of found references (called "hits"), but you are interested only in the first 10 to 20. Look at the universal resource locators (URLs), that is, the addresses of the sites that are returned by your search, and try to decipher what they mean. Pay attention to the domains: .com is commercial; .edu is an educational institution; .gov is the government. Quickly visit a few sites. Look for the information you need, or useful links. If a site is not relevant, use the Back button on your browser to return to your search results and go to the next site. After you find a site that appears to be useful, begin to explore the site. Many sites will connect you to other sites, using links, or hot buttons. If you click on a link, it will take you to a related site. If the site you are looking at has links (most do), use them to connect to other relevant sites. This process—quick search, quick review, clicking, and linking—can provide a starting point for finding useful information in a relatively short period of time. You then can evaluate the information further using the evaluation method discussed later in this chapter.

BRUTE FORCE

Brute force searching is another alternative. To do this, type in an address in the URL box (the address box at the top of the browser window) and see what happens. The worst outcome is an annoying error message, but you may land on a site that is exactly what you want. To be effective, think how URLs work: they usually start with www (for World Wide Web). Then there is the "thing in the middle" followed by a domain. Perhaps you are trying to find a school of nursing at a certain university. What is the common name for the university? WWW.unh.edu is the very logical URL for the University of New Hampshire. Organizations are also quite logical in their URLs: www.aorn.org is the Association of periOperative Registered Nurses (AORN); www.aone.org is the American Organization of Nurse Executives (AONE).

LINKS AND BOOKMARKS

As noted earlier, just about every single Website has links to other Websites of related interest. Take advantage of these links because the site developer has already done some of the work of finding other useful resources. Combine quick and dirty searching or brute force with links to get the information you need. Each site you visit will have more links, and in this way, the resources keep building. Visiting a variety of sites will open up the vistas of information that are available. When you find a site of interest, "bookmark" it or add it to your list of favorites. A bookmark list, or list of favorites, is like a personal address book. Each time you find a site that is particularly useful, you can add it to your list of favorites, using the appropriate feature in your browser. Eventually, you will have a comprehensive list of sites that are relevant to your work and interests. By having this list, you will be able to quickly return to sites during future Internet sessions.

RESOURCES FOR PROFESSIONALS AND CONSUMERS

The preceding discussion has focused on strategies to use when you are faced with a "needle in a haystack" searching situation—just dive in and see what you find. The advantage of this method is that it is fast and easy. There are disadvantages though: sites of dubious quality may be obtained, and the process, while fast, is not terribly efficient.

Another approach is to develop a "short list" of well-known, well-researched sites that can be used as starting points for further exploration. Such a list is useful to share with others so that they can begin their own exploration. These should be sites that you have determined

are trustworthy and reliable. Examples of such sites include organizations and associations with which we are all familiar, such as the American Cancer Society (ACS). The ACS has patient education and consumer information materials that can be obtained by a virtual, Internet visit to www.cancer.org. In addition to the traditional types of resources available from the ACS, at the Website, it is also possible to send an e-mail requesting more information, sign up for regular updates and news, read news items, and obtain updated statistical information. The Website is truly a "value-added" version of the ACS. Practically any health organization you can think of has created a virtual storefront on the Web. Professional associations, in nursing, medicine, and other disciplines, are also becoming comprehensive resource sites on the Web. NursingCenter.com (www.nursingcenter.com) is a handy source of information.

Other resources include U.S. government agencies, such as the Agency for Healthcare Research and Quality (www.ahrq.gov) and the National Institutes of Health (www.nih.gov). Once again, all these agencies have been busy creating virtual institutes on the Web. A useful resource is Healthfinder (www.healthfinder.gov), which can point you to news, information, tools, and databases.

While these resources are the Web versions of known and useful organizations, there are also virtual resources that exist only on the Web. One such site that is particularly impressive is MEDLINE*plus* (www.medlineplus.gov), developed by the National Library of Medicine. A similar resource, specific to oncology, is OncoLink at the University of Pennsylvania (www.oncolink.org). OncoLink was created in 1994 and was the first multimedia oncology information resource placed on the Internet. It continues to be true to its original mission to "help cancer patients, families, health care professionals and the general public get accurate cancer-related information at no charge" (About Oncolink, 2001).

If you are searching for scientific-, technical-, or research-oriented information, then you must search online literature databases. In this case, the first places to turn to are CINAHL (www.cinahl.com) for nursing, and the National Library of Medicine (NLM) (www.nlm.nih.gov) for the PubMed and MEDLINE online bibliographical databases. You may search the databases either to produce a list of bibliographic citations of publications or to retrieve factual information on a specific question. MEDLINE covers the fields of medicine, nursing, dentistry, veterinary medicine, and the preclinical sciences. Journal articles are indexed for MEDLINE, and their citations are searchable, using NLM's controlled vocabulary, MeSH (Medical Subject Headings). MEDLINE contains all citations published in Index Medicus and corresponds in part to the International Nursing Index and the Index to Dental Literature. Citations include the English abstract when published with the article. This is approximately 76% of the current file. MEDLINE contains over 11 million records from 4,000 health science journals. The file is updated weekly. You can search MEDLINE for free, using PubMed (www.pubmed.gov).

Another literature resource to investigate is the National Guideline Clearinghouse (NGC) (www.ngc.gov). While MEDLINE includes citations to articles in professional journals, the NGC is a comprehensive database of evidence-based clinical practice guidelines and related documents produced by the Agency for Healthcare Research and Quality (AHRQ) in partnership with the American Medical Association (AMA) and the American Association of Health Plans (AAHP). The NGC mission is to provide practitioners, nurses, and other health professionals and health care providers; health plans; integrated delivery systems; purchasers; and others an accessible mechanism for obtaining objective, detailed information on clinical practice guidelines and to further their dissemination, implementation, and use.

A variety of other literature resources are also available on the Web, some of which have fees attached. However, do not automatically assume that you must pay the fee. Your workplace or school may have licensing agreements in place with different vendors, and as an employee or student, you may have access to the literature

resources. Check with your library or information services department to see if this applies to you and how you can access them from your computer at home or work. Your librarian can be very helpful to you in your searches also.

Another element of searching for literature online is finding full-text articles. The databases so far discussed (MEDLINE and so on) do not contain full text—they include only literature citations. Finding full-text online at the present time is an unorganized situation. Options include journals that have full-text available either for free or for a fee, or you can do things the old-fashioned way, that is, take a trip to the library and photocopy articles by hand. Given the state of confusion that exists, your best approach is to begin exploring, using quick and dirty or brute force methods. You can also visit the publisher's Website to see whether access to the journal is available. Another option is to use a document delivery service, such as UnCover (www.ulib.iupui.edu/erefs). This resource allows you to conduct a search. It identifies which articles can be sent to you, and what the fees will be (including article fees, service charges, and copyright fees). If you elect to order the article, you can identify how you want to have it sent to you (mail, fax, or other).

You can also use a search engine, for example, www.google.com. Search for full text nursing journal articles and see what you get. A final option is to use Google Scholar (http://scholar.google.com), which allows you to conduct a search, to identify the articles needed, and search the publisher's site for delivery costs, including article fees, service charges, and copyright fees. If you elect to order the article, you can identify how you want to have it sent to you, that is, by e-mail, fax or other.

RESOURCES FOR PATIENTS

A major problem with using the Internet is that information on the Internet lacks the conventional standards by which traditional published resources are evaluated. Though many general instruments can be used in evaluating health-related Websites, most of them are incomplete, and many do not measure what they claim to measure (Silberg, Lundberg, & Musacchio, 1997). In addition, they are geared toward professional and regulatory organizations. Yet, it is critical that nonclinicians be able to evaluate health information on the Internet. Health care consumers also need a way to judge the quality and relevance of the information provided on the Internet. Helping patients determine this quality and relevance becomes a key responsibility for clinicians.

Criteria to evaluate Internet health information have developed over the years. However, these criteria often assume knowledge of medical content and some familiarity with traditional standards for evaluating such resources.

EVIDENCE FROM THE LITERATURE

Citation: Fox, S. (2005). Health Information Online [Electronic Version]. *PEW Internet & American Life Project.* Retrieved March 1, 2006 from http://www.pewinternet.org/pdfs/PIP_Healthtopics_May05.pdf.

Discussion: The Pew Internet & American Life Project's previous survey has suggested that previous online health information seekers were often motivated to search out information that related to actions they might need to take for specific medical issues in their lives. For instance, they, or people they love, might have experienced health symptoms that worried them or Internet users might search for information about whether they would be wise to visit a doctor. They might have just received a diagnosis and want to learn more about their medical condition. They might have had a new medical treatment or new medicine prescribed, and they want to learn more about it. In many cases, online health information seekers were action-oriented and highly purposeful because there was a pressing medical issue for them to address.

In the current survey, those concerns remain reflected in many respondents' answers. At the same time, there are also notable changes that relate to specific kinds of health searches. Online investigations for information about diet, fitness, exercise, and over-the-counter drugs have grown. This suggests that online health information seekers are increasingly interested in wellness information and material that could be unconnected to worrisome symptoms, a doctor's diagnosis, or another kind of health crisis. Two other notable categories of growth were seen in searches related to health insurance and material about specific doctors and hospitals. This suggests that health seekers are doing more health homework online before they make big decisions about health care. The article asks, what is the best approach to online, information-seeking health care consumers?

Suggested answers are the following:

- Keep in mind that you can turn this behavior into an opportunity to teach. Encourage the patient to take the time to research and learn more about his/her health condition.
- React in a positive manner about information from the Internet but remind the patient that its quality and reliability may be unknown.
- Inform patients that time constraints will not permit you to read the information on-the-spot but that you will gladly read it if they send it to you via e-mail, perhaps before a scheduled appointment.
- Accept patient's contributions and acknowledge that they may have valuable information that you may not have come across yet.

Things you should not do include the following:

- Be dismissive or paternalistic.
- Be derogatory about others' comments on the Internet.
- Refuse Internet material.
- Try to "one-up" the patient or family members regarding the information.
- Break normal rules of patient confidentiality.

Implications for Practice: Clinicians may improve their care delivery by acknowledging Internet information gathered by patients. It is also important to help patients evaluate the validity of any information they find on the Internet.

None of them focus on helping patients filter the information found on the Web. Based on these published criteria and taking into account patient context and needs, the nurse can provide the patient with a simple set of criteria, subjective and objective, to evaluate Website content, design, navigation, and credibility (Jones, 1999) using the Health on the Net (HON) principles (www.hon.ch). Health information Websites adhering to the HON principles are accredited with the HON code and can be verified at www.hon.ch.

EVALUATION OF INFORMATION FOUND ON THE INTERNET

As mentioned earlier, traveling through the Internet, one must always use critical thinking skills to evaluate the information that is found. The "wide open" nature of the Internet means that just about anyone with a computer and online access can create a home page and post it for the world to see. Although there are many excellent health-

and nursing-related sites, there are others that just do not measure up in terms of accuracy, content, or currency.

In recent years, criteria for Website evaluation have proliferated. They range from the simple and cursory to the elaborate and expansive. I have found a simple mnemonic, "Are you PLEASED with the site?" to be very helpful (Table 6-1).

The mnemonic makes the seven criteria very easy to remember, but I have found, in hundreds of hours of surfing and evaluating, they are extremely comprehensive (Nicoll, 2000, 2001). To determine whether you are PLEASED, consider the following:

■ *P—Purpose:* What is the author's purpose in developing the site? Are the author's objectives clear? Many people will develop a Website as a hobby or way of sharing information they have gathered. It should be immediately evident to you what the true purpose of the site is. At the same time, consider your purpose; that is, think back to your P-F-A assessment. There should be congruence between the author's purpose and yours.

■ *L—Links:* Evaluate the links at the site. Are they working? Links that do not take you anywhere are called "dead links." Do they link to reliable sites? It is important to critically evaluate the links at sites hosted by organizations, businesses, or institutions because these entities are usually presenting themselves as authorities on the subject at hand. Some pages, such as those created by individuals, are really nothing more than a collection of links. These can be useful as a starting point for a search, but it is still important to evaluate the links that are provided at the site.

■ *E—Editorial (site content):* Is the information contained in the site accurate, comprehensive, and current? Is there a particular bias, or is the information presented in an objective way? Who is the consumer of the site: is it designed for health professionals, patients, consumers, or other audiences? Is the information presented in an appropriate format for the intended audience? Look at details, too. Are there misspellings and grammatical errors? "Under construction" banners that have been there forever?

TABLE 6-1   WEBSITE EVALUATION

Ask yourself, is this site accredited by Health On the Net(HON)? If no, "Are you PLEASED with the site?"

P — Purpose

L — Links

E — Editorial (site content)

A — Author

S — Site navigation

E — Ethical disclosure

D — Date site last updated

Source: The search or verification tool of HONcode aceredited websites at www.hon.ch/HONcode/Hunt, accessed on March 1, 2006.

CASE STUDY 6-1

You are working in a women's health clinic with a number of nursing and medical practitioners. The clinic receives at least two to three telephone calls a day from women with a urinary tract infection (UTI). The question comes up: do all these women need to be seen by a practitioner or is there a way to manage some of the cases by telephone? You are asked to be on a committee to explore this issue and possibly come up with a protocol. Where do you begin? Is a protocol for telephone management of UTI realistic?

These types of errors can be very telling about the overall quality of the site.

- **A—Author:** Who is the author of the site? Does that person or group of people have the appropriate credentials? Is the author clearly identified by name and is contact information provided? One suggestion is to double-check an author's credentials by doing a literature search in MEDLINE. When people advertise themselves as "the leading worldwide authority" on such and such a topic, they should have a few publications to their credit that establish their reputations. It is surprising how many times this search brings up nothing.

  Be wary of how a person presents his or her credentials, too. Consider a site where "Dr. X" is touted as an expert. Upon further exploration, you may find that, in fact, Dr. X does have a PhD (or MD or EdD), but the discipline in which this degree was obtained has nothing to do with the subject matter of the site. Remember that there is no universal process of peer review on the WWW, and people can present themselves in any way they want. Be suspicious.

  Keep in mind that the Webmaster and the author may be two (or more) different people. The Webmaster is the person who designed the site and is responsible for its upkeep. The author is the person who is responsible for the content and is the expert in the subject matter provided. In your evaluation, make sure you determine who these people are.

- **S—Site:** Is the site easy to navigate? Is it attractive? Does it download quickly or have too many graphics and other features that make it inefficient? A site that is pleasing to the eye will invite you to return. Sites that cause your computer to crash should be viewed with a skeptical eye.

- **E—Ethical:** Is there contact information for the site developer and author? Is there full disclosure of who the author is and the purpose of the site? Is this information easy to find or is it buried deep in the Website? There are many commercial services, particularly pharmaceutical companies, that have excellent Websites with very useful information. But some of them exist only to sell their product, although this is not immediately evident on evaluation.

- **D—Date:** When was the site last updated? Is it current? Does the information need to be updated regularly? Generally, with health and nursing information, the answer to that last question is yes. You should be concerned with sites that have not been updated within 12 to 18 months. The date the site was last updated should be prominently displayed on the site. Keep in mind that different pages within the site may be updated at different times. Be sure to check the date on each of the pages that you visit.

As you become more proficient at evaluating Websites, you may have additional criteria that you would add to this list or criteria that are important to you for a specific purpose, but, in general, this simple group of seven is surprisingly comprehensive. Test them for yourself. Do a quick search on a topic of interest, visit a number of sites, and determine just how PLEASED you are with what you find.

Key Concepts

- Computers and the Internet are no longer a novelty but a fact of life, with exponential growth on a worldwide basis.

- Within nursing, the combination of computer science and information science with clinical expertise allows us to develop systems that have the ultimate goal of improving patient outcomes.

- Nursing informatics is the specialty that integrates nursing science, computer science, and information science in identifying, collecting, processing, and managing data and information to support and expand nursing practice, administration, education, research, and nursing knowledge.

- Nurses can pursue formal education in nursing informatics at both the graduate and undergraduate levels.

- Informal education in informatics can be pursued through self-study, attendance at conferences, and reading the informatics literature.

- Certification in nursing informatics is voluntary and recognizes superior achievement and excellence in the specialty.

- Virtual reality simulations have been used in education and patient care. Minimally invasive surgery has been developed in large part through the technology of virtual reality.

- Telehealth applications are developing rapidly in nursing.

- Effective searching for information on the Internet requires that you target your search.

- PubMed is a digital archive of health journals developed by the National Library of Medicine (NLM) that allows you to search the NLM databases, including professional ones such as MEDLINE but also several ones geared toward health care consumers.

- It is important to evaluate information found on the Internet and to educate your patients about the importance of evaluating the information found on the Internet.

- Several Institute of Medicine reports have highlighted the need for health care technology.

KEY TERMS

clinical information system (CIS)
computer literacy
computerized patient
  record (CPR)
data capture

information
  communication
information literacy
nursing informatics
storage

REVIEW QUESTIONS

1. E-health includes which of the following activities?
   A. Obtaining health information online
   B. Shopping for health products online
   C. Online case management
   D. All of the above

2. A person who is HIV positive and chooses not to reveal this information to a nurse during an admission assessment is keeping this information
   A. anonymous.
   B. secure.
   C. confidential.
   D. private.

3. If a patient came to you asking for an Internet site where he could learn more about diabetes, which of the following would be appropriate for you to suggest?
   A. MEDLINE at the National Library of Medicine
   B. OncoLink
   C. MEDLINE*plus*
   D. All of the above

4. You are interested in learning more about amyotrophic lateral sclerosis (ALS). You find a Website where the author states that he is a worldwide leading researcher into causes for this disease. As part of your evaluation of the author's credentials, you
   A. take him at his word.
   B. e-mail him and ask for a list of references.
   C. ask several colleagues whether they are familiar with his research.
   D. do an author search on MEDLINE.

5. Decipher the following URL: www.noah-health.org This is the URL for which of the following Websites?
   A. The National Library of Medicine
   B. A local health organization for immigrants
   C. A consumer health Website
   D. A Website published by medical librarians

REVIEW ACTIVITIES

1. The EHR and health information exchanges between health care agencies are supported by the government, insurers, and many health care organizations. Do you think consumers will encourage the development of such systems or not? Why?

2. A popular area of research in nursing informatics has been the integration of information technology in all areas of nursing practice. Another topic that has been studied widely is the development and implementation of terminologies to document and communicate nursing practice. As we move into the era of EHR, do you think that we need to refocus on more generic health care terminologies such as SNOMED-CT, which serve the health care community rather than nursing alone? Why or why not?

EXPLORING THE WEB

- Pick a specialty area in nursing that interests you. Visit the American Nurses Credentialing Center (*www.ana.org*) to determine whether the ANCC certifies nurses in this specialty. If yes, what are the requirements? If no, is there another organization that credentials nurses in this specialty? Do a Web search to find the organization and the requirements for certification.

- Search for Books, then PDA at: *www.barnesandnoble.com*

- The Unified Medical Language System (*http://umlsks.nlm.nih.gov*) is developed to compensate for differences in concepts in several biomedical terminologies.

  How many nursing languages are incorporated in the UMLS?

  How are the languages used in clinical practice?

  How would you obtain more information on each of the approved languages?

Check these sites:

PEW Health Professions
www.futurehealth.ucsf.edu

IBM: Planet Blue project
www.research.ibm.com

Massachusetts Institute of Technology Project Oxygen
www.oxygen.lcs.mit.edu

Softscape, Inc.
www.softscape.com

Duke University
www.duke.edu

Fred Hutchinson Cancer Research Center
www.fhcrc.org

Argonne National Laboratory
www.library.anl.gov

University of Southern California
www.usc.edu

University of Virginia
www.virginia.edu

University of Wisconsin-Madison
www.wisc.edu

■ The Nursing Information and Data Set Evaluation Center of the ANA was established "to review, evaluate against defined criteria, and recognize information systems from developers and manufacturers that support documentation of nursing care within automated Nursing Information Systems (NIS) or within computer-based Patient Record systems (CPR)." Visit the center at *www.nursingworld.org* to find answers to the following questions:

How many nursing languages have been recognized by the ANA?

Why have these languages been developed?

What are they designed to do?

How would you obtain more information on each of the approved languages?

REFERENCES

About Oncolink (2001). University of Pennsylvania Cancer Center. Retrieved November 27, 2001, from http://www.oncolink.com/templates/about/index.cfm

American Nurses Association (ANA). (2001). *Scope and standards of practice for nursing informatics.*

American Nurses Credentialing Center (ANCC). (1993). *Statement of philosophy.* Washington, DC: American Nurses Association.

Ball, M. J., & Hannah, K. J. (1984). *Using computers in nursing.* Reston, VA: Reston Publishers.

Ball, M. J., Hannah, K. J., Newbold, S. K., & Douglass, J. V. (2000). *Nursing informatics: Where caring and technology meet* (3rd ed.) New York: Springer Verlag.

Beyea, S. C., & Kobokovich, L. J. (2004, Oct.). Human patient simulation: A teaching strategy. *AORN Journal,* 719–724.

Blois, M. S. (1986). What is medical informatics? *The Western Journal of Medicine, 145*(6), 776–777.

Brailer, D. (2005). Healthcare information and management systems society, National conference. February 13–17. Washington, DC.

Buckert-Donelson, A. (1995). Heads up projects: Disabled learn to use public transportation. *VR World, 3*(3), 4–5.

Cannon, D. S., & Allen, S. N. (2000). A comparison of the effects of computer and manual reminders on compliance with a mental health clinical practice guidelines. *Journal of American Medical Informatics Association, 7*(2), 196–203.

Carroll, K., Bradford, A., Foster, M., Cato, J., & Jones, J. (2007). An emerging giant: Nursing Informatics. *Nursing Management, 38*(3), 38–42.

CPRI Work Group on Confidentiality, Privacy & Security. (1995). *Guidelines for establishing information security policies at organizations using computer-based patient records.* Schaumburg, IL: Computer-based Patient Record Institute.

Eysenbach, G. (2001). What is e-health? *Journal of Medical Internet Research, 3*(2), e20.

Fox, S. (2005). Health Information Online [Electronic Version]. *PEW Internet & American Life Project.* Retrieved March 1, 2006 from http://www.pewinternet.org/pdfs/PIP_Healthtopics_May05.pdf

Goossens, W. T. F. (1996). Nursing information management and processing: A framework and definition for systems analysis, design and evaluation. *International Journal of Biomedical Computing, 40,* 187–195.

Graves, J. R., & Corcoran, S. (1989). The study of nursing informatics. *Image—The Journal of Nursing Scholarship, 21*(4), 227–231.

Grobe, S. J. (1988). Introduction. In H. E. Petersen & U. G. Jelger (Eds.), *Preparing nurses for using information systems: Recommended informatics competencies* (p. 4). New York: National League for Nursing.

Hannah, K. J. (1985). Current trends in nursing informatics: Implications for curriculum planning. In K. J. Hannah, E. J. Guillemin, & D. N. Conklin (Eds.), *Nursing uses of computer and information science* (pp. 181–187). Amsterdam: Elsevier.

Hersher, B. (2000). New roles for nurses in health care information systems. In M. Ball, K. Hannah, S. Newbold, & J. Douglas (Eds.), *Nursing informatics: Where caring and technology meet* (3rd ed., pp. 80–87). New York: Springer-Verlag.

Hiltzik, M. (2000). *Dealers of lightning: Xerox PARC and the dawn of the computer age.* New York: Harper Business.

Hoch, I., Heymann, A. D., Kurman, I., Valinsky, L. J., Chodick, G., & Shalev, V. (2003). Countrywide computer alerts to community physicians improve potassium testing in patients receiving diuretics. *Journal of American Medical Informatics Association, 10*(6), 541–546.

Hodges, L., Rothbaum, B., Kooper, R., Opdyke, D., Meyer, T., North, M., et al. (1995). Virtual environments for treating the fear of heights. *IEEE Computer, 28*(7), 27–34.

Horrigan, J., & Rainie, L. (2006). When facing a tough decision, 60 million Americans now seek the Internet's help. Observation Deck: Analysis of public opinion, demographic and policy trends. Retrieved May 3, 2006, from http://pewresearch.org/obdeck/?ObDeckID=19

Institute of Medicine (IOM). (2001). *Crossing the quality chasm: A new health system for the 21st century.* National Academy Press: Washington, DC.

Institute of Medicine (IOM). (2003). *Health professions education: A bridge to quality.* Washington, DC: National Academies Press.

International Medical Informatics Association (IMIA)—Special Interest Group of International Medical Informatics Association, Nursing Informatics, Helsinki, Finland, 1997.

Jacobs, S. K., Rosenfeld, P., & Haber, J. (2003). Information literacy as the foundation for evidence-based practice in graduate nursing education: A curriculum-integrated approach. *Journal of Professional Nursing, 19*(5), 320–328.

Jenkins, S. (2000). Nurses' responsibilities in the implementation of information systems. In M. Ball, K. Hannah, S. Newbold, &

J. Douglas (Eds.), *Nursing informatics: Where caring and technology meet* (pp. 207–223). New York: Springer-Verlag.

Johnston, D., Pan, E., Walker, J., Bates, D. W., & Middleton, B. (2003). *The value of computerized provider order entry in ambulatory settings: Executive preview.* Wellesley, MA: Center for Information Technology Leadership.

Joint Commission (JC). (2007). Hospital/Critical Access Hospital National Patient Safety Goals. Retrieved July 27, 2006 from http://www.jointcommission.org/PatientSafetyNational PatientSafetyGoals/07hap_cahnpsgs.htm

Jones, J. (1999). *Development of a self-assessment method for patients to evaluate health information on the Internet.* Paper presented at the AMIA, 1999 Fall Symposium, Washington, DC.

Jones, J. (2003). Patient education and the WWW. *Clinical Nurse Specialist, 17*(6), 281–283.

Joos, I., Whitman, N., Smith, M., & Nelson, R. (1996). *Computers in small bytes: The computer workbook* (2nd ed.). New York: National League for Nursing Press.

Levine, C. (2006). HIPAA and Talking with Family Caregivers. *American Journal of Nursing, 106*(8), 51–53.

Littlejohns, P., Wyatt, J. C., & Garvican, L. (2003). Information in practice, evaluating computerized health information systems: hard lessons still to be learnt. *British Medical Journal, 326*, 860–863.

Madden, M., & Fox, S. (2006). Finding Answers Online in Sickness and in Health. Retrieved May 15, 2006, from http://www. pewinternet.org/pdfs/PIP_Health_Decisions_2006.pdf

McNeil, B. J., Elfrink, V. L., Pierce, S. T., Beyea, S. C., Bickford, C. J., & Averill, C. (2005, Dec.). Nursing informatics knowledge and competencies: A national survey of nursing education programs in the United States. *International Journal of Medical Informatics, 74*(11–12), 1021–1030.

Medical Records Institute (2006). Retrieved July 25, 2006, from http://www.medrecinst.com

Miller, J., Shaw-Kokot, J. R., Arnold, M. S., Boggin, T., Crowell, K. E., Allegri, et al. (2005). A study of personal digital assistants to enhance undergraduate clinical nursing. *Nursing Outlook, 44*(1), 19–24.

National Institute of Nursing Research (NINR). (1997). Nursing Informatics: Enhancing Patient Care. Retrieved August 25, 1998, from http://www.nih.gov/ninr/research/vol4

Nicoll, L. H. (2000). *Nurses' Guide to the Internet* (3rd ed.). Philadelphia: Lippincott, Williams & Wilkins.

Nicoll, L. H. (2001). Quick and effective Website evaluation. *Lippincott's Case Management, 6*(4), 220–221.

North, M. M., North, S. M., & Coble, J. R. (1996). Effectiveness of virtual environment desensitization in the treatment of agorophobia. *Presence, Teleoperators, and Virtual Environments, 5*(3), 127–132.

Oh, H., Rizo, C., Enkin, M., & Jadad, A. (2005). What is eHealth: A systematic review of published definitions. *Journal of Medical Internet Research, 7*(1), e1.

Overhage, J. M., Evans, L., & Marchibroda, J. (2005). Communities' Readiness for Health Information Exchange: The National Landscape in 2004. *Journal of the American Medical Informatics Association, 12*(2), 107–112.

Raymond, B., & Dold, C. (2001). *Clinical information systems: Achieving the vision.* Prepared for the Meeting, The Benefits of Clinical Information Systems. Sponsored by the Kaiser Permanent Institute for Health Policy.

Satava, R. (1993). Virtual reality surgical simulator: The first steps. *Surgical Endoscopy, 7,* 203–205.

Satava, R. (1995). *Medicine 2001: The king is dead: Interactive technology and the new paradigm for healthcare* (pp. 334–339). Washington, DC: IOS Press.

Semancik, M. (1997). *The history of clinical information systems: Legacy systems, computer-based patient record and point of care.* Seattle, WA: SpaceLabs Medical.

Sequist, T. D., Gandhi, T. K., Karson, A. S., Fiskio, J. M., Bugbee, D., Sperling, M., et al. (2005). A Randomized Trial of Electronic Clinical Reminders to Improve Quality of Care for Diabetes and Coronary Artery Disease. *Journal of the American Medical Informatics Association, 12*(4), 431–437.

Shop.org. (1999). Statistics: Holiday 1999, Transactions and spending. Retrieved July 19, 2001 from http://www.shop.org/learn/ stats_hol1999_spending.html

Silberg, W. M., Lundberg, G. D., & Musacchio, R. A. (1997). Assessing, controlling, and assuring the quality of medical information on the Internet. *Journal of the American Medical Association, 277*(15), 1244–1245.

Smith, D., & Alexander, R. (1988). *Fumbling the future: How Xerox invented, then ignored, the first personal computer.* New York: W. Morrow.

Stevens, K. R., & Staley, J. M. (2004). The Quality Chasm reports, evidence-based practice, and nursing response to improve healthcare. *Nursing Outlook, 54*(2) 94–101.

Watts, J. (1999). The healthy home of the future comes to Japan. *Lancet, 353*(9164), 1597–1600.

Weaver, C. A., Warren, J. J., & Delaney, C. (2005). Bedside, classroom and bench: Collaborative strategies to generate evidence-based knowledge for nursing practice. *International Journal of Medical Informatics, 74*(11–12), 989–999.

Weiser, M. (1991). The computer for the 21st century. *Scientific American, 265*(3), 94–102.

Weiser, M., & Brown, J. (1996, October 5). The coming age of calm technology. Retrieved July 19, 2001, from http://www.ubiq.com/ hypertext/weiser/acmfuture2endnote.htm

Wickham, V., Miedema, F., Gamerdinger, K., & DeGooyer, J. (2006). Bar-coded patient ID: Review an organizational approach to vendor selection. *Nursing Management, 37*(12), 22–26.

Work Group on Confidentiality Privacy & Security. (1995). *Guidelines for establishing information security policies at organizations using computer-based patient records.* Schaumburg, IL: Computer-based Patient Record Institute.

SUGGESTED READINGS

Artinian, N. T. (2007, Jan.–Feb.). Telehealth as a tool for enhancing care for patients with cardiovascular disease. *Journal of Cardiovascular Nursing, 22*(1), 25–31.

Bowles, K. H., & Baugh, A. C. (2007, Jan.–Feb.). Applying research evidence to optimize telehomecare. *Journal of Cardiovascular Nursing, 22*(1), 5–15.

Demiris, G. (2007). Interdisciplinary innovations in biomedical and health informatics graduate education. *Methods in Infectious Medicine, 46*(1), 63–66.

Doebbeling, B. N., Vaughn, T. E., McCoy, K. D., & Glassman, P. (2006). *Informatics implementation in the Veterans Health Administration (VHA) healthcare system to improve quality of care.* American Medical Informatics Association Annual Symposium Proceedings, 204–208.

Gurses, A. P., Hu, P., Gilger, S., Dutton, R. P., Trainum, T., Ross, K., et al. (2006). *A preliminary field study of patient flow management in a trauma center for designing information technology.* American Medical Informatics Association Annual Symposium Proceedings, 937.

Hao, A. T., Chang, H. K., & Chong, P. P. (2006). *Mobile learning for nursing education.* American Medical Informatics Association Annual Symposium Proceedings, 943.

Palm, J. M., Colombet, I., Sicotte, C., & Degoulet, P. (2006). *Determinants of user satisfaction with a clinical information system.* American Medical Informatics Association Annual Symposium Proceedings, 614–618.

Poon, E. G., Keohane, C., Featherstone, E., Hays, B., Dervan, A., Woolf, S., et al. (2006). *Impact of barcode medication administration technology on how nurses spend their time on clinical care.* American Medical Informatics Association Annual Symposium Proceedings, 1065.

CHAPTER 7

Population-Based Health Care Practice

Patricia M. Schoon, MPH, RN

The selection of groups for care should be based on the questions: What difference might nursing care be expected to make in this situation? Is it more or less than would be expected in other groups (Ruth B. Freeman, 1957)?

OBJECTIVES

Upon completion of this chapter, the reader should be able to:

1. Discuss the social mandate to provide population-based health care at the global, national, state, and local levels.

2. Describe how population-based nursing is practiced within the community and the health care system.

3. Identify vulnerable and high-risk population groups for whom specific health promotion and disease-prevention services are indicated.

4. Outline a multidisciplinary population-based planning and evaluation process that includes partnerships with the community and health care consumers.

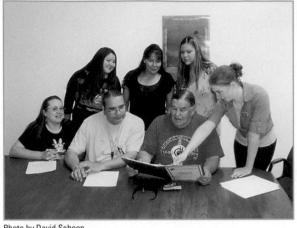

Photo by David Schoon

You are completing a clinical experience in an elementary school located in a large metropolitan area. This school has 600 students from kindergarten through sixth grade; 95% of them are from families living at or below the poverty level. Seventy-five percent of the student body transfers in or out of the school during each school year. Of these children, 40% are Southeast Asian, 25% are Hispanic, 10% are African-American, 10% are white, 10% are Somali refugees, and 5% are Native Americans. Sixty percent of the students speak English as a second language. Although 95% of the students are eligible for state-sponsored health insurance, only 30% of the children have health insurance, and only 10% have dental insurance. You observe that many children have significant dental problems and many are below the fifth percentile in height and weight on the standardized growth grid. The school nurse encourages you to think about what nursing actions you might take with these two groups of children.

> *What health problems can you identify in this group of schoolchildren?*
>
> *What social and environmental factors might contribute to these health problems?*
>
> *What actions directed at groups of children, rather than individuals, could you take to help these children?*
>
> *How can this be addressed at the population level?*

Nurses have acted to improve the health of populations and communities since the time of Florence Nightingale. Nightingale's actions to improve the health care of soldiers on the battlefields of the Crimean War and of the poor and infirm in London were directed at vulnerable population groups (Falk-Rafael, 2005). Nightingale's actions were based on the recognition that vulnerable population groups were not able to advocate effectively for themselves. She became their advocate. Nightingale was able to intervene to improve the health status of disenfranchised groups of people by influencing the health policies of the English government and changing the health care delivery systems in London and on the battlefield. That same spirit of advocacy and call to action is alive today among nurses throughout the world.

The primary thrust of this advocacy is directed at population groups that are at greatest risk for a decrease in health status and those groups that are most vulnerable to the socioeconomic forces that interfere with access to affordable quality health care. Nurses are united in partnership with other health care disciplines, the community, and health care consumers to achieve population-based global, national, state, and local health care goals related to access, cost, and quality. This chapter provides readers with an understanding of how population-based health care is practiced in the public and private health care sectors.

Population-based care requires active partnership of both providers and recipients of care. The phrase *health care consumers* includes current recipients of care, potential or past recipients of care, and other interested parties within the community.

This chapter introduces the reader to the application of the nursing process to population-based nursing practice. Collaboration with other health and social service providers and partnership with community members are key strategies to improve population-based health outcomes particularly among disenfranchised and vulnerable population groups. The diverse health care needs of the twenty-first century will require innovation in how health care is delivered. Nurses can take the lead in creating culturally inclusive population-based health care services and interventions that meet the needs of diverse population groups in the community.

POPULATION-BASED HEALTH CARE PRACTICE

Population-based health care practice is the development, provision, and evaluation of multidisciplinary health care services to population groups experiencing increased health risks or disparities, in partnership with health care consumers and the community, to improve the health of the community and its diverse population groups. Vulnerable population groups are subgroups of a community that are powerless, marginalized, or disenfranchised, and are experiencing health disparities.

Health risk factors are variables that increase or decrease the probability of illness or death. Health risk factors may be modifiable (that is, they can be changed), for example, health care prevention practices, or nonmodifiable (cannot be changed), for example, age, sex, race, or other inherent physical characteristic.

Health determinants are variables that include biological, psychosocial, environmental (physical and social), and health systems factors or etiologies that may cause changes in the health status of individuals, families, groups, populations, and communities. Health determinants may be assets (positive factors) or risks (negative factors). **Health assets** are health-promoting attributes of individuals/families, communities, and systems.

Individuals, families, population groups, and communities may experience health disparities. **Health disparities** are differences in health risks and health status measures that reflect the poorer health status that is found disproportionately in certain population groups. Health disparities lead to unequal burdens in disease morbidity and mortality rates borne by racial and ethnic groups in comparison to the dominant racial or ethnic group in a society (Baldwin, 2003). The Office of Minority Health, Center for Disease Control (CDC) describes the increasing disease burden and risk factors experienced by people of color and American Indians (www.cdc.gov/omh, click About Minority Health, and then click Disease Burden & Risk Factors). Significant health disparities persist in the United States among population groups representing racial, ethnic, socioeconomic, and geographic differences (American College of Physicians, 2004; Eberhardt & Parnuk, 2004; Hartley, 2004; Institute of Medicine [IOM], 2002).

Health care systems disparities are differences in health care system access and quality of care for different racial, ethnic, and socioeconomic population groups that persist across settings, clinical areas, age, gender, geography, and health needs and disabilities. These health care system disparities result in poorer health care outcomes. Significant health care disparities exist in the U.S. health care system (Agency for Healthcare Research and Quality [AHRQ], 2005, IOM, 2002). Social and economic factors, including health care system disparities, are the primary cause of health disparities among people of color and American Indians in the United States. The Health Disparities Collaborative was created to improve primary care access and quality and reduce disparities in health care outcomes for the poor, minorities, and other underserved people. Their Website (www.healthdisparities.net, search for Health Care Outcomes) is a resource for health care providers who want to improve practice outcomes for these populations. Global measures of health status of population groups include morbidity (illness) and mortality (death) rates as well as measures of quality of life. Population health status is measured by health status and health indicators (behaviors) at the national level. In 1979, the Surgeon General released a report on health promotion and disease prevention for the United States. Ten-year evidence-based health objectives for the nation were established in 1980, 1990, and 2000. The current objectives found in Healthy People 2010 (www.phpartners.org, search for Healthy People 2010, and research Healthy People 2010) are related to the primary causes of

---

CRITICAL THINKING 7-1

Review the major health indicators:

- Physical activity
- Overweight/obesity
- Tobacco use
- Substance abuse
- Responsible sexual behavior
- Mental health
- Injury and violence
- Environmental quality
- Immunizations and access to health care

How do you and your family score on achievement of them? How does your community score?

---

death in the United States as well as other major health concerns.

Progress toward achievement of these objectives is measured by nine major health indicators: physical activity, overweight and obesity, tobacco use, substance abuse, responsible sexual behavior, mental health, injury and violence, environmental quality, immunizations and access to health care. The Partners in Information Access for the Public Health Workforce (http://phpartners.org/hp) Website helps you search for published research on Healthy People 2010 and evidence-based strategies that help to improve the health of population groups.

The goals of population-based health care include: (1) improvement of access to health care services, (2) improvement of quality of health care services, (3) reduction of health disparities among different population groups, and (4) reduction of health care delivery costs. Population-based interventions are provided at three levels: (1) individuals, families, and groups; (2) systems within the community such as health care systems; and (3) community systems. Outcomes of these interventions are measured in three domains: population health status, quality of life, and functional health status.

Health status is the level of health of an individual, family, group, population, or community. It is the sum of existing health risk factors, level of wellness, existing diseases, functional health status, and quality of life. **Quality of life** is the level of satisfaction one has with the actual conditions of one's life, including satisfaction with socioeconomic status, education, occupation, home, family life, recreation, and the ability to enjoy life, freedom, and independence. Quality of life assessment reviews the perceived and actual ability to be autonomous and independent in making life choices; one's sense of happiness, satisfaction, and security; and the ongoing ability to strive to reach one's potential. **Health-related quality of life** refers to one's level of satisfaction with those aspects of life that are influenced either positively or negatively by one's health status and health risk factors.

Functional health status is the ability to care for oneself and meet one's human needs. Functional abilities are the combined abilities to be independent in both activities of daily life and in the instrumental activities of daily living. **Activities of daily living** are activities related to toileting, bathing, grooming, dressing, feeding, mobility, and verbal and written personal communication. **Instrumental activities of daily living** (IADLs) are activities related to food preparation and shopping; cleaning; laundry; home maintenance; verbal, written, and electronic communications; financial management; and transportation, as well as activities to meet social and support needs, manage health care needs, access community services and resources, and meet spiritual needs. Functional health status affects health-related quality of life.

Addressing the priority health needs of the most vulnerable population groups at the population level rather than the individual level challenges nurses to target finite health care resources more effectively. Vulnerable population groups are often underserved. These vulnerable groups may have decreased health status and increased risk for morbidity and mortality because of multiple and complex medical and social problems. They may be marginalized, meaning they exist at the margins of mainstream society without access to the majority of community resources and networks. They may be disenfranchised, meaning they do not have the ability to participate in or influence decisions that affect their health care status.

CULTURALLY INCLUSIVE HEALTH CARE

The U.S. population is becoming more diverse. According to U.S. census data, more than 25% of the population was comprised of ethnic minority groups in 2000 (Baldwin, 2003). The U.S. ethnic minority population in 2004 was reported to be 32.1% (Health Resources and Services Administration [HRSA], 2005). If immigration and birth patterns continue, the number of Hispanics, Asians, and African-Americans in the U.S. population will increase far more rapidly than the White population. Nurses graduating in 2006 and beyond will experience significantly more diversity in the workplace than older nurses experienced. Ethnic minorities in the United States who have been marginalized from mainstream society experience more health care disparities in increased rates or morbidity, mortality, and burden of disease (Keltner, Kelly, & Smith, 2004). Increased health care disparities among racial and ethnic minorities are primarily a result of social and economic structures rather than genetic racial and ethnic factors (Tashiro, 2005). Due to these health care disparities, the proportion of ethnic minorities seeking health care services will increase in comparison to the White population (Baldwin, 2003).

The proportion of ethnic minorities in the RN workforce in 2004 (HRSA, 2005) continues to lag behind the proportion of ethnic minorities in the U.S. population (Table 7-1). Nurses need to play a key role in reshaping the health care system to be more culturally inclusive, increasing the ethnic diversity of the nursing profession, and becoming more culturally inclusive in their nursing

TABLE 7-1	RACE/ETHNICITY OF REGISTERED NURSE WORKFORCE COMPARED TO U.S. POPULATION		
	Registered Nurses	**U.S. Population**	**Difference**
White Non-Hispanic	88.4%	67.9%	+20.5%
Black, African American (Non-Hispanic)	4.6%	12.2%	−7.6%
Asian/Pacific Islander (Non-Hispanic)	3.3%	4.1%	−0.8%
Hispanic	1.8%	13.7%	−11.9%
American Indian/Alaskan Native	0.4%	0.7%	−0.3%
Two or More Racial Backgrounds	1.5%	1.3%	+0.2%

Source: Compiled from HRSA. (2005). *National sample survey of registered nurses—preliminary findings, March 2004.* Retrieved June 26, 2006, from ftp://ftp.hrsa.gov/bhpr/nursing/rnpopulation/theregisterednursepopulation.pdf.

practice. Barriers to cultural competence and cultural inclusivity in the health care workplace include lack of awareness of differences; lack of time; ethnocentrism, bias and prejudice; lack of skills to address differences; and lack of organizational support (Taylor, 2005).

A culturally inclusive health care system is one in which health care is population based. This system includes multiple methods of providing cultural health care that reflects the diverse history and cultures of the population groups served. A culturally inclusive health care system promotes positive health outcomes using a variety of intervention strategies to achieve outcome measures tailored to the diversity of the population groups served. The U.S. health care system demonstrates significant disparities in the provision of just and equitable health care. It tends to be more culturally exclusive than inclusive (Gustafson, 2005). The development of a culturally inclusive health care system requires significant change in the current health care system. To start this change, nurses and other health care providers need to work together to create it. Increased awareness of the injustice of existing health care systems may lead to both individual and system change (Giddings, 2005). Individual and systems change will require increased diversity in the health care workforce. Increasing the proportion of bicultural and bilingual health care providers to fit the diversity of the U.S. population will increase the probability that health care will be delivered in a culturally inclusive manner that is truly population-based. This is a start!

A community-based action research model in which the community or population group is an active part of the research process is another effective strategy in developing culturally inclusive health care programs (Garwick & Auger, 2003; Giachello et al., 2003). Student nurses of similar racial and ethnic origins and with ties to the ethnic community can play a significant role in contributing to a culturally inclusive health care system by participating in community-based action research. All health care providers must work together to develop this research and other strategies to achieve a culturally inclusive health care system.

REAL WORLD INTERVIEW

The Experience of Hmong Women Living with Diabetes Community-Based Collaborative Action Research (CBCAR) includes the community in the definition of the research question, data analysis, dissemination, and action planning (Pharris et al., 2002). One example of a culturally sensitive use of CBCAR occurred when the advisory council of a community clinic identified diabetes as a health disparity among Hmong women that needed to be addressed. Female Hmong nursing researchers from the clinic's academic partner wondered if clinic health care providers were labeling Hmong women with diabetes as noncompliant without understanding the women or their culture.

CBCAR using Dr. Margaret Newman's nursing theory of health as expanding consciousness (Newman, 1999) was the framework used to engage Hmong women with diabetes in a dialogue to understand their life patterns and to envision health promoting actions. Five Hmong women with Type 2 diabetes and HgbA1c levels over 7.0 were recruited from the clinic and interviewed in their homes by female Hmong nursing researchers to identify common patterns. Researchers worked with a female Hmong playwright to weave common patterns into a play. Hmong women were invited via Hmong radio and community advertisements to a dinner, performance, and dialogue. Two senior female Hmong nursing students performed the play for the Hmong women. After the play, the Hmong women were grouped into four small dialogue circles facilitated by female Hmong students and female Hmong community leaders. The dialogue focused on what needed to be added so that the play could better reflect the women's life experiences. It also focused on what actions needed to be taken so that Hmong women with diabetes could live healthy, happy lives in the United States.

Avonne A. Yang, RN, BSN
Faculty Assistant/Director of Community Health
Nursing Student Internship Program (CHNSIP)
Department of Nursing
College of St. Catherine
St. Paul, Minnesota

HEALTH DETERMINANT MODELS

Health determinant models provide conceptual tools to use in assessing and addressing the priority health needs of at-risk population groups. Assessment and intervention models take into account the importance of community systems such as health, social service, government, and economics in influencing the health outcomes in population groups as well as individuals. (U.S. Department of Health and Human Services [USDHHS], 2000; Falk-Rafael, 2005). Health determinant models are holistic and reflect the multiple causes of health disparities in diverse population groups. Existing health determinants models identify income inequality in concert with social, cultural, and political conditions as a key health determinant influencing population health outcomes such as morbidity and mortal-

ity rates globally (Falk-Rafael, 2005). Some health determinants have a greater impact on health outcomes and health status. Pawlak (2005) proposes a health determinants model in which health literacy, the ability to find and use health information to make decisions, is a key determinant of population health. The Healthy People Health Determinants Model, A Systematic Approach to Health Improvement (U.S. DHHS, 2000), is a systems approach to organizing health determinants that reviews the behaviors and biology of the individual/population group, the social and physical environment of the population group, the health policies and interventions of government and private organizations, and access to quality health care (Figure 7-1). Examples of selected community level, health systems level, and population level health determinants are provided in Table 7-2. This schema can be used to identify those at greatest risk for specific health events and diseases.

Data sources used for population based assessment are seen in Table 7-3.

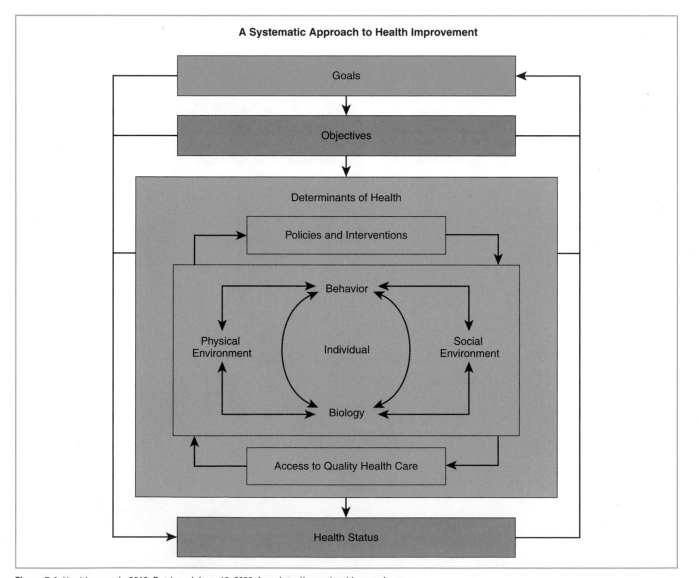

Figure 7-1 Healthy people 2010. Retrieved June 18, 2006, from http://www.healthypeople.gov.

TABLE 7-2	**POPULATION-BASED HEALTH DETERMINANTS ASSESSMENT TEMPLATE—EXCERPT**

Community Level

Physical Environment

- Housing and geographic location, safety of neighborhoods, community, and school quality
- Environmental quality: air, water, ground, chemical, physical, and biological hazards
- Availability of transportation, communication systems, parks, and recreation facilities

Social Environment

- Community norms, values, and patterns of behavior; political structures within community
- Incidence of crime and violence within the population group and the larger community
- Employment opportunities within community, economic viability of community

Policies and Interventions

- National, state, county, and city health and social policies
- Policies of public, private, and voluntary organizations that provide health and social services
- Policies of health insurance companies, health maintenance organizations, health systems, and health care provider groups

Health Systems Level

Access to Quality Health Care

- Appropriate primary, secondary, and tertiary health services and providers
- Health and social services workforce (numbers, diversity, interdisciplinary mix, deployment, sustainability); educational institutions offering health care provider education and training
- Availability of health and social services resources 24 hours a day, seven days per week

Population Level

Biological

- Demographic data (age, gender, racial/ethnic patterns)
- Biological and genetic factors, patterns of health and disease (morbidity and mortality data)

Behavioral

- Education patterns and levels, cultural patterns (lifestyle, languages, religion)
- Socioeconomic status (employment patterns, housing, health and dental insurance)
- Cultural health patterns (health beliefs and self-care practices, nutrition, fitness, previous experiences with health care system, current health providers, family and intergenerational health patterns)

Data Analysis

- Prioritize the health needs of the community and prioritize the vulnerable and at-risk population groups based on need and health status.
- Identify the modifiable and nonmodifiable health risks of the at-risk population.
- Identify the biological, psychosocial, environmental, cultural, political, financial, and iatrogenic causes of the identified health risks.

TABLE 7-3   DATA SOURCES FOR POPULATION-BASED ASSESSMENT

Common Sources of Primary Data

- Key informant interviews and surveys of health and social services providers, community leaders, media, and governmental agency officials and personnel
- Key informant interviews, surveys, and observations (participant and nonparticipant) of members of at-risk or vulnerable population groups (may require formal approval process if research done on human subjects)
- Windshield and walk-through surveys of the community and organizations involved

Common Sources of Secondary Data

- Health data, vital statistics, and census data obtained from governmental sources
- Community planning documents
- Health reports on subpopulations from governmental, voluntary, private organizations, and consumer groups
- Scientific and professional literature and databases
- Proprietary client/member population data from health care insurers and providers—may be available only to employees of the organization
- The news and communications media, including newspapers, journals, television, radio, and the Internet

Data utilized may be primary (collected by group conducting assessment) or secondary (collected from other sources).

REAL WORLD INTERVIEW

Last April, a 12-year-old boy from a nearby village was brought to our clinic at Nuestros Pequeños Hermanos (NPH). He had fallen out of a tree about 30 feet. He was unresponsive and vomiting. His head was bleeding, and there was blood coming from both ears. On the 45-minute drive to the hospital in our clinic ambulance, I sat in the back of the pick-up with the boy, trying to physically immobilize him with my own body until we got to the hospital. I left the hospital that night feeling sure the little boy wasn't going to make it.

Two weeks later, the boy was discharged to his home to die so we brought him to our clinic. He could not speak, had casts on his left arm and leg, and couldn't sit on his own. Within two weeks, he was eating food and sitting up. After the boy went home, he came back to our clinic for homeopathic treatments. Several months later, I saw the little boy in the clinic waiting room. When he saw me, his eyes lit up and he broke into a big smile. He hadn't remembered me until now and hadn't been able to speak more than a few words. Tears welled in my eyes when the little boy looked at me with eyes that had been so full of fear that April night, as he asked me for water to share with his little brother.

The children that live at NPH have lived through unimaginable horrors. Their parents have been killed in front of them. Some parents have died from AIDS or cancer. Many children have been abandoned and left to survive on their own, children caring for children. Some have been beaten, abused, or neglected. It means the world to me to see these kids enjoying a happy and loving life. Every step I took as a volunteer has brought me to a better place with a greater outlook and understanding of life.

Annie Kautza, BSN
2004 Graduate and Volunteer
Nuestros Pequeños
Hermanos, Honduras

TABLE 7-4	HEALTH DETERMINANTS OF CHILDREN AT RISK FOR FEMUR FRACTURES

Health Determinant Risk Factors	Examples of Risk Factors That Can Be Modified
Environmental Determinants of Health: Social ■ Low socioeconomic status ■ Large family size ■ Presence of older children who are used as babysitters ■ Children living in crowded households ■ Children of single parents	■ Increase safety practices of children who are babysitters. ■ Improve health care access of families.
Environmental Determinants: Physical ■ Living in rural areas, for example, farm equipment injury ■ Recreation areas and playgrounds close to place of residence, for example, playground injury ■ Lack of safe children's furniture ■ Lack of safety gear ■ Access to farm machinery	■ Strengthen safety features of recreational areas and playgrounds. ■ Increase availability of safety gear and safe children's furniture. ■ Increase use of protective gear when riding bikes and farm machinery.
Individual Biological and Behavorial Determinants ■ Young maternal age ■ Children age 0–3 years ■ Children with car and access to outdoor recreational areas ■ Inadequate knowledge about child safety ■ Lack of caregiver supervision ■ Unsafe or risk-taking behavior	■ Improve safety and car riding habits. ■ Increase knowledge level of parents and caregivers. ■ Improve home safety practices (safety straps in high chairs and booster seats, safety gates on stairs, don't leave child alone on changing table, or don't allow climbing on furniture).
Health System Determinants ■ Lack of awareness of primary health care providers about risk factors and need for patient teaching.	■ Increase knowledge level of health care providers.

Source: Compiled with information from Rewes et al. (2005). Childhood femur fractures, associated injuries, and sociodemographic risk factors: A population-based study. *Pediatrics, 115*(5), e543–e552. Retrieved March 20, 2006, from http://www.pediatrics.org

CRITICAL THINKING 7-2

Assess your community using the template in Table 7-2 and Table 7-3. How does your community score? Do you have any suggestions to improve your community's health based on this assessment?

Selected health determinants for children at risk for femur fractures (Rewes et al., 2005) and the health determinants that may be modified are outlined in Table 7-4.

An analysis every 10 years of U.S. health statistics provides the direction for national priorities (U.S. Department of Health and Human Services, 2000). The Healthy People 2010 Model in Figure 7-1 emphasizes the use of four key elements to achieve health improvement: goals, objectives, determinants of health, and health status. This model lends itself to a partnership approach between health consumers, the community, and health care providers in addressing health needs.

REAL WORLD INTERVIEW

The Native American Community Clinic (NACC) is a nonprofit clinic established in 2003 to provide health services to low-income Native Americans and others in this inner-city Minneapolis community. We have enrolled over 4,800 patients and have had over 30,000 patient visits since opening. Eighty-five percent of our patients are Native American. NACC health providers, including nursing and medical practitioners, have 66 years of combined experience in the community. These practitioners have established relationships with many families, groups, and organizations, and are well connected to services and organizations serving the Native American community. All of the NACC's Governing Board are Native American community members and many of them are directors of Indian organizations and leaders in the community.

NACC's mission is to promote wellness and regular health maintenance in Native American families, decrease health disparities in Native Americans in the metropolitan area, and provide access to care regardless of ability to pay. We are committed to serving Native Americans because of their significant health disparities and because they do not have any clinic other than NACC in the metropolitan area that they can say is "theirs." Although all are welcome, we are committed to preserving NACC as a place where Native Americans feel welcome and respected. Our vision is centered on involving the Indian community in the work of disease prevention, health promotion, and the elimination of health disparities. We believe in spending time out in the community, involved in projects, activities, and other efforts to make the issue of health disparities more understandable and practical for individuals.

Despite years of funding and services from governmental sources such as the Indian Health Service, Indian people have many of the worst health disparities of any racial group in the state and nation. American Indians experience rates of disease and premature death significantly greater than Whites and other racial and ethnic groups. Significant health disparities exist across the lifespan. The rate of inadequate or no prenatal care is almost six times higher than the rate for Whites. American Indian babies die at a rate more than three times higher than White babies. The teen pregnancy rate is five times higher than the White rate. Disease rates for heart disease, diabetes, cervical cancer, HIV/AIDS, and sexually transmitted diseases are two to five times higher than for Whites. Less than 50% of American Indian elders are vaccinated against pneumococcal disease, one of the leading causes of death in American Indians. American Indian males have a suicide rate sixteen times higher than Whites. Child maltreatment is three times higher, and Native American people suffer from significant mental health disorders such as depression, posttraumatic stress disorder, and chemical dependency (MDH, 2005).

Many NACC patients suffer from poverty and chronic medical conditions. Many have a history of physical and/or sexual abuse during childhood. Domestic abuse is common among women of childbearing age. Forty to sixty percent of pregnant women use alcohol during the first trimester of their pregnancy, and alcohol dependency is a common struggle in many families. Forty seven percent of our diabetic patients had a positive depression screen. NACC provides comprehensive primary health care services to all with major emphasis on health disparities across the lifespan.

Lydia Caros, DO
Executive Director
Native American Community Clinic
Minneapolis, Minnesota

CASE STUDY 7-1

Think about the health assets and health barriers that exist for one group of immigrants in your community. See if you can list ten health assets and ten health barriers. Analyze your lists. What is the most important health priority for immigrant health that you believe your community should address? Identify one action you could take to bring this health priority to the attention of the community. Can you identify any potential community partners?

POPULATION-BASED NURSING PRACTICE

Population-focused nursing practice and *population-based nursing practice* are terms that are used interchangeably in contemporary community health nursing literature. Population-focused practice has been an integral part of nursing since the profession began. Florence Nightingale's use of aggregated statistics as population-based indices and outcome measures demonstrates her population-focused practice. Lillian Wald established population-focused nursing practice in the United States in the early 1900s. Her population-focused efforts included founding the Henry Street Nurses' Settlement; helping to establish the Children's Bureau; and advocating for the rights of children, the mentally ill, the indigent, and immigrants. Wald's vision of nurses was that they would be "carriers of health" (Peters, 1995). According to Wald (1915), nurses were "part of the community plan for the attainment of communal health" (p. 60). As nursing in the community became more organized, particularly in public health agencies, nursing leaders like Ruth Freeman encouraged nurses to consider the health needs of the total community as their mission (Freeman, 1957).

In the future, both nursing education and nursing practice will place a greater emphasis on use of population-based mortality and morbidity statistics for assessment of community health needs. They will focus on maximizing health status, functional abilities, and improving the quality of life of groups of health care consumers.

The American Nurses Association (ANA) (1995) states that population-focused nursing practice is "defined by nursing activities that focus on all of the people and reflects responsibility to and for the people." Furthermore, "provision of services to those who appear for service are not population focused without actions to gain participation of the entire population who might benefit from that service."

In 1920, the National Organization for Public Health Nursing (NOPHN) identified three levels of public health nursing practice: individual, family, and community (Abrams, 2004). In 1949, NOPHN redefined public health nursing (PHN) based on the understanding that it was a population-based autonomous nursing practice in the community. Public health nurses were expected to work with individuals, families, health care providers within systems of care and communities. The PHN Competencies delineated by the Quad Council of Public Health Nursing Organizations in 2003 are based on the premise that PHN is population-focused, and that provision of care to individuals and families occurs within the content of the community (Abrams, 2004; Quad Council of Public Health

Organizations, 2004). Contemporary public health nursing leaders have consistently stressed the need for nurses in the community to be population-focused in their practice (Keller, Shaffer, Lia-Hoagberg, & Strohschein, 2002). More recent discussions have included the need for nurses across all health care settings to be population-focused.

Population-based nursing practice is defined as the practice of nursing in which the focus of care is to improve the health status of vulnerable or at-risk population groups within the community by employing health promotion and disease prevention interventions across the health continuum. Health care consumers are involved as full partners in the planning and evaluation of the nursing services provided. Population-based nursing practice is holistic in nature, taking into account cultural and ethnic diversity, religious and spiritual uniqueness, economic disparities, and geographic and regional differences. It seeks to empower population groups by enhancing their protective factors and resiliency. **Protective factors** are client strengths and resources that clients can use to combat health threats that compromise core human functions. **Resilience** is the social and psychosocial capacity of individuals and groups to adapt, succeed, and persevere over time in the face of recurring threats to psychosocial and physiologic integrity. Population groups that experience greater threats to health based on biological, physical, or social environmental risk factors will experience poorer health and safety outcomes. The level of resilience in the population group or the ability of the population group to thrive despite the presence of risk factors will help to reduce the groups health and safety risks (Davis, Cook, & Cohen, 2005). Promoting resilience in marginalized and disenfranchised population groups and simultaneously working to reduce the barriers to health care are dual responsibilities for nurses practicing population-based nursing.

The goals of population-based nursing practice are consistent with the health goals identified by the World Health Organization (WHO Task Force, 2005) and Healthy People 2010 (U.S. DHHS, 2000). Population-based nursing practice goals address the health needs of individuals, families, communities, and population groups, and focus on the goals of health care access, quality, cost, and equity.

POPULATION-BASED NURSING PRACTICE INTERVENTIONS

A population-based public health interventions model for public health nursing practice, developed by the Minnesota Department of Health (2001), is in concert with the public mandate that directs public health agencies to protect the health of the public they serve. A primary principle of population-based nursing practice is that it is initiated with a community health assessment. Multidisciplinary interventions are developed based on the community health priorities identified in the assessment process.

Population-based interventions encompass three levels of practice: (1) the community; (2) systems within the community; and (3) individuals, families, and groups. Population-based community-focused practice changes community norms, attitudes, practices, and behaviors. Population-based systems-focused practice changes laws, power structures, policies, and organizations. Population-based individual-focused practice changes the knowledge, attitudes, beliefs, practices, and behaviors of individuals, families, and groups (Keller, Strohschein, Lia-Hoagberg, & Schaffer, 2004a; Keller, Strohschein, Schaffer, & Lia-Hoagberg, 2004b). Figure 7-2 depicts the Minnesota Department of Health Public Health Interventions II Wheel developed by the section of public health nursing.

These interventions have a logical sequence. For example, to provide health services to underserved and vulnerable population groups, outreach (finding the people at risk in the community) and screening must precede referral, teaching, counseling, and consultation.

Nursing interventions need to be provided in a culturally sensitive and appropriate manner to be effective with culturally diverse population groups.

TRADITIONAL VERSUS NONTRADITIONAL MODEL

The traditional model of population-based public health nursing practice starts with public health and community health agencies working in partnership with the community to carry out a community assessment. Priorities are established, and a plan is developed in partnership with community members. After the plan is implemented, evaluation is also conducted in partnership with the community. In recent years, private health care organizations have launched population-based health care initiatives to improve the health status of their members and to

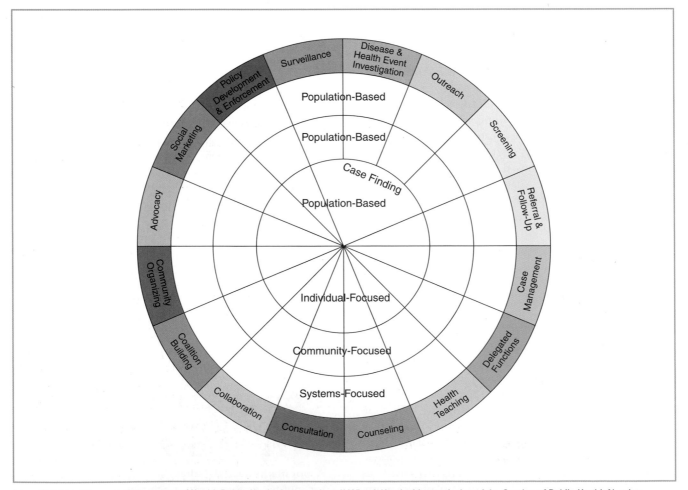

Figure 7-2 The Minnesota Department of Health Public Health Interventions II Wheel. Used with permission of the Section of Public Health Nursing, Minnesota Department of Health. (Retrieved December 17, 2006, from http://www.health.state.mn.us.)

REAL WORLD INTERVIEW

The Hmong Health Care Professionals Coalition received a grant to do community education for the elderly Hmong population regarding depression. Depression was considered a risk for Hmong elders because there had been several suicides in that population. Many Hmong elders were isolated and did not view depression as a disease. In addition, other agencies serving this population had also identified depression as an issue for the elders.

In doing outreach to the target population, several adaptations specific to the Hmong culture were made. One was in regard to eligibility criteria. Even though the program targeted persons over 50, people were allowed to determine their own eligibility. That is, if they "felt old," they qualified. Second, although the coalition had a booth at the annual Hmong Health Fair, the coalition members considered it unlikely that the elders would come to the booth. Therefore, the interviewers decided to walk around and talk with elders in a more relaxed setting. They approached elders while sitting under shade trees, selling products at the market booth, and the like. Third, interviews were done entirely in the Hmong language. Elderly persons were screened, provided information about depression, and given a list of community resources.

Ma Her, PHN
St. Paul-Ramsey County Department of Public Health
St. Paul, Minnesota

From Her, M. (2001) "Outreach" in Getting Behind the Wheel, *Public Health Nursing Online Newsletter,* 15. Section of Public Health Nursing, Minnesota Department of Health. Retrieved July 13, 2001, from http://www.health.state.mn.us/divs/chs/ phn/phnnews15.html. St. Paul Ramsey County Department of Public Health, Hmong Health Professionals Coalition.

---

reduce the health systems' costs. The nontraditional initiatives generally start with an assessment of specific population groups within the health systems membership that have complex health care problems. These might include older adults with multiple chronic diseases who are experiencing significant health disparities, such as Native Americans with diabetes, or patients with complex health and social problems, for example, pregnant adolescents. Health services such as outreach and case management are commonly used. For example, a hospital might undertake a survey of frequent nonacute visitors to its emergency department (ED) to determine if other more appropriate and less expensive health services could be developed to better meet the health needs of these frequent visitors.

Public Health Nursing (PHN) Agencies and many Visiting Nurse Associations provide the traditional model of population-based health care. These nursing agencies work with other health and social service organization to provide comprehensive health services to population groups in their communities who are at-risk for or experiencing health disparities. Public health nurses and community health nurses use a variety of independent nursing interventions in their population-based practice. Interventions most commonly used are displayed in Figure 7-2 in the Minnesota Public Health Intervention Wheel (Minnesota Department of Health, 2001). PHN Agencies throughout the United States provide these interventions. A recent Public Health workforce Study (HRSA, 2005) of four states documented the importance of these public health interventions to public health nursing agencies as well as the percentage of agencies providing these interventions (Table 7-5).

A nontraditional model of population-based nursing practice is also emerging. This model is being developed by private for-profit and nonprofit health care organizations. In this model, the vulnerable or at-risk population group is identified before community assessment occurs, and the subsequent community assessment process focuses on health determinants related to the at-risk group. The organizations generally focus on the population groups within their service areas, their market niche, and current membership. The primary goal of these organizations is usually to contain or reduce health care costs. The secondary goal is to improve the quality of care provided to their membership to improve health outcomes. Generally, the population groups who have the highest health risks, the poorest health outcomes, and the highest service costs are the groups targeted for additional services. Population groups with

TABLE 7-5	POPULATION-BASED PUBLIC HEALTH NURSING (PHN) INTERVENTIONS IN FOUR STATES

Prevalence of Selected Population-Based PHN Interventions in Four State PHN Agencies (HRSA, 2005)

Population-Based PHN Interventions From Minnesota Department of Health (2001)	PHN Roles Found in Four State Public Health Counties or Departments by Percent*			
	CA	GA	MO	NM
Surveillance				
Community Level**	100	100	80	100
System Level	100	NR	NR	NR
Disease Investigation				
Individual Level	83	100	80	100
Community Level	83	NR	NR	NR
Outreach				
Individual Level	100	100	20	88
Screening				
Individual Level	83	100	80	100
System Level	67	100	NR	100
Referral and Follow-up—Not reported in HRSA Study				
Case Management				
Individual Level	83	100	40	100
Delegated Medical Function/Treatment				
Individual Level	83	100	40	75
Health Education				
Individual Level	100	100	100	100
Community Level	100	100	80	100
Staff Development				
Systems Level	17	NR	NR	NR
Counseling & Advocacy				
Community Level	67	100	80	100
Individual Level	100	100	60	88
Collaboration				
Community Level	17	NR	NR	NR
Consultation—Not reported in HRSA Study				
Coalition Building				
System Level	83	100	40	100

TABLE 7-5	POPULATION-BASED PUBLIC HEALTH NURSING (PHN) INTERVENTIONS IN FOUR STATES (CONTINUED)			
Population-Based PHN Interventions From Minnesota Department of Health (2001)	**PHN Roles Found in Four State Public Health Counties or Departments by Percent***			
	CA	**GA**	**MO**	**NM**
Community Organizing				
Community Level	50	100	80	100
Social Marketing				
Systems/Community Merged Levels	83	100	40	75
Public Policy Development				
System Level	100	100	60	100
Community Level	67	NR	NR	NR
Enforcement (Identified only as Facility Licensing in HRSA Study)				
Systems (Facility Licensing) Level	NR	100	20	NR
Program Evaluation***				
Community Level	100	100	40	100

*NR = Not reported

**Some states collected intervention data by levels of practice: individual, system, community, and others did not. Where data have been collected by level of practice, the findings are presented by level of practice.

***Not Separate PHN Intervention (MDH, 2001).

Note on significance of interventions: State PHN agencies rated 84% of interventions with a score of 3 or higher on scale of 1–4 (4 highest).

Source: Table compiled from data in HRSA (2005). Public Health Workforce Study. USDHHS. Accessed June 26, 2006 from ftp://ftp.hrsa.gov/bhpr/nationalcenter/publichealth2005.pdf

multiple diagnoses, called comorbidities, as well as complex therapeutic treatment regimes and a pattern of noncompliance and missed visits, are also targeted for services.

APPLICATION OF NURSING PROCESS TO POPULATION-BASED NURSING PRACTICE

Population-based nursing practice involves the application of the nursing process in working with communities, organizations, and population groups. Depending on the focus of a project, nurses may spend more of their time and effort on different components of the nursing process. Assessment, diagnosis, planning, implementation, and evaluation may take different forms depending on the nature of the project.

Assessment methods using the assets approach identified in Table 7-6 provide more opportunity for an egalitarian relationship between health providers and community members and are more consistent with the partnership model recommended by most community and public health professionals. The assessment phase may focus on the total health resources and needs of a community or may be limited to one population group or one health concern. Use of community-based action research in which the community is an equal partner throughout the assessment, diagnosis planning, implementation, and evaluation phase is becoming more common. This method enhances the ability of diverse communities to manage their own health care needs.

Population-based health care is interdisciplinary and involves participation of community members and population groups experiencing health disparities. Use of a nursing diagnosis may be a barrier to collaboration on an interdisciplinary team. One option would be a community-impact or goal statement that reflects the community's concerns about a specific health issue or population group and that reflects the culture and lifestyle of the community

REAL WORLD INTERVIEW

Gillette Lifetime Specialty Clinic in St. Paul, Minnesota, was started in 2001 to provide a continuum of care for adolescents and adults with disabilities. At that time, the community had interdisciplinary pediatric services for children with disabilities but no interdisciplinary specialty care for adults with disabilities. The clinic's primary service area includes Minnesota, Wisconsin, Iowa, South Dakota, and North Dakota, but we also serve patients from all over the United States. Our mission is to help those we serve realize greater well-being, independence, and enjoyment in life. We combine medical, nursing, physical, occupational and orthotic therapies, social work, and other specialty services in family-centered programs. These services are provided at our clinics and hospital and throughout the region in response to community needs and often in collaboration with other organizations. We expect to quadruple our 2006 outpatient clinic population visits, currently at 2,000 visits, as more young adult patients transition to our adult specialty providers.

Gillette Lifetime Specialty Clinic uses a rehabilitative and interdisciplinary approach to care delivery to promote independence and community integration. We work with local, regional, and national resources to enhance the continuum of care for adolescents and adults. We work as a team with our patients, their families, caregivers, and primary care physicians, and serve as a bridge to our clients' primary care physicians. We provide specialty care, yet assure that our clients receive ongoing care in their communities. Building strong relations within the community to provide comprehensive services for our unique clients' health care needs is a priority. Gillette Lifetime Specialty Healthcare provides unique client services to a complex patient population, underserved by most health care systems and not duplicated anywhere.

Holly Cain, BSN, RN
Clinic Nursing Supervisor and Clinic Coordinator
St. Paul, Minnesota

TABLE 7-6	**NURSING PROCESS APPLIED TO POPULATION-BASED NURSING—ASSESSMENT EXAMPLES**

Assets Approach to Community Health Assessment: Assessment process begins with an assessment of the assets, that is, strengths and resources, of a community or population group. An assets-based approach lends itself to identifying how the community can manage its own health needs by building on community and population group strengths and resources.

Community Mapping: Community mapping involves identifying the strengths and resources of the community, including its natural and built physical environment and its social environment, such as social systems, networks, formal and informal organizations, and cultural and lifestyle patterns.

Holistic Community Assessment: An assessment of the total community is carried out to identify population and community assets, health needs, vulnerable and at-risk population groups, community health priorities, existing health services, and service gaps.

Focused Community Assessment: An assessment of a specific at-risk population group with a specific health concern is carried out to identify population group assets, priorities, health needs, existing health services, and service gaps.

Community-Based Action Research: An assessment is completed in partnership with the community or specific population group. The assessment goals, data collection tools, methods of data analysis, reporting, and documentation are determined and designed in partnership with the community.

Health Determinants Analysis: This health determinants (USDHHS, Healthy People 2010) assessment process combines community assessment and population group assessment in assessing a specific population group. Health determinants include community and population assets, health promoting factors and health limiting factors, for example, barriers and risks to health.

as understood by all members of the partnership. Another option is use of an interdisciplinary collaborative diagnosis (Table 7-7).

Goal setting and implementation should be culturally and developmentally specific to the population group served (Table 7-8).

Community members should be involved in planning how, what, when, and where health care services will be delivered so that systems are not created that produce barriers to health care access. Evaluation methods and measures need to be developed or selected during the planning process. It is important to realize that many global health status measures are directed toward population changes in morbidity, mortality, longevity, and lifestyle (Table 7-9).

Changes in morbidity, mortality, longevity, and lifestyle may take years to occur, thus intermediate health status measures may be used to begin to evaluate the success of a specific program. Intermediate measures include factors such as changes in health behaviors and health risk factors, increased program participation and patient satisfaction, and changes in community norms and values, health policies, and health funding.

Examples of population-based public health intervention programs developed by both public and private health care organizations are found in Table 7-10.

TABLE 7-7	**POPULATION-BASED PRACTICE DIAGNOSIS EXAMPLES**

Nursing Diagnosis: Ineffective therapeutic management of mental health needs of community homeless related to lack of community awareness, lack of funding, and lack of community mental health workers as evidenced by a 20% increase in homeless people visiting the emergency departments of local hospitals for psychotropic medications, and an increase in police calls to attend to homeless people exhibiting psychotic behavior.

Community Impact Statement: Community concern that homeless people have mental health needs that are not being addressed by community mental health professionals because of lack of funding and staff resulting in the community's fear of the homeless and increased calls to police to manage homeless people exhibiting frightening behaviors.

Collaborative Diagnosis: Unmet mental health needs of community homeless due to lack of funding, staffing, and outreach as identified by 20% increase in homeless people visiting the emergency department for psychotropic medications, an increase in police calls to attend to homeless people exhibiting psychotic behavior, and an increase in incarceration of homeless people with psychiatric diagnoses.

TABLE 7-8	**NURSING PROCESS APPLIED TO POPULATION-BASED NURSING—PLANNING AND IMPLEMENTATION EXAMPLES**

Planning: Planning always involves a collaborative process. When working with the community, key community or population group representatives, members of the interdisciplinary health team, and representatives of community organizations and agencies all participate in the planning process. Nurses or other members of the health team may be functioning as consultants to the community, project managers, or coordinators for a specific community or population-based initiative, or be part of an interdisciplinary service team working with the community or local health care agency.

Implementation: Implementation is designed to fit the specific culture and lifestyle of the community or population group. Goals and outcomes demonstrate joint planning in partnership with the community. Interventions are interdisciplinary, build on community or population group assets, take into account existing resources and services, do not duplicate existing services and fill gaps in service needs, allocate resources based on need, and improve the health of the community or population group in a cost-effective manner. Interventions may be at the population group, system, or community levels of practice. Interventions are public health-oriented such as the 17 public health interventions found in the Minnesota Public Health Intervention Wheel (MDH, 2002), see Figure 7-2. Interventions should be evidence-based. This may be difficult to achieve if complementary therapies and culture-specific interventions that have not been studied are employed.

TABLE 7-9	**NURSING PROCESS APPLIED TO POPULATION-BASED NURSING—EVALUATION ELEMENTS**

Partnership: The evaluation process and outcome should be a joint effort with the community and/or population group and the interdisciplinary health care team.

Global Measures of Health Outcomes or Health Status: Global measures of health outcomes or the health status of population groups or communities may include morbidity, mortality, birth and death rates, life satisfaction inventories, and lifestyle functioning measures.

Intermediate Measures of Health Outcomes of Health Status: Intermediate measures may include changes in health determinants such as reduction in health risks, changes in health behaviors, development and implementation of programs and services, changes in community beliefs and values, changes in policy, laws, regulations, and funding.

REAL WORLD INTERVIEW

In January of 2005, I began a 13-month commitment, volunteering as a registered nurse at Nuestros Pequeños Hermanos (NPH), Our Little Brothers and Sisters, an orphanage outside of Tegucigalpa, Honduras. A Catholic priest who wanted to improve the lives of orphaned children in Central America and the Caribbean founded NPH in Mexico in 1954. I work with nurses, social workers, physical therapists, occupational therapists, speech therapists, physicians, and pharmacists. Social workers find the children that live in our home. A Honduran doctor, responsible for the overall health care of the children, works with all of us to provide the children with the best care possible.

NPH has two clinics located at the Tegucigalpa orphanage. The internal clinic serves the needs of the resident children, staff, and volunteers. Six hundred children live here. Eighteen children are HIV positive. There is at least one lay nurse on duty 24 hours a day. Two employees have studied health in high school and have on-the-job training. There are also three young men and women who grew up at NPH and who are completing their obligatory years of service in the clinics. Two will start medical school next year. One will continue her education in nursing. The external clinic serves the community of surrounding villages. The majority of our clinic patients have chronic problems such as hypertension, diabetes, or asthma. The clinic has a laboratory and is equipped for emergencies.

I had the opportunity to go on a medical brigade to a village six hours away from our house. A team of U.S. doctors, nurses, and medical students came to provide care to people living in remote areas. Some had never seen a physician before. We saw nearly 900 patients in two weeks. What an awesome experience!

Annie Kautza, BSN
2004 Graduate, College of St. Catherine
St. Paul, Minnesota

Senior nursing students at the College of St. Catherine, St. Paul, Minnesota, completed these population-based public health nursing projects using the nursing process approach (Table 7-11).

Student teams functioned as consultants to community agencies, including public health nursing agencies, community centers, schools, community clinics, non-profit health-related community organizations, and departments and committees within their college to complete these projects. An example of population-based nursing intervention plan created by a group of nursing students is found in Figure 7-3.

TABLE 7-10	EXAMPLES OF POPULATION-BASED PUBLIC HEALTH INTERVENTION PROGRAMS*

Individual/Family Level of Practice

Case Finding: PORSCHE, New Jersey State Department of Health and Senior Services	Case finding initiated this multiphasic public health nursing home visiting program to families with at-risk children (Worobey, Pisuk, & Decker, 2004).
Counseling: Peer counselors	Smoking cessation in African American women in subsidized housing was facilitated by peer counselors (Anderson, Felton, Wewers, Waller, & Humbles, 2005).
Health Teaching: Lifestyle Education for Activity Program (LEAP)	Health teaching was used effectively to promote physical activity in high school girls (Pate et al., 2005).
Outreach: Public Health Nursing Agencies	This study looked at strategies to make public health nursing outreach more effective (Tembreull & Schaffer 2005).
Referral and Follow-Up: Discharge referral from Emergency Department	Vulnerable older adults discharged from emergency department to home were referred for public health nursing home visits (Kelly, 2005).
Social Marketing: College campus initiative	Social marketing with a "grateful head" theme was used to increase helmet use among cyclists on a college campus (Ludwig, Buchholz, & Clarke, 2005).

Community Level of Practice

Advocacy and Community Organizing: Mobilization of community group	Minority women were mobilized to advocate for health services as a social justice issue for their community (Littlefield, Robinson, Engelbrecht, Gonzalez, & Hutcheson, 2002).
Counseling: Community resilience building	Community counseling strategies were used to build resilience and reduce ethnic and racial health disparities in a community of color (Davis, Cook, & Cohen, 2005).
Coalition building: Chicago southeast diabetes community action coalition	Coalition building was used as a strategy to reducing diabetic health disparities in a Chicago community (Giachello et al., 2003).
Disease and health event investigation: Public high school students in New York	Health event investigation identified changes in use of cigarettes and alcohol among public high school students after their exposure to the World Trade Center attack (Wu et al., 2006).
Policy Development: Public Health Nursing Directors	Factors strengthening public health nursing directors' abilities to affect public health policy development process were identified (Deschaine & Schaffer, 2003).
Screening: County of San Diego TB Control Program	County-level screening of recent immigrants and refugees for pulmonary tuberculosis is used to identify those with a positive Mantoux (LoBue & Moser 2004).
Surveillance and Disease: Health event investigation	Community-level surveillance methods were used to measure health effects in World Trade Center survivors exposed to collapsed and damaged buildings (Brackbill et al., 2006).

Systems Level of Practice

Case Management and Coordination: Medically Coordinated Care Demonstration (MCCD)	Interdisciplinary care management and care coordination of elders with comorbidities was improved using the chronic care model in a vertically integrated health care system (Schraeder et al., 2005).
Collaboration: Health disparities collaborative	Collaboration among health care providers improved diabetic care in community health centers (Chin et al., 2004).
Consultation and Delegated Functions: School-based health clinics	Use of POTS (plain old telephone system) to link school nurses with other health care providers improved school health services (Young & Ireson, 2003).

*Interventions from Minnesota Department of Health. (2001). Public Health Interventions.

TABLE 7-11	NURSING STUDENT POPULATION-BASED PUBLIC HEALTH NURSING PROJECTS

Assessment Focus

Assets-Approach
- Assessment of an urban Native American community to identify community assets, values, beliefs, and health lifestyle practices

Community-Mapping
- Assessment of an urban community of East African Somali and Oromo refugees to identify health and fitness resources and gaps for East African born women and girls
- Assessment of Hispanic community assets, health resources, and health service gaps

Holistic Community Assessment
- Assessment of health resources and unmet health needs of students, teachers, and staff at a K-12 grade school for children with significant learning disabilities

Focused Community Assessment
- Assessment of health screening needs of K-12 students in a Native American charter school
- Assessment of health needs of homeless and poor clientele of a drop-in homeless shelter
- Assessment of health needs of immigrant Hmong children recently relocated from a refugee camp in Thailand to Minneapolis-St. Paul

Community-Based Action Research
- Assessment of health lifestyle practices and needs of Hmong women with diabetes

Focus Group
- Development of a focus group for adolescents at-risk for Methamphetamine use

Health Determinants Analysis
- Analysis of health determinants (Healthy People 2010) is a component of all forms of population-based health assessment student projects.

Planning, Implementation, and Evaluation Focus

Development of the following:
- Asthma Education Health Fair Module with Tool Kit for an Elementary School
- Radon Gas Community Health Education Module and Tool Kit for Community at High-Risk for Radon Poisoning
- Health Education Module for Prevention of Methamphetamine Use for Adolescent Hmong Girls with a History of Sexual Exploitation
- Alcohol Awareness Health Education Module and Tool Kit for Female College Students
- All About Me Prototype Kit for Children with Disabilities to take with them when transported from school to hospital or clinic for urgent or emergency care. Second student group evaluated effectiveness of Kit
- Dental Health Education Module and Tool Kit with Dental Health Resources for Children and Families in Poverty
- Fitness Module for East-African Immigrant Adolescent Girls at a Community Center
- Nutrition module for East African Women Immigrants with or at-risk for Diabetes
- Health Education Resource Guide and Resources for Primary Care Providers at a Native American Community Clinic

NURSING DIAGNOSIS: Female students, ages 13 to 15, in Data Middle School at risk for altered nutrition: less than body requirements related to nutritional habits, body image disturbance, sense of powerlessness, and lack of screening and outreach services as evidenced by:

■ 10% of the female students are below the 5th percentile in weight but above the 25th percentile in height on standardized growth and development charts.

■ 75% of the female students report that they routinely skip breakfast on three or more school days per week, and 50% routinely eat snacks from the vending machines for lunch.

■ 90% of the female students agree with the statement, "I do not like my body the way it is."

■ 80% of the female students agree with the statement, "It is very important to me and my friends to be thin."

■ 20% of the female students report that their lives are out of control, and one of the only things they have control over is their eating behavior.

■ The school staff has not been trained to refer girls who appear extremely thin or are not eating meals to the school nurse.

GOAL: Reduce the risk for altered nutrition among 13-to-15-year-old female students at Data Middle School.

MODIFIABLE RISK FACTORS: Nutrition habits, body image disturbance, powerlessness, lack of screening and outreach services

PROTECTIVE FACTORS: Friendship and peer network, school nurse, social worker, and counseling staff, school breakfast and lunch program, primary care clinic open at school

STRENGTHS, ASSETS, RESILIENCE: Most of the girls have parents they are willing to talk to about nutrition; students like health and fitness class and instructor at school; school district has small amount of money to start intervention program; most at-risk females visit health office often and appear motivated to improve their health and fitness.

Outcomes	Interventions	Providers	Evaluation
1. 75% of the students will obtain lunch from cafeteria rather than vending machines by 1/1/02. (P)	1.1 Health teaching: nutrition 1.2 Collaboration: redesigning how and where students eat lunch 1.3 Policy development: change school policies about use of vending machines during lunch hour	School nurse, health teachers Administration, food services, student council, school nurse School board	Student survey Cafeteria register count
2. 50% of students at risk will agree with the statement, "I like my body the way it is" by 5/01/02. (P)	2.1 Counseling: support group for at-risk students, peer counseling	Social workers, psychologist, school nurse, peer helpers, and peer helper instructor	Survey or interview
3. 100% of the students at risk will agree with the statement, "I am more in charge of my life than I was six months ago" by 5/01/02. (P)	3.1 Counseling: support group for at-risk students, peer counseling	Social workers, psychologist, school nurse, peer helpers, and peer helper instructor	Survey or interview
4. A screening and outreach program to identify and refer students at risk for eating disorders will be implemented by 1/30/02. (S)	4.1 Outreach and referral: program implemented school-wide for outreach and referral 4.2 Screening: process for screening at-risk students will be developed and implemented 4.3 Provider education: workshop and information sheets will be provided to school staff 4.4 Social marketing: parents association and school board will be targeted for informational meetings	Administration, school staff, peer counselors Administration, school nurse, social workers, psychologist Administration, school staff, health education teacher, school nurse Administration, PTA, school nurse, health education teacher, school board	Provider survey Log of students referred analyzed Evaluation at end of meeting of school board

C: community-focused outcome; P: population-focused outcome related to individuals, families, small groups; S: system-focused outcome.

(continues)

Figure 7-3 Population-based nursing intervention plan.

Outcomes	Interventions	Providers	Evaluation
5. 25% of students with weight below the 5th percentile and height above the 25th percentile on a standardized growth grid will weigh above the 5th percentile by 6/1/02. (P)	5.1 Surveillance: a monitoring program for at-risk students will be developed and implemented	School nurse, administration	Review of student progress records
6. 75% of participants on community health education will agree at end of session that adolescents with eating disorders are an important health priority in their community. (C)	6.1 Social marketing and health teaching: Community education department will hold a community meeting on eating disorders and adolescence in June 2002	Panel: health educator, school psychologist, social worker, school nurse, nutritionist, physician	Exit survey

C: community-focused outcome; P: population-focused outcome related to individuals, families, small groups;
S: system-focused outcome.

Figure 7-3 Population-based nursing intervention plan (continued).

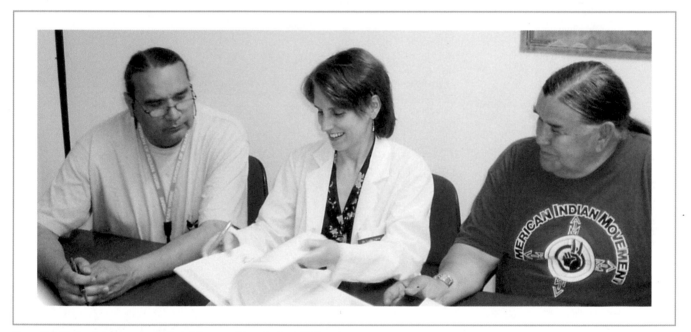

Figure 7-4 Native American community clinic team. (Photo by David Schoon)

EVALUATION

Outcomes of population-based nursing practice focus on health status, functional abilities, and quality of life of at-risk population groups. Data are collected that reflect the aggregated response of the total at-risk group for each specified outcome. Descriptive statistics, such as mean, range, and percentages as well as biometric measures such as rates are used in the analysis of group data. Case studies illustrating how services are provided to clients are also very effective. The evaluation process involves the multidisciplinary team, health consumers, and community partnerships (Figure 7-4). After the evaluation of population outcomes is completed, the unmet needs of the at-risk population groups are determined to identify whether further interventions are necessary.

PROGRAM EVALUATION

Program evaluation is an integral part of the evaluation process when providing population-based care. Justification of resources and budget is necessary. A cost-benefit analysis, comparing improvements in health status, functional abilities, and quality of life of the targeted at-risk population with expenditures of human and material resources, is appropriate. Ethical guidelines, as well as guidelines for culturally competent care, should be used to evaluate the efficacy of health provider interactions with vulnerable or marginalized population groups. A set of questions that may be used to focus program evaluation is found in Figure 7-5.

Program Evaluation of Population Based Nursing Practice

Access

Did we find the high-risk, underserved, vulnerable population groups in the community/service area and provide timely and accessible services?

Did we offer service regardless of age, gender, race, ethnicity, health care status, or location?

Quality

Did our services meet the greatest unmet health needs of the community or the at-risk, vulnerable, underserved population groups?

Did their health status improve?

Were their health risks reduced?

Were they satisfied with the services they received?

Cost

Were patients able to afford what we had to offer?

Did we manage to stay within our budget?

Are we reducing the cost of care over time?

Equity

Did we use our resources in a way that met the priority health needs of all of our high-risk patient groups?

Did we target our services and use our resources to improve the health status of those who were the most underserved?

Did we have enough resources left over to meet the essential health needs of lower-risk population groups?

Figure 7-5 Program evaluation of population-based nursing practice.

CRITICAL THINKING 7-3

Consider the implications of the following situation. Your community is experiencing a measles epidemic. You are asked to forgo your home visits to your hospice clients for one day so that you can staff a measles immunization clinic. You have three hospice visits scheduled, including one to a family with a child near death. By staffing the immunization clinic, you would be able to vaccinate and protect 150 children.

What decision would you make? What alternative choices might you have in resolving this dilemma?

REAL WORLD INTERVIEW

I work with pregnant and parenting teens at an alternative high school program that provides educational options for teens whose lives don't fit the traditional school day. Our program includes teens from a variety of cultures and backgrounds. The program currently has eight young women who will deliver their babies during the school year. This year, we also have four young fathers enrolled. The program has an on-site child care center, so these students bring their children to school with them and are able to visit their child during the school day.

Another public health nurse and I share this assignment. We teach weekly prenatal classes in conjunction with the life skills class that all our students are required to take for graduation. Each student spends time working in the child care rooms, both in their own child's room as well as the next age group's room. This provides us with the opportunity to discuss growth and development, health care, and to role model parent-child interactions.

We also work with each student to look at family planning options for him or her and are very proud of a program we started called The Pregnancy Free Club. This is a voluntary "club" that allows each student to have private time with a public health nurse to talk about how to use birth control correctly and look at barriers that prevent the student from effectively using birth control.

Peer support has also become an unexpected part of this program, making it easier and more acceptable for the students to talk about their birth control choice or their choice of abstinence. Our program currently has a repeat pregnancy rate significantly lower than the national average.

Barbara Reilly, PHN
City of Bloomington Health Department
Bloomington, Minnesota

From Reilly, B. (2001). "Health Teaching" in Getting Behind the Wheel, *Public Health Nursing Online Newsletter, 13.* Section of Public Health Nursing, Minnesota Department of Health. Retrieved July 13, 2001, from http://www.health.state.mn.us/divs/chs/phn/phnnews13.html

CASE STUDY 7-2

You are caring for a 72-year-old client, Mrs. Ramone, in her home. She lives mainly off her Social Security pension. She is getting weaker each time you visit her, yet she wants to stay in her home as long as she can.

What nursing advocacy initiatives might you undertake to ensure the provision of safe home care services to Mrs. Ramone? How might you justify the distribution of resources to assist Mrs. Ramone to stay in her home longer?

INNOVATIONS IN POPULATION-BASED HEALTH CARE PRACTICE

Nurses in the twenty-first century will be continuously challenged to look for new solutions to health care needs for populations at risk. The elderly, the poor, and marginalized population groups continue to grow nationally and globally. We must continue to find ways to partner with local communities in finding solutions and in providing services. Nurses must take the lead in working collaboratively within a variety of health care and social service disciplines and agencies within the community. There is growing evidence that interdisciplinary and community partnerships are more effective in reducing health disparities in populations at risk.

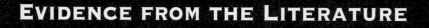

EVIDENCE FROM THE LITERATURE

Citation: Fowler, B., Rodney, M., Roberts, S., & Broadus, L. (2005). Collaborative breast health intervention for African-American women of lower socioeconomic status. *Oncology Nursing Forum, 32*(6), 1207–1216.

Discussion: A collaborative community program using specially trained community health advisors was developed to increase the rate of mammography in African-American women of low socioeconomic status. African-American women leaders in the community were influential in encouraging community women to participate in the mammography screening project. Outreach, case finding, referral, monitoring, follow-up, and health education interventions were provided by the community health advisors. Of the women recruited, 90 (81%) met the study inclusion criteria, and 68 (76%) followed through and received mammography screening. Health education provided at the time of the mammogram resulted in the African-American women demonstrating increased knowledge about breast health and increased sharing about their health concerns.

Implications for Practice: Collaboration with community members is an effective way to reach population groups at risk who may not be comfortable participating in health care programs provided by the established health care system. Nurses should consider collaboration with community members as well as other health care providers when trying to reach at-risk and marginalized population groups within the community.

REAL WORLD INTERVIEW

On August 29, 2005, Hurricane Katrina slammed into the Gulf Coast of eastern Louisiana and Mississippi. Katrina, a Category Four storm when it made landfall with wind speeds of 140 mph, was the largest storm to ever hit the United States. Hundreds of thousands of residents were evacuated before and after the storm and went to motels, homes of relatives, or shelters. On September 5, the American Refugee Committee (ARC) sent a seven-member advance team to Louisiana to determine how to deploy Minnesota Lifeline, a volunteer consortium of Minnesota health care professionals. The ARC advance team included the Director of International Operations, the International Programs Manager, a Medical Director, and a Registered Nurse. The team worked with the Office of Public Health (OPH) to develop a plan for providing primary health care to evacuees that would be sustainable after the volunteer consortium left.

Minnesota Lifeline was an interdisciplinary group of physicians, physician's assistants, advance practice nurses, RNs, psychologists, social workers, respiratory care therapists, phlebotomists, health information managers, and clinic assistants from the College of St. Catherine, the University of Minnesota Health Corps, and the Mayo Clinic. Minnesota Lifeline made a 60-day commitment to OPH to work in Region Four, which encompassed seven parishes near Lafayette, that is, Acadia, Evangeline, Iberia, Lafayette, St. Martin, St. Landry, and Vermillion parishes. The 60-day commitment was divided into four two-week waves of workers. The first wave included about 95 persons. The following groups were smaller. The final group focused on integrating the primary care services for the evacuees into the local health care delivery systems.

Interdisciplinary teams were dispatched to one of the approximately 68 sanctioned shelters in Region Four. The shelters primarily housed New Orleans area residents and were located in churches, campgrounds, American Legion halls, community centers, and indoor sports facilities. Truckloads of supplies arrived with the first wave of workers and included personal care kits, medications, nebulizers, blood glucose monitors, dressings, gloves, blood pressure cuffs, and everything else needed to run a primary care clinic. The Mayo Foundation donated most of the supplies. Clinic supplies and medications were packed into large totes and brought to whichever shelter was in need of care. A recreational vehicle provided by the Northwest Medical Team was first used as a mobile clinic and later as a mobile pharmacy.

(continues)

REAL WORLD INTERVIEW (CONTINUED)

Prior to participating in a clinic, permission had to be obtained from multiple levels of governmental and community organizations, including the Region Four OPH Medical Director, the Public Health Nursing Director, the Parish Emergency Preparedness Coordinator, the City Emergency Preparedness Coordinator, and the Shelter Manager. Clinics were also set up in churches, motels, and parking lots to serve those who were living at those sites. Teams participated in community meetings to assess health needs, to gain community trust, and to help the team learn how to fit into the community culture.

The Minnesota Consortium provided primary health care for longstanding health needs as well as acute health care needs. The budget for providing public health in Louisiana had been severely cut many years ago, and little public health care was available. Most parishes had a clinic facility, which was used during weekday work hours to provide immunizations, reproductive health, and Women, Infant, and Children (WIC) clinics. Uninsured Louisiana residents received health care through the Charity Hospital system. Emergency care was provided at Charity Hospitals, but diagnostic workups and preventative care were provided on a sliding fee scale and required cash upfront prior to receiving care. Only about 15% of children in Region Four were up to date on immunizations.

A three-page health form was developed by combining The CDC forms with OPH forms. Vaccines were administered to tens of thousands of evacuees and residents. Tetanus-diphtheria, hepatitis A, hepatitis B, and influenza vaccines were administered to persons who had been or would be in contact with the floodwaters or would be working on demolition of buildings. Most medications prescribed were for chronic illnesses such as diabetes and hypertension. Antibiotics, asthma and allergy medications, blood glucose monitors, and nebulizers were given out. Reproductive health care needs were common. Those who had contact with floodwaters often experienced skin rashes and a dry cough coined the "Katrina Cough." Psychological trauma from separation of family members and flight from the hurricane were common. Those with mental health illnesses without their medications experienced symptoms of medication withdrawal and increased severity of symptoms.

The arrival of Hurricane Rita required evacuation of the first wave of relief workers into northern Mississippi to wait out the storm. Many New Orleans evacuees who had just gotten permanent housing and jobs and whose children were adjusting to new schools in their newly adopted towns had to again pack up belongings and evacuate. Some were later able to return. Many evacuees had to adjust to another new setting. The economically depressed area of the Gulf Coast has received a devastating blow. The development of a viable private-public health care infrastructure will be slow.

Pam Hamre, RN, MS, CNM
Associate Professor, Nursing College of St. Catherine
St. Paul, Minnesota

Nurses are being challenged to expand their professional boundaries by participating in the political process, working within their professional organizations and working as volunteers with disenfranchised populations. Nurses will continue to participate in local, national, and international rescue and humanitarian efforts using population-based nursing practice interventions.

KEY CONCEPTS

- Health status of population groups is measured by global measures such as morbidity, mortality, and quality of life. These are the vital signs of population groups.

- Health determinants give us a holistic picture of both the health assets and the health risks of population groups within the community. When nurses identify the health determinants of population groups, they can build on population strengths and target the most significant health risks to help improve the health status of population groups.

- There are significant health disparities within the U.S. population. The causes for these disparities are complex and involve societal factors such as governmental health policies, lack of insurance, poverty, health literacy, barriers to health access, culture, and ethnicity. Societal interventions are necessary to reduce health disparities. Traditional nursing and medical care alone will not reduce health disparities significantly.

- The U.S. health care system provides unequal access, treatment, and quality to people of different ethnic and cultural groups. These disparities persist over time, geography, and different health care systems. Nurses need to take the lead in creating culturally inclusive health care systems that meet the needs of diverse population groups.

- Population-based health care starts with community assessment, identifies health disparities among population groups within the community, and establishes community health priorities. The unequal needs of diverse populations within the community require an unequal division of available resources. Nurses need to be able to use ethical principles in determining how to use resources in an ethical and equitable manner.

- Population-based nursing practice is the application of the nursing process to population groups and communities. It focuses on the priority health needs in a community or specific population groups. Nurses practice population-based care at three levels: individual, system, and community, across the prevention continuum. This includes primary, secondary, and tertiary health care. A set of population-based public health nursing interventions has been identified as specific to this area of nursing practice. Almost all of the interventions are independent nursing functions within the scope of practice of the baccalaureate nursing graduate.

- Empowering communities and population groups to manage their own health care needs is an important aspect of population-based nursing practice. To empower these populations, nurses must develop egalitarian partnerships with the population groups they wish to help. Using an assets-based approach, in which community and population group strengths and resources are identified first before health needs, facilitates the development of partnerships.

- Health needs of vulnerable population groups are complex and require the combined resources of the interdisciplinary team, including paraprofessionals. Nurses need to be skilled in communications, group processes, care coordination, and collaboration to work effectively within the interdisciplinary team.

KEY TERMS

activities of daily living
functional health status
health assets
health care systems disparities
health determinants
health disparities
health-related quality of life
health risk factors
health status

instrumental activities
 of daily living
population-based health
 care practice
population-based
 nursing practice
protective factors
quality of life
resilience

REVIEW QUESTIONS

1. Your have just attended a community hearing about the increasing rate of sexually transmitted infections (STIs) among adolescents in your community. The community is divided on what actions to take. You want to help the community reach some consensus on a plan of action. What intervention would be the most appropriate to do first?
   A. Develop a social marketing campaign to increase awareness of STIs.
   B. Talk to adolescents at a local high school about their concerns.
   C. Encourage the passage of a new law funding a free condom program.
   D. Form a coalition of community leaders and interest groups to take action.

2. The *best* indication that a community clinic is interested in providing culturally inclusive care is that the clinic does which of the following?
   A. Provides care for people from all cultures in the community
   B. Recruits board members that reflect community diversity
   C. Provides cultural diversity training for its staff annually
   D. Conducts a health survey of the community annually

REVIEW ACTIVITIES

1. What are the health determinants for students on your college campus? Consider using an assets-based approach. Use the health determinants model to identify the health promoting social and physical environmental factors that influence the holistic health of students: body, mind, and spirit. Then identify the social and physical environmental barriers to holistic health. Consider college policies and access to health and social services on campus.

2. What are the major health risks for the people in your community? Take a walk in your community and see what physical and environmental health risks you can identify for one or more vulnerable groups in the community.

3. Think about a service project that your nursing class could do to improve the health of one vulnerable group within your community. What might you want to do before you launch any initiative?

EXPLORING THE WEB

Where could you find information to help you search the health needs of immigrants and refugees?

- Center for Cross Cultural Health: *www.crosshealth.com*

- National Institute of Health: *www.nih.gov*

- Office of Minority Health: *www.cdc.gov*
  Search for Office of Minority Health.

- Office of U.S. Surgeon General:
  www.surgeongeneral.gov

- United Nations: *www.un.org*

- U.S. Department of Health and Human Services:
  www.dhhs.gov

- U.S. Committee for Refugees and Immigrants:
  www.refugees.org

- World Health Organization: *http://who.org*

What sites could you search for health information on your community and the nation?

- Centers for Disease Control and Prevention: *www.cdc.gov*

- FEDSTATS: *www.fedstats.gov*

- Governmental health initiatives: *www.health.gov*

- Healthy People 2010: *www.healthypeople.gov*

- National Institute of Environmental Health Services: *www.niehs.nih.gov*

REFERENCES

Abrams, S. (2004). From function to competency in public health nursing, 1931 to 2003. *Public Health Nursing, 21*(5), 507–510.

Agency for Health Care Research and Quality (AHRQ). (2005). *National Healthcare Disparities Report 2005.* USDHHS. Retrieved June 18, 2006, from http://www.ahrq.gov/qual/nhdr05/nhdr05.pdf

American College of Physicians. (2004). Racial and ethnic disparities in health care. *Annals of Internal Medicine, 141*(3), 221–225.

American Nurses Association. (1995). Position Statements: Promotion and Disease Prevention. Retrieved March 30, 2002, from http://nursingworld.org/readroom/position/social/seprmo.htm

Anderson, J., Felton, G., Wewers, M., Waller, J., & Humbles, P. (2005). Sister to sister: A pilot study to assist African-American women in subsidized housing to quit smoking. *Southern Online Journal of Nursing Research, 1*(6), 1–23. Retrieved June 1, 2006, from http://www.snrs.org

Baldwin, D. (2003). Disparities in health and health care: Focusing efforts to eliminate unequal burdens. *Online Journal of Issues in Nursing, 8*(1), 113–122. Retrieved June 1, 2006, from EBSCOhost at http://sas.epnet.com.pearl

Brackbill, R., Thorpe, L., DiGrande, L., Perrin, M., Sapp, J., Wu, D., et al. (2006). Surveillance for world trade center disaster health effects among survivors of collapsed and damaged buildings. *Morbidity and Mortality Weekly Report,* (55), SS-2, 1-18. Retrieved May 1, 2006, from http://www.cdc.gov

Chin, M., Cook, S., Drum, M., Guillen, J., Humikowski, C., Koppert, J., et al. (2004). Improving diabetes care in midwest community health centers with the health disparities collaborative. *Diabetes Care, 27*(1), 2–8.

Davis, R., Cook, D., & Cohen, L. (2005). A community resilience approach to reducing, ethnic and racial disparities in health. *American Journal of Public Health, 95*(12), 2168–2173.

Deschaine, J., & Schaffer, M. (2003). Strengthening the role of public health nurse leaders in policy development. *Policy, Politics, & Nursing Practice, 4*(4), 266–274.

Eberhardt, M., & Parnuk, E. (2004). The importance of place of residence: Examining health in rural and nonrural areas. *American Journal of Public Health, 94*(10), 1682–1686.

Falk-Rafael, A. (2005). Speaking truth to power—nursing's legacy and moral imperative. *Advances in Nursing Science, 28*(3), 212–223.

Fowler, B., Rodney, M., Roberts, S., & Broadus, L. (2005). Collaborative breast health intervention for African-American women of lower socioeconomic status. *Oncology Nursing Forum, 32*(6), 1207–1216.

Freeman, R. B. (1957). *Public health nursing practice* (2nd ed.). Philadelphia: Saunders.

Garwick, A., & Auger, S. (2003). Participatory action research: The Indian family stories project. *Nursing Outlook, 51*(6), 261–266.

Giachello, A., Arrom, J., Davis, M., Sayad, J., Ramirez, D., Nandi, C., et al. (2003). Reducing diabetes health disparities through community-based participatory action research: The Chicago southeast diabetes community action coalition. *Public Health Reports, 118*(4), 309–323.

Giddings, L. (2005). A theoretical model of social consciousness. *Advances in Nursing Science, 28*(3), 224–239.

Gustafson, D. (2005). Transcultural nursing theory from a critical cultural perspective. *Advances in Nursing Science, 28*(1), 2–17.

Hartley, D. (2004). Rural health disparities, population health, and rural culture. *American Journal of Public Health, 94*(10), 1675–1678.

Health Resources and Services Administration (HRSA). (2005). *National sample survey of registered nurses—Preliminary findings, March 2004.* USDHHS. Retrieved June 26, 2006, from ftp://ftp.hrsa.gov/bhpr/nursing/rnpopulation/theregisterednursepopulation.pdf

Her, M. (2001). Case study: Target population, Hmong elderly at risk for depression-intervention, outreach in Behind the Wheel, *Public Health Nursing Newsletter, 13.* Retrieved July 13, 2001, from http://health.state.mn.us/divs/chs/phn/phnnews15.html (no longer available).

Institute of Medicine (IOM). (2002). *Unequal treatment confronting racial and ethnic disparities in healthcare.* Institute of Medicine Report. Washington, DC: National Academy Press.

Keller, L., Schaffer, M., Lia-Hoagberg, B., & Strohschein, S. (2002). Assessment, program planning, and evaluation in population-based public health practice. *Journal of Public Health Management and Practice, 8*(5), 30–43.

Keller, L., Strohschein, S., Lia-Hoagberg, B., & Schaffer, M. (2004a). Population-based public health interventions: Practice-based and evidence-supported. Part I. *Public Health Nursing, 21*(5), 453–468.

Keller, L., Strohschein, S., Schaffer, M., & Lia-Hoagberg, B. (2004b). Population-based public health interventions in practice, teaching, and management. Part II. *Public Health Nursing, 21*(5), 469–487.

Kelly, D. (2005). From the emergency department to home. *Journal of Clinical Nursing, 14,* 776–785.

Keltner, B., Kelley, F., & Smith, D. (2004). Leadership to reduce health disparities: A model for the nursing leadership in American Indian communities. *Nursing Administration Quarterly, 28*(3), 181–190.

Littlefield, D., Robinson, C., Engelbrecht, L., Gonzalez, B., & Hutcheson, H. (2002). Field action report. Mobilizing women for minority health and social justice in California. *American Journal of Public Health, 92*(4), 576–579.

LoBue, P., & Moser, K. (2004). Screening of immigrants and refugees for pulmonary tuberculosis in San Diego County, California. *Chest, 126*(6), 1777–1782. Retrieved June 15, 2006, from http://www.chestjournal.org

Ludwig, T., Buchholz, C., & Clarke, S. (2005). Using social marketing to increase the use of helmets among bicyclists. *Journal of American College Health, 4*(1), 51–58.

Newman, M. A. (1999). *Health as expanding consciousness.* New York: National League for Nursing Press.

Minnesota Department of Health (MDH). (2005). *Background information. Priority health areas for elimination of health disparities in Minnesota.* St. Paul, MN: Author. Retrieved May 10, 2006, from http://www.health.state.mn.us/divs/chs/pdf/gdlinebkgrd9.pdf

Minnesota Department of Health, Section of Public Health Nursing. (2001). *Public health interventions: Application for public health nursing practice.* St. Paul, MN: Minnesota Department of Health. Retrieved April 12, 2006, from http://www.health.state.mn.us/divs/cfh/ophp/resources/docs/ph-interventions_manual2001.pdf

Pate, R., Ward, D., Saunders, R., Felton, G., Dishman, R., & Dowda, M. (2005). Promotion of physical activity among high-school girls: A randomized controlled trial. *American Journal of Public Health, 95*(9), 1582–1587.

Pawlak, R. (2005). Economic considerations of health literacy. *Nursing Economics, 23*(4), 173–180.

Peters, R. M. (1995). Teaching population-focused practice to baccalaureate nursing students: A clinical model. *Journal of Nursing Education, 34*(8), 378–383.

Pharris, M. D., Sankofa, P., Amaikwu-Rushing, L., Fitzgerald, D., & Ollom, K. (2002). *Racism, health, and well being: The experience of women and girls of color in North Minneapolis, Centers of Excellence in Women's Health.* St. Paul, MN: College of Catherine.

Quad Council of Public Health Nursing Organizations. (2004). Public health nursing competencies. *Public Health Nursing, 21*(ss), 443–452.

Rewes, A., Hedegaaard, H., Lezotte, D., Meng, K., Battan, K., Emery, K. et al. (2005). Childhood femur fractures, associated injuries, and sociodemographic risk factors: a population-based study. *Pediatrics, 115*(5), e543–e552. Retrieved March 20, 2006, from http://www.pediatrics.org

Reilly, B. (2001). Health teaching in Getting Behind the Wheel, *Public Health Nursing Newsletter, 13.* Retrieved July 13, 2001, from http://health.state.mn.us/divs/chs/phn/phnnews13.html (no longer available).

Schraeder, C., Dworak, D., Stoll, J., Kucera, C., Waldschmidt, V., & Dworak, M. (2005). Managing elders with comorbidities. *Journal Ambulatory Care Management, 28*(3), 201–209.

Tashiro, C. (2005). Health disparities in the context of mixed race—challenging the ideology of race. *Advances in Nursing Science, 28*(3), 203–211.

Taylor, R. (2005). Addressing barriers to cultural competence. *Journal for Nurses in Staff Development, 21*(4), 135–142.

Tembreull, C., & Schaffer, M. (2005). The intervention of outreach: Best practices. *Public Health Nursing, 22*(4), 347–353.

U.S. Department of Health and Human Services. *Healthy People 2010.* 2nd ed. With Understanding and Improving Health and Objectives for Improving Health. 2 vols. Washington, DC: U.S. Government Printing Office, November 2000.

Wald, L. D. (1915). *The house on Henry Street.* New York: Dover Publications.

WHO Task Force on Research Priorities for Equity in Health & WHO Equity Team. (2005). Priorities for research to take forward the health equity policy agenda. *Bulletin of the World Health Organization, 83*(12), 948–953.

Worobey, J., Pisuk, J., & Decker, K. (2004). Diet and behavior in at-risk children: Evaluation of an early intervention program. *Public Health Nursing, 21*(2), 122–127.

Wu, P., Duarte, C., Mandell, D., Fan, B., Liu, X., Fuller, et al. (2006, May). Exposure to the World Trade Center attack and the use of cigarettes and alcohol among New York City public high-school students. *American Journal of Public Health, 96*(5), 804–807. Epub 2006 Mar 29.

Young, T., & Ireson, C. (2003). Effectiveness of school-based telehealth care in urban and suburban elementary schools. *Pediatrics, 112*(5), 1088–1094.

SUGGESTED READINGS

Baker, M. (2005). Creation of a model of independence for community-dwelling elders in the United States. *Nursing Research, 54*(5), 288–295.

Baltrus, P., Lynch, J., Everson-Rose, S., Raghunathan, T., & Kaplan, G. (2005). Race/ethnicity, life-course socioeconomic position, and body weight trajectories over 34 years: The Alameda County study. *American Journal of Public Health, 95*(9), 1595–1601.

Barr, V., Robinson, S., Marin-Link, B., Underhill, L., Dotts, A., Ravensdale, D., et al. (2003). The expanded chronic care model: An integration of concepts and strategies from population-health promotion and the chronic care model. *Hospital Quarterly, 7*(1), 73–82.

Bent, K. (2003). Culturally interpreting environment as determinant and experience of health. *Journal of Transcultural Nursing, 14*(4), 305–312.

Harrison, K., & Marske, A. (2005). Nutritional content of foods advertised during the television programs children watch most. *American Journal of Public Health, 95*(9), 1568–1574.

Hinton, A., Downey, J., Lisovicz, N., Mayfield-Johnson, S., & White-Johnson, F. (2005). The community health advisor program and the deep south network for cancer control: Health promotion programs for volunteer community health advisors. *Family & Community Health, 28*(1), 20–27.

Kara, M. (2005). Preparing nurses for the global pandemic of chronic obstructive pulmonary disease. *Journal of Nursing Scholarship, 37*(2), 127–133.

Katz, D., O'Connell, M., Yeh, M., Nawaz, H., Njike, V., Anderson, L., et al. (2005). Public health strategies for preventing and controlling overweight and obesity in school and worksite settings. *Morbidity and Mortality Weekly Report,* (54), RR-10, 1–11. Retrieved May 1, 2006, from http://www.cde.gov

Kim, J., Must, A., Fitzmaurice, G., Gillman, M., Chomitz, V., Kramer, E., et al. (2005). Incidence and remission rates of overweight among children aged 5 to 13 years in a district-wide school surveillance system. *American Journal of Public Health, 95*(9), 1588–1594.

Kim, S., Flaskerud, J., Koniak-Griffin, D., & Dixon, E. (2005). Using community-partnered participatory research to address health disparities in a Latino community. *Journal of Professional Nursing, 21*(4), 199–209.

Kolb, S., Gillilard, I., Deliganis, J., & Light, K. (2003). Ministerio de Salud: Development of a mission-driven partnership for addressing health disparities in a Hispanic community. *Journal of Multicultural Nursing & Health, 9*(3), 6–12.

Lavery, S., Smith, M., Esparza, A., Hrushow, A., Moore, M., & Reed, D. (2005). The community action model: A community-driven model designed to address disparities in health. *American Journal of Public Health, 95*(4), 611–616.

Lewis, L., Sloane, D., Nascimento, L., Diamart, A., Guinyard, J., Yancey, A., et al. (2005). African americans' access to healthy food options in south Los Angeles restaurants. *American Journal of Public Health, 95*(4), 668–673.

McNaughton, D. (2004). Nurse home visits to maternal-child clients: A review of intervention research. *Public Health Nursing, 23*(3), 207–219.

Pavlish, C. (2005). Action responses of Conglolese refugee women. *Journal of Nursing Scholarship, 37*(1), 10–17.

Reid, L., Hatch, J., & Parrish, T. (2003, Nov.). The role of a historically black university and the black church in a community-based health initiatives: The project DIRECT experience. *Journal of Public Health Management Practice,* S70–S73.

Rovi, S., Chin, P. H., & Johnson, M. (2004). The economic burden of hospitalizations associated with child abuse and neglect. *American Journal of Public Health, 94*(4), 586–590.

Schultz, A., Senk, S., Odoms-Young, A., Hollis-Neely, T., Nwankwo, R., Lockett, M., et al. (2005). Healthy eating and exercising to reduce diabetes: Exploring the potential of social determinants of health frameworks within the context of community-based participatory diabetes prevention. *American Journal of Public Health, 95*(4), 645–651.

Welch, D., & Kneipp, S. (2005). Low-income housing policy and socioeconomic inequalities in women's health: The importance or nursing inquiry and intervention. *Policy, Politics, & Nursing Practice, 6*(4), 335–342.

UNIT II
Leadership and Management of the Interdisciplinary Team

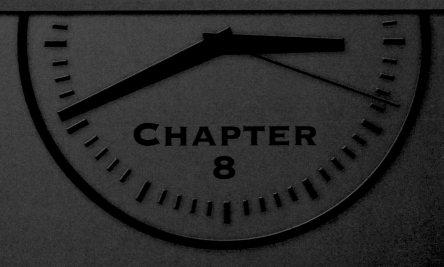

CHAPTER 8

Personal and Interdisciplinary Communication

Jacklyn Ludwig Ruthman, PhD, RN

Fundamentally who we are and how we work together is what our patients receive (Nancy Moore, 2000).

OBJECTIVES

Upon completion of this chapter, the reader should be able to:

1. Analyze how current trends in society affect communication.
2. Focus on the elements of the communication process.
3. Describe the Health Insurance Portability and Accountability Act.
4. Use various modes of communication.
5. Identify common communication networks.
6. Describe organizational communication and communication skills in the workplace.
7. Identify barriers to communication and strategies to overcome them.
8. Identify linguistically appropriate communication strategies.
9. Describe the SBARR communication tool.

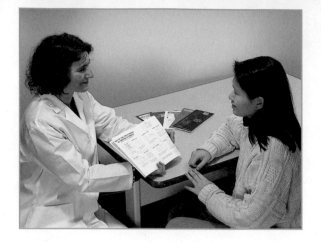

As a newly licensed RN working on a medical unit in a community hospital, Steve begins the shift by making rounds on patients to perform initial assessments. He enters the room of Mr. Mason, who has a long history of chronic obstructive pulmonary disease. He was admitted yesterday with pneumonia. Mr. Mason is well known to the experienced staff. As Steve assesses Mr. Mason's breath sounds, he says, "I don't think I'm going to make it this time." His wife, who is at his bedside, replies, "Don't talk like that."

> *What nonverbal cues might be used to help Steve interpret this message?*
>
> *What communication skills will Steve use to respond appropriately?*

Today's nurses use basic principles of communication to facilitate interactions with patients, family members, peers, and other disciplines. These principles allow nurses to adapt to trends that affect the profession of nursing and its practice. Nurses rely on communication skills to effectively promote patient care and professionalism in a variety of settings for an increasingly diverse society. These skills enable nurses to engage in the complex, interactive process of communication that uses both verbal and nonverbal modes. Nurses are aware of the context in which communication occurs. Nurses must be aware of potential barriers to communication to be able to overcome them. Awareness of principles and skills of communication empowers nurses to manage a variety of communication demands in the workplace.

TRENDS IN SOCIETY THAT AFFECT COMMUNICATION

Good communication will grow in importance because of trends in our culture. Among the trends affecting nursing practice is the increasing diversity in society. The United States has been called the melting pot, and that has never been more true than now when we see the influence of many different ethnic, racial, cultural, and socioeconomic backgrounds. Increased diversity causes once-dominant values and beliefs to be replaced or diluted with different values and beliefs. These differences become a source of possible misunderstanding that can be bridged by effective communication.

Another trend is our aging population. It is estimated that 20% of the population will be 65 years of age or older by 2020. Our aging society will challenge nurses to maintain effective communication to compensate for the diminished sensory abilities that typically accompany aging. Multiple sensory deficits can occur simultaneously so that patients may experience losses in a variety of combinations that include hearing, seeing, smelling, tasting, and touching. The potential diminished input challenges nurse and patient alike to creatively compensate for these deficits. At the same time that the population is aging, it is also shifting to an electronic mode, with computer technology playing an increasingly dominant role. As electronic communication assumes a greater role, the nurse's ability to effectively communicate in writing will grow in importance. Reliance on written communication using electronic input shifts the source of input away from traditional visual, auditory, and kinesthetic modes to the written word. To use electronic tools effectively, tomorrow's nurses will require keen writing skills. These trends have influenced nursing today.

ELEMENTS OF THE COMMUNICATION PROCESS

Communication is an interactive process that occurs when a person (the sender) sends a verbal or nonverbal message to another person (the receiver) and receives feedback. The communication process is influenced by emotions, needs, perceptions, values, education, culture, goals, literacy, cognitive ability, and the communication mode (Figure 8-1).

Communication in health care is used to coordinate patient care. Several studies of ICUs indicate that effective communication and coordination among clinical staff results in more efficient and better quality of care (Baggs, Ryan, Phelps, Richeson, & Johnson, 1992; Knaus, Draper, Wagner, & Zimmerman, 1986; Shortell et al., 1994). More recent studies of other health care delivery settings also indicate that effective coordination of staff leads to better clinical outcomes (Gittell et al., 2000; Young et al., 1997; Young et al., 1998). Additionally, research suggests that ineffective coordination and communication among hospital staff contributes substantially

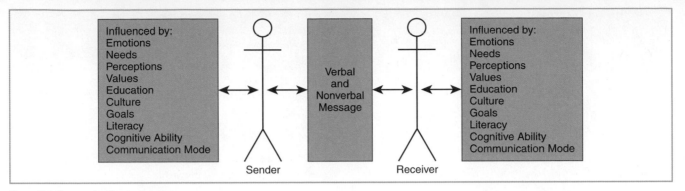

Influenced by:
Emotions
Needs
Perceptions
Values
Education
Culture
Goals
Literacy
Cognitive Ability
Communication Mode

Verbal
and
Nonverbal
Message

Influenced by:
Emotions
Needs
Perceptions
Values
Education
Culture
Goals
Literacy
Cognitive Ability
Communication Mode

Sender   Receiver

Figure 8-1 Communication process.

to adverse events. For example, one study of the care of 1,047 patients in a large tertiary care hospital found that approximately 15% of the 480 adverse events identified, for example, failure to order indicated tests and misplaced test results, had causes related to the interaction of staff, such as the failure of a consultant team to communicate adequately with the requesting team (Andrews et al., 1997).

For many types of health care organizations, staff communication and coordination is also relevant to their ability to comply with the requirements of accrediting bodies. In particular, both the Joint Commission (JC), formerly the Joint Commission on the Accreditation of Health Care Organizations (JCAHO; www.jointcommission.org), and the National Committee on Quality Assurance (web.ncqa.org), two leading accrediting bodies in the health care industry, have adopted standards that address coordination among professional groups, patient care units, and service components within health care organizations. While setting standards obviously cannot ensure good communication and coordination, it does symbolize the growing recognition among accrediting and other oversight bodies that communication and coordination is highly important to the performance of health care organizations (Munoz & Luckmann, 2005). Another important area of communication involves following patient privacy guidelines.

HEALTH INSURANCE PORTABILITY AND ACCOUNTABILITY ACT (HIPAA) OF 1996

As nurses communicate today, they must increasingly be aware of patient privacy. The Department of Health and Human Services (HHS) has issued regulations known as the Privacy Rule that were required by April 14, 2003. The Privacy Rule protects all individually identifiable health information held or transmitted by a covered entity or its business associate, in any form or media, whether electronic, paper, or oral. It applies to all health care plans, health care clearinghouses, and to any

health care provider who transmits health information. The law introduced new standards for protecting the privacy of individuals' identifiable health information. There are 18 personal health identifiers. This law also may apply to health information that is shared for research purposes (www.hhs.gov); see Table 8-1.

MODES OF COMMUNICATION

Two traditional modes of communication, verbal and nonverbal, are exemplified in the nurse–patient scenario that follows in the Real World Interview. Because face-to-face encounters usually allow for verbal and nonverbal exchange, they have been regarded as the most effective modes of communication and hence have been preferred. Verbal communication is a conscious process, so the sender has the ability to control what is said. While it is generally accepted that tone of voice is more important than the words spoken, it has long been suggested that nonverbal facial expression is even more important than either tone of voice or the words used. Nonverbal communication tends to be unconscious and more difficult to control.

When face-to-face encounters are not possible or practical, other approaches are used. Historically, the next most effective approach is the telephone, followed by voice messages, electronic pages, e-mail messages, and written documents. These electronic methods comprise the third mode of communication, and they will grow in importance as nurses increasingly rely on technology, particularly computers, to communicate interpersonally. One example of a wireless e-mail device is the BlackBerry.

ELECTRONIC COMMUNICATION

Electronic communication is playing an increasingly dominant role. This transition in health care communication is slowly inching its way into the twenty-first century.

TABLE 8-1	ELEMENTS THAT ARE CONSIDERED PATIENT IDENTIFIERS UNDER HIPAA

- Names
- All geographic subdivisions smaller than a state, including street address, city, county, precinct, ZIP code
- All elements of dates (except year) for dates directly related to an individual, including birth date, admission date, discharge date, date of death; all ages over 89
- Telephone numbers
- Fax numbers
- E-mail addresses
- Social security numbers
- Medical record numbers
- Health plan beneficiary numbers
- Account numbers
- Certificate/license numbers
- Vehicle identifiers and serial numbers
- Device identifiers and serial numbers
- Web universal resource locators (URLs)
- Internet Protocol (IP) address numbers
- Biometric identifiers, including fingerprints and voiceprints
- Full face photographic images and any comparable images
- Any other unique identifying number, characteristic, or code unless otherwise permitted

Source: Compiled with information from U.S. Department of Health and Human Services. (2003). *Protecting personal health information in research: Understanding the HIPAA privacy rule.* NIH Publication Number 03-5388.

CRITICAL THINKING 8-1

Upon entering a patient's room, you identify yourself as his nurse and greet the patient. You then ask the patient how he is feeling. He responds with a whisper and a grimace, "I've never felt better." You notice the patient is slightly cyanotic. The patient is supporting himself with his elbows so that he is sitting upright over the bedside table. You note he is using pursed lip breathing. Respirations are 36 per minute and shallow.

What kinds of problems occur when verbal and nonverbal communications are incongruent? How will you handle the incongruent verbal and nonverbal communications? Which message, the verbal or nonverbal, is easier to identify?

Some new nurses find this frustrating, because they grew up with the technology and expect it to be available in their work settings (Greene, 2005). Patients are being monitored long distance and connecting to their health care providers using a variety of technologies, including telephones, voice mail, and e-mail. Handheld devices such as BlackBerry allow for rapid connections. These methods, where caregiver and care receiver interact using technology rather than the traditional face-to-face or voice-to-voice encounter, require careful communication. For example, e-mail now allows almost instantaneous communication around the world, but it also accommodates individual preferences with respect to the timing of the response. This allows a patient to provide an update on a condition early in the day and affords the caregivers the opportunity to respond as their schedules permit. Using e-mail may save a patient and caregiver from travel or loss of work. However, using e-mail requires that nurses acting in such a caregiver role have keen writing skills. An explanation of all the considerations that are important to effective writing is beyond the scope of this text. However, a few tips are worth sharing. The speed with which exchanges can now be made using technology has reduced the acceptable response time. Therefore, the first tip when communicating using technology is that it is important that both parties have an understanding about the circumstances under which different modes of communication will be used. Although one practitioner who is "connected" may be comfortable receiving urgent patient information such as an elevated potassium level electronically, perhaps by e-mail, most practitioners

REAL WORLD INTERVIEW

I view my primary responsibility as a nurse to be that of patient advocate. As a team leader, I am responsible for coordinating patient care for a group of patients. I am responsible for setting patient care goals and then directing my team to achieve the goals. I make those patient care goals the focus of my team's efforts. Patient care is rendered with the assistance of subordinates, including certified nurse assistants (CNAs), nursing student externs, and occasional high school student volunteers. Communication is the key to a successful team. A recent patient typifies how I interact with my team.

An elderly nonverbal patient with a history of schizophrenia was admitted to our surgical unit for dehydration. She was in need of total care, especially with respect to hygiene, which had been neglected. She was dependent on staff to turn and position her. Her level of awareness suggested she was unable to use a call light for help.

This patient challenged staff for a variety of reasons. First, due to multiple other health problems, she was not a candidate for surgery. This placed her among the patients who don't really "fit" the surgical unit where she was admitted. Nonetheless, my goal was to advocate for comfort care with her physician while also encouraging subordinates to provide quality care even though the goal was not for cure with this particular patient. The patient's inability to communicate verbally added to the challenge. It was unclear how aware the patient was of the care she was receiving. Her nonverbal status blocked her ability to dialogue. This caused us to rely on nonverbal cues. Respect for patients with or without their verbal feedback is essential. The CNA and I tackled the needed bed bath together. Teamwork kept the focus on the goal for the patient, which was to optimize comfort and maintain skin integrity. It allowed me to complete a thorough assessment and to model desired communication with the patient, whom I addressed by name. I inquired whether she was in pain, to which she responded with twisting motions. I continued the one-way conversation, attempting to clarify what her nonverbal responses meant. She pointed to her shoulder, so we repositioned her and she settled down, resting quietly. As is often the case, the CNA willingly returned to reposition the patient with confidence the remainder of the shift. The patient's inability to verbalize needs was perceived as less of a barrier once we were successful in overcoming it together.

I find that CNAs will often volunteer to complete entire tasks they feel capable of performing independently. They also need to be assured that they will not be expected to handle clinical situations for which they do not feel qualified. This mutual respect for each other is essential to an ongoing working relationship. They honor my standard of care and will often complete tasks, going above and beyond what I ask. For example, later in the afternoon, the CNA returned to the patient and washed and braided her hair. Since this same patient would not likely use the call light, I also explained our goal to the high school student volunteer and I asked her to check the patient's position whenever she went by the room. I instructed her to let me know if the patient appeared uncomfortable, assuring her that I would reposition the patient as needed. The student expressed that she thought it was cool how nurses communicate with patients who can't talk. I believe through effective communication our team achieved the goal of optimizing this patient's comfort in spite of many potential barriers.

Lari Summa, RN, BSN
Team Leader
Peoria, Illinois

expect a telephone call if the data being shared is potentially life-threatening. Practitioners may be satisfied to receive a fax if the data are not urgent. Often, organizations have policies that guide under what circumstances a particular mode of communication is used, so be sure to understand your institution's policy for communicating urgent information.

Another tip is to respond in a timely manner. Timeliness is defined by what information is being shared and the route being used. A fax delivered to a practitioner's office over the weekend will likely not generate a reply before Monday. E-mail, in general, provides greater immediacy, but the telephone remains the primary tool for communicating urgent information. Other tips for communicating on e-mail include the following:

- NO CAPITAL LETTERS—this looks like you are shouting.
- Be brief and reply sparingly, as appropriate.
- Use clear subject lines.
- Cool off before responding to an angry message. Answer tomorrow.

- Forward e-mail messages from others only with their permission.
- Forward jokes selectively, if ever.
- Use good judgment; e-mail may not be private.

Keep in mind that accurate spelling, correct grammar, and organization of thought assume greater importance in the absence of verbal and nonverbal cues that are given in face-to-face encounters. Always proofread correspondences prior to sending them. Imagine yourself the recipient of the document. Look for complete sentences, logical development of thought and reasoning, accuracy, and appropriate use of grammar such as punctuation and capitalization.

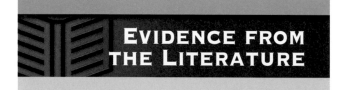

EVIDENCE FROM THE LITERATURE

Citation: Cleary, M., & Freeman, A. (2005). Email etiquette guidelines for mental health nurses. *International Journal of Mental Health Nursing, 14,* 62–65.

Discussion: Most practitioners have e-mail addresses. E-mail provides greater immediacy than traditional modes of communication. Used correctly, e-mail is a fast and effective mode of communication.

1. Ask yourself, is e-mail the best route for communicating? If yes, does the subject line match the content?
2. While e-mail does not necessitate the same level of social interchange as a telephone call, nurses consider courtesy and respect for others to be important principles. Use an appropriate level of formality. Is it readable, concise, and professional?
3. E-mail is about as private as putting a message on the back of a postcard. Limit information and get patient's permission prior to using e-mail.
4. Avoid common pitfalls by keeping e-mails brief and arranging for how communication will be managed during periods of absences.
5. Use standard font. Avoid forwarding e-mail that could be construed as attacking. Use the high priority feature sparingly.
6. Copy information prudently so that only those in need of information receive it.
7. Open attachments only from known sources to avoid viruses. Forward attachments sparingly.
8. Acknowledge important e-mail when it is received.

Implications for Practice: Nurses can avoid communication problems by following these e-mail guidelines.

Electronic record keeping is increasingly being adopted by health care systems, particularly acute care settings. However, these systems are expensive to implement, so there is a lag between what's available to improve record keeping and what is actually being used. The types and features of the systems adopted are almost as numerous as the institutions using them so specific details will not be elaborated here. Orientation to each institution likely includes an introduction to the system(s) in use. In general, as with all patient records, issues of confidentiality are of utmost importance, so nurses must be mindful of their important role in maintaining privacy and accessing and granting access to the system appropriately.

LEVELS OF COMMUNICATION

The level of communication involves who the audience is when communicating. Consequently, communication can be thought of as having three levels: public, intrapersonal, and interpersonal.

PUBLIC COMMUNICATION

Nurses rely primarily on interpersonal communication. However, they also use the other levels, so brief descriptions will be given for them. First, there is public communication. The nurse educator presenting a workshop on signs and symptoms of menopause to a room full of middle-aged women engages in public communication. Her audience is a group of people with a common interest. As presenter, she acts primarily as a sender of information. By design, feedback is typically limited in public speaking, though it does occur. Strategies abound to enhance public speaking skills, but it is beyond the scope of this text to discuss them.

INTRAPERSONAL COMMUNICATION

Another level is **intrapersonal communication**, which can be thought of as self-talk. As the name suggests, it is what individuals do within themselves and can present as doubts or affirmations. Complex mechanisms are involved in understanding how subconscious beliefs drive behavior, and what is needed to change them is based on social learning theory and social cognitive theory. A new nurse may engage in intrapersonal communication as he simultaneously doubts and affirms his ability to complete a procedure. For example, the first time the newly licensed RN has to catheterize a patient, he may simultaneously doubt his ability to insert a Foley catheter with one message, "I haven't done this before," while affirming his ability to insert a Foley catheter with an "I can do this" message to himself. He is engaging in

CRITICAL THINKING 8-2

A diabetic patient who lives in the rural West is excited to have recently become "connected" to the World Wide Web with the acquisition of a computer and Internet services. His wife, who accompanies him to the office visit, wonders whether some of the monitoring that currently occurs during office visits might not be accomplished using e-mail. They reason that winters are hard and travel is difficult, the patient's circulation is poor, he fatigues easily, and it could save them the six-hour round-trip. Furthermore, they're hoping to spend several weeks in the South this winter. They reason that using e-mail, they can maintain contact as needed without the drawbacks they identified.

What are the advantages of this suggestion for the patient? The caregiver? What safeguards can you think of to facilitate communicating using e-mail and to assure quality care?

intrapersonal communication. The so-called competing voices within himself act as sender and receiver in this intrapersonal conversation whose outcome will be influenced by the feedback that follows.

Communication with self or intrapersonal communication is the first important element in developing a sphere of communication. From self-awareness and understanding of oneself, a nurse can move confidently into one-to-one interactions with others, and then into interactions with smaller and larger groups. See Figure 8-2 for some spheres of communication and their related skills.

INTERPERSONAL COMMUNICATION

The last level, **interpersonal communication**, involves communication between individuals, person-to-person or in small groups. Not surprisingly, nurses engage in this level regularly. Interpersonal communication allows for a very effective level of communication to occur and incorporates all of the elements, channels, and modes previously discussed. The nurse, who observes a patient grimace when he moves, interprets the nonverbal cue as indicating that the patient is experiencing pain. Using verbal communication, she clarifies her perception by asking the patient to describe and rate his pain. He describes it as tolerable and states he is expecting a visitor and he does not want to be drowsy. The communication goes back and forth until, ideally, both parties' understanding of the message match. This is the goal of communication. Note that good nursing care and effective nursing and medical practitioner communication has been linked to patient survival in ICUs (Arford, 2005).

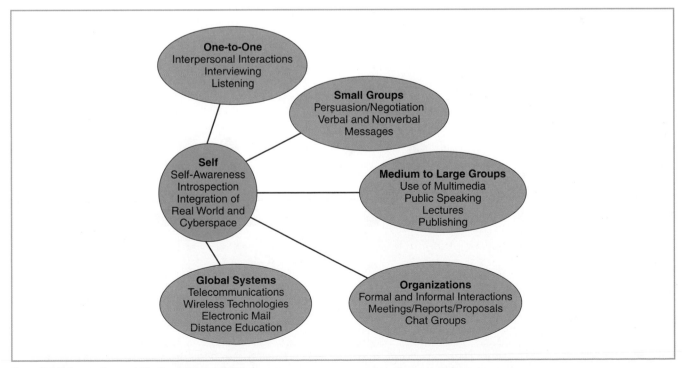

Figure 8-2 Spheres of communication and related skills.

ORGANIZATIONAL COMMUNICATION

Avenues of communication are often defined by an organization's formal structure. The formal structure establishes who is in charge and identifies how different levels of personnel and various departments relate within the organization. These relationships are typically depicted by an organizational chart. When the chief executive officer of an organization announces that the company will adopt a new policy that all employees will follow, that is downward communication. The message starts at the top and is usually disseminated by levels through the chain of communication (Figure 8-3). Upward communication is the opposite of downward communication. The idea originates at some level below the top of the structure and moves upward. For example, when a nurse recommends a more efficient approach to organizing care to his nurse manager, who takes the recommendation to her superior, who uses the recommendation to develop a new policy, that is upward communication. The Y pattern of communication shows two people reporting to another person who reports to others. An example is two staff nurses who report to the nursing unit director, who reports to the vice president for nursing, who reports to the president. The wheel pattern shows a situation in which four nurses report to one nurse manager. There is no interaction among the four nurses, and all communications are channeled through the nurse manager at the center of the wheel. This pattern is rare in health care organizations. Even though this network pattern is not used routinely, it may be used in circumstances in which urgency or secrecy is required. For example, the president of an organization who has an emergency might communicate with the vice presidents in a wheel pattern because time does not permit using other modes.

The circle pattern allows communicators in the network to communicate directly only with two others, but since each communicates with another communicator in the network, the effect is that everyone communicates with someone, and there is no central authority or leader. The all-channel network is a circle pattern except that each communicator may interact with every other communicator in the network.

Communication networks vary along several dimensions. The most appropriate pattern depends upon the situation in which it is used. The wheel and all-channel networks tend to be fast and accurate compared with the

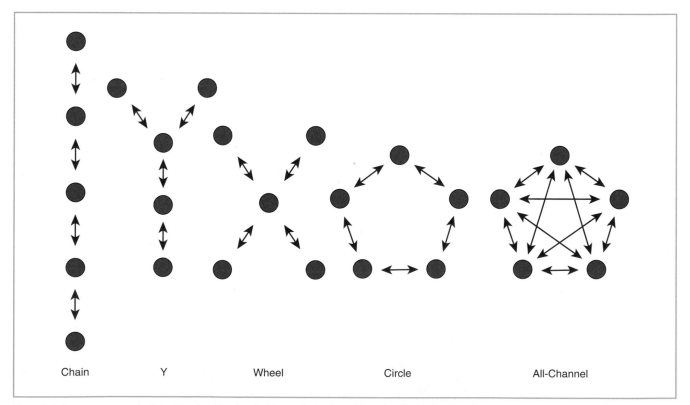

Chain   Y   Wheel   Circle   All-Channel

Figure 8-3 Common communication networks. (Reprinted with permission from *Managing Health Services Organizations and Systems* [4th ed.] by B. B. Longest Jr., J. S. Rakich, & K. Darr, 2000, Baltimore, MD: Health Professional Press.)

REAL WORLD INTERVIEW

In the future world of work and service, one of the most important things that you can do for yourself and others is to take responsibility for creating and sustaining high-quality connections. Develop a reputation as someone who energizes people at work rather than someone who de-energizes people at work. High-quality connections (HQCs) foster admiration, appreciation, support, challenge, and hope for the future. Low-quality connections (LQCs) foster distrust, alienation, and regret in work environments.

How do you tell the difference between a high- and low-quality connection? Think of the people who energize you. Use them as role models, and pay attention to how they act and what they say. Develop a plan to model their behavior and interactions with others.

At the same time, pay attention to those people who de-energize you. Think about what they say and do. Pay attention to how co-workers react when these de-energizers are around. Researchers Dutton and Heaphy (2003) believe HQCs are like strong, flexible, resilient, and healthy blood vessels that feed connective tissue to sustain health and nourish vitality.

In contrast, LQCs block the positive flow of life-giving energy in interpersonal relationships. Dutton and Heaphy observe, "with a low quality connection there is a little death in every interaction." Develop a reputation for being affirming and life giving rather than negative and de-energizing. People skilled at creating and maintaining HQCs create more meaningful work for themselves and the organizations within which they work.

Daniel J. Pesut, PhD, APRN, BC, FAAN
Professor and Associate Dean for Graduate Programs
President of the Honor Society of Nursing, Sigma Theta Tau International, 2003–2005
Indianapolis, Indiana

---

chain or Y-pattern networks. The chain or Y patterns promote clear-cut lines of authority and responsibility. The circle and all-channel networks enhance morale among those in the networks better than other patterns, but these patterns result in relatively slow communication. This is a serious problem if an immediate decision or response is needed. Nurses must construct communication networks to fit the various communication situations they face (Shortell & Kaluzny, 2006). Note that E-mail has had the effect of flattening some organizational communications to sometimes allow more direct access between levels that were formerly controlled through middle managers.

A final avenue worth mentioning, which is not a formal avenue, is the grapevine. The **grapevine** is an informal avenue in which rumors circulate. It ignores the formal chain of command. The major benefit of the grapevine is the speed with which information is spread, but its major drawback is that it often lacks accuracy. For example, nurses who inform an oncoming shift about a rumor that layoffs or mandatory overtime is imminent in the absence of any information from the hospital's administration are participating in grapevine communication.

CRITICAL THINKING 8-3

How does your organization use formal and informal communication? How does the organization assure effective communication within the organization? How does the organization communicate with other organizations in the community?

COMMUNICATION SKILLS

Because nurses are often placed in positions of leadership and are responsible for representing nursing's concerns to others, including the patient, it is important they have the requisite skills to be effective communicators. There is no one correct way to ensure effective communication. Rather, effective communication requires that

TABLE 8-2	COMMUNICATION SKILLS

Skill	Description
Attending	Active listening for what is said and how it is said as well as noting nonverbal cues that support or negate congruence, for example, making eye contact and posturing.
Responding	Verbal and nonverbal acknowledgement of the sender's message, such as "I hear you."
Clarifying	Restating, questioning, and rephrasing to help the message become clear, for example, "I lost you there."
Confronting	Identifying the conflict, for example, "We have a problem here" and then clearly delineating the problem. Confronting uses knowledge and reason to resolve the problem.
Supporting	Siding with another person or backing up another person: "I can see that you would feel that way."
Focusing	Centers on the main point: "So your main concern is. . . ."
Open-ended questioning	Allows for patient-directed responses: "How did that make you feel?"
Providing information	Supplies one with knowledge she did not previously have: "It's common for people with pneumonia to be tired."
Using silence	Allows for intrapersonal communication.
Reassuring	Restores confidence or removes fear: "I can assure you that tomorrow. . . ."
Expressing appreciation	Shows gratitude: "Thank you" or "You are so thoughtful."
Using humor	Provides relief and gains perspective; may also cause harm, so use carefully.
Conveying acceptance	Makes known that one is capable or worthy: "It's okay to cry."
Asking related questions	Expands listener's understanding: "How painful was it?"

both parties engaged in communicating use skills that enhance that particular interaction. In general, the most important considerations for facilitating communication are to be open, assertive, and willing to give and receive feedback. Some of the most important skills upon which nurses rely to do this are listed in Table 8-2.

BARRIERS TO COMMUNICATION

Barriers are obstacles to effective communication. The nurse who can identify potential barriers to communication will be better equipped to avoid them or to compensate for them. Some barriers can be physical barriers, such as trying to communicate with someone on a poor phone connection. Some of the most common other barriers are language, gender, culture, anger, generational differences, illiteracy, and conflict. Conflict

management is so central to good patient care that it will be discussed in another chapter.

USE OF LANGUAGE

Language is the primary means we use to communicate with each other. Humans have developed written, sign, and oral languages to share messages. We use language to express ideas, feelings, and emotions and to communicate information, reactions, and directions to each other and to negotiate with each other.

Oral language is a feature of every society. In a health care setting, oral language is used to verbally communicate with patients and other health care professionals. Individuals also communicate nonverbally with body language. It is important to remember that there are many cross-cultural similarities in body language, but there are also key differences. The meaning of different gestures varies from culture to culture. Never assume that a gesture holds the same meaning for you and your patient, especially if your patient is from another culture.

As you work with patients, you will encounter a great diversity in spoken languages. For instance, more than 6,000 languages and dialects are spoken today. Mandarin Chinese is spoken by approximately 836 million people. In the late 1990s, there were nearly as many Spanish speakers, who number 332 million, as there are Hindi speakers, who number 333 million worldwide (Microsoft, 1996). There are 322 million English speakers. If we include individuals who speak English as a second language, with approximately 418 million speakers, then English is the second most widely spoken language, with Mandarin Chinese being the most widely spoken (Munoz and Luckmann, 2005).

LINGUISTICALLY APPROPRIATE SERVICES

Any individual who is seeking health care services and who has limited English proficiency (LEP) has the right, based on Title VI of the Civil Rights Act of 1964, to have an interpreter available to facilitate communication within the health care system. Open and clear communication is essential to develop an appropriate diagnosis and treatment. Potential errors in this area can occur when the health care provider is unable to obtain accurate information from the patient with LEP. These individuals must be able to access language services, such as using an interpreter and translated materials for information necessary to understand the health care services and benefits available. It is important to note that some patients may not be literate even in their native language; therefore, they may not benefit from translated material that requires them to read instructions or health information.

Recognizing the challenge of obtaining an interpreter twenty-four hours a day, the Office of Civil Rights suggests the need for the availability of interpreter services during the hours of operation. Language assistance services need to be comprehensive in that the patient should receive these services from the initial point of contact with the provider, during the initial health interview, while receiving health care services, and during planning for discharge and home care. Furthermore, the health care provider must ensure that the trained interpreter follows ethical practices and guidelines. This means that strict confidentiality and privacy of information must be ensured and maintained at all times. It is the responsibility of the health care organization to ensure that the interpreters are competent and properly trained in the medical and health context. Unfortunately, use of family members or friends as interpreters is convenient and continues to be common practice in some health care settings. This practice is discouraged and can be acceptable only when the patient expresses the preference to have a family member or friend be the interpreter. Clearly, there may be situations in which a formally trained interpreter is unavailable and the use of telephone interpretation is not practical; family members may then be used with permission from the patient. Although telephone interpreter services are permissible, the use of a face-to-face in-person interpretation is desirable, acceptable, and appropriate.

Health care organizations are expected to make known to all their patients and families the availability of interpreter services at no cost to the patient. Information about available bilingual staff can also help the patient access these services. Posting translated signs in the agency that are clearly visible will be very helpful to the patient. Linguistically and culturally appropriate services may be posted in community newspapers and radio stations to inform the community of the available service. To maintain the quality-improvement process, the health care organizations are also encouraged to share with the public and the recipients of their services how they have implemented culturally and linguistically appropriate services. An annual report may be one way to inform the public. Although these standards are directly addressed to the health care organizations, their application and relevance are clearly an expectation in all professional practice (Munoz & Luckmann, 2005).

GENDER

Gender interferes with communication when men and women lack the understanding that they may process information differently. In general, some men are more interested in using reason, where some women want to be heard and validated through communication (Gray, 1992). Gender differences and patterns do not preclude working together. Rather, both sides must realize the other's preference and make accommodations so that effective communication results.

CRITICAL THINKING 8-4

Nurses who practice assertiveness are direct, honest, and appropriate. They say, "I need you to do . . ." rather than, "You should do. . . ." The next time you work in the clinical area, note how nurses interact with other staff and nursing and medical practitioners. Do the nurses and other staff always speak assertively? Do they become aggressive or passive instead? Is assertiveness always easy to do? Is being assertive part of being a professional nurse? Is it possible to meet your patient's needs if you are not assertive?

Gender differences have been attributed, in part, to gender socialization in which males are provided with more opportunities to develop confidence and assertiveness than females. Fortunately, the feminist movement and increased sexual equality in Western society, in general, have lessened traditional sociological patterns of competitiveness and decisiveness in men and passivity and nurturing in women. However, remnants of the traditional model persist, particularly in health care settings. Nurses who lack assertiveness and confidence are encouraged to acquire the requisite skills to be assertive and confident to be an effective patient advocate and also to communicate in a confident manner.

CULTURE

As was stated previously, our culture grows increasingly diverse. This diversity reduces the likelihood that patients and nurses will share a common cultural background. In turn, the number of safe assumptions about beliefs and practices decreases, and the probability for misunderstanding increases. For example, shortly after delivering a baby, women are often hungry and thirsty. Some cultures believe that for women to restore their energies appropriately, women are to eat hot foods and beverages while others believe cold foods and beverages are appropriate. A well-intentioned nurse who does not consult with the patient about her preferences may arrange culturally inappropriate nourishment. Broadly defined, culture encompasses different groups' beliefs and practices by gender, race, age, economic status, health, and disability. Sanders and Ewart (2005) stress that developing communication that is culturally competent requires respect for each individual's unique mix of values and beliefs. These values and beliefs can only be identified by carefully listening to each individual. Culture and communication are intrinsically intertwined. Culture is discussed more in Chapter 25. Nurses are responsible for bridging gaps between themselves and their patients through first being accepting of differences. They can also overcome cultural differences by learning about other cultures. Nurses bridge cultural differences by vigilantly using the skills previously described to facilitate communication.

GENERATIONAL DIFFERENCES

Generational differences can create tensions among workers because of the divergent outlooks on life. Different generations can have different values about work, motivation, lifestyle, and communication. It is important to be aware that even though generalizations can be misleading and unfair, four generations make up the current workforce. Awareness of generational differences allows you as a nurse to use this information as a tool to maximize strengths and deal with conflicts (Greene, 2005). This is discussed more in Chapter 25.

EVIDENCE FROM THE LITERATURE

Citation: Greene, J. (2005). What nurses want. *Hospitals and Health Networks, 79*(3), 34–42.

Discussion: The author discusses four distinct generations working together in the workforce today:

- *Matures, Veterans (Born 1922–1946):* They believe in hard work, paying dues, conformity, and long-term commitment to one employer.
- *Baby Boomers (Born 1946–1964):* They define selves through employment, that is, self worth = work. They are willing to work long hours and like to change things.
- *Generation X (Born 1964–1980):* They are independent and may change employment places often. They seek connection with managers on an equal footing and are very comfortable with technology.
- *Generation Y (Born 1980–2000):* They are optimistic, street smart, expect diversity, crave structure, and are technologically savvy.

Implications for Practice: Awareness of generational differences helps the nurse work well with coworkers. Learning styles, work habits, beliefs about family and work balance, computer literacy, and comfort with technology may all vary in the different generations.

ILLITERACY

Nurses need to be mindful that many individuals lack the literacy skills to navigate the health care system and function successfully as health care consumers. The World Health Organization (WHO) offers the following definition:

> **Health literacy** represents the cognitive and social skills which determine the motivation and ability of individuals to gain access to, understand, and use information in ways that promote and maintain good health (WHO, 1998, p. 10).

This definition encompasses the elements of personal empowerment and action and views health literacy as an outcome of health promotion and health education efforts that have both personal and social benefits. Patients, families, and even subordinates simply do not always understand what nurses and other health care providers are trying to communicate. For example, while most health care materials are written at the tenth-grade level or higher, most adults read between an eighth and ninth grade level (Safeer & Keenan, 2005). Almost a quarter of the adult population in the United States is functionally illiterate, and nearly half have limited literacy skills. Literacy challenges are increased for patients whose primary language is not English. It is also increased for patients from some racial or ethnic backgrounds, patients from certain areas of the country, patients with low-income levels, patients who have been in prison, and patients older than 60 years of age (Safeer & Keenan, 2005).

The Health Literacy of America's Adults is the first release of the National Assessment of Adult Literacy (NAAL) health literacy results. The results are based on assessment tasks designed specifically to measure the health literacy of adults living in the United States. Health literacy was reported using four performance levels: Below Basic, Basic, Intermediate, and Proficient. The majority of adults (53%) had Intermediate health literacy. About 22% had Basic and 14% had Below Basic health literacy. Relationships between health literacy and background variables (such as educational attainment, age, race/ethnicity, where adults get information about health issues, and health insurance coverage) were also examined and reported. For example, adults with Below Basic or Basic health literacy were less likely than adults with higher health literacy to get information about health issues from written sources (newspapers, magazines, books, brochures, or the Internet) and more likely than adults with higher health literacy to get a lot of information about health issues from radio and television.

Assessing patients' literacy is one way that you as the nurse can decide what patient education material to use and how to best present it. It is a mistake to rely on patients' self report of their reading skills because the majority of patients who have low health literacy say they read "well." The Rapid Estimate of Adult Literacy in Medicine is a quick assessment that takes two to three minutes to complete (Davis et al., 1991). Always try to communicate in short, clear and simple ways with patients using pictures if possible to aid understanding.

Focus on the patient's experience of the condition rather than elaborating on the patient's pathophysiology (Safeer & Keenan, 2005).

ANGER

Anger is a universal, strong feeling of displeasure that is often precipitated by a situation that frustrates or prevents a person from attaining a goal or getting what is wanted from life. Anger is influenced by one's beliefs. Ellis (1997) describes anger as an irrational response that arises from one of four irrational ideas: (1) that the treatment one received was awful (awfulizing), (2) feeling that one can't stand having been treated so irresponsibly and unfairly (can't-stand-it-itis), (3) believing that one should not, must not behave as he did (shoulding and musting), and (4) because one acted in a terrible manner, he is a terrible person (undeservingness and damnation). Ellis maintains that beliefs remain rational as long as the evaluation of the action does not involve an evaluation of the person. Rational and appropriate responses are feelings of disappointment. Anger, on the other hand, can be unmanageable and self-defeating. He believes that we all have the ability to choose our response to anger.

Anger can be dealt with in one of several ways. Three methods that may work from time to time but that may have serious and potentially destructive drawbacks are denying and repressing anger, which may lead to resentment; expressing anger, which may lead to defensiveness on the part of the respondent; and turning the other cheek, which may lead to continued mistreatment and lack of trust. Because anger stems from carrying things further and viewing the situation as awful, terrible, or unfair, Ellis (1997) advocates disputing irrational beliefs. Anger can stem from deep-seated feelings of unassertiveness. Assertion involves taking a stand, where aggression involves putting another down. If unassertiveness is the source of anger, then a solution is to learn to act assertively.

Additional barriers to communication are seen in Table 8-3. Ways to overcome these communication barriers are seen in Table 8-4.

CRITICAL THINKING 8-5

Nurses need to be aware that different staff in the workforce may see things differently based on their age differences. For example, some staff often do only exactly what is asked. They work primarily to earn money to spend. Other staff may believe it is important to save, save, save. They work hard to eliminate a task. Some staff like to buy now, pay later, and work very efficiently. Some other staff work fast, sacrifice, and are very thrifty. These various staff members may have a hard time working together toward a goal. Do you see any of these age differences affecting the clinical area where you work? How can nurses bridge these differences?

TABLE 8-3	ADDITIONAL BARRIERS TO COMMUNICATION

Barrier	Description
Offering false reassurance	Promising something that cannot be delivered.
Being defensive	Acting as though one has been attacked.
Stereotyping	Unfairly categorizing someone based on his or her traits.
Interrupting	Speaking before other has completed her message.
Inattention	Not paying attention.
Stress	A state of tension that gets in the way of reasoning.
Unclear expectations	Ill-defined direction to perform tasks or duties that make successful completion of them unlikely.
Incongruent responses	When words and actions in a communication don't match the inner experience of self and/or are inappropriate to the context. This response commonly presents itself as blaming, placating, being super reasonable, or using irrelevant information when communicating with another person.

WORKPLACE COMMUNICATION

It is probably clear by now that how individuals communicate depends, in part, on where communication occurs and in what relationship. Patterns of communication in the workplace are sensitive to organizational factors that define relationships. Nurses have diverse roles and relationships in the workplace that call for different communication patterns with supervisors, coworkers, subordinates, practitioners and other health care professionals, patients, families, and mentors. Nurses need to keep in mind what the educational levels are of the people with whom they are communicating. Using medical terminology is appropriate with another practitioner who shares a common understanding. Discussions with others such as LPNs, nurse aides, patients, and family members will more likely result in understanding when language is adjusted to their level of understanding. Always remember that the goal is to communicate effectively.

SUPERVISORS

Communicating with a supervisor can be intimidating, especially for a new nurse. Observing professional courtesies is an important first step. For instance, begin by requesting an appointment to discuss a problem when it arises. This demonstrates respect and allows for the conversation to occur at an appropriate time and place. Dress professionally. Arrive for the appointment on time, and be prepared to state the concern clearly and accurately. Provide supporting evidence, and anticipate resistance to any requests. Separate out your needs from your desires. State a willingness to cooperate in finding a solution and then match behaviors to words. Persist in the pursuit of a solution (Table 8-5).

COWORKERS

Nurses depend on their coworkers in many ways to collectively provide quality patient care. Nowhere is this more important than in the acute care setting where nursing services are nonstop around the clock. Transfer of patient care from nurse to nurse is one of the most important and frequent communications between coworkers. It depends on fluid communication in end of shift handoff reports to achieve quality nursing care. However, time constraints demand that the change of shift handoff report be accurate, informative, and succinct. How the nursing care is organized influences who gets the report. Nursing handoff reports are discussed in Chapter 18. Tips for communicating with coworkers include remembering professional courtesies and being mindful of an

TABLE 8-4	OVERCOMING COMMUNICATION BARRIERS

Method	Actions
Understand the receiver	Ask yourself what's in it for the other person.
	Work to develop understanding of the other person's needs.
Communicate assertively	Be direct.
	Explain ideas clearly and with feeling.
	Repeat important messages.
	Use various communication channels, for example, written, e-mail, verbal, and so on.
Use two-way communication	Ask questions.
	Communicate face-to-face.
Unite with a common vocabulary	Define the meaning of important terms, such as high quality, so that everyone understands their meaning.
Elicit verbal and nonverbal feedback	Request and offer verbal feedback often.
	Document important agreements.
	Observe nonverbal feedback.
Enhance listening skills	Pay attention to what is said, what is not said, and to the nonverbal signals.
	Continue listening carefully even when you don't like the message.
	Give summary reflections to assure understanding, for example, "You say you are late giving medications because the pharmacy did not deliver meds on time."
	Engage in concluding discussions, such as, "Has your unit been late with medications due to problems with pharmacy deliveries before?"
	Ask questions to explore problems.
	Paraphrase a speaker's words to decrease miscommunication rather than blurting out questions as soon as the other person finishes speaking.
Be sensitive to cultural differences	Know what cultural communication barriers exist.
	Show respect for all workers.
	Minimize use of jargon specific to your culture.
	Be sensitive to cultural etiquette, such as use of first names, eye contact, hand gestures, personal appearance.
Be sensitive to gender differences	Be aware that men and women may have some differences in communication style, for instance, men may call attention to their accomplishments, and women may tend to be more conciliatory when facing differences.
	Know that male-female stereotypes often don't fit the person you are working with.
	Avoid barriers by knowing that differences exist and don't take things personally.
	Males can improve communication by showing more empathy and females by becoming more direct.
Engage in metacommunication	Communicate about your communication to resolve a problem, such as, "I'm trying to get through to you, but either you don't react to me or you get angry. What can I do to improve our communication?"

Source: Adapted from DuBrin, A. J. (2000). *The active manager.* United Kingdom: South-Western Pub.

TABLE 8-5	**HOW TO IMPROVE YOUR ABILITY TO WORK WITH YOUR BOSS**

Know your boss's:
- Goals and objectives
- Pressures
- Strengths, weaknesses, and blind spots
- Working style

Understand your own:
- Objectives
- Pressures

- Strengths and weaknesses
- Working style
- Predisposition toward dependence on authority figures

Develop a relationship that:
- Meets both your objectives and styles
- Keeps your boss informed
- Is based on dependability and honesty
- Selectively uses your boss's time and resources

Source: Adapted from Gabarro, J. & Kotter, J. P. (1993, May–June). Managing your boss. *Harvard Business Review,* 150–157.

CRITICAL THINKING 8-6

You are having a coffee break with another nurse who mentions a problem she is having with care delivery. The nurse is not sure how to solve it. You want to be helpful and supportive and yet avoid giving advice. Ask the nurse if she can describe the problem fully for you. Do not interrupt. Then, ask the nurse some questions about the problem, and seek clarification until you are clear on the problem and the nurse has fully described it. Do not give advice. Use your communication skills, such as attending, clarifying, and responding, and ask the nurse such things as, tell me more about that, what did you think about it, and so forth, until you are both clear on the issue. At the end of this process, you can just finish by relaxing for the rest of your break or you can ask the nurse, "Do you want advice about your problem?"

Many times, this process will help the nurse solve the problem by himself or herself. If the nurse does want advice, you can give some suggestions if you are comfortable doing so. Do you think this process can strengthen people's ability to find answers to their problems? Do you think this process would be helpful to you in working with others on the unit? Do you think this approach honors people's integrity and ability to solve their own problems?

Source: Adapted from M. Parsons (personal communication, 2003). San Antonio, Texas.

appropriate time and place to share your concerns. Stay focused on what is needed to get the job done and seek a win-win solution to conflicts, where all parties are satisfied with the outcome.

An excellent guide for directing communication with coworkers is the golden rule: "Do unto others as you would have them do unto you." As a nurse who will be responsible for overseeing others' work, a valuable perspective for you to maintain is that all members of the team are important to successfully realize quality patient care. Communication between nurses and coworker, will most likely involve delegating. This important topic is covered in Chapter 16, and you are encouraged to review this material as it relates to coworkers. In addition to delegating, a few other communications skills are worth mentioning. Offering positive feedback such as, "I appreciate the way you interacted with Mr. T. to get him to ambulate twice this shift," goes a long way toward team building, and it

REAL WORLD INTERVIEW

A second shift occupational health nurse working in a factory setting was presented with a patient who entered the nursing office complaining that he didn't feel good. The nurse's initial assessment, including vital signs, revealed that the only abnormality was an elevated blood pressure. In this situation, like in any clinical situation, it is important to distinguish the urgent from the nonurgent. With hypertensive patients, it is important to realize that an urgent situation is suggested by evidence of acute end organ damage from the elevated BP. Specifically, in this situation, it was important to know whether the patient was experiencing altered sensorium, headache, visual disturbance, chest pain, or dyspnea. The presence of any of these findings should be communicated to the physician and would dictate urgent transport to the hospital. In their absence, the patient can be referred for more elective blood pressure control.

In any clinical situation, such as the one above, the nurse can check the patient, and if there is evidence of any signs or symptoms, the nurse can facilitate communications by being organized and objective. Discuss the basics such as the patient's chief complaint, his vital signs, his medications, and any changes from baseline. Know why you are worried about observed changes and communicate this to the practitioner.

John C. Ruthman, MD
Peoria, Illinois

improves coworkers' sense of worth. Nurses also have an opportunity to act as teachers to coworkers. Often in a hospital setting, nurses teach by example. Demonstrating the desired behavior allows the coworker the opportunity to copy the behavior. It is important to allow time for return demonstrations to evaluate that the coworker has learned the intended skill. For example, as the nurse, you may demonstrate how to position a patient with special needs, encouraging the coworker to assist and ask questions.

CRITICAL THINKING 8-7

Sometimes you may work with staff who are difficult. These staff can include staff who usually work in another setting; staff who are more knowledgeable than you; staff who are older than you; staff who think they are better than they are; and staff who are defensive when you ask them to do something. With all these staff members, it can help to develop strategies that identify your performance expectations clearly and involve them in the work that needs to be done. This is useful with all types of staff, those who are easy to work with and those who are difficult. How can you work to improve your ability to communicate your performance expectations clearly to the staff you work with?

The next time repositioning is indicated, accompany the coworker and observe his or her ability to successfully complete the task. Offer constructive feedback. Be patient. Remember your own learning curves when mastering new skills and behaviors and allow those you supervise the opportunity to grow. Be open to the possibility that coworkers, particularly those with experience, may have a few pearls of wisdom to share with you as well. For example, this author is forever indebted to a nurse aide who shared how to really position patients comfortably. Likewise, a veteran LPN who knew the politics of the institution willingly shared her knowledge with a batch of new graduates as they began to work on the evening shift.

MEDICAL PRACTITIONERS, NURSE PRACTITIONERS, AND OTHER HEALTH CARE PROFESSIONALS

One of the most intimidating experiences for new nurses may be to communicate with medical or nurse practitioners (NP), or physician assistants. Despite gender and role challenges that have already been discussed, this need not be a stressful event. The nurse's goal is to strive for collaboration, keeping the patient goal central to the discussion. Collaboration allows all parties to be satisfied, improves quality, and is an attribute of magnet hospitals (Arford, 2005). It involves seeking creative, integrative solutions while also working through emotions. To communicate effectively with the practitioner, the nurse presents information in a straightforward manner, clearly delineating

EVIDENCE FROM THE LITERATURE

Citation: Haig, K. M., Sutton, S., & Whittington, J. (2006). The SBARR Technique: Improves Communication, Enhances Patient Safety. *Joint Commission's Perspectives on Patient Safety, 5*(2), 1–2.

Discussion: Communication failures are the root cause of nearly two-thirds of sentinel events in hospitals. This is due, in part, because nursing and medical practitioners and nurses are trained to communicate differently. The SBAR technique (Situation, Background, Assessment, Recommendation) is designed to improve communication between these health care personnel:

- *Situation:* What is going on with the patient? Identify self, unit, patient, room number. Briefly state the problem, when it started, and its severity.
- *Background:* Provide background information related to the situation, as needed. Be aware of patient's admitting diagnosis, date of admission, current medications, allergies, IV fluids, most recent vital signs, lab results with date and time each was performed, other clinical information, and patient code status. The practitioner may ask you for these when you call.
- *Assessment:* What is your assessment? Do you think the patient's condition is deteriorating? Do you think the patient needs medication?
- *Recommendation:* What is your recommendation or what do you want? Know what you want from the practitioner before you call. Don't hang up without communicating this to the practitioner and assuring that your patient's needs are met, e.g., patient needs to be admitted, or patient needs to be seen. Order needs to be changed, or medication needs to be added.
- *Response:* Document response of practitioner.

Implications for Practice: Nursing and medical practitioners who use the SBARR technique will improve their communications. Patients will be the beneficiaries.

---

the problem, supported by pertinent evidence. This is especially important when reporting changes in patient conditions. Nurses are responsible for knowing classic symptoms of conditions, orally apprising the practitioner of changes, and recording all observations in the chart. It is important that the nurse remain calm and objective even if the practitioner does not cooperate. Calfee (1998) offers suggestions for handling telephone miscommunications. For example, if a practitioner hangs up, document that the call was terminated and fill out an incident report. If the practitioner gives an inappropriate answer or gives no orders, for example, for a patient complaint of pain, document the call, the information relayed, and the fact that no orders were given. In addition, document any other steps that were taken to resolve the problem, for example, notifying the nursing supervisor. If a practitioner cannot be reached, first follow the institution's procedure for getting the patient treated and then document the actions taken (Table 8-6).

PATIENTS AND FAMILIES

Communication with patients and families is optimized by the many skills previously described in this chapter. There are a few additional skills that have not yet been mentioned. The first is touch. Nurses routinely use touch as a way to communicate caring and concern. Occasionally, language barriers will limit communication to the nonverbal mode. For instance, a stroke patient who cannot process words can still interpret a gentle hand on his shoulder.

Communication requires an openness and honesty with concurrent respect for patients and families. In addition, it is important to honor and protect patients' privacy with the nurse's actions and words. Information that patients share with nurses and other health care providers is to be held in confidence. Verbal exchanges regarding patient conditions are private matters that should not occur in the hallway or just outside a patient's room where others will hear them. Nurses are obligated to not discuss patient conditions with others, even family members, without patient permission.

MENTOR AND PRODIGY

The final pattern of communication that occurs in the workplace that will be discussed is between mentor and prodigy. Mentoring may be an informal process that occurs between an expert nurse and a novice nurse, but it may also be an assigned role. This one-on-one relationship focuses on professional aspects and is mutually beneficial. The optimal novice is hardworking, willing to learn, and anxious to succeed. Communication entails using the skills previously described in this chapter to help the novice develop expert status and career direction. The novice accomplishes this by gleaning the mentor's

TABLE 8-6	SBARR TOOL TO ORGANIZE INFORMATION FOR CALLING ANOTHER NURSING OR MEDICAL PRACTITIONER FOR ASSISTANCE

Situation:
Identify date and time of call.
Identify self, unit, patient, room number, admitting diagnosis.
State the problem: What it is, when it started, and the severity of it.

Background:
Review background information related to the situation. What are current medications, allergies, IV fluids, vital signs, level of consciousness, urine output, status of airway, breathing, circulation, pain level, pulse oximeter, cardiac rhythm, lab results, patient code status, and other clinical information?

Assessment:
What is your assessment of patient? Is the patient's problem severe? Is his condition deteriorating? Does the patient need medication?

Recommendation:
What is needed from the practitioner? Know what you want from the practitioner before you call. Don't hang up without communicating this to the practitioner and assuring that your patient's needs are met, for example, patient needs to be admitted, patient needs to be seen, patient needs medication, and so on.

Response:
Document response of practitioner. Document all calls to practitioner and messages left. Notify supervisor when needed for follow up.

Source: Adapted from Haig, K. M., Sutton, S., & Whittington, J. (2006).

CASE STUDY 8-1

As a new graduate, you have finished orientation and received notice that you have passed your NCLEX exam. The nursing care manager is relieved because two of the other regular nurses are pregnant and will soon be off on maternity leave. One of them is your preceptor. These absences will create a staffing crunch. Therefore, the nursing care manager is anxious to acclimate you to the role of team leader because you will soon be expected to assume those responsibilities.

How can your preceptor help you to take on this additional responsibility?

What techniques will you use to enhance your communication with all staff and your manager to assure the care you oversee is safe?

wisdom. This wisdom is typically shared through listening, affirming, counseling, encouraging, and seeking input from the novice. A strategy that facilitates mentoring is to share the same work schedule so that the novice is exposed to the mentor. This allows for sharing and shadowing opportunities. The mentor can also anticipate added challenges that will likely occur with increasing responsibility.

Outlining these challenges with suggestions for how to manage them prepares the novice for his expanding responsibilities (Ihlenfeld, 2005). Role-playing, in which the expert preceptor nurse describes a theoretical situation and allows the novice to practice his response to new and sometimes challenging situations, is another strategy that can be used.

KEY CONCEPTS

- Nurses rely on basic principles of communication.

- Trends such as increasing diversity, an aging population, generational differences, illiteracy, and changing technology affect nursing practices.

- At the most basic level, communication involves a sender, a message, a receiver, and feedback. The input comes from visual, auditory, and kinesthetic stimuli.

- There are three levels of communication: intrapersonal, interpersonal, and public.

- Nurses may participate in chain, Y, wheel, circle, and all-channel communication, and/or communicate through the grapevine.

- Nurses use linguistically appropriate services.

- Barriers to effective communication exist.

- Communication happens with patients, families, supervisors, coworkers, medical practitioners, nurse practitioners, other health care workers, and mentors.

KEY TERMS

communication
grapevine
health literacy

interpersonal communication
intrapersonal communication

REVIEW QUESTIONS

1. An RN asks the UAP to take a set of vital signs on a patient who has just had an arterial venous shunt placement. The RN reminds the UAP not to take the blood pressure (BP) on the operative side. An hour later, the RN finds the deflated blood pressure cuff on the operative arm of the patient. The UAP has done this before and has been counseled about it. What should the RN do first?
   A. Assess the patient's condition.
   B. Avoid asking the UAP to take BPs in the future.
   C. Discuss the situation with the UAP and the supervisor.
   D. Find the UAP and review the importance of taking the blood pressure on the nonoperative side.

2. A new graduate RN received an unfamiliar treatment order from the practitioner. How should the nurse proceed?
   A. Refuse to do the treatment.
   B. Do the treatment to the best of the nurse's ability.
   C. Inform the practitioner and then proceed to do the treatment.
   D. Inform the practitioner and ask the practitioner or charge nurse for assistance in doing the procedure.

3. What part of the communication process returns input to the sender?
   A. Feedback
   B. Message
   C. Receiver
   D. Sender

4. Which of the following characteristics is most relevant to to verbal communication?
   A. Eye contact
   B. Nodding
   C. Smiling
   D. Tone of voice

5. All but which of the following are steps to improve communication using the SBARR technique?
   A. Share the situation.
   B. Provide background information.
   C. Assure patient safety.
   D. Ask for a recommendation from the practitioner.

6. Which of the following skills involves active listening and is a very important skill used by nurses to gain an understanding of the patient's message?
   A. Attending
   B. Clarifying
   C. Confronting
   D. Responding

REVIEW ACTIVITIES

1. Your nursing care manager has asked you to serve on a committeee to explore how your unit might communicate more effectively. What elements of communication might affect the group's plan?

2. The charge nurse apologizes as she informs you that your assignment includes the "problem patient" on the unit. What communication skills will you use to enhance communication with this patient? How will you avoid barriers of communication with this patient?

3. You found out that you passed your licensure exam last month. When you report for your evening shift, you discover you are assigned to be the team leader. What considerations will you give as you communicate with coworkers?

EXPLORING THE WEB

- What sites would you consider to improve your communication skills? Google identifies 8,330,000 sites for communication for nurses. Try it at *www.google.com,* and look at the incredible possibilities online.

■ Would you like to keep up with what is happening in the field of nursing and technology? Visit *www.ania.org.* What did you find?

■ Search this site, accessed March 29, 2007, to order articles from over 1,700 journals indexed in the CINAHL database, *www.cinahl.com.*

■ Note this site for links to various cultural sites to improve your communication awareness, *www.diversityrx.org.*

REFERENCES

Andrews, L. B., Stocking, C. T., Krizek, T., Gottlieb, L., Krizek, C., Vargish, T. et al. (1997, Feb.). An alternative strategy for studying adverse events in medical care. *Lancet, 349,* 309–313.

Arford, P. H. (2005). Nurse-physician communication: An organizational accountability. *Nursing Economics, 23*(2), 72–77.

Baggs, J. G., Ryan, S. A., Phelps, C. E., Richeson, J. F., & Johnson, J. E. (1992). The association between interdisciplinary collaboration and patient outcomes in a medical intensive care unit. *Heart and Lung, 21*(1), 18–24.

Calfee, B. E. (1998). Making calls to the physician. *Nursing 98,* 10, 17.

Cleary, M., & Freeman, A. (2005). Email etiquette guidelines for mental health nurses. *International Journal of Mental Health Nursing, 14,* 62–65.

Davis, T. C., Crouch, M. A., Long, S. W., Jackson, R. H., Bates, P., George, R. B., & Bairnsfather, L. E. (1991). Rapid assessment of literacy levels of adult primary care patients. *Family Medicine, 23*(6), 433–435.

Dutton, J., & Heaphy, E. (2003). The power of high quality connections. In K. Cameron, J. Dutton, & R. Quinn, (Eds), *Positive organizational scholarship: Foundations of new discipline* (pp. 263–279). San Francisco: Berrett-Koehler.

Ellis, A. (1997). *Anger: How to live with it and without it.* New York: Citadel Press, Kensington.

Gittell, J. H., Fairfield, K. M., Bierbaum, G., Head, W., Jackson, R., Kelly, M., et al. (2000). Impact of relational coordination of quality of care, postoperative pain and functioning, and length of stay: A nine-hospital study of surgical patients. *Medical Care, 38*(8), 807–819.

Gray, J. (1992). *Men are from Mars, women are from Venus.* New York: HarperCollins.

Greene, J. (2005). What nurses want. *Hospitals and Health Networks, 79*(3), 34–42.

Haig, K. M., Sutton, S., & Whittington, J. (2006). The SBARR Technique: Improves Communication, Enhances Patient Safety. *Joint Commission's Perspectives on Patient Safety, 5*(2), 1–2.

Ihlenfeld, J. T. (2005). Hiring and mentoring graduate nurses in the intensive care unit. *Dimensions of Critical Care Nursing, 24*(4), 175–187.

Knaus, W. A., Draper, E. A., Wagner, D. P., & Zimmerman, J. E. (1986). An evaluation of outcome from intensive care in major medical centers. *Annals of Internal Medicine, 104*(3), 410–418.

Microsoft (1996). *Microsoft Encarta 97 Encyclopedia,* Microsoft Corporation.

Munoz, C., & Luckmann, J. (2005). *Transcultural Communication in Nursing* (2nd ed.). Clifton Park, NY: Delmar Learning.

Safeer, R. S., & Keenan, J. (2005). Health literacy: The gap between physicians and patients. *American Family Physician, 72*(3), 463–468.

Sanders, J. & Ewart, B. (2005). Developing cultural competency for healthcare professionals through work based learning. *Work Based Learning in Primary Care, 3,* 99–105.

Shortell, S. M., & Kaluzny, A, D. (2006). *Health Care Management.* Clifton Park, NY: Thomson Delmar Learning.

Shortell, S. M., Zimmerman, J. E., Rousseau, D. M., Gillies, R. R., Wagner, D. P., Draper, E. A. et al. (1994). The performance of intensive care units: Does good management make a difference? *Medical Care, 32*(5), 508–525.

World Health Organization (WHO). (1998). Division of Health Promotion, Education and Communication. Health Education and Health Promotion Unit. *Health Promotion Glossary.* Geneva: World Health Organization.

Young, G. J., Charns, M. P., Daley, J., Forbes, M. G., Henderson, W., & Khuri, S. F. (1997). Best practices for managing surgical services: The role of coordination. *Health Care Management Review, 22*(4), 72–81.

Young, G. J., Charns, M. P., Desai, K., Khuri, S. F., Forbes, M. G., Henderson, W. et al. (1998). Patterns of coordination and surgical outcomes: A study of surgical services. *Health Services Research, 33*(5).

SUGGESTED READINGS

Joint Commission. (2005). Focus on five strategies to improve hands-off communication. *Joint Commission on Perspectives on Patient Safety, 5*(7), 11.

Joint Commission. (2005). The SBAR technique: Improves communication, enhances patient safety. *Joint Commission's Perspectives on Patient Safety, 5*(2), 1–2.

Kirsch, I., Jungeblut, A., Jenkins, L., & Kolstad, A. (1993). *Adult literacy in America: A first look at the findings of the national adult literacy survey.* Washington DC: National Center for Education Statistics, US Department of education.

Office of Minority Health. (2001). *National standards for culturally and linguistically appropriate services in health care: Final Report.* Washington DC. Office of Minority Health.

National Institutes of Health (NIH). (2003). *Protecting personal health information in research: Understanding the HIPAA Privacy Rule.* NIH Publication Number 03-5388.

Simms, L. M., Price, S. A., & Ervin, N. E. (2000). *The professional practice of nursing administration* (3rd ed.). Clifton Park, NY: Thomson Delmar Learning.

Speros, C. (2005). Health literacy: Concept analysis. *Journal of Nursing Administration, 50*(6), 633–640.

Stoddard, D. A., & Tamasy, R. J. (2003). *The heart of mentoring.* Colorado Springs, CO: NavPress.

Politics and Consumer Partnerships

Terry W. Miller, PhD, RN ✦ Patsy Maloney, RN, BC, EdD, MSN, MA, CNAA ✦
Richard J. Maloney, BS, MA, MAHRM, EdD

For the nursing profession to flex its collective political muscle and get involved with the redesign of the nation's health care system, we have to use our leadership to get the professional organizations to think and act collaboratively (Pierce, 2004, p. 115).

OBJECTIVES

Upon completion of this chapter, the reader should be able to:

1. Relate how politics defines health care services and affects nursing practice.
2. Explain the need for nurses to be politically involved with the consumer movement in health care.
3. Identify the role of a nurse as a consumer advocate and political force.
4. Plan a political strategy for strengthening nurse-consumer relationships.
5. Devise a service-oriented plan for providing nursing services to a selected consumer interest group.
6. Analyze the impact of demographic changes on nurses and nursing practice.

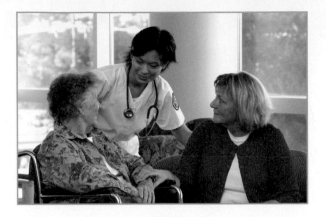

A 60-year-old man lying in a hospital bed, pushing a call button and waiting for a nurse, is not thinking about insurance, Medicare, Medicaid, or any other payer for the service. All he knows is that he is not getting the care that he expected, and what little care he is receiving is costing far more than he or his family can afford. He is imagining losing his home and his meager savings. Because he had lost his job and his health insurance, he ignored his headaches and dulled thinking as long as he could, hoping that his very treatable symptoms would resolve. He probably does not know that he is one of more than 43 million uninsured Americans (Mills & Bhandari, 2003). Nor does he know that care for the uninsured exceeds $100 billion dollars annually (Hadley & Holahan, 2003).

> *How does a new graduate approach the care of adults like these?*
>
> *How do politics play a role in health care?*
>
> *Should a new graduate work with a consumer group to improve the care of this man and others like him? If you answered yes, what consumer group or groups would you choose to work with?*

Politics is predominantly a process by which people use a variety of methods to achieve their goals. These methods inherently involve some level of competition, negotiation, and collaboration for the power to achieve desired outcomes, as well as to protect and enhance the interests of groups or individuals. Nurses who can effectively compete, negotiate, and collaborate with others to get what they want or need develop strong political skills. They have the greatest ability to build strong bases of support for themselves, patients, and the nursing profession. Nurses consistently show up as rated number one in consumer opinion polls asking who are considered to be trusted professionals. Nurses can garner consumer support for professional nursing positions to help patients and help the profession of nursing by tapping into this strong support. Nursing is important as a profession only as it meets its societal mandate for professional nursing service. Nurses must garner political support to do this most effectively.

Politics exist because resources are limited, and some people control more resources than others. **Resources** include people, money, facilities, technology, and rights to properties, services, and technologies. Individuals, groups, or organizations that have the ability to provide or control the distribution of desirable resources are politically empowered. The consumer movement in health care is a political movement about health care resources. It reflects consumer perceptions and values and influences patient care delivery.

The purpose of this chapter is to support the need for nurses as the largest health care group to be politically active for the good of patients and the health care system. A major focus is how the consumer movement in health care creates new opportunities for nurses to advance nursing services by giving patients, including all people who receive health care, a stronger voice in their health care as consumers. Nurses are encouraged to develop strong political skills and partner with their professional nursing organization and with consumer groups to take the lead to improve health care.

STAKEHOLDERS AND HEALTH CARE

Control of health care resources is spread among a number of vested interest groups called **stakeholders**. Everyone is a stakeholder in health care at some level, but some people are far more politically active about their stake in health care than others. See Table 9-1 for a list of Washington's most powerful lobbying groups. These lobbyists are stakeholder groups and include insurance companies; consumer groups; professional organizations, such as the American Nurses Association; health care groups, such as nursing and medical, practitioners, pharmacists, dieticians, physical therapists, administrators, and educational groups. These stakeholders exert political pressure on health policy makers—local, state, and federal legislative bodies—in an effort to make the health care system work to the economic advantage of the stakeholder.

Not all stakeholders in health care support the consumers' potentially dominant role in health care politics, for a variety of reasons. Some contend that consumers do not necessarily know what is best for them. Instead, they support the idea that health care experts, such as practitioners, are better able to direct health care policy. Others maintain that only those directly paying for the services should make policy decisions and that health care is not necessarily a right because services should be based on ability to pay.

Nolin and Killackey note that "increased consumer expectations and rising health care costs are exerting enormous pressure on the American health care system" (2004, p. 1). This has led to increasing political activism

TABLE 9-1	**WASHINGTON'S TOP 15 MOST POWERFUL LOBBYING GROUPS**

1. National Rifle Association
2. American Association of Retired Persons
3. National Federation of Independent Business
4. American Israel Public Affairs Committee
5. Association of Trial Lawyers
6. AFL-CIO
7. Chamber of Commerce
8. National Beer Wholesalers Association
9. National Association of Realtors
10. National Association of Manufacturers
11. National Association of Home Builders
12. American Medical Association
13. American Hospital Association
14. National Education Association
15. American Farm Bureau Federation

Source: From Birnbaum, J. H., & Newell, R. (2001, May 28). Fat & happy in D.C. *Fortune,* 94.

EVIDENCE FROM THE LITERATURE

Citation: McDonald, L. (2006). Florence Nightingale as a social reformer. *History Today, 56*(1), 9–15.

Discussion: The purpose of this historical research on the work of Florence Nightingale is to illuminate her work as a social reformer of a public health system. She advocated health promotion and disease prevention based on evidence. Ms. Nightingale extended the use of nurses that she had trained in hospitals to the care of the poor in pauper houses. She not only placed nurses in these workhouses for the poor, but she lobbied the powerful for passage of laws for the poor. She persuaded key figures to support her ideas for reform. Due to her hard work, the Metropolitan Poor Bill was passed by Parliament in 1867 and followed by other reforms that improved the lot of the poor and infirmed in Britain. Ms. Nightingale was able to obtain the support of such powerful and influential people due to her meticulous attention to detail and careful, methodical preparation. Florence Nightingale used what is now dubbed "Nightingale Methodology." First, study the best information in print, especially government reports and statistics. Second, interview experts, and if the available information is inadequate, survey others with a questionnaire. When you have a proposed plan, test it at one institution, consult with the practitioners that implemented it, and send out the draft reports for comment before sending the final report out for publication and dissemination to the influential.

Implications for Practice: New nurses often believe that their responsibilities begin and end at the bedside. But historical research demonstrates that from the very beginning of modern nursing, nurses have not only given care but partnered with others to influence public opinion and to change legislation for the benefit of the consumer of health care, especially the vulnerable—the poor, the mentally ill, the soldier, and children. So as a new nurse, you may view yourself as a patient advocate who is willing to join with others through professional associations or consumer groups to improve health care and the system within which it is delivered.

by third-party payers. Third-party payers include the government, business, and health insurance companies. Exposure of Medicare/Medicaid fraud has led to the very nature and control of professional practice being questioned by government payers. Nurses have come to understand how the control and distribution of resources in health care can drastically affect their incomes, workloads, work environments, and patients. Nurses across the country have reported that the patient load per nurse provider has increased significantly. However, these nursing concerns without political influence do little to change health care at any level.

Nurses must work to strengthen the long tradition of pulling together the various stakeholders of health care, such as patients, practitioners, administrators, pharmacists, physical therapists, dieticians, and so on. These stakeholders are needed to coordinate health care services and ensure that patients obtain the health services they need. Although unknown by many of today's practicing nurses, this tradition began with Florence Nightingale and her "Nightingale methodology" (McDonald, 2006). New nurses who recognize their critical role in addressing the major issues in health care delivery at the bedside will ensure that nursing enters into a partnership with agency executives who have control in the wider health care system of which the agency is a part. As partners, they will be able to compete, negotiate, and collaborate with other stakeholders at the system level to be politically effective. These nurses also must be concerned with the price of health care at the system level and understand that resources are controlled and distributed through health policy decisions.

Many authors of nursing articles, some books, and a few research studies support nurses' involvement in public policy and health care politics (Grindel, 2005; Mason & Leavitt, 2002; Milstead, 2004; Ortner, 2004; Steele, Rocchiccioli & Porche, 2003; Wakefield, 2004). Several other authors promote greater inclusion of policy content and political process in nursing curricula (Byrd, Costello, Shelton, Thomas, & Petrarcha, 2004; Deschaine & Schaffer, 2003; Harrington, Crider, Benner, & Malone, 2005; Keepnews, 2005; Yoho, Sridaromont, Tuong-Vi, & Decker, 2004). Nurses' involvement in policy arenas, such as policy-making committees and institutional boards,

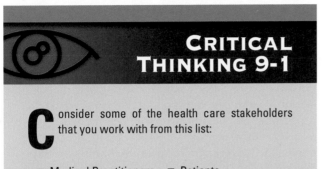

CRITICAL THINKING 9-1

Consider some of the health care stakeholders that you work with from this list:

- Medical Practitioners
- Pharmacists
- Nurse Aides
- Nurse Practitioners
- Dieticians
- Patients
- Physical Therapists
- Hospital Administrators
- Social Workers

How might each of these stakeholders see the importance of efficient, high-quality care to patients on a clinical unit? How might they define the need for patient access to services differently?

REAL WORLD INTERVIEW

Nurses serve as advocates and allies for consumers by helping consumers obtain what they perceive they need. Nurses have the opportunity to help consumers better understand what is available to them, as well as what they can legitimately expect to get from both the provider and system. Competent nurses need to work at understanding how the system works because that is "where they live." The consumer moves in and out of the system, so he is not acclimated to the limitations or pathways of the system. The consumer and the nurse become natural allies whether it is a patient care setting or a public policy setting. One of my biggest frustrations is when nurses fail to see themselves connected to the patient and the whole health care system. Nurses become myopic in their approach to problems in direct patient care because they do not see that they are a piece of something bigger. No nurse's practice occurs in isolation. We are all part of an interdependent, highly complex system with governing economic and political relationships. I found consumer partnerships to be most useful when working as a lobbyist for the Washington State Nurses' Association because, as nurses, we were able to build politically powerful coalitions with consumer groups and subsequently define the direction of long-term health care policy, specifically, state policies governing the long-term care industry. Because we were successful in partnering with selected consumer interest groups, we were able to assure passage and funding of seven significant legislative bills. These bills included the AIDS Omnibus legislation, a long-term care reform act, and an act enabling nurses to declare a patient dead for the purpose of preventing unnecessary stress, care, and cost to consumers.

Robert S. Ball, MSN, RN
Nursing Care Manager
Tacoma, Washington

includes advocating for recipients of health care when those in need have little or no voice and advocating for those who need a stronger voice. Any professional nurse should understand and be able to articulate the relevance of politics to nursing practice. Making a difference in health care arenas is an outcome of involvement in policy making. As Margaret Mead said, "Never doubt that a small group of thoughtful committed citizens can change the world, indeed it's the only thing that ever has."

THE POLITICS AND ECONOMICS OF HUMAN SERVICES

Many nurses want to avoid the political nature of their work because they believe that human service should not be politically motivated. They also may ignore the business aspects of health care until they find themselves responsible for a budget. Yet all health care is inextricably linked to politics and economics as well as to the availability and services of providers. As a human service, health care has yielded remarkable returns in terms of improving overall quality of life as well as in extending life spans. As a business, health care has afforded millions of people, including nurses, with economic opportunities and lifelong careers.

Health care in the United States depends heavily on a continuous supply of resources from both public and private sectors. These resources include people such as the providers of health care services and the money to educate and pay these providers. Buildings, technology, administration, and equipment are just some of the other resources needed for the health care system to be serviceable. With health care requiring so many resources on such a large economic scale, thousands of people are directly involved in the allocation of those resources, hence, the politics of health care. Most of those people have good intentions, but they often disagree about how the resources can best be used to support health care.

Many consumers are aware that the ongoing redistribution of health care resources may not meet their health care needs, especially as they age and become more dependent upon related services. They are frightened by media reports of increasing national health care expenditures. Although most consumers do not directly pay for the majority of their health care, their individual portions of expenses incurred are rapidly increasing.

Health policy is formulated, enacted, and enforced through political processes at the local, state, or federal levels. For example, at the local level, policies would be established and implemented by an individual hospital board or by directors of a total health care system regarding whether or when flu injections would be available to high-risk populations being served by those institutions. At the state level, policies govern nurses within a state by defining nursing practice, nursing education, and nursing licensure. These policies are often governed by a state nurse practice act that designates a state nursing commission or health professions board as the authority for enforcing the policies. Federal policies are evident in the rules and regulations governing Medicare and Medicaid funding.

When bills affecting health care are being developed in state and federal legislative bodies, it is important that nurses be aware of those actions and obtain copies of those bills, thus adding to their political knowledge base.

Ultimately, health care will be defined and controlled by those wielding the most political influence. If nurses fail to exert political pressure on the health policy makers, they will lose ground to others who are more

CASE STUDY 9-1

Maria is a maternity support nurse for First Steps, a specific state-funded program designed to provide care to underserved and underinsured pregnant women. Maria is in her third year of professional practice and has become highly resourceful as well as able to work in new situations with minimal supervision. Many of her case referrals come through a partnership with the local hospital's Teen Parent Resource Center, targeting girls under 20 who have dropped out of school during their pregnancy. Many of Maria's patients are from families at high risk for domestic violence and substance abuse. Recently, she was informed that the Teen Parent Resource Center will be discontinuing its partnership with First Steps because of funding issues.

What does Maria need to know to continue to serve her high-risk population?

What are her options?

How could you use the Nightingale Methodology (see McDonald Evidence from the Literature discussed earlier in this chapter) to study the best information in print, especially government reports and statistics; interview experts and survey others with a questionnaire if the information is inadequate; propose and test a plan; consult with the practitioners who proposed it; and send out draft reports for comment before sending out the final report for publication and dissemination to the influential?

politically active. It is unrealistic to believe that other stakeholders will take care of nursing while the competition for health care resources increases. Historically, some stakeholders in health care have never supported nursing as a profession or acknowledged professional roles for nurses. Nurses, like other health care providers, must compete, negotiate, and collaborate with others to ensure their future in health care.

CULTURAL DIMENSIONS OF PARTNERSHIPS AND CONSUMERISM

By 2005, the U.S. minority population was one-third of the total population, that is 98 million people out of the nation's 296.4 million people. These numbers identify the increasing racial and ethnic diversity of the U.S. population. The largest minority group continues to be Hispanics at 42.7 million. Hispanics increased 3.3% in one year from July 2004 to July 2005 to clearly become the fastest-growing minority group. Black African Americans are the second largest minority group with 39.7 million people, followed by Asians at 14.4 million, 4.5 million

Alaska Natives and American Indians, and almost 1 million native Hawaiian and other Pacific Islanders. Non-Hispanic Whites totaled 198.4 million (Bernstein, 2006). Non-Hispanic Whites have decreased from 70% of the population in 2000 to 66.9% in 2005. The minority population increased from 30% of the total population to 33.1%.

If nurses intend to form partnerships with consumer groups distinguished by cultural heritage, racial makeup, or ethnic background, they must understand and value diversity. Strong partnerships will frame nursing services in ways that respect cultural differences.

POLITICS AND DEMOGRAPHIC CHANGES

Certainly not all consumers agree about what health care should be, who should provide it, or how it should be paid for. The social, cultural, economic, psychological, and demographic characteristics of consumers largely determine their attitudes and inclination toward the health care system, its providers, and its services. Consumers also recognize some level of personal risk when changes are made in the system, especially involving payment for services and providers. If consumers, such as retired persons, perceive that their out-of-pocket cost for health care extends beyond their capacity to pay or will increase in the future, they are highly motivated to exert political pressure on their legislators to reverse the perceived trend.

The fastest growing consumer group for years to come is the elderly—persons 65 and older—because of the unprecedented reproductive growth rate in the United States between 1946 and 1964 (U.S. Bureau of the Census, 2004). An estimated 76 million Baby Boomers will be turning 65 by 2011. The number of elderly people, 85 years of age, is growing at an explosive rate and is expected to reach 27 million by 2050 (Lanser, 2003). People over age 50 control approximately one-half of the country's disposable income as well as three quarters of its financial assets and 80% of its savings. Yet most elderly Americans are not wealthy, with 20% of them projected as qualifying for Medicare benefits by the year 2020 (Shi & Singh, 2004).

Without doubt, this aging of the U.S. population will profoundly affect health care at every level. The dramatic increase in the number of elderly people in the Western world means that about one-half of all people who have ever reached age 65 are alive today (Roszak, 1998). Studies of voting behavior of U.S. citizens show that the elderly have no predictable political orientation on anything except obvious threats to perceived entitlements, the most widely recognized entitlement being Social Security benefits.

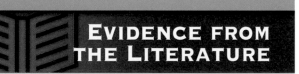

EVIDENCE FROM THE LITERATURE

Citation: Wakefield, M. (2003). Change drivers for nursing and health care. *Nursing Economics, 21*(3), 150–151.

Discussion: There are exciting opportunities and challenges for the latest crop of new nurses as well as for experienced nurses. Changes in health care delivery are being driven by multiple catalysts both external and internal to the health care delivery system. Some of these catalysts include the aging population, cultural diversity, and technology.

Implications for Practice: As new nurses graduate, they face a complex health care system that needs to change to meet the needs of the ever growing population of older adults, the increasing diversity of patients, an epidemic of patients without health care, and technology that can preserve life but not necessarily quality of life. New nurses will need to join with experienced nurses and answer the call to both individually and collectively influence policy to improve health care to meet the needs of the changing population.

CRITICAL THINKING 9-2

Demographic changes present multiple challenges to health care. Of the additional 185,000 nurses that joined the nursing workforce in 2002 and 2003, 70% were age 50 and over (Norman et al., 2005). By 2005, the nursing shortage had entered its eighth year "making it the longest lasting nursing shortage in half a century" (Buerhaus, Donelan, Ulrich, Norman, & Dittus, 2005, p. 62). It is predicted that by 2010, 40% of the nursing workforce will be over 50 years old, and by 2020, the Registered Nurse workforce will be 20% below need (Cooper, 2003). Sister Rosemary Donley (2005) believes that it is time to think outside the box for new solutions to the nursing shortage. Doing business as we have in the past will not work.

How do you anticipate that the aging workforce coupled with the aging population will affect your nursing practice?

What are the political implications?

Many seniors are joining consumer groups to have a greater political voice, influence health policy decisions, and ensure that they receive the health care services they will need for years to come. A growing number are bridging the gap of social isolation, prominent in the past, through the Internet as well as through involvement in consumer groups. They are establishing closer contact with the outside world and are managing to successfully strengthen their relationships with other stakeholders in health care.

The American Association of Retired Persons (AARP), with more than 15 million members, constitutes a growing political powerhouse and an ideal consumer partner for nursing in many ways. A large percentage of nurses are 50 years of age or older and qualify for membership in the AARP. Few other consumer groups appear to have the potential that the AARP has for defining the health care system of the future.

NURSE AS POLITICAL ACTIVIST

Nurses are the largest health care group, and nurses who are politically active have a definitive voice in their work environments for patient welfare as well as for themselves. Nurses must set their political goals as individual nurses, nurse citizens, nurse activists, and nurse politicians for the future (Table 9-2). Nurses must study the issues, garner political support, and contact policy makers such as the chairperson of the hospital board or legislators through phone calls, letters, and e-mail messages. Nurses join professional organizations and actively participate to ensure a more collective, unified voice supporting health care issues and policies that have value for consumers and nursing. Nurses who are most involved will be seen supporting political activities and candidates, assisting during campaigns, helping to draft legislation, and running for political office.

As nurses develop politically, they come to understand the need for political strategy. The purpose of developing political strategies is to understand different ways to achieve your goals, or the goals you are advocating for, while identifying the other stakeholders and their goals. Political strategy attempts to persuade those people supporting an issue, formulating a policy, or taking an action to take the position in support of those using the political strategy. To be feasible, a political strategy requires commitment by those using it, as well as their awareness of the other stakeholders. Effective political strategy implies considerable forethought and clarity of purpose in even the most ambiguous situations. Nurses who are most likely to wield political influence operate with strategy in mind before taking political action, voicing concerns, making demands, or even advocating for others. It is important to study the political issues and the major stakeholders' positions regarding the issue prior to becoming involved and seek opportunities for collaboration.

Every nurse should be cognizant of what other involved groups think regarding any relevant political health issue. It is critical that nurses listen to other policy perspectives and understand as many facets of the issue as possible when making health policy proposals. Proposals need to include a rationale to neutralize opposing views. This ensures that unnecessary political fights can be avoided and that more collaboration will occur prior to any policy proposal being made to policy-making bodies such as hospital boards or state legislatures. The more support obtained from the various stakeholders in any policy arena, the better chance of a workable policy being developed and implemented.

To be most politically effective, nurses must be able to clearly articulate several dimensions of nursing to any audience or stakeholder: what nursing is; why nursing is important to society; what distinctive services nurses provide to consumers; how nursing benefits consumers including the prevention of nurse-sensitive outcomes, such as pneumonia, cardiac arrest, and so on; and what nursing services cost in relation to other health care services. Although anecdotal stories and emotional appeals may be effective with certain audiences, it is far more powerful to present research-based evidence to support the political position of the nursing profession. Table 9-3 details essential dimensions of nursing.

TABLE 9-2   POLITICAL ROLES FOR NURSES

Role	Activities
Nurse individual	■ Highlights important role of nurse to prevent nursing-sensitive outcomes, for example, pneumonia, cardiac arrest, and so on.
	■ Sets goals to strengthen nursing as a profession (Chapter 31).
	■ Highlights the essential dimensions of nursing (Table 9-3).
	■ Participates as a member in health care consumer groups, for example, the American Association for Retired Persons, and so on.
Nurse citizen	■ Votes and writes members of Congress and state legislators on issues of interest.
	■ Educates patients on how to evaluate Website sources of health care information.
Nurse activist	■ Active member of professional organization that lobbies and influences state and federal legislation.
	■ Notifies hospital Board of Trustees of any quality issues.
Nurse politician	■ Runs for a political office and serves society as a whole.
	■ Collaborates with other health care professionals to improve care at the local-, state-, and national levels.

TABLE 9-3   ESSENTIAL DIMENSIONS OF NURSING

■ Establishing a caring relationship that enhances healing and health

■ Focusing on the full range of experiences and human responses to illness and health within both the physical and social environments

■ Appreciating the subjective experience and the integration of such experience with objective data

■ Diagnosing and intervening in care by using scientific knowledge, judgment, and critical thinking

■ Advancing nursing knowledge through scholarly inquiry

■ Influencing social and public policy to promote social justice

Source: From American Nurses Association. (2003). *Nursing's social policy statement* (2nd ed.). Washington, DC: American Nurses Publishing.

POLITICS AND ADVOCACY

The concept of patient advocacy has been a fundamental aspect of nursing since nursing's beginning. The role of a nurse as a patient advocate has changed as nursing has evolved. Originally nurses acted as an intermediary and pleader for the patient, and now they act to insure that the patient's rights to self-determination and free choice are not violated (Rudolph, 2005). Advocacy can be seen as representing the patient to others in the health care organization, which has extended into what has been referred to as cultural brokering or interpreting the health care environment for the patient. There is a strong argument that advocacy actually stems from patient power and consumerism rather than a lack of power or vulnerability as some authors have implied (O'Conner & Kelly, 2005). If a nurse is to act as a patient advocate that interprets the health care environment to the patient and actually guides the patient through the maze, the nurse needs knowledge of the system. Sometimes a nurse's advocating for a patient's rights may be contrary to the wishes of another health care provider or to the organization as a whole. This can be risky for a nurse. Nurses from the beginning of the profession have served as patient advocates. They have acquired the necessary knowledge, and they have taken on the risk. Some early nurses were even jailed for taking unpopular stands. Entry-level nurses need knowledge of the health care organization and the courage of their convictions to act as patient advocates.

Interestingly, some patients have begun advocating for nurses, a role reversal. Those patients perceived nurses as overextended by the nature of the work environment and contended that something had be done to improve the working conditions of nursing. Nurses in California used consumer support to build their case for counteracting significant staffing cuts affecting nursing practice in their state. With strong consumer support, California nurses developed a legislative proposal in 1999 that has been enacted into state law. This law mandates a minimal staffing level of registered nurses for patient care. The intent is to protect patients from unqualified or dangerous staffing levels while receiving nursing services.

ADVOCACY AND CONSUMER PARTNERSHIPS

Nurses must understand the political forces that define their relationships with consumers. Consumers expect the best people to be health care providers, but they are confused about what the roles and responsibilities of professional nurses are. Informed consumers understand how health policy directly affects them but are less likely to recognize how health policy affects nurses. Consumers may expect nurses to be their advocates only in the context of providing direct patient care.

Working through their professional organizations, nurses can collaborate with consumer groups by creating formal partnerships, which serve to promote the role of nurses as consumer advocates in health policy arenas and strengthen the political position of both partners. These partnerships have a stronger political voice than either group has alone. The partners gain power when interacting with any policy-making body because they represent (1) a larger **voting block**—a group that represents the same political position or perspective; (2) a broader funding base—a source of financial support; and (3) a stronger **political voice**—an increase in the number of voices supporting or opposing an issue—to any policy-making body. Increasingly, professional organizations in nursing recognize the value of partnering with consumers to build a better health care system. See Table 9-4 for steps in establishing a partnership with a consumer group.

CONSUMER DEMANDS

As recipients of health care are required to pay a larger portion of the cost for health care services, consumers are demanding to be treated as something more than passive recipients of health care. They are very vocal in their requests to providers, payers, and agencies that they be more consumer friendly and service oriented, and they are seriously requesting a voice in how health care is regulated.

Nurses, working through professional organizations such as the American Nurses Association (ANA), have been strong, early supporters for patients' rights, regardless of the patient's ability to pay. Other professional groups, such as the American Medical Association (AMA) and the American Hospital Association (AHA), have received far more media recognition for their support of patients' rights. This is an indication that the AMA and AHA are better funded, wield more political power, and may do a better job of presenting their positions on consumer issues to the media than the ANA.

Any political vision to make health care more consumer friendly and service oriented must address cost, access, choice, and quality. Perhaps the vision starts with the formula: the highest quality of care for all people at the least cost. Yet defining—much less evaluating—quality is culturally bound and very complicated. Many people cannot afford minimal health care services. Other people are increasingly unwilling to subsidize the care of other patients by paying increased costs for their health care.

CRITICAL THINKING 9-3

Political conflict occurs because people may hold significantly different or conflicting opinions about any given topic. Consumers may disagree about what health care should be, who should provide it, how much it should cost, and/or who should pay for it. As a new nurse, you have a professional responsibility to promote consumer dialogue and offer creative, thoughtful, and evidence-based solutions to health care problems. Yet nurses, like consumers, disagree with each other in regard to the same issues consumers may have about health care.

What do you think your responsibility is as a consumer of health care?

What is your responsibility as a health care provider?

Do you think your responsibility as a consumer could conflict with your responsibility as a provider?

TABLE 9-4 — STEPS IN ESTABLISHING A PARTNERSHIP WITH A CONSUMER GROUP

Step	Description
1. Listen	Become sensitized to the health care needs and political nature of the potential consumer partner.
2. Study	Seek both representative and opposing perspectives from consumer group meetings, focus groups, relevant literature, and interviews.
3. Assess	Determine the need, value, context, and boundaries for establishing the partnership.
4. Focus	Mutually identify the purpose, and articulate the goals and specific, realistic objectives for the partnership.
5. Compromise	Work through nonessential and noncritical points and issues.
6. Negotiate	Agree on your position and responsibilities in the partnership.
7. Plan	Develop a political strategy for achieving the goals and fulfilling the objectives.
8. Test	Test the political waters. Gather feedback on the plan from key people before taking action.
9. Model	Model the political work. Define the structure for working the political strategy with partners.
10. Direct the political action	Understand the bigger picture and concentrate on what can be changed.
11. Implement	Line up political support and take action.
12. Network	Be committed to the mutually recognized goal, and consistently work to have an adequate base of support in terms of people, money, and time.
13. Build political credibility	Participate in local, state, and national policy-making efforts that support the partnership and its political agenda.
14. Soothe and bargain	Downplay rivalry, and address conflict in a timely, constructive manner.
15. Report, publicize, and lobby	Report, publicize, and lobby the group's political cause. Draw public attention to the needs of the consumer group.
16. Reaffirm, redefine, or discontinue	Regularly evaluate work with consumer group.

CRITICAL THINKING 9-4

The American public has become increasingly aware of and interested in health promotion (Hood & Leddy, 2006). The relationship between personal lifestyle and the incidence of several diseases has been demonstrated through the mainstream media with public education campaigns. Many health promotion programs include the expectation that people invest in themselves, but people who live in poverty lead precarious lives. How do you think people in the lowest socioeconomic class perceive their health care? Do you assume most people will invest in themselves by living a lifestyle that promotes higher education, planned savings, healthy eating, regular exercise, deferred gratification, avoidance of smoking and excessive alcohol consumption, planned birth control, and regular physical checkups? Do you know people who seem to live only from one day to the next because their perspective of time is in the immediate, and they do not seem to recognize the benefits of long-term planning?

REAL WORLD INTERVIEW

Gary, age 46, and Laurie, age 42, have been married seven years and have two daughters, ages 4 years and 6 years. Gary is a practicing commercial architect recently diagnosed with Ménière's disease. Laurie is a professional photographer working from home. She was recently diagnosed with sarcoidosis. Gary said the effectiveness of the U.S. health care system is "very restricted by the dictates of insurance companies and by what health care providers want. It's like doing the minimum for whatever reason. There's a reluctance to take a holistic approach." Laurie agreed, adding that "as it stands, service providers are needlessly competing with each other. As a consumer, I do not feel comfortable with how they collaborate with each other, much less the consumer. Nursing has been channeled into a corporate culture because so many nurses fail to think or practice as professionals." Gary said, "Nursing is taken for granted; we really do not see nurses as providers as much as technicians. There is a missed opportunity to meet the expanding needs of consumers. Create a system that is more accessible from a daily living or health maintenance standpoint." Consumers need their "concerns addressed openly and should be able to get answers or at least options without going through so many gatekeepers. I have come to believe that health care is a very inexact science. They are just guessing, or don't seem concerned enough to do more than what the provider wants or will get paid for." Laurie said, "Information is lost between service providers, hospitalizations, and clinic visits. You provide the same information several times and you wonder if anyone is really using or thinking about the information they are gathering. If nurses were better educated, they could be stronger advocates for the consumer." Gary adds, "Health care is becoming more inaccessible unless you are dying. Nurses certainly have the opportunity to do more and be first-level providers. We think that nurses did more to shape our hospital experiences to be a positive experience than anyone. They can be the worker bees of health care. They are vital, but they could do a better job of working with consumers of health care. We are willing to pay more if we trust the competence of the provider and can understand the need for the service. This includes nursing."

Gary and Laurie Maples
Consumers
Tacoma, Washington

A vision for high-quality, low-cost care will require multiple stakeholders collaborating with one another to develop a workable philosophy, to include a mechanism for checks and balances to minimize abuse and misuse and encourage intelligent, ethical decisions by those wielding the most political power.

TURNING A CONSUMER-ORIENTED VISION INTO REALITY

Nurses have opportunities to be more than supporters of a consumer-oriented vision for health care; they can be cocreators. To make this vision real, nurses will need to be more educated and articulate about what value they add to the overall health care system. Getting other stakeholders and the policy makers to understand and promote the value of nursing to consumers will take considerable political work. This work will have to be more than anecdotal pleas, arguments in support of some consumer cause, or reactions to some particular health care issue or workplace

injustice. Believing in a vision and working hard are not enough. Nurses must have a clear image of the vision; develop a sound philosophy; demonstrate intelligent, strategic thinking; and wield more political influence.

Although nurses may think they are the ones primarily affected by the changes in health care, it is more powerful and therefore strategic to understand that everyone, especially consumers, is affected.

As patient advocates, nurses need to seize the opportunity to make a difference. New nurses can make a difference by implementing the strategies outlined in Table 9-5.

THE CONSUMER DEMAND FOR ACCOUNTABILITY

The vigilance of government, payers, and even attorneys is understandable when you look at the behavior of some providers (Kavaler & Spiegel, 2003). Some providers focus on "What's good for the agency, my interest group, or me?" rather than "What is going to work for the consumers and all the other stakeholders over the long run?"

When stakeholders are motivated and directed solely by their own perceived needs, competitive political strategies replace more collaborative approaches to addressing the consumer's health care needs. Accountability

TABLE 9-5	POLITICAL STRATEGIES FOR MOUNTING CONSUMER CAMPAIGNS

- Lobbying at state and federal levels for health care regulations and guidelines that serve a consumer group's interest
- Consulting with representatives from a consumer group when health care regulations and guidelines are being debated or written
- Monitoring the enforcement of health care regulations and exacting corrective or punitive action when noncompliance occurs
- Encouraging providers and payers to make changes in delivery of services voluntarily to meet changing consumer demands
- Changing consumer perceptions and behaviors through the distribution of educational materials or other media

becomes a serious issue because the goal of overtaking the competition supersedes the goal of offering the highest-quality services. People who will own the future of health care must address this growing problem of accountability. They will have to establish and sustain their credibility during a time when more people are distrustful of the health care system, its providers, third-party payers, and legislators.

Most people comprehend that being accountable requires being held responsible for one's behavior, decisions, and affiliations with others. Not withstanding, some nurses claim they are not culpable for their actions because they are merely doing what they must do as defined by their employer or some other larger entity. These nurses fail to understand that professional accountability goes beyond responsibility in a particular employment situation. The practice of nursing is based on a social contract with society that gives nurses certain rights and responsibilities and requires that nursing is accountable to the public (ANA, 2003). In addition, the individual nurse practice acts of each state address these concepts.

Increasingly, consumers are more educated and have more access to the internet, for example, www.webMD.com. Consumers are demanding positive results and are holding those in the health care system accountable for better health care outcomes. If the trend in increased litigation related to professional negligence and medical malpractice is any indication, just having an ethical process for providing care will not satisfy the consumer who experiences negative health outcomes. The strongest potential for litigation in health care comes from too few health care professionals accepting personal responsibility for ensuring that health care services are provided in a safe, competent manner at a system level as well as at a personal level. Health care professionals, including nurses, depend upon each other to ensure the quality, consistency, and overall effectiveness of health care within their work environments.

CASE STUDY 9-2

Juan and Casey are study partners in the final semester of a nursing program. Juan has served as a medical corpsman and worked as an emergency medical technician for several years, whereas Casey entered college right out of high school, starting as a business major. One of their class assignments was to develop a strategy for reducing malpractice risks in a hospital setting. Casey proposes redefining the patient as the customer of health care services because adopting a more customer-oriented approach to health care services in hospitals would improve patient satisfaction and subsequently reduce malpractice claims. Juan opposes that strategy because he thinks that too many health care providers are adopting the culture of corporate America when they define patients as customers. He views patients as something more than customers but also thinks that patients do not know what is best for them in most health care situations.

Do you think patients should be defined as health care customers?

Would patients be less likely to sue health care providers if they were approached as customers instead of patients?

PATIENT SAFETY: AN IMPORTANT PARTNERSHIP

Historically, patients have been passive recipients of health care, but with the consumer movement, this is changing. Readily available information through Internet resources, such as www.pubmed.org, www.webMD.com, and www.askanurse.com, has facilitated this move from patient to consumer of health. Patients who have chronic diseases may be active members in organizations that educate and advocate for those with the disease. No longer do the health care providers have all the information. This information is widely disseminated (Ballard, 2003). Informed consumers are important partners in ensuring safe care. Consumers can demand competent, educated care providers as emphasized in ANA's campaign, entitled "Every Patient Deserves a Nurse." Consumers can require information about statistical indicators of care quality, such as medical error rates, nosocomial infection rates, morbidity and mortality rates, lengths of stays for patients with certain conditions, and incidents of malpractice (Ballard, 2003). Individual consumers can ask questions when given prescriptions, treatments, and diagnostic tests. Collectively, educated consumers can partner with nursing organizations or other health care organizations to support policies and legislation that facilitate safe care (Table 9-6).

Professional nursing organizations have a major role in promoting patient safety. The role includes but is not limited to developing policy statements, lobbying for regulations and legislation that serve and protect the consumers of nursing care, and advocating for patients. There are times when a professional organization's need to advocate for its members conflicts with its usual purpose of advocating for the welfare of the public. The organization must balance these conflicting roles and promote patient safety (Rowell, 2003).

Since the shift from a service focus to a business focus within health care, nurses have found themselves working to maintain quality care and patient safety when the powers that be are focused on income generation (Rowell, 2003). Where do nurses turn when they have concerns but no power to change the situation? Both new nurses and experienced nurses need to turn to their professional organizations. Alone, a nurse is only one voice, but together, nurses are powerful. There are many professional organizations that speak for nurses. Most are specialty organizations with small memberships. Some of the specialty organizations, such as Emergency Nurses Association and the Association of Critical Care Nurses, have large memberships (Table 9-7).

The American Nurses Association (ANA) is the largest representative of registered nurses in the United States. ANA is not specialty focused and it represents nurses from all specialties, all work sites, and all levels of education. ANA has many goals, but one of them is to promote patient safety (Rowell, 2003). To achieve its patient safety goal, ANA develops and disseminates documents such as the *Nursing's Social Policy Statement* and the *Code of Ethics for Nurses*. These documents define nurses' contract with society and each nurse's obligation to act ethically.

CRITICAL THINKING 9-5

Access, quality, and timing of information available to the public have greatly enhanced the consumer health care movement. Using the Internet, people can do customized searches on practically any health care concern; garner input from a wide audience; and do comparative shopping for services, providers, and products. Several uniform sources of information have been developed for the U.S. health care delivery system. These data sets offer information requested by the decision makers about some predetermined dimension of health care. They also establish standard definitions, classifications, and measurements for making evidence-based decisions. Nursing has been relatively absent from the data sought, collected, and disseminated to the decision makers.

Is there a need for nursing-sensitive consumer outcome measures that can be used by decision makers? What steps could be taken to make such information available to the public?

Patient safety is part of the contract as well as an ethical responsibility of nurses. ANA lobbies for regulations and legislation that ensure patient safety. This is done largely through state nursing associations, state nursing boards, and state legislatures that define nursing practice in each state. ANA advocates for the consumers of health care by pushing for evidence-based patient outcome data and encouraging certification and credentialing (Rowell, 2003). Educated consumers can choose facilities with improved patient outcomes and well prepared nurses.

CREDIBILITY AND POLITICS

To have credibility, nurses must demonstrate professional competence and a degree of professional accountability that exceeds consumer expectations. Nurses who are most able to successfully overcome these challenges assert their professional credibility in several ways. They are lifelong learners and demonstrate professional growth throughout their careers in nursing. They approach their vocation as a service to the public and to the nursing profession and an honorable way to make a living. They take ownership of the situations in which they find themselves and work to resolve problems and overcome obstacles to

TABLE 9-6	**HOW A BILL BECOMES LAW**

Step 1: A Bill Is Born

Anyone may draft a bill; however, only members of Congress can introduce legislation, and, by doing so, become the sponsor(s). The president, a member of the cabinet, or the head of a federal agency can also propose legislation, although a member of Congress must introduce it.

Step 2: Committee Action

As soon as a bill is introduced, it is referred to a committee. At this point, the bill is examined carefully and its chances for passage are first determined. If the committee does not act on a bill, the bill is effectively "dead."

Step 3: Subcommittee Review

Often, bills are referred to a subcommittee for study and hearings. Hearings provide the opportunity to put on the record the views of the executive branch, experts, other public officials and supporters, and opponents of the legislation.

Step 4: Mark up

When the hearings are completed, the subcommittee may meet to "mark up" the bill, that is, make changes and amendments prior to recommending the bill to the full committee. If a subcommittee votes not to report legislation to the full committee, the bill dies. If the committee votes for the bill, it is sent to the floor.

Step 5: Committee Action to Report a Bill

After receiving a subcommittee's report on a bill, the full committee votes on its recommendation to the House or Senate. This procedure is called "ordering a bill reported."

Step 6: Voting

After the debate and the approval of any amendments, the bill is passed or defeated by the members voting.

Step 7: Referral to Other Chamber

When the House or Senate passes a bill, it is referred to the other chamber, where it usually follows the same route through committee and floor action. This chamber may approve the bill as received, reject it, ignore it, or change it.

Step 8: Conference Committee Action

When the actions of the other chamber significantly alter the bill, a conference committee is formed to reconcile the differences between the House and Senate versions. If the conferees are unable to reach agreement, the legislation dies. If agreement is reached, a conference report is prepared describing the committee members' recommendations for changes. Both the House and Senate must approve the conference report.

Step 9: Final Action

After both the House and Senate have approved a bill in identical form, it is sent to the president. If the president approves of the legislation and signs it, it becomes law. Or, if the president takes no action for 10 days, while Congress is in session, it automatically becomes law. If the president opposes the bill, the president can veto it; or if the president takes no action after the Congress has adjourned its second session, it is a "pocket veto," and the legislation dies.

Step 10: Overriding a Veto

If the president vetoes a bill, Congress may attempt to override the veto. If both the Senate and the House pass the bill by a two-thirds majority, the president's veto is overruled, and the bill becomes a law.

Source: www.genome.gov/pfv.cfm?pageID=12513982

TABLE 9-7 **NURSING ORGANIZATIONS**

Organization	Website
Academy of Medical-Surgical Nurses	www.medsurgnurse.org
Air & Surface Transport Nurses Association	www.astna.org
American Academy of Nurse Practitioners	www.aanp.org
American Academy of Ambulatory Care Nursing	www.aaacn.org
American Assembly for Men in Nursing	aamn.org
American Association for the History of Nursing	www.aahn.org
American Association of Colleges of Nursing	www.aacn.nche.edu
American Association of Critical-Care Nurses	www.aacn.org
American Association of Legal Nurse Consultants	www.aalnc.org
American Association of Managed Care Nurses	www.aamcn.org
American Association of Neuroscience Nurses	www.aann.org
American Association of Nurse Anesthetists	www.aana.com
American Association of Nurse Life Care Planners	aanlcp.org
American Association of Occupational Health Nurses	www.aaohn.org
American Association of Spinal Cord Injury Nurses	www.aascin.org
American College of Nurse-Midwives	www.acnm.org
American Forensic Nurses	www.amrn.com
American Holistic Nurses Association	www.ahna.org
American Nephrology Nurses' Association	www.annanurse.org
American Nurses Association	www.ana.org
American Nursing Informatics Association	www.ania.org
American Organization of Nurse Executives	www.aone.org
American Pediatric Surgical Nurses Association	www.apsna.org
American Psychiatric Nurses Association	www.apna.org
American Radiological Nurses Association	www.arna.net
American Society of Ophthalmic Registered Nurses	webeye.ophth.uiowa.edu
American Society of PeriAnesthesia Nurses	www.aspan.org
American Society of Plastic Surgical Nurses	www.aspsn.org
Association of Camp Nurses	www.campnurse.org
Association of Child Neurology Nurses	www.acnn.org
Association of Nurses in AIDS Care	www.anacnet.org
Association of Operating Room Nurses (Same as Association of PeriOperative Registered Nurses)	www.aorn.org
Association of Pediatric Gastroenterology and Nutrition Nurses	apgnn.org
Association of Pediatric Hematology/Oncology Nurses	www.apon.org
Association of PeriOperative Registered Nurses	www.aorn.org
Association of Rehabilitation Nurses	www.rehabnurse.org
Association of Women's Health, Obstetric and Neonatal Nurses	www.awhonn.org
Chi Eta Phi Sorority, Inc	www.chietaphi.com
Dermatology Nurses' Association	dna.inurse.com

TABLE 9-7 CONTINUED	
Organization	**Website**
Developmental Disabilities Nurses Association	*www.ddna.org*
Emergency Nurses Association	*www.ena.org*
Family Medicine Residency Nurses Association	*www.fmrna.org*
Home Healthcare Nurses Association	*www.hhna.org*
Hospice and Palliative Nurses Association	*www.hpna.org*
Infusion Nurses Society	*www.ins1.org*
International Association of Forensic Nurses	*www.iafn.org*
National Organization of Nurse Practitioner Faculties	*www.nonpf.com*
National Association of Clinical Nurse Specialists	*www.nacns.org*
National Association of Hispanic Nurses	*thehispanicnurses.org*
National Association of Nurse Practitioners in Women's Health	*www.npwh.org*
National Association of Neonatal Nurses	*www.nann.org*
National Association of Orthopedic Nurses	*www.orthonurse.org*
National Association of Pediatric Nurse Practitioners	*www.napnap.org*
National Association of School Nurses	*www.nasn.org*
National Association of School Nurses for the Deaf	*www.nasnd.org*
National Conference of Gerontological Nurse Practitioners	*www.ncgnp.org*
National Council of State Boards of Nursing	*www.ncsbn.org*
National Black Nurses Association	*www.nbna.org*
National Gerontological Nursing Association	*www.ngna.org*
National League for Nursing	*www.nln.org*
National Nursing Staff Development Organization	*www.nnsdo.org*
Nurses Organization of Veterans Affairs	*www.vanurse.org*
Oncology Nursing Society	*www.ons.org*
Nurses for a Healthier Tomorrow	*www.nursesource.org*
Pediatric Endocrinology Nursing Society	*www.pens.org*
Preventive Cardiovascular Nurses Association	*www.pcna.net*
Sigma Theta Tau International	*www.nursingsociety.org*
Society of Gastroenterology Nurses and Associates, Inc.	*www.sgna.org*
Society of Otorhinolaryngology and Head-Neck Nurses, Inc.	*www.sohnnurse.com*
Society of Pediatric Nurses	*www.pedsnurses.org*
Society of Urologic Nurses and Associates	*www.suna.org*
Wound, Ostomy and Continence Nurses Society	*www.wocn.org*

providing the best care possible. Nurses strengthen their political position by sharing accountability for health care problems with other health care providers. When nurses point fingers at others such as supervisors, administrators, politicians, or practitioners for health care problems, or look to others for improvement, their power is weakened. Nursing's accountability to the public is part of their professional responsibility. This means that nurses must work cohesively with partners to assure quality care (Hood & Leddy, 2006).

Nursing ownership, however, is not enough to guarantee the political credibility of nursing in the future. This is because others see the political gains to be made from identifying themselves as consumer advocates.

As other service providers board the consumer bandwagon, nurses will need to continuously demonstrate that they are more valuable to the consumer than providers of alternative services that cost less. Consumers increasingly will demand tangible evidence from nurses that their services are worth it.

KEY CONCEPTS

- Individuals or groups take political action to get what they want or prevent others from getting something they do not want them to have.

- Entry-level nurses can join organizations that influence policy such as gun control, tobacco sales, and mandatory helmets for certain activities.

- Politics are inherent in any system in which resources are absolutely or relatively scarce and where there are competing interests for those resources.

- Nurses have a critical role in addressing the major system-level issues in health care delivery.

- Political, economic, and social changes such as aging, diversity, and the costs of technology in the United States are transforming the health care system.

- Nurses must articulate what nursing is, what distinctive services they provide, how these services benefit consumers, and how much these services cost in relation to other health care services.

- If nursing is defined through politics to be less than critical or professional, nurses will be less empowered and paid less.

- The aging of the U.S. population constitutes a growing political force and affords nursing a wonderful opportunity to become stronger in health policy arenas.

- Consumer partnerships will become more critical for all stakeholders in health care.

- When a consumer group forms a political coalition with other groups, such as nurses, in a given community, the political influence of both is strengthened.

KEY TERMS

political voice   stakeholders
politics   voting block
resources

REVIEW QUESTIONS

1. Political methods inherently involve which of the following? Choose all that apply.
   _____ A. Competition
   _____ B. Naiveté
   _____ C. Negotiation
   _____ D. Collaboration

2. Politics exist because of which of the following statements?
   A. They are required by law.
   B. Resources cannot be limited by political process.
   C. Some people want to control more resources than others.
   D. Resources must be equally distributed among stakeholders.

3. The consumer movement in health care is characterized by which of the following statements?
   A. It is a socialist movement about health care resources.
   B. It is growing because of the Internet and organizations such as the American Association for the Advancement of Retired People (AARP).
   C. It is supported by all stakeholders in the health care system.
   D. It is inclusive of only people who are not health care providers.

4. In that the national expenditures on health care for the uninsured exceeds $100 billion annually, which of the following is true?
   A. All Americans receive adequate health care.
   B. Forty-three million Americans are uninsured.
   C. Medicaid provides insurance for the working poor.
   D. Medicare insures that all patients over 60 receive health care.

5. Many consumers are concerned about media reports of health care expenditures rising because of which of the following?
   A. They are uninsured.
   B. Their individual share of expenses is rising.
   C. They pay the entire cost of health care out of pocket.
   D. Rationing is inevitable.

6. Which of the following is true concerning the minority population in the United States? Choose all that apply.
   A. It includes 98 million racially and ethnically diverse people.
   B. It makes up one-third of the U.S. population.
   C. It has resisted the consumer movement.
   D. It is a well organized, cohesive group of consumers.

7. Which of the following is true regarding the consumer movement in the United States?
   A. It is a passing fad.
   B. It challenges nurses to be more professionally accountable.
   C. It is sustainable only through partnerships with the nursing profession.
   D. It is encouraged by all health care systems and providers.

8. ANA describes the essential elements of nursing. Which of the following is not an essential element?
   A. Establishing a caring relationship
   B. Delivering problem-focused care
   C. Focusing on the full range of experiences and human responses
   D. Appreciating the patient's subjective experience and integrating such experience with objective data

9. As a new school nurse, you become aware of some state laws that actually get in the way of providing the best care for your students. What are the best steps in becoming politically active and changing this? Choose all that apply.
   _____ A. Join the state school nurse organization, become active, and partner with parent groups.
   _____ B. Vote in the next election, and encourage all your friends to do so.
   _____ C. Study politics, and run for political office.
   _____ D. Write your state legislators, describe your problem, and ask them to initiate laws that will resolve the problem.

REVIEW ACTIVITIES

1. Find out who your Congressional representatives are. Write or e-mail them to find out what health care legislation they are supporting.

2. Notice who is supporting current health care legislation. Are consumer protections being emphasized in any proposed legislation?

3. Identify a consumer group in which you are interested. Use the steps identified in Table 9-4 to establish a partnership with the group. What did you learn?

EXPLORING THE WEB

- Identify some Websites for consumer groups:
  American Association of Retired Persons (AARP): *www.aarp.org*

  Citizen's Council on Health Care: *www.cchc-mn.org* and *www.cchconline.org*

- Go to the consumer site for combating health-related fraud: *www.quackwatch.org*

- Note the consumer tips at this site: *www.consumertips.com*

- Search for *health care* on this Consumers for Quality Care (CQC) site: *www.consumerwatchdog.org*

- Search for *health* on this site for consumer reports: *www.consumersunion.org*

- Identify some sites for government offices and health care agencies:
  U.S. Congress: *www.congress.org*

U.S. Department of Health and Human Services: *www.hhs.gov*

Government consumer health Website: *www.healthfinder.gov*

Medicare and Medicaid Programs: *www.cms.hhs.gov*

- Read about the Milbank Memorial Fund whose purpose is to improve health by helping the decision makers: *www.milbank.org*

- Identify some Websites that new nurses should know concerning policy:

  ANA keeps nurses abreast of legislative issues that involve them: *www.nursingworld.org* Search for government.

  The Electronic Policy Network provides up-to-date information on politics of global issues: *www.movingideas.org*

  The Library of Congress Thomas provides a searchable database of Federal legislation: *http://thomas.loc.gov*

  The Library of Congress State Government Information provides state and local government links: *www.loc.gov* Search for state and local government news.

REFERENCES

American Nurses Association. (2003). *Nursing's social policy statement* (2nd ed.). Washington, DC: American Nurses Publishing.

Ballard, K. (2003, September 30). Patient safety: A shared responsibility. *Online Journal of Issues in Nursing, 8*(3), manuscript 4. Retrieved September 30, 2003, from http://www.nursingworld.org/ojin/topic22/tpc22_4.htm

Bernstein, R. (2006, May 10). Immediate news release: Nation's population one-third minority. U.S. Census Bureau. Retrieved June 29, 2006, from http://www.census.gov/Press-Release/www/releases/archives/population/006808.html

Birnbaum, J. H., & Newell, R. (2001, May 28). Fat & happy in D.C. *Fortune,* 94.

Buerhaus, P., Donelan, K., Ulrich, B., Norman, L., & Dittus, R. (2005). Part one: Is the shortage of hospital registered nurses getting better or worse? Findings from two recent national surveys of RNs. *Nursing Economics, 23*(2), 61–71, 96.

Byrd, M. E., Costello, J., Shelton, C. R., Thomas, P. A., & Petrarcha, D. (2004). An active learning experience in health policy for baccalaureate nursing students. *Public Health Nursing, 21*(5), 501–506.

Cooper, E. E. (2003). Pieces of the shortage puzzle: Aging and shift work. *Nursing Economics, 21*(2), 75–79.

Deschaine, J. E., & Schaffer, M. A. (2003). Strengthening the role of public health nurse leaders in policy development. *Policy, Politics & Nursing Practice, 4*(4), 266–275.

Donley, R. (2005). Challenges for nursing in the 21st century. *Nursing Economics, 23*(6), 312–318.

Grindel, C. (2005). Influencing health care policy with our children in mind. *MedSurg Nursing, 14*(5), 277–278.

Hadley, J., & Holahan, J. (2003). How much medical care do the uninsured use, and who pays for it? *Health Affairs-Web Exclusive.* Retrieved July 1, 2006, from http://content.healthaffairs.org/cgi/reprint/hlthaff.w3.66v1.pdf

Harrington, C., Crider, M., Benner, P. E., & Malone, R. (2005). Advanced nursing training in health policy, designing, and implementing a new program. *Policy, Politics & Nursing Practice, 6*(2), 99–108.

Hood, L. J., & Leddy, S. (2005). *Conceptual bases of professional nursing* (6th ed.). Philadelphia: Lippincott.

Kavaler, F., & Spiegel, A. D. (2003). *Risk management in health care institutions: A strategic approach* (2nd ed.). Boston: Jones and Bartlett.

Keepnews, D. M. (2005). Health policy—A nursing specialty? *Policy, Politics & Nursing Practice, 6*(4), 275–276.

Lanser, E. G. (2003). Our aging population. *Healthcare Executive, 18*(1), 6–11.

Mason, D., & Leavitt, J. K. (2002). *Policy and politics in nursing and health care* (4th ed.). W. B. Saunders.

McDonald, L. (2006). Florence Nightingale as a social reformer. *History Today, 56*(1), 9–15.

Mills, R. J., & Bhandari, S. (2003). Health insurance coverage in the United States: 2002. Washington, DC: U.S. Department of Commerce, Economics, and Statistics Administration, Bureau of the Census.

Milstead, J. A. (2004). *Health policy & politics: A nurse's guide* (2nd ed.). Gaithersburg, MD: Aspen.

Nolin, J., & Killackey, J. (2004). Redirecting health care spending: Consumer directed health care. *Nursing Economics, 22*(5), 251–253, 257.

Norman, L., Donelan, K., Buerhaus, P., Willis, G., Williams, M., Ulrich, B., & Dittus, R. (2005). Part five: The older nurse in the workforce: Does age matter? *Nursing Economics, 23*(6), 282–289.

O'Conner, T., & Kelly, B. (2005). Bridging the gap: A study of general nurses' perceptions of patient advocacy in Ireland. *Nursing Ethics, 12*(5), 453–467.

Ortner, P. M. (2004). The nurse as change agent: An approach to environmental health advocacy. *Policy, Politics, & Nursing Practice, 5*(2), 125–130.

Pierce, K. M. (2004). Insights and reflections of a congressional nurse detailee. *Policy, Politics & Nursing Practice, 5*(2), 113–115.

Roszak, T. (1998). *America the wise: The longevity revolution and the true wealth of nations.* Boston: Houghton Mifflin.

Rowell, P. (2003, September 30). The professional nursing association's role in patient safety. *Online Journal of Issues in Nursing, 8*(3), manuscript 3. Retrieved September 30, 2003, from http://www.nursingworld.org/ojin/topic22/tpc22_3.htm

Rudolph, B. J. (2005). *How nurses define the role of patient advocacy.* Unpublished master's thesis, Division of Nursing, Wilmington College, Wilmington, DE.

Shi, L., & Singh, D. A. (2003). *Delivering health care in America* (3rd ed.). Gaithersburg, MD: Aspen.

Steele, S., Rocchiccioli, J., & Porche, D. (2003). Analyzing and promoting issues in health policy: Nurse manager's perspective. *Nursing Economics, 21*(2), 80–83.

U.S. Bureau of Census. (2004). *Global population at a glance: 2002 and beyond.* Retrieved http://www.census.gov/ipc/prod/wp02/wp02-1.pdf

Wakefield, M. K. (2004). A call to arms. *Nursing Economics, 22*(3), 166–167.

Wakefield, M. (2003). Change drivers for nursing and health care. *Nursing Economics, 21*(3), 150–151.

Yoho, M. J., Sridaromont, K., Tuong-Vi, H., & Decker, S. (2004). Student perspectives on the George Mason University 12th Annual Washington Health Policy Summer Institute. *Policy, Politics & Nursing Practice, 5*(4), 263–271.

SUGGESTED READINGS

Aaron, H. J. (2006). Longer life spans: Boon or burden? *Daedalus, 135*(1), 9–19.

Buerhaus, P., Donelan, K., Ulrich, B., Norman, L., & Dittus, R. (2005). State of the Registered Nurse workforce in the United States. *Nursing Economics, 23*(2), 6–12.

Buerhaus, P., Donelan, K., Ulrich, B., Norman, L., & Dittus, R. (2005). Six part series on the state of the Registered Nurse workforce in the United States. *Nursing Economics, 23*(2), 58–60.

Buerhaus, P., Donelan, K., Ulrich, B., Norman, L., Williams, M., & Dittus, R. (2005). Hospital RNs' and CNOs' perceptions of the impact of the nursing shortage on the quality of care. *Nursing Economics, 23*(5), 214–221.

Cohen, E., & DeBack, V. (1999). *The outcomes mandate: Case management in health care today.* St. Louis: Mosby.

Donlan, K., Buerhaus, P. I., Ulrich, B. T., Norman, L., & Dittus, R. (2005). Awareness and perceptions of the Johnson & Johnson campaign for nursing's future. *Nursing Economics, 23*(4), 150–156, 180.

Jones, A. (2004). U.S. faces oncoming aging boom. *National Catholic Reporter, 40*(26), 10–11.

Mundinger, M. O., Thomas, E., Smolowitz, J., & Honig, J. (2004). Essential health care: Affordable for all? *Nursing Economics, 22*(5), 239–244.

Siegel, E., & Bennett, P. (2006). Creating partnership through patient safety awareness week. *Nursing Economics, 24*(3), 162–165.

Smith, S. P., & Flarey, D. L. (1999). *Process-Centered Health Care Organizations.* Gaithersburg, MD: Aspen.

Smith, A. P. (2004). Patient advocacy: Roles for nurses and leaders. *Nursing Economics, 22*(2), 88–90.

Wetle, T., Wallace, S., Fortinsky, R., & Salsberg, E. (2004). Aging of America: A crisis for the health care workforce. *The Gerontologist, 44*(1), 131.

Strategic Planning and Organizing Patient Care

Amy Androwich O'Malley, MSN, RN ✛ Ida M. Androwich, PhD, RN, BC, FAAN

Strategic planning is a process by which we can envision the future and develop the necessary procedures and operations to influence and achieve that future (Clark Crouch, Management Consultant and Principal, The Resource Network).

OBJECTIVES

Upon completion of this chapter, the reader should be able to:

1. Understand the importance of an organization's mission and philosophy and the impact of these on the structure and behavior of the organization.

2. Define the purpose and identify the steps in the strategic planning process.

3. Articulate the importance of aligning the organization's strategic vision both with its mission, philosophy, and values and also with the goals and values of the communities and stakeholders served by the organization.

4. Apply a basic understanding of common organizational structures and the advantages and the disadvantages of each in identifying which structures would be best suited to meeting differing organizational objectives.

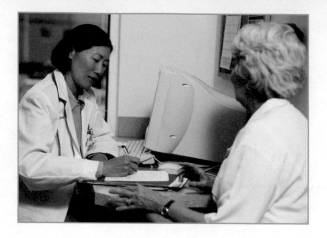

A friend is discussing her plans to step down as the Assistant Unit Coordinator on 3 West. You recall how pleased and excited she was to be offered the position only a few months ago and wonder what has changed. She begins to describe her frustration with never feeling that she had sufficient information for decision making nor receiving the information in a timely manner. She feels that this puts her in a poor position to be a staff and patient advocate for her unit. She states, "I feel as if my manager has so many areas that are taking up all her time, and she really can't concentrate on our unit's needs. It seems as if we are always putting out fires and never have a chance to step back and actually plan programs and operational processes that could make a big improvement on the unit. The organization's mission statement says that we value education, but I continually have to turn down requests from staff to go to educational programs because of inadequate staffing. We are not recruiting and hiring nurses for all our budgeted positions. There are plenty of nurses routinely scheduled on days and not nearly enough on evenings when most patients are now discharged. Consequently, we have our major needs for discharge planning and patient education in the evening and there is no plan for providing this necessary information in a consistent manner. The result is dissatisfied patients, staff, and physicians."

What are your thoughts about this situation?

What advice do you have for your friend?

Is this situation unusual and can it be improved? How?

There are increasing opportunities for nurses to become involved in strategic and tactical planning for the delivery of health care services in their organizations and communities. Yet, to be effective in leadership roles, nurses need a basic understanding of the way in which organizations are structured, how organizational systems function, and how to engage in the strategic planning process. In the past, many health care organizations were structured in a highly formal, top-down, militaristic manner. These bureaucratic organizations worked well in a relatively stable environment when communication channels could be hierarchical.

They tend not to be as useful in a dynamic health care system in which information needs and practice are rapidly changing. In addition, workers in today's health care systems are considered knowledge workers—professionals hired for their knowledge, skills, and expertise. They need a system that supports their ability to practice to the full extent of their professional accountability.

Leadership in the health care organizations of the twenty-first century demands competent nurses with different skill sets than in the past. That is because performance in a leadership role in today's highly complex health care environment requires a good understanding of how systems function and how to improve health care delivery. Yet health care providers, including professional nurses, have been slow to integrate this information into their clinical practice. Planning for continuous improvement of quality, service, and cost-effectiveness is a critical competency for nurses in twenty-first century health care organizations.

The seminal (1999) Institute of Medicine (IOM) report *To Err Is Human* states that preventable adverse events cause between 44,000 and 98,000 deaths each year at an annual cost of between $37.6 billion to $50 billion. That report and the follow-up IOM report, *Crossing the Quality Chasm* (2001), have changed the way we view quality and patient safety. It is now generally understood that patient safety is dependent on the implementation of collaborative teams and interdisciplinary focused care-delivery systems that address the realities of practice and patient care. Recent research studies stress that the way a nurse's work is organized is a major determinant of patient welfare. Consequently, nurses in leadership positions must be educationally prepared to be able to develop and implement sound models for the effective delivery of patient care. Although many health care organizations collect large sets of data and are beginning to use scientific methods to improve the services they render, these activities are typically fragmented, isolated from day-to-day nursing management, and lack alignment with organizational strategy. The American Nurses Association (ANA) concurs with the IOM (1999) that errors occur as a result of system failure rather than human failure.

This chapter will discuss the strategic planning process and the importance of aligning the organization's strategic vision with the mission, philosophy, and values of the organization and the communities served by the organization. Also, because the manner in which organizations are structured has an impact on their ability to be effective in providing care, it is important for nurses to have a good understanding of the structures that support and promote health care delivery.

Generally, the organization starts with a defined vision, purpose, and mission. The strategic planning process allows the organization to scan the environment and develop strategic goals based on changes in the environment. This is a process that occurs within the defined vision, purpose, and mission of the organization. The March of Dimes is a good example of an organization that was able to revise its mission in response to an environmental change. In 1938, the March of Dimes was established as the National Foundation for Infantile Paralysis (Polio). With funding provided by the organization, Dr. Jonas Salk was able to develop an experimental polio vaccine in 1952, and, in 1962, Dr. Sabin, also with funding from the March of Dimes, developed the oral polio vaccine. Today, virtually all American babies receive the vaccine to prevent polio, and there has not been a new case since 1991 in the United States. Consequently, since 1958, the March of Dimes has changed its mission to funding cutting-edge research and innovative programs to save babies from birth defects, premature births, and low birth weight (March of Dimes, 2006). Most organizations do not have such a dramatic need for mission change.

ORGANIZATIONAL VISION, PURPOSE, MISSION, PHILOSOPHY, VALUES

Every organization has a guiding vision and mission. Most often, the purpose and philosophy are explicitly stated and detailed in a formal mission statement. Typically, this mission statement reflects the organization's values and provides the reader with an indication of the behavior and strategic actions that can be expected from that organization. Most health care organizations have mission statements that speak to providing high quality or excellence in patient care. Some mission statements focus exclusively on providing care, whereas others assume a broader view and consider the education of health care professionals and the promotion of research as contributing to their broader mission. The mission of other organizations may be community based, and these organizations consequently will focus on providing community outreach and population-based services to a specific community or population within a community.

MISSION STATEMENT

The **mission statement** is a formal expression of the purpose or reason for existence of the organization. It is the organization's declaration of its primary driving force or its vision of the manner in which it believes care should be delivered. (For examples of actual mission statements, refer to the "Exploring the Web" section at the end of the chapter.)

PHILOSOPHY

The **philosophy of an organization** is typically embedded in the mission statement. It is, in essence, a value statement of the principles and beliefs that direct the organization's behavior. A careful reading of the mission statement will usually provide a good understanding of

---

CRITICAL THINKING 10-1

Examine these two mission statements and then respond to the questions that follow.

Hospital A: "Our mission is to ensure the highest quality of care for the patients in our community. We believe that each patient has the right to the most innovative care that current science and technology can provide. To that end, we have assembled a world-renowned medical staff who will strive to ensure that the latest developments in medical science are used to combat disease."

Hospital B: "Our mission is to provide excellence in care to all. Our health care staff, nurses, practitioners, and other professionals believe that care can best be provided in an atmosphere of collaboration and partnership with our patients and community. We believe in education—for our patients, for our staff, and for future health care providers. At all times, we strive for optimal health promotion and the prevention of disease and disability."

Which of these institutions do you think would be more likely to have a patient lecture series on, "Living with Diabetes"? Value the contributions of nursing? Provide experimental therapy for cancer? Be open to scheduling routine patient care visits for uninsured patients?

the institutional philosophy or value system. Mission statements with phrases such as "without consideration for ability to pay," "with respect for the dignity of each elderly resident," "a brighter future for all children," or "vigorous rehabilitation to maximize each individual's utmost potential" provide clues to the type of service that you could expect from an organization. In the best of worlds, there is congruence among the stated mission vision philosophy values, and the behavior of the organization.

Sometimes, this consequence is not the case. For example, does the mission statement read, "Our patients are our highest priority," only to organize the environment and services in such a manner that there are inadequate directional signs and registration staff? The result is that these "highest priority" patients are often not able to find their way around the health care organization and have unduly long waits for registration.

When a mission is formally stated, quality can be measured (Table 10-1).

It is always important to assess an organization's mission, vision, and values prior to considering employment because when important individual and organizational values collide, it is likely to be a constant source of frustration for the employee and employer.

EXAMINING A MISSION STATEMENT

In 1956, the United Mine Workers of America (UMWA) dedicated the Miners Memorial Hospital Association's (MMHA) facilities, which consisted of ten hospitals in Kentucky and West Virginia and included services to patients from Appalachia. This hospital system soon became a model for similar health care organizations across the country. The MMHA system was such a rarity

that one publication described the newly opened hospital locations as "ten places where hospital and medical care history will be written." Today, the health care system, now known as Appalachian Regional Healthcare (ARH), to more accurately describe its far-ranging activities, continues its mission by offering residents of Eastern Kentucky and Southern West Virginia a local option for state-of-the-art technology and advanced quality health care services. Since its inception, ARH has been committed to growing and meeting the needs of their communities (Table 10-2).

STRATEGIC PLANNING

As Lewis Carroll observed in *Alice's Adventures in Wonderland*, "If you don't know where you are going, any road will do." A health care organization needs to have a good idea of where it fits into its environment and what types of programs and services are needed and demanded by its customers or stakeholders. This is true at a broad organizational level as well as at a unit level. It is important that a nurse manager have an understanding of which programs and services are valued by a patient population and plan for how the unit's ongoing activities fit in with the overall strategy of the larger organization.

STRATEGIC PLANNING DEFINITION

A **strategic plan** can be defined as the sum total or outcome of the processes by which an organization engages in environmental analysis, goal formulation, and strategy

REAL WORLD INTERVIEW

Strategic planning and organizing patient care are critical issues in the field of clinical information systems. The strategic planning process consists of several phases, each of which requires specific activities to design and implement an electronic health record. One important area to consider is the selection of a standardized coded terminology for documenting patient care. I recommend that the Clinical Care Classification (CCC) System or another similar system be selected as the terminology of choice. It is important to select a research-based and ANA-recognized documentation terminology, such as CCC, Systematized Nomenclature of Medicine (SNOMED), North American Nursing Diagnosis Association (NANDA), Nursing Intervention Classification (NIC), and Nursing Outcomes Classification (NOC), Omaha, or the International Classification for Nursing Practice. These allow nurses to document nursing diagnoses, nursing interventions and actions, and patient outcomes. This documentation is critical in the development of a computerized information system that supports and informs nursing practice.

Virginia K. Saba, EdD, RN, FAAN, FACMI
Developer and Consultant, CCC System
Arlington, Virginia
Distinguished Scholar, Adjunct
Georgetown University
Washington, DC

TABLE 10-1   MISSION, GOALS, AND QUALITY MEASURES

Mission

The Peoples Choice Healthcare Center provides excellent health care to all patients through partnerships with patients and the community and collaboration with nursing and medical, practitioners, and other health care staff. We believe in continuous education for patients, health care staff, and future health care providers. We are committed to optimal health care promotion and prevention of disease and disability.

Goals

1. Collaborate with all health care staff to improve patient care
2. Increase customer satisfaction scores
3. Increase number of emergency room visits
4. Increase patient days
5. Increase use of computers by all staff
6. Increase funding for staff's continued education
7. Encourage all staff to attend one education program yearly
8. Increase number of specialty certifications of staff
9. Monitor nurse-sensitive patient outcomes, such as incidence of cardiac arrest, UTI, upper GI bleeding, thrombophlebitis, failure to rescue, and so forth
10. Decrease medication errors

Quality Measures for Emergency Department

Customer/Patient
1. Increase in patient satisfaction
2. Increase in customer return
3. Decrease in patient complaints
4. Increase in market share
5. Decrease in repeat asthma patient visits
6. Develop patient education materials explaining norms for ER stays, well and ill child care, and so on
7. Develop evidence-based standards for care of patients with cardiac arrest, UTI, upper GI bleeding, and thrombophlebitis
8. Review all Emergency Department deaths

Financial
1. Increase use of computers on all units
2. Monitor budget compliance
3. Improve nurse staffing ratios
4. Develop computerized order-entry system for medications

Internal Processes
1. Achieve 90% on key Performance Improvement measures
2. Decrease sick time and overtime by 10%
3. Increase number of nursing research projects
4. Achieve magnet status
5. Increase use of Best Practice Educational Materials for all patients and staff
6. Increase participation of nursing, medicine, unlicensed assistive personnel, and pharmacy staff in quality improvement activities
7. Arrange for all staff to attend one outside conference yearly
8. Set up nursing journal club meetings monthly
9. Set up interdisciplinary committee on medication administration safety

Employee Growth and Learning
1. 50% of the nursing department join a nursing professional association
2. All nurses working in the ED are certified in ACLS and PALS trauma nursing
3. One-third of nurses are continuing their nursing education
4. 50% of all staff are cross-trained and can work in ICU and ER
5. 90% of employees are very satisfied
6. 90% of staff are retained
7. All nurses are able to use the computer for patient information, to search literature, and so forth
8. 20% of nursing staff present a community program on topics such as stroke and so forth annually

Source: Kelly, P. (2004). *Essentials of nursing leadership and management.* Clifton Park, NY: Thomson Delmar Learning.

TABLE 10-2	MISSION, VISION, AND VALUES OF APPALACHIAN REGIONAL HEALTHCARE (ARH)

ARH Mission: To improve the health and promote the well-being of all the people in Central Appalachia in partnership with our communities.

ARH Vision: To become the most respected and admired health care organization in Kentucky and West Virginia.

ARH Values: Compassion, integrity, respect and trust are the values that guide ARH. The system also values the safety of patients and employees while providing excellent facilities and clinical and administrative quality for the residents of Central Appalachia.

Source: www.arh.org.

development with the purpose of organizational growth and renewal. Drucker (1973) defines strategic planning as "a continuous, systematic process of making risk-taking decisions today with the greatest possible knowledge of their effects on the future" (p. 125). Strategic planning is ongoing and is especially needed whenever the organization is experiencing problems or internal/external review problems.

PURPOSE OF STRATEGIC PLANNING

The purpose of strategic planning is twofold. First, it is important that everyone has the same idea or vision for where the organization is headed, and second, a good plan can help to ensure that the needed resources are available to carry out the initiatives that have been identified as important to the unit or agency. In addition, a clear plan allows the manager to select among seemingly equal alternatives based on the alternatives' potential to move the organization toward the desired end goal.

STEPS IN STRATEGIC PLANNING PROCESS

In any strategic planning process, there are steps to be followed. This process is similar to the nursing process. You assess and plan before implementing a nursing treatment. It is equally important when developing an organizational-, unit-, or program plan to progress in a systematic manner. Table 10-3 lists the steps in the strategic planning process.

ENVIRONMENTAL ASSESSMENT

An environmental or a situational assessment requires a broad view of the organization's current environment. For example, an environmental analysis of the type of undergraduate nursing education that would be needed for the twenty-first century professional nurse led one school of nursing to begin planning a curriculum revision that would incorporate the increasing emphasis on community-focused care. In addition, this analysis of the environment led faculty to understand that new models

REAL WORLD INTERVIEW

The pivotal value of strategic planning is that it requires an organization to focus on its raison d'être, its mission, and to test how its operations are leading to accomplishment of that mission. Determined by the degree of dynamic change present in both its internal and external environments, an organization's strategic planning may extend years, or only months, into the future. However, at least annually, the strategic plan must be examined, reasserted as appropriate, and used as the standard against which short-term initiatives are measured for congruency with mission accomplishment.

Laura J. Nosek, PhD, RN
Health Care Consultant
Auborn, Ohio

TABLE 10-3	**STEPS IN STRATEGIC PLANNING PROCESS**
1. Perform environmental assessment. 2. Conduct stakeholder analysis. 3. Review literature for evidence-based best practices. 4. Determine congruence with organizational mission. 5. Identify planning goals and objectives. 6. Estimate resources required for the plan.	7. Prioritize according to available resources. 8. Identify timelines and responsibilities. 9. Develop a marketing plan. 10. Write and communicate the business plan/strategic plan. 11. Evaluate.

for clinical education will be needed to promote improved and expanded linkages between education and practice.

It is important that the internal environment as well as the external environment be carefully appraised. Whereas the external environmental assessment is broad based and attempts to view trends and future issues and needs that could impact the organization, the internal assessment seeks to inventory the organization's assets and liabilities.

SWOT ANALYSIS

A **SWOT analysis** is a tool that is frequently used to conduct these environmental assessments. SWOT stands for strengths, weaknesses, opportunities, and threats. A SWOT analysis identifies both strengths and weaknesses in the internal environment and opportunities and threats in the external environment. The SWOT analysis is useful both for initial brainstorming and for a more formal planning document. Figure 10-1 is an example of a SWOT analysis that could be conducted by a university health care center (Jones & Beck, 1996).

COMMUNITY AND STAKEHOLDER ASSESSMENT

A frequently overlooked but highly important area for analysis is the stakeholder assessment. A **stakeholder** is any person, group, or organization that has a vested interest in the program or project under review. A **stakeholder assessment** is a systematic consideration of all potential stakeholders to ensure that the needs of each of these stakeholders are incorporated in the planning phase.

For a program to be successful, the involvement of those who will be affected is essential. This is true whether the stakeholders are in the community or the stakeholders are the unit staff who will be affected by a proposed strategic plan. When stakeholders are not involved in the project planning, they do not gain a sense of ownership and may accept a program or strategic goals only with limited enthusiasm, or not at all.

REAL WORLD INTERVIEW

The Electronic Health Record (EHR) plays an essential role in achieving the quality, safety, and efficiency goals that are defined in our strategic plan. Automation of the EHR is an evolutionary process whereby specific application implementations are sequenced and timed in accordance with the priorities established within the strategic plan. For this reason, the plan for automating the EHR is closely connected to the strategic plan. The financial and clinical indicators used for evaluating success of the strategic plan are similar to the indicators used for evaluating the success of the EHR implementation plan. These indicators include improvement in quality patient outcomes, reduction in adverse events, and increases in efficiency, along with many other desired outcomes as defined by the organization. An effective model in deriving value from both the strategic plan and the use of information technology is one where nursing takes the lead in setting the critical foundation for success. Nursing has a critical role in leading the process and ultimately driving the creation of new paradigms in improving healthcare.

Rosemary Kennedy, RN, MBA
Chief Nursing Informatics Officer, Siemens Medical Solutions
Philadelphia, Pennsylvania

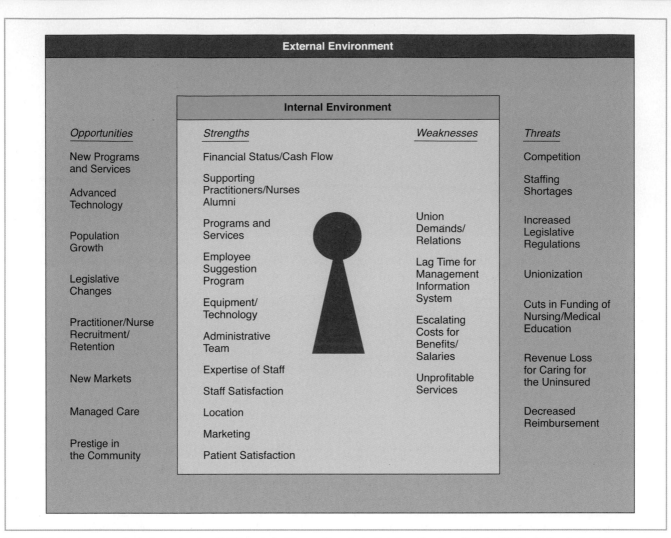

External Environment

Internal Environment

Opportunities	*Strengths*	*Weaknesses*	*Threats*
New Programs and Services	Financial Status/Cash Flow		Competition
Advanced Technology	Supporting Practitioners/Nurses Alumni		Staffing Shortages
Population Growth	Programs and Services	Union Demands/ Relations	Increased Legislative Regulations
Legislative Changes	Employee Suggestion Program	Lag Time for Management Information System	Unionization
Practitioner/Nurse Recruitment/ Retention	Equipment/ Technology	Escalating Costs for Benefits/ Salaries	Cuts in Funding of Nursing/Medical Education
New Markets	Administrative Team		Revenue Loss for Caring for the Uninsured
	Expertise of Staff	Unprofitable Services	
Managed Care	Staff Satisfaction		Decreased Reimbursement
	Location		
Prestige in the Community	Marketing		
	Patient Satisfaction		

Figure 10-1 Key to success in strategic planning: SWOT analysis. (*Source:* Compiled with information from *Decision Making in Nursing* by R. Jones and S. Beck, 1996, Clifton Park, NY: Thomson Delmar Learning.)

OTHER METHODS OF ASSESSMENT

A number of methods can be used to support involvement in the strategic planning process. Thoughtful planning is required to determine the method and when to use the method.

SURVEYS AND QUESTIONNAIRES Frequently, surveys or questionnaires are used when there are a large number of stakeholders and there is a general idea of the options available. For example, staff might be polled to see whether they would attend continuing education and which days and times would be most desirable.

FOCUS GROUPS AND INTERVIEWS Focus groups are small groups of individuals selected because of a common characteristic, such as a recent diagnosis of diabetes. The focus group is invited to meet in a group and respond to questions about a topic in which they are expected to have interest or expertise. An example of a

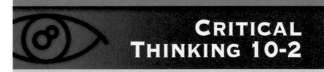

CRITICAL THINKING 10-2

Think about a community organization with which you are familiar. What is the mission of your organization? Compare it to the mission in Table 10-1. Is it clearly communicated to the stakeholders? Are the activities of your organization reflective of its mission? If not, why do you think this is so?

focus group would be a group of patients who have recently had experiences with childbirth. They might be asked to come together to discuss their obstetric experiences at the institution in the hope that the discussion will lead to insights or information that could be used for improving care or marketing services in the future. Focus groups are usually more time-consuming and expensive to conduct than questionnaires or surveys. They work best when the topic is broad and the options are not clear. For example, an organization might conduct patient focus groups to determine what programs would be of most interest to a community.

ADVISORY BOARD   Large projects often benefit from the formation of an advisory board, selected from various constituencies affected by a proposed program. The advisory board does not have formal authority over a pro-

gram, but it is instrumental in reviewing the planned program and making recommendations and suggestions. Because the advisory board is deliberately selected to reflect representation from various stakeholders and areas of expertise, it is expected that the board will be able to identify potential concerns and provide sound guidance for the program.

REVIEW OF LITERATURE ON SIMILAR PROGRAMS   A review of the literature should be completed prior to strategic planning or beginning any new project or program. This allows the project team to identify similar programs, their structures and organization, potential

EVIDENCE FROM THE LITERATURE

Citation: Atencio, B., Cohen, J., & Gorenberg, B. (2003). Nurse retention: Is it worth it? *Nursing Economic$, 21*(6), 262–268, 299.

Discussion: The predicted nursing shortage is anticipated to reach one million by the year 2010. This is due to multiple reasons, including the aging of the nursing workforce, nursing faculty shortages, perceived stress and low job satisfaction, the economy, and an increased number of opportunities for nurses. As a result of the nursing shortage, it is essential for hospitals to evaluate current retention strategies to keep valued employees. The primary reason for the aging of the RN workforce is the decline in the number of younger women choosing nursing. Unless this trend is reversed, long-term workforce needs will not be met. It is essential to retain nurses during the current nursing shortage. Extensive research has been done on the importance of nursing turnover in an organization and its costs. Job satisfaction is closely linked with retaining nurses. It is essential for hospitals to find ways to retain current nurses or the turnover cycle will continue. If an institution is not successful in retaining nurses, nurses will leave the institution for a new hospital with such attractions as salary sign-on bonuses. It is essential that a hospital develop new and different ways to keep nursing staff.

Although there are many reasons for retaining current nursing staff, the fact that increased nursing satisfaction and nursing retention leads to increased patient satisfaction is an important one. The latest research shows that not only is the cost of orientation lost when a nurse leaves a position prematurely, but there is also a loss to the hospital in terms of lost productivity. In the past, nurses have often been viewed as replaceable widgets, that is, if some leave, recruit more. In the future, the successful institution will understand that nurses need to be seen as human capital and a valuable institutional resource. No longer will the past measures be adequate to retain nurses. Innovative ways to retain nurses must be attempted. The role of nurse recruiter must be changed to focus on retaining current employees. This new role of nurse recruiter/nurse retainer (NR) will focus on the human capital of nursing and will help keep this nursing capital within an institution.

One of the main focuses of the NR will be to track nursing turnover data and conduct exit interviews. In the past, there has not been enough review of the causes of nurse turnover and ways to prevent nurse turnover. The NR can be expected to work with nurse managers to address unit-based issues, including promoting early employee intervention to keep nurses and facilitating potential transfers in and out of the unit. The NR can help to facilitate this transfer process, including using "the right fit" interview to ensure employee transfers to the best area. The NR can provide in-services on the clinical ladder to draw more nurses into an institution's clinical ladder. In the past, clinical ladders had proven to be an effective way to retain staff and provide greater nursing satisfaction. The NR can work to help decrease the total number of nursing vacancies. In the recruitment role, the NR can continue to attract external candidates. In the retaining role, the NR can focus on increasing the satisfaction of current nursing staff. This reduces the number of external positions being recruited for. As the latest nursing shortage emerges, it is essential that recruitment and retention efforts remain focused and work together to decrease nursing vacancies. Because all hospitals are facing the same shortage, new and different techniques must be applied to retain staff.

Implications for Practice: The dual role of nurse recruiter/nurse retainer has the potential to show not only an increase in nursing staff satisfaction but also significant savings from orientation costs.

REAL WORLD INTERVIEW

Loyola University Chicago is a national, independent, urban Catholic University. The Marcella Niehoff School of Nursing is one of over 60 departments. The School of Nursing is housed in Chicago at the Lake Shore campus but also maintains about half of all faculty offices, nursing classrooms, and laboratory space in suburban Maywood at Loyola University Health System facilities. The School of Nursing has recently changed its reporting structure to report to the President of the Health System. Loyola University Health System is an academic medical center that includes Foster McGraw Hospital, a 536-bed facility that is a major referral center for the Chicago metropolitan area and the Midwest. It also includes Mulcahy Outpatient Department, the Cardinal Bernadin Cancer Center, and the Stritch School of Medicine. Both Loyola University Chicago and the Loyola University Health System are dedicated to higher education, and emphasize excellence in teaching, research, and community service. Prior to the early 1990s, there was little involvement with the community in which the Medical Center is located. At that time, members of the professional schools and the health system met with representatives of the Maywood community to determine major health issues and concerns. At a conference, they identified teen pregnancy, hypertension, sexually transmitted diseases, HIV, substance abuse, and access to health professions for minority youth as major concerns. Since many of these concerns centered on issues of youth, the concept of Healthy Teens 2000 was established. In 1993, the School of Nursing and the Stritch School of Medicine received a grant funding the Healthy Teens 2000 program. The award was from the Pew Foundation's Health of the Public Initiative, a national award supporting academic health professionals who partner with local communities to identify and intervene in community health concerns. The Healthy Teens 2000 program coordinator wanted to build an infrastructure that would provide widespread support for the project from the community, the University, and the health system. Consequently, volunteers from each of these areas were sought for an advisory board. Representatives from public offices, faith-based organizations, schools, parents, youth, the local Chamber of Commerce, the police department, educators, the University, the School of Nursing, the School of Medicine, and the health care system were invited to take an active role. Everyone was to be aware of the Healthy Teens Program and what it hoped to accomplish, and to participate in reaching those goals.

Throughout its many years of operation, high school students mentored younger youth on healthy lifestyle choices. During this period, the unmet health needs of high school students surfaced, as did the need to establish a school-based health center at Proviso East High School, located in Maywood. To begin the process of strategic planning and generating funding for the site, a survey was administered in 1999 to a sample of Proviso East students to determine health needs and feelings toward the creation of a school-based health center. In November of 2000, the School of Nursing was awarded over $2 million in grants from the Health Resources Services Administration and the Illinois Department of Human Services to develop a School-based Health Center at Proviso East High School. The School-based Health Center was successfully established and as a result of positive program outcomes, it received additional federal funding to support the ongoing project in 2006. Members of the Healthy Teens Advisory Board were the first to envision such a project and continued to meet until recently, when the program was incorporated into the School-based Health Center.

Carolyn Johnson, MSN
Program Coordinator—Healthy Teen 2000
Maywood, Illinois

problems and pitfalls, and successes. This is an ongoing process that includes tentatively identifying programs, searching the literature for successes and issues, and then refining the program ideas.

BEST PRACTICES Identifying best practices or evidence-based innovations that have been adopted with success by other organizations can facilitate strategic planning. Consequently, nurses planning to develop a new program need to carefully examine the existing evidence and practices prior to beginning planning.

RELATIONSHIP OF STRATEGIC PLANNING TO THE ORGANIZATION'S MISSION

All strategic planning, goals, and objectives must be examined with an eye to the purpose or mission of the organization. Sometimes, organizations get into trouble when they move too far afield of their core mission. Consequently, each new project needs to be evaluated in light of its congruence with the main mission that

CRITICAL THINKING 10-3

You have just read about the Healthy Teens 2000 project in the Real World Interview. Use the description of that program to answer the following questions.

Do you think that community involvement was important in the success of this program? Why? Why weren't the health problems identified earlier by the Health Care System and health professionals?

What do you think would have been the response of the community if Loyola attempted to tell the community members their problems instead of working collaboratively to identify major health issues? What kinds of strategies did the project use for building community support?

Are there any stakeholders who you think could have been included but were not? What do you see as key ingredients for making a community program such as this one successful?

has been identified. It is fine for an organization to move to another project, but only if the new project is in line with the mission. Otherwise, there is a risk that the new programs will drain energy from the main mission. Figure 10-2 depicts the relationship of strategic planning to the organization's vision and mission.

PLANNING GOALS AND PRIORITIZING OBJECTIVES

After all strategic goals and objectives have been identified, they need to be prioritized according to strategic importance, resources required, and time and effort involved. A timeline should be set. This will allow a thoughtful evaluation of each goal and objective and the degree to which each can be implemented in the specified time frame and with the available resources.

SETTING A TIME LINE WITH RESPONSIBILITIES IDENTIFIED

Setting a time line for completion of a strategic plan is similar to the prioritization process in that the strategic importance, resources, and effort required are major considerations. Realistic timelines and individual responsibilities must be developed, specified, clarified, and communicated to all stakeholders. This will help to avoid misunderstandings and unmet expectations.

DEVELOPING A MARKETING PLAN

If a part of the strategic planning involves new programming for external audiences or if only internal redesign or restructuring is involved, the strategic plan, goals, and objectives will need to be communicated to all involved constituencies. Such communication will be needed, for example, when an institution is planning to implement a

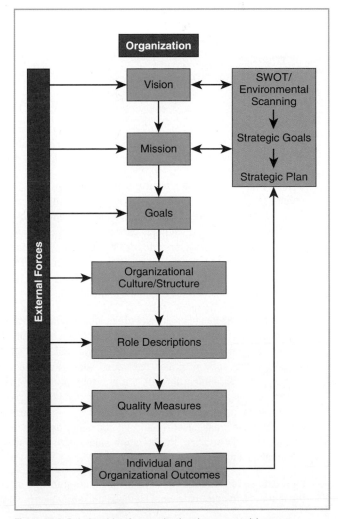

Figure 10-2 Relationship of strategic planning to organizing care.

new information system to ensure that it remains competitive in the market. Designing, implementing, training, and evaluating this new system will require substantive changes in work flow and in the way that employees carry out their day-to-day work processes. If there has not been adequate thought to communication across the organization about the project, there is less chance of success and a greater risk of poor cooperation.

A marketing plan insures that all stakeholders have the needed information. A solid marketing plan is especially important when there are proposed new programs for consumers. Depending on the program and the target audience, marketing approaches will need to be matched with an understanding of desired consumer behaviors (Thomas, 2004).

ORGANIZATIONAL STRUCTURE

Organizations are structured or organized to facilitate the execution of their mission, goals, reporting lines, and communication within the organization. This is true of entire organizations as well as individual nursing units. There are a number of ways to describe organizational structures that involve classifying them by identifying selected characteristics. Each of these characteristics tends to exist on a continuum. For example, under the category of type or level of authority in an organizational structure, a highly bureaucratic, highly authoritarian structure is at one end of the continuum and a highly democratic, participative structure is at the other end. The highly authoritarian model is seen in the military and is well suited for the purpose of the military. When decisions need to be made quickly, with clarity and not with challenges or discussion, as in a battle situation, a highly authoritarian organizational structure works well.

An example at the other end of the continuum would be a multidisciplinary group of professionals meeting to determine the care management of a patient or patient population. An example of this group might be a hospice team task force made up of nurses, social workers, practitioners, home care aides, bereavement specialists, and chaplains, all meeting to discuss the care planning for a dying patient. In this situation, it will be important for team members of each discipline to freely

EVIDENCE FROM THE LITERATURE

Citation: Ortiz, J., McGilligan, K., & Kelly, P. (2004). Duration of breast milk expression among working mothers enrolled in an employer-sponsored lactation program. *Pediatric Nursing, 30*(2), 111–119.

Discussion: An institution, aware of the impending nursing shortage, identified a strategic planning goal of increasing nurse employee satisfaction in the organization. The institution determined that one method of supporting the large number of staff currently breastfeeding was to improve the work environment in this area. The positive benefits of breastfeeding are well documented in the literature, yet many barriers are associated with successful breastfeeding in the workplace. Many nurses, as employed health care providers and breastfeeding mothers, face these challenges in their work environments. Although protocols exist to support breastfeeding in general, none were found that were designed to support successful breastfeeding in the working mother. As the institution was interested in increasing nurse satisfaction and improving retention, it developed the following protocol based on the evidence found in the literature.

The protocol was based on the two areas focused on in most of the literature, available support in the work environment and education for the mother. Staff members requesting a maternity leave would receive informational materials outlining the types of physical and emotional support available in the workplace as well as the educational resources. This is consistent with evidence suggesting that early education, motivation, support, and planning promotes successful breastfeeding. Support was demonstrated in the work environment through the provision of a comfortable, appealing, private room for pumping milk. Refrigeration and needed supplies were made available. Unit managers were expected to provide break coverage for nurses to pump milk in the same manner as for work breaks and lunch hours. A business case can be made for the cost-effectiveness of the program in that the costs of the break coverage and environmental adaptations would be expected to be balanced positively by lower absenteeism and turnover. In addition, the literature supports that breast-fed infants have fewer illnesses, which are associated with less maternal absenteeism.

Implications for Practice: When planning a program that involves workplace redesign, it is important to assess the evidence in the literature to determine what methods and strategies have worked well in the past.

contribute according to their particular area of knowledge and expertise. An organizational structure such as this can function successfully only in a participative, democratic manner.

TYPES OF ORGANIZATIONAL STRUCTURES

Most often, the existing organizational structures are communicated by means of an organizational chart. Figure 10-3 is an example of an organizational chart for a typical acute-care general hospital (Shortell & Kaluzny, 2006). This organization has a tall bureaucratic structure with many layers in the hierarchy or chain of command and a centralized formal authority in the board of trustees. It represents a formal, top-down reporting structure.

For example, three middle managers report to the nursing vice president, two first-line unit nurse managers (NMs) report to each middle manager. Two service providers report to each first-line unit NM.

MATRIX STRUCTURE

Today, given the greater complexity of the health care system, more organizations are using matrix structures. Figure 10-4 shows a matrix design (Shortell & Kaluzny, 2006).

FLAT VERSUS TALL STRUCTURE

Organizations are considered flat when there are few layers in the reporting structure. A tall organization would have many layers in the chain of command. An example of a flat organizational structure in a hospital would be one director of nursing with two head nurses reporting to her, one for maternal and child patient care units and one for medical-surgical patient care units (Figure 10-5). Contrast this flat type of structure in Figure 10-5 with Figure 10-6, which has many layers.

DECENTRALIZED VERSUS CENTRALIZED STRUCTURE

The terms *centralized* and *decentralized* refer to the degree to which an organization has spread its lines of authority, power, and communication. A tall, bureaucratic design like that in Figure 10-6 would be considered highly centralized. A matrix design like that in Figure 10-4 would be on the decentralized end of the continuum. As can be seen in Figure 10-4, the nursing manager can interface with the Alzheimer's disease program manager without going through a central, hierarchical core, as would happen in a bureaucratic structure like that in Figure 10-3.

Other characteristics or attributes can be used to assess organizations. Many typologies exist that may be used

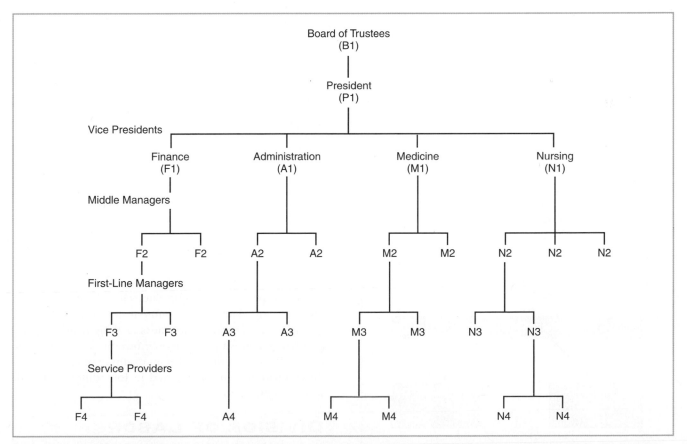

Figure 10-3 Organizational chart, formal tall bureaucratic, multilayered authority structure: Acute care general hospital. (From *Health Care Management: Organization Design and Behavior* by S. Shortell & A. Kaluzny, 2006 (5th ed). Clifton Park, NY: Thomson Delmar Learning.)

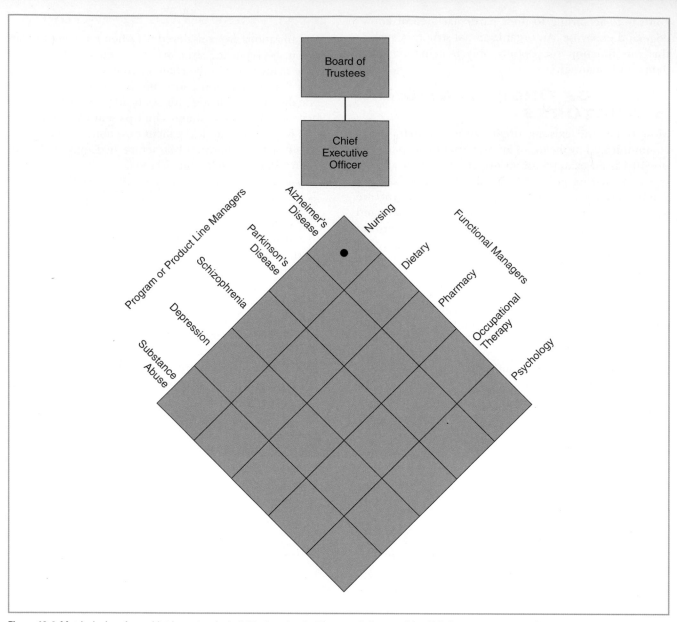

Figure 10-4 Matrix design: A psychiatric center. An individual worker in this example is part of the Alzheimer program as well as a member of the nursing department. (From *Health Care Management: Organization Design and Behavior* by S. Shortell & A. Kaluzny, 2006 (5th ed). Clifton Park, NY: Thomson Delmar Learning.)

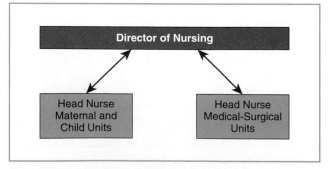

Figure 10-5 Example of a flat organizational structure.

for this purpose. For example, Shortell and Kaluzny (2006) suggest using external environment, mission/goals, work groups/work design, organizational design, interorganizational relationships, change/innovation, and strategic issues. Refer to Table 10-4 for an example of how some of these attributes can be assessed in four different health service organizations.

DIVISION OF LABOR

The way that the labor force is divided or organized has an impact on how the mission is accomplished. The

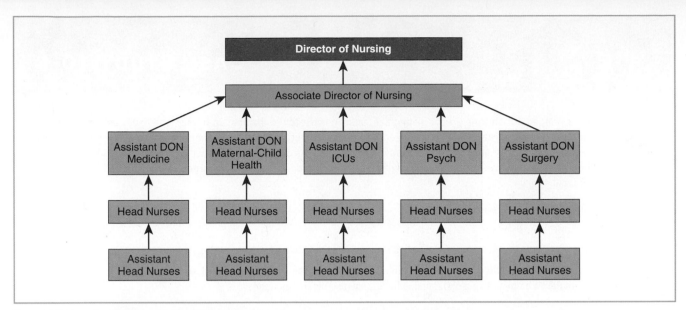

Figure 10-6 Example of a tall organizational structure.

	TABLE 10-4	**ATTRIBUTES OF FOUR HEALTH SERVICES ORGANIZATIONS**		
Attribute	**Health Maintenance Organizations (HMOs)**	**Home Health Care Agencies**	**Hospitals**	**Pharmaceutical Companies**
Mission/goals	Primary care emphasis; keep people well	Quality of life; maintaining functional status	Acute care emphasis; curing illness	Research and development (R&D) emphasis; new product development
Work group/ work design	Primary care teams; coordinated referrals	Simple design: primary nursing; one-on-one patient contact	Departmental and across departmental teams; high need for coordination	Separation of functions possible; R&D vs. sales; relatively low need for coordination
Organizational design	Functional and divisional	Functional	Divisional, product line, or matrix	Divisional and strategic business units
Change innovation	Creates and responds to new patient care management approaches	Respond to demographic and social changes	Respond to the new paradigm; implement new role within vertically integrated systems	Respond to new product development demands
Strategic issues	Expand the concept of managed care	Demonstrate continuing value, and therefore, reimbursement for services	Fit into an expanded and changing delivery system	Decrease time to develop new drugs

Source: Compiled with information from Shortell, S. & Kaluzny, A. (2006). *Health care management: Organization design and behavior.* Clifton Park, NY: Thomson Delmar Learning.

A patient developed a rash from a new medication, unbeknownst to the medication nurse, who never asked about any signs of problems. The treatment nurse noticed the rash during a routine dressing change but never thought to inquire about any new dietary or medication changes. It was not until the time of discharge when the patient read the drug information sheet advising that any skin changes be reported that the patient asked the discharge planning nurse if the week-old rash was significant.

What could have been done differently?

Was anyone at fault? Who?

Why is good communication especially important in a situation in which there is a functional division of labor?

What types of problems could you expect if staff members focused on their own tasks and failed to communicate with each other about the patient's emotional, psychosocial, educational, and discharge needs?

organizational chart in Figure 10-7 graphically depicts a functional design of how the formal authority in this organization is structured. At the highest level, the board of trustees delegates authority to the chief executive officer, who delegates to the two vice presidents. The vice president of Patient Care Services has five directors, that is, directors of Social Work, Rehabilitation, Pharmacy, Nursing, and Health Records departments. The nurse managers (NMs) of Unit A and Unit B report to their department director of nursing. The charge nurse reports to the NM of Unit B. The treatment nurse and the medication nurse report to the charge nurse. In this functional design, the division of labor is efficient and specialized. A danger with functional division of labor is that each individual may be so focused on a specific area that he or she has little perspective about the overall picture. For example, a treatment nurse may focus only on treatments and have little information about the total patient.

In the matrix structure shown in Figure 10-4, the structure was less important, and the workforce roles and reporting relationships are based on the project or task to be accomplished, rather than on a rigid hierarchy. An example of this is the planning involved in the preparation for a Joint Commission (JC), formerly Joint Commission on Accreditation of Healthcare Organization (JCAHO), review. The JC team could be composed of various individuals at varying levels of responsibility and from programs across the organization, but they could interact with staff at all levels and report as a task force at a high level in the organization.

SPAN OF CONTROL

The term *span of control* is used to designate the number of individuals that report to one person. If the span of control is too narrow, an organization may become "top heavy," and much time may be wasted in unnecessary communications up and down the chain of command, resulting in lost efficiency. On the other hand, if the span of control is too broad, it is difficult for one manager to give adequate attention to the support and development of all the individuals that report to him or her.

ROLES AND RESPONSIBILITIES

Note that exact roles and responsibilities within each level and division are not defined on the organizational charts beyond specifying the given division, for example, nursing. Scope of responsibilities, specific duties, and specific job requirements are found in documents such as individual job or position descriptions.

REPORTING RELATIONSHIPS

An organizational chart, such as the one in Figure 10-7, allows you to determine the formal reporting relationships, which are shown with a solid line. Sometimes dotted lines are used in an organizational chart to depict dual or secondary reporting relationships. An example of this might be the role of the director of performance improvement. This individual might directly report to the chief executive officer but also have position accountabilities to the board of trustees. The formal reporting relationships may or may not reflect the actual communications that occur within the institution.

BASIS FOR DIVISION OF LABOR

There are a number of ways to divide the workload in an organization. The important consideration is that the

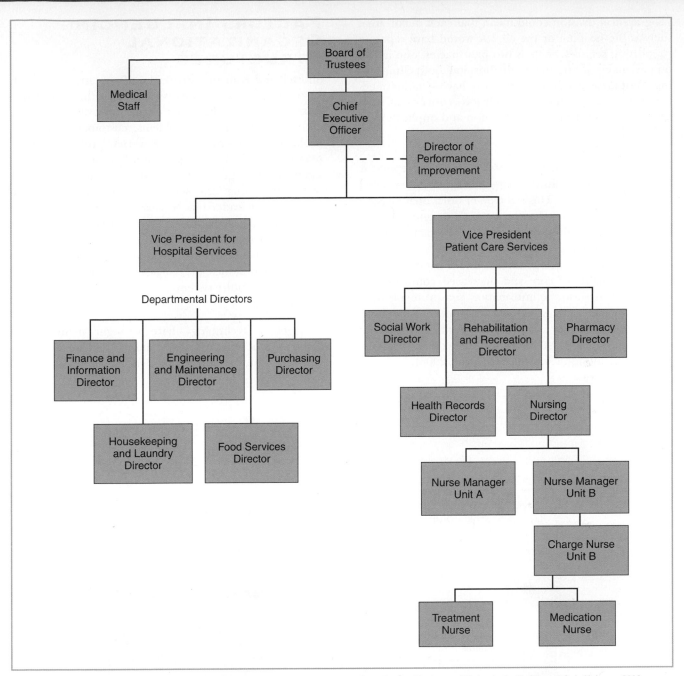

Figure 10-7 A functional design: Nursing home. (From *Health Care Management: Organization Design and Behavior* by S. Shortell & A. Kaluzny, 2006 (5th ed). Clifton Park, NY: Thomson Delmar Learning.)

manner in which the work is distributed should match the goals of the organizational unit and should contribute maximally to the efficient, effective attainment of the desired outcomes.

FUNCTIONAL DIVISION OF LABOR In a functional division of labor, work is divided by job activity. Nursing care that would be distributed in this manner might consist of a medication nurse role, a treatment nurse role, and an education or a discharge planner role.

Each nurse would be specialized and would potentially become highly proficient in a given functional role.

DIVISION OF LABOR BY GEOGRAPHIC AREA Care delivery divided according to geography or location can be efficient. It might consist of the hospital and ambulatory care, or at smaller unit levels, the North Team and the West Team. Frequently, care provided by home health agencies is divided by geographic district for efficiency in travel. At the health care system level, geographical division could mean that each major area, such as the hospital or the clinics, would have separate supporting services, such as two pharmacies, one in the outpatient clinic and one in the hospital. Both clinic and inpatient areas could, and often do, have separate medical records departments. An obvious concern in such arrangements is lack of coordination and duplication of services.

DIVISION OF LABOR BY PRODUCT OR SERVICE

Sometimes, care delivery is organized around product lines or service lines. This is a type of functional division of work, but it is based on a patient's diagnosis or the specialty care required by a patient. For example, there might be a cardiology service line, a woman's health service line, and an oncology service line. This can lead to improved quality of care and decreased confusion for the patient because the information and protocols used in the outpatient side would be consistent with the information and protocols used in the hospital and across the entire health care system. Figure 10-8 demonstrates a product line design (Shortell & Kaluzny, 2006).

FACTORS INFLUENCING ORGANIZATIONAL STRUCTURES

Shortell and Kaluzny (2006) identify situations in which an organization's structure should be rethought. These situations include the experiencing of severe problems, either in performance problems, customer satisfaction problems, or internal/external review problems. Other reasons to rethink an organization's structure include a significant change in the internal or external environments; new programs, services, or product lines; or a change in the leadership. It is also important to note that design changes can be made in many levels. These range from changes in individual positions, to changes in work groups, to changes in clusters of work groups, to changes in total organizations, to changes in networks, and, finally, to changes in entire systems.

TECHNOLOGY

Changes in technology have wrought many design changes in health care organizations. The ability to provide safe same-day surgery has led to patients staying in

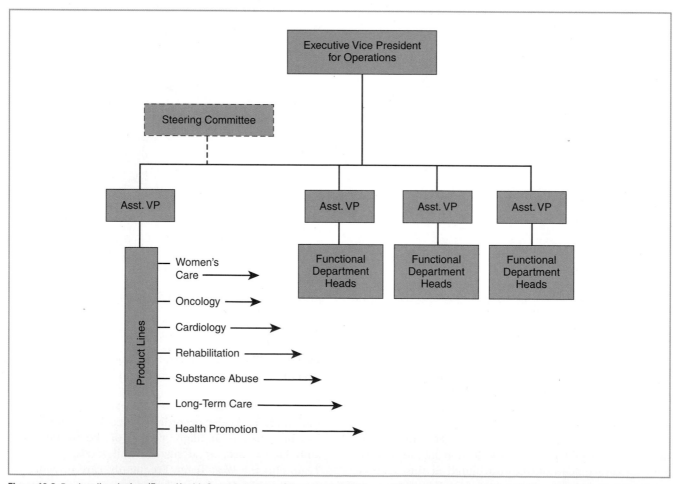

Figure 10-8 Product line design. (From *Health Care Management: Organization Design and Behavior* by S. Shortell & A. Kaluzny, 2006 (5th ed). Clifton Park, NY: Thomson Delmar Learning.)

SOCIOCULTURAL ENVIRONMENT

We are working in an increasingly diverse workforce. Educational, language, ethnic, cultural, age, and values divisions are greater than ever before. Nurses entering the health care field will need to be increasingly sensitive and skilled in dealing successfully with the differences that are likely to exist among their coworkers, patients, and themselves.

SIZE

Often the size of an organization, system, or department will determine the organizational structure that is used. The larger an organization, the more complex structures are needed. In a smaller, rural hospital, one Nursing department with a director and assistant director of nursing may be adequate to provide leadership resources. However, in an urban, multihospital health care system, there may need to be a corporate Nursing department, headed by a system-wide chief nurse executive, and separate Nursing departments at each hospital in the system.

REPETITIVENESS OF TASKS

Another factor that determines organizational structure is the repetitive nature of the tasks to be accomplished. It is possible to manage a larger number of individuals, units, or departments if they are all engaged in similar activities and processes. If there is a great deal of differentiation among their tasks, more levels of management are usually needed.

TRENDS IN ORGANIZATIONS

There is a need for a leadership culture that promotes sound ethical values and quality assurance. In turn, cultures with strong leadership promote productivity and performance. One nurse leader can help to make this difference. Consequently, transformational nurse leaders are needed who can create ethically sound environments and assist nurses to strive for quality outcomes and personal mastery. There is a need for concerted efforts to reconnect nursing education and nursing service and assure that nurses employed in leadership positions are educationally prepared to function in management and clinical decision-making roles.

CRITICAL THINKING 10-4

You, as a nurse, have been asked to take a leadership role in identifying potential depression management programs that could be implemented in the community-based psychiatric center where you work. Suppose that you would normally report to the depression product line manager, but for this project you are designated as the coordinator of depression management programs. As you begin your assessment of potential programs, you will need to interact with a number of functional departments across the organization, such as dietary, pharmacy, occupational therapy, and psychology. In addition, you will have to examine the other product lines to be sure that you are not duplicating services.

Given this situation, what would be some advantages of working in an institution that had a matrix design such as that depicted in Figure 10-4? What might be disadvantages?

---

hospitals for less than 24 hours. This means that there is an increased need for nurses to provide discharge planning with patients that they may have just met and in a very rapid time frame. Information Technology or Medical Information Systems departments in most institutions were relatively small 10 to 15 years ago. Today, there may be numerous employees involved in information technology throughout the organization. Communication and information exchange is instant and broad-based with e-mail and other technologic advances. This has had tremendous impact on the information flow in an organization. Information can rapidly be in more than one place at a time. Nurses and practitioners can update their nursing and medical care and medications quickly. Treatment plans may be revised instantaneously. In general, nurses and practitioners are less dependent on old communication patterns, which is changing the way we deliver care.

KEY CONCEPTS

- There are increasing opportunities for nurses to become involved in strategic planning for the delivery of health care services in their organizations and communities. To do so effectively, however, they will need a basic understanding of the way in which organizations are structured, how organizational systems function, and how to engage in the strategic planning process.

- The mission statement reflects the organization's values and provides the reader with an indication of the behavior and strategic actions that can be expected from that organization.

■ A health care organization needs to have a good idea of where it fits into its environment and what types of programs and services are needed and demanded by its customers or stakeholders.

■ The pivotal value of strategic planning is that it requires an organization to focus on its raison d'être and its mission and to test how its operations are leading to accomplishment of that mission.

■ The purpose of strategic planning is twofold. First, it is important that everyone has the same idea or vision of where the organization is headed; second, a good plan can help to ensure that the needed resources are available to carry out the initiatives that have been identified as important to the unit or agency.

■ A stakeholder assessment is a systematic consideration of all potential stakeholders to ensure that the needs of each of these stakeholders are incorporated in the planning phase. For a program to be successful, the involvement of those who will be affected is essential.

■ Organizations are structured or organized in a manner that is designed to facilitate the execution of their mission and their strategic plans.

■ There are a number of ways to describe organizational structures that involve classifying them by identifying selected characteristics.

KEY TERMS

focus groups	stakeholder assessment
mission statement	stakeholder
philosophy of an	strategic plan
organization	SWOT analysis

REVIEW QUESTIONS

1. A document that describes the institution's purpose and philosophy is
   A. the organizational chain of command.
   B. the organizational chart.
   C. the mission statement.
   D. the strategic plan.

2. Which of these statements is true about a strategic plan? Choose all that apply.
   ____ A. Requires focus on its mission and vision
   ____ B. Should not be attempted during turbulent times
   ____ C. Requires an assessment of the environment
   ____ D. Needs to be revisited periodically

3. The most formal and hierarchical organizational structure would be expected to have an organizational chart with
   A. a matrix design.
   B. many layers of command.

C. a product line design.
D. a number of dotted lines representing reporting relationships.

4. SWOT means
   A. strengths, weaknesses, opportunities, threats.
   B. strengths, worries, outcomes, threats.
   C. strengths, weaknesses, opportunities, treatment.
   D. structures, worries, outcomes, threats.

5.
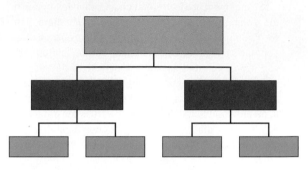

The above figure is an example of what type of organizational structure?
   A. Tall
   B. Matrix
   C. Product Line
   D. Flat

6. Which of the following are steps of the strategic planning process? Choose all that apply.
   ____ A. Stakeholder analysis
   ____ B. Developing organizational charts
   ____ C. Identifying planning goals and objectives
   ____ D. Hiring well-prepared individuals

7. A small hospital with 25 beds would probably be best served by which of the following organizational structures?
   A. Matrix
   B. Tall
   C. Flat
   D. Product Line

REVIEW ACTIVITIES

1. Identify a situation where a strategic plan could guide an organization in its choices among alternative actions.

2. Write a beginning mission statement and strategic plan for your professional nursing career.

3. You are asked to plan for the advisory board for your institution's proposed hospice program. How would you go about determining who to include on the advisory board? What groups of professionals and consumers would you want to see represented in a hospice advisory board? Identify several candidates and the stakeholder group that they might represent.

4. Examine the organizational structure of an organization or institution with which you are familiar. How would you characterize it using the types of structures that were discussed in this chapter?

EXPLORING THE WEB

Upon completion of your nursing degree, you are planning to interview for a position at an area hospital. In preparation for your interview, you want to understand the mission as well as other information about that institution. Today that information is readily available on the Web. For example, if you were planning to apply at Loyola University Chicago (*www.luc.edu*) you would go to *www.luhs.org*. Another example is Children's Memorial Hospital in Chicago at *www.childrensmemorial.org*.

Look at above Web pages, paying particular attention to the descriptions they provide of the organizations' missions. What impressions do you form about these organizations and their missions? Does the stated mission seem to fit with the general "feel" that you get from the Website? Could you easily find information about positions available? About the institution? Try this exercise with your local hospital or medical center.

REFERENCES

Atencio, B., Cohen, J., & Gorenberg, B. (2003). Nurse retention: Is it worth it? *Nursing Economic$, 21*(6), 262–268, 299.

Drucker, P. (1973). *Management tasks, responsibilities, and practices*. New York: Harper and Row.

Institute of Medicine. (1999). *To err is human*. Washington, DC: National Academies Press.

Institute of Medicine. (2001). *Crossing the quality chasm*. Washington, DC: National Academies Press.

Jones, R., & Beck, S. (1996). *Decision making in nursing*. Clifton Park, NY: Thomson Delmar Learning.

March of Dimes. (2006). The March of Dimes Story. Retrieved September 6, 2006, from http://www.marchofdimes.com/printableArticles/789_821.asp

Ortiz, J., McGilligan, K., & Kelly, P. (2004). Duration of breast milk expression among working mothers enrolled in an employer-sponsored lactation program. *Pediatric Nursing, 30*(2), 111–119.

Shortell, S., & Kaluzny, A. (2006). *Health care management: Organization design and behavior* (5th ed). Clifton Park, NY: Thomson Delmar Learning.

Thomas, R. (2004). *Marketing healthcare services*. Chicago: Health Administration Press.

SUGGESTED READINGS

Aiken, L. H., Clarke, S. P., & Sloane, D. M. (2002). Hospital staffing, organization, and quality of care: Cross-national findings. *International Journal for Quality in Health Care, 14*(1), 5–13.

Arnold, L., Campbell, A., Dubree, M., Fuchs, M. A., Davis, N., Hertzler, B., et al. (2006). Priorities and challenges of health system chief nursing executives: Insights for nursing educators. *Journal of Professional Nursing, 22*(4), 213–220.

Brewer, C. S. (2005). Health services research and the nursing workforce: Access and utilization issues. *Nursing Outlook, 53*(6), 281–290.

Buerhaus, P., Donelan, K., Ulrich, B., Norman, L., Williams, M., & Dittus, R. (2005). Hospital RNs' and CEOs' perceptions of the impact of the nursing shortage on the quality of care. *Nursing Economic$, 23*(5), 214–221.

Clancy, C., Sharp, B. A., & Hubbard, H. B. (2005). Guest editorial: Intersections for mutual success in nursing and health services research. *Nursing Outlook, 53*(6), 263–265.

Covaleski, M. A. (2005). The changing nature of the measurement of the economic impact of nursing care on health care organizations. *Nursing Outlook, 53*(6), 310–316.

Jones, C. B., & Mark, B. A. (2005). The intersection of nursing and health services research: Overview of an agenda setting conference. *Nursing Outlook, 53*(6), 270–273.

Jones, C. B., & Mark, B. A. (2005). The intersection of nursing and health services research: An agenda to guide future research. *Nursing Outlook, 53*(6), 324–332.

Mick, S. S., & Mark, B. A. (2005). The contribution of organization theory to nursing health services research. *Nursing Outlook, 53*(6), 317–323.

Ricketts, T. C., & Goldsmith, L. J. (2005). Access in health services research: The battle of the frameworks. *Nursing Outlook, 53*(6), 274–280.

Spetz, J. (2005). The cost and cost-effectiveness of nursing services in health care. *Nursing Outlook, 53*(6), 305–309.

Effective Team Building

Crisamar Javellana-Anunciado, MSN, APRN, BC

Teamwork is the ability to work together toward a common vision, the ability to direct individual accomplishments toward organizational objectives. It is the fuel that allows common people to attain uncommon results (Andrew Carnegie, 1984).

OBJECTIVES

Upon completion of this chapter, the reader should be able to:

1. Identify advantages and disadvantages of teamwork.
2. Review key concepts of creating an effective team.
3. Relate the stages of a team process.
4. Relate ways to create a conducive environment for teamwork
5. Identify the qualities of an effective team leader.
6. Identify elements of groupthink.

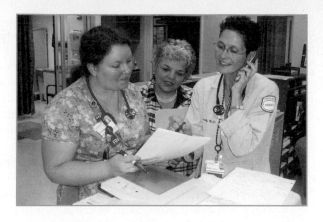

You are a new graduate nurse who has six months clinical experience working on an oncology unit. Your nurse manager observed your skill and compassion for terminally ill patients and your warm interaction and interpersonal relationship with the other staff nurses on the unit. Complimenting you on your skills and personal work ethic, the nurse manager also asked if you would be interested in joining the Interdisciplinary Cancer Support Committee to help address pain management and other issues to improve patient care. If you accept this responsibility, this will be your first committee membership.

How would you respond to this request?

Would you be ready at this point to accept the responsibility?

How would you prepare yourself for this unfamiliar role?

What qualities or skills do you need to possess to become a productive member of the team?

In today's health care environment, great demands are placed on each health care professional to provide the best quality of care efficiently, safely, and cost-effectively to optimize patient care outcomes. Many administrators and nurse managers recognize that effective interprofessional communication and collaboration through teamwork is needed to do this. In the interest of creating a safe patient care environment, health care professionals recognize that each discipline can no longer work alone. However, collaboration among health care professionals with varying specialties and focuses is a complex process. It requires careful planning, time, and effort to achieve the common goal of positive patient care outcomes.

A popular trend in human resource development is team training. Team training is well developed by many in the airline industry, major businesses, large corporations, bank institutions, and health care organizations. The demand for team training is so great that in the last few decades, there has been an explosion of team training companies providing tool kits, seminars, and conferences to improve teamwork and collaboration among executives, administrators, and employees. Collaboration

and teamwork among staff nurses and other disciplines in the health care setting is so critical to optimizing patient care safety and outcomes that it is a priority for most health care administrators, directors, and managers (Amos, Hu, & Herrick, 2005).

This chapter focuses on the different aspects of effective team building. It discusses the advantages and disadvantages of teams and the various types of teams and committees using the Tuckman and Jensen Conceptual Model of the team process (1977). The chapter also dissects the components of a successful team.

DEFINITION OF A TEAM

According to Buchholz and Roth (1987), authors of *Creating a High Performance Team*, "Wearing the same T-shirt doesn't make you a team." If a collection of T-shirts does not make a team, what then makes a team? What characteristics of people make a team? What is a team?

An often-quoted definition of a team is by Katzenbach and Smith (1993), authors of *Creating a High-Performance Team:* "A **team** is a small number of people with complementary skills who are committed to a common purpose, performance goals, and approach for which they are mutually accountable." There are several types of teams, and these teams exist for specific purposes. Thomas Edison, the inventor, said when asked why he had a team of 20 first assistants, "If I could solve all the problems myself, I would!"

TYPES OF TEAMS

A multidisciplinary or interdisciplinary team is comprised of varied disciplines contributing to an individual patient's care. For example, a critically ill patient after coronary artery bypass graft surgery may have a team of medical and nursing practitioners, and other disciplines, such as respiratory therapy, pharmacy, dietary, and physical therapy, as part of the team working to deliver care to the patient. The team works together closely and communicates frequently to optimize patient care. This close and frequent communication allows each discipline to work together collaboratively, complementing each other's specialty to provide a more holistic management of the patient's complex health care needs (Hall & Weaver, 2001).

COMMITTEES

In the health care setting, teams serve on standing committees, advisory committees, and ad hoc committees, which are created for specific goals or tasks. An example of a standing committee is the Nursing Policy and Procedure

Committee, which meets routinely to review, revise, and approve nursing-related policies and procedures. Other types of standing committees may be created to help meet requirements of federal regulatory agencies such as the Department of Health and Human Services (DHHS) or national accreditation agencies such as the Joint Commission (JC), formerly the Joint Commission on Accreditation of Healthcare Organizations (JCAHO). Examples of these standing committees are the Bioethics Committee, Medication Safety Committee, and the Quality Improvement Council. An example of an ad hoc committee is a Hypoglycemia Treatment Policy and Procedure Committee, which will meet only until the policy and procedure is developed, approved, and adopted by the institution. An example of an advisory committee is the Nursing Clinical Leadership Committee. This committee may be overseen by the chief nursing officer and include nurse managers and other members of the interdisciplinary team who meet to discuss and advise on concerns pertaining to the professional nursing staff.

The central goal of all of these health care teams is improving patient care for individuals or groups across the continuum of health and illness. The person, patient, or community and their holistic health needs are central (Naish, 2004).

ADVANTAGES OF TEAMWORK

Teams do not evolve by happenstance nor is the path to effective teamwork easy. Developing an effective team requires ample planning, with conscious and deliberate intentions focused on building its foundation through an organized system. Teamwork has both advantages and disadvantages.

Teamwork promotes safe and efficient patient care delivery. Effective interprofessional team communication is the central factor in the efficient delivery of safe health care (Lingard et al., 2005). Collaboration among health care professionals with increasingly diverse specialization optimizes safe patient care outcomes.

Teamwork equalizes power through shared governance. Porter-O'Grady (2005) advocates shared governance, where power is more evenly distributed among the nursing staff and leaders, as an effective tool to promote empowerment, ownership of one's own clinical practice, and responsibility and accountability among nursing staff members. Shared governance affirms that the patient is the center of care and formalizes and demands collaboration among members of the health care team (Caramanica, 2004).

Teamwork improves interpersonal relationships and job satisfaction. Effective collaboration on a team promotes free exchange of ideas, team cohesion, trust, mutual respect, and personal satisfaction of health care providers (Lindeke & Sieckert, 2004). Teamwork increases job satisfaction. In a study conducted among medical-surgical nursing staff on the factors improving job satisfaction, the authors noted that team building decreased the employee turnover rates from 13.42% to 6.56%. It also improved productivity, decreased absenteeism, and stabilized the workforce. This stability in employee turnover allowed the hospital to improve quality of care and provided positive economic benefits for the hospital (Amos et al., 2005).

EVIDENCE FROM THE LITERATURE

Citation: Caramanica, L. (2004). Shared Governance: Hartford Hospital's experience. *Online Journal of Issues in Nursing, 9*(1), 2. Retrieved April 23, 2006, from http://www.nursinworld.org/ojin/topic23/tpc23_2.htm

Discussion: The concept of shared hospital governance by administrative and hospital staff is not a new one. Shared governance encourages administrators and hospital staff to work together to improve patient outcomes. Many hospitals have not adopted this concept and may use other methods to improve outcomes. Hospitals that practice shared governance as opposed to authority-based bureaucratic governance have met many successes in improving collaboration and teamwork through increased accountability, responsibility, partnership, ownership, and equity.

Implications for Practice: With or without systemwide adoption of shared governance, certain concepts of the shared governance model may be adopted in patient care areas to improve collaboration and teamwork. This has a positive effect on patient outcomes.

DISADVANTAGES OF TEAMWORK

Teams may take longer to achieve a goal than one individual. On a team composed of varied disciplines, or even on a team with all members from the same discipline but with various levels of experiences and backgrounds, one may expect that one patient care situation may produce very diverse solutions. The team members may have disagreements on the best course of action to take for a specific situation. Another disadvantage is that teams develop through time, going through predictable stages of selecting the right members for the team, organizing team goals and manpower, and collaborating as a team. This team process takes time, effort, and resources.

Some team members may lack interest, motivation, ability, or skill to participate in the team process. These members may have been appointed or self-appointed for whatever reason, but they may not do the work as expected. Factors such as personality differences, personal work ethics, and varied perceptions of team goals may impede effective team collaboration. This, in turn, may create tension among other team members, cause delay in achieving goals, and cause frustration (Polifko-Harris, 2003).

INFORMAL TEAMS

Anyone working in an organization needs to be aware of the informal teams that influence the organization. Shortell and Kaluzny (2006) state that the importance of informal workgroup structure and group processes has been recognized for many years. The Hawthorne experiments firmly established the proposition that an individual's performance is determined in large part by informal relationship patterns that emerge within workgroups (Roethlisberger & Dickson, 1939). The workgroup has an impact on individual behaviors and attitudes because it controls so many of the stimuli to which the individual is exposed in performing organizational tasks (Hasenfeld, 1983).

Informal groups are not directly established or sanctioned by the organization but often form naturally by individuals in the organization to fill a personal or social interest or need. Shortell and Kaluzny (2006) identify a number of circumstances under which informal groups can have a negative impact on an organization. Groups may become overly exclusionary and lead to interpersonal conflict. In other cases, informal groups can become so powerful that they undermine the formal authority structure of the organization.

Informal groups can assume a change agent role. Informal groups are often responsible for facilitating improvements in working conditions. Such informal groups sometimes evolve into formal groups. Informal groups may also emerge to deal with a particular organizational problem or to work toward changes in organizational policies and procedures. In sum, informal groups play a unique role in organizations. These roles may be positive or negative.

STAGES OF A TEAM PROCESS

Teams evolve through a predictable development process. A widely used theory of the team development process was introduced by Tuckman (1965) and then modified by Tuckman and Jensen (1977). They identified five stages of team development: Forming, Storming, Norming, Performing, and Adjourning. Teams develop at various paces depending on the team's composition, experiences, relationships, and type of tasks. Understanding the phases of the team development process may help improve team development and participation (Amos et al., 2005); (Table 11-1).

FORMING STAGE

The first phase of the team process is the Forming stage. This stage occurs when the group is created, and they meet as a team for the first time. The team members come to the meeting with zest and a sense of curiosity, adventure, and even apprehension as they orient themselves to each other and get to know each other through personal interaction and perhaps team-building activities. With the help of the team leader or facilitator, they will explore the purpose of the team, why they are called to be a part of the team, and what contribution they can bring to the table. When the purpose of the team is clearly identified, they may proceed to establishing their team goals and expectations and setting boundaries for the teamwork.

STORMING STAGE

The second phase of the team process is the Storming stage. As the group relaxes into a more comfortable team setting, interpersonal issues or opposing opinions may arise that may cause conflict between members of the team and with the team leader. This may cause feelings of uneasiness in the group. It is important at this stage to understand that conflict is a healthy and natural process of team development. When members of the team come from various disciplines and specialties, there is always a tendency to approach an issue from several completely different standpoints. These differences need to be openly confronted and addressed so that effective resolution of the issue may occur in a timely manner. Real teams don't emerge unless individuals on them take risks involving conflict, trust, interdependence and hard work (Katzenbach & Smith, 2003).

TABLE 11-1	TUCKMAN AND JENSEN'S STAGES OF TEAM PROCESS

Stages	Description
Forming	*Relationship development:* Team orientation, identification of role expectations, beginning team interactions, explorations, and boundary setting occurs.
Storming	*Interpersonal interaction and reaction:* Dealing with tension, conflict, and confrontation occurs.
Norming	*Effective cooperation and collaboration:* Personal opinions are expressed and resolution of conflict with formation of solidified goals and increased group cohesiveness occurs.
Performing	*Group maturity and stable relationships:* Team roles become more functional and flexible, structural issues are resolved leading to supportive task performance through group-directed collaboration and resources sharing.
Adjourning	*Termination and consolidation:* Team goals and activities are met leading to closure, evaluation, and outcomes review. This may also lead to reforming when the need for improvement or further goal development is identified.

Source: Compiled with information from Tuckman & Jensen, 1977; Hall & Weaver, 2001; Polifko-Harris, 2003; Amos et al., 2005.

NORMING STAGE

The third stage is called Norming. After resistance is overcome in the Storming stage, a feeling of group cohesion develops. Team members master the ability to resolve conflict. Although complete resolution and agreement may not be attained at all times, team members learn to respect differences of opinion and may work together through these obstacles to achieve team goals. Communication of ideas, opinions, and information occurs through effective cooperation among the team members. Overcoming barriers to performance is how groups become teams (Katzenbach & Smith, 2003).

PERFORMING STAGE

The fourth phase of the team development process is the Performing stage. In this stage, group cohesion, collaboration, and solidarity are evident. Personal opinions are set aside to achieve group goals. Team members are openly communicating, know each other's roles and responsibilities, are taking risks, and trusting or relying on each other to complete assigned tasks. The group reaches maturity at this stage. One of the biggest strengths of this stage is the emphasis on maintaining and improving interpersonal relationships within the team as each member functions as a whole. Kenneth Blanchard, author of the *One Minute Manager,* sums it up with his comment, "None of us is as smart as all of us."

ADJOURNING STAGE

The fifth and final stage of team process development is the Adjourning stage. Termination and consolidation occur in this stage. When the team has achieved their goals and assigned tasks, the team closure process begins. The team reviews their activities and evaluates their progress and outcomes by answering the questions: Were the team goals sufficiently met? Was there anything that could have been done differently? The team leader summarizes the group's accomplishments and the role played by each member in achieving their goals. It is important to provide closure or feedback regarding the team process to leave each team member with a sense of accomplishment.

ANATOMY OF A WINNING TEAM

Henry Ford once said, "Coming together is a beginning. Keeping together is progress. Working together is success." Effective teamwork is essential in any setting, whether it be in a large business corporation, a complex health care system, dynamic social assemblies, and even within the close network of a family unit. People cannot avoid interacting with others. This is deeply ingrained in our culture and society. In today's health care setting, effective teamwork is not considered an option. It is a

CRITICAL THINKING 11-1

Mrs. Zenaida Corpuz, an 85-year-old female patient of Dr. Porter, is admitted with an acute myocardial infarction. She has a past history of multiple hospital admissions for congestive heart failure, hypertension, dyslipidemia, renal insufficiency, and type 2 diabetes. Mrs. Corpuz has been admitted to the hospital four times in the past six months for recurring chest pain, exacerbation of her congestive heart failure, and severe hyperglycemia with blood glucose levels >400 mg/dL. Her beta-natriuretic peptide (BNP) levels, troponin levels, glomerular filtration rate, and glycosylated A_1C levels are all elevated. She has received patient teaching on congestive heart failure and diabetes management during each of her previous admissions. You schedule a patient care conference to involve the patient's family, case manager, social worker, nursing and medical practitioners, diabetes educator, dietitian, and yourself.

What are some of the key patient care issues that concern you as the primary nurse?

How can you enlist the team's support on behalf of Mrs. Corpuz?

What contribution does each member of the care team conference bring to the table?

How would you proceed to develop or update Mrs. Corpuz's plan of care?

---

necessity. Patient welfare and safety depends on health care professionals collaborating together.

Effective teamwork is achieved when there is synergy. Mark Twain defines synergy as, the bonus that is achieved when things work together harmoniously. Steven Covey identifies that synergy means that the whole is greater than the sum of its parts (1989). The American Association of Critical Care Nurses has a Synergy Model of Professional Caring & Ethical Practice that guides the nurse and results in Synergy, where the needs and characteristics of a patient, clinical unit, or system are matched with a nurse's competencies (Hardin, 2005). Effective nurses and teams achieve this synergy. They develop the ingredients for creating a winning team where people with different ideas, backgrounds and beliefs work together synergistically and harmoniously.

To comprehend the teamwork process as a whole, you must examine the intricacies of each part that makes the whole. An effective team is composed of several parts. These parts are a conducive environment for teamwork to flourish, a collection of effective team members, and an effective team leader.

CASE STUDY 11-1

You are a nurse in a busy 42-bed telemetry unit. Both the staff nurses and unlicensed assistive personnel (UAP) work 12-hour shifts. Change of shift hand-off report occurs at 0700 and 1900 daily. During the staff meeting, the nurse manager charges everyone to think of ways to improve patient satisfaction. You note that patients are dissatisfied during the change-of-shift hand-off report times when the unit hallways become crowded and noisy. Most nurses and UAP are not available to answer call lights and attend to patient needs during this time.

What are some suggestions you can make to improve patient care during the change of shift hand-off report?

If you are asked to lead a team to problem-solve and identify solutions to these issues, what qualities do you possess that will be essential in this team leadership role?

What qualities would you look for in selecting your team members?

How can you use the five stages of team development—Forming, Storming, Norming, Performing, and Adjourning—to develop your team?

CONDUCIVE ENVIRONMENT FOR TEAMWORK

Developing a supportive and conducive environment for teamwork to succeed requires ongoing time and effort. The physical environment as well as the social and political climate must be considered.

Lindeke and Siekert (2006) point out that physical facility design can impact teamwork by influencing productivity, work attitudes, confidentiality, and the professional image of the health care personnel. Facility design that allows for adequate allotted space enhances team collaboration and interaction. Factors to consider in facility design include noise control, privacy, seating space, and convenience.

Social factors affecting the team environment need to be examined carefully. These social factors are related to human relationships and interaction. For teams to succeed, there are several crucial factors to consider. These factors are clear identification and ownership of the team goal; clear definition and acceptance of each person's role and responsibilities; clear delineation of team processes such as decision making, conflict resolution, communication, and participation; clear opportunities to build trust between participants; and finally, clear acceptance of each other's strengths and limitations in a manner that encourages positive working relationships. Javitch (2003) emphasizes the word, *clear*. When the team trusts each other, its environment promotes clear goals, clear role delineation, and clear work processes. More trust and better relationships, and success will follow. The team must know each person's role and know who resolves conflicts and makes decisions. They must accept the strengths and weaknesses of each other. This leads to quality team decisions.

The type of communication that occurs between a team and those outside the team is also important. Ancona and Caldwell (1992) use the following classification to describe the range of communication activities seen on a team and observed in their research:

- *Ambassador activities:* Members carrying out these activities communicate frequently with those above them in the organizational hierarchy. This set of activities is used to protect the team from outside pressures, to persuade others to support the team, and to lobby for resources.
- *Task-coordinator activities:* Members carrying out these activities communicate frequently with other groups and persons at lateral levels in the organization. These activities include discussing problems with others, obtaining feedback, and coordinating and negotiating with outsiders.
- *Scout activities:* Members carrying out these activities are involved in general scanning for ideas and information about the external environment. These

activities differ from the other two in that these activities relate to general scanning instead of specific coordination issues (Shortell & Kaluzny, 2006).

Another key factor to team success is its political environment. Is there sufficient support and buy-in from the administrative level from the staff? Are there enough resources available to the team, that is, financial, support staff, time allotted, and so on? Administrative support means leadership support for team efforts. Does administration empower staff by encouraging decision making at the team level? Does administration allow for individual creativity and self-governance? Is the role of the team clear from the beginning of the team's work on who has the final power to make a decision? (Table 11-2).

TEAM SIZE

It is believed that team size affects performance in that too few or too many members reduce performance (Cohen & Bailey, 1997). As teams become larger, communication and coordination problems tend to increase, and a climate of fairness and cohesiveness decreases (Colquitt, Noe, & Jackson, 2002; Liberman, Hilty, Drake, & Tsang, 2001). However, teams have to be large enough or small enough to accomplish the task assigned. Probably, smaller groups are less cumbersome, with fewer social distractions. Smaller teams also have lower incidences of social loafing (Liden, Wayne, Jaworski, & Bennett, 2004). Individuals in large teams are able to maintain a sense of anonymity and gain from the work of the group without making a suitable contribution (Shortell & Kaluzny, 2006).

STATUS DIFFERENCES

Status is the measure of worth conferred on an individual by a group. Status differences are seen throughout organizations and serve some useful purposes (Shortell & Kaluzny, 2006). Differences in status motivate people, provide them with a means of identification, and may be a force for stability in the organization (Scott, 1967).

Status differences have a profound effect on the functioning of teams. Research findings are fairly consistent in showing that high-status members initiate communication more often, are provided more opportunities to participate, and have more influence over the decision-making process (Owens, Mannic, & Neale, 1998). Thus, an individual from a lower-status professional group may be intimidated or ignored by higher-status team members. The group, as a result, may not benefit from this person's expertise. This situation is very likely in health care, where status differences among the professions are well entrenched (Topping, Norton, & Scafidi, 2003). Often, multidisciplinary teams are idealistically expected to operate as a company of equals, yet the reality of

TABLE 11-2	TEAM EVALUATION CHECKLIST	Yes	No
1. Is the environment/climate conducive to team building?		_____	_____
2. Do the team members have mutual respect for and trust of one another?		_____	_____
3. Are the team members honest with one another?		_____	_____
4. Does everyone actively participate in the decision making and problem solving of the team?		_____	_____
5. Are the purpose, goals, and objectives of the team obvious to all participants?		_____	_____
6. Are the goals met?		_____	_____
7. Are creativity and mutual support of new ideas encouraged by all team members?		_____	_____
8. Does the team work to avoid groupthink?		_____	_____
9. Is the team productive, and does it see actual progress toward goal attainment?		_____	_____
10. Does the team begin and end its meetings on time?		_____	_____
11. Does the team leader provide vision and energy to the team?		_____	_____
12. Do any persons on the team serve as ambassador, task coordinator, or scout?		_____	_____

Source: Compiled with information from Polifko-Harris (2003) and Ancona & Caldwell (1992).

the situation makes this difficult (Shortell & Kaluzny, 2006). In a study of end-stage renal disease teams, in which the equal participation ideology was accepted by most team participants, it was clear that the medical practitioners, who were perceived as having higher professional status than other groups, had greater involvement in the actual decision-making process (Deber & Leatt, 1986). The mismatch between expectations and reality made many team members, particularly staff nurses, feel a sense of role deprivation, with accompanying implications for morale and job satisfaction. This problem is exacerbated in teams characterized by sex diversity. In one study, men were more likely to want to exit teams that were female-dominated for those that were male-dominated or homogenous. Following from this, men have historically been perceived as having higher status in managerial roles in organizations, thereby affecting the men's satisfaction with the team (Chatman & O'Reilly, 2004).

Status differences may have very significant impacts on patient outcomes. According to the recent report, *Keeping Patients Safe: Transforming the Work Environment of Nurses,* "counterproductive hierarchical communication patterns that derive from status differences" are partly responsible for many medical errors (Institute of Medicine, 2003, p. 361). Further, a review of medical malpractice cases from across the country found that medical practitioners, perceived by some as the higher-status members of the team, often ignored important information communicated by nurses, perceived by some as the lower-status members of the team. Nurses in turn were found to withhold relevant information for diagnosis and treatment from medical practitioners (Schmitt, 2001). In this status-consciousness environment, opportunities for learning and improvement can be missed because of unwillingness to engage in quality-improving communication.

Shortell and Kaluzny (2006) suggest that if status inequality exists, it is advisable to build a trust-sensitive environment in which members can disagree with the leader and others on the team without repercussions. The use of training with nonmember team facilitators early in the team-development process may be able to help a team cope with any problems brought about by status differences. In well-managed multidisciplinary groups, all individuals are encouraged to contribute to the team goals. It is important to develop a team where all members of the team are highly regarded and respected if the team's goals are to be fully achieved.

PSYCHOLOGICAL SAFETY

Psychological safety describes individuals' perceptions about the consequences of interpersonal risks in their work environment, that is, largely taken-for-granted beliefs about how others will respond when one puts oneself on the line, such as by asking a question, seeking feedback, reporting a mistake, or proposing a new idea in the team context (Shortell & Kaluzny, 2006). In psychologically safe teams, people believe that if they make a mistake, other team members will not penalize or think less of them for it. This belief fosters the confidence to experiment, discuss mistakes and problems, and ask others for help. Psychological safety is created by mutual respect and trust among team members, and leader behavior is a powerful influence on the level of psychological safety in teams (Edmondson, 1999; 2003).

It is important to note that psychological safety is distinct from group cohesiveness. As noted, team cohesiveness can lead to groupthink, a reduction in willingness to disagree and challenge others' views (Janis, 1972). Groupthink leads to a lack of interpersonal risk-taking and is discussed later in this chapter. Psychological safety describes instead a climate that fosters productive discussion enabling early prevention of problems and accomplishment of shared goals because people feel less need to focus on self-protection (Shortell & Kaluzny, 2006).

QUALITIES OF EFFECTIVE TEAM MEMBERS

To be an effective team member, you need to possess certain characteristics conducive to team collaboration. You must be proactive, motivated, have a certain personal sense of purpose or mission, and possess personal and time management skills (Covey, 1989).

Being proactive and motivated means taking charge of your life and the circumstances around you. Proactive, motivated people are not easily affected by situations in their surroundings because they avoid being reactive. Being proactive and motivated is to take full responsibility for your own actions, decisions, and behavior. People who end up with the good jobs are the proactive and motivated ones who are the solutions to the problems, not the problems themselves. They seize the initiative to do whatever is necessary, consistent with correct principles, to get the job done (Covey, 1989).

To succeed in nursing as a new graduate and as a member of a team, you need to develop a personal sense of purpose, mission, and professional goals early on and work toward meeting them. Covey (1989) calls this "working toward goals and beginning with the end in mind." When joining a team, the nurse needs to examine their own skills, what contributions they can provide, and be confident in their role as a team member. Knowing your

REAL WORLD INTERVIEW

I find the Tahari Window beneficial because it deals with projecting your personality and receiving feedback. Let me explain the Tahari Window to you. Imagine a square window divided into quarters. This is a representation of the different aspects of yourself, i.e., the four aspects of your personality. The first quarter, the Open Quarter, is the window open to the rest of the world. It is your attitudes, behavior, motivation, and values that you are aware of and which are known to others. The second quarter of the window, called the Mask, is that part of you that you don't want others to know about unless you allow them to do so. This quarter of the window covers beliefs, feelings, and impulses that you control. You need a "Chicken Soup Squad" to help you get rid of the Mask, i.e., people you can trust who won't use information from this Mask Quarter against you. The third quarter of the window is the Blindspot. This Blindspot Quarter represents the things about you that you don't know but that others can see, i.e., mannerisms and unconscious behavior. When others give you feedback in a supportive, responsible way and you listen, you can see some of this Blindspot Quarter of the window and test the reality of who you are and grow. The fourth quarter of the window is the Unknown Quarter. This quarter is your true depth. It is what motivates you, what influences you, and holds your deepest beliefs and feelings. This Unknown Quarter represents your potential and is your source of uniqueness, that which makes you different from those around you.

Knowing these different sides of your personality can help you understand others, their mannerisms, and their behavior. This can help you in your relationships with others. It allows you to work better with them ideally for mutual benefit.

Mary Kay Slowikowski
Darien, Illinois

priorities and managing personal and professional time wisely and efficiently will go a long way towards teamwork.

QUALITIES OF EFFECTIVE TEAM LEADERS

A team leader will organize, facilitate, and manage the entire team. Nurse leaders need to examine their own leadership styles, strengths, and weaknesses, and learn to capitalize on their strengths. Effective team leaders must understand how various learning styles, cultural diversity, and personality differences play into the dynamics of teamwork. Qualities of a good team leader should include good communication skills, conflict resolution skills, and leadership skills (Hall & Weaver, 2001).

Open and honest communication is an essential skill to develop as a team leader. Respectful negotiations, clear and tactful expression of ideas and messages, and empathetic listening must occur. The team leader must work to develop these skills. Empathetic listening allows a leader to seek first to understand the other person, become truly interested and attentive in what the other person has to say, and place him or herself in the other person's shoes (Covey, 1989).

Conflict resolution skill is also an important quality of a good team leader. In interdisciplinary practice collaboration, people come to the table with varying ideas about the goal, as well as with different levels of commitment and diverse attitudes. These differences are the breeding ground for conflict. Conflict may be minimized if the team learns conflict-resolution skills early on. The team leader can help by providing a clear statement of goals, setting team guidelines, and identifying role delineations to avoid or minimize conflict (Hall & Weaver, 2001).

GUIDELINES FOR MEETINGS

A fundamental skill in effectively working with a team is leadership. The leader must implement appropriate leadership or guidance through the stages of the team process. For example, when the team is just forming, members may need more guidance and highly directive leadership during meetings (Table 11-3).

As the team matures and begins working on the goals, the leader may need to take a step back from directive leadership and become a facilitator, mentor, and guide. The leader focuses on encouraging and guiding the team's sense of self-direction, ownership, and responsibility to accomplish desired goals (Hall & Weaver, 2001). The leader reinforces teamwork by focusing the team on outcome improvement, visually tracking results, and recognizing members who make significant contributions (Cox, 2003). In one study, leadership in ICUs was positively related to efficiency of operation, satisfaction, and lower turnover of nurses (Shortell et al., 1994). Successful leaders adopted a supportive formal or informal leadership style, emphasizing standards of excellence, encouraging interaction, communicating clear goals and expectations, responding to changing needs, and providing support resources when possible. Successful leaders communicate a compelling rationale for change, motivate others to exert the necessary effort, and also minimize the status difference between themselves and other members of the team to facilitate others' ability to speak up with questions, observations, and concerns (Shortell & Kaluzny, 2006).

In deciding upon a leadership style, group leaders need to consider in realistic terms their formal and informal authority within the group. Use of a coercive or forceful style may backfire when the individual does not have

---

TABLE 11-3	**GUIDELINES FOR MEETINGS**

In managing meetings, leaders should be aware of the following principles:

- Set a time frame for meetings, and stick to it.
- At the beginning of the meeting, review the progress made to date and establish the task facing the group.
- Help group members feel comfortable with one another.
- Establish ground rules governing group discussions.
- As early in a meeting as possible, get a report from each member who has been preassigned a task.
- Sustain the flow of the meeting by using informational displays.
- Manage the discussion to achieve equitable participation.
- Work to avoid groupthink by using critical appraisal of all ideas.
- Close the meeting by summarizing what has been accomplished and reviewing assignments.
- Identify a time frame for future meetings.

the power to back up decisions. Such a leader may find that the informal leader is able to veto, modify, or sabotage demands. It is best for the formal leader not only to consider the views of informal leaders but also to collaborate with them, if possible (Shortell & Kaluzny, 2006).

AVOIDING GROUPTHINK

Effective leaders work to avoid groupthink. The concept of groupthink emerged from Janis's studies of high-level policy decisions by government leaders, including decisions about Vietnam, the Bay of Pigs, and the Korean War. Groupthink occurs when the desire for harmony and consensus overrides members' rational efforts to appraise the situation. In other words, groupthink occurs when maintaining the pleasant atmosphere of the team implicitly becomes more important to members than reaching a good decision (Shortell & Kaluzny, 2006). There is a reduced willingness to disagree and challenge other's views in groupthink. Some of all of the following symptoms may indicate the presence of groupthink (Janis, 1972):

- *The illusion of invulnerability:* Team members may reassure themselves about obvious dangers and become overly optimistic and willing to take extraordinary risks.
- *Collective rationalization:* Teams may overlook blind spots in their plans. When confronted with conflicting information, the team may spend considerable time and energy refuting the information and rationalizing a decision.
- *Belief in the inherent morality of the team:* Highly cohesive teams may develop a sense of self-righteousness about their role that makes them insensitive to the consequences of decisions.
- *Stereotyping others:* Victims of groupthink hold biased, highly negative views of competing teams. They assume that they are unable to negotiate with other teams, and rule out compromise.

- *Pressures to conform:* Group members face severe pressures to conform to team norms and to team decisions. Dissent is considered abnormal and may lead to formal or informal punishment.
- *The use of mindguards:* Mindguards are used by members who withhold or discount dissonant information that interferes with the team's current view of a problem.
- *Self-censorship:* Teams subject to groupthink pressure members to remain silent about possible misgivings and to minimize self-doubts about a decision.
- *Illusion of unanimity:* A sense of unanimity emerges when members assume that silence and lack of protest signify agreement and consensus.

Shortell and Kaluzny (2006) state that the consequences of groupthink are that teams may limit themselves, often prematurely, to one possible solution and fail to conduct a comprehensive analysis of a problem. When groupthink is well entrenched, members may fail to review their decisions in light of new information or changing events. Teams may also fail to consult adequately with experts within or outside the organization, and fail to develop contingency plans in the event that the decision turns out to be wrong.

Team leaders can help avoid groupthink. First, leaders can encourage members to critically evaluate proposals and solutions. Where a leader is particularly powerful and influential, yet still wants to get unbiased views from team members, the leader may refrain from stating his or her own position until later in the decision-making process. Another strategy is to assign the same problem to two separate work teams. Most importantly, groupthink can be avoided by proactively engaging in a process of critical appraisal of ideas and solutions, and by understanding the warning signs of groupthink (Shortell & Kaluzny, 2006).

KEY CONCEPTS

- Effective teamwork and collaboration is essential to improving patient care outcomes.

- Teams and committees are formed for a variety of reasons depending on the level of collaboration required or the specific purpose desired.

- Each team goes through the stages of a team process.

- Successful teamwork requires a conducive physical, social, and political environment for it to succeed.

- An effective team member must be proactive, motivated, have a certain personal sense of purpose or mission, and possess personal and time-management skills.

- Teams are affected by team size, status differences, and psychological safety.

- Guidelines for conducting meetings are useful when managing meetings.

- Successful teams work to avoid groupthink, which can cause the group to fail to analyze a problem.

- The team leader must possess effective communication skills, conflict-resolution skills, and leadership skills.

- Great teams have clear goals, well-defined role delineation, organized processes that are outcomes-oriented, and open and honest interpersonal relationships.

KEY TERM

team

REVIEW QUESTIONS

1. Based on the Tuckman and Jensen Team Process, what stage of team development is it when team members work harmoniously together, have open communication, take risks, and trust each other to complete assigned tasks?
   A. Forming
   B. Storming
   C. Norming
   D. Performing

2. A good leader does all except which of the following?
   A. Encourages open communication and interpersonal relationship
   B. Uses only an authoritative leadership style
   C. Actively listens to team members' concerns and opinions
   D. Clearly identifies goals, roles and the team process

3. Which of the following is not a characteristic of groupthink?
   A. Use of mindguards
   B. Illusion of unanimity
   C. Free discussion of ideas
   D. Pressure to conform

4. Which of the following communication roles is used to protect the team from outside pressures from those above them in the organizational hierarchy?
   A. Ambassador
   B. Task-coordinator
   C. Scout
   D. Leader

5. Which of the following showed that an individual's performance is often determined in large part by the work group?
   A. Kaluzny Study
   B. Dickson Research
   C. Carnegie Study
   D. Hawthorne Experiments

REVIEW ACTIVITIES

1. Ask to attend a team meeting in your clinical agency. Who is the formal leader of the group? What does the leader do to facilitate the team's attaining their objectives?

2. Note a team of which you are a member. Have you ever seen groupthink operate in the team? What did you do?

3. Note the communication roles of ambassador, task coordinator, and scout. Have you seen these roles operate on any teams to which you belong?

EXPLORING THE WEB

Check these sites for information on teams:

- American College of Health Care Administrators (ACHCA): *www.achca.org*

- Belbin Team-role Theory, products, conferences, and free online newsletter: *www.belbin.com*

- Free online newsletter on leadership: *www.injoy.com*

- Healthcare Teams information: *www.learningcenter.net*

- Tuckman and Jensen Stages of the Team Process: *www.infed.org*

  Search for Tuckman and Jensen.

REFERENCES

Amos, M., Hu, J., & Herrick, C. A. (2005). The impact of team building on communication and job satisfaction of nursing staff. *Journal for Nurses in Staff Development, 21*(1), 10–16.

Ancona, D. G., & Caldwell, D. F. (1992a). Briding the boundary: External activity and performance in organizational teams. *Administrative Science Quarterly, 37,* 634–665.

Buchholz, S., & Roth, T. (1987). *Creating the high performance team.* New York: John Wiley & Sons, Inc.

Caramanica, L. (2004). Shared Governance: Hartford Hospital's experience. *Online Journal of Issues in Nursing, 9*(1), 2. Retrieved April 23, 2006, from http://www.nursinworld.org/ojin/topic23/tpc23_2.htm

Carnegie, D. (1984). *How to win friends and influence people.* New York: Galahad books.

Chatman, J., & O'Reilly, C. (2004). Asymmetric effects of work group demographics on men's and women's responses to work group composition. *Academy of Management Journal, 47*(2), 193–208.

Cohen, S. G., & Bailey, D. E. (1997). What makes teams work: Group effectiveness research from the shop floor to the executive suite. *Journal of Management, 23,* 239–290.

Colquitt, J. A., Noe, R. A., & Jackson, C. L. (2002). Justice in teams: Antecedents and consequences of procedural justice climate. *Personnel Psychology, 55,* 83–100.

Covey, S. (1989). *The 7 habits of highly effective people.* New York: Fireside.

Cox, S. (2003). Nursing management: Building dream teams. Retrieved April 18, 2006, from http://www.findarticles.com/p/articles/mi_qa3619/is_200303/ai_n9221079/print

Deber, R. B., & Leatt, P. (1986). The multidisciplinary renal team: Who makes the decisions? *Health Matrix, 4*(3), 3–9.

Edmondson, A. C. (1999). Psychological safety and learning behavior in work teams. *Administrative Science Quarterly, 44,* 350–383.

Edmondson, A. C. (2003). Speaking up in the operating room: How team leaders promote learning in interdisciplinary action teams. *Journal of Management Studies, 40*(6), 1419–1452.

Hall, P., & Weaver, L. (2001). Interdisciplinary education and teamwork: A long and winding road. *Medical Education, 35,* 867–875.

Hardin, S. R., & Kaplan, R. (2005). *Synergy for Clinical Excellence, American Association of Critical Care Nurses.* Boston: Jones & Bartlett.

Hasenfeld, Y. (1983). *Human service organizations.* Englewood Cliffs, NJ: Prentice-Hall.

Huber, G. (1980). *Managerial decision making.* Glenview, IL: Scott, Foresman.

Institute of Medicine (2003). *Keeping patients safe: Transforming environment of nurses.* Washington, DC: National Academics Press.

Janis, L. (1972). *Victims of groupthink.* Boston: Houghton-Mifflin.

Javitch, D. (2003). *How to foster effective teamwork.* Retrieved April 18, 2006, from http://www.entrepreneur.com/article/0,4621,308367,00.html

Katzenbach, J. R., & Smith, D. K. (2003). *The wisdom of teams: Creating the high-performance organization.* New York: HarperCollins Publishers Inc.

Liberman, R. P., Hilty, D. M., Drake, R. E., & Tsang, H. (2001). Requirements for multidisciplinary teamwork in psychiatric rehabilitation. *Psychiatric Services, 52*(10), 1331–1342.

Liden, R. C., Wayne, S. J., Jaworski, R. A., & Bennett, N. (2004). Social loafing: A field investigation. *Journal of Management, 30,* 285–305.

Lindeke, L. L., & Siekert, A. M. (2004). Nurse-physician workplace collaboration. Retrieved April 18, 2006, from http://www.nursingworld.org/mods/mod775/nrsdrfull.htm#team

Lingard, L., Regehr, G., Espin, S., Devito, I., Whyte, S., Buller, D., et al. (2005). Perceptions of operating room tension across professions: Building generalizable evidence and educational resources. *Academic Medicine, 8*(10), S75–S79.

Naish, J. (2004). The evolving nurse. *Nursing Standard, 19*(5), 13.

Owens, D. A., Mannic, E. A., & Neale, M. A. (1998). Strategic formation of groups: Issues in task performance and team member selection. In D. H. Gruenfeld (Ed.), *Research on managing groups and teams* (pp. 149–165). Stamford, CT: MAI Press.

Polifko-Harris, K. (2003). Effective team building. In P. Kelly-Heienthal, *Nursing Leadership and Management.* Clifton Park NY: Thomson Delmar Learning.

Porter-O'Grady, T. (2005). Strong leaders or empowered staff: Where is real empowerment? Retrieved April 18, 2006, from http://www.tpogassociates.com/considerthis/fall2005.htm

Roethlisberger, F. J., & Dickson, W. J. (1939). *Management and the worker.* Cambridge, MA: Harvard University Press.

Schmitt, M. H. (2001). Collaboration improves the quality of care: Methodological challenges and evidence from health care research. *Journal of Interprofessional Care, 15,* 47–66.

Scott, W. G. (1967). *Organization theory.* Homewood, IL: Irwin.

Shortell, S. M., & Kaluzny, A. D. (2006) *Health care management* (5th ed.). Clifton Park, NY: Thomson Delmar Learning.

Shortell, S. M., Zimmerman, J. E., Rousseau, D. M., Gillies, R. R., Wagner, D. P., Draper, E. A., et al. (1994). The performance of intensive care units. Does good management make a difference? *Medical Care 32,* 508–525.

Topping, S., Norton, T., & Scafidi, B. (2003). Coordination of services: The use of multidisciplinary, interagency teams. In S. Dopson & A. L. Mark (Eds.), *Leading Health Care Organizations* (pp. 100–112). New York: Palgrave Macmillan.

Tuckman, B. W. (1965). Developmental sequences in small groups. *Psychological Bulletin, 63,* 384–399.

Tuckman, B. W., & Jensen, M. A. C. (1977). Stages of small group development revisited. *Group and Organizational Studies, 2,* 419–427.

SUGGESTED READINGS

Batson, V. (2004). Shared governance in an integrated health care network. *Association of Operating Room Nurses Journal, 80*(3), 493–520.

Buchbinder, S. B. (2006). Building an effective team. Retrieved April 18, 2006, from http://community.nursingspectrum.com/MagazineArticles/article.cfm?AID=20377

Hardin, S., & Hussey, L. (2003). AACN synergy model for patient care: Case study of a CHF Patient. *Critical Care Nurse, 23*(1), 73–76.

Hinkle, J. L., Steffen, K. A., Heck, C. E., McBride, J., & Wenograd, D. (2006). A team approach to neuroscience nursing critical care orientation. *Journal of Neuroscience Nursing, 38*(5), 390–394.

Leonard, M., Graham, S., & Bonacum, D. (2004). The human factor: The critical importance of effective teamwork and communication in providing safe care. *Quality and Safety in Health Care 2004, 13,* 85–90.

Murray, T., & Kleinpell, R. (2006). Implementing a rapid response team: Factors influencing success. *Critical Care Nursing Clinics of North America, 18*(4), 493–501.

Pronovost, P. J., Holzmueller, C. G., Clattenburg, L., Berenholtz, S., Matinez, E. A., Paz, J. R., et al. (2006). *Current Opinions in Critical Care, 12*(6), 604–608.

Smith, M. K. (2005). Bruce W. Tuckman—forming, storming, norming and performing in groups. *Encyclopedia of Informal Education.* Retrieved April 23, 2006, from http://www.infed.org/thinkers/tuckman.htm

Williamson, S. (2006). Training the team: Talk is cheap—but vital in keeping patients safe. *Inside: Duke University Medical Center & Health System Newsletter, 15*(5).

CHAPTER 12

Power

Terry W. Miller, PhD, RN ⊕ Richard J. Maloney, BS, MA, MAHRM, EdD ⊕
Patsy Maloney, RN, BC, EdD, MSN, MA, CNAA

The sole advantage of power is
that you can do more good
(Baltasar Gracian,
17th Century).

OBJECTIVES

Upon completion of this chapter, the reader should be able to:

1. Define power, and describe it at the personal, professional, and organizational levels.

2. Describe each of the following sources of power, and analyze its likely relative strength for an entry-level nurse: coercion, reward, legitimate, expert, referent, information, and connection.

3. Apply an understanding of power to help nurses improve their effectiveness.

4. Analyze how new nurses can increase their power.

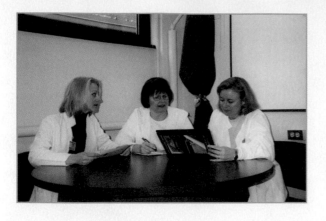

Nurse Pat, a new graduate who just finished her medical-surgical nursing orientation, is working with a patient for whom a surgical consult has been written. The unit clerk and a long-time nurse on the unit remark that Dr. Killian, the practitioner doing the surgical consultation, should be named Dr. Killjoy because she humiliates new nurses to try to put them in their place. Based on previous reports by other nurses on the unit, Pat knows Dr. Killian has the reputation of being demeaning and inappropriately demanding when interacting with new nurses. Two hours later, Dr. Killian appears on the unit and asks to see the nurse who did the surgical admission sheet.

What would you do if you were Pat?

How would you approach Dr. Killian?

Effective nurses are powerful. They show objectivity, creativity, and knowledge throughout their practice and regardless of their work setting. They have and exert power by understanding the concept of power from multiple perspectives; they then use this understanding to motivate others; accomplish organizational goals; and provide safe, competent care. The political process, discussed in Chapter 9, is another venue through which effective nurses achieve desired outcomes and protect their own as well as their patients' interests.

This chapter will discuss power and how nursing power affects patient care. It looks at sources of power, levels of power and how nurses can increase their power.

DEFINITIONS OF POWER

Power has been defined in multiple ways. Commonly, **power** is described as the ability to create, get, and use resources to achieve one's goals. Goals within an organization vary widely across departments, health care groups, and individuals. It is a goal of nurses to gain knowledge of the distribution of power in their organization, the circumstances under which power is used, and strategies associated with the use of power. Power can be defined at various levels: personal, professional, or organizational. Personal power derives from characteristics in the individual. For example, parents and teachers are often seen as personally powerful because of the trust or knowledge they possess. Professional power is conferred on members of a profession by one another and the larger society to which they belong. This power comes from offering a service that society values. Organizational power comes from one's position in an organizational hierarchy, as well as from understanding the organizational structure and function, and from being authorized to function powerfully within an organizational culture. Power, regardless of level, comes from the ability to influence others or affect others' thinking or behavior.

Power at the personal level is closely linked to how an individual perceives power, how others perceive the individual, and the extent to which an individual can influence events. Nurses who feel empowered at a personal level are likely to manifest a high level of self-awareness. They are more likely to understand nursing as a profession because it represents a group to which they belong. They also understand the structure and operations of health care because it represents their work environment.

People who are perceived as experts in health care have a significant amount of authority and influence, which makes them more effective than those not perceived as experts. There are at least two ways to wield the influence of an expert. The first way is to be introduced and promoted to a group as an expert, which validates one's expertise; the second way is to actually become an expert based on knowledge, skills, and abilities that are consistently demonstrated in practice settings. Remarkably, nurses are sometimes reluctant to be identified as experts to patients, practitioners, administrators, other nurses, other health care workers, and the public in general. This lack of identification must be addressed if the nursing profession is to achieve the status and degree of empowerment it seeks and become more visible.

The personal power of nurses is evident in the decisions they make on a daily basis about how their lives and work are organized to accomplish what they want and obtain what they need for themselves and their patients. The more nurses believe they can influence events through personal effort, the greater their sense of power. Many nurses believe they can make a difference and influence events in their lives. These nurses are likely to participate actively in trying to get what they want. This participation will make them feel more powerful even if their efforts are not always successful.

CRITICAL THINKING 12-1

The work and contributions of some nurses are so significant that they change the world. To be effective, these nurses conceptualize themselves in terms far more powerful than society may expect. Such an empowering self-image begins for entry-level nurses on day one. When we consider the relevance and significance of nursing history, we realize the contributions made by nurses who saw themselves as powerful and acted on that empowered self-image to improve the lives of others. A lack of historical awareness within the nursing profession empowers others to discount nursing's importance to society. Ultimately, we limit our own future as nurses by hindering our potential for making even greater contributions to the future of health care.

Can you name two nurses who represent powerful figures in modern history and tell why their contributions are so significant? See Exploring the Web in this chapter.

Can you identify some obstacles they experienced because they were nurses?

REAL WORLD INTERVIEW

I try to use power in a positive manner in the pain management clinic that I manage. I attempt to get people to move without them necessarily knowing they are being helped. I think that power at the bedside is a personal thing. Confidence, authenticity, and genuineness are qualities I most value and see as empowering nurses in practice. I feel that the middle manager in nursing gets power by developing staff, building self-confidence on a personal level, and delegating authority in a way that supports others. In higher levels of management I found, through my military experience, that the best leaders almost give power away with the caveat that the persons are being delegated to represent the leader and are accountable for the decisions they make. I believe that the tighter a person holds onto power, the less powerful she or he becomes. I also believe that nurses run the risk of losing power when they look for power outside nursing to direct them. New graduates should seek experiences and input from a variety of people and glean what they can from each experience. It is somewhat like a smorgasbord. Ultimately, the new nurse has to decide what she or he wants because there is no one answer or approach to power. No one really has *the* answer; instead, they have *an* answer.

Nancy Safranek, MSN, RN
RN Director, OPS, PACU, SP, PMC
Puyallup, Washington

POWER AND ACCOUNTABILITY

Effective nurses see power as positive and view their ability to understand and use power as a significant part of their responsibilities to patients, their coworkers, the nursing profession, and themselves. Nurses therefore have a professional obligation not to view power as a negative concept, thus avoiding power struggles and those who seem to savor power.

Traditionally, accountability has been considered one of the major hallmarks of the health care professions. Nursing is a profession and, as such, nurses have the primary responsibility for defining and providing nursing services. Yet some nurses appear to have a difficult time

EVIDENCE FROM THE LITERATURE

Citation: Buresh, B., & Gordon, S. (2006). *From Silence to Voice*. Ithaca & London: Cornell U. Press.

Discussion: This book discusses the fact that not enough nurses are willing to talk about their work. When nurses and nursing organizations do talk about their work, too often they unintentionally project an inaccurate picture of nurses using a virtue script instead of a knowledge script to highlight what nurses do. They discuss the virtuous and caring acts of nurses. They do not discuss the expert knowledge that nurses bring to patient care. When nursing groups give voice to nursing, they sometimes bypass, downplay, or even devalue the basic nursing work that occurs in direct care of the sick, while elevating the image of elite nurses in advance practice, administration, or academia. This contributes to social stereotypes that deride anyone who is "just a nurse."

Implications for Practice: If nursing is misunderstood by the public or by those with influence, it will be vulnerable to the budget axe, and new resources for nursing education and practice won't happen. A focus on the virtues of nurses is an invitation to seek not the best and brightest but rather the most virtuous, meekest, and self-sacrificing.

understanding the underlying accountability that comes with this powerful claim. Inherent in the role of the nurse are professional accountability and direct responsibility for decisions made and actions rendered.

SOURCES OF POWER

Most researchers agree that the sources of power are diverse and vary from one situation to another. They also agree that these **sources of power** are a combination of conscious and unconscious factors that allow an individual to influence others to do as the individual wants (Fisher & Koch, 1996). Articles and textbooks about nursing administration, educational leadership, and organizational management commonly include references to the work of Hersey, Blanchard, and Natemeyer (1979), an expansion of the power typology originally developed by French and Raven in 1959 (cited in Hersey, Blanchard, & Natemeyer, 1979). The typology helps nurses understand how different people perceive power and subsequently relate to others in the work setting and in attempts to achieve their goals. Power is described as having a basis in expertise, legitimacy, reference, reward, coercion, or connection. More recently, another power source—information—has been added to the typology (Wells, 1998). Generally speaking, nurses exert influence derived from one or a combination of these power sources. Some of these power sources may be from the organization, and other power sources may be from the individual. Power that an organization confers on someone, for example, the ability to work as

a staff RN, is not necessarily transportable to another organization unless the second organization agrees to confer power.

Power derived from the knowledge and skills nurses possess is referred to as **expert power**. There are, however, special considerations to keep in mind about expertise and power. The geometric explosion of knowledge has made expertise more valuable, and technological advances for accessing information have enabled more people to acquire expertise on any given subject. Knowing more about a subject than others, combined with the legitimacy of holding a position, gives an individual a decided advantage in any situation. But the less acknowledged that experts are in a group, the less effective their expert powers become. Visible reciprocal acknowledgment of expertise among group members balances power and enhances productivity, whereas lack of reciprocal acknowledgment has the opposite effect. Combining expertise with high position is most powerful if the person consistently demonstrates expertise. Entry-level nurses will enhance their expert power and their ability to get the patient care mission accomplished if they add to their current knowledge through professional reading and seek additional training to improve their clinical skills.

Legitimate power is power derived from the position a nurse holds in a group, and it indicates the nurse's degree of authority. The more comfortable nurses are with their legitimate power as nurses, the easier it is for them to fulfill their role. Nurses in legitimate positions are expected to use what authority they have and may be punished for not doing so. Sometimes, too little legitimacy or authority is delegated to nurses who are given the responsibility for leading. People generally follow legitimate leaders with whom they agree. Although legitimacy is a significant part of influence and control, it is not universally effective and is not sufficient as one's only source of power. New nurses may be placed in positions of legitimate power and authority relatively quickly following their orientation. For example, they may be assigned as charge nurses, supervising paraprofessionals on the shift. They must be aware of the limits of their legitimate authority so they don't overstep their bounds and should seek guidance in situations in which they must act. Appropriate and timely use of legitimate power assures positive patient care outcomes.

Power derived from how much others respect and like any individual, group, or organization is referred to as **referent power**. Nurses who are identified with respected, trustworthy individuals or groups will benefit from referent power by virtue of such identification. A nurse identified as a graduate of a respected university gains prestige and power from such identification, regardless of the personal qualities such nurse may possess. New nurses often start the job with a blank slate as far as referent power is concerned but can quickly gain influence among coworkers by identifying with other individuals or groups for which the coworkers have respect. Through identification with their university, church membership, or some other agent of influence, the entry-level nurse taps into referent power. Even dressing and looking like a nurse who has earned respect can confer referent power.

The ability to reward or punish others, as well as to create fear in others to influence them to change their behavior, is commonly termed reward power and coercive power. Meaningful rewards exist other than money, such as formal recognition before one's nursing peers at an awards ceremony. The manner in which rewards are distributed is important. Rewards seldom motivate as effectively as a vision that unifies the members of the group, thus reward power is an uncertain instrument for long-term change. New nurses may lack a direct ability to dispense rewards, but they can often indirectly exercise reward power by giving appropriate positive feedback to supervisors about the performance of others with whom they work. Rewards are not likely to permanently change attitudes. Withholding rewards or achieving a goal by instilling fear in others often results in resentment.

People who have the ability to administer punishment or take disciplinary actions against others have coercive power. This type of power is often considered the least desirable tactic to be used by people in positions of authority. Typically, people do not enjoy being coerced into doing something other than what they choose to do, and often perceive punishment as humiliating. A new nurse can indirectly influence others' behavior by reporting incidents that require disciplinary action. This course of action should not be taken lightly for it affects working relationships and should therefore be sparingly employed because of possible unintended consequences.

The extent to which nurses are connected with others having power is called **connection power**. Leaders can dramatically increase their influence by understanding that people are attracted to those with power and their associates. As a new nurse, when you go to the office of the director of nursing services or the vice president for patient care services, do not forget that the clerical workers in the outside office have relationships with their boss—thus they have connection power. If you try to go around them and take their power lightly, and insult or patronize them, you have risked your own power base in relation to the director or vice president. Similarly, if an entry-level nurse bypasses a person who is directly responsible for a situation, the attempted circumvention reflects negatively on the nurse. Nurses should work to resolve issues at the appropriate level before they take their concerns to a higher level of authority. Nurses are expected to understand the structure and policies of the organizations in which they provide services.

Nurses who influence others with the information they provide to the group are using **information power**. Regardless of a nurse's leadership style, information plays an increasingly critical role. Legitimate power, reward power, and coercive power tend to be bestowed on individuals by their organizations. They tend to be effective only for a short period of time unless they are accompanied by another form of power, such as information power. Information power is especially important because, to be functional, health care teams and organizations require accurate and timely information that is shared. To be seen by others as having information power, nurses must share knowledge that is both accurate and useful. Information sharing can improve patient care, increase collegiality, enhance organizational effectiveness, and strengthen one's professional connections. New nurses who value team membership will empower coworkers and themselves by giving and receiving information with which to do the job more effectively. See Table 12-1 for a summary of the different sources of power.

Effective nurses use the sources of power covered thus far: expertise, legitimacy, reference, reward, coercion, connection, and information. They have the ability to combine referent (charismatic) power and expert power from a legitimate power base, adding carefully measured portions of reward power and little or preferably no coercive power (Fisher & Koch, 1996). These emerging leaders gather and use information in new and creative ways. They understand that power should be a means to accomplish a goal rather than a goal in itself.

TABLE 12-1	UNDERSTANDING AND USING SOURCES OF POWER

Type	Source	Examples for Nursing
Expert	Power derived from the knowledge and skills nurses possess. The more proficiency the nurse has, the more the nurse is received as an expert.	Communicating information from current evidence-based journals and bringing expert knowledge to patient care.
Legitimate	Power derived from an academic degree, licensure, certification, experience in the role, and job title in the organization.	Wearing or displaying symbols of professional standing, including license and certification.
Referent	Power based on the trust and respect that people feel for an individual, group, or organization with which one is associated.	Gaining power by affiliating with nurses and others who have power in the organization.
Reward	Power that comes from the ability to reward others to influence them to change their behavior.	Using a hospital award to alter other's behavior.
Coercive	Power that comes from the ability to punish others to influence them to change their behavior.	Using the hospital disciplinary evaluation system to alter another's behavior.
Connection	Power that comes from personal and professional relationships that enhance one's resources and the capacity for learning and information sharing.	Developing good working relationships and mentoring with your boss and other powerful people.
Information	Power based on information that someone can provide to the group.	Sharing useful knowledge gleaned from the Internet and other sources with coworkers.

Source: Developed with information from Hersey, Blanchard, & Natemeyer (1979); French and Raven (1959); and Wells (1998).

POSITIVE PERSONAL ORIENTATION TO POWER

A person's desire for power, takes one of two forms. One form is an orientation toward achieving personal gain and self-glorification. Another form is an orientation toward achieving gain for others or the common good. Orientation to personal gain and power as a bad thing and therefore something to be avoided is reflected in a quotation from Lord Acton (Seldes, 1985, p. 234): "Power tends to corrupt, and absolute power corrupts absolutely." People having this orientation tend to believe that those wielding or afforded power ultimately should not have power because of their potential to misuse it, that people desiring power should not be trusted because their motivation for acquiring power is inherently wrong—they want power for personal gain at any cost.

The other point of view, that power is a good thing, that is, a force that is used for good purposes, is reflected in Gracian's (1892, p. 172) saying: "The sole advantage of power is that you can do more good." Nurses today are likely to see power as a positive thing and are more inclined to use this positive power to help others.

EMPOWERMENT

Empowerment is a popular term in the nursing literature related to management, leadership, and politics. Authors describing empowerment usually view it as something positive or highly desirable to be aspired to, advocated for, or attained. Kelly and Joel (2005) described empowerment in nursing as a process of power sharing by involvement in the decision-making process. Kuokkanen (2003) describes empowerment as a process of personal growth and development. Using the basis of power of French and Raven (1959), we can conceive of empowerment as a form of capacity building, in which one's capacity to influence others is enhanced by an increase in any of the sources of power.

Nurses empower themselves and others in many ways. At the most basic level, they empower others because they perceive them to be powerful. If an individual, a group, or an organization is perceived as being powerful, that perception can empower that individual, group, or organization. Some health care provider groups are viewed as more powerful than others because of the alliances they have formed with associations such as the American Medical Association (AMA), known to be powerful. Nurses disempower themselves if they see nurses or nursing as powerless.

POWER AND THE MEDIA

People who work in the media recognize the relationship between power and perception. Those who work in advertising, marketing, and public relations understand how media can be used to create or change perceptions. They have long recognized that the public's perception can be created or changed through advertising and marketing campaigns, damage control, timely press releases, and well-orchestrated media events.

The way the media present nursing to the public will empower or disempower nursing. Nurses must work to consistently use the media as effectively as other more powerful occupational groups. To date, the media have failed to recognize nursing as one of the largest most trusted groups in health care. The media's presentation of the rapidly growing nursing shortage over the next decade can improve the public's perceptions of nursing as a career and human service. The media can show

nurses as decision makers, coordinators of care, and primary care providers in health care. Too often, the media has presented a stereotypical, insignificant view of nurses (Kalisch & Kalisch, 1986). According to the Woodhull Study on Nursing and the Media (Sigma Theta Tau International, 1998), nurses are nearly invisible to the media. Sometimes, even nurses fail to view nursing as the honorable profession it is. One strategy for empowering nursing

---

CRITICAL THINKING 12-2

Think about the challenges you will face as a new nurse on a busy medical-surgical unit. How will you fit into the group? Who can you rely on among your new coworkers? What is the status of nursing vis-à-vis the medical practitioners, pharmacy service, and food service? What sources of power do you bring into the work setting? How might you establish and enhance your knowledge and skills as a competent member of the team? Are you able to appropriately assert yourself in this new environment? What additional assets do you bring to the job?

REAL WORLD INTERVIEW

Ms. Cox is 38 years old and has been hospitalized four times. She underwent surgery this past spring and has encountered nursing care and nurses in various roles throughout the health care system. Ms. Cox is articulate and reflective, having earned a degree in English and holding a position at a selective liberal arts university as an admissions counselor. She states, "I don't think nurses know they are powerful. . . . Nurses can take on more than they think they can. They have the power to change the system in which they work. Yet I see nurses as the most overworked, underpaid, and underachieving professions also. There is so much more they could be doing if they didn't spend so much time railing against the machine. They are telling the wrong people—each other—that they are frustrated. They should be telling the ones with real power, or, better yet, more of them should become the ones in power. Instead, they suffer with each other and stay angry. It appears almost passive-aggressive how nurses deal with power. My concern is that it can affect patient care in such a negative way. Believe me when I say patients value nurses, but the people writing the paycheck for nurses must value nurses. Patients need nursing far more than they need anything else. The better nurses that have cared for me have been instrumental in my healing. Beyond knowing when I need medication or doing some procedure, it is the smile, the touch, and the well-placed word of encouragement that has gotten me through. This is where nurses have power because no one but a real nurse can provide it. It comes from the heart."

Audrey Cox
Patient
University Place, Washington

is to employ the media to create a stronger, more powerful image of nursing, for example, by writing opinion editorial (op-ed) pieces and letters to the editor for the local newspaper. Examples on a larger scale include a series of television spots promoting a positive nursing image, such as that recently sponsored by the Johnson and Johnson Corporation as part of its Campaign for Nursing's Future (Johnson and Johnson, 2006). Advocacy for nursing on a national scale requires more nurses to become active participants in some formal part of their profession, that is, the American Nurses Association (ANA), the National League for Nursing (NLN), or one of the nursing specialty organizations, for example, Emergency Nurses Association.

PERSONAL POWER DEVELOPMENT

Understanding power helps the novice nurse to become more effective, to make better decisions, and to better help others. Understanding power from a variety of perspectives is not just important for nurses professionally, it is important for them personally as well. It allows nurses to gain more control of their work lives and personal lives. There are three ways to imagine the future: (1) what is possible, for example, brainstorming various scenarios about what could be; (2) what is probable, for example, making a judgment about the likelihood of a given scenario; and (3) what is preferred, for example, choosing a desired scenario, even one that may be less likely to happen than the probable future. A nurse who wants to experience a preferred future should think about what is happening to him or her as a person and as a nurse, consider what possibilities he or she faces as a person and as a nurse, and then take action to create the future.

CRITICAL THINKING 12-3

Personal empowerment for a beginning nurse requires imagining the future; setting concrete, achievable goals that represent the imagined future; and then creating that future by taking specific action steps that are likely to result in each desired goal. Think for a moment about the kind of nurse you might become. What kind of skills and expert knowledge are needed by someone who meets that description?

What are the possibilities? Are you really imagining all possible scenarios? What is probable at this time knowing what you know now? What do you prefer? Finally, what would it take, in steps, for you to achieve your preference?

CASE STUDY 12-1

Maria and Haley work on the same nursing unit in a large, metropolitan hospital. Both predominantly work the evening shift and have less than one year's experience since graduating from nursing school. Maria has been offered increasingly difficult patient assignments, given charge duties, and recently was selected for a two-week leadership training program. Haley has not adapted as well and has withdrawn from what was once a close relationship with Maria. Haley seeks consolation with the nurses she and Maria claimed they would never emulate. Haley takes her breaks and eats dinner with two nurses who complain that the best nurses are undervalued in the organization, yet these same nurses were not supportive of Maria or Haley or any other new nurses oriented to their unit. Maria seeks out others she perceives to be knowledgeable and more satisfied in their professional roles. She strives to participate in nonmandatory meetings as well as clinical rounds, using them as an opportunity to ask questions, thus she is beginning to increase her personal level of power by connecting with the other staff and gathering information. One night after a difficult shift, Haley accuses Maria of abandoning her, and playing up to administration and states that Maria is being used by the unit's nurse manager. Haley tells Maria that the other nurses are planning to file a complaint against the unit supervisor for selecting Maria over the nurses that have been on the unit longer to attend the leadership training program.

What does Haley's behavior tell you about her personal orientation toward power?

How should Maria react to Haley in this situation?

Apply your understanding of power to suggest how Maria can empower Haley.

POWER AND THE LIMITS OF INFORMATION

Even if nurses could fully trust the completeness and accuracy of information they have in their practice, they would have insufficient data. "There is no end to information just as there is no end to what we could know about something" (Wells, 1998, p. 29). To make good decisions, nurses must be able to gather enough information and realistically interpret its value, as well as share and apply information in a safe, competent manner. Effective nurses understand time constraints and set priorities to ensure that what is most important receives the most attention. These nurses are willing to take the inherent risk of making a decision, while understanding there will always be more information to gather and analyze. They recognize that choosing to make no decision is a decision in itself and that information is never complete. Table 12-2 presents a framework for becoming empowered.

EVIDENCE FROM THE LITERATURE

Citation: DeCicco, J., Laschinger, H., & Kerr, M. (2006, May). Perceptions of empowerment and respect: Effect on nurses' organizational commitment in nursing homes. *Journal of Gerontological Nursing,* 49–56.

Discussion: This study supported Kanter's theory of structural empowerment by finding that access to empowering work structures, such as information support, opportunity, and resources, empowers individuals to get their work accomplished and thus contributes to overall organizational effectiveness.

Implications for Practice: Access to empowering work structures lead to empowerment and respect and are strong predictors of organizational commitment. Entry-level nurses should be able to recognize and value such conditions as access to information, opportunity, support, and resources as means that enable them and their coworkers to get the job done. They will be better prepared to act and thus to increase their success and that of the organization with self-reinforcing intermediate benefits such as feeling respected and increasing their commitment to the organization.

REAL WORLD INTERVIEW

Power is the ultimate responsibility to care for the patient. Our assessment and subsequent actions can determine whether a patient will live or die. I feel confident in my abilities for the future, but as a new nurse, it is difficult to feel powerful because there is so much to learn. I believe that nurses tend to perceive power as being able to stand up to those above or higher up in the work setting. I think nursing is changing for the better because of the power gained with nurses having more autonomy. There is more trust put into the nurse's judgment because women's roles in society have changed. Equal opportunity programs have created the structure to protect women and others who have been vulnerable to those in positions of greater power. I have learned that you do not have to be afraid to advocate for your patient. If you need to call the attending physician during the night, then you do it. I have come to realize that power is not abusing the people working under you. Also, to understand power, it is important to understand people's roles and where they are coming from.

Julie Bergman
New Nursing Graduate
Tacoma, Washington

TABLE 12-2	A FRAMEWORK FOR BECOMING EMPOWERED
Personal power	Find a mentor.
	Notice who holds power in your personal, professional, and organizational life. Introduce yourself to them.
	Find and maintain good sources of evidence-based information.
	Seek answers to questions.
	Make a plan to develop all sources of personal, professional, and organizational power.
	Evaluate the plan.
Professional power	Assess patient's condition using relevant, objective measurements.
	Collaborate with administrators and other nursing and medical practitioners and health care workers involved in the care of your patients.
	Join your professional nursing organization.
	Consult with significant others, friends, and members of the patient's family.
	Monitor and improve patient care quality.
Organizational power	Get involved beyond direct patient care.
	Volunteer for committee assignments that will challenge you to learn and experience more than what is expected of you in a staff nurse role.
	Think about the following when involved with committees:
	1. What is the committee trying to do?
	2. What specific information does the committee use to operate and make decisions?
	3. How does the committee apply to my practice, to my colleagues, to my patients, to my organizational unit, and to the organization as a whole?
	Continually improve and add to the knowledge you have in relation to your patients, your colleagues, your organizational unit, to the organization as a whole, and to the profession of nursing.
	Readily share appropriate knowledge with others who will value it and use it to a good end.
	Evaluate your plans. Did you achieve the expected outcomes? If not, why? Were there staffing problems or patient crises? Were the activities that were necessary for outcome achievement carried out?
	How can you apply lessons learned from this evaluation to the future?
	Periodically review Table 12-1. Continue to develop all your sources of power.
	Volunteer to be involved with health care at the local, state, and national level.

MACHIAVELLI ON POWER

It would be naive to think that one can necessarily expect easy acceptance, understanding, or even support for what one is attempting to do. Machiavelli, an early authority on power, is reported to have said:

There is nothing more difficult to take in hand, more perilous to conduct than to take a lead in the introduc-

tion of a new order of things, because the innovation has for enemies all those who have done well under the old conditions, and lukewarm defenders in those who may do well under the new (Machiavelli & Rebhorn, 2003).

The entry-level nurse will do well to heed Machiavelli's warning. Machiavelli recognized the fact that the power to innovate even small changes should be employed thoughtfully.

CRITICAL THINKING 12-4

As an entry-evel nurse you empower yourself not only by using information for providing patient care but also by using information in areas beyond direct patient care. Think about the following when involved with committees:

What is the committee trying to do?

What specific information does the committee use to make decisions?

How does the committee's work apply to your practice, your colleagues, your organizational unit, and the organization as a whole?

What is the strength of the information you have in relation to your patients, your colleagues, your organizational unit, and the organization as a whole?

Are you readily sharing information with others who will value it and use it to good end?

KEY CONCEPTS

- Power can be described as the ability to get and use resources to achieve goals.

- Power can be defined at personal, professional, and organizational levels.

- Sources of power include coercion, reward, legitimate, expert, referent, and connection.

- A significant additional source of power comes from information.

- Effective nurses have a positive orientation toward power.

- Effective nurses understand power from multiple perspectives.

- Effective nurses increase their own power sources and use power for safe, competent care.

- The personal power of effective nurses is evident in the decisions they make.

KEY TERMS

connection power   power
expert power   referent power
information power   sources of power
legitimate power

REVIEW QUESTIONS

1. If, as a new nurse, you propose a change in a longstanding unit routine. You can expect:

A. support from the head nurse.
B. resistance from your coworkers.
C. resistance from anyone who is comfortable with the status quo.
D. support from your coworkers.

2. Which of the following can interfere with a new nurse's ability to influence his or her peers?
A. Seeking knowledge of recent advances in nursing practice
B. Viewing the acquisition and use of power as a bad thing
C. Sharing helpful information about patients with coworkers
D. Interacting with nonnursing hospital staff

3. Which of the following sources of power should a new nurse expect to increase during the first few months on the job?
A. Expert power
B. Legitimate power
C. Referent power
D. Coercive power

4. The most effective nurses use power
A. in one primary way.
B. to influence others or affect others' thinking or behavior.
C. predominantly at an organizational level.
D. only to gain the necessary resources to be a better nurse.

5. When a person fears another enough to act or behave differently than he would otherwise, the source of the other person's power is called
A. coercive power.
B. reward power.

C. expert power.

D. connection power.

6. A nurse's personal power can be enhanced by
   A. collaborating with colleagues on special projects outside the work setting.
   B. developing skills that do not apply directly to patient care.
   C. volunteering to serve on organizational committees led by nonnurses.
   D. All of the above.

7. Three levels of power include all but which of the following?
   A. Personal
   B. Professional
   C. Organizational
   D. Unit

8. Power has been described in the literature
   A. consistently as a negative concept.
   B. most often as a manifestation of personal ambition.
   C. as maintained through one's position in society, a work setting, or family.
   D. in multiple ways, some not so positive.

REVIEW ACTIVITIES

1. Identify a nursing leader. Observe the nurse and note what type of power the nurse uses to meet objectives.

2. Watch a television show that portrays nurses. Note how nurses use or do not use the different types of power available to them. What do you observe?

3. Observe our national leaders. What examples of the use of power do you see? Is power used in helpful or unhelpful ways? Explain.

4. Observe a nursing unit during a shift. How do nursing coworkers use various types of power to influence one another?

EXPLORING THE WEB

- This site critiques and advocates for accuracy in the media's portrayal of the role of nursing and of nurses. www.nursingadvocacy.org

- This site has a funny, not scholarly, synopsis of nursing power. www.NursingPower.net

- This site supports political power for patients. www.healthcarereform.net

- This site discusses a variety of nursing resources and issues, including collective power. www.nursingworld.org

- Go to the site for the Center for Health Policy, Research and Ethics, College of Nursing & Health Science, George Mason University. Note the seminars and internships offered to nurses interested in health policy. hpi.gmu.edu

- On the Google search engine, perform a search using the term "nursing leaders." www.google.com

- Find two nurses identified on the following site: www.distinguishedwomen.com

REFERENCES

Buresh, B., & Gordon, S. (2006). *From Silence to Voice*. Ithaca & London: Cornell U. Press.

DeCicco, J., Laschinger, H., & Kerr, M. (2006, May). Perceptions of empowerment and respect: Effect on nurses' organizational commitment in nursing homes. *Journal of Gerontological Nursing*, 49–56.

Fisher, J. L., & Koch, J. V. (1996). *Presidential leadership: Making a difference*. Phoenix, AZ: American Council on Education and The Oryx Press.

French, J. P. R. Jr., & Raven, B. (1959). The bases of social power. In D. Cartwright and A. Zander (Eds.), *Group Dynamics* (pp. 607–623). New York: Harper and Row.

Gracian, B. (1892). *The art of worldly wisdom*. (J. Jacobs, Trans.) Boston: Dover Publications, 2005. (Original work published 1647).

Hersey, P., Blanchard, K., & Natemeyer, W. (1979). Situational leadership, perception and impact of power. *Group and Organizational Studies, 4,* 418–428.

Johnson and Johnson. (2006). Campaign for nursing's future. Retrieved July 3, 2006, from http://www.jnj.com/our_company/advertising/discover_nursing

Kalisch, G., & Kalisch, P. (1986). A comparative analysis of nurse and physician characters in the entertainment media. *Journal of Advanced Nursing, 11,* 179–195.

Kelly, L. Y., & Joel, L. A. (2005). *The nursing experience: Trends, challenges, and transitions* (5th ed.). New York: McGraw-Hill.

Kuokkanen, L., Leino-Kilpi, H., & Katajisto, J. (2003). Nurse empowerment, job-related satisfaction, and organizational commitment. *Journal of Nursing Care Quality, 18*(3), 184–192.

Machiavelli, N., & Rebhorn, W. A. (2003). *The prince and other writings*. New Providence, NJ: Barnes & Noble.

Seldes, G. (1985). *The Great Thoughts*. New York: Ballantine Books.

Sigma Theta Tau International. (1998). Woodhull Study on Nursing and the Media. Retrieved September 11, 2003, from http://www.nursingsociety.org/media/woodhullextract.html

Wells, S. (1998). *Choosing the future: The power of strategic thinking*. Boston: Butterworth-Heinemann.

SUGGESTED READINGS

American Nurses Association. (1985). *Nursing's social policy statement*. Washington, DC: American Nurses Publishing.

Benner, P. E. (2000). *From novice to expert: Excellence and power in clinical nursing practice* (Commemorative edition). Upper Saddle River, NJ: Prentice Hall.

Buresh, B., & Gordon, S. (2005). *From silence to voice: What nurses know and must communicate to the public.* Cornell, NY: ILR Press.

Christman, L.. (2002). Women and leadership in health care: The journey to authenticity and power. *Nursing Administration Quarterly, 26*(2), 87–89.

Government Technology (any recent issue). (Available free online at www.govtech.net or by writing to Government Technology at 100 Blue Ravine Road, Folsom, CA 95630.)

Addresses the information age and the power of information.

Hanna, L. A. (1999). Lead the way. *Nursing Management, 30*(11), 36–39.

Leddy, S., & Pepper, J. M. (1998). *Conceptual bases of professional nursing* (4th ed.). Philadelphia: Lippincott.

Schira, M. (2004). Reflections on "About Power in Nursing." *Nephrology Nursing Journal, 31*(5), 583–584.

Short, P. M. (1998). Empowering leadership. *Contemporary Education, 69*(2), 70–72.

Spitzer, K. L., Eisenbery, M. B., & Lowe, C. A. (1998). *Information literacy essential skills for the information age.* Syracuse, NY: ERIC Clearinghouse on Information & Technology.

Strasen, L. (1987). *Key business skills for nurse managers.* Philadelphia: Lippincott.

Change, Innovation, and Conflict Management

Kristine E. Pfendt, RN, MSN ✛ Margaret M. Anderson, EdD, RN, CNAA

Change and innovation are closely related concepts. In our society, change is inevitable and innovation is a necessary component of our culture (Lillian Sims, 2000).

OBJECTIVES

Upon completion of this chapter, the reader should be able to:

1. Explain change from personal, professional, and organizational perspectives.
2. Identify the change theorists.
3. Explain the concept of the learning organization.
4. Identify driving and restraining forces of change within a structured setting context.
5. Relate change strategies.
6. Explain the role and characteristics of a change agent in the change process.
7. Plan, implement, and evaluate a change project using the change process.
8. Apply the concept of innovation to health care.
9. Identify conflict situations.
10. Identify steps in the conflict management process.

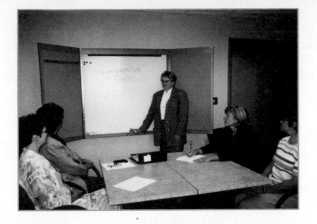

Dwayne is working on a patient care unit as a new computerized charting system is introduced. He notices that several of the staff start using the system quickly. Other staff are resistant and angrily say they want no part of the new system. Dwayne feels comfortable with the system and quickly begins to use it.

How can Dwayne contribute to the staff's smooth transition to the new charting system?

How can Dwayne's nurse manager help staff with the transition to the new system?

What knowledge and tools would help a new graduate adapt to the changing environment?

Living organisms must constantly adapt to changes in their environment in order to thrive. In this same way, human beings must also successfully adapt and manage change in order to maintain homeostasis and equilibrium. Rapid changes and innovations occurring in the world today require continuous human responses. How these changes and innovations are perceived by the individual can mean the difference between successful adaptation and maladaptation, survival and extinction.

Today's health care environment is also constantly changing. Luthans and Jensen (2005) state that "the health care industry is suffering from an unprecedented shortage of qualified nurses as well as increasing demands and complexity due to technological innovations and changing consumer expectations" (p. 304). Access to information has transformed the relationship between the patient and health care provider. Individuals in many cases are better informed about their medical conditions and treatment options. These same individuals view themselves as partners in their health care rather than just consumers of it.

Evidence-based practice is changing the way that decisions are made regarding health care treatment and how nursing care is delivered. Interventions such as surgery and diagnostic testing that once required lengthy and costly stays in hospitals are often provided now in outpatient settings. The length of stay in hospitals has

been shortened both by the impact of enhanced technology and the requirements of managed care.

Changing demographics within the population has resulted in a diversity of cultures and languages as well. Challenges continue for nursing and others involved with health care delivery to understand these cultures and to communicate effectively. The aging of the Baby Boom generation and the continuous need for nurses to care for them will also impact health care in the future.

The rising costs of health care services have had a major impact on society as well. Premiums are continuously rising for those consumers who are fortunate enough to have health care insurance. Cost of Medicare and Medicaid also continue to rise, and the nation continues to grapple with payment. For those without any access to health care, the costs continue to soar. Delays in seeking care because of an individual's inability to pay for services and medications often results in more seriously ill patients with life-altering consequences.

Issues regarding patient safety can be translated into the cost of care. The Institute of Medicine (IOM) Report states that there are staggering consequences to unsafe care and medication errors. "Medication errors alone, occurring either in or out of the hospital, are estimated to account for over 7,000 deaths annually . . . One recent study conducted at two prestigious teaching hospitals, found that about 2 out of every 100 admissions experienced a preventable adverse drug event, resulting in average increased hospital costs of $4,700 per admission or about $2.8 million annually for a 700-bed teaching hospital" (IOM, 2002).

All of these factors affect the ways that nurses function in the health care environment and how they care for their patients. How nurses manage these changes and innovations will impact quality of care, the health care system of the future, and the lives of all health care consumers. This chapter discusses the change process, innovation, and conflict management. This information will enhance the nurse's ability to manage future change and innovation successfully.

CHANGE

There are many definitions of change, and there are many types of change. For simplicity, **change** can be defined as "making something different from what it was" (Sullivan & Decker, 2005, p. 217). The outcome may be the same, but the actions performed to get to the outcome may be different. For instance, because of road closures, how you get to work may have to change. The goal of getting to work remains the same, but the method may be different, perhaps by bus rather than automobile or by use of a different route. In the professional nursing setting, new patient admission forms may necessitate a different method of assessing the patient or change the number of people involved in the admission process. Rather than one registered nurse conducting the entire admission process, the process may be broken down so that individuals with different skill levels conduct parts of the process. The goal is still the admission of the patient to a unit; how it is done may be different. Most change is implemented for a good or reasonable purpose. Beason (2005) states that to be effective, change should affect all levels of the health care organization, and communication throughout all levels is essential.

For purposes of discussion, **personal change** is a change made voluntarily for your own reasons, usually for self-improvement. This may include changing your diet for health reasons, taking classes for self-improvement, or removing yourself from a destructive or unhealthful environment or situation. **Professional change** may be a change in position or job such as obtaining education or credentials that will benefit you in a current position or allow you to be prepared for a future position. Professional change is often planned and involves extensive change in both personal and professional lives. Although either personal or professional change may be stressful, if it is voluntary and carries intrinsic or extrinsic rewards, it is often considered important and worth the stress.

Organizational change often causes the most stress or concern. Generally speaking, **organizational change**, which is a planned change in an organization to improve efficiency, is thrust upon employees. Sometimes there is a lot of preparation and prior discussion. Change that is unexpected causes a great deal of consternation and stress. Organizational change that is planned and purposeful is generally better accepted. It is used to improve efficiency or improve financial standing or for some other organizational purpose. Change is planned to meet organizational goals. One of the goals most organizations have is to maintain a positive financial balance. Change to ensure a healthy financial standing maintains jobs and increases the organization's capability to meet its mission. Improved efficiency is good for the organization's capability to get goods and services to the customer. Improved efficiency in health care provides better quality care for patients and improves the workload of the employees.

Organizations that adapt successfully to change are able to adapt quickly to new market conditions. These are the organizations that will survive in a competitive environment. Employees who are educated about the need for change and who embrace new ideas are key to the achievement of successful outcomes (Recklies, 2006). Organizational change must be embraced by all levels of employees, including managers, to be effective (Beason, 2005).

Budget changes may be a necessary change for the survival of a health care institution. Nurses caring for patients are often impacted by staff reductions due to budget cuts. Nursing staff may believe that the quality of patient care will diminish as a result. As staffing levels are cut, those nurses who are left to care for patients often face increased workloads. Staff burnout may result, and attrition rates may rise as turnover increases. In the larger picture, the increased costs of hiring and orienting new nurses to replace the ones who have left may exceed the cost of savings from the initial staff layoffs (Ponte, Kruger, & DeMarco, 2004).

Effective communication to nursing staff about why budget changes are necessary is essential to adaptation to changes that impact the quality of patient care. Education is needed about the current marketplace and how nursing units are impacted. For example, changes in third-party payment practices may influence the number of nurses that a patient care unit can have. Nurse leaders and managers often have the responsibilities for communicating and educating staff concerning why these changes are necessary (Heath, Johnson, & Blake, 2004).

At times, when organizational change is planned, the employees may be the last to know what the anticipated change is but may be the ones most affected by it. The staff nurse is expected to implement the new care delivery system, but he may also be the last one to know about the change until it is to be implemented. For example, in an organization in which primary nursing has been the care delivery system for several years, the implementation of modified team nursing is a major change in philosophy and thinking. It is important that proper care and planning of the change process be used, so that the staff will not resist the change and make the implementation much more stressful than necessary. Table 13-1 summarizes the types of change.

TRADITIONAL CHANGE THEORIES

The classic change theories discussed here are Lewin's Force-Field Model (1951), Lippitt's Phases of Change (1958), Havelock's Six-Step Change Model (1973), and Rogers' Diffusion of Innovations Theory (1983). These are classic change theories based on Lewin's original model.

Lewin's model has three simple steps. The steps are unfreezing, moving to a new level, and refreezing. Unfreezing means that the current or old way of doing is flawed. People begin to be aware of the need for doing things differently, that change is needed for a specific reason. In the next step, the intervention or change is introduced and explained. The benefits and disadvantages are discussed, and the change—the move to a new level—is implemented. In the third step, refreezing occurs. This means that the new way of doing is incorporated into the routines or habits of the affected people. Although these steps sound simple, the process of change is, of course, more complex.

Lippitt's Phases of Change are built on Lewin's model. Lippitt defined seven stages in the change process. These steps include: (1) diagnosing the problem,

TABLE 13-1	TYPES OF CHANGE
Personal	A change made voluntarily for one's own reasons, usually for self-improvement.
Professional	A change in position or job such as obtaining education or credentials that will benefit one in a current position or allow one to be prepared for a future position.
Organizational	A planned change in an organization to improve efficiency.

EVIDENCE FROM THE LITERATURE

Citation: Haase-Herrick, K. (2005). The Opportunities of Stewardship. *Nursing Administration Quarterly, 28*(2), 115–118.

Discussion: This article discusses goals for improving the current health care system that were first recommended by the Institute of Medicine. These were published in *Crossing the Quality Chasm: A New Health System for the 21st Century* in 2002. The recommendations were that health care should be safe, effective, patient-centered, efficient, and equitable. Haase-Herrick challenges nurses to strive to change the health care delivery system as it currently exists and to change the status quo. She recommends that nurses do this by increasing their knowledge level of health care economics, health care financing, and statistical and financial analysis.

Nurses are applying these strategies and are in fact changing the way that health care is delivered. Through the establishment of new nurse-run centers, care is being provided that is cost effective and patient centered. These centers are meeting the needs of many underserved populations in their respective communities. (See the article "Nurse-Managed Health Centers Are Changing the Face of Health Care" at www.nncc.us/about/nmhc.html.)

The author also advocates for nurses to become more actively involved in the political process to ensure that the most current standards of practice are used by professional organizations, licensing, and accrediting agencies. The profession of nursing can impact the quality of care through continuous involvement in these processes.

Implications for Practice: Nurses must ask themselves in what way can they become involved in the political processes that are changing health care continuously. Change is inevitable!

(2) assessing the motivation and capacity for change, (3) assessing the change agent's motivation and resources, (4) selecting progressive change objectives, (5) choosing an appropriate role for the change agent, (6) maintaining the change after it has been started, and (7) terminating the helping relationship. Lippitt emphasized the participation of key personnel and the change agent in designing and planning the intended change project. Lippitt also emphasized communication during all phases of the process.

Havelock designed a six-step model of the change process. This model is based on Lewin's model, but Havelock included more steps in each stage. The planning stage includes: (1) building a relationship, (2) diagnosing the problem, and (3) acquiring resources. This planning stage is followed by the moving stage, which includes (4) choosing the solution, and (5) gaining acceptance. The last stage, the refreezing stage, includes (6) stabilizing and self-renewing. Havelock emphasized the planning stage. He believed that resistance to change can be overcome if there is careful planning and inclusion of the affected staff. Havelock also believed that the change agent, the person responsible for planning and implementing the change, encouraged participation on the part of the people. The more the people affected by the change participate in the change, the more they are likely to make the change successful and to support the necessity for the change (Sullivan & Decker, 2005).

In 1983, Rogers published his Diffusion of Innovations Theory. Though based on Lewin's model, this theory is much broader in scope and approach. He developed a five-step innovation/decision-making process. Rogers believes that the change can be rejected initially and then adopted at a later time. He believes that change is a reversible process and that initial rejection does not necessarily mean the change will never be adopted. This also works in reverse—the change may initially be adopted and then rejected at a later time. Rogers' approach emphasized the capriciousness of change. Timing and format take on new meaning and importance. Rogers meant that as the time involved in change implementation grows longer, the more the change process takes on a life of its own, and the original change and reasons for it may be lost. The change process must be carefully managed and planned to ensure that it survives mostly intact.

COMMONALTIES AND DIFFERENCES

These change theories, models, and phases are helpful in understanding change and the dynamics involved in change. They do have similarities and differences as shown in Table 13-2.

All of these theorists relate to Lewin's three simple steps of unfreezing, moving, and refreezing. Table 13-2 also identifies the situations in which each theorist is most useful. The theories described in Table 13-2 are linear in nature in that they more or less proceed in an orderly manner from one step to the next. This linearity

TABLE 13-2	**COMPARISON CHART OF CHANGE THEORIES AND THEIR USES**			
Theorist and Year	Lewin (1951)	Lippitt (1958)	Havelock (1973)	Rogers (1983)
Title of Model	Force-Field Model	Seven Phases of Change	Six-Step Change Model	Diffusion of Innovations Theory
Steps in Model	1. Unfreeze. 2. Move. 3. Refreeze.	1. Diagnose problem. 2. Assess motivation and capacity for change. 3. Assess change agent's motivation and resources. 4. Select progressive change objective. 5. Choose appropriate role of change agent. 6. Maintain change. 7. Terminate helping relationship.	1. Build relationship. 2. Diagnose problem. 3. Acquire resources. 4. Choose solution. 5. Gain acceptance. 6. Stabilize and self-renew.	1. Awareness 2. Interest 3. Evaluation 4. Trial 5. Adoption
Use in Change Projects	General model for most situations and organizations.	Good for changing a process and general change.	Often used for educational change or cultural change.	Used in organizational change, individual change, and group change.

Source: Compiled with information from Lewin, K. (1951). *Field history in social science.* New York: Harper & Row; Lippitt, R. (1958). *The dynamics of planned change.* New York: Harcourt Brace; Havelock, R. G. (1973). *The change agent's guide to innovation in education.* Englewood Cliffs, NJ: Educational Technology; Rogers, E. M. (1983). *Diffusion of Innovations* (3rd ed.). New York: Free Press.

and the fact that they are all based on Lewin's theory make them similar in complexity and in use. These theories work well for low-level uncomplicated change. They may not always work well in highly complex and nonlinear situations. Havelock's theory is often applied to educational change, whereas Rogers' is useful for individual change. Health care organizations are very complex and require more sophisticated theories of change that will be presented next.

CHAOS THEORY

Two often-used and emerging theories of change are much more complex in breadth and depth than the theories previously discussed. These theories are *Chaos theory* and *Learning Organization theory*. Chaos theory hypothesizes that chaos actually has an order. That is, although the potential for chaos appears to be random at first glance, further investigation reveals some order to the chaos. Health care organizations have experienced chaos at times repeatedly during the past twenty years. Chaos theory would say that this is normal. Most organizations go through periods of rapid change and innovation and then stabilize before chaos erupts again. Even though each chaotic occurrence is similar to the one that occurred before, each is different. The political, scientific, and behavioral components of the organization are different from before, so the chaos looks different. Order emerges through fluctuation and chaos. Thus, the potential for chaos means that nurses and the organization must be able to organize and implement change quickly and forcefully. There is little time for orderly linear change.

THEORY OF LEARNING ORGANIZATIONS

Peter Senge (1990) first described his classic Learning Organization theory, which focused on ways organizations learn and adapt. Learning organizations demonstrate responsiveness and flexibility. Senge believed that because organizations are open systems, they could best respond to unpredictable changes in the environment by using a learning approach in their interactions and interdisciplinary workings with one another. The whole cannot function well without a part regardless of how small that part may seem. An example in health care is that the billing department cannot submit an accurate bill to the insurance company without the cooperation of the nursing staff. If the patient is not charged appropriately for items used in his care, then the biller cannot prepare an accurate invoice. Without this invoice, the organization cannot be paid for the actual services and supplies used. The learning organization understands these interrelationships and responds quickly to improve relationships. This may be through dialogue or team problem solving, but all parties must understand what is at stake for cooperation and working together to occur.

Health care has been suffering from continuous and unrelenting change since the early 1980s. Senge believes that institutional change is essential for many industries, including health care, though prospective payment and managed care have certainly taken their toll. Several positive outcomes have resulted from these changes. Most health care agencies have implemented some of the latest business methods for improving efficiency, increasing financial health, and doing their best to reduce the cost of health care. Most health care organizations have reduced management layers, cut nonessential employees, and reordered how patient care is delivered at the bedside. Most organizations have determined what their best patient service lines are and have concentrated on excellence in those areas. Patient service or product lines are the health needs the organization is best prepared to meet in the community it serves. Rather than being all things or "full service" to all patients, patient service lines are selected where a health care organization already has a market niche, that is, a market niche where the organization is already known. For example, acute care health care organizations with small numbers of patients in obstetrics may get out of the obstetrical business and expand in another area such as orthopedics or oncology, areas where the organization has large, robust numbers of patients and a healthy market niche in which to expand. In most markets, health care has undergone a series of acute care organizational mergers and agency closures in an effort to economize on labor and expenses.

However, even with all the mergers and closures, chaos still exists in many areas of health care. Many organizations have not incorporated the need to work together or the need to build a multidisciplinary approach to problem solving as recommended by the Institute of Medicine.

Senge has developed five disciplines that he believes are necessary for organizations to achieve the "learning organization status" to deal effectively with chaos. These disciplines are using systems thinking, developing personal mastery, developing mental models, building shared vision, and developing team learning. In health care, these five disciplines may be the ones necessary to provide high-quality patient care as efficiently as possible. Most experts agree that few, if any, health care organizations have evolved to learning organization status. This is a goal to work toward so that health care workers can react quickly and proactively to chaos and a rapidly changing environment. In the learning organization, each individual has something to offer that melds with what others have to offer to determine the right steps to take in sorting out the causes of chaos and responding positively to it. The goals of the organization and individual are mutually related so that quick response to chaos occurs, with positive results for both the organization and individual. Communication is key.

THE CHANGE PROCESS

Planned change in the work organization is similar to planned change on a personal level. The major difference is that more people are involved, the scale is larger, and more opinions must be considered. There are three basic reasons to introduce a change: (1) to solve a problem, (2) to improve efficiency, and (3) to reduce unnecessary workload for some group (Marquis & Huston, 2006). To plan change, one must know what has to be changed. Change for the sake of change is unnecessary and stressful (Bennis, Benne, & Chin, 1969).

STEPS IN THE CHANGE PROCESS

The change process can be related to the nursing process. Using the nursing process as a model, the first step in the change process is assessment.

ASSESSMENT   In assessment, you identify the problem or the opportunity for improvement through change by collecting and analyzing data. Sometimes, the change is planned to meet a previously determined goal. The current methods to meet that goal may not be working, so a new plan needs to be developed. Often the change is needed to take advantage of an opportunity rather than to solve a problem. Assessment must be aimed at the perceived problem or opportunity, and then the plan is focused on that. For example, if the nurse manager observes that the evening shift is not able to finish its work on time or within a reasonable time, then what is the problem? It could be the staff is not very experienced, or maybe there are too many transient staff. Perhaps there is a new patient service offered, and the care for these patients is taking more time than is anticipated. Is there a structural problem? For example, maybe the supplies or care products are stored too far away for the number of staff members working this shift. Maybe the supply stations should be less far apart. Are supplies or drugs not delivered in an appropriate time frame? Is new or old technology slowing down the staff response time? These are the issues to be assessed to identify the problem. A quick examination or a hasty decision will not accurately diagnose the problem.

After assessment to determine the problem has been completed, attention must be paid to data collection and data analysis. This may be different from data with which the nurse is familiar. The data collection and analysis should be from several sources: structural, technological, and people. A structural problem is one of physical space or the configuration of physical space. For instance, a med-surg unit in a hospital may move to the space vacated by the old obstetrics unit. The problem may be that the space is large enough, but it is not configured to be conducive to the care of med-surg patients. Assessment of structural components may include examination of the location of elevators, supply stations, patient charts, telephones, call lights, or any other physical or structural components. If nurses have not been included in the space configuration, then more expensive remodeling may be necessary. Structural components often mandate how the work is done or the process of doing the work. Poor structural configuration may require extra steps or work to accomplish the goals of the work team.

Technological problems may include a lack of wall outlets for necessary equipment, poorly situated computer locations, and lack of computer systems capability to interface with one another. Often, technology lags behind the goals of a work team and therefore slows the team down. The team spends more time troubleshooting technology to meet their needs than in providing care.

People problems may include personnel with inadequate training, willingness, commitment, or understanding to change and meet any new goals.

A work process problem (how the work is done), an equipment problem, or a people problem may be the cause of the need to change. Data collection must focus on the work, equipment, or people problem, in order to reach desired goals.

Assessment data are collected from internal and external sources. Lewin identified forces that were supportive of as well as barriers to change. He called these driving and restraining forces. If the restraining forces outweigh the driving forces, then the change must be abandoned because it cannot succeed. Driving and restraining forces include political issues, technology issues, cost and structural issues, and people issues. The political issues include the power groups in favor of or against the proposed change. This may include practitioners, administrators, civic and community groups, or state or federal regulators. The technology issues include whether to update old equipment, computer systems, or methods for accounting for supply use. Structural issues include the costs, desirability, and feasibility of remodeling or building new construction for the change project. People issues include the commitment of the staff, their level of education and training, and their interest in the project. The most common people issue is fear of job loss or fear of not being valued. It bears repeating that if the restraining forces outweigh the driving forces, then the change will not succeed, and it should be abandoned or rethought.

During data analysis, potential solutions may be identified, sources of resistance may come to light, determination of strategies may become apparent, and some areas of consensus may become evident. Statistical analysis is an important component of analysis. This should be done whenever possible to provide persuasive information in favor of the change, especially if meeting cost or mission objectives is the issue. The goal of data analysis is to support the need to change and offer data to support the potential solution selected. The people who are potentially going to be most affected by the change need to be involved in the assessment, data collection, and data analysis. They have a vested interest in the change and must not only support the change but also be willing to implement change (Bennis, Benne, & Chin, 1969).

PLANNING

The next step is the planning step. In this step, the who, how, and when of the change is determined. All of the potential solutions are examined. The driving and resisting forces are again examined, and strategies are determined for implementing the change. The target date for implementation and the outcomes or goals are clearly determined and stated in measurable terms. Although these items were examined in the assessment step, they are now made more specific. The potential for error is reduced, and the forces for success are marshaled. Again, the individuals who will be most affected must be involved. The most successful plan for change is one in which the affected people are involved, satisfied, and committed. Change cannot be thrust upon people without expecting resistance. Most of the time, resistance can be overcome with planning and involvement of those most affected by the change.

As you plan the change, consider, for instance, how many work groups or units will implement the change at once? Will the change implementation be staggered from month to month or week to week? Will the supports necessary to manage the change go into effect first? Just how will this change be implemented? Finally, the overall plan includes plans for evaluation. It is crucial that evaluation be built in. Expected outcomes must be identified in measurable terms, and the plan to evaluate those outcomes and a timetable for evaluation must be evident. Unevaluated change will not succeed. The status quo will seep back into play, and all the efforts directed at change will be for naught. Planned evaluation keeps the project in the forefront of people's minds. In health care, there is no change that does not involve people. Patients and staff are affected by any changes.

IMPLEMENTATION OF CHANGE STRATEGIES

The next step is the implementation step. In this step the plan actually goes live! There are several ways to implement change. The most common method to encourage change by individuals is to provide information. Information regarding the change and its anticipated advantages must be disseminated early and often. The change should be viewed by those who designed it and those who must implement it as a positive solution to a problem or a wonderful method for addressing an opportunity. Optimism is the key to a higher success rate.

Another method used to change individuals is competency-based education. The educator provides information and practice. This is especially useful for equipment or technology change. The individual is shown how to use the equipment and when to use it. The information provides useful data for incorporating the equipment into daily work life. Large groups of individuals can be taught together for the best results. They help each other achieve the goals of safe practice and appropriate use of the product. Bennis, Benne, & Chin (1969) identified three strategies to promote change in groups or organizations. Different strategies work in different situations. The power or authority of the change agent has an impact on the strategy selected. Most change agents use a variety of strategies to promote successful change. The power-coercive strategy is very simple—"do it or get out." This is a strategy based on power, authority, and control. This is a strong indication of the political clout of the change agent. There is very little effort to encourage participation of employees, and there is little concern about their acceptance or resistance to the proposed change. Sullivan and Decker (2005) use the federal government's decision to impose prospective payment on Medicare hospital clients as an example of the power-coercive strategy—no discussion, simply, this is what will be. This group of strategies is generally reserved for situations in which resistance is expected but not important to the power group.

The second group change strategy is normative-reeducative. This strategy is based on the assumption that group norms are used to socialize individuals. This strategy assumes that because people are social beings, social relationships are important, and they will go along with a change if the social group sanctions it. The change agent uses satisfactory interpersonal relationships rather than power to gain compliance with the desired change. This strategy uses noncognitive methods of inducing compliance by focusing on social relationships and perceptual orientations. This means that information and knowledge are not used to gain compliance but rather the individual's need for satisfying social relationships in the workplace is used. Very few individuals can withstand social isolation or rejection by the workgroup. So compliance and support for a change is garnered by focusing on the perceived loss of social relationships in the workplace. Although some resistance to change may be expected, this strategy assumes people are interested in preserving relationships and will go along with the majority.

The third group of strategies is rational-empirical. This group of strategies assumes that humans are rational people and will use knowledge to embrace change. It is assumed that once the self-interests of a group are evident, they will see the merit in a change and embrace that

TABLE 13-3	STRATEGIES FOR CHANGE
Strategy	**Description**
Power-coercive approach	Uses authority and threat of job loss to gain compliance with change.
Normative-reeducative approach	Uses social orientation and the individual's need to have satisfactory relationships in the workplace as a method of inducing support for change. Focuses on the majority rule to induce change.
Rational-empirical approach	Uses knowledge as power base. Once workers understand the organizational need for change or understand the meaning of the change to them as individuals and the organization as a whole, they will change.

change. Knowledge is the component used to encourage compliance with change. This is a very successful strategy when little resistance is anticipated. Table 13-3 summarizes the strategies for change.

These strategies are important to the success of the change and are often used together to effect a necessary change. The implementation phase is very important to success. When compliance is gained, implementation will be smoother. The project has a greater chance of being successful.

Two characteristics indicate successful implementation of a project. The most important is that the people affected by the change begin to own the change and speak well of it. The benefits stated as positive outcomes of the change actually begin to materialize. The importance of the change is apparent, and those involved demonstrate interest and enthusiasm for the change. The communication about the change supports its value, benefits, and usefulness. The second characteristic of successful implementation is that the change is perceived as an improvement and is received with positive regard and anticipation throughout the organization.

EVALUATION OF CHANGE In the evaluation step, the effectiveness of the change is evaluated according to the outcomes identified during the planning and implementation steps. This is the most overlooked step, and it is considered by some experts to be the most important. Usually enough time is not allowed for the change to be effective or stable. This is especially true in health care. The learning curve is not identified and, therefore, the change is prematurely assumed to be ineffective. This is a terrible error. The time intervals for evaluation should be identified and allowed to elapse before modifications and declarations of failure are asserted. A certain period of confusion and turmoil accompanies all changes, whether large or small. If the outcomes are achieved, then the

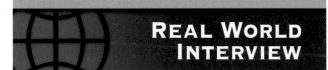

REAL WORLD INTERVIEW

One of the things I have learned about change is that fear of the change is worse than the change itself. Now I concentrate on assisting my staff to focus on the reasons why the change is necessary and involve them in the process of finding solutions to the problem.

Joy Churchill, RN
Team Leader
Highland Heights, Kentucky

change was a success. If not, then some revision or modification may be necessary to achieve the anticipated outcomes. Note that although it is important to understand why a change was not successfully implemented, it is equally important to understand why a change was successful.

STABILIZATION OF CHANGE After the effectiveness of the change is determined, then stabilization of the change is completed. The project is no longer a pilot or experiment but is a part of the culture and function of the organization. This is when the change agent bows out, and the affected employees own the change. Although there is no magical time frame for stabilization to occur, it should be encouraged as soon as possible to make the change project complete. Often, reevaluation is planned after the first six months or year of implementation to assure that stabilization has occurred.

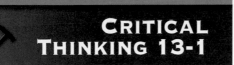

CRITICAL THINKING 13-1

Nirmala was nearing the end of her 12-hour day shift and looking forward to attending her son's final high school soccer game after work. Just when she was ready to leave the unit, a new patient unexpectedly arrived and needed to be admitted. Judy, the nurse on the next shift, asked Nirmala to admit the new patient before she left. Nirmala refused, and a heated interchange occurred. What were the conditions leading to this conflict? What was the core of the conflict? Who was right? How can conflicts like this be avoided in the future?

RESPONSES TO CHANGE

People do have responses to change. In health care, there has been such chaos and confusion at times, that employees are often resistant to change simply because it is a change. The most typical response to change is resistance. Human beings like order and familiarity. Humans enjoy routine and the status quo, so it is common for humans to resist change. The more the relationships or social mores are challenged to change, the more resistance there is to change. Marquis and Huston (2006) point out that nurses are more likely to accept a change in an intravenous pump rather than a change in who can administer the intravenous fluid. This suggests that the social mores of a group are more important than technology in a change. The social mores dictate the roles and responsibilities of groups of workers such as registered nurses, licensed practical nurses, nurse aides, and so on. Registered nurses are often less concerned with technology and more concerned with maintaining traditional roles and responsibilities. The trick to successful change is to manage the resistance rather than try to eliminate it.

Several factors affect resistance to change. The first is trust. The employee and employer must trust that each is doing the right thing and that each is capable of producing successful change. In addition to capability, predictability is important. The employee wants a predictable work environment and security. When change is introduced, predictability begins to come into question. Another factor is the individual's ability to cope with change. Silber (1993) points out four factors that affect an individual's ability to cope with change:

1. Flexibility for change, that is, the ability to adapt to change

2. Evaluation of the immediate situation, that is, if the current situation is unacceptable, then change will be more welcome
3. Anticipated consequences of change, that is, the impact change will have on one's current job
4. Individual's stake or what the individual has to win or lose in the change, that is, the more individuals perceive they have to lose, the more resistance they will offer

Change is a frightening prospect for those who have not had much experience with change or have had negative experiences with change. It is important to help individuals remember that change is inevitable and ever present. Developing an attitude of embracing and accepting change is desirable.

Bushy and Kamphius (1993) have identified six behavioral responses that individuals have to planned change. These responses may be categorized as the following:

1. *Innovators:* Change embracers. Enjoy the challenge of change and often lead change.
2. *Early adopters:* Open and receptive to change but not obsessed with it.
3. *Early majority:* Enjoy and prefer the status quo but do not want to be left behind. They adopt change before the average person.
4. *Late majority:* Often known as the followers. They adopt change after expressing negative feelings and are often skeptics.
5. *Laggards:* Last group to adopt a change. They prefer tradition and stability to innovation. They are somewhat suspicious of change.
6. *Rejectors:* Openly oppose and reject change. May be surreptitious or covert in their opposition. They may hinder the change process to the point of sabotage.

Regardless of the importance and necessity of change, the human response is very important and cannot be dismissed. So often, in the zeal to respond to a need, the change agent forgets that the human side of change must be dealt with. People have a right to their feelings and a right to express them. The important point is that the change agent helps people respond and then move on to the goal of implementing the change. Gently, but firmly, people must be guided toward acceptance.

THE CHANGE AGENT

Throughout this discussion of change, the term **change agent**, has been used instead of manager, leader, or administrator. The change agent leads and manages change. This person may be from inside or outside an organization. The change agent may be a leader or manager or may have become a leader or manager because he or she is an innovator and likely to enjoy change. The change agent is the person who is ultimately responsible for the success of the change project, large or small. The role of the change agent is to manage the dynamics of the change process. This role requires knowledge of the organization, knowledge of the change process, knowledge of the participants in the change process, and understanding of the feelings of the group undergoing change. Probably the most important role of the change agent is to maintain communication, momentum, and enthusiasm for the project while still managing the process. Table 13-4 summarizes the roles and characteristics of the change agent.

The change agent should possess some important characteristics. These include trust and respect from the recipients of change as well as from the chief executives in the organization. The recipients of change must trust not only the change agent's interpersonal skills to provide information and manage change but also the change agent's personal integrity and standing as an honest, principled individual. The executives in the organization must trust that the change agent will accomplish the established goals given the proper support. Credibility and flexibility are also important characteristics for the change agent to possess. The change agent cannot be temperamental or rigid. The ability of the change agent to compromise and negotiate is also important.

An essential characteristic of the change agent is the ability to maintain and communicate the vision of the change. No matter how small or large the project is, the vision or picture of that change must be maintained and kept in the forefront of everyone's memory. The ability to articulate the vision and to mold disparate concepts into that vision is paramount to success. The astute change agent recognizes that those affected by the change may not have the same vision, so the change agent must paint a vivid mental picture of the change and how it will work during change implementation. The change agent will also have to recognize that those developing the project have some definite inclusion concepts that must be folded in to the vision for success. Inclusion concepts are those ideas or concepts that the affected parties believe are absolutely necessary for their peace of mind or moral value. Including these concepts in the change process helps people feel ownership and value, that is, a piece of them or their idea is in the plan.

Perhaps the outstanding skill the change agent needs is the ability to communicate and have good interpersonal skills. Communication throughout the change process cannot be emphasized enough. Each stage must be communicated to all who want or need to know about the project. The ability to establish trusting relationships, interact with others, and manage conflict is of utmost importance to the success of the project. Honesty is the key to truly excellent communication. People are better able to deal with the truth rather than a half-truth or a lie. If a project team member's ideas are not acceptable for whatever reason, let them know immediately so there are no misunderstandings later. Communication includes using positive, concise, clear words that communicate accurately and responsibly. Ambiguity in communication is an error that leads to conflict and distrust later in the

REAL WORLD INTERVIEW

Good communication is essential to "buy in" of nursing staff to the change process. It is very important for nurses to understand why a change is necessary in order for them to embrace change.

Caron Martin, RN
Staff Nurse
Highland Heights, Kentucky

TABLE 13-4	ROLES AND CHARACTERISTICS OF THE CHANGE AGENT
■ Leads the change process	■ Communicates change, progress, and feelings
■ Manages the change process and group dynamics	■ Knowledgeable about the organization
■ Understands feelings of the group experiencing change	■ Trustworthy
■ Maintains momentum and enthusiasm	■ Respected
■ Maintains vision of change	■ Intuitive

project. Credible communication maintains open communication lines and helps to manage the process. The change agent must be sensitive to the project team members' feelings and involvement with the way things were. Do not denigrate or disrespect what was. Concentrate on how much better things can be.

Another important characteristic of the change agent is the ability to empower people to control the change project as it affects their lives. Those most affected by the change must be involved in assessing, planning, implementing, and evaluating the change. Without this support, the change cannot be successful. The change agent needs to be open and empowering about the selection of people to work on this project. Empowerment and participation in the project help people own the project and support its successful implementation. It is important for the change agent to respond appropriately to people's responses to change and not dismiss or be disrespectful of those reactions. Empowerment is a powerful tool in helping people realize that although something is changing, they have some control and input into that change. The change agent needs to use that empowerment to move the change along and to help people respond positively to the change.

The change agent must have some intuition during the evaluation steps so that he or she can bow out of the change and allow those affected accept ownership of the change. This is a matter of timing and insight into when the staff is ready to accept and incorporate the change as its own. Bennis (1989) warns that to not step away from the project and cut the ownership bonds means that it remains the change agent's project for many years to come, even after the change agent might leave the organization. During evaluation, the change agent must support modifications and revisions that help transfer project ownership.

CHANGE AGENT STRATEGIES

Following are some strategies the change agent can use in managing the process:

1. Begin by articulating the vision clearly and concisely. Use the same words over and over. Constantly remind people of the goals and vision.
2. Map out a tentative time line and sketch out the steps of the project. Have a good idea of how the project should go.
3. Plant seeds or mention some ideas or thoughts to key individuals from the first step through the evaluation step so that some idea of what is expected is under consideration.
4. Select the change project team carefully. Make sure it is heavily loaded with those who will be affected and other experts as needed. Select a variety of people. For example, an innovator, someone from the

late majority group, a laggard, and a rejector are probably good to include. These people provide insight into what others are thinking.
5. Set up consistent meeting dates and keep them. Have an agenda and constantly check the time line for target activities.
6. For those not on the team but affected by the project, give constant and consistent updates on progress. If the change agent does not, someone on the project team will, and the change agent wants to control the messages.
7. Give regular updates and progress reports both verbally and in writing to the executives of the organization and those affected by the change.
8. Check out rumors and confront conflict head on. Do not look for conflict, but do not back away from it or ignore it.
9. Maintain a positive attitude, and do not get discouraged.
10. Stay alert to political forces both for and against the project. Get consensus on important issues as the project goes along, especially if policy, money, or philosophy issues are involved. Obtain consensus quickly on major issues or potential barriers to the project from both executives and staff.
11. Know the internal formal and informal leaders. Create a relationship with them. Consult them often.
12. Having self-confidence and trust in oneself and one's team will overcome a lot of obstacles (Lancaster, 1999).

As has been reiterated over and over, change is an inevitable part of life and will continue to affect the health care system for several years to come. It is important to maintain an attitude that change is preferable to stagnation. This will help leaders to identify opportunities for change and embrace those changes for a better quality work life or for better care for the patient. Nothing can ever stay the same for long.

INNOVATION

Innovation can be defined as the process of creating new services or products. Shortell & Kaluzny (2006) state that change and innovation are different. Change is a generic concept that deals with any modification. Innovation is more restricted to new modifications in ideas or practices. Tom Kelly, author of the *The Ten Faces of Innovation* (2005), stresses that the innovative process is now recognized as a pivotal management tool in all industries, including health care. Kelly emphasizes that innovation is a team event that is made up of individuals who possess different strengths and points of view. This team approach results in new innovative ways to effectively solve problems (Figure 13-1).

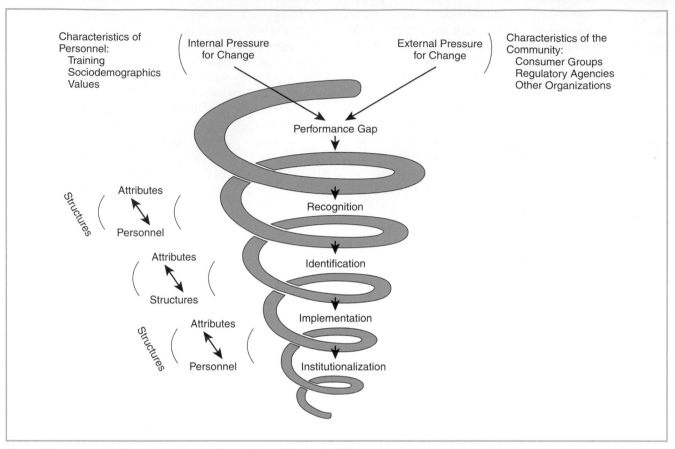

Figure 13-1 Change/innovation process. (Adapted from Kaluzny & Hernandez, 1988.)

Two of the biggest problems in health care today are related to patient safety and soaring costs. The nursing profession can find practical solutions in both of these areas. Through ongoing research, application of evidence-based practice, safe care initiatives, and innovation, nurses can improve the quality of patient care (Manojlovich, 2005).

An example of innovation in health care has been applied to the problem of medication errors. Injuries and death from medication errors have been identified by internal and external groups creating pressure for change in performance. Once the medication performance gap was recognized and identified by interdisciplinary health care groups, nurses, working in collaboration with practitioners, pharmacists, and other team members, analyzed why medication errors were occurring. Rather than blaming the person who administered the medication, an innovative "systems" analysis revealed why the errors were occurring. Systems errors included illegible handwriting, unfamiliar medications, dosage calculation errors, food/drug interactions, and lack of documentation of patient allergic reactions.

By applying a systems approach to problem solving, new safety structures and health care processes were implemented and institutionalized. Health care structures and processes were developed to include a computerized medication order-entry system and education of all personnel on the system. This system changed the process of how health care orders are written. Handwritten orders that are prone to interpretation errors are replaced by clear, concise, computer-generated orders. Multiple checks and balances were incorporated into the computer system that document patient allergies, health care conditions, and current height and weight to assist in appropriate medication ordering and dosing. Nurses and dietitians review the computerized patient information profiles for possible food/drug allergies and interactions. Pharmacists review orders using this computer system before dispensing medications to analyze whether the medication dosage is indeed correct based on the patient's height and weight. Nurses review computer-generated Medication Administration Records (MARS). Bar-coding systems are used now to ensure that the right drug is being administered to the right patient at the right time.

Centralized computerized charting for nurses and other health care providers now aid in the accurate and timely flow of information. Patient histories and current laboratory results can be accessed quickly. Home care nurses access this same database from their portable laptop computers. This use of portable technology speeds the flow of information from the medical practitioner or nurse practitioner to the nurse caring for the patient in the community. By improving the flow of essential information, patient safety is enhanced. Hopefully, ongoing evaluations of these innovative measures will indicate that medication errors are occurring less frequently and that patient outcomes are improving.

Challenges for the future include encouraging continued innovative approaches to solve other problems in health care. Nurses play an important role in this process through their professional knowledge, clinical expertise, leadership, and conflict-management skills.

CONFLICT

An important part of the change process is the ability to resolve **conflict**. Conflict management skills are leadership and management tools that all registered nurses should have in their repertoire. Conflict itself is not bad. Conflict is healthy. It, like change, allows for creativity, innovation, new ideas, and new ways of doing things. It allows for the healthy discussion of different views and values and adds an important dimension to the provision of quality patient care.

DEFINITION OF CONFLICT

There are a variety of definitions of conflict. Conflict can be defined as two or more parties holding differing views about a situation (Tappen, Weiss, & Whitehead, 2004), or as the consequence of real or perceived differences in mutually exclusive goals, values, ideas, and so on within one person or among groups of two or more (Sullivan & Decker, 2005). As can be surmised from these definitions, conflict can be defined as a disagreement about something of importance to each person involved. Not all disagreements become conflicts, but all disagreements have the potential for becoming conflicts, and all conflicts involve some level of disagreement. It is the astute manager who can determine which disagreements might become conflicts and which ones will not. This discussion of conflict management does not include professional communication skills. These are discussed elsewhere in this book.

SOURCES OF CONFLICT

Whenever there is the opportunity for disagreement, there is a potential source of conflict. The common sources of conflict in the professional setting include disputes over resource allocation or availability, personality differences, differences in values, threats from inside or outside an organization, cultural differences, and competition. In recent years, organizational, professional, and unit goals have served as a major source of conflict. Nurses frequently see financial goals and patient care goals as being in direct conflict with one another.

Sources of conflict in personal arenas include differences in values, threats to security or well-being, financial problems, and cultural problems. Living conditions and social contacts can increase or decrease the sources of conflict in someone's personal life. When people believe they have control over their living conditions and their social contacts, they can work to minimize conflict. Family relationships may present sources of conflict because of the complexity of these relationships.

TYPES OF CONFLICT

There are three broad types of conflict: intrapersonal, interpersonal, and organizational. Intrapersonal conflict occurs within the individual. When opposing values or differences in priority arise within an individual, they may suffer intrapersonal conflict. For example, if Marilyn is not granted her requested day off, she may have internal conflict about whether or not to call in sick or to take the day off without pay or to go to work. Or Marilyn may have conflict about priorities. Should she attend her daughter's softball game or write her paper for school? Individuals often have internal conflict about values. For example, in Marilyn's case, the requested day off may have been to attend the softball game, so the values in conflict were the values of family versus the values of the work ethic.

In interpersonal conflict, the source of disagreement may be between two people or groups or work teams. There may be disagreement in philosophy or values, or policy or procedure. It may be a personality conflict; for example, two people just rub each other the wrong way. This type of conflict is not unusual in the work situation. People new to a team may bring ideas with them that are not totally acceptable to the members in place. Individuals who transfer from one unit to another often stir up a certain amount of conflict over processes and procedures. For example, the nurse transferring from the intensive care unit (ICU) to the coronary care unit (CCU) may be comfortable with one way of making assignments and then try to encourage his new peers to adopt that methodology without sharing the rationale for why his way is better.

On occasion, there may be some interpersonal conflict between ICU nurses and medical-surgical nurses when they are required to work in one another's areas. Little regard is sometimes offered to each other about differences among patients, equipment, or required organizational skills. This lack of regard may sometimes lead to conflict based on preconceived notions rather than fact.

Organizational conflict is often referred to as inter-group conflict. It is at times a healthy way of introducing new ideas and encouraging creativity. Competition for resources, organizational cultural differences, and other sources of conflict help organizations identify areas for improvement. Conflict helps organizations identify legitimate differences among departments or work teams based on corporate need or responsibility. When organizational conflict is highlighted, corporate values and differences are aired and resolved.

In today's health care environment, conflict between the organizational goals of quality patient care and the need for a healthy financial bottom line can occur. These are both important values to the organization. Organizational conflict may help individual workgroups or teams clarify goals and become more cohesive, hopefully with few interpersonal disagreements. This process may also work for organizations in direct competition with one another as they unite against an outside threat to their well-being.

THE CONFLICT PROCESS

In 1975, Filley suggested a process for conflict management that is widely accepted. In this process, there are five stages of conflict: (1) antecedent conditions, (2) perceived and/or felt conflict, (3) manifest behavior, (4) conflict resolution or suppression, and (5) resolution aftermath. In Filley's model, conflict and conflict management proceed along a specific process that begins with specific preexisting conditions called antecedent conditions. The situation develops so that there is perceived or felt conflict by the involved parties that initiate a behavioral response or manifest behavior. The conflict is either resolved or suppressed, leading to the development of new feelings and attitudes, and may create new conflicts. Conflict management is vital in change. The antecedent conditions that Filley suggests may or may not be the cause of the conflict, but they certainly move the disagreement to the conflict level. The sources of these conditions include those discussed earlier: disagreement in goals, values, or resource utilization. Other issues may also serve as antecedent conditions such as the dependency of one group on another. For instance, the nursing department is dependent on the pharmacy department to provide drugs for the nursing unit in a timely fashion. The goals and priorities of pharmacy and nursing may be different at the time the nurse requests the drugs, and so a source of disagreement arises. If the circumstances for disagreement continue, a conflict will develop. According to Sullivan and Decker (2005), goal incompatibility is the most important antecedent condition to conflict.

An example of this is the incompatibility of quality nursing care and financial goal setting. There is often suspicion on the part of nurses that cutting costs in any area of nursing will lead to poor quality nursing care, and the antecedent condition of goal disagreement is established. If the cost cutting occurs too often, patient care may or may not be negatively affected. There is no way of actually knowing the exact impact of financial cuts on quality, but there is some predictability that at some point, continual financial cuts will negatively affect the quality of care provided for the patient. The point here is that the antecedent condition or preexisting condition for conflict is present with apparently incompatible goals; that is, financial goals and quality-care goals are not always compatible.

The antecedent conditions lead to frustration, and a conflict is born. The frustration is often described as a felt conflict, that is, when one party feels in conflict with another and perceives conflict and when each party believes they know what the other party's position is in the conflict. Of course, in the case of groups, one group or person may not be aware of another person's or group's feelings of conflict. This adds to the frustration. In the case of intrapersonal conflict, the frustration surrounds the internal conflict and how to resolve it. Once frustration has been felt, then resolution of some kind is necessary. The emotional components of frustration are anger and resignation. Both of these are powerful emotions that require some kind of action. For example, if Julio is not aware of the conflict between him and Tamika, Tamika may feel frustrated and upset. She is then obligated to let Julio know of her feelings so the conflict can be managed. If Tamika does not let Julio know of her feelings, then the frustration builds to anger, and Tamika will not be able to resolve the issues with Julio until that frustration is alleviated. This often results when frustration erupts into anger over some little thing rather than over the actual conflict.

MEANING OF THE CONFLICT

Conceptualization of the meaning of a conflict develops when individuals form an idea or concept of what the conflict is about, such as a conflict over control, professional standards, values, goals, and so on. Each party may or may not be aware of the other's conceptualization of the meaning of the conflict, but the parties do have what they believe is a clear concept of the conflict in their own minds. To determine the accuracy of the beliefs about the conflict, both parties need to sit down and determine the existence and nature of the conflict and the reasons it exists. According to Keenan and Hurst (1999), people may disagree on four aspects of a conflict. These include facts, goals, methods of goal achievement, and the values or standards used to select the goals or methods. This means that the actual facts of the dispute may be in question, the goals each side wishes to achieve may not be the same, how to achieve the agreed upon goal is not acceptable to one side or the other, or values are in dispute. After the nature of the conflict or the points of disagreement are known, then conflict management can begin.

The actions taken to resolve the conflict can take many forms:

- Discussion of the conflict may move it toward resolution.
- Someone in power may take steps to end the conflict or at least suppress it.
- One or both parties may decide to do nothing to resolve the conflict.

Successful conflict management will be discussed later. The important point here is that failure to successfully manage the conflict leads to more frustration and a further heightening of the conflict. Communication breaks down, and fighting spreads to the pettiest of issues. After it is apparent that a conflict is occurring, conflict management of some type must occur. People simply do not get over it and move on. The conflict is a source of friction and pain that must be resolved.

Outcomes are, of course, the result of any action taken. Positive resolution of conflict leads to positive outcomes; negative resolution or no resolution of conflict leads to negative or angry consequences. To determine if successful outcomes were achieved, you can ask whether or not important goals were achieved to some degree and what the relationships are between the parties at this point. Although the relationships may not be affectionate, it is hoped the parties can at least be cordial and collegial with one another. The hope is that each side has gained some measure of trust and respect, but if they are at least still talking, progress has been made. The best outcome is one in which both sides feel something is won, and their self-respect is intact.

CONFLICT MANAGEMENT

There are essentially seven methods of conflict management. These methods dictate the outcomes of the conflict process. Although some methods are more desirable or produce more successful outcomes than others, there may be a place in conflict management for all the methods, depending on the nature of the conflict and the desired outcomes. Table 13-5 is a summary of these methods, highlighting some of their advantages and disadvantages. The five techniques most commonly acknowledged are avoiding, accommodating, competing, compromising, and collaborating. Other techniques are negotiating and confronting.

Avoiding is a very common technique. The parties involved in the conflict ignore it, either consciously or

CRITICAL THINKING 13-2

Recall a time of conflict in your life. Looking at it with a different perspective, what antecedent conditions led to the conflict? What was the core of the conflict? Were personal goals or values at stake? How would you look at the same conflict now?

unconsciously. Use of this is common where there is interpersonal conflict in a highly cohesive group. The threat to cohesiveness is greater than the potential gains from the conflict. There may be circumstances where avoidance is appropriate such as (1) one of the parties is leaving so the conflict will resolve itself; (2) the conflict is not solvable and not all that important; (3) there are other more important issues at stake and conflict management is not worth the time and energy at this point. An example of avoiding is when two members of a highly cohesive nursing team disagree on some minor treatment modality or the amount of initial pain relief medication. The cohesiveness of the group is more important than the issue, so the two nurses agree to disagree, avoid discussing the issue, and monitor patient outcomes for more information. Each nurse uses the treatment or provides the pain relief according to his or her own values until outcomes are clear.

Accommodating is often called smoothing or cooperating. In this technique, one side of the disagreement decides or is encouraged to accommodate the other side by ignoring or sidestepping their own feelings about the issue. This is often done when the stakes are not all that high, and the need to move on is pressing. Frequent use of this method, however, can lead to feelings of frustration or being used—one person is "used" to get the cooperation of another. This can be an effective technique as long as the losing side is agreeable to the situation. This is clearly a technique where one party gains or wins and the other loses. The losing side often agrees to this method to gather "credits" that can be called in at another time. The leader/manager who uses this technique needs to do so prudently and sparingly. An example of this method is when one nurse will agree to last-minute schedule changes to accommodate other team members. This nurse will then call in these credits at a later date to use for an extended vacation or leave of absence.

TABLE 13-5 — SUMMARY OF CONFLICT MANAGEMENT TECHNIQUES

Conflict Management Technique	Advantages	Disadvantages
Avoiding—ignoring the conflict	Does not make a big deal out of nothing; conflict may be minor in comparison to other priorities	Conflict can become bigger than anticipated; source of conflict might be more important to one person or group than others
Accommodating—smoothing or cooperating; one side gives in to the other side	One side is more concerned with an issue than the other side; stakes not high enough for one group and that side is willing to give in	One side holds more power and can force the other side to give in; the importance of the stakes are not as apparent to one side as the other
Competing—forcing; the two or three sides are forced to compete for the goal	Produces a winner; good when time is short and stakes are high	Produces a loser; leaves anger and resentment on losing side
Compromising—each side gives up something and gains something	No one should win or lose but both should gain something; good for disagreements between individuals	May cause a return to the conflict if what is given up becomes more important than the original goal
Negotiating—high-level discussion that seeks agreement but not necessarily consensus	Stakes are very high, and solution is rather permanent; often involves powerful groups	Agreements are permanent, even though each side has gains and losses
Collaborating—both sides work together to develop the optimal outcome	Best solution for the conflict and encompasses all important goals to each side	Takes a lot of time; requires commitment to success
Confronting—immediate and obvious movement to stop conflict at the very start	Does not allow conflict to take root; very powerful	May leave impression that conflict is not tolerated; may make something big out of nothing

Competing is a conflict management technique that produces a winner and loser. The concept is that there is an all-out effort to win at all costs. This technique may be used when time is too short to allow other techniques to work or when a critical, though unpopular, decision has to be made quickly. This is often called forcing because the winner forces the loser to accept his stance on the conflict.

Some authorities see negotiation and compromise as the same; others see them as separate. They will be discussed separately here. Compromising is a method used to achieve conflict management in situations where both sides can win, and neither side should lose. Compromise is rampant in our society and is useful for goal achievement when the stakes are important but not necessarily critical. Compromise is often seen as appeasement; each side gives up something and each side gains something. Compromise is a good technique for minor conflicts or conflicts that cannot be resolved satisfactorily for both sides. Both parties win and lose. An example of compromise is when two nurses want the same shift off on the same day. One way to compromise is to split the shift so each nurse has part of the shift off.

Negotiating is an advanced skill that requires careful communication techniques and highly developed skills.

The optimum solution for the conflict may not be reached, but each side has some wins and some losses.

The term *negotiation* is often used in reference to collective bargaining or politics. It is, however, a very useful technique for conflict management at all levels. Negotiating is used when the stakes are high or when return to the conflict cannot occur. Return to the conflict may not be possible for a variety of reasons, such as a union contract, permanent change in policy or governance, or career or life changes. The idea of negotiation is that each party will gain something, so general agreement is reached, but consensus is not necessarily the goal. Consensus means that the negotiating parties reach an agreement that all parties can support, even if it is not completely what they want. Consensus does not satisfy everyone completely, but reaching a consensus indicates that all parties to a decision will accept the conditions of the agreement. Negotiating a consensus among staff nurses may be done when doing scheduling. Each nurse may negotiate his or her best, though not necessarily optimum, schedule.

According to Lewicki, Hiam, and Olander (1996), there are five basic approaches to negotiating: collaborative (win-win), competitive (win at all costs), avoiding (lose-lose), accommodating (lose to win), and compromise (split the difference). These five approaches to negotiation are influenced by the importance of maintaining the relationship relative to the importance of achieving desired outcomes (Figure 13-2).

Collaborating occurs in conflict management when both sides work together to develop the optimal outcome. It is a creative endeavor designed to find the best solution to the conflict so that all of the perceived important goals are achieved. Often this involves the creation of new higher goals that encompass the goals of both sides. This is a very high-level technique that requires maturity and a spirit of cooperation to reach each other's goals. To achieve collaboration is a very time-consuming process. Of course, in most conflicts, collaboration is preferred. An example of collaboration is the merger of two nursing teams. Instead of one team's methods of operation being forced on the other team, the two teams work together to create an even better environment than each had separately. This is accomplished by collaborating to pick the best policies, methods of operation, and so on.

One other technique used in conflict resolution is *confronting*. This technique heads off conflict as soon as the first symptoms appear. Although most commonly used between supervisor and employee, it can be used very successfully with conflict management. Both parties are brought together, the issues are clarified, and some outcome is achieved. Often conflict is the result of people misunderstanding or testing if the new policy is really going to be enforced. Confrontation heads off both situations early and quickly. The danger to confrontation is that when used extensively, it would appear that there is little tolerance for conflict. As mentioned earlier, conflict is often healthy and encourages creativity and open discussion and debate. The technique of

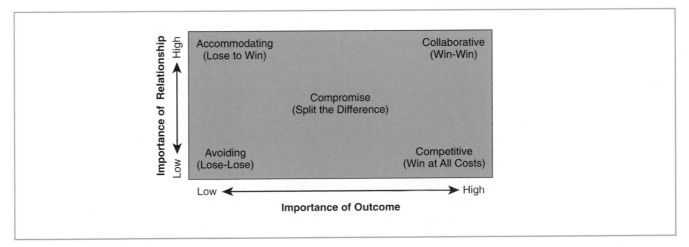

Figure 13-2 Negotiation strategies.

confrontation should be used judiciously to avoid the impression of intolerance.

Success of the techniques presented here depends on several factors. The importance of the issue in the conflict to the various sides has an enormous impact on the technique selected and the degree of success that will be achieved. Conflict management is never really permanent because new issues will always arise. The trick for the nurse is to determine what conflicts require intervention and what techniques stand the best chance of success. If one technique does not work, try another. Conflicts should be suppressed or avoided only under special circumstances that are dependent on the issues involved and the importance of the issues to the parties. Keep in mind that little problems become big problems later if the stakes are high and the issue is important to someone.

STRATEGIES TO FACILITATE CONFLICT MANAGEMENT

Open, honest, clear communication is the key to successful conflict management. The nurse and all parties to the conflict must agree to communicate with one another openly and honestly. Courtesy in communicating is to be encouraged. This includes listening actively to the other side. This does not include interrupting, being aggressive, or being overbearing in demeanor. Most importantly, use of derogatory language or gestures is not acceptable or tolerable. Voice level should be calm and at a normal tone. This sounds easy, but it may not always be easy to do.

The setting for the discussions for conflict management should be private, relaxed, and comfortable. If possible, external interruptions from phones, pagers, overhead speakers, and personnel should be avoided or kept to a minimum. The setting should be on neutral territory so that no one feels overpowered. The ground rules, such as not interrupting, who should go first, time limits, and so on, should be agreed upon in the beginning. Adherence to ground rules should be expected.

The management of conflict should be entered into by both sides in the spirit of expectation of compliance to the results. Threats on either side of the conflict should not be tolerated. Conflict management cannot be achieved if the nurse or either party is threatening one another. If one party cannot agree to comply with the decisions or outcomes, there is no point to the conflict-management process. A tool for assessing conflict is identified in Figure 13-3. This tool can be used to determine interpersonal or intergroup conflict within an organization and whether a given conflict is functional or dysfunctional.

LEADERSHIP AND MANAGEMENT ROLES

Marquis and Huston (2006) have identified some leadership and management roles in conflict management. Leadership roles include the role modeling of conflict management methods as soon as the conflict is evident. This strategy demonstrates awareness of and works to resolve intrapersonal or interpersonal conflict and sets the goal of conflict management so that both parties win. The leader also works to lessen the perceptual differences of the conflicting parties about the conflict and tries to encourage each side to see the other's view. The nurse assists the conflicting parties to identify techniques that may resolve the conflict and accepts differences between the parties without judgment or accusation. The leader fosters open and honest communication.

The nursing manager role includes the creation of an environment conducive to conflict management. The manager uses his or her authority to solve conflicts including the use of competition for immediate or unpopular decisions. The manager facilitates conflict resolution in a formal manner when necessary. The manager competes and negotiates for available resources for unit needs when necessary. The manager can compromise unit goals when necessary to achieve another more important unit goal. The manager negotiates consensus or compliance to conflict resolution outcomes or goals. Although the roles of leader and manager often appear in the same person, the leadership roles in conflict management are often more important to resolution and compliance. The manager has formal power that can be used when necessary, but it should be reserved for truly unmanageable or important issues.

CONFLICT MANAGEMENT AND CHANGE

Conflict management is an important part of the change process. Change can often threaten individuals and groups, so conflict is an inevitable part of the process. It is important to keep in mind that some conflicts resolve themselves, so the change agent should not be too quick to jump into an intervention mode. Figure 13-4 provides a guide for assessment of the level of conflict. If the level of conflict is too high, the nurse manager must apply conflict management strategies. Both change and conflict are positive processes that promote creativity, idea exchange, and innovation. Leaders, managers, and staff should be encouraged to embrace them and explore them as opportunities for positive growth development and professional expansion.

Interpersonal or intergroup?

1. Who?
   - Who are the primary individuals or groups involved? Characteristics (values; feelings; needs; perceptions; goals; hostility; strengths, past history of constructive conflict management; self-awareness)?
   - Who, if anyone, are the individuals or groups that have an indirect investment in the result of the conflict?
   - Who, if anyone, is assisting the parties to manage the conflict constructively?
   - What is the history of the individuals' or groups' involvement in the conflict?
   - What is the past and present interpersonal relationship between the parties involved in the conflict?
   - How is power distributed among the parties?
   - What are the major sources of power used?
   - Does the potential for coalition exist among the parties?
   - What is the nature of the current leadership affecting the conflicting parties?

2. What?
   - What is (are) the issues(s) in the conflict?
   - Are the issues based on facts? Based on values? Based on interests in resources?
   - Are the issues realistic?
   - What is the dominant issue in the conflict?
   - What are the goals of each conflicting party?
   - Is the current conflict functional? Dysfunctional?
   - What conflict management strategies, if any, have been used to manage the conflict to date?
   - What alternatives in managing the conflict exist?
   - What are you doing to keep the conflict going?
   - Is there a lack of stimulating work?

3. How?
   - What is the origin of the conflict? Sources? Precipitating events?
   - What are the major events in the evolution of the conflict?
   - How have the issues emerged? Been transformed? Proliferated?
   - What polarizations and coalitions have occurred?
   - How have parties tried to damage each other? What stereotyping exists?

4. When/Where?
   - When did the conflict originate?
   - Where is the conflict taking place?
   - What are the characteristics of the setting within which the conflict is occurring?
   - What are the geographic boundaries? Political structures? Decision-making patterns? Communication networks? Subsystem boundaries?
   - What environmental factors exist that influence the development of functional versus dysfunctional conflict?
   - What resource persons are available to assist in constructive conflict management?

Functional or dysfunctional?

	YES	NO
Does the conflict support the goals of the organization?	[ ]	[ ]
Does the conflict contribute to the overall goals of the organization?	[ ]	[ ]
Does the conflict stimulate improved job performance?	[ ]	[ ]
Does the conflict increase productivity among work group members?	[ ]	[ ]
Does the conflict stimulate creativity and innovation?	[ ]	[ ]
Does the conflict bring about constructive change?	[ ]	[ ]
Does the conflict contribute to the survival of the organization?	[ ]	[ ]
Does the conflict improve initiative?	[ ]	[ ]
Does job satisfaction remain high?	[ ]	[ ]
Does the conflict improve the morale of the work group?	[ ]	[ ]

A yes response to the majority of the questions indicates that the conflict is probably functional. If the majority of responses are no, then the conflict is most likely a dysfunctional conflict.

Figure 13-3 Guide for the assessment of conflict. (From *Nursing Leadership & Management* by G. McFarland, & M. Morris, 1984. Clifton Park, NY: Thomson Delmar Learning.)

Is conflict too low?

	YES	NO
Is the work group consistently satisfied with the status quo?	[ ]	[ ]
Are no or few opposing views expressed by workgroup members?	[ ]	[ ]
Is little concern expressed about doing things better?	[ ]	[ ]
Is little or no concern expressed about improving inadequacies?	[ ]	[ ]
Are the decisions made by the workgroup generally of low quality?	[ ]	[ ]
Are no or few innovative solutions or ideas expressed?	[ ]	[ ]
Are many workgroup members "yes-men"?	[ ]	[ ]
Are workgroup members reluctant to express ignorance or uncertainties?	[ ]	[ ]
Does the nurse manager seek to maintain peace and group cooperation regardless of whether this is the correct intervention?	[ ]	[ ]
Do the workgroup members demonstrate an extremely high level of resistance to change?	[ ]	[ ]
Does the nurse manager base the distribution of rewards on "popularity" as opposed to competence and high job performance?	[ ]	[ ]
Is the nurse manager excessively concerned about not hurting the feelings of the nursing staff?	[ ]	[ ]
Is the nurse manager excessively concerned with obtaining a consensus of opinion and reaching a compromise when decisions must be made?	[ ]	[ ]

A yes response to the majority of these questions can be indicative of conflict level in a workgroup that is too low.

Is conflict too high?

	YES	NO
Is there an upward and onward spiraling escalation of the conflict?	[ ]	[ ]
Are the conflicting parties stimulating the escalation of conflict without considering the consequences?	[ ]	[ ]
Is there a shift away from conciliation, minimizing differences, and enhancing goodwill?	[ ]	[ ]
Are the issues involved in the conflict being increasingly elaborated and expanded?	[ ]	[ ]
Are false issues being generated?	[ ]	[ ]
Are the issues vague or unclear?	[ ]	[ ]
Is job dissatisfaction increasing among workgroup members?	[ ]	[ ]
Is the work-group productivity being adversely affected?	[ ]	[ ]
Is the energy being directed to activities that do not contribute to the achievement of organizational goals (e.g., destroying opposing party)?	[ ]	[ ]
Is the morale of the nursing staff being adversely affected?	[ ]	[ ]
Are extra parties getting dragged into the conflict?	[ ]	[ ]
Is a great deal of reliance on overt power manipulation noted (threats, coercion, deception)?	[ ]	[ ]
Is there a great deal of imbalance in power noted among the parties?	[ ]	[ ]
Are the individuals or groups involved in the conflict expressing dissatisfaction about the course of the conflict and feel that they are losing something?	[ ]	[ ]
Is absenteeism increasing among staff?	[ ]	[ ]
Is there a high rate of turnover among personnel?	[ ]	[ ]
Is communication dysfunctional, not open, mistrustful, and/or restrictive?	[ ]	[ ]
Is the focus being placed on nonconflict-relevant sensitive areas of the other party?	[ ]	[ ]

A yes response to the majority of these questions can be indicative of a conflict level in a workgroup that is too high.

Figure 13-4 Guide for the assessment of level of conflict. (From *Nursing Leadership & Management* by G. McFarland, & M. Morris, 1984. Clifton Park, NY: Thomson Delmar Learning.)

CASE STUDY 13-1

Jane's staff was about three weeks into the latest change in care delivery when one of the staff nurses, Linda, returned from maternity leave. Linda tended to be negative about change, but she had terrific clinical skills and often served as a preceptor for new staff. Jane knew that if she could control Linda's tendency toward the negative, then not too much would happen to get the change off course. Linda's first words to Jane were "Whose brilliant idea is this? I do not want to work with Kathy. She is an idiot." Jane smiled and said, "Welcome back, Linda. We have missed you. How is the baby? Got any pictures?"

What do you think Jane should do to help Linda adjust to the change? Should Jane explore Linda's feelings about Kathy? Which is most stressful for Linda, the change or working with Kathy? Should Jane have done something to prepare Linda for this change and her assignment to work with Kathy? What is the source of the conflict?

KEY CONCEPTS

- Change is inevitable, exciting, and anxiety provoking.

- Change is defined as making something different from what it was.

- Major change theorists include Lewin; Lippitt; Havelock; and Rogers.

- Senge's model of five disciplines describes the learning organization. This model describes organizations undergoing continuous and unrelenting change.

- The change process is similar to the nursing process. The steps in the change process include assessment; data collection; and analysis, planning, implementation, and evaluation.

- Strategies for change include the power-coercive approach, the normative-reeducative approach, and the rational-empirical approach.

- Evaluation of change is a very important part of determining success and cannot be overlooked or skimmed.

- The change agent must be honest, open, optimistic, and above all, trustworthy.

- The change agent is an important part of the change process. The change agent is responsible and accountable for the project.

- Chaos theory says that most organizations go through periods of rapid change and innovation and then stabilize before chaos erupts again.

- Innovation is the process of creating new services or products.

- Conflict is a normal part of any change project and is often healthy and positive.

- Conflict comes from many sources, including values differences, fear, goal disagreement, and cultural differences.

- The four steps in the conflict-management process are frustration, conceptualization, action, and outcomes.

- There are several strategies for conflict management. Clear, open communication is key. There must be commitment to conflict management.

- Useful tools for conflict management include a guide for the assessment of conflict and a guide for the assessment of the level of conflict.

- The techniques for conflict management include avoiding, accommodating, compromising, competing, negotiating, confronting, and collaborating.

- Conflict can move the change process along if it is handled well. Conflict can stop the change process if it is handled poorly or allowed to get out of control.

KEY TERMS

change	organizational change
change agent	personal change
conflict	professional change
innovation	

REVIEW QUESTIONS

1. What is often the most desirable conflict resolution technique?
   A. Avoiding
   B. Competing
   C. Negotiating
   D. Collaborating

2. The change agent and the person responsible for conflict management have what characteristic in common?
   A. Secretive and willful
   B. Trustworthy and a good communicator
   C. Ambitious and avoiding
   D. Powerful and dictatorial

3. Select the best reason why change is necessary.
   A. To maintain the status quo
   B. To enhance the quality of health care
   C. To encourage staff turnover
   D. To increase the cost of patient care

4. Identify the theorist who first proposed the original change theory model.
   A. Rogers
   B. Havelock
   C. Lewin
   D. Lippitt

5. Identify the least reliable form of communication on a nursing unit.
   A. The grapevine
   B. Minutes from a staff meeting
   C. A memo from the unit director
   D. A medical center newsletter

REVIEW ACTIVITIES

1. Select a change project that either you have personally achieved or you have experienced in a clinical situation, and discuss with your classmates how you felt and how the change agent maintained momentum and enthusiasm for the project. If this is a personal change, how did you maintain enthusiasm?

2. Recall a conflict with which you have been involved in the clinical situation. Discuss each of the methods of conflict management identified in the chapter. Identify which ones would have worked. Did the conflict ever get resolved? How?

3. Discuss with a nurse manager how they determine whether a conflict is occurring and what steps they take to bring it out in the open. Share the information with your classmates.

4. Discuss with a nurse manager how they feel about constant change on a personal level. How did the nurse present an impending change to the staff? Did the nurse use any of the techniques discussed in this chapter? Was the change successful?

EXPLORING THE WEB

- Look up the Journal of Conflict Resolution (*http://jcr.sagepub.com*) and describe its purpose. Would this journal be useful to the new nurse manager? A new nurse? Anyone else in health care?

- Use a search engine to look up change and conflict management. What did you find? Were any of the sites helpful in understanding either subject?

- Explore the following Websites to learn more about change, conflict management, and innovation.
  www.embracechange.com.au
  A Beginners Guide to Change Management
  www.iacm-conflict.org
  The International Association of Conflict Management
  www.nln.org
  National League for Nursing
  Search for position statement and innovation.

REFERENCES

Beason, C. F. (2005). The nurse as investor: Using the strategies of Sarbanes-Oxley corporate legislation to radically transform the work environment of nurses. *Nursing Administration Quarterly, 29*(2), 171–178.

Bennis, W. (1989). *On becoming a leader.* Reading, MA: Addison-Wesley.

Bennis, W., Benne, K., & Chin, R. (Eds.). (1969). *The planning of change* (2nd ed.). New York: Holt, Rinehart, Winston.

Bushy, A. (1993). Managing change: Strategies for continuing education. *The Journal of Continuing Education in Nursing, 23,* 197–200.

Bushy, A., & Kamphius, J. (1993, March). Response to innovation: Behavioral patterns. *Nursing Management, 24*(3), 62–64.

Filley, A. C. (1975). *Interpersonal conflict resolution.* Glenview, IL: Scott Foresman.

Haase-Herrick, K. (2005). The opportunities of stewardship. *Nursing Administration Quarterly, 29*(2), 115–118.

Havelock, R. G. (1973). *The change agent's guide to innovation in education.* Englewood Cliffs, NJ: Educational Technology.

Heath, J., Johnson, W., & Blake, N. (2004). Health work environments: a validation of the literature. *Journal of Nursing Administration Quarterly, 34*(11), 524–530.

Institute of Medicine. (2002). *To err is human: Building a safer health care system.* Washington, DC: The National Academies Press.

Kaluzny, A. D., & Hernandez, S. (1988). Organizational change and innovation. In S. Shortell & A. Kaluzny, *Health care management.* New York: John Wiley and Sons.

Keenan, M. J., & Hurst, J. B. (2006). Conflict: The cutting edge of change. In P. S. Yoder-Wise, *Leading and managing in nursing* (4th ed.) (pp. 318–334). St. Louis, MO: Mosby.

Kelly, T. (2005). *The ten faces of innovation.* New York: Doubleday.

Kelly, T., Peters, T., & Littman, J. (2001). *The art of innovation.* Garden City, NJ: Doubleday.

Lancaster, J. (1999). *Nursing issues in leading and managing change.* St. Louis, MO: Mosby.

Lewicki, R., Hiam, A., & Olander, K. (1996). *Think before you speak: The complete guide to strategic negotiation.* New York: John Wiley & Sons.

Lewin, K. (1951). *Field theory in social science.* New York: Harper & Row.

Lippitt, R. (1958). *The dynamics of planned change.* New York: Harcourt, Brace.

Luthans, K. W., & Jenson, S. M. (2005). The linkage between psychological capital and commitment to organizational mission: A study of nurses. *Journal of Nursing Administration, 35*(6), 304–310.

Manojlovich, M. (2005). Promoting nurses' self-efficacy. *Journal of Nursing Administration, 35*(5), 271–278.

Marquis, B. L., & Huston, C. J. (2006). *Leadership roles and management functions in nursing: Theory applied* (5th ed.). Philadelphia: Lippincott.

McFarland, G., Skipton Leonard, H., & Morris, M. (1984). *Nursing leadership and management contemporary strategies.* Clifton Park, NY: Thomson Delmar Learning.

Ponte, P., Kruger, N., & DeMarco, R. (2004). Reshaping the practice environment—the importance of coherence. *Journal of Nursing Administration, 34,* 173–179.

Recklies, O. (2006). Managing Change—Definitions and Phases in Change Processes. Retrieved September, 2006, from http://www.themanager.org/Strategy/ Change_Phases.htm

Rogers, E. M. (1983). *Diffusion of innovations* (3rd ed.). New York: Free Press.

Senge, P. M. (1990). *The fifth discipline: The art and practice of the learning organization.* New York: Doubleday.

Shortell, S., & Kaluzny, A. D. (2000). *Health care management-organization design and behavior* (4th ed.). Clifton Park, NY: Thomson Delmar Learning.

Shortell, S. M., & Kaluzny, A. D. (2006). *Health Care Management* (5th ed.). Clifton Park, NY: Thomson Delmar Learning.

Silber, M. B. (1993, September). The "C"s in excellence: Choice and change. *Nursing Management, 24*(9), 60–62.

Simms, L. et al. (2000). *The Professional Practice of Nursing Administration* (3rd ed.). Clifton Park, NY: Thomson Delmar Learning.

Sullivan, E. J., & Decker, P. J. (2005). *Effective leadership & management in nursing* (6th ed.). Upper Saddle River, N.J.: Pearson Education Inc.

Tappen, R. M., Weiss, S. A., & Whitehead, D. K. (2004). *Essentials of Nursing Leadership and Management* (3rd ed.). Philadelphia: F. A. Davis.

SUGGESTED READINGS

Ball, M. J. (2005, Feb.). Nursing informatics of tomorrow. One of nurses' new roles will be agents of change in the health care revolution. *Healthcare Informatics, 22*(2), 74, 76, 78.

Begun, J., Zimmerman, B., & Dooley, K. (2006). *Health care organizations as complex adaptive systems.* Retrieved September 8, 2006, from http://www.change-ability.ca/ComplexAdaptive.pdf

Diekelmann, N. (2004, Oct.). Class evaluations: Creating new student partnerships in support of innovation. *Journal of Nursing Education, 43*(10), 436–439.

Institute of Medicine. (2003). *Health professions education: A bridge to quality.* Washington, DC: The National Academies Press.

Kotter, J. P. (1996). *Leading change.* Boston: Harvard Business School Press.

MacGuire, J. M. (2006, Jan.). Putting nursing research findings into practice: Research utilization as an aspect of the management of change. *Journal of Advanced Nursing, 53*(1), 65–71.

McCartney, P. (2006, Nov.–Dec.). The International Council of Nurses innovations database. *American Journal of Maternal Child Nursing, 31*(6), 389.

McDaniel, R. R. (1997). Strategic leadership: A view from quantum and chaos theories. *Health Care Management Review, 22*(1), 21–37.

National Nursing Centers Consortium. (2006). Nurse-managed health centers are changing the face of health care. Retrieved February 16, 2006, from http://www.nncc.us/about/nmhc.html

Pfeffer, J., & Sutton, R. (2006, January). Evidence-based management. *Harvard Business Review, 63*–74.

Porter-O'Grady, T., & Malloch, K. (2003). *Quantum leadership: A textbook of new leadership.* Sudbury, MA: Jones and Bartlett Publishers.

Senge, P., Flowers, B. S., & Scharmer, C. O. (2005). *Presence: An exploration of profound change in people, organizations, and society.* New York: Doubleday.

Thomas, L. M., Reynolds, T., & O'Brien, L. (2006, Sept.). Innovation and change: Shaping district nursing services to meet the needs of primary health care. *Journal of Nursing Management, 14*(6), 447–454.

UNIT III
Leadership and Management of Patient-Centered Care

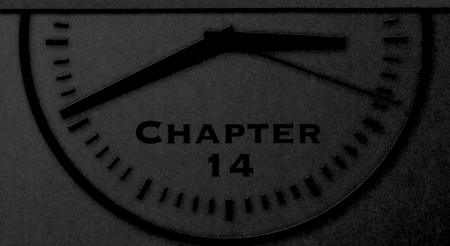

CHAPTER 14

Budget Concepts for Patient Care

Corinne Haviley, RN, MS

A higher proportion of nursing care provided by registered nurses (RNs) and a greater number of hours of care by RNs per day are associated with better care for hospitalized patients (Jack Needleman, 2002).

OBJECTIVES

Upon completion of this chapter, the reader should be able to:

1. Identify the budget-preparation process for health care organizations.
2. Illustrate commonly used types of budgets for planning and management.
3. Select key elements that influence budget preparation and monitoring.
4. Illustrate a scope of service.
5. Identify expenses associated with the delivery of service.

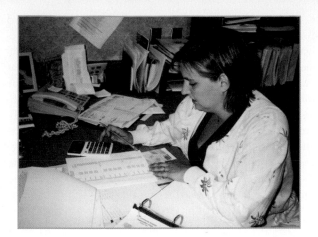

You are assigned to a patient care unit for your clinical experience. You are wondering what types of services are provided to patients on this unit. You talk with your instructor and the nursing manager of the unit to review unit staffing. You review the unit's scope of service and budget.

What kinds of patients are cared for on this unit?

What kinds of services are provided to patients on this unit?

How does the staffing model help ensure provision of care for patients on this unit?

How would a nurse shortage affect the model?

A key factor that influences patient care is the cost involved in the delivery of service. Resources—people, equipment, and time—are required to support the services delivered by nurses. These resources cost money. The economic success of a health care organization depends on those who are involved with service delivery. The decline in health care reimbursement as well as escalating costs and increasing competition, have required hospitals to improve operational efficiency and to make economically sound decisions. The challenge in health care is to ensure that the quality of care and the caliber of the staff are not compromised in this ever-changing, cost-controlled environment.

Nurses need to understand how to manage the cost of patient care as it relates to their own clinical practice. Nurses are accountable for the distribution and consumption of resources, whether that equates to time, supplies, drugs, or staff. It is essential that appropriate decisions be made regarding cost-effective practices. Cost containment affects the patient's bill and the financial viability of a nursing department or unit. Hence, nurses need to be informed and partner with the management team to generate revenue and control expenses in relation to patient care. According to regulatory and accrediting health care organizations, departmental budgets need to be developed in collaboration with staff from respective services involved in care.

The purpose of this chapter is to provide an overview of the operational budget process, including budget development, implementation, performance, and evaluation. Common financial language and tools are discussed so nurses can understand the process involved in cost-effective care.

TYPES OF BUDGETS

Hospitals use several types of budgets to help with future planning and management. These include operational, capital, and construction budgets.

OPERATIONAL BUDGET

An **operational budget** accounts for the income and expenses associated with day-to-day activity within a department or organization. Revenue generation is based upon billable services and expenses associated with equipment, supplies, staffing, and other indirect costs. Revenue may be based on the number of days that a patient stays on an inpatient unit or the number of hours spent in a procedure room. Revenue may be also based on the types of procedures delivered to a patient. Depending on reimbursement rates and requirements, expenses are sometimes bundled or included into a procedure or room charge, for example, an admission packet that includes a washbasin, cup, soap holder, and so on. In other situations, supply items may be billed separately, such as IV start kits, leukocyte removal filters, and so on.

CAPITAL BUDGET

A **capital budget** accounts for the purchase of major new or replacement equipment. Equipment is purchased when new technology becomes available or when older equipment becomes too expensive to maintain because of age-related problems such as inefficiencies resulting from the speed of the equipment or downtime (amount of time it is out of service for repairs). Sometimes the expense and availability of replacement parts make it prohibitive to maintain equipment. Finally, equipment may become antiquated because of its inability to deliver service consistently, meet industry or regulatory standards, or provide high-quality outcomes.

Because a significant expense is associated with equipment acquisition, organizations want to make the best and most economical and informed decisions. Staff members from a variety of areas, including materials management, clinical experts, legal counsel, biomedical engineering, information technology, finance, and management, often participate in planning for equipment purchases because they may have important input. Substantial analysis is required because equipment features, benefits, and limitations have to be understood as they relate to a department or institution's needs and goals.

Often multiple vendors or companies sell similar or varying products with different terms, conditions, and warranty and maintenance agreements that can have short- and long-term effects.

Some organizations may differ regarding the dollar amount that is considered a capital purchase. Capital purchases are based upon the equipment cost and the life expectancy (also known as shelf life) or how long the equipment is expected to perform over time. Generally, capital purchases cost more than $500 and last five years or longer. For example, in one organization, a stent costing $2,000 is a supply item used during a surgical procedure. This supply is considered an operational expense because its life expectancy is two years, whereas a CT scanner costing more than $500 with a life expectancy of seven years is considered a capital expense.

CONSTRUCTION BUDGET

A **construction budget** is developed when renovation or new structures are planned. The construction costs generally include labor, materials, building permits, inspections, equipment, and so on. If it is anticipated that a department will need to close during construction, then projected lost revenue is accounted for in the budget. Revenue and expenses may also be shifted to another department that absorbs the services on a temporary basis.

BUDGET OVERVIEW

An operational budget is a financial tool that outlines anticipated revenue and expenses over a specified period. A process called **accounting**, which is an activity that managers engage in to record and report financial transactions and data, assists with budget documentation. The budget translates operational plans into financial and statistical terms so that income can be projected with associated costs. Budgets serve as standards to plan, monitor, and evaluate the performance of a health care system. Details regarding a budget are specific to the area governed. Budgets account for the income generated as compared to the expenses needed to deliver the service. **Profit** is determined by the relationship of income to expenses. Profitability results when the income is higher than the expenses.

Budgets make the connection between operational planning and allocation of resources. This is especially important because health care organizations measure multiple key indicators of overall performance. For example, along with financial performance, organizations routinely evaluate quality patient outcomes and customer and staff satisfaction. All these indicators are intertwined and hold value in terms of patient care. Collectively, they reflect organizational success.

Figure 14-1 is a balanced scorecard or dashboard showing a variety of indicators that illustrate the connectivity between performance and quality outcomes. A **dashboard** is a documentation tool providing a snapshot image of pertinent information and activity at a particular point in time. A dashboard or balanced scorecard identifies any of four perspectives about an organization: finances, customer satisfaction and services, internal operating efficiency, and learning and growth (Norton & Kaplan, 2001). Figure 14-1 shows two separate units, the gastrointestinal laboratory (GI lab) and a medical nursing unit. These dashboards display measurable unit activity such as the number of procedures delivered in the GI lab and the number of patient days accrued on the medical nursing unit. They illustrate the amount of revenue generated and the expenses incurred. **Variance**, or the difference between what was budgeted and the actual result, can be tracked. A key activity that affects the number of patients that can be cared for, such as the room turnaround time, is also monitored. Finally, specific patient satisfaction indicators are visualized to determine whether the goals are met in high-priority areas.

Similar to controlling personal funds, such as managing a checking or savings account, budgeting helps to define services by projecting how much cash is generated (revenue) and how much services will cost to operate (expenses). Budgeting requires forward thinking so that problems can be planned for, and ways to work around any obstacles can be anticipated. Budgets also serve as a benchmark to measure whether the planning expectations are being met. Typically, budgets are monitored monthly, so that if deficiencies arise throughout the year, financial improvement plans can be instituted early. Corrective action is often initiated to prevent long-term effects in a particular area, such as wastage or loss of supply items. The budget functions as a tool to foster collaboration because individuals within departments must work together to achieve its goals.

BUDGET PREPARATION

Formulating a budget begins with preparation and planning. Budgets are generally developed for a 12-month period. The yearly cycle can be based on a fiscal year as determined by the organization (e.g., September 1 through August 31) or a calendar year (e.g., January 1 through December 31). Shorter- or longer-term budgets may also be developed depending upon the organizational planning process.

Prior to the beginning of the budget year, most organizations devote approximately six months to preparing and developing the operational budget. To prepare a

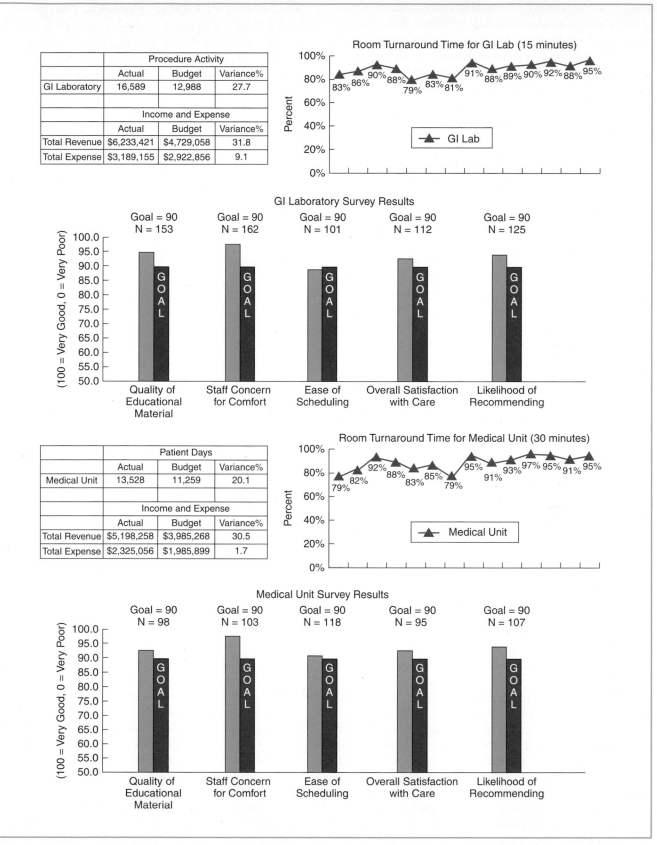

Figure 14-1 Patient satisfaction, room turnaround time, and budget activity dashboard. (Adapted with permission of Northwestern Memorial Hospital, Chicago, IL)

budget, organizations gather fundamental information about a variety of elements that influence the organization, including demographic and marketing information, competitive analysis, regulatory influences, and strategic plans. Additionally, it is helpful to review the department's scope of service, goals, and history.

DEMOGRAPHIC INFORMATION AND MARKETING

Pulling together demographic information relative to the population that the organization serves is most helpful because it identifies unique market characteristics, such as age, race, sex, income, and so on, that influence patient behavior. For example, an obstetrical practice would be expected to attract women of childbearing age rather than an older male population. Therefore, understanding the demographics and capture rate (the percent of the population that has been "captured" by the organization as a consumer) of the immediate or distant market region helps paint a clear picture regarding the patient population.

It is important to understand demographics as it relates to determining what type of patients are consumers that institutions target. Marketing strategies are built around the population types that an organization is attempting to attract. For example, if a hospital is opening an open heart or transplant department, then outreach activities might be developed to attract those patients that can benefit from the specialty screening, prevention, or treatment services.

Marketing is the process of creating a product or health care service for patients. Health care facilities use the four P's of marketing, that is, Patient, Product, Price, and Placement, to place desirable health care services or products in desirable locations at a price that benefits both patients and the health care facility. In this way, the health care facility, the patient, and the community benefit. Marketing of services does have a price tag such as the cost of advertising campaigns on television and radio. Using printed materials, mailing information to patient residences, and advertising in journals, magazines, and newspapers are all examples of ways to educate and stimulate the public for future referrals for health care services. Once marketing strategies are implemented, most organizations attempt to measure the effectiveness or return on investment of marketing strategies. Hospitals can begin to measure the effectiveness of advertising for new cardiovascular patient care services by reviewing the number of new patient referrals to the hospital that are made resulting from the marketing and media exposure. Sometimes the measurement is not clear cut because results cannot always be clearly attributed to the marketing efforts.

COMPETITIVE ANALYSIS

A competitive analysis is important because it probes into how the competition is performing as compared to other health care organizations. A competitive analysis examines other hospitals or practices' strengths and weaknesses, in addition to other details such as location and new or existing services and technology. Having this knowledge can influence decisions regarding the implementation of new programs, hiring of specialty staff, and purchasing of equipment. Figure 14-2 presents a competitive analysis of three different hospitals.

REGULATORY INFLUENCES

Regulatory requirements and reimbursement rates have an effect on financial performance. Regulatory changes are influenced by several governing bodies. A government agency that has high visibility in the area of reimbursement is the Centers for Medicare and Medicaid Services (CMS), whose mission is to ensure health care security for beneficiaries. CMS (www.cms.hhs.gov) administers federal control, quality assurance, and fraud and abuse prevention for Medicare, Medicaid, and the State Children's Health Insurance Program (SCHIP). Under the aegis of the Department of Health and Human Services, it is also responsible for coordinating health care policy, planning, and legislation.

Other regulatory bodies play a role in reimbursement by ensuring that federal and state laws are adhered to through approval and accreditation. For example, the Food and Drug Administration (www.fda.gov) regulates the use of drugs, food products, and medical devices in the United States. If equipment or drugs under its jurisdiction are not approved, then organizations cannot bill for their use, by law. The Joint Commission (JC) formerly known as the Joint Commission on Accreditation of Healthcare Organizations (JCAHO) (www.jointcommission.org) accredits hospitals and ambulatory care and home health agencies and departments to ensure that organizations meet specific standards. Medicare and Medicaid will not reimburse for services unless a hospital is accredited by the JC.

Regulatory requirements may change regarding who may deliver a specific service and in what type of setting; for example, a procedure may have to be done in the hospital rather than in a practitioner's office if it is to be reimbursed by the insurance company. Medicare and Medicaid change their reimbursement rates periodically. Total and partial coverage of specific procedures can change and may not be predictable from year to year.

Managed care organizations and insurance companies typically negotiate rates on a yearly basis, which can affect hospital revenue. Consumers' willingness to pay out of pocket when not covered by insurance affects revenue as well.

Competitive Analysis: Hospital A

Location: Rural—100 miles from metropolitan area

Affiliation: Currently negotiating with three academic hospitals

General clinical description:

- Scattered bed approach to inpatient oncology
- Ambulatory chemotherapy clinic
- Many of the same physicians on staff at Hospital J

Radiation capability: None—refers to Hospital J

Support services: Cancer screenings offered sporadically

Miscellaneous:

- Tumor board
- Cancer committee

Competitive Analysis: Hospital B

Location: Suburb of large metropolitan city

Affiliation: University hospital

General clinical description:

- Dedicated oncology inpatient unit
- Ambulatory chemotherapy department
- Comprehensive breast center
- Head and neck oncology team

Radiation therapy:

- Linear accelerator—two units
- High dose rate
- Intraoperative radiation therapy
- Stereotactic radiosurgery

Support services:

- Home infusion and home care program
- Hospice care program
- Annual cancer awareness fair
- Support group—general cancer patients

Miscellaneous:

- Tumor registry
- Tumor board
- Committee on cancer
- Head and neck patient conferences
- Stereotactic radiosurgery conferences

Competitive Analysis: Hospital C

Location: Urban city with a population of 150,000

Affiliation: For-profit corporation

- Medical oncology affiliation with University K
- Radiation Therapy Department affiliation with University K Radiation Therapy Department

General clinical description:

- Dedicated inpatient medical oncology unit
- Dedicated inpatient surgical oncology unit
- Four-bed autologous and stem cell bone marrow transplant unit (Eastern Cooperative Oncology Group Referral Center for autologous bone marrow transplants)
- Coagulation laboratory
- Therapeutic pheresis
- Pain clinic
- Oncology clinic
- Oncology rehabilitation
- Breast cancer rehabilitation program
- Ambulatory care chemotherapy unit
- Medical oncologist on staff at two hospitals

Radiation therapy:

- Linear accelerator
- Stereotactic radiosurgery
- Hyperthermia
- Brachytherapy

Support services:

- Home health and hospice program
- Cancer registry
- Cancer committee
- Physician update—quarterly cancer newsletter
- Cancer information line
- Cancer advisory council
- Cancer Survivor's Day offered annually
- Cancer screenings offered routinely
- Cancer support group—general cancer patients

Figure 14-2 Competitive analysis of three hospitals.

STRATEGIC PLANS

Generally, hospitals have strategic plans that map out the direction for the organization over several years. Strategic plans guide the staff at all levels so that the entire organization can have a shared mission and vision with clearly defined steps to meet the goals.

Each department develops unit-specific plans to help the organization follow its overall strategic plan. For example, a goal may be to become the most preferred GI lab or site for inpatient hospital care in the surrounding region. To meet the goal, one department may focus on patient satisfaction and room turnaround time to increase volume and decrease patient wait time for a procedure appointment. This goal is part of the organization's overall plan.

SCOPE OF SERVICE AND GOALS

During the budget-preparation phase, it is important to examine the individual nursing or hospital department or section thoroughly. Hospital systems are frequently divided into sections, departments, or units to compartmentalize them for organizational purposes. These subsections or units, commonly called **cost centers**, are used to track financial data.

Each department or cost center defines its own scope of service (Figure 14-3 and Figure 14-4 provide examples of scope of service). The scope of service is helpful because it provides information related to the types of

REAL WORLD INTERVIEW

In order to be successful, all health care organizations need to strategize regarding financial performance. Nursing managers receive training to develop unit budgets based on long-range financial planning and organizational goals. Staff nurses, as well, need to have input into the budget process. The budget is developed based upon a projected average daily census or number of procedures. Patient acuity is also taken into consideration, along with the patient population. Patient acuity is based on the severity of the patient's illness and the nursing time that is needed to meet the patients needs, that is, monitoring of frequent vital signs, intake and output, and the need for additional nursing support, such as care of the patient with feeding tubes, frequent suctioning, and so on. Many organizations compare their operations against national benchmarks using the daily nursing care hours required for different types of nursing units and patient populations as a benchmark. Organizations may rely on the finance department to forecast increased volume, and need for growth in patient care programs and patient service lines.

The nurse at the bedside is very valuable in providing input into the budgetary process. This is accomplished by evaluating appropriate nurse/patient ratios for their patient populations, examining patient acuity, and assisting in projecting appropriate staffing levels for various work shifts and days of week. Nurses at the bedside can also identify additional support needs as well as equipment needs, which all help with budget planning.

The use of staffing guidelines, that is, the number of nurses needed to care for a specific quantity of patients, patient acuity levels, and reports that measure nursing productivity, help the staff nurse to participate in managing the staffing budget on a daily basis. Giving nurses at the bedside the autonomy to flex the number of staff either up and down as appropriate, using patient census and patient acuity as key measures, promotes accountability and ownership of appropriate staffing decisions. Based on the census and patient acuity on the unit as well as on the patient expected admissions, transfers, and discharges, nurses can plan staffing patterns for the oncoming work shift. This is called flexing up and down. It includes floating staff to units that need more help, utilizing a float pool of both available staff and agency or registry staff if needed to get additional staff when needed for patient care. Nursing productivity measures the direct patient care hours and the indirect hours, which include education time, orientation time, and sick and vacation time. This also needs to be calculated at budget time.

Carol Payson, MSN, RN
Director of Surgical Services
Northwestern Memorial Hospital
Chicago, Illinois

The gastrointestinal (GI) laboratory may be defined as a specialized department that performs major procedures that are both diagnostic and therapeutic in nature such as upper endoscopies, colonoscopies, flexible sigmoidoscopies, and endoscopic retrograde cholangiopancreatography (ERCP). Conscious sedation is typically delivered to patients to provide comfort during the procedures. The gastrointestinal laboratory is operational Monday through Friday from 7 A.M. to 5 P.M. and provides after-hours service for emergent cases. Preprocedure, intraprocedure, and postprocedure care, including full recovery, is provided on site. Services are provided to critical in-house patients at the bedside via the staff assigned to travel to inpatient units. The department employs nurses, technicians, and receptionists, who work with gastroenterologists and surgeons to provide care. The unit is equipped with 10 procedure rooms, 25 recovery bays, and a GI scope cleaning facility on site.

Figure 14-3 Gastrointestinal laboratory scope of service.

A medical nursing unit provides primarily inpatient care to patients with acute or chronic medical problems, such as congestive heart failure, diabetes, pulmonary disease, cancer, and so on. The unit, equipped with 30 private beds, a full kitchen, a lounge, and conference/consultation rooms, is operational 24 hours per day, seven days per week. Patient education and support groups are held routinely in the library located directly on the unit. Team nursing is employed as the model of care. Nurses, patient care technicians, and unit secretaries are employed, with a social worker and diabetes educator providing additional patient support. Patients admitted to the unit for longer than 48 hours are discussed during daily multidisciplinary rounds. The rounds include case-management personnel; psychosocial counselors; and nutrition, nursing, and medical staff. Staff discuss patient problems to facilitate future care, including discharge planning.

Figure 14-4 Medical nursing unit scope of care.

CASE STUDY 14-1

The manager from an inpatient unit asks for staff input into identifying ways to decrease use of medical supply and paper items. These items have been identified as in excess of the budget by 10% to 20% during the past three months. This is the first time that the staff members have been involved in helping with cost containment. Clinical nurses and assistants have been invited to participate.

When approaching an analysis of health care supply use, what might be the first step in the process? If you were to break the staff into workgroups, which members should be chosen to analyze the use of clerical supplies? How would you proceed if you were trying to determine the supply costs associated with starting an IV with continuous infusion?

service and the sites at which services are offered, including the usual treatments and procedures, hours of operation, and the types of patient/customer groups.

Departmental goals may include the introduction of new technology or treatments, patient education, and creation of a special patient care environment. Staff members are generally queried to determine whether they have any proposed quality initiatives that should be included in the plans for the upcoming year. Generally, new treatments, patient education materials, and documentation tools require different types or amounts of supplies. Technically trained staff members are often needed to implement new services. Both the staff and supplies can have varying costs during the early induction phase through full implementation. Creating a new environment or "best patient" experience may require additional funding that must be identified early in the planning stages. If new services are offered that are billable to the insurance company, then a method for charging patients has to be established to ensure that the hospital can receive appropriate payment. The manager is responsible for identifying the expenses associated with patient care upfront so that they are covered by the charges. A charge is the dollar amount that the patient is responsible for paying as a result of service.

HISTORY

Organizations typically use history or past performance as a baseline of experience and data to better understand activity in a department or unit. These data are used to assist in interpreting associated expenses with staff productivity and unit performance. Most often, adjustments are made to planned budgets because of the ever-changing cost of products, supplies, and buying contracts. Buying contracts are negotiated so that predetermined reduced rates can be realized when organizations purchase large quantities of supplies. For example, if a hospital purchases a large quantity of one product, the vendor may reduce the price below the list price as an incentive. If a hospital can demonstrate that a particular product is used in a certain percentage, in 60% of all procedures or departments (called penetration rate), for example, then a reduced rate may be offered.

Additionally, knowledge about historical volume (e.g., procedures, admissions, or patient visits and average length of stay) provides a perspective as to how a department has grown or declined over time. This information may help with anticipating future demand and capacity. The story behind a unit and its heritage related to how the department developed is equally important because the financial numbers are tracked over time. Often the culture and complexity of a unit unfold by interviewing staff that may have been involved in the unit during the past, including practitioners, nurses, technologists, assistants, housekeeping, dietary counselors, and so on. This information may provide further insight into why and how decisions were made in the past. Hence, multiple phases of data gathering are imperative to building a budget with a full knowledge base.

BUDGET DEVELOPMENT

Once background data have been gathered, the development of the budget can follow. This includes projecting revenue and expenses.

REVENUE

Revenue is income generated through a variety of means, including billable patient services, investments, and donations to the organization. Specific unit-based revenue is generated through billing for services such as x-rays, invasive diagnostic or therapeutic procedures, drug therapy, surgical procedures, physical therapy, and so on. Revenue can also be generated through the delivery of multiple services over time, such as hourly rates for chemotherapy administration or blood transfusions. The specific number and types of services and procedures have to be projected for the budget. Each type of service may have varying volume associated with it. For example, projecting the volume and type of procedures to be conducted in a gastrointestinal laboratory is based upon feedback from referring physicians and technical staff, in addition to conclusions from historical data.

Similarly, the same types of projections occur for inpatient units, including the number of patients anticipated to be admitted, along with the average length of stay (e.g., three to five days) and the projected occupancy rate. The type and amount of services and patient days can be measured. The number of patient days or the services delivered are commonly called service units or primary statistics so that productivity and efficiency can be tracked.

It is important to note that the reimbursement rates of third-party payers affect revenue and can change from year to year. Uniform rates are often used, which transfers significant financial risk to the provider. Medicare, Medicaid, managed care companies, and insurance companies dictate or negotiate rates with health care organizations that may include discounts or allowances. Payers determine what costs are allowable for procedures, visits, or services. Payment schedules vary from state to state and among plans. Additionally, the rates can change monthly such as with the ambulatory payment classification (APC) system from Medicare, which applies to the outpatient setting. The reimbursement rates or payments received by hospitals often do not equal the actual hospital or unit charges for the services rendered. For example, there may be a fixed or flat reimbursement rate per case regardless of how long the patient stays in the hospital or how much the hospital pays for the service. If the costs exceed the reimbursement rate, then the provider absorbs the remaining costs.

Another payment classification system called diagnosis-related groups (DRGs) is used to group inpatients into categories based upon the number of inpatient days, age, complications, and so on. Reimbursement covers room and board, tests, and therapy during a predetermined length of stay.

Some patients will not have health care insurance nor the ability to pay their bills. Therefore, the hospital may receive only a portion of the payment for services, if any.

Typically, organizations will review their payer mix to determine the percentage of patients carrying different types of health care coverage (Figure 14-5). The proportions help measure the anticipated dollars to be received for services delivered and projections for the coming year.

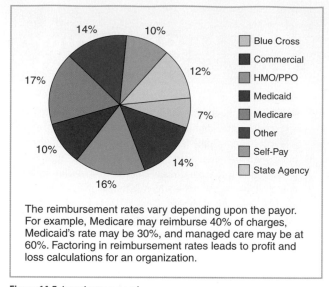

The reimbursement rates vary depending upon the payor. For example, Medicare may reimburse 40% of charges, Medicaid's rate may be 30%, and managed care may be at 60%. Factoring in reimbursement rates leads to profit and loss calculations for an organization.

Figure 14-5 Inpatient payer mix.

If charges for patient care are negotiated with a third-party payer, such as insurance companies and managed care corporations, they are preestablished and are not negotiable once established. Third-party payers often impose a penalty fee, as a disincentive, if a health care organization changes a charge under contract. The penalty often exceeds the charge amount and will usually create a loss for the organization.

The following illustrates the differences in reimbursement related to a procedure. The charge for a central line placement is $2,500, which includes the use of the fluoroscopy equipment, supplies, nursing, and technical time. If a hospital places 200 central lines per year, then the anticipated total revenue is $500,000. The breakdown of third-party payers becomes important because the total revenue does not mean that the hospital will be reimbursed for the full amount of $500,000. Third-party payers typically contract with health care organizations for the amount that the third-party payer is willing to pay or reimburse. Table 14-1 demonstrates the potential reimbursement rates based upon varying third-party payers.

TABLE 14-1	TOTAL CHARGES—CENTRAL LINE PLACEMENT $500,000	
Third Party Payer Reimbursement	**Rate (Measured in Percent of Charges)**	**Expected Reimbursement**
Managed Care	60%	$300,000
Medicare	40%	$200,000
Medicaid	30%	$150,000

EVIDENCE FROM THE LITERATURE

Citation: Hendrich, A. L., & Lee, N. (2005, July–Aug.). Intra-Unit Patient Transports: Time, Motion and Cost Impact Upon Hospital Efficiency. *Nursing Economics, 23*(4), 157–164, 147.

Discussion: Intrahospital transport of patients between patient care units can produce detrimental effects on patients. Accuracy in monitoring, patient stress, and potential nursing shift report hand-off errors have been cited as risk factors. Patients are moved to different patient care units during hospitalization primarily due to changing clinical requirements. Appropriate units are determined based upon the technical capacity, for example, availability of oxygen in the head wall, cardiac monitoring, clinical caregiver skill level, and nursing ratio or hours per patient day. These authors initiated a study to examine the cost of patient transfer between patient care units, including the transfer process, time, and personnel required. Delays, disruptions, communication gaps, administrative work, and resource availability were factors identified that negatively affected productivity. Of the patient transfer process, 87% was quantified as inefficient due to the previously stated reasons.

The authors recommend re-evaluation of facility design and patient models of care to accommodate fluctuations in patient acuity so that patients do not need to be transferred. Lack of progressive care beds covering multiple levels of care causes bottlenecks within hospital systems and excess resource requirements.

The strength of this article was the creative analysis of the transfer process highlighting inefficiencies. Although every organization may have differences in the process, it appears that by using this valuable exercise, organizations might bring forward opportunities to rethink the cost and safety of transfers. Reducing the contributing causes for transfer delays may prove to improve financial, clinical, and operational management and outcomes.

Implications for Practice: Many factors can be identified that influence operations. Using the workforce can potentially bring to light new ideas. Imagine the potential if a workgroup were continually analyzing patient scheduling, transport, and discharge to improve operations and decrease cost. Different team members have different perspectives. It is important to have empowered workgroups address problems and challenges to create constructive measures for improvement.

EXPENSES

Expenses are determined by identifying the costs associated with the delivery of service. Expenditures are resources used by an organization to deliver services and may include supplies, labor, equipment, utilities, and miscellaneous items.

It is important to understand what it takes to deliver patient care services so that there are appropriate charges in place to pay for or cover the services. Expenses are commonly broken down into line items that represent specific categories that contribute to the cost of the procedure or activity such as paper supplies, medical supplies, drugs, and so on. This breakdown helps identify where the significant expenses lie related to a service. For example, a colonoscopy may have a high medical supply cost, whereas chemotherapy administration may have a high drug cost associated with it.

SUPPLIES

As new procedures are introduced, or when a manager wants to ascertain the actual supply expenses associated with a procedure or activity, zero-based budgeting may be instituted. Zero-based budgeting is a process used to drill down into expenses by detailing every supply item and the quantity of items typically used. A list of supplies is developed, including large and small items, along with the itemized expense. Often supplies are packaged in bulk and sold in quantity. Hence, the expense of the items has to be calculated and backed out of the bulk figure to accurately depict the expense.

Figure 14-6 illustrates the zero-based budgeting that may be necessary to understand all of the expenses associated with delivering a procedure. This example can be expanded further to calculate the total expense associated with the anticipated number of procedures. This calculation can be achieved by multiplying the number of anticipated procedures by the total expense per procedure, which leads to authentic projections.

LABOR

Labor is another significant expense associated with medical and nursing care. Health care services are very labor intensive. It is estimated that salaries and benefits account for 50% to 60% of operational costs. Hence, it is very

General Supplies	Quantity	Price	Drugs	Quantity	Price
4 Chux	4	$ 3.00	Fentanyl	1	$ 0.25
Tri Pour Container	1	$ 0.20	Versed	1	$ 2.10
Sterile Water 1,000ml	1	$ 0.40	**Total**		**$ 2.35**
Normal Saline Vial	2	$ 0.10			
Cannister/Lid	2	$ 3.25			
Tubing	2	$ 0.50			
02 Cannula	1	$ 0.05	**Printed Forms**	**Quantity**	**Price**
Suction Catheter	1	$ 0.02			
Disposable Gowns	2	$ 3.80	Hospital Consent	1	$ 0.10
Gloves	6	$ 0.35	Procedure Consent	1	$ 0.75
4X4's	10	$ 0.25	Nursing Form	1	$ 0.75
Surgilube	2oz.	$ 0.15	Vital Sign Sheet	1	$ 0.05
Photos	2	$ 4.30	Doctors Orders	1	$ 0.15
Syringe 10cc	2	$ 0.15	History/Physical	1	$ 0.10
Syringe 60cc	1	$ 0.35	Discharge Instruction	1	$ 0.20
Emesis Basin	1	$ 0.10	Education Sheet	1	$ 0.80
Denture Cup	1	$ 0.15	Charge Voucher	1	$ 0.10
Recording Paper	1	$ 0.05	Procedure Education	1	$ 0.10
Alcohol Pads	2	$ 0.05	**Total**		**$ 3.10**
Slippers	1	$ 0.75			
Mask	2	$ 0.25			
Goggles/Face Shield	1	$ 1.20	**Clerical Supplies**	**Quantity**	**Price**
Cetacaine Spray	1	$ 0.10			
Bite Block	1	$ 2.00	Patient File	1	$ 0.80
Patient Bag	1	$ 0.20	Labels	2	$ 0.05
Cleaning Brush	1	$ 2.20	Xerox Paper	6	$ 0.05
	Totals	**$23.72**	Pen	1	$ 0.05
			Pencil	1	$ 0.05
			Marker	1	$ 0.05
IV Start	**Quantity**	**Price**	Highlighters	1	$ 0.05
			Total		**$ 1.10**
Tourniquet	1	$ 0.15			
Alcohol Wipes	2	$ 0.05			
Angiocath	1	$ 0.05			
IV Solution	1	$ 0.60			
IV Primary Set	1	$ 4.00			
Tegaderm	1	$ 0.15			
Tape	6 inches	$ 0.05	**Grand Total**		
Band-Aid	1	$ 0.05			
4X4	4	$ 0.10			
	Totals	**$ 5.20**			

Figure 14-6 Zero-based budgeting for gastrointestinal laboratory. (Adapted with permission of Northwestern Memorial Hospital, Chicago, IL.)

CRITICAL THINKING 14-1

Staff working day to day handling patient care activities are in an optimal position to identify the best practices that impact efficiency and cost-effectiveness. Managers can learn from staff and organize processes to assist with unit-based improvement. Think back on the steps taken by a nurse during the first hour of a shift. Reflect on communication and how information is received. Examine the amount of time spent in patient care versus other activities. Create a journal of activity from different time increments during a shift. Discuss your observations with your coworkers and manager. What problems in flow of activity and gaps in communication or efficiency did you find? How can you drill down further into understanding how the unit operates and ways to increase productivity? How could you improve your team's functioning?

TABLE 14-2	TIME AND SALARY EXPENSE ANALYSIS PER PROCEDURE

Reception Staff, Average Salary per Hour = $12.00	Preprocedure Care	Time (Minutes)
	Appointment schedule	5
	Registration	10
	Escort to changing room	5
$4.00	**Subtotal**	**20**

Staff Nurse, Average Salary per Hour = $22.00	Direct Patient Preparation	Time (Minutes)
	History	5
	Patient education and consent	15
	IV start	10
$11.00	**Subtotal**	**30**

Staff Nurse, Average Salary per Hour = $22.00	Intraprocedure Care	Time (Minutes)
	Positioning	5
	Initiation of conscious sedation	10
	Procedure	15
$11.00	**Subtotal**	**30**

Staff Nurse, Average Salary per Hour = $22.00	Postprocedure Care	Time (Minutes)
	Recovery	120
	Education	10
	Discharge	10
$51.33	**Subtotal**	**140**

Grand Total Salary Expense = $77.33 per procedure   **Grand Total = 220 minutes per procedure**

Source: Used with permission of Northwestern Memorial Hospital, Chicago, IL.

important to calculate the amount of time the staff members are involved with the service. This analysis includes professional, technical, and support staff. For example, the time that it takes to schedule an appointment, register a patient, and take a patient to a procedure room or unit needs to be calculated into the overall cost of care for the patient.

In the ambulatory area, staff time is calculated relative to the delivery of a specific procedure, including preparation for the procedure, intraprocedure care, and postprocedure care. Preprocedure preparation entails gathering of supplies, assembling equipment, and preparing the environment. Preparing the patient may involve taking a history, completing a physical, administering medication or taking specimens, placing tubes or establishing an intravenous line, and positioning the patient. Intraprocedure care is the actual care delivered after the procedure has been initiated. Postprocedure care may require activity such as educating and discharging a patient, or extensive recovery activity requiring several hours of direct nursing care and removal of equipment and supply items. Refer to Table 14-2 for a sample time analysis.

STAFFING The amount of staff and types of staff are often accounted for in a staffing model. The model outlines the number of staff required based upon the primary statistic such as procedures or patients. An outpatient model may focus on the number of procedure

CRITICAL THINKING 14-2

When you walk onto a patient care unit, ask a staff member what key quality initiatives the unit is working on that reflect process improvement. Ask what the goals are for the unit and how staff is participating in decisions so that the goals may be achieved. Think about how these initiatives may increase productivity, increase staff or patient satisfaction, or decrease expenses. Ask the staff what impact their efforts are having.

How are the staff involved in helping the organization to meet its goals?

rooms, that require staff. One nurse may be required to staff a gastrointestinal laboratory procedure room, and one shared technician may staff two procedure rooms.

Models may help in analyzing productivity as illustrated in the following:

■ *Scenario 1:* One nurse is assigned to a procedure room during a four-hour period in which eight patients are treated.

■ *Scenario 2:* One nurse and a technical assistant are assigned to a procedure room for four hours, and sixteen patients are treated.

The second scenario depicts greater productivity because the number of procedures delivered doubled by using two staff, recognizing that the assistant staff member will cost the organization less in terms of salary expense. Because labor is one of health care's greatest operational costs, enhancing productivity will likely produce savings.

For an inpatient unit, nurses may be assigned to a fixed number of patients during all three shifts. The ratios vary depending upon the shift and patient acuity. The nurse-to-patient ratio on a medical nursing unit may be one nurse to six (1:6) patients during the day and evening shift, whereas it may be 1:8 during the night shift. The nurse-to-patient ratio may be 1:2 for all shifts on a critical care unit. Figure 14-7 and Figure 14-8 illustrate sample staffing models.

Staffing ratios and salary data are particularly important because of the cost factor. Specialty salaries fluctuate, depending upon supply and demand. When there are shortages of certain staff, the salary tends to increase. Additionally, a health care organization may change its benefits, offering a more attractive package that includes continuing education, paid time off for education purposes, or professional membership expenses. Institutions may also look for alternative ways to supplement or deliver services during staff shortages. This means that

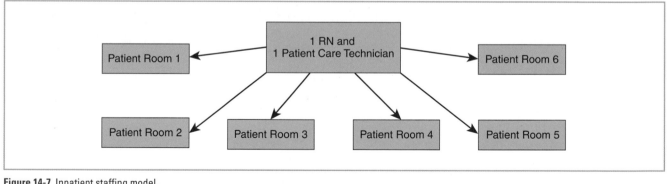

Figure 14-7 Inpatient staffing model.

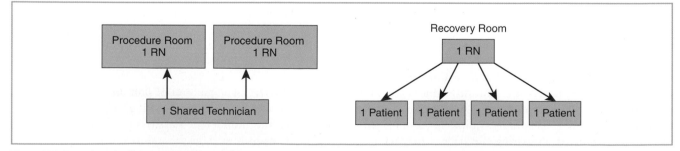

Figure 14-8 Gastrointestinal laboratory staffing model.

REAL WORLD INTERVIEW

Nurses need to have a good understanding of the financial aspects of the business, which includes the budget process. In addition, they also need to know how their everyday actions affect the bottom line. I also think that staff on a unit or outpatient clinic needs to "own" their budgets. It is not just the manager's budget; it is everyone's budget. I also think it is the role of nursing leaders to make the budget "real" for staff by education and implementing tools to aid in the process. For example, there are a number of staffing guideline tools that can be implemented to help staff calculate the cost of the shift, as well as the cost of the day. I have found these tools to be very beneficial in helping staff make better and more cost-conscious staffing decisions.

The most important factor in developing an annual operating budget is to assess your current environment in light of the department's goals and objectives. Where am I now, and where do I plan to be a year from now? Determining services and programs that are going to be added, as well as eliminated, is essential information needed to establish an annual budget. Analyzing historical data related to patient volume, patient days/visits, patient type, and acuity are also important factors to consider. In addition, assessing equipment and supply needs based on current as well as projected future needs is also essential.

There are a number of ways that staff can assist in controlling costs. One way that I have found to be extremely useful is to have staff "own" certain line items. For example, I have had my staff responsible for ordering office supplies and forms and become responsible and accountable for the variances (positive and negative). I believe that using this approach has helped staff make more economical supply choices. In addition, it has also helped reduce supply usage because they become much more actively involved in monitoring the use of supplies.

Beth Kelly-Hayden, RN, BSN, MBA
Director of Nursing and Clinic Operations
Chicago, Illinois

supplemental staff—professional agency nurses, nurses from in-house registries, or patient care technicians—may be hired at a different salary rate. It is important to note whether a unit has had historical difficulty retaining or recruiting staff. Recruitment and retention, especially attracting, interviewing, hiring, and orienting staff, require dollars. For example, it has been estimated that the turnover cost per nurse, including advertising, recruitment, orientation, and time to fill the vacancy, can equate to $67,000 (Jones, 2005). The average cost to educate a nurse during a six-week orientation period is more than $5,000. Not only the salary but also benefits are frequently factored into a salary package, and they need to be included in the budget.

UNPRODUCTIVE TIME Unproductive time is also calculated into a budget because there has to be staff coverage when nurses or other staff members are not working. Unproductive time usually includes sick-, vacation-, personal-, holiday-, and education time. For example, Table 14-3 illustrates average number of days that a nurse at one institution may take off from work during a 12-month period. These days off may require coverage by another nurse, depending on the unit.

CRITICAL THINKING 14-3

Calculate the added expense that a nursing unit will need to budget based upon the addition of five nurses (five full-time equivalents, [FTE] taking into account a salary increase over each year). Instruction: Multiply the average hourly rate times the total FTE worked per year times the total paid FTE hours per year to get the salary expense.

	Last Year	This Year	Next Year
Total FTE	50	55	60
Average hourly rate	$25.10	$25.45	$26.00
Salary expense	$2,616,675.00	$2,918,478,75	$3,252,600.00

*FTE (full-time equivalent) works 2,085 hours per year.

What would the salary expense be on a clinical unit that you have recently worked on?

TABLE 14-3   UNPRODUCTIVE TIME

Unproductive Time	Number of Days	Salary*
Vacation	21	$4,200
Holiday	7	$1,400
Sick	5	$1,000
Personal	3	$ 600
Education	1	$ 200
Total	37	$7,400

*Salary dollars are based upon an average rate of $25.00 per hour. Remember to calculate the number of days times eight hour shifts. The salary dollars change depending upon pay rate and shifts, for example, day shift versus evening shift differential or ten and twelve hours shift rates.

EVIDENCE FROM THE LITERATURE

Citation: Needleman, J., Buerhaus, P., Mattke, S., Stewart, M., & Zelevinsky, K. (2002). Nurse-Staffing Levels and the Quality of Care in Hospitals. *New England Journal of Medicine, 346*(22), 1714–1722.

Discussion: Administrative data from 799 hospitals in 11 states (covering 5,075,969 discharges of medical patients and 1,104,659 discharges of surgical patients) was examined to note the relation between the amount of care provided by nurses at the hospital and patients' outcomes.

The mean number of hours of nursing care per patient day was 11.4, of which 7.8 hours were provided by registered nurses, 1.2 hours by licensed practical nurses, and 2.4 hours by nurses' aides. Among medical patients, a higher proportion of hours of care per day provided by registered nurses and a greater absolute number of hours of care per day provided by registered nurses were associated with a shorter length of stay ($P = 0.01$ and $P < 0.001$, respectively), and lower rates of both urinary tract infections ($P < 0.001$ and $P = 0.003$, respectively) and upper gastrointestinal bleeding ($P = 0.03$ and $P = 0.007$, respectively). A higher proportion of hours of care provided by registered nurses was also associated with lower rates of pneumonia ($P = 0.001$), shock or cardiac arrest ($P = 0.007$), and "failure to rescue," which was defined as death from pneumonia, shock or cardiac arrest, upper gastrointestinal bleeding, sepsis, or deep venous thrombosis ($P = 0.05$). Among surgical patients, a higher proportion of care provided by registered nurses was associated with lower rates of urinary tract infections ($P = 0.04$), and a greater number of hours of care per day provided by registered nurses was associated with lower rates of "failure to rescue" ($P = 0.008$). No associations existed between increased levels of staffing by registered nurses and the rate of in-hospital death or between increased staffing by licensed practical nurses or nurses' aides and the rate of adverse outcomes.

Implications for Practice: A higher proportion of hours of nursing care provided by registered nurses and a greater number of hours of care by registered nurses per day are associated with better care for hospitalized patients and improved outcomes.

DIRECT AND INDIRECT EXPENSES

Expenses can be further broken down into direct and indirect. **Direct expenses** are those expenses directly associated with the patient, such as medical and surgical supplies and drugs. **Indirect expenses** are expenses for items such as utilities—gas, electric, and phones—that are not directly related to patient care. Other support functions frequently charged to a department that are not specifically related to patient care delivery are housekeeping, maintenance, materials management, and finance.

NET EXPENSE WORKSHEET
2003 BUDGET

DESCRIPTION	GI Lab	Medical Unit
Out Patient	8,290,564	33,450
In Patient	3,400,678	10,162,875
CORPORATE BILLING REVENUE	17,806	10,419
TOTAL OPERATING REVENUE	**11,709,048**	**10,206,744**
EXPENSES		
Salary Expense		
BUDGET REDUCTION SLALARY	0	24,932
SALARIES	1,398,630	2,098,150
SALARIES OVERTIME	219,878	142,359
PROFESSIONAL AGENCY FEE	106,608	166,456
TOTAL SALARY	**1,725,116**	**2,431,879**
TRANSPORTATION EXPENSE	4,190	3,870
TOTAL	**4,190**	**3,870**
NON-SALARY EXPENSE		
NONMEDICAL SUPPLIES		
SUPPLIES CLERICAL	12,924	8,524
PRINTED FORMS	31,486	28,854
SOAP AND CLEANING	6,092	8,950
PAPER GOOD SUPPLIES	1,192	930
FILM SUPPLY PHOTO	3,836	
PACKAGING SUPPLIES	94	
TOTAL	**55,624**	**47,258**
FOODS		
MEETING AND LUNCHEONS BANQUETS	0	495
SUNDRY FOOD ISSUES	5,872	8,990
TOTAL	**5,872**	**9,485**

MEDICAL SUPPLIES		
MEDICAL SUPPLIES	1,480,840	865,872
DIAG TEST CTR/IONIC CONTRST	2,798	
SUTURES	4,064	
DRUG SUPPLIES	120,120	569,088
IV & IRRIGATION SOLUTIONS	13,994	11,431
IV & IRRIGATION SETS	56,280	30,649
MEDIA	48	
PHLEBOTOMY SUPPLIES	680	
LAB GLASSWARE & INSTRUM	3,948	
LABORATORY SUPPLIES	156	
CHEMICALS	158	
TOTAL	**1,683,086**	**1,477,040**
TOTAL SUPPLIES	**1,744,582**	**1,533,783**
PURCHASE SERVICES		
PURCHASED SERVICES	41,436	15,678
TOTAL	**41,436**	**15,678**
UTILITIES		
TELEPHONE CHARGES-Long Distance	1,480	1,500
TELEPHONE CHARGES	13,608	15,238
TOTAL	**15,088**	**16,736**
OTHER EXPENSES		
CONTINUING ED	6,715	4,127
AUDIO VISUAL	500	0
TRAVEL EXPENSE	6,120	5,100
DISCOUNTED PARKING	190	150
MISCELLANEOUS	730	500
SM FIXTURES & EQUIPMENT	728	410
EQUIP RENTAL GENERAL	1,342	1,071
COPY MACHINE EXPENSES	13,440	6,424
BOOK LIBRARY	250	320
SUBSCRIPTION MAGAZINE	200	150
REPAIR REPL PARTS EQUIP	1,070	125
REPAIRS & REPL PARTS MED EQUIP	146,498	
FILM PROCESSING EXPENSE	220	
TOTAL	**178,003**	**18,377**
TOTAL NON-SALARY EXPENSE	**1,983,299**	**1,588,446**
TOTAL EXPENSE	**3,708,415**	**4,020,343**
TOTAL NET EXPENSES	**1,983,299**	**1,588,446**

Figure 14-9 Net expense worksheet. (Adapted with permission of Northwestern Memorial Hospital, Chicago, IL.)

FIXED AND VARIABLE COSTS

Fixed costs are those expenses that are constant and are not related to productivity or volume. Examples of these costs are building and equipment depreciation, utilities, fringe benefits, and administrative salaries. **Variable costs** fluctuate depending upon the volume or census and types of care required. Medical and surgical supplies, drugs, laundry, and food costs often increase with the volume. Figure 14-9 shows sample worksheets used to calculate expenses.

BUDGET APPROVAL AND MONITORING

Once developed, budgets are submitted to administration for review and final approval. The approval process may take several months as the unit budgets are combined to determine the overall budget for the health care organization. Senior management, representing finance and operations, often makes the final decisions regarding acceptance of a budget.

The unit or department manager is responsible for controlling the budget. Budget monitoring is generally carried out on a monthly basis. The purpose of monitoring is to ensure that revenue is generated consistent with projected productivity and standards. Organizations often recognize a flexible budget, which allows for adjustments if the volume or census increases or decreases. If the volume increases, it is likely that expenses will increase. If the volume decreases, and expenses increase, then the manager needs to determine what actions are necessary to control or bring costs down. Many organizations require managers to complete a budget variance report, which is a tool used to identify when categories

	Budget	Actual	% Variance	Comments/Actions
Revenue				
Inpatient	21,171,760	22,011,344	4	Patient days increasing
Outpatient	393,863	412,318	4.7	Clinic visits are increasing
		List all line items over or under budget		
Overall Expenses	3,370,828	3,400,795	(.1)	Expenses in line with budget
Salary	3,071,298	3,034,483	(1.2)	Salary is over budget consistently with added FTEs
Full-time equivalent employees (FTEs)	56.5	55.5	(1.2)	Increasing FTEs to accommodate volume and census
RN	46.6	45.4	(1.2)	
Assistive Staff	10.1	10.0	0.0	
Overall Medical Supplies	120,223	129,742	(9)	Supplies are over budget due to volume
IV Sets	80,000	85,000	(9)	Higher acuity patients requiring multiple IVs
Surgical Instruments	20,000	18,008	9	
Phlebotomy Supplies	21,742	17,722	8	
Clerical Supplies	1,629	2,460	(6.6)	Implementation of electronic medical record delayed Increasing paper expense
Paper Supply	1,300	1,800	(7.2)	Patient education materials are increasing causing higher expense
Purchased Service	183,752	193,790	(5.5)	Consultant expense for bed and board
Transportation	75,000	72,000		
Maintenance	150,800	125,700	8.3	
Continuing Education	1,500	1,500	0	
Staff Training	1,985	1,900	9	

*Figures are for instructional purposes only

Figure 14-10 Cardiovascular nursing step down unit budget (CVT step down). (Used with permission of Northwestern Memorial Hospital, Chicago, IL.)

are out of line and to identify the need for corrective action. Figure 14-10 illustrates a variance report.

The entire health care team is responsible for ensuring that expenses are kept within the budgeted amount and that the volume or census is maintained. The manner in which this is accomplished depends on the organization. Some institutions request that budget dashboards (see Figure 14-11) be developed reflecting departmental activity at a glance. Variance reports or dashboards may be posted so that all staff members have an opportunity to review the budget and participate in any improvement needed.

Staff can meet to discuss implementation or reinforcement of strategies that can positively affect the budget. Following are examples of such strategies:

■ Analyze time efficiency of staff involved in patient care.
■ Understand the process for entering patient charges.
■ Educate coworkers regarding the charging process.
■ Plan for supplies needed for every patient encounter and consciously eliminate unnecessary items.
■ Learn how a department is reimbursed for services delivered, identifying covered and excluded expenses.
■ Input charges in a timely manner.
■ Discuss quality and cost differences in supplies with other staff and management.
■ Evaluate staff and equipment downtime.

Year to Date						
Volume/Access						
Department	**Cost Center**	**Volume Year to Date**	**Percentage Budget Variance**	**Percentage Variance from Last Year**	**Days to Next Appointment/ Available Bed**	
GI Laboratory	1265	6,706	16	23	3	
Medical Unit	7095	9,705	18	28	1	
Patient Satisfaction						
	Overall Score		**Percentile**	**Percentile**	**Results Reporting**	
Department	**Actual**	**Target**	**Actual**	**Target**	**Average Report Turnaround Time**	**Reports > 24**
GI Laboratory	90.5	91.70	90	95	28	20%
Medical Unit	89	90.00	88	92	NA	NA
Human Resources						
					Employee Performance	
		Actual	**Vacancies**	**Turnover**	**Staff Performance Reviews on Time**	
Department	**Manager**	**FTEs Year to Date**	**Year to Date**	**Rate**	**> 30 Days**	
GI Laboratory	1	33.00	0.4	8%	0	
Medical Unit	1	45.00	6	12%	1	
Expenses						
				Supply	**Productivity**	
		Percentage of Budget Compared to Actual	**Percentage Variance from Budget Year to Date**	**Variance from Budget Year to Date**	**Variance from Last Year**	
Department						
GI Laboratory	250	(5.00)	11.00	Unfavorable	Unfavorable	
Medical Unit	118	8.00	12.00	Favorable	Unfavorable	
Capital Budget						
Line Items	**Number**	**Year**	**Budgeted**	**Expensed**	**Balance**	
GI Lab						
7 Video Endoscopes	10002895	2001	112,550.00	109,389.19	14,226.00	
Endoscopy Travel Cart	30256409	2001	2,750.00	0.00	32,750.00	
Scopes	89756452	2001	38,255.00	35,225.00	1,199.00	
Comments						
Financial improvement plan ongoing in GI lab: Interventional charges have been adjusted and cost reduction/inventory control is being explored with materials management.						
Medical nursing unit has achieved highest overall patient satisfaction goal. Multidisciplinary conferences are being held every other day to focus on patient care issues.						

Figure 14-11 Gastrointestinal laboratory and medical unit dashboard. (Adapted with permission of Northwestern Memorial Hospital, Chicago, IL.)

- Analyze cause of schedule delays, canceled cases, and extended procedure times.
- Explore new products with vendor representatives and network with colleagues who have tried both new and modified products.
- Reduce the length of stay by troubleshooting early.
- Assist staff in organizational planning.
- Enhance productivity through rigorous process improvement.
- Post overtime and high/low productivity analysis.
- Explore how time and motion studies may increase efficiencies by identifying gaps or duplication in effort.
- Ensure that staff have the right tools and that the tools are ready when needed.

- Analyze patient supplies and review cost per patient encounter (e.g., chemotherapy administration, dialysis, insertion of indwelling or peripheral catheter).
- Track various steps in patient care that are time consuming or problematic for a unit (e.g., communication from front desk to recovery room, staff response to patient call lights, number of staff responding to an emergency code).
- Acquire a working knowledge of how a department/unit monitors financial and quality indicators, and participate in the development of action plans to increase patient satisfaction or to create the "best patient experience."

KEY CONCEPTS

- Nurses play an integral role in the preparation, implementation, and evaluation of a unit or department budget.

- If nurses are not conscious of revenue and expenses, then deviation from financial performance will occur.

- Overall, organizational performance is dependent upon the insight and skills of staff members regarding patient care quality and financial outcomes.

- Hospitals use several types of budgets to help with future planning and management. These include operational-, capital-, and construction budgets.

- The budget preparation phase is one of data gathering related to a variety of elements that influence an organization, including demographic information, competitive analysis, regulatory influences, and strategic initiatives. Additionally, it is helpful to understand the department's scope of service, goals, and history.

- During the budget-preparation phase, it is important to examine the individual nursing or hospital department or section thoroughly. Hospital systems are frequently divided into sections, departments, or units to compartmentalize them for organizational purposes. These subsections or units, commonly called cost centers, are used to track financial data.

- Organizations typically use history or past performance as a baseline of experience and data to better understand activity in a department or unit.

- Once background data have been gathered, the development of the budget can follow. This includes projecting revenue and expenses.

- Expenses are determined by identifying the cost associated with the delivery of service.

- Expenditures are resources used by an organization to deliver services. They may include labor, supplies, equipment, utilities, and miscellaneous items.

- Once developed, budgets are submitted to administration for review and final approval. The approval process may take several months as the unit budgets are combined to determine the overall budget for the health care organization.

KEY TERMS

accounting	dashboard
capital budget	direct expenses
construction budget	fixed costs
cost centers	indirect expenses
operational budget	variable costs
profit	variance
revenue	

REVIEW QUESTIONS

1. An operational budget accounts for
   A. the purchase of minor and major equipment.
   B. construction and renovation.
   C. income and expenses associated with daily activity within an organization.
   D. applications for new technology.

2. Revenue can be generated through
   A. billable patient services.
   B. donations to service organizations.
   C. use of generic drugs.
   D. messenger and escort activities.

3. Cost centers are used to
   A. develop historical and demographic information.
   B. track expense line items.
   C. plan for strategic growth and movement.
   D. track financial data within a department or unit.

4. The purpose of monitoring a budget is to
   A. keep expenses above budget.
   B. maintain revenue above the previous year's budget.
   C. ensure revenue is generated monthly.
   D. generate revenue and control expenses within a projected framework.

5. Productivity can be measured by the
   A. number of beds in a hospital.
   B. reimbursement rates for services rendered.
   C. past performance and history regarding revenue.
   D. volume of services delivered.

6. Revenue and expenses are typically tracked using which of the following tools:
   A. Strategic planning
   B. Competitive analysis
   C. Operational budget
   D. Construction budget

7. Identify which of the following are indirect expenses.
   A. Salary of staff providing care
   B. Gas, electric, phones
   C. Medical supplies
   D. Monitoring equipment

8. The following should be reviewed immediately after an operational budget has been put into place:
   A. Demographic information
   B. Regulatory influences
   C. Competitive analysis
   D. Budget monitoring

REVIEW ACTIVITIES

1. Look around your clinical agency. Do you see any dashboard displays of quality measures? What do they reveal about your agency?

2. Using the tables in this chapter as a guideline, construct a competitive analysis of one or more of the agencies in your community. Note whether the agencies have a Website at www.google.com.

3. Using the zero-based budgeting figure in this chapter, construct an analysis of one of the clinical procedures in your agency.

EXPLORING THE WEB

- Go to the site for the Joint Commission. What information did you find there?
  www.jointcommission.org

- Review the site for the American Organization of Nurse Executives. Was the information helpful?
  www.aone.org

- Review these sites for helpful information. What did you find there?

  Healthcare Financial Management Association:
  www.hfma.org

  American College of Healthcare Executives:
  www.ache.org

  The Advisory Board Company:
  www.advisory.com

  Centers for Medicare and Medicaid Services:
  www.cms.hhs.gov

Agency for Healthcare Research and Quality:
www.ahrq.gov

Food and Drug Administration: *www.fda.gov*

REFERENCES

Hendrich, A. L., & Lee, N. (2005). Intra-unit patient transports: Time, motion, and cost impact on hospital efficiency. *Nursing Economics, 23*(4), 157–164.

Jones, C. B. (2005). The Costs of Nurse Turnover, Part 2. *Journal of Nursing Administration, 35*(1), 41–49.

Needleman, J., Buerhaus, P., Mattke, S., Stewart, M., & Zelevinsky, K. (2002). Nurse-Staffing Levels and the Quality of Care in Hospitals. *New England Journal of Medicine, 346*(22), 1714–1722.

Norton, D., & Kaplan, R. (2001). *The strategy-focused organization: How balanced scorecard companies thrive in the new business environment.* Boston: Harvard Business School Press.

SUGGESTED READINGS

Joint Commission. (2006). Comprehensive Accreditation Manual for Hospitals (CAMH): The Official Handbook. Oakbrook Terrace, IL: Joint Commission.

Vonderheid, S., Pohl, J., Schafer, P., Forrest, K., Poole, M., Barkauskas, V., et al. (2004). Using FTE and RVU performance measures to assess financial viability of academic nurse-managed centers. *Nursing Economics, 22*(3), 124–134.

Wagner, C., Budreau, G., & Everett, L. (2005). Analyzing fluctuating unit census for timely staffing intervention. *Nursing Economics, 23*(2), 85–90.

CHAPTER 15

Effective Staffing

Anne Bernat, RN, MSN, CNAA ⊕ Mary L. Fisher, PhD, RN, CNAA, BC

Best practice staffing provides timely and effective patient care while providing a safe environment for both patients and staff, as well as promoting an atmosphere of professional nursing satisfaction (Carl Ray, et al., 2003).

OBJECTIVES

Upon completion of this chapter, the reader should be able to:

1. Calculate full-time equivalents (FTEs) needed to staff a typical inpatient nursing unit.

2. Analyze the impact of patient volume and work intensity on the demand for nursing care.

3. Discuss appropriate units of service used to measure nursing need by unit type.

4. Critique organizational, regulatory, staff, and patient dynamics underlying the development of a staffing plan.

5. Analyze scheduling issues that impact the matching of nursing resources to patient needs.

6. Compare and contrast models of care delivery and their impact on patient outcomes.

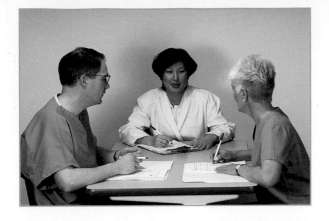

You are a new nurse manager of a 30-bed medical unit that uses primary nursing as the care delivery model. You have 40 employees who work full and part time with vacancies for eight additional full-time staff. The current schedule does not accommodate any 12-hour shifts. You have five long-term staff members who threaten to leave if they are forced to work 12-hour shifts. You have interviewed several new graduates who will come to work for you only if you offer them 12-hour shifts.

How can you accommodate the needs of all groups of staff?

What effect will the 12-hour shifts have on your care delivery model?

The ability of a nurse to provide safe and effective care to a patient is dependent on many variables. These variables include the knowledge and experience of the staff, the severity of illness of the patients, patient dependency for daily activities, complexity of care, the amount of nursing time available, the care delivery model, care management tools, and organizational supports in place to facilitate care. This chapter will explore these factors, how they affect planning for staffing, scheduling staff, and patient outcomes associated with staffing factors. By the end of this chapter, you will understand how to plan staffing and measure the effectiveness of a staffing plan. You will also be able to critique the models of care delivery that are applicable to your environment and patient population.

DETERMINATION OF STAFFING NEEDS

Historically, patient census was used to determine staffing needs. This resulted in fixed nurse-to-patient care ratios. This method of patient census staffing proved to be highly inaccurate because patient care needs vary greatly (Gran-Moravec & Hughes, 2005). As nursing salaries rose and became a larger part of the health care budget, better matching of patient needs to nursing resources became an important financial quest in health

care institutions. In today's rapidly changing health care environment, many variables are considered in determining nurse staffing requirements. The effectiveness of the staffing pattern is only as good as the planning that goes into its preparation.

CORE CONCEPTS

Gaining an understanding of the key terms—full-time equivalents (FTEs), productive time, nonproductive time, direct and indirect care, nursing workload, and units of service—is necessary to understand staffing patterns.

FTES

A **full-time equivalent (FTE)** is a measure of the work commitment of an employee who works five days a week or 40 hours per week for 52 weeks a year. This amounts to 2,080 hours of work time (Figure 15-1).

A full-time employee who works 40 hours a week is referred to as a 1.0 FTE. An employee who works 36 hours (three 12-hour shifts) is considered full time for benefit purposes in many agencies but is assigned 0.9 FTE for budgeting purposes (36/40 = 0.9 FTE). A part-time employee who works five days in a two-week period is considered a 0.5 FTE. FTE calculation is used to mathematically describe how much an employee works (Figure 15-2). Understanding FTEs is essential when moving from a staffing plan to the actual number of staff required.

FTE hours are a total of all paid time. This includes worked time as well as nonworked time. Hours worked and available for patient care are designated as **productive hours**. Benefit time such as vacation, sick time, and education time is considered **nonproductive hours**. When considering the number of FTEs needed to staff a unit, count only the productive hours available for each staff member because this represents the amount of time required to meet patient needs. Available productive time can be easily calculated by subtracting benefit time from the time a

| 5 days per week | × | 8 hours per day | = | 40 hours per week |
| 40 hours per week | × | 52 weeks per year | = | 2,080 hours per year |

Figure 15-1 Calculation of full-time equivalent hours.

1.0 FTE = 40 hours or five 8-hours shifts per week
0.9 FTE = 36 hours or three 12-hour shifts per week
0.8 FTE = 32 hours or four 8-hour shifts per week
0.6 FTE = 24 hours or two 12-hour or three 8-hour shifts per week
0.4 FTE = 16 hours or two 8-hour shifts per week
0.3 FTE = 12 hours or one 12-hour shift per week
0.2 FTE = 8 hours or one 8-hour shift per week

Figure 15-2 FTE calculation for varying levels of work commitment.

Vacation time	15 days	or	120 hours
Sick time	5 days	or	40 hours
Holiday time	6 days	or	48 hours
Education time	3 days	or	24 hours
Total nonproductive time		=	232 hours

2,080 − 232 = 1,848 hours of productive work time available for each staff member with these benefits.

Figure 15-3 Calculation of productive and nonproductive time.

Unit Type	Unit of Service
In-patient Unit	Nursing Hours Per Patient Day (NHPPD)
Labor and Delivery	Births
Operating Room	Surgeries/Procedures
Home Care	Patient Visits
Emergency Services	Patient Visits

Figure 15-4 Units of service—volume measures by unit type.

20 patients on the unit

5 staff × 3 shifts = 15 staff

15 staff each working 8 hours = 120 hours available in a 24-hour period

120 nursing hours ÷ 20 patients = 6.0 NHPPD

Figure 15-5 Calculation of nursing hours per patient day (NHPPD).

full-time employee would work (Figure 15-3). These figures vary greatly depending on institutional policy and availability of human resource benefits. In this case, a full-time registered nurse (RN) would have 1,848 hours per year of productive time available to care for patients.

Employees who work with patients can be classified into two categories: those who provide direct care and those who provide indirect care. **Direct care** is time spent providing hands-on care to patients. **Indirect care** is time spent on activities that support patient care but are not done directly to the patient. Documentation, order entry, time consulting with people in other health care disciplines, and time spent following up on outstanding issues are good examples of indirect care. Even though RNs, licensed practical nurses (LPNs), and unlicensed assistive personnel (UAP) engage in indirect care activities, the majority of their time is spent providing direct care, therefore, they are classified as direct care providers. Nurse managers, clinical specialists, unit secretaries, and other support staff are considered indirect care providers because the majority of their work is indirect in nature and supports the work of the direct care providers.

UNITS OF SERVICE

Nursing workload is dependent on the nursing care needs of patients. Both patient volume and work intensity—that is, severity of illness, patient dependency for activities of daily living, complexity of care, and amount of time needed for care—contribute to nursing workload. **Units of service** include a variety of volume measures that are used to reflect different types of patient encounters as indicators of nursing workload (Figure 15-4). Volume measures are used in budget negotiations to project nursing needs of patients and to assure adequate resources for safe patient care.

The majority of nurses practice on in-patient units, therefore, further calculations for this chapter's examples will be in Nursing Hours Per Patient Day (NHPPD). **Nursing Hours Per Patient Days (NHPPD)** is the amount of nursing care required per patient in a 24-hour period and is usually based on midnight census and past unit needs, expected unit practice trends, national benchmarks, professional staffing standards, and budget ne-

gotiations. NHPPD reflects only productive nursing time needed. Calculation of NHPPD is displayed in Figure 15-5.

NURSE INTENSITY

Nurse intensity is "a measure of the amount and complexity of nursing care needed by a patient" (Adomat & Hewison, 2004, p. 304). Nurse intensity is dependent on many factors that are difficult to measure: severity of illness, patient dependency for activities of daily living, complexity of care, and amount of time needed for care (Beglinger, 2006). It is vital that nurses measure nurse intensity because staffing needs vary not only with the number of patients being cared for but also with the type of care provided for each of those patients (Unruh & Fottler, 2006).

Patient turnover affects nurse intensity. **Patient turnover** is a measure reflecting patient admission, transfer, and discharge; all of which entail RN-intensive procedures. As the health care industry pushes to reduce costs through shorter lengths of stay, these RN-intensive procedures related to patient turnover consume an increasing proportion of the hospital stay. As length of stay shortens, the intensity and need for NHPPD increases. What is not known at this time is the exact nature of this inverse relationship (Unruh & Fottler, 2006).

PATIENT CLASSIFICATION SYSTEMS

A **patient classification system (PCS)** is a measurement tool used to articulate the nursing workload for a specific patient or group of patients over a specific period of time. The measure of nursing workload that is generated for each patient is called the **patient acuity**. Classification data can be used to predict the amount of nursing time needed based on the patient's acuity. As a patient becomes sicker, the acuity level rises, meaning the patient requires more nursing care. As a patient acuity level decreases, the patient requires less nursing care. In most patient classification systems, each patient is classified once a day using weighted criteria that then predict the nursing care hours needed for the next 24 hours. Because patient care is dynamic, it is impossible to capture future patient care needs using a one-time measure (Gran-Moravec & Hughes, 2005). The criteria reflects care needed in bathing, mobilizing, eating, supervision, assessment, frequent observations, treatments, and so on. The ideal PCS produces a valid and reliable rating of individual patient care requirements, which are matched to the latest clinical technology and caregiver skill variables. These systems are generally applied to all inpatients in an organization. Other PCS systems exist to measure the workload associated with patient visits in the Emergency Department (ED) or in clinic environments based on relative weights for visit lengths as well as complexity of care. There are two different types of classification systems: factor and prototype.

FACTOR SYSTEM

The factor classification system uses units of measure that equate to nursing time. Nursing tasks are assigned time or are weighted to reflect the amount of time needed to perform the task. These systems attempt to capture the cognitive functions of assessment, planning, intervention, and evaluation of patient outcomes along with written documentation processes. There are many factor systems that have been home grown or built for a specific organization. There are also many factor systems available for purchase on the open market. This is the most popular type of classification system because of its capability to project care needs for individual patients as well as patient groups. The time assigned or the weighted factor for different nursing activities can be changed over time to reflect the changing needs of the patients or hospital systems.

ADVANTAGES AND DISADVANTAGES   In the factor classification system, data are generally readily available to managers and staff for day-to-day operations. These data provide a base of information against which one can justify changes in staffing requirements. A disadvantage to this system type is the ongoing workload for the nurse in classifying patients every day. There are also documented problems with classification creep, whereby acuity levels rise as a result of misuse of classification criteria. These systems do not holistically capture the patient's needs for psychosocial, environmental, and health management support. And finally, these systems calculate nursing time needed based on a typical nurse. A novice nurse may take longer to perform activities than the average nurse.

Recommended nursing time needed may differ from the actual time needed based on the expertise of the staff.

PROTOTYPE SYSTEM

The prototype classification system allocates nursing time to large patient groups based on an average of similar patients. For example, specific **diagnostic-related groups (DRGs)** have been used as groupings of patients to which a nursing acuity is assigned based on past organizational experience. DRGs are patient groupings established by the federal government for reimbursement purposes. DRGs are sorted by patient disease or condition. This model assumes that, on average, this will reflect the nursing care required and provided. The data are then used by hospitals in determining the cost of nursing care and negotiating contracts with payers for specific patient populations.

ADVANTAGES AND DISADVANTAGES   The distinct advantage of this classification system is the reduction of work for the nurse because daily classification is not needed. A major disadvantage of this system is that DRGs do not accurately reflect patients' nursing needs because medical diagnosis alone does not adjust for variances in patients' self-care ability and severity of illness. There is no ongoing measure of the actual nursing work required by individual patients. There are also no ongoing data to monitor the accuracy of the preassigned nursing care requirements. The prototype system is much less common than the factor system.

UTILIZATION OF CLASSIFICATION SYSTEM DATA

Patient classification data are valuable sources of information for all levels of the organization. On a day-to-day basis, acuity data can be utilized by staff and managers in planning nurse staffing over the next 24 hours. Acuity data and NHPPD are concrete data parameters that are used to educate staff on how to adjust staffing levels. Experienced staff have the knowledge to manage staffing to acuity given the information, boundaries, and authority to do so. In many organizations, a central staffing office monitors the census and acuity on all units and deploys nursing resources to the areas in most need using the classification system data and recommended staffing levels. The manager reviews the results of staffing over the past 24 to 48 hours to adjust staffing performance to patient requirements. At the unit level, acuity data are also essential in preparing month-end justification for variances in staff utilization. If your average acuity has risen, then there should be an expected rise in NHPPD to accommodate the increased patient needs.

At an organization level, acuity data have been used to cost out nursing services for specific patient populations and global patient types. This information is also very helpful in negotiating payment rates with third-party payers such as insurance companies to ensure that reimbursement reflects nursing costs. In most organizations, the classification or acuity data are also used in preparation of the nursing staffing budget for the upcoming fiscal year. The data can be benchmarked with other organizations to lend credence to any efforts to change nursing hours. Finally, patient acuity data and NHPPD can be used to develop a staffing pattern. Patient classification and NHPPD data provide an enormous amount of information that serves a multitude of needs.

CONSIDERATIONS IN DEVELOPING A STAFFING PLAN

Developing a staffing plan is a science and an art. The following sections will consider other areas in addition to the acuity data and NHPPD just discussed. Each of these areas should be reviewed and the findings incorporated into development of the staffing plan.

BENCHMARKING

Benchmarking is a tool used to compare productivity across facilities to establish performance goals. Note, however, that "being the best performer in a group does not necessarily indicate best practice" (Ray, Jagim, Agnew, Inglass-Mckay, & Sheehy, 2003, p. 246). Often, benchmarking data provides only comparable unit-of-service performance and does not reflect quality-of-care indicators that can link quality patient care outcomes to productivity measures. In developing a staffing pattern that leads to a budget, it is important to benchmark your planned NHPPD against other organizations with similar patient populations as part of evidence-based decision-making (EBD-M). Purchased patient classification systems often offer acuity and NHPPD benchmarking data from around the country as part of their system. This kind of data can be helpful in establishing a starting point for a staffing pattern or as part of justification for increasing or reducing nursing hours. Caution must be used, however, because each organization has varying levels of support in place at the unit level for the nurse. For example, a nursing unit that has dietary aides from the Dietary department distribute and pick up meal trays would need less nursing time than a unit that had no external support for this activity. Practice differences such as these contribute significantly to differences in hours of care from one organization to another.

REGULATORY REQUIREMENTS

Generally speaking, there are few regulatory requirements related to nurse staffing. This is changing, however, as the nursing shortage heightens. Eight states have mandated nurse staffing plans (White, 2006). Note that staffing plans are different from staffing ratios. In 1999,

California became the first state to mandate development of nurse-to-patient ratios. By January, 2005, California hospitals were required to meet a 1:5 ratio in all medical-surgical units. Similar legislation is pending in Massachusetts. In both cases, the State Nurses Associations were central to the legislation. There is considerable controversy within the nursing profession over this issue. There are nurses who are adamant that they need to be protected by law with stipulated staffing levels. There are nurse leaders who are concerned that the mandated staffing levels would soon become the maximum staffing levels rather than the minimum.

The Joint Commission (JC), formerly known as the Joint Commission on Accreditation of Healthcare Organizations (JCAHO), surveys hospitals on the quality of care provided. The JC does not mandate staffing levels but does assess staffing effectiveness. The JC standards (2006) regarding staffing require organizations to monitor at least four indicators, including two human resource indicators and two clinical indicators. An example of a human resource indicator is NHPPD. An example of a clinical indicator is skin breakdown occurrence. There are 21 indicators from which to choose. Those indicators chosen must be analyzed and staffing levels adjusted based on the information (White, 2006).

SKILL MIX

Skill mix is another critical element in nurse staffing. **Skill mix** is the percentage of RN staff compared to other direct care staff (LPNs). For example, in a unit that has 40 FTEs budgeted, with 20 of them being RNs and 20 FTEs of other skill types, the RN skill mix would be 50%. If the unit had 40 FTEs, with 30 of them being RNs, the RN skill mix would be 75%. The skill mix of a unit should vary according to the care that is required and the care delivery model utilized. For example, in a critical care unit, the RN skill mix will be much higher than in a nursing home where the skills of an RN are required to a much lesser degree. It is important to note that RN hours of care are more costly than those of lesser skilled workers, but there is evidence that RNs are a very productive and efficient type of labor. As nurses become more scarce, it will become even more important to evaluate the patient care required and who can perform necessary functions. For instance, if many patients require feeding, UAP may be most appropriate. As you consider skill mix, however, you need to clearly understand the activities in which each level of staff can engage within the scope of practice in your state. In some states, UAP may catheterize patients if they have received training and are competent. In other states, UAP may not perform this function regardless of their training and expertise. RNs are always required for patient assessment, monitoring changes in patient status, evaluation, teaching, and patient treatments requiring judgment.

CASE STUDY 15-1

Y ou are the manager of a critical care unit that has 16 beds in a state that does not mandate nurse-to-patient ratios. The nurse-to-patient ratio is budgeted at one nurse to two patients. Medical-surgical beds are not available for your patients who have improved. Of the sixteen patients in your unit, four are well enough to go to a general-floor bed. On the medical-surgical units, the nurse-to-patient ratio is one RN to six patients. You are planning staffing for the next two shifts. What is the budgeted NHPPD for this unit? What would the typical NHPPD be for a medical-surgical unit where the nurse-to-patient ratio was 1:4?

To adjust staffing to the current situation, what factors should you consider? After consideration of these factors, what is your plan for staffing? What would you communicate to your staff?

STAFF SUPPORT

Another important factor to consider in developing a staffing pattern is the supports in place for the operations of the unit or department. For instance, does your organization have a systematic process to deliver medications to the department or do unit personnel have to pick up patient medications and narcotics? Does your organization have staff to transport patients to and from ancillary departments? The less support available to your staff, the more nursing hours have to be built into the staffing pattern to provide care to patients. Nursing areas such as critical care that have a significant amount of equipment to track and supply may benefit greatly from adding a materials coordinator. This kind of support for staff allows staff to spend their precious available time with patients rather than looking for equipment or supplies. An additional important unit-based need is secretarial support. If the unit has admissions, discharges, and transfers, it makes sense to provide unit secretarial support for the peak periods of the day. In ICUs, unit secretaries are commonly scheduled around the clock to provide support for the unit staff as well as for other disciplines.

HISTORICAL INFORMATION

As you consider the many variables that affect staffing, it helps to ask the following questions: What has worked in the past? Were the staff able to provide the care that was needed? How many patients were cared for? What kind of patients were they? How many staff were utilized and what kind of staff were they? This kind of information can help to identify operational issues that would not be apparent otherwise. For example, in an older part of a facility, there may not be a pneumatic delivery tube system, a system that is available in most other parts of the facility. Because it is generally available, you may overlook its absence. But its absence means a significant amount of time will be required to collect needed items, affecting the staffing plan you develop. It also would be important to review any data

on quality or staff perceptions regarding the effectiveness of the previous staffing plan. This information will allow you to calculate previous NHPPD and outcomes for comparison to your staffing plan. History is a valuable tool that we often overlook as we plan for the future.

ESTABLISHING A STAFFING PLAN

A **staffing plan** articulates how many and what kind of staff are needed by shift and day to staff a unit or department. There are basically two ways of developing a staffing plan. It can be generated by determining the required ratio of staff to patients; nursing hours and total FTEs are then calculated. It can also be generated by determining the nursing care hours needed for a specific patient or patients and then generating the FTEs and staff-to-patient ratio needed to provide that care. In most cases, you would use a combination of methods to validate your staffing plan. We will start with development of a plan from the staff-to-patient ratio.

INPATIENT UNIT

An **inpatient unit** is a hospital unit that provides care to patients 24 hours a day, seven days a week. Establishing a staffing pattern for this kind of unit utilizes all the data discussed in the previous areas. Using data from all your sources, you can build a staffing plan that you believe will meet the needs of the patients, the staff, and the organization. To illustrate the concept of calculating a staffing plan, we will use a typical medical unit with 24 beds and an average daily census (ADC) of 20. **Average daily census (ADC)** is calculated by taking the total numbers of patients at census time, usually midnight, over a period of time, for example, weekly, monthly, or yearly, and dividing by the number of days in the time period. Many institutions budget their staffing based on ADC and then adjust for patient census and acuity changes. Utilizing the staffing plan (Figure 15-6),

Scenario: A 24-bed medical unit where the ADC is 20 and NHPPD is budgeted at 8.

Step 1:

Formula: Number of patients $\times$ NHPPD = care hours per day = shifts needed per 24 hours staff productive hours per shift

Example: $20 \times 8 = \dfrac{160 \text{ care hours per 24 hour day}}{8} = 20$ eight-hour shifts needed per 24 hours

Step 2:

Allocate 20 staff to the unit by shift and skill mix

	% of Staff Per Shift	# of Staff	RN	Tech/Unit Clerk
Days	40	8	4	4
Evenings	35	7	4	3
Nights	25	5	4	1
			12	8 (Total 20)

Step 3:

Calculate FTE to cover staff days off. (Calculations are in parentheses in the matrix below.)

Formula: $\dfrac{\text{number of staff needed per shift} \times \text{Days of needed coverage}}{\text{Number of shifts each FTE works}}$

Example: $\dfrac{4 \times 7}{5} = 5.6$

	% of Staff Per Shift	# of Staff	RN	Tech/Unit Clerk
Days	40	8	4 (5.6)	4 (5.6)
Evenings	35	7	4 (5.6)	3 (4.2)
Nights	25	5	4 (5.6)	1 (1.4)
			12 (16.8)	8 (11.2) = 20 (28)

Step 4:

Provide coverage for benefit time off.

Formula: Productive hours/budgeted nonproductive hours = percent of nonproductive hours $\times$ total FTE = additional FTE needed to cover benefits;

Productive + nonproductive FTE to cover each week = Grand Total FTE

Example: $2080/232 = 0.11 \times 28 = 3.08$;

       $3.08 + 28 = 31.08$ Grand Total FTE

Figure 15-6 Staffing plan template for an inpatient unit.

plot out the number and type of staff needed during the week and on weekends for 24 hours a day for the number of patients on a clinical unit.

Step 1: To develop a staffing plan using NHPPD, you would start with a target NHPPD. If your target NHPPD were 8, for example, and you expected to have 20 patients on your 24-bed unit, you would multiply 8 NHPPD times 20 patients to get 160 productive hours needed every day. Dividing 160 by 8-hour shifts worked by each staff member gives you 20 staff members needed per day.

Step 2: Now that you know how many 8-hour shifts are needed in 24 hours, the next step is to allocate staff to the plan based on how care is delivered on the unit. To fully understand the complexity of decisions involved in this step, you must review the "Models of Care Delivery" section later in this chapter. Allocating FTEs cannot be separated from an intelligent understanding of how patient care is delivered and how to use the right mix of staff to accomplish that patient care. In our example, the medical unit uses team nursing to provide care.

Taking the twenty shifts that are needed for patient care in our example, the nurse manager must determine the mix of staff, the weighting of staff per shift, and whether this changes by day of the week. The census on this unit does not lower on the weekends, so we calculate the staffing for the entire week. If the unit had reduced census on specific days of the week, those days would be calculated separately. The result of Step 2 is a snapshot of the staffing plan for 24 hours (see Figure 15-6).

You have now determined a staffing plan for your unit. The staffing plan calculates the number of FTEs needed per day.

Step 3: You must now calculate the amount of additional staff that will be needed to provide for days off. Direct caregivers will need to be replaced, but some other support staff may not need to be replaced for days off or benefited time off. Managers typically are not replaced on days off. The formula for calculating coverage for staff days off is the number of staff needed per shift multiplied by the number of days of needed coverage, usually 7, divided by the number of shifts each FTE works per week. For each 8-hour staff member needed in the daily plan, the unit must hire 1.4 FTEs ($1 \times 7/5 = 1.4$). In a 12-hour staffing model, the manager must hire 2.3 FTEs for each 12-hour staff member needed in the daily plan ($1 \times 7/3 = 2.3$). This is true because each 12-hour staff member works only 3 days per week.

In our example for Step 3, the calculations for seven-day coverage are in parenthesis in the staffing plan. To have 4 RNs on day shift, for example, you need to hire 5.6 FTEs. In total, you need to hire 28 FTEs to have 20 staff working 7 days per week.

Step 4: The next step is to provide additional FTEs for coverage for benefited time away from work. This includes vacations, educational time, orientation time, and so on.

The amount of time away from work varies by organization. If every employee receives the benefits outlined in Figure 15-3, 232 benefit hours are needed per person. We then need to determine what percent of each FTE's productive time that the benefits represent. In our example, 232 is 11% of 2,080. We then take our total FTEs from Step 3 and multiply by 0.11 ($28 \times 0.11 = 3.08$). Thus, we need an additional 3.08 FTEs to work when other staff are taking benefit time. This figure is then added to our total from Step 3 to get our grand total FTEs for the budget ($28 + 3.08 = 31.08$).

DETERMINING THE FTES NEEDED TO STAFF AN EPISODIC CARE UNIT

An **episodic care unit** refers to a unit that sees patients for defined episodes of care; dialysis or ambulatory care units are good examples. In these units, patients tend to be more homogenous and have a more predictable path of care. Determining staffing needs for an episodic unit starts with an assessment of the hours of care required by the patients and an understanding of unit needs based on how care is delivered. For example, in an ambulatory care clinic, staffing may be done to cover the number of rooms used by practitioners to see patients because volume is dependent on efficiently moving patients through the care process and keeping the practitioner engaged and not waiting on the next patient. Nurses in these settings must be masters at providing the nursing care needed within this constraint. If the clinic has nine rooms that are used by three practitioners, the staffing may be set at one nurse per practitioner and an additional secretary to handle scheduling and paper work. If the clinic is open only Monday through Friday, we can skip Step 3 of the staffing pattern template, but we would still need to calculate benefit replacement (Step 4).

SCHEDULING

Scheduling of staff is the responsibility of the nurse manager, who must ensure that the schedule places the appropriate staff on each day and shift for safe, effective patient care. There are many issues to consider as you schedule staff: the patient type and acuity, the number of patients, the experience of your staff, and the supports available to the staff. The combination of these factors should guide the number of staff scheduled on each day and shift. These factors must be reviewed on an ongoing basis as patient types and patient acuity drive different patient needs and staff expertise.

PATIENT NEED

Patient classification systems do not tell you when the nursing activity will take place over the next 24 hours. In addition to planning for the acuity of the patients, the staffing plan must support having staff working when the

REAL WORLD INTERVIEW

Given the need for staffing and financial accountability, I used spreadsheet software to improve the development of staffing patterns in our facility. We had been using a pencil and paper template for managers to use to develop staffing patterns. This manual template concentrated on the weekday staffing needs and applied an overall factor to calculate weekend and benefit time. The FTE number provided did not address orientation and education needs for any of the staff or benefit needs for the weekend staff. Although these staffing patterns were used to project the number of FTEs needed and the distribution of employees to staff the nursing unit, they were not used to drive the budgeted quota for the unit.

Using a computer software program, I developed a spreadsheet template the managers could use to accurately project FTEs needed to meet the staffing pattern. This computerized approach allows for weekday and weekend staffing to be considered independently considering any differences in census or direct NHPPD. A benefit time factor, tailored to our organization's specific benefit package for each skill level, was used to calculate the number of FTEs needed to staff for benefit time. Benefit time was now calculated for weekday and weekend staffing, coverage for a 24/7 operation. Additionally, an orientation and education factor is used to calculate the FTEs needed to provide coverage. For the first time, benefited time off and orientation time were built into each unit's staffing pattern. Additionally, direct and indirect NHPPD are automatically calculated as the staffing pattern is changed, and the calculated FTE needs can be compared to the current budgeted quota for variances. I also worked with Finance to use this template as the basis for a Budgeted Quota Sheet, which is used during the budget process for determining the unit quota for the next year, a quota that now includes benefited time off and orientation time.

One of the biggest assists has been the ability of the nurse managers to use the template for what-if scenarios. When they are planning for a census or patient program change, FTE needs can be quickly calculated and compared to their current budgeted quota. This tool has become part of our business planning process.

Overall, this template has been accepted as a valid management tool, has standardized inclusion of nonproductive time into FTE budgets, and has given managers a simple tool to develop new staffing patterns. It has also helped in raising the accountability of managers to develop workable staffing patterns for which they can be held accountable.

Barbara Leafer, RN, BS
Fiscal Administrator for Patient Care
Albany, New York

---

work needs to be done. A good example of this would be an oncology unit in which chemotherapy and blood transfusions typically occur on the evening shift. In this scenario, staffing in the evening may need to be higher than for other shifts to support these nurse-intensive activities. As patient types change, so do patients' needs and staffing requirements. Adding a population of step-down patients from the ICU would likely require additional FTEs on a medical-surgical unit. Anytime patient populations change, staffing and NHPPD should be assessed. A general rule is that the higher the patient acuity, the more consistent the staffing needs are across shifts. A critical care unit is continuously monitoring patients around the clock, whereas a surgical unit has activities concentrated before and after surgeries each day with somewhat less activity on the late evening and night shifts.

EXPERIENCE AND SCHEDULING OF STAFF

Each nurse differs regarding knowledge base, experience level, and critical thinking skills. A novice nurse takes longer to accomplish the same task than an experienced nurse. An experienced RN can handle more in terms of workload and acuity of patients. If your area requires special skills or competencies of the staff, you would also want to plan so that staff with the special skills are scheduled when the patient care need may arise. Remember, the underlying principle of good staffing is that those you serve come first. This may dictate some undesirable shifts, but your responsibility is to ensure that there are appropriate numbers and kinds of staff on hand to care for the patients you serve. Staff are plotted out across a staffing sheet (Figure 15-7).

	Monday 04	Tuesday 05	Wednesday 06	Thursday 07	Friday 08	Saturday 09	Sunday 10	Monday 11	Tuesday 12	Wednesday 13	Thursday 14	Friday 15	Saturday 16	Sunday 17
Melinda	D		D	D		D	D	D		D	D	D		
Carlos		8.00 1900			N	N	N	D	8.00 1900		D			
Tabitha	12.00 0900		12.00 0900		D	12.00 0900	12.00 0900	12.00 0900		12.00 0900		N		
Maria	D	8.00 1100		E	E	E		vac		8.00 1100	E	E	E	
Barbara		14.00 2400	13.00 2400	13.00 2400	D				14.00 2400	13.00 2400	13.00 2400		D	D
Nirmala	D	D	D	D		E	D		D	N	N		E	N
Robert	N	N	N	N	N		N	N	N	N	N		E	
Jacqueline	E	E	E		E		E	E	E	E	E	E		E
Irma		D		D	D	D	D		D			D		
Sara	E		E	E	8.00 0800	N	E	E			E	8.00 0800		E
Gary			N					E	E	E		12.00 1500		
Cynthia	N	N	N		N	P	P	N	N	P		P		
Jose	8.00 0730	8.00 0730	8.00 0730	8.00 0730	8.00 0730			8.00 0730	8.00 0730		8.00 0730	8.00 0730	N	

The first number in a square is the number of hours scheduled, the second number is the shift start time in military time.

Standard Work Assignments

D 0700–1500
E 1500–2300
N 2300–0700
A 0700–1900
P 1900–0700

Figure 15-7 Excerpt from the schedule for an emergency department showing great variation in shift design.

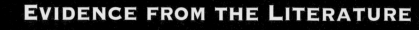

EVIDENCE FROM THE LITERATURE

Citation: Currie, V., Harvey, G., West, B., McKenna, H., & Keeney, S. (2005). Relationship between quality of care, staff levels, skill mix, and nurse autonomy: Literature review. *Journal of Adanced Nursing, 51*(1), 73–82.

Discussion: This integrative literature review attempts to confirm the expected links between quality of care, staffing, and nurse autonomy issues. One trend in the literature is a disenchantment with patient satisfaction monitors as a measure of quality of care because the tools used usually find high satisfaction levels, have doubtful validity, are general in nature, and do not point to specific patient issues that might lead to improved care. Later studies have begun monitoring quality through measures of nurse-sensitive patient outcomes, such as patient mortality, failure to rescue, urinary tract infections, and pneumonia, instead of using patient satisfaction. Studies have found significant links between nurse staffing and these patient outcome measures. It is difficult to attribute these outcomes directly to nursing care alone, however, because patient care involves many disciplines.

Research in 1983 led to our understanding of magnet hospitals. Magnet hospitals give excellent care and are successful in attracting and retaining nurses, in part, through their dedication to adequate staffing, flexible work schedules, and nurse autonomy. Further studies in the 1990s indicated significantly lower mortality rates for magnet hospitals. In the new millennium, the American Nurses Credentialing Center (ANCC) began a national accreditation program for magnet hospitals. Staffing, scheduling, and patient quality are all still key indicators of a magnet facility. The literature does call for more research on magnet facilities to assure that the link between patient outcomes and magnet status continues to be affirmed.

Implications for Practice: There continues to be a gap in our understanding of patients' perspectives on how they "define and experience quality care" (p. 79). Significant work needs to be done in this area so we can have a valid and reliable measure of patient satisfaction that helps us to improve care. We need to continue analyzing all the parameters that impact quality patient care and nurse staffing.

Staff members should be scheduled for the number of days for which they are committed: five days a week for a full-time eight-hour employee and less for part-time employees as determined by their hiring commitment. When staff are hired, there is an agreement between the manager and the employee as to the shift, schedule, and work commitment. If the unit workload is consistent, the scheduled days should be assigned so that there are equal numbers of staff available through the week. Typically, the spread of FTEs across the 24-hour period falls within the following guidelines: days 33% to 50%, evenings 30% to 40%, and nights 20% to 33%. The spread should be based on patient need.

SHIFT VARIATIONS

To attract and retain employees, organizations offer traditional schedules and flexible schedules to meet organizational and employee needs.

TRADITIONAL STAFFING PLANS Traditional staffing plans are generally eight-hour shifts, 7 A.M. to 3:30 P.M., 3 P.M. to 11:30 P.M., and 11 P.M. to 7:30 A.M. A full-time employee works 10 eight-hour shifts in a two-week

period. The start time of eight-hour shifts may vary by organization or by nursing unit and patient need. For example, EDs are typically busiest during the evening into the night hours. An eight-hour shift for the ED may be 7 P.M. to 3 A.M. to cover the peak activity times. After you have determined what numbers of staff are necessary, it is important to attempt to schedule staff in a way to meet their needs. Some prefer to work long stretches to have several days off in a row. Others prefer to work short stretches.

NEW OPTIONS IN STAFFING PLANS As the nursing shortage deepens, there will be an increasing need to develop schedules that meet the needs of both the patients and the worker. In recent years, there have been more new options in scheduling to meet both of these needs. Twelve-hour shifts have become very popular across the country. In many organizations, employees can work 36-hours per week and get full-time benefits. In this situation, a nurse could work three 12-hour shifts per week, have four days off, and be full time. Another popular option is weekend programs. Weekend program staff work two 12-hour shifts every weekend and are paid a rate that would make the 24 hours of work equal to 40 hours of work during the week. Some of these programs include full-time benefits as well. The purpose of this kind of program is to improve weekend staffing and allow full-time staff members who usually work 26 weekends a year to work fewer weekends for staff retention purposes.

IMPACT ON PATIENT CARE   Any time you implement a scheduling plan, it is critical to assess what the effect will be on the care of patients. For example, workweeks made up of three 12-hour shifts have in many units disrupted continuity of care. **Continuity of care** is generally defined as the follow-through in patient care that is inherent in having the same nurse return to care for patients in subsequent shifts on sequential days of the week. Disruptions in continuity of care are especially true when 12-hour shifts are not scheduled on sequential days. To mediate this impact, 12-hour staff can be paired so that the patient has the same pair of nurses every day for three days, and then the patient can be transitioned to a new pair of 12-hour staff. Units that have short patient lengths of stay may have fewer continuity problems than units with longer lengths of stay. The number of staff shift

handoff reports per day also affect continuity of care. A **handoff** occurs any time the nurse caring for a group of patients reports off to the nurse on an oncoming shift. Such shift handoff reports are opportunities for missed communication and errors in patient care. In eight-hour shifts, there are three shift handoffs per 24 hours; whereas, in twelve-hour shifts, there are only two shift handoffs. This is another type of continuity of care issue that must be balanced with the number of shifts per week that each nurse works. When implementing staffing plans, you must ensure that there are always staff scheduled who are familiar with the patients and the events that have transpired previously.

FINANCIAL IMPLICATIONS   New staffing plans or program changes may have significant financial implications. Because of the nursing shortage, a number of new programs are being put into place to recruit staff and encourage staff to work more hours. Weekend programs are more expensive than traditional staffing plans because of the higher rate of hourly pay, but they are a recruitment and retention tool for nursing leadership. For example,

REAL WORLD INTERVIEW

As a manager of an intensive care unit, I can say that self-scheduling has greatly increased my staff's satisfaction with their schedules. I think the biggest factor in the success of our process was the initial buy-in from the staff. Before implementing, staff were surveyed to assess their commitment to making the process work. I was looking for 60% to 75% staff buy-in before implementation and found greater than 70%. A second critical factor was having clear guidelines for the process. These included time lines for how and when staff can sign up for time and how time off is prioritized.

During implementation, we learned many things. One key factor was that staff needed to have confrontation and negotiation skills in order for this process to work. Inevitably there were situations when someone had to change their schedule. When confrontation and negotiation didn't take place, there were periods of short staffing and patient care needs not being met. We also learned that this is a time-consuming process. It takes about 16 hours per month for the self-scheduling committee to put the schedule together.

Another key element I found was the manager had to maintain accountability for staffing. I meet with the scheduling committee regularly and oversee the orientation of new staff to the self-scheduling process. I sign off on every schedule to ensure that the schedule maintains appropriate staffing levels at all times. I found that I needed to identify trends that may be affecting staffing and assist the staff in addressing the trends. I also work with the staff on the implementation of any new program that affects the schedule. The weekend program is a good example of this. I worked with the staff to ensure there were appropriate guidelines for staff receiving a reduced weekend commitment. And finally, the most important role I play is to be very clear about the expectations for all—the committee, the staff, and myself. This scheduling process has been one of the most positive quality of work life efforts for my staff.

Rob Rose, BSN, MSN
Nurse Manager, Cardiopulmonary Surgery Intensive Care Unit
Albany, New York

Weekend staff working at $42 an hour × 24 hours = $1,008 per weekend

Regular staff working at $25 an hour × 24 hours = $600 per weekend
_____

Difference in cost = $408 per weekend option FTE

Six weekend option staff members at $1,008 would cost $2,448 more than regular staff per weekend;

$2,448 × 52 weekends a year would cost $127,296 more than regular staff annually.

Figure 15-8 Annual cost of a weekend option program for one nursing unit.

note the financial impact of a weekend option program (Figure 15-8). Reduced turnover of nurses must also be considered in evaluating the financial impact of a weekend option program.

To implement a similar program or other new programs, collaboration with the Finance and Human Resources department of the organization is necessary. This collaboration must be used to develop a financial analysis to measure the dollar and human resource impact of the program.

SELF-SCHEDULING

Self-scheduling is a process in which unit staff take leadership in creating and monitoring the work schedule while working within defined guidelines. Often, there is a staffing committee that is part of unit-shared governance, which is a unit model where staff manage professional practice through unit committees. Increasing staff control over their schedule is a major factor in nurse job satisfaction and retention and has been associated with reductions in sick time usage. The nurse manager retains an important role in self-scheduling through mentoring, providing open communication, and holding everyone to equal expectations.

BOUNDARIES OF SELF-SCHEDULING   To implement self-scheduling, responsibilities and boundaries need to be established that clearly state expectations of staff. This is best done by a unit committee, made up of staff, that reports to the nurse manager. It is important to spell out the roles and responsibilities of all—the unit-based committee, the chairperson (if there is one), the staff, and the manager. Generic boundaries need to be established regarding fairness, fiscal responsibility, evaluation of the self-scheduling process, and the approval process. Table 15-1 spells out specific issues that must be addressed. During the self-scheduling process, the unit staff should be included and educated about the guidelines as they are being developed. For this process to be successful, all staff members must under-

stand the process, their responsibilities, and the effect of their decisions on staffing. All personnel must also be committed to providing safe staffing on all shifts for their patients.

EVALUATION OF STAFFING EFFECTIVENESS

Many patient outcomes are driven by the available hours of care delivered and the competence of staff delivering the care. The nurse manager and the organizational nurse leader have the ongoing responsibility to monitor the effectiveness of the staffing plan. To ensure objectivity, staffing outcomes must be delineated, measured, and reviewed.

PATIENT OUTCOMES AND NURSE STAFFING

The American Nurses Association (ANA) (Lichtig, Knaug, Rison-McCoy, & Wozniak, 2000) commissioned two studies to determine whether there was a relationship between nurse staffing and patient outcomes. The results of these studies did confirm there is a relationship. Specifically, one study found five patient outcomes showing a consistent significant relationship with nurse staffing. The outcomes found to be affected by nurse staffing are length of stay and incidence of pneumonia, postoperative infections, pressure ulcers, and urinary tract infections. These outcomes are negatively affected when nurse staffing or the skill mix is inadequate. Tracking these outcomes over time will give you data to judge whether your staffing pattern is adequate or inadequate.

Other professional organizations are weighing in on staffing and patient outcomes. For example, the American Association of Critical Care Nurses (AACN) considers appropriate staffing to be one of six key measures of

TABLE 15-1	ISSUES TO BE SPELLED OUT IN SELF-SCHEDULING GUIDELINES

- *Scheduling period:* Is the scheduling period two-, four-, or six-week intervals?
- *Schedule time line:* What are the time frames for staff to sign up for regular work commitment, special requests, overtime, and per diem workers?
- *Staffing pattern:* Will eight- or twelve-hour shifts be used? a combination?
- *Weekends:* Are staff expected to work every other weekend? If there are extra weekends available, how are they distributed?
- *Holidays:* How are they allocated?
- *Vacation time:* Are there restrictions on the amount of vacation during certain periods?
- *Unit vacation practices:* How many staff from one shift can be on vacation at any time?
- *Requests for time off:* What is the process for requesting time off?
- *Short-staffed shifts:* How are shifts that are short staffed handled?
- *On call, if applicable:* How do staff get assigned or sign up for on-call time?
- *Cancellation guidelines:* How and when do staff get canceled for scheduled time if they are not needed?
- *Sick calls:* What are the expectations for calling in sick, and how are these shifts covered?
- *Military/National Guard leave:* What kind of advance notice is required?
- *Schedule changes:* What is the process for changing one's schedule after the schedule has been approved?
- *Shifts defined:* What are the beginnings and endings of available shifts?
- *Committee time:* When does the self-scheduling committee meet and for how long?
- *Seniority:* How does it play into staffing and request decisions?
- *Staffing plan for crisis/emergency situations:* What is the plan when staffing is inadequate?

sustaining healthy work environments for nurses (AACN, 2005), and the Emergency Nurses Association (ENA) has issued guidelines for determining appropriate ED nurse staffing (Ray et al., 2003).

NURSE STAFFING AND NURSE OUTCOMES

In the previous section, we reviewed outcome measures for patients directly affected by staffing. In addition to patient outcomes, nurse outcomes should also be measured. Staff's perception of the adequacy of staffing should be tracked. Kramer and Schmalenberg (2005) recommend an instrument to measure Perception of Adequacy of Staffing (PAS) as a proxy measure of acceptable staffing levels. Nurse perception of staffing effectiveness must be monitored by hospitals seeking magnet status. Initiating such measures might lead to comparisons for benchmarking

best practice in the future and linking RN staffing perception to patient outcomes (Shirey & Fisher, in press).

There should be the ability for staff to communicate both in written and verbal form regarding staffing concerns. Nurses have the obligation to report to their supervisor their concerns regarding staffing, and every manager has the responsibility to follow up on staffing issues identified by staff. Formalizing this communication process says that you take the issues seriously and gives you data on which to act. In addition, actual staffing compared to recommended staffing should be tracked. This will identify changes in patient acuity and give you clues to other staffing issues. Medication errors is another measure that has been linked with inadequate NHPPD. When resources are scarce, data are imperative to drive needed changes. The outcomes of ineffective staffing patterns and nursing care can be devastating to both patients and staff.

REAL WORLD INTERVIEW

We have developed a nursing practice quality scorecard. The scorecard is a tool to display data on our three organizational priorities: mission, customer orientation, and cost-effectiveness. By looking at measures in all three arenas, we can see how we are doing in these areas. We also can see if changes made in one arena positively or negatively affect the other measures. To look at nursing's mission for nursing practice, we track and trend several of the American Nurses Association national indicators. We track medication errors, patient falls, restraints, nosocomial pressure ulcers, and urinary tract infections. For customer satisfaction, we measure overall satisfaction with nursing care provided and how well patients' pain was controlled. For cost-effectiveness, we track nursing hours per patient day. All of these measures are tracked and trended on control charts every three months. The specific data is trended, and measures that are greater than two standard deviations from the target are identified as potential points to be reviewed for identification of opportunities for improvement.

One of the areas we chose to target for improvement was medication errors. It became evident that the most prominent reason for medication errors was delayed and omitted medications. Further investigation proved that the procedures for obtaining medications were unclear and outdated. We have written new procedures to specify responsibilities of the nursing staff and the pharmacy staff. We are now monitoring our rate of medication errors to see if our changes have made any improvement in the error rate.

Another example of use of the scorecard was in review of our pressure ulcer rate. We found there was an increase in the incidence of pressure ulcers.

In review of causes, we found that the reporting system had been revised to include all stages of skin breakdown. Since the reporting change, we have seen an increase in the number of pressure ulcers reported. This is a positive change as we now have accurate data on which to target our improvement efforts.

Lessons that we have learned in the development of the scorecard is that we needed to set improvement targets earlier in the process to push the search for opportunities for improvement. We also learned that many of these measures are not well defined and therefore benchmarking to other organizations is difficult. We continue to strive for further improvement and utilize the scorecard to measure our success and look for opportunities for improvement. Reviewing nursing outcome data for the entire nursing division has been a powerful tool to ensure that care provided is meeting expected outcomes, and it allows us to benchmark our outcomes to other organizations.

Louann Villani, RN, BSN
Nursing Quality Specialist
Albany, New York

MODELS OF CARE DELIVERY

To ensure that nursing care is provided to patients, the work must be organized. A care delivery model organizes the work of caring for patients. Over the history of nursing, there have been many models of care delivery. The decision of which care delivery model is used is based on the needs of the patients and the availability of competent staff in the different skill levels. The model of care delivery utilized is often determined by the nurse leader and applied across an organization. Managers have the responsibility to implement models and evaluate the outcomes in their area. Staff have the responsibility to engage in the implementation and evaluation process. Each model has strengths and weaknesses that should be considered when deciding which to implement. Several different care delivery models are explored in the following sections.

CASE METHOD

The case method is the oldest model for nursing care delivery. As nurse training programs began to turn out educated nurses, these nurse were found working in the homes of the sick, taking care of one individual patient. In this model of care, the nurse cares for one patient exclusively. Total patient care is the modern-day version of the case method.

CRITICAL THINKING 15-1

Recently, you have been able to access data on your unit's pressure ulcer rates. In researching further, you uncover that your unit's rates are significantly higher than those of other units. Your staffing has been stable and in accordance with your staffing plan. Your staff are experienced, and in fact, you have the longest tenured staff in the hospital.

What are possible explanations for why your pressure ulcer rates are higher than other units? What would you do?

TOTAL PATIENT CARE

In **total patient care**, the nurse is responsible for the total care for assigned patients for the shift worked. The RN has several patients for whom she is responsible. The nurse may have some support from LPNs or UAP, but they are not assigned to a specific group of patients.

ADVANTAGES AND DISADVANTAGES

The advantage of total patient care and the case method for the patient is the consistency of one individual caring for patients for an entire shift. This enables the patient, nurse, and family to develop a relationship based on trust. This model provides a higher number of RN hours of care than other models. The nurse has more opportunity to observe and monitor progress of the patient. A disadvantage is that these models utilize a high level of RN hours to deliver care and are more costly than other models of delivery. This model works well in a specialized unit, such as hospice, where patient/family needs are unstable and require frequent RN assessment and intervention.

FUNCTIONAL NURSING

This model of care delivery became popular during World War II when there was a significant shortage of nurses in the United States. This method allowed LPNs and UAP to take on tasks that were previously carried out by the RN in the case method. **Functional nursing** divides the nursing work into functional roles that are then assigned to one of the team members. In this model, each care provider has specific duties or tasks for which they are responsible. For instance, a typical division of labor for RNs is medication nurse, admission/assessment nurse, and so on. Decision making is usually at the level of the charge nurse (Figure 15-9).

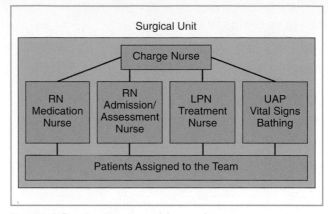

Figure 15-9 Functional nursing model.

ADVANTAGES AND DISADVANTAGES

In this model, care can be delivered to a large number of patients. This system utilizes other types of health care workers when there is a shortage of RNs. Patients are likely to have care delivered to them in one shift by several staff members. To a patient, care may feel disjointed. A risk of this model is that patients become the sum of the tasks of care they require rather than an integrated whole. Technical rather than professional nursing care often results from a functional model of care, and communication blocks across functional roles can put the patient at peril.

TEAM NURSING

During World War II, multilevel training programs were developed to teach auxiliary personnel how to perform simple care and technical procedures. In the military, these trained workers were called corpsmen. Outside of the military, there were one-year programs developed to teach technical nursing care. On-the-job training programs were established to produce what would today be called nursing assistants. The model of team nursing was developed after the war in an effort to utilize these trained workers and to ease the shortage of nurses that most hospitals were experiencing.

Team nursing is a care delivery model that assigns staff to teams that then are responsible for a group of patients. A unit may be divided into two or more teams, and each team is led by an RN. The team leader supervises and coordinates all the care provided by those on the team. The team is most commonly made up of LPNs and UAP. The team leader is responsible for safely delegating specific duties to the team. The larger the team, the more the RN is stretched to safely monitor and care for the patients (Figure 15-10).

A **modular nursing** delivery system is a kind of team nursing that divides a geographic space into modules of patients, with each module cared for by a team of staff led by an RN. The modules may vary in size, but center in a

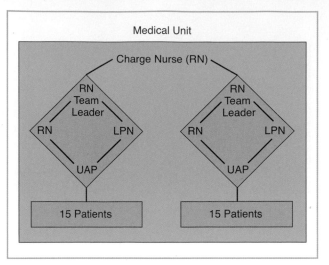

Figure 15-10 Team nursing model.

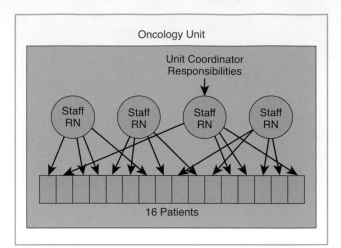

Figure 15-11 Primary nursing model.

geographical location and may be associated with a decentralized nursing station.

ADVANTAGES AND DISADVANTAGES

In team nursing and modular nursing, the RN is able to get work done through others, but patients often receive fragmented, depersonalized care. Communication in these models is complex. The shared responsibility and accountability can cause confusion and lack of accountability. These factors contribute to RN dissatisfaction with these models. These models require the RN to have very good delegation and supervision skills.

PRIMARY NURSING

Primary nursing is a care delivery model that clearly delineates the responsibility and accountability of the RN and designates the RN as the primary provider of care to patients. The primary nurse retains 24-hour accountability for care coordination for a set of patients throughout the patients' hospital stay. Patients are assigned a primary nurse, who is responsible for developing with the patient a plan of care that is followed by other nurses caring for the patient. Nurses and patients are matched according to needs and abilities. Patients are assigned to their primary nurse regardless of unit geographic considerations. Daily care is provided by associate nurses who enact the plan of care in collaboration with the primary nurse when the primary nurse is not working (Figure 15-11).

ADVANTAGES AND DISADVANTAGES

An advantage of this model is that patients and families are able to develop a trusting relationship with the nurse. There is defined accountability and responsibility for the nurse to develop a plan of care with the patient and family. A holistic approach to care facilitates continuity of care rather than a shift-to-shift focus. Nurses, when they have adequate time to provide necessary care, find this model professionally rewarding because it gives the authority for decision making to the nurse at the bedside. Disadvantages include a high cost because there is a higher RN skill mix. The person making out the assignments needs to be knowledgeable about all the patients and the staff to ensure appropriate matching of nurse to patient. With no geographical boundaries within the unit, nursing staff may be required to travel long distances at the unit level to care for their primary patients. Nurses often perform functions that could be completed by other staff. And finally, nurse-to-patient ratios must be realistic to ensure that enough nursing time is available to meet the patient care needs.

PATIENT-CENTERED CARE OR PATIENT-FOCUSED CARE

Patient-centered care or **patient-focused care** is designed to focus on patient needs rather than staff needs. In this model, required care and services are brought to the patient. In the highest evolution of this model, all patient services are decentralized to the patient area, including radiology and pharmacy services. Staffing is based on patient needs. In this model, there is an effort to have the right person doing the right thing. Care teams are established for a group of patients. The care teams may include other disciplines such as respiratory or physical therapists. In these teams, disciplines collaborate to ensure that patients receive the care they need. Staff are kept close to the patients in decentralized work stations. For example, on a rehabilitation unit, physical therapists may be members of the care team and work at the unit level rather than in a centralized physical therapy department (Figure 15-12).

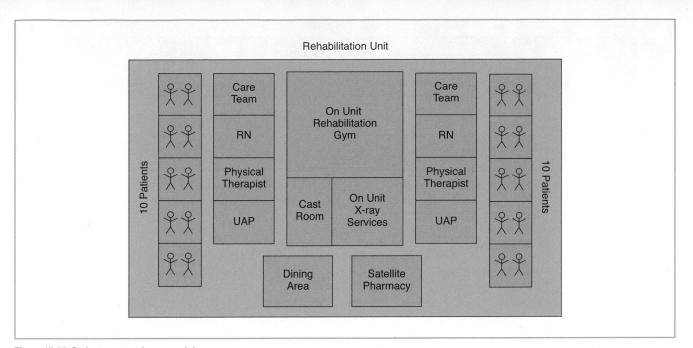

Figure 15-12 Patient-centered care model.

EVIDENCE FROM THE LITERATURE

Citation: Aiken, L. H., Clarke, S. P., Cheung, R. B., Sloane, D. M., & Silber, J. H. (2003). Education levels of hospital nurses and surgical patient mortality. *Journal of the American Medical Association, 290*(12), 1617–1623.

Discussion: This study looked at whether the proportion of RNs with a baccalaureate or higher level of nursing education is associated with risk-adjusted mortality and failure to rescue of surgical patients in Pennsylvania. "Nurses constitute the surveillance system for early detection of complications and problems in care, and they are in the best position to initiate actions that minimize negative outcomes for patients" (p. 1617). It stands to reason that the level of education of an RN might impact the nurse's clinical judgement and ability to serve as a detector and minimizer of complications, although impact on patient outcomes has not been studied before.

Outcomes data from hospital discharges of 168 adult acute-care hospitals were compared to American Hospital Association (AHA) administrative data on the hospitals and a survey of Pennsylvania nurses. There was a statistically significant relationship to the proportion of RNs with baccalaureate or higher level of nursing education and patient mortality and failure to rescue. Each 10% increase in the RN BSN or higher proportion resulted in a 5% reduction of mortality and failure to rescue, after adjusting for both patient and hospital characteristics. Nurses' years of experience were not found to be a significant factor in the statistical models developed by the team.

Implications for Practice: The conventional idea that nursing experience is more important than the underlying educational preparation for the RN role is refuted by this study. These findings are additive to our knowledge that nurse-to-patient staffing ratios for medical-surgical nursing of more than 1:4 are associated with increased mortality and failure to rescue. Although further studies are needed to control for additional variables, this study strongly supports the need for leaders to encourage RNs to advance their education for the sake of patients and to set goals that increase the proportion of their nurses who hold a BSN or higher level degree.

REAL WORLD INTERVIEW

We consider several key elements when we make staffing decisions. First, we have developed an activity ratio which monitors the RN-sensitive tasks associated with patient movement. The formula is the number of admissions, discharges, and transfers divided by the midnight census for each unit.

Next, we look at trends in average length of stay (ALOS). For example, in one of our surgical units, we tracked a change in ALOS from seven days down to four days. This type of change dramatically impacts RN work by compressing the care into fewer days. This may necessitate a change in delivery model so the nurse can maintain appropriate surveillance of patients. Failure to rescue patients is directly related to the nurse's ability to monitor the patient closely.

The third element in staffing decisions is the level of care needed by patients. We base the intensity of care needed on frequency of patient assessments needed. If there is a significant change in the level of care, then we may need to change the RN mix or the staffing numbers. If we can keep units pure as to the level of care, then we will not be as likely to overstaff them. This is important for productivity and to assure that all of our patients receive the correct level of care. For that reason, it is important to place patients who need observation, who are postprocedure, or who are postcatheterization in one area because their numbers on an inpatient unit really impact the level of care needs.

Since adopting this model of evidence-based staffing, I believe we have achieved a more rational and appropriate staffing level that assures optimal outcomes for our patients and supports our nurses' practice.

Janet M. Bingle, MS, RN
Chief Nursing Officer, Community Health Network
Indianapolis, Indiana

ADVANTAGES AND DISADVANTAGES

The pros of the system are that it is most convenient for patients and expedites services to patients. But it can be extremely costly to decentralize major services in an organization. A second disadvantage is that some staff have perceived the model as a way of reducing RNs and cutting costs in hospitals. In fact, this has been true in some organizations, but many other organizations have successfully used the patient-centered model to have the right staff available for the needs of the patient population.

PATIENT CARE REDESIGN

In the 1990s, there was significant pressure to reduce health care costs. Hospitals bore the brunt of this pressure. During this decade, patient care redesign was an initiative to redesign how patient care was delivered. The industry learned a lot about how care is delivered as it struggled with the redesign process. In addition to cost reduction, the redesign movement goals included making care more patient centered and not caregiver centered. This was accomplished by reducing the number of caregivers with which each patient had to interface and by organizing care around the patients, thus encouraging greater patient satisfaction. The concept is one of having caregivers cross-trained so they can intervene in more

patient situations without having additional resources from outside the care team to assist. Examples include having the team members, for example, RNs and cross-trained care technicians, draw lab specimens instead of having a phlebotomy team come to the unit, or team members doing their patients' breathing treatments instead of calling respiratory therapy to come to the unit. Team control of these functions allowed the functions to occur when patients needed them and not at the convenience of outside departments. Work flow analysis is a tool used to determine what activities are value-added and how to streamline or eliminate those that do not contribute to improved patient outcomes (Capuano, Bokovoy, Halkins, & Hitchings, 2004). Value-added refers to activities that possess the following characteristics:

- The customer is willing to pay for this activity.
- The activity must be done right the first time.
- The activity must somehow change the product or service in some desirable manner (Six Sigma, 2006).

Many of these value-added changes in care attributed to the patient care redesign movement of the 1990s continue to this day as good practices within patient-centered care. Other aspects of redesign have not survived. Those redesign projects that failed to assist caregivers to change their roles or failed to consider unit culture in the patient care redesign were frequently not successful.

CARE DELIVERY MANAGEMENT TOOLS

In 1983, the federal government established diagnostic-related groups (DRGs) as a payment system for hospitals. In DRGs, the national average length of stay (LOS) for a specific patient type is used to determine payment for that grouping of medicare patients. **Length of stay (LOS)** refers to the average number of days a patient is hospitalized from day of admission to day of discharge. In DRGs, hospitals are paid the same amount for caring for a DRG patient group regardless of the actual LOS of the specific patient. This prompted initiatives in hospitals to reduce LOS and reduce hospital costs. There

are further adjustments to costs based on patient co-morbidities, that is, additional conditions that add to the complexity of care needed by a patient with heart disease, for example, diabetes or hypertension. Hospitals were able to benchmark their LOS for specific patient populations against a national database published through the Medicare DRG system. As hospitals looked for opportunities to reduce costs through reduction in the LOS, clinical pathways and case management surfaced as significant strategies.

CLINICAL PATHWAYS

Clinical pathways were a major initiative to come out of the efforts to reduce LOS and are widely used to enhance outcomes and contain costs. **Clinical pathways** are care-management tools that outline the expected clinical course and outcomes for a specific patient type. Clinical pathways should be evidence-based, reflecting the best

REAL WORLD INTERVIEW

In my role as a case manager, I work exclusively with the pediatric population at our hospital. I facilitate the care of patients while they are in the hospital and plan for their home care needs. Our main goal is to ensure that there is a safe transition between hospital and home. As an example of how this goal is achieved, we have met with the cardiac surgery patients and families prior to surgery to identify and proactively address insurance, equipment, or other issues that may arise during hospitalization and at discharge. We have found that patients, families, and staff find our function very helpful. For the staff RN, case managers take on the burden of complex discharge planning, which is enormously time consuming. Patients and families find it comforting to know there is someone who can help them plan for postdischarge.

As the pediatric case manager, I meet with the social worker and the RN staff on the pediatric unit weekly to go over each patient and their specific discharge and social work needs. We have found the work of the case managers and social workers to be complementary, and working together allows us to both have more information and help the patient get through our system more efficiently. All of these functions help to reduce the patient's length of stay.

As case managers, we also perform some utilization management functions for our organization. We review admission charts, assessing for evidence of meeting admission criteria that the patient's insurer will accept. In addition, we review charts daily to ensure that the patient's acuity warrants continued hospitalization. On occasion, we have to inform the patient and family that the patient's stay is no longer covered by their insurance and they will be responsible for paying the remaining portion of their hospital bill. This can be a difficult situation, and we sometimes get caught between the patient and the patient's insurer. In these cases, we sometimes refer the patients back to their insurer and sometimes we advocate for the patient to have their continued hospital stay approved.

As a case manager, I find that my diverse clinical background has enabled me to better anticipate the patient's clinical course and be proactive to support the patient's needs. This is a role that is supportive of patients, families, and staff and one I find very challenging and rewarding.

Linda Zeoli, RN
Pediatric Case Manager
Albany, New York

knowledge to date for patient care. Typically pathways outline the normal course of care for a patient and for each day, expected outcomes are articulated. Patient progress is measured against expected outcomes.

Any variance in outcome can then be noted and acted upon to get the patient back on track. In some facilities, pathways have practitioner orders incorporated into

the pathway to facilitate care. In some organizations, the pathways include multidisciplinary orders for care, including orders from nursing, medicine, and other allied health professionals such as physical therapy and dietary services. This serves to further expedite care for patients. Figure 15-13 provides an excerpt from a clinical pathway that identifies expected outcomes.

Clinical Pathway: Lower Extremity Revascularization
Page 21 of 22

ADDRESSOGRAPH

DAILY ANTICIPATED OUTCOMES

POD2	Date/Time /Init When met	POD3	Date/Time /Init When met	POD4	Date/Time /Init When met	POD5	Date/Time /Init When met
Patient rates pain 0-2 on pain scale 0-10 using po analgesia.		Graft signal present with doppler.		Graft signal present with doppler.		Graft signal present with doppler.	
Graft signal present with doppler.		Incisional edges will be approximated without drainage.		Able to participate in self-care and adjunct therapies.		Ambulates independently.	
Patient will verbalize knowledge of plan of care, testing, and treatment.		Site of invasive devices without signs of infection.		Patient viewed diet video.		Patient/significant other will verbalize understanding of activity/diet restrictions, medication use, wound management.	
Ambulate in hall QID.		Ambulates in hall QID.				Completed nutrition posttest.	
Tolerates po solids.		Patient/significant other will describe appropriate problem solving skills to decrease anxiety.					
Voiding without difficulty.		Rehab referral started: _yes _no					
		Family support available at discharge, specify _____					

TO BE KEPT IN PROGRESS NOTE SECTION OF CHART AT ALL TIMES.

Figure 15-13 Example of a clinical pathway (excerpt). (*Source:* Courtesy of Albany Medical Center, Albany, NY.)

ADVANTAGES AND DISADVANTAGES

By articulating the normal course of care for a patient population, clinical pathways are a powerful tool for managing care. They are very instructive for new staff, and they save a significant amount of time in the process of care. In most cases, the implementation of a clinical pathway will improve care, reduce variability and shorten the LOS for the patient population on the pathway. Pathways also allow for data collection of variances to the pathway. The data can then be used to continuously improve hospital systems and clinical practice.

Some practitioners perceive pathways to be cookbook medicine and are reluctant to participate in their development. Practitioner participation is critical. Development of multidisciplinary pathways also requires a significant amount of work to gain consensus from the various disciplines on the expected plan of care. For patient populations that are nonstandard, pathways are less effective because the pathway is constantly being modified to reflect the individual patient's needs.

CASE MANAGEMENT

Case management is a second strategy to improve patient care and reduce hospital costs through coordination of care. Typically, a case manager is responsible for coordinating care and establishing goals from preadmission through discharge. In the typical model of case management, a nurse is assigned to a specific high-risk patient population or service, such as cardiac surgery patients. The case manager has the responsibility to work with all disciplines to facilitate care. For example, if a postsurgical hospitalized patient has not met ambulation goals according to the clinical pathway, the case manager would work with the practitioner and nurse to determine what is preventing the patient from achieving this goal. If it turns out that the patient is elderly and is slow to recover, they may agree that physical therapy would be beneficial to assist this patient in ambulating. In other models, the case-management function is provided by the staff nurse at the bedside. This works well if the population requires little case management, but if the patient population requires significant case-management services, there needs to be enough RN time allocated for this activity. In addition to facilitating care, the case manager usually has a data function to monitor and improve care. In this role, the case manager collects aggregate data on patient variances from the clinical pathway. The data are shared with the responsible practitioners and other disciplines that participate in the clinical pathway and are then used to explore opportunities for improvement in the pathway or in hospital systems.

KEY CONCEPTS

- To plan nurse staffing, you must understand and apply the concepts of full-time equivalents (FTEs) and units of service such as nursing hours per patient day (NHPPD).

- Patient classification systems predict nursing time required for groups of patients; the data can then be utilized for staffing, budgeting, and benchmarking.

- Determination of the number of FTEs needed to staff a unit requires review of patient classification data, units of service, regulatory requirements, delivery systems, skill mix, staff support, historical information, and the physical environment of the unit.

- The number of staff and patients in your staffing plan drives the amount of nursing time available for patient care.

- In developing a staffing plan, additional FTEs must be added to a nursing unit budget to provide coverage for days off and benefited time off.

- Scheduling of staff is the responsibility of the nurse manager, who must take into consideration patient need and intensity, volume of patients, and the needs and experience of the staff.

- Whatever staffing plans are chosen, it is critical to assess the effect of staffing decisions on patient care and finances.

- Self-scheduling can increase staff morale and professional growth, but success requires clear boundaries and guidelines.

- Evaluating the outcomes of your staffing plan on patients, staff, and the organization is a critical activity that should be done daily, monthly, and annually.

- Case management and clinical pathways are care-management tools that have been developed to improve patient care and reduce hospital costs and should be evidence based.

KEY TERMS

average daily census (ADC)
benchmarking
case management
clinical pathways
continuity of care

diagnostic-related groups (DRGs)
episodic care unit
direct care
full-time equivalent (FTE)

functional nursing
handoffs
indirect care
inpatient unit
length of stay (LOS)
modular nursing
nonproductive hours
nurse intensity
nursing hours per patient day (NHPPD)
patient acuity
patient-centered care

patient classification system (PCS)
patient-focused care
patient turnover
primary nursing
productive hours
self-scheduling
skill mix
staffing plan
team nursing
total patient care
units of service

REVIEW QUESTIONS

1. Patient classification systems measure nursing workload needed to care for patients. The higher the patient's acuity, the more care that is required by the patient. Which of the following statements is a *weakness* of classification systems?
    A. Patient classification data are useful in predicting the required staffing for the next shift and for justifying nursing hours provided.
    B. Patient classification data can be utilized by the nurse making assignments to determine what level of care a patient requires.
    C. Classification systems typically focus on nursing tasks rather than a holistic view of a patient's needs.
    D. Aggregate patient classification data are useful in costing out nursing services and developing the nursing budget.

2. If your full-time staff members receive four weeks of vacation and 10 days of sick time per year, how many productive hours would each FTE work in that year if they utilized all of their benefited time?
    A. 2,080 productive hours
    B. 1,840 productive hours
    C. 1,920 productive hours
    D. 1,780 productive hours

3. Patient outcomes are the result of many variables, one being the model of care delivery that is utilized. From the following scenarios, select which is the *worst* fit between patient need and care delivery model.
    A. Cancer patients cared for in a primary nursing model
    B. Rehabilitation patients cared for in a patient-centered model
    C. Medical intensive care patients being cared for in a team nursing model
    D. Ambulatory surgery patients with a wide range of illnesses being cared for using a functional practice model

4. When calculating paid nonproductive time, the nurse manager considers
    A. overtime pay and evening and night shift differential.
    B. total hours available to work.

C. insurance benefits and educational hours.
D. all hours that are paid, but not worked on the assigned unit.

5. The most important variable that affects staffing patterns and schedules should be which of the following?
    A. Organizational philosophy
    B. Budget allocation and restrictions
    C. Delivering safe, quality patient care
    D. Personnel policies regarding shift rotation

6. The medical-surgical unit provides 200 hours of care daily to 20 patients. Their NHPPD is which of the following?
    A. 1
    B. 10
    C. 20
    D. 200

7. Benchmarking is which of the following?
    A. A comparison of productivity data for similar nursing units
    B. A method to measure cost of care
    C. A comprehensive measure of good quality
    D. A set of written standards of care

REVIEW ACTIVITIES

1. How do you know whether the outcomes of your staffing plan are positive? What measures do you have available in your organization that indicate your staffing is adequate or inadequate?

2. You are a nurse manager of a new unit for psychiatric patients. What would you consider in planning for FTEs and staffing for this unit?

3. You are a new nurse, and you have increasing concerns regarding the staffing levels on your unit. You are becoming increasingly anxious each time you go to work. What would you do?

EXPLORING THE WEB

■ To get more information on mandated staffing levels, go to *www.ana.org*. Go to Core Initiatives on the menu and click on Appropriate Staffing. Follow related links on staffing and patient outcomes.

■ To get more information on staffing effectiveness, go to *www.jointcommission.org*. Type *staffing effectiveness* into the search box, and read about staffing effectiveness standards issued by the JC.

■ To get more information on staffing and quality, go to *www.ahrq.gov*. This government site of the Agency for Healthcare Research and Quality provides evidence-based analysis of clinical issues. Look in the section for Quality and Patient Safety. You can also search using the term *safe staffing*.

REFERENCES

Adomat, R., & Hewison, A. (2004). Assessing patient category/dependence systems for determining the nurse/patient ratio in ICU and HDU: A review of approaches. *Journal of Nursing Management, 12*(5), 299–308.

Aiken, L. H., Clarke, S. P., Cheung, R. B., Sloane, D. M., & Silber, J. H. (2003). *Journal of the American Medical Association, 290*(12), 1617–1623.

American Association of Critical-Care Nurses. (2005). *AACN standards for establishing and sustaining healthy work environments.* Aliso Viego, CA: AACN.

Beglinger, J. E. (2006). Quantifying patient care intensity: An evidence-based approach to determining staffing requirements. *Nursing Administration Quarterly, 30*(3), 193–202.

Capuano, T., Bokovoy, J., Halkins, D., & Hitchings, K. (2004). Work flow analysis: Eliminating nonvalue-added work. *Journal of Nursing Administration, 34*(5), 246–256.

Currie, V., Harvey, G., West, B., McKenna, H., & Keeney, S. (2005). Relationship between quality of care, staff levels, skill mix and nurse autonomy: Literature review. *Journal of Adanced Nursing, 51*(1), 73–82.

Gran-Moravec, M. B., & Hughes, C. M. (2005). Nursing time allocation and other considerations for staffing. *Nursing & Health Science, 7*(2), 126–133.

Joint Commission. (2006). Staffing standards. Retrieved November 9, 2006, from http://www.jointcommission.org

Kramer, M., & Schmalenberg, C. (2005). Revising the essentials of magnetism tool: There is more to adequate staffing than numbers. *Journal of Nursing Administration, 35*(4), 188–198.

Lichtig, L. K., Knaug, R. A., Rison-McCoy, R., & Wozniak, L. M. (2000). *Nurse staffing and patient outcomes in the inpatient hospital setting.* Washington, DC: American Nurses Association.

Ray, C. E., Jagim, M., Agnew, J., Inglass-McKay, J., & Sheehy, S. (2003). ENA's new guidelines for determining emergency department nurse staffing. *Journal of Emergency Nursing, 29*(3), 245–253.

Shirey, M., & Fisher, M. L. (in press). Leadership agenda for change: Toward healthy work environments for the 21st century. *AACN Journal.*

Six Sigma. (2006). Value added. Retrieved December 1, 2006, from http://www.sixsigma.com/dictionary/value-added-134.htm

Unruh, L. Y., & Fottler, M. D. (2006). Patient turnover and nursing staff adequacy. *Health Services Research, 41*(20), 599–612.

White, K. M. (2006). Policy spotlight: Staffing plans and ratios. *Nursing Management, 37*(4), 18–24.

SUGGESTED READINGS

Anthony, M. K. (2004). Shared governance models: The theory, practice, and evidence. *Online Journal of Issues in Nursing, 9*(1), 13.

Frith, K., & Montgomery, M. (2006). Perceptions, knowledge, and commitment of clinical staff to shared governance. *Nursing Administration Quarterly, 30*(3), 273–284.

Harrison, J. (2004). Addressing increasing patient acuity and nursing workload. *Nursing Management (Harrow), 11*(4), 20–25.

Lang, T. A., Hodge, M., Olson, V., Romano, P. S., & Kravitz, R. L. (2004). Nurse-patient ratios: A systematic review on the effects of nurse staffing on patient, nurse employee, and hospital outcomes. *Journal of Nursing Administration, 34*(7–8), 326–337.

Mangold, K. L., Pearson, K. K., Schmitz, J. R., Loes, J. L., & Specht, J. P. (2006). Perceptions and characteristics of registered nurses' involvement in decision making. *Nursing Administration Quarterly, 30*(3), 266–272.

Rischbieth, A. (2006). Matching nurse skill with patient acuity in the intensive care units: A risk management mandate. *Journal of Nursing Management, 14*(5), 397–404.

Spence, K., Tarnow-Mordi, W., Duncan, G., Jayasuryia, N., Elliott, J., King, J., & Kite, F. (2006). Measuring nursing workload in neonatal intensive care. *Journal of Nursing Management, 14*(3), 227–234.

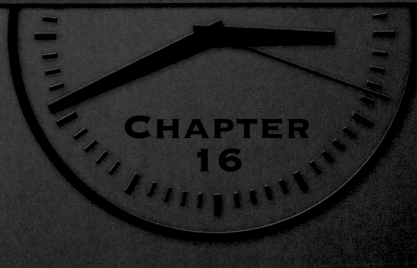

CHAPTER 16

Delegation of Patient Care

Maureen T. Marthaler, RN, MS ⊕ Patricia Kelly, RN, MSN

The authority was delegated to me to care for this patient and, by assuming this responsibility for the patient, I will then be accountable for this patient's care (Phyllis Franck and Marjorie Price, 1980).

OBJECTIVES

Upon completion of this chapter, the reader should be able to:

1. Identify delegation, accountability, responsibility, authority, assignment, and supervision.
2. Identify organizational responsibility for delegation and the chain of command.
3. Support the National Council of State Boards of Nursing Delegation Decision-Making Tree.
4. Identify responsibilities of the health care team in delegation.
5. Relate the five rights of delegation.
6. Identify potential delegation barriers.
7. Outline six cultural phenomena that affect transcultural delegation.
8. Categorize direct and indirect patient care.

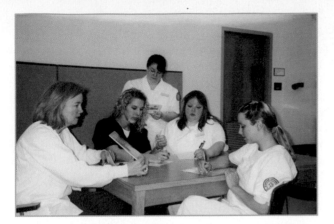

Delegation to the appropriate personnel is an important responsibility in nursing. Iuappropriate delegation can be life threatening as in the following instance.

A patient was admitted to 3C with the diagnosis of transient ischemic attack (TIA). She required neurological assessments to be performed at the onset of every shift and whenever necessary as indicated by a change in the patient's condition. The night nurse assessed the patient at the beginning of her shift, noting that the patient's neurologic status was fully intact. During the night, the nurse periodically checked on the patient every two hours but did not awaken the patient. A sitter was in the room with the patient. The sitter had assured the nurse that the patient was "doing fine." The sitter did not report that when the patient had been assisted to the bathroom initially, she had no difficulty. Upon assisting the patient a second time, the sitter noted that the patient was leaning to one side so badly that she could not stand and required help from two additional nursing assistive personnel. No one reported this to the nurse. When the nurse checked the patient at 6 A.M., she noted that the patient was not able to move her right side.

Should the nurse have checked the patient more carefully during the night?

What are the responsibilities of the nurse and the sitter?

How could delegation have been appropriately performed in this situation?

On the National Council of State Boards of Nursing Licensure Examination (NCLEX), a student may often encounter test questions that assess the ability of the nurse to delegate care. Safeguarding patients is a number one patient care priority. To ensure that this responsibility is met, nurses are accountable under the law for care rendered by both themselves and other personnel. Multiple levels of unlicensed assistive personnel (UAP) give care to patients. UAP include nurse aides, nurse technicians, patient care technicians, personal care attendants, unit assistants, nursing assistants, and other nonlicensed personnel. In support of the role of the UAP and the licensed practical nurse (LPN) in delivering patient care, the National Council of State Boards of Nursing (1995) states, "there is a need and a place for competent, appropriately supervised, unlicensed assistive personnel in the delivery of affordable, quality health care. However, it must be remembered that unlicensed assistive personnel are equipped to assist—not replace—the nurse" (p. 2). As the nursing shortage continues and health care facilities continue to seek more cost-effective ways to provide care, RNs must learn new ways to manage care and delegate and supervise tasks. As the use of UAPs and LPNs has increased in today's health care system, RNs have become increasingly responsible for delegation and supervision. It is imperative that RNs have confidence with delegation skills and understand the legal responsibility that they assume when delegating to and supervising licensed personnel and UAPs. RNs must know what aspects of nursing can be delegated and what level of supervision is required to ensure that the patient receives safe, high-quality care. RNs must always be able to ensure patient safety with delegated care.

With increased opportunities to delegate care, nurses will be able to meet the duty of safe, quality care to their patients only by delegating properly. Without delegation skills, nurses caring for patients in today's health care community will not be able to complete the necessary duties, tasks, and responsibilities. They will find themselves stressed and exhausted by the many activities their nursing role requires. An inability to delegate can engender feelings of frustration, poor self-esteem, and lack of control. As nurses develop appropriate delegation skills, they become more productive and enjoy their work more.

PERSPECTIVES ON DELEGATION

As the history of nursing shows, Florence Nightingale had foresight regarding how nurses would function. Nightingale is quoted as saying, "But again, to look at all these things does not mean to do them yourself. . . . But can you not ensure that it is done when not done by yourself" (Nightingale, 1859). Thus, delegation in nursing formally was recognized in the 1800s with Nightingale and has continued to evolve as health care delivery models have evolved.

Today, delegation is a must for the new nurse as well as the experienced nurse. Delegating to personnel with different educational levels from a variety of nursing programs requires nurses to be vigilant in ensuring that safety is maintained for the patient. Efficient delegation of care protects the patient and provides desirable outcomes. The RN coordinates all nursing care, including the care ordered by all nursing and medical practitioners. The RN delegates nursing care and supervises the care of the LPN, Licensed Vocational Nurse (LVN), and UAP based on the RN's evaluation of the patient's condition; the level of the skill and knowledge that the LPN and UAP have; the state legal scope of practice of the RN, LPN, and UAP; and the nature of the task being delegated to the LPN or UAP.

DELEGATION DEFINED

Different organizations and experts define delegation in different ways. The American Association of Critical-Care Nurses (AACN) states that delegation is not a skill that is simply learned in a classroom. It requires a discussion of concerns related to delegation, and then clinical assistance or mentorship in delegation responsibilities. The process also includes discussion of how to handle situations where tasks were not accomplished when delegated. The National Council of State Boards in Nursing (NCSBN) defines **delegation** as transferring to a competent individual the authority to perform a selected nursing task in a selected situation. The nurse retains accountability for the delegation (NCSBN, 1995).

Delegation, as defined by the American Nurses Association (ANA, 1996), is the "transfer of responsibility for the performance of an activity from one individual to another while retaining accountability for the outcome" (p. 4). RNs can transfer the responsibility and authority for the performance of an activity, but they remain accountable for overall nursing care. Timm (2003) states that delegation is a legal and management concept and a process that involves assessment, planning, intervention, and evaluation in which selected nursing tasks are transferred from one person in authority to another person, involving trust, empowerment, and the responsibility and authority to perform the task. In delegation, communication is succinct, guidelines are clearly delineated in advance, and progress is constantly monitored in which the person in authority remains accountable for the final outcomes. The ANA's position statement, *Registered Nurse Utilization of Unlicensed Assistive Personnel* (1996), states that as an accepted standard of care, the RN should use professional judgment to determine activities that are appropriate to delegate based on the concept of providing safe and effective patient care and protecting the patient. In delegation, the RN will consider the assessment of the patient condition; capabilities of the nursing and assistive staff; complexity of the task to be delegated; amount of clinical oversight (supervision) the RN will be able to provide; and staff workload. The RN cannot delegate activities that include the core of the nursing process and that require specialized knowledge, judgment, or skill.

The ANA (1996) has also delineated direct or indirect patient care activities that can be delegated by the nurse. Direct-care activities assist the patient to meet basic human needs and include activities related to feeding, drinking, positioning, ambulating, grooming, toileting, dressing, and socializing. They may involve the collecting, reporting, and documenting of data related to these activities. The patient-related data are reported to the RN, who uses the information to make clinical judgments about patient care. Indirect-care activities that may be delegated by the RN focus on maintaining a clean, safe, efficient environment in which to practice nursing. Indirect-care activities, which only incidentally involve patient contact, include activities involved in housekeeping, transporting, record keeping, stocking, and maintaining supplies. Activities that the nurse may not delegate include the initial nursing assessment and any subsequent assessment that requires professional nursing knowledge, judgment, and skill; determination of nursing diagnoses, establishment of nursing care goals, development of the nursing plan of care, evaluation of the patient's progress with the nursing plan of care; and any nursing intervention that requires professional knowledge, judgment, and skill (ANA, 1996).

Delegation is a communication process in which the RN requests that a qualified staff member, such as the LPN or UAP, perform a specific task. When a task is delegated to the UAP or LPN, the RN shares with them the ultimate responsibility and authority for the accomplishment and outcome of the task. However, the RN remains accountable for the nursing care outcomes. When delegating, the RN is accountable for the act of delegation; supervising the performance of the delegated task; assessment and follow-up evaluation; and any intervention or corrective actions that may be required to ensure safe, high-quality care. The LPN and UAP are accountable for their actions, accepting delegation within the parameters of their education and experience, communicating the appropriate information to the delegate, and completing the task. Effective delegation contributes to the accomplishment of cost-effective, high-quality care.

All delegation involves at least two individuals as well as specifying duties to be accomplished with or through others via a transfer of authority. The authority has to be delegated along with the ability to direct others. To be effective in accomplishing goals, the individual delegating must take on the leadership role. With successful delegation, the patient's personal health needs are addressed, and the nurse's professional goals are achieved. Communication techniques facilitate the delegation process for the RN.

It is frustrating for RNs to have to accomplish all of their duties single-handedly. Many new graduate nurses become overwhelmed by the large number of duties to be learned and implemented. In nursing school, students typically perform total patient care for one or two patients. Students might occasionally ask another student to help them, or perhaps they might pitch in to help others on their unit. Rarely will they have the opportunity to delegate to another nurse or UAP. So it can be a shock to new nurses that delegation is now an expected part of their behavior. It is required in the health care setting, and the NCLEX also tests them on it.

Delegation is not meant to intimidate or isolate the new nurse. The sole purpose of delegation is to get the job done in the most efficient way utilizing appropriate resources. The job must be delegated to personnel who can handle it and who understand the goal. Delegation can be done to spark interest and prevent personnel from becoming bored, nonproductive, and ineffective. Finding the duties or tasks that best suit the personnel can help them feel as if they are part of the team, regardless of their position. Personnel want to feel they are making a difference in the well-being of the patient, whether through a bath, medications, or even a simple smile. To delegate, the nurse takes into account the personnel's personal and professional position within the health care team, including ability, education, and experience as well as the patient's needs. Infection control and patient safety are high priorities in making assignments. The NCSBN developed a Delegation Decision-making Grid that is available at its Website. A Decision Tree is illustrated later in this chapter.

ACCOUNTABILITY AND RESPONSIBILITY

Nurses are legally liable for their actions and are accountable for the overall nursing care of their patients. **Accountability** is being responsible and answerable for actions or inactions of self or others in the context of delegation (NCSBN, 1995). There are different levels of accountability.

Licensed nurse accountability involves compliance with legal requirements as set forth in the jurisdiction's laws and rules governing nursing. The licensed nurse is also accountable for the quality of the nursing care provided; for recognizing limits, knowledge, and experience; and for planning for situations beyond the nurse's expertise (NCSBN, 2004). Licensed nurse accountability includes the preparedness and obligation to explain or justify to relevant others (including the regulatory authority) the relevant judgments, intentions, decisions, actions, and omissions . . . and the consequences of those decisions, actions, and behaviors. Nurses are accountable for following their state nurse practice act, standards of professional practice, the policies of their health care organization, and ethical-legal models of behavior. RNs are accountable for monitoring changes in a

patient's status, noting and implementing treatment for human responses to illness, and assisting in the prevention of complications.

The RN assesses the patient; makes a nursing diagnosis; and develops, implements, and evaluates the patient's plan of care. The RN uses nursing judgment and monitors unstable patients with unpredictable outcomes. The monitoring of other more stable patients cared for by the LPN and UAP may involve the RN's direct continuing presence, or the monitoring may be more intermittent. As stated by the AACN in 2004, the delegation of direct and indirect patient care to other caregivers is reasonable, relevant, and practical. Nursing tasks that do not involve direct patient care can be reassigned more freely and carry fewer legal implications for RNs than delegation of direct nursing practice activities. The assessment, analysis, diagnosis, planning, teaching, and evaluation stages of the nursing process may not be delegated to UAP. Delegated activities usually fall within the implementation phase of the nursing process.

Responsibility involves reliability, dependability, and the obligation to accomplish work when an assignment is accepted. Responsibility also includes each person's obligation to perform at an acceptable level—the level to which the person has been educated. For example, a nurse aide is expected to provide the patient with a bed bath. She does not administer pain medication or perform invasive or sterile procedures. After the nurse aide performs the assigned duties, she provides feedback to the nurse about the performance of the duties and the outcome of her actions. This feedback is given to the nurse within a specified time frame. Note that feedback works two ways. It is also the RN's responsibility to follow up with ongoing supervision and evaluation of activities performed by nonnursing personnel. The nurse transfers

CRITICAL THINKING 16-1

A major responsibility of nurses is to keep patients safe. This responsibility is tested on the NCLEX-RN. This responsibility means not only keeping side rails up on patients who are at risk for falls but also means such things as monitoring patients' vital signs and level of consciousness. Maintaining safety also includes implementing safety devices such as a "keep open" IV line on patients who are at risk for poor outcomes. How have you seen nurses monitor patients? Have you noted any strategies nurses use to prevent negative nurse-sensitive patient outcomes?

CRITICAL THINKING 16-2

Note this assignment sheet excerpt. Which patients are complex and unstable and need RN monitoring constantly? Which patients are stable and can be delegated?

Room	Patient	Staff	Assignment
211	Mr. W.	RN	Trach care 8 A.M. and prn (Patient with new trach)
213	Mrs. R.	LPN	Colostomy care 8 A.M. and prn (Patient with old colostomy)
215	Mr. L.	UAP	Ambulate at 8 A.M. and 12 noon (Patient is postop day 3 and has been walking)

*All patients—complete bath with A.M. care.
Report problems to RN stat.
Report patient status to RN at 2 P.M.

responsibility and authority for the completion of a delegated task, but the nurse retains accountability for the delegation process. Whenever nursing activities are delegated, the RN is to follow federal regulations, state nursing practice acts, state boards of nursing rules and regulations, and the standards of the hospital.

AUTHORITY

The right to delegate duties and give direction to unlicenced assistive personnel (UAP) places the RN in a position of authority. Authority identifies the source of the power to act (NCSBN, 1995). **Authority** occurs when a person who has been given the right to delegate, based on the state nurse practice act, also has the official power from an agency to delegate. Authority comes with the job as authority given by an agency legitimizes the right of a nurse to give direction to others and expect that they will comply. An understanding of the level of authority at the time the task is delegated and the level of authority that is identified by the state nurse practice act and the agency's job description prevents each party from making inaccurate assumptions about authority for delegated assignments (Kelly-Heidenthal & Marthaler, 2005).

ASSIGNMENT

An assignment is the distribution of work that each staff member is to accomplish on a given shift or work period. The RN retains accountability for the assignment. It is

necessary to ensure that the education, skill, knowledge, and judgment levels of the personnel being assigned to a task are commensurate with the assignment. For example, administration of intravenous solutions to patients on a nursing unit would initially best be assigned to an RN who has received education about intravenous solutions and who has been performing these duties on a regular basis rather than to someone who has little or no experience in administering intravenous solutions. When an assignment is made, the RN should specify the expected outcome of the assignment, the time frame for completion, and any limitations on the assignment.

ASSIGNMENT VERSUS DELEGATION

Note that there is a significant difference between assigning care to another RN and delegating to an LPN/LVN or UAP. Assignment is the process of designating nursing activities to be performed by an individual consistent with the person's licensed scope of practice (NCSBN, 1995). Assignment is defined by the ANA as "the downward or lateral transfer of both the responsibility and accountability of an activity from one individual to another" (1996, p. 4). An assignment designates those activities that a staff member is responsible for performing as a condition of employment and is consistent with the staff member's job position and description, legal scope of practice, and education and experience. Scope of practice refers to the parameters of the authority to practice granted to a nurse through licensure (NCSBN,

2004). Experienced RNs are expected to work with minimal supervision of their nursing practice. The RN who assigns care to another competent RN who then assumes responsibility and accountability for that patient's care, does not have the same obligation to closely supervise that person's work as when the care is delegated to an LPN/LVN or UAP. The RN can delegate responsibility to the LPN/LVN or UAP, but the RN retains accountability for the patient's care. LPN/LVNs and UAPs work under the direction of the RN, although they must complete their assignments.

It may be useful to assign UAP to work with the RN. Typical assignments for UAP include passing trays, assisting with transfers, transporting patients, and stocking supplies. The LPN may be assigned specific patients for whom to perform care, but the RN remains responsible for all nursing care. When the RN assigns care to the LPN or the UAP, the RN must consider the patient ABCs, safety and infection control needs, and the degree of supervision required. For example, in considering patient ABCs, the RN would assess the patient's level of consciousness, vital signs, physical status, changing needs, complexity, stability, multisystem involvement, and technology requirements such as the need for cardiac monitoring and so on. The RN would also consider patient teaching needs and emotional support needs.

In considering patient safety and infection control needs, the RN would assess patient isolation needs and cross-contamination protections and try to avoid assigning infected patients and immuno-suppressed patients to the same caregiver.

In considering the degree of supervision involved, the RN considers the level of supervision, direct or indirect, required based on the staff member's education, experience, skill level, and competence. It is useful to also use assignments to develop staff. Assigning a less experienced nurse to a more complex patient, but at the same time increasing the level of supervision, increases the less experienced nurse's skill level, competence, and confidence while maintaining safe, high-quality patient care.

Assigning full care responsibility and accountability to a new graduate or to a nurse working in an unfamiliar specialty may be unsafe at times. In these instances, the supervising nurse may have a greater responsibility and accountability to evaluate the abilities and performance of the new nurse.

Certain actions may be delegated to an LPN/LVN in keeping with the scope of practice as designated by state regulation. If the LPN is certified in IV therapy, and the policy of the state and the employing institution permits LPNs/LVNs to provide IV treatment, the RN should not have an inordinate duty to supervise the work of the LPN after the LPNs skills in this are verified. Note that prior competency certification of the LPN may have been done through a skills day or through a competency validation that ensures that the LPN has been observed inserting a nasogastric tube or an IV line successfully three times under direct supervision of an RN in states where this practice by an LPN is allowed. The RN cannot assign responsibility and accountability for total nursing care to UAP or LPNs, but the RN can delegate certain tasks to them in keeping with the state law, the job description, their knowledge base, and the demonstrated competency of these individuals. The RN is then responsible for adequate supervision of the person to whom the task is given.

COMPETENCE

Competence is the ability of the nurse to apply knowledge and interpersonal decision making, and psychomotor skills expected for the practice role of a licensed nurse in the context of public health safety and welfare (NCSBN, 1995). Competence is required to practice safely and ethically in a designated role and setting. Licensed nurse competence is built upon the knowledge gained in a nursing education program, orientation to specific settings, and the experiences of implementing nursing care. Nurses must know themselves first, including strengths and challenges; assess the match of their knowledge and experience with the requirements and context of a role; gain additional knowledge as needed; and maintain all skills and abilities needed to provide safe nursing care.

UAP competence is built upon formal training and assessment, orientation to specific settings and groups of patients, interpersonal and communication skills, and the experience of the nurse aide in assisting the nurse to provide safe nursing care.

Health care organizations require employees to demonstrate that they are competent to perform certain technical procedures and apply specific knowledge to safely care for patients. Written documentation of these competencies is maintained in the employee's personnel file. Most health care organizations require employees to undergo annual competency training for elements of care unique to their practice setting. Annual competency testing for RN, LPN, and UAP may include: patient safety, infection control, code blue, medication safety, IV skills, glucose testing, chain of command, HIPAA policies, and restraints.

SUPERVISION

Supervision is the provision of guidance or direction, evaluation, and follow up by the licensed nurse for accomplishment of a nursing task delegated to UAP (NCSBN, 1995). ANA (1996) states that supervision is

CRITICAL THINKING 16-3

Steve, RN, is working with a new RN, Nirmala. Steve tells Nirmala that when she assigns patient care to another RN, that RN assumes both responsibility and accountability for the care. When Nirmala delegates to UAP, she delegates responsibility but keeps the accountability for that patient's care. When Nirmala asks Jill, the UAP, to give a bath, what does Nirmala retain responsibility and accountability for? What is Jill responsible for?

CRITICAL THINKING 16-4

The RN continuously monitors unstable, complex patients who have threats to their airway, breathing, circulation, or safety. Examples of these patients might include a patient on a ventilator and an unconscious patient. The RN can delegate care of stable patients to the LPN or UAP. What are some examples of unstable patients?

"the active process of directing, guiding, and influencing the outcome of an individual's performance of an activity" (p. 20). Supervision can be categorized as on-site, in which the nurse is physically present or immediately available while the activity is being performed, or off-site, in which the nurse has the ability to provide direction through various means of written, verbal, and electronic communication (ANA, 1996). On-site supervision generally occurs in the acute care setting where the RN is immediately available. Off-site supervision may occur in community settings.

As a result of the rapidly increasing use of technology in patient care, some operational guidelines for supervision from the ANA are helpful. Ask yourself, who is in control of the activity? If the RN is responsible, the nurse should incorporate measures to determine whether an activity has been completed to meet the expectations. Also ask yourself, how should controls be instituted? Controls must be in place that allow the RN delegating an activity to stop the task when inappropriately done, review the measures taken, and take back control of the task (ANA, 1996).

A nurse who is supervising care will provide clear direction to the staff about what tasks are to be performed for specific patients. The supervisor nurse must identify when and how the task is to be done and what information must be collected as well as any patient-specific information. The nurse must identify what outcomes are expected and the time frame for reporting results. The nurse will monitor staff performance to ensure compliance with established standards of practice, policy, and procedure. The supervisor nurse will obtain feedback from staff and patients, and intervene, as necessary, to ensure quality nursing care and appropriate documentation.

Hansten and Washburn (2004) identify three levels of supervision based on the task delegated and the educa-

tion, experience, competency, and working relationship of the people involved:

- Unsupervised occurs when one RN works with another RN. Both are accountable for their own practice. When an RN is in a management position, for example, charge nurse, nurse manager, and so on, the RN will supervise other RNs.
- Initial direction and periodic inspection occurs when an RN supervises licensed or unlicensed staff, knows the staff's training and competency level, and has a working relationship with the staff. For example, an RN who has worked with UAP for several weeks is now comfortable giving initial directions to ambulate two new postoperative patients. The RN follows up with UAP once and as needed during the shift.
- Continuous supervision occurs when the RN determines that the delegate needs frequent-to-continuous support and assistance. This level is required when the working relationship is new, the task is complex, or the delegate is inexperienced or has not demonstrated competency.

RESPONSIBILITIES OF HEALTH TEAM MEMBERS

The new graduate nurse may feel overwhelmed by the amount of patient care required and the lack of time to complete the care. The new graduate may be consumed by feelings of inadequacy and failure. Thoughts of not knowing how to answer the phone or find a washcloth, as well as not finding time to eat lunch, can be exhausting. All of these feelings and behaviors may be a result of trying to do it all and not asking for help. New graduate nurses may quickly realize that if they do not delegate, the patient's care will not be completed in a timely and effective manner. The consequences and likely effects must be considered when delegating patient care. The AACN (2004) suggests assessment of five factors that must occur before deciding to delegate:

1. *Potential for Harm:* Determine if there is a risk for the patient in the activity delegated.
2. *Complexity of the Task:* Delegate simple tasks. These tasks often require psychomotor skills with little assessment or judgment proficiency.
3. *Amount of Problem Solving and Innovation Required:* Do not delegate simple tasks that require a creative approach, adaptation, or special attention to complete.
4. *Unpredictability of Outcome:* Avoid delegating tasks in which the outcome is not clear, causing volatility for the patient.
5. *Level of Patient Interaction:* Value time spent with the patient and the patient's family to develop trust, and so on.

Attention to these five factors will improve patient safety associated with delegation.

In addition, Parkman (1996) has identified the following areas in which UAP need training and skill development:

- Basic care procedures, including vital sign measurement, transfer and body mechanics, infection control procedures, basic emergency procedures, privacy and confidentiality, and documenting care activities
- Communication skills, including greeting patients and facilities, handling complaints, resolving conflicts, and reporting to the supervisor
- Decision-making skills, including prioritizing tasks and deciding when and what to report
- Critical thinking skills, including recognizing abnormal vital signs, identifying risks to patient safety, and reporting appropriately to the RN

The RN should create an environment that encourages teaching and learning by all staff. The RN should be willing to teach and demonstrate how to perform a task rather than just telling how it should be done. The RN should strive to earn a reputation for exceptional training and mentoring, involving everyone on the health care team, including LPNs and UAPs.

NURSE MANAGER RESPONSIBILITY

The nursing manager is responsible for developing staff members' ability to delegate. Guidance in this area is necessary because new graduates, wanting to be regarded favorably, may not ask too much of UAP. Delegation is a skill that requires practice. Graduate nurses are often sent to classes conducted by the Education department in the hospital. Topics may include policies and procedures,

health team member's roles, and nursing delegation to name a few. This is where the graduate nurses often learn the job descriptions of health care team members. This information is needed to determine what and to whom to delegate.

The nurse manager will determine the appropriate mix of personnel on a nursing unit. The nurse manager may have personnel with a variety of skills, knowledge, and educational levels. The acuity and needs of the patients usually determine the personnel mix. From this personnel mix, the new graduate nurse will begin to identify who can best perform assigned duties. The non-nursing duties are shifted toward clerical personnel, UAP, or housekeeping personnel to make the best use of individual skills.

NEW GRADUATE RESPONSIBILITY

New graduate nurses need to focus on the duties for which they are directly responsible. What duties can they delegate and to what extent? What do UAP do? What do LPNs/LVNs do? Reviewing the Nurse Practice Act for a nurse's individual state applies to all licensed nurses regardless of whether the nurse is a new graduate or not. The Nurse Practice Act is the legal authority for nursing practice in each state. In the individual states, the definitions, regulations, or directives regarding delegation may be different. The RN also reviews any other applicable state or federal laws; patient needs; job descriptions and competencies of the RNs, LPNs, and UAPs; the agency's policies and procedures; the clinical situation; and the professional standards of nursing in preparation for delegation. Table 16-1 includes delegation suggestions for RNs.

REGISTERED NURSE (RN)

The RN is responsible and accountable for the provision of nursing care. The RN is always responsible for patient assessment, diagnosis, care planning, evaluation, and teaching. Although UAP may measure vital signs, intake and output, or other patient status indicators, it is the RN who interprets this data for comprehensive assessment, nursing diagnosis, and development of the plan of care. UAP may perform simple nursing interventions related to patient hygiene, nutrition, elimination, or activities of daily living, but the RN remains responsible for the patient outcome. Having UAP perform functions outside their scope of practice is a violation of the state Nursing Practice Act and is a threat to patient safety.

Inconsistent facility or agency expectations regarding UAP duties or tasks coupled with minimal, if any, training can lead to an unstable and, in some cases, a less qualified workforce, according to the American Nurses Association (ANA) publication, *Principles for Delegation* (2005).

As the RN prepares to care for the patient, they should describe the health care team to the patient. For

TABLE 16-1   DELEGATION SUGGESTIONS FOR RN

Delegation Suggestions	Examples
■ Consider qualifications of all personnel in the delegation process when making assignments.	■ The charge nurse will assign a new graduate nurse a team of patients less complex than the assignment of an RN who has several years of experience.
■ Assess what is to be delegated and identify who would best complete the assignment.	■ The RN will ask a nursing assistant to pick up specific equipment, that is, a pediatric pulse oximeter from a stock room. This assistant has worked on this unit for five years and is familiar with the type of equipment the nurse needs.
■ Communicate the duty to be performed, and identify the time frame for completion. The expectations for personnel should be clear and concise.	■ The charge nurse tells another nurse, "While I am at lunch, Mr. Jones, the patient in bed 34-2 may ask for a pain shot. Please make him comfortable and tell him that it is too early for another shot for 60 more minutes."
■ Avoid changing duties once they are assigned. Changing duties should be considered only when the duty is above the level of the personnel, as when the patient's care is in jeopardy due to a change in status.	■ A patient sent to surgery for a knee replacement is now experiencing atrial fibrillation postoperatively. The patient will probably be transferred to a telemetry floor for cardiac monitoring.
■ Evaluate the effectiveness of the delegation of duties. Monitor care and check in with UAP frequently. Ask for a feedback report on the outcomes of care delivery.	■ After the patient was assisted to the bathroom, the nurse asked the UAP, what amount of assistance did the patient require? Is the patient safely back in bed?
■ Accept minor variations in the style in which the duties are performed. Individual styles are acceptable as long as the duty is performed correctly within the scope of practice and there is a good outcome.	■ Both nurses below are successful at providing care using different and acceptable methods. One nurse assesses the assigned patients, documents care, and then passes medications. Another nurse assesses the patients while passing medications and then documents care.

example, "Hello Mrs. Jones, my name is Luke Ellingsen. I am a registered nurse, and I will be responsible for your care until 3 P.M. today. Thelma Marks, a nursing assistant, is working with me and will be in to take your vital signs and help with your bath. Please call me if you have any questions."

UNLICENSED ASSISTIVE PERSONNEL (UAP)

The increase in numbers of UAP in acute care settings poses a degree of risk to the patient. The Patient Safety and Quality Improvement Act of 2005 requires health care institutions to make public specified information on staffing levels, patient mix, and patient outcomes, including the number of RNs providing direct care; the numbers of unlicensed personnel utilized to provide direct patient care; the average number of patients per RN

providing direct patient care; the patient mortality rate; the incidence of adverse patient care incidents; and the methods used for determining and adjusting staffing levels and patient care needs.

In addition, health care institutions have to make public their data regarding complaints filed with the state agency, the Health Care Financing Administration, or an accrediting agency related to Medicare Conditions of Participation. The agency would then have to make public the results of any investigations or finding related to the complaint. Recent studies have demonstrated a direct relationship between RN staffing levels and positive patient outcomes. This legislation is intended to allow consumers and researchers to have ready access to information on this issue. UAP are trained to perform duties such as bathing, feeding, toileting, and ambulating patients (Figure 16-1). UAP are also expected to document

Elements to Consider

- Federal, state, and local regulations and guidelines for practice, including the State Nurse Practice Act
- Nursing Professional Standards
- Agency policy, procedure, and standards

- Job description of Registered Nurse, Licensed Practical Nurse/Licensed Vocational Nurse, Unlicensed Assistive Personnel
- Five rights of delegation

- Knowledge and skill of personnel
- Documented personnel competency, strengths, and weaknesses (select the right person for the right job)

↓

RN accountable for application of the Nursing Process
Assessment and Nursing Judgment*
Nursing diagnosis
Planning care
Implementation and teaching
RN delegates as appropriate.
RN retains accountability.
Note that LPN/LVNs and UAP are also responsible for their actions**

↓

RN assesses, monitors, and evaluates all patients, especially complex, unstable patients with unpredictable outcomes.

Administer medications, including IV Push and IVPBs.

Start and maintain IVs and blood transfusions.

Perform sterile or specialized procedures, for example, Foley catheter and nasogastric tube insertion, tracheostomy care, suture removal, and so on.

Educate patient and family.

Maintain infection control.

Administer cardiopulmonary resuscitation.

Interpret and report laboratory findings.

Triage patients.

Prevent nurse-sensitive patient outcomes, for example, cardiac arrest, pneumonia, and so on.

Monitor patient outcomes.

LPN/LVN cares for stable patients with predictable outcomes. They work under the direction of the RN and are responsible for their actions within their scope of practice.

Gather patient data.

Implement patient care.

Maintain infection control.

Provide teaching from standard teaching plan.

Depending on the state and with documented competency, may do the following:**

- Administer medications.
- Perform sterile or specialized procedures, for example, Foley catheter and nasogastric tube insertion, tracheostomy care, suture removal, and so on.
- Perform blood glucose monitoring.
- Administer CPR.
- Perform venipuncture and insert peripheral IVs, change IV bags for patients receiving IV therapy, and so on.

UAP assists the RN and the LPN and gives technical care to stable patients with predictable outcomes and minimal potential for risk. They work under the direction of an RN and are responsible for their actions within their scope of practice.

Assist with activities of daily living.

Bathe, groom, and dress.

Assist with toileting and bed making.

Ambulate, position, and transport.

Feed and socialize with patient.

Measure intake & output (I&O).

Document care.

Weigh patient.

Maintain infection control.

Depending on the state and with documented competency, may do the following:**

- Perform blood glucose monitoring.
- Collect specimens.
- Administer CPR.
- Take vital signs.
- Perform twelve lead EKGs.
- Perform venipuncture for blood tests.

↓

Evaluation
RN uses judgment and is responsible for evaluation of all patient care.

*Nursing Judgment is the process by which nurses come to understand the problems, issues, and concerns of patients, to attend to salient information, and respond to patient problems in concerned and involved ways. Judgment includes both conscious decision making and intuitive response (Benner, Tanner, & Chesla,1996).

**Some variation from state to state and agency.

Figure 16-1 Considerations in delegation.

REAL WORLD INTERVIEW

I use delegation now that I have completed school. I began working as a graduate nurse immediately after graduating nursing school. Prior to graduation, I worked as a nurse technician. I feel that I do understand how it feels to be at both ends of patient care delivery. I vowed that when I became a registered nurse, I would delegate appropriately and fairly to others.

As a registered nurse, I make a point to delegate appropriately to certified nursing assistants (CNAs). I delegate duties like vital signs, changing beds, bathing patients, feeding patients, and performing an accurate intake and output. I delegate these things after giving my CNA a complete report of my patients.

I work on a medical-surgical floor where our CNAs use an automated DYNAMAP to take blood pressures, pulses, and temperatures. I will take my own manual blood pressure when I am assessing my patient if the readings from the DYNAMAP were high or low. My CNAs bring me their vital signs as soon as they are done so that I can determine what more I need to evaluate.

It is important to mention that I never delegate patient assessments or patient education. These duties are reserved for the registered nurse. I will never delegate to a CNA to watch over a patient while they take their medication. I never delegate the insertion or removal of Foleys. I do believe my CNAs take me seriously as I do not delegate anything that I am not willing to do myself and have not done myself in the past. In essence, I do not give the impression that I am "beyond" or "better" than anyone else.

I get concerned when I see a fellow nurse walk out of a patient's room who has just requested a bedpan and go to find a CNA to get him that bedpan. I would never make my patient wait to perform such a necessary and often immediate task. Like I said earlier, I have been on both ends of patient care delivery, and I know what it feels like to be unappreciated. So far, I have stuck to my promise to delegate appropriately and fairly. I truly believe my CNAs would agree.

Shelly A. Thompson
New Graduate Nurse
Dyer, Indiana

and report information related to these activities. The RN will delegate to the UAP and is liable for those delegations. According to the ANA (2005), if the RN knows or reasonably believes that the assistant has the appropriate training, orientation, and documented competencies, then the RN can reasonably expect that the UAP will function in a safe and effective manner.

Reasons for using UAP in acute care settings include cost control; freeing RNs from duties, primarily nonnursing duties; and allowing time for RNs to complete assessments of patients and their potential responses to treatments. UAP cannot be assigned to assess or evaluate responses to treatment because that is the role of the RN. It is more cost-effective to have UAP perform nonnursing duties than to have nurses perform them. UAP can deliver supportive care. They cannot practice nursing or provide total patient care. The RN has an increased scope of liability when tasks are delegated to UAP. The RN must be aware of the job description, skills, and educational background of the UAP prior to the delegation of duties.

If the LPN or UAP performs poorly, the RN should tell them about mistakes privately, as much as possible, in a supportive manner with a focus on learning from mistakes. If they perform in an inappropriate, unsafe, or incompetent manner, the RN must intervene immediately and stop the unsafe activity, counsel the LPN or UAP, document the facts, and report to the nurse manager, as appropriate.

LICENSED PRACTICAL/ VOCATIONAL NURSE

Licensed practical/vocational nursing caregivers who have undergone a standardized training and competency, and licensing evaluation are licensed practical nurses/licensed vocational nurses (LPNs/LVNs). Even though LPNs/LVNs are able to perform duties and functions that UAP are not allowed to do, LPNs/LVNs are held to a higher standard of care and are responsible for their actions. LPN/LVNs usually care for stable patients with predictable outcomes, though they may help the RN with seriously ill patients in ICU. Common duties of the LPN include the duties of the UAP plus data collection, sterile dressing changes, colostomy irrigations, respiratory suctioning, insertion of Foley catheters, and teaching from a standard patient care plan. In some states, passing medications, including the administration and initiation of IV fluids, monitoring of IV sites, and passing of nasogastric tubes is part of the LPN role. In other states, IV therapy under the supervision of an on-site RN is allowed. The LPN does not do initial patient assessment, but after the RN has completed the patient's initial assessment and the plan of care, the LPN does the ongoing head-to-toe assessment, monitoring vital signs, IV sites, IV fluids, breath sounds, and so on. In some states in nursing homes, the LPN may assume the charge nurse role with an on-site supervising RN. LPNs report their findings to the RN. The RN is still primarily responsible for overall patient assessment, nursing diagnosis, planning, implementation, and evaluation of the quality of care delegated. Table 16-2 (NCSBN, 1997) lists five rights of delegation to be considered.

DIRECT PATIENT CARE

As mentioned earlier in this chapter, **direct patient care activities** include activities such as assisting the patient with feeding, drinking, ambulating, grooming, toileting, dressing, and socializing. Direct patient care activity may also involve collecting, reporting, and documenting related to these activities. Activities delegated to UAP do not include health counseling or teaching or activities that require independent, specialized nursing knowledge, skill, or judgment.

INDIRECT PATIENT CARE ACTIVITIES

Indirect patient care activities are often necessary to support the patient and their environment, and only incidentally involve direct patient contact. These activities

TABLE 16-2	THE FIVE RIGHTS OF DELEGATION
Right Task	Does the delegated task confirm to agency established policies, procedures, and standards consistent with the state Nurse Practice Act, federal and state regulations and guidelines for practice, nursing professional standards, and the ANA Code of Ethics?
Right Circumstance	Does the delegated task require independent nursing management? Do the personnel have the education, experience, resources, equipment, and supervision needed to complete the task safely?
Right Person	Is a qualified, competent person delegating the right task to a qualified, competent person to be performed on the right patient? Is the patient stable with predictable outcomes? Is it legally acceptable to delegate to this patient? Do health care personnel have documented knowledge, skill, and competency to do the task?
Right Direction/Communication	Does the RN communicate the task clearly with directions, specific steps of the tasks, any limitations, and expected outcomes? Are times for reporting back to the RN specified? Is staff understanding of the task clarified? Are staff encouraged to say "I don't know how to do this and I need help," as needed?
Right Supervision	Is there appropriate monitoring, intervention, evaluation, and patient and staff feedback as needed? Are patient and staff outcomes monitored? Does the RN answer staff questions and problem solve as needed? Does the staff report task completion and patient response to the RN? Does the RN provide follow-up teaching and guidance to staff as appropriate? Is there continuous quality improvement of the delegation process and patient care? Are problems, particularly any sentinel events, reported via the chain of command and as needed to the State Board of Nursing and the Joint Commission (JC)?

Source: Adapted from National Council of State Boards of Nursing (NCSBN). (1997). *The Five Rights of Delegation.*

CRITICAL THINKING 16-5

It was just about 6:30 P.M. on the 3 P.M. to 11 P.M. shift on 2 East. Most of the practitioners had made their rounds, so the evening was calming down. The UAP, Jill, was picking up the dinner trays from the patient's rooms. Steve, the RN, had just sat down to document his patient assessments when he heard the UAP, Jill, yell "I need some help in Room 2510, Mr. Olson is not breathing." As several of the nurses ran to Room 2510, another UAP ran for the Emergency Crash Cart. The cart was wheeled into the patient's room during the overhead announcement by the operator, "CODE BLUE, Room 2510." The nurses initiated CPR. The UAP plugged the cart into the wall, turned the suction machine on, and then assisted the family out of the room and stayed with them until the nurse was able to talk with them.

How does completion of these tasks by the UAP contribute to patient care?

Does the UAP relieve the pressure on the nurse to complete everything?

REAL WORLD INTERVIEW

Upon evaluating delegation on several, varied nursing units, I arrive at one conclusion; we as professional nurses just do not do it well. There is the exception, of course, that being the individual who has developed an outstanding ability to delegate nearly all of his or her responsibilities to others in an authoritative or diplomatic manner with the recipients either loving or hating it.

Part of the problem may lie with the job description, that black-and-white document that delineates a role in great detail right up to the final statement of "inclusive of duties as assigned." The latter statement is too vague and the delegated task should be clearly stated somewhere in the job description.

On a nursing unit, it generally falls on the staff nurse to function in the assigning and delegating role. For this role, he or she is often criticized, most frequently behind the scenes, though occasionally they are blasted right out in the open. "What do you mean I am getting the next admission; I already have gotten two!" At best, one becomes apprehensive when assigning *anything*, from an admission to cleaning up the break room. I wonder, if that is the fate of the charge nurse, just how well would one expect the staff RN to delegate?

Perhaps our failures with delegation stem from our predominantly female, motherly gender. Moms can do it! Moms can do it all. Often, Mom finds the route of least resistance: "It's just easier to do it myself!" It is the same thing with RNs; RNs can do it, RNs can do it all.

I believe that the fine art of delegation needs to be taught more in the educational process, along with the concept of teamwork. The team is hindered when we become ineffective at delegation. The challenges in contemporary health care are tremendous, only to become even more challenging in the future. We as professional nurses would do well to acquire advanced skills in delegation, team building, and diplomacy, for these skills will become tools of survival in the very near future.

Suzanne Kalweit, RN, MS
Charge Nurse
Dyer, Indiana

TABLE 16-3	DELEGATION CHECKLIST		

Question	Yes	No
Do you recognize that you retain ultimate responsibility for the outcome of delegated assignments?	____	____
Do you spend most of your time completing tasks that require an RN?	____	____
Do you trust the ability of your staff to complete job assignments successfully?	____	____
Do you allow staff sufficient time to solve their own problems before interceding with advice?	____	____
Do you clearly outline expected outcomes and hold your staff accountable for achieving these outcomes?	____	____
Do you support your staff with an appropriate level of feedback and followup?	____	____
Do you use delegation as a way to help staff develop new skills and provide challenging work assignments?	____	____
Does your staff know what you expect of them?	____	____
Do you take the time to carefully select the right person for the right job?	____	____
Do you feel comfortable sharing control with your staff as appropriate?	____	____
Do you clearly identify all aspects of an assignment to staff when you delegate?	____	____
Do you assign tasks to the lowest level of staff capable of completing them successfully?	____	____
Do you support your staff, even when they are learning?	____	____
Do you allow your staff reasonable freedom to achieve outcomes?	____	____

Source: Compiled with information from Harvard ManageMentor® Delegating Tools. (2004). *Delegation skills checklist.* Boston: Harvard Business School Publishing.

are often designated "unit routines" and assist in providing a clean, efficient, and safe patient care milieu. They typically encompass chore services, companion care, housekeeping, transporting, clerical, stocking, and maintenance tasks (ANA, 1996).

UNDERDELEGATION

Personnel in a new job role, such as nurse manager, RN, or nursing graduate, often underdelegate. Believing that older, more experienced staff may resent having someone new delegate to them, a new nurse may simply avoid delegation. Or, new nurses may seek approval from other staff members by demonstrating their ability to complete all assigned duties without assistance. In addition, new nurses may be reluctant to delegate because they do not know or trust individuals on their team or are not clear on the scope of their duties or what they are allowed to do. New nurses can become frustrated

and overwhelmed if they fail to delegate appropriately. They may fail to establish appropriate controls with staff or fail to follow up properly; they may fail to delegate the appropriate authority to go with certain responsibilities. Perfectionism and a refusal to allow mistakes can lead a new nurse in over her head in patient-care responsibilities. More-experienced staff members can help new personnel by intervening early on, assisting in the delegation process, and clarifying responsibilities (Table 16-3).

OVERDELEGATION

Overdelegation of duties can also place the patient at risk. The reasons for overdelegation are numerous. Personnel may feel uncomfortable performing duties that

TABLE 16-4	OBSTACLES TO DELEGATION

- Fear of being disliked
- Inability to give up any control of the situation
- Fear of making a mistake
- Inability to determine what to delegate and to whom
- Inadequate knowledge of delegation process
- Past experience with delegation that did not turn out well
- Poor interpersonal communication skills
- Lack of confidence to move beyond being a novice nurse
- Lack of administrative support for nurse delegating to LPN and UAP
- Tendency to isolate oneself and choosing to complete all tasks alone

- Lack of confidence to delegate to staff members who were previously one's peers
- Inability to prioritize using Maslow's hierarchy of needs and the nursing process
- Thinking of oneself as the only one who can complete a task the way "it is supposed" to be done
- Inability to communicate effectively
- Inability to develop working relationships with other team members
- Lack of knowledge of the capabilities of staff, including their competency, skill, experience, level of education, job description, and so on

are unfamiliar to them, and they may depend too much on others. They may be unorganized or inclined to either avoid responsibility or immerse themselves in trivia. Overdelegation leads to delegating duties to personnel who are not educated for the tasks such as LPNs and UAP. Delegating duties that are inappropriate for personnel to perform because they have been inadequately educated is dangerous and against the state Nurse Practice Act. Overdelegating duties can overwork some personnel and underwork others, creating obstacles to delegation (Table 16-4).

ORGANIZATIONAL RESPONSIBILITY FOR DELEGATION

Certain elements must be in place in an organization for efficient nursing delegation to occur. These elements help assure nursing and medical quality. They also help clarify all health care staff's roles within the organizational system (Table 16-5).

Organizations fulfill their responsibility to staff and patients by developing these organizational elements and maintaining a clear chain of command.

CHAIN OF COMMAND

The RN, including the new graduate nurse, is accountable to the charge nurse and nurse manager of the unit. The nurse manager is accountable to the chief nursing executive, for example, the vice president for nursing. The chief nursing executive is accountable to the chief executive officer. The hospital's chief executive officer is accountable to the board of directors. The board of directors is accountable to the community it serves and often to another larger hospital corporation, as well as to state nursing and medical licensing boards and the Joint Commission. All are accountable for their actions to the patients and the communities that they serve.

DELEGATION OF NURSING PROCESS

Ultimately, some professional activities involving the specialized knowledge, judgment, or skill of the nursing process can never be delegated. These include patient assessment, triage, nursing diagnosis, nursing plans of care, extensive teaching or counseling, telephone advice, outcome evaluations, and patient discharges (Zimmermann, 1996). Delegated tasks are typically those tasks that occur frequently, are considered technical by nature, are considered standard and unchanging, have predictable results, and have minimal potential for risks (Westfall, 1998). As a professional standard for all nurses in all states, the assessment, analysis, diagnosis, planning, teaching, and evaluation stages of the nursing process may not be delegated. Delegated activities usually fall within the implementation phase of the nursing process.

TABLE 16-5	**ORGANIZATIONAL ELEMENTS NEEDED FOR EFFICIENT DELEGATION**

- Follow professional standards for education, licensure, and competency in all hiring decisions, orientation, and ongoing continuing education programs.

- Have clear job descriptions and ongoing licensing and credentialing policies for RNs, MDs, LPN/LVNs, UAP, and other health care staff. The organization must ensure that all staff members are safe, competent practitioners before assigning them to patient care. Orient staff to their duties, chain of command, and the job descriptions of RN, LPN, and UAP.

- Facilitate clinical and educational specialty certification and credentialing of all health care practitioners and staff.

- Provide standards for ongoing supervision and periodic licensure/competency verification and evaluation of all staff.

- Provide access to professional health care standards, policies, procedures, library, Internet, and medication information with unit availability and efficient library and Internet access.

- Facilitate regular evidence-based reviews of critical standards, policies, and procedures.

- Have clear policies and procedures for delegation and chain of command reporting lines for all staff from RN to charge nurse to nurse manager to nurse executive and, as appropriate to risk management, the hospital ethics committee, the hospital administrator, nursing and medical practitioners, the chief of the medical staff, the board of directors, the State Licensing Board for Nursing and Medicine, and the Joint Commission. See Figure 16-2 for illustration of one such organizational chain of command.

- Provide administrative support for supervisors and staff who delegate, assign, monitor, and evaluate patient care.

- Clarify health care provider accountability, for example, if a medical or nursing practitioners or physician assistant delegates a nursing task to UAP, the health care provider is responsible for monitoring that care delivery. This must be spelled out in hospital policy. If the RN notes that the UAP is doing something incorrectly, the RN has a duty to intervene and to notify the ordering practitioner of the incident. The RN always has an independent responsibility to protect patient safety. Blindly relying on another nursing or health care provider is not permissible for the RN.

- Provide education and standards for regular RN evaluation of UAP and LPN/LVN, and reinforce the need for UAP and LPN/LVN accountability to the RN. RNs must delegate and supervise. They cannot abdicate this professional responsibility.

- Develop a physical, mental, and verbal "No Abuse" policy to be followed by all professional and nonprofessional health care staff. Follow up on any problems.

- Consider applying for magnet status for your facility. This status is awarded by the American Nurses Credentialing Center to nursing departments that have worked to improve nursing care, including the empowering of nursing decision making and delegation in clinical practice.

- Monitor patient outcomes, including nurse-sensitive outcomes, staffing ratios, and other quality indicators, as well as developing ongoing clinical quality improvement practices. Benchmark with national groups.

- Maintain ongoing monitoring of incident reports, sentinel events, and other elements of risk management and performance improvement of the process and outcome of patient care.

- Develop systematic, error-proof systems for medication administration that ensure the six rights of medication administration, that is, the right patient, right medication, right dose, right time, right route, and right documentation. Develop safe computerized order-entry systems.

- Provide documentation of routine maintenance for all patient care equipment.

- Attain the JC Patient Safety Goals (www.jointcommission.org).

- Develop intrahospital and intraagency safe transfer policies.

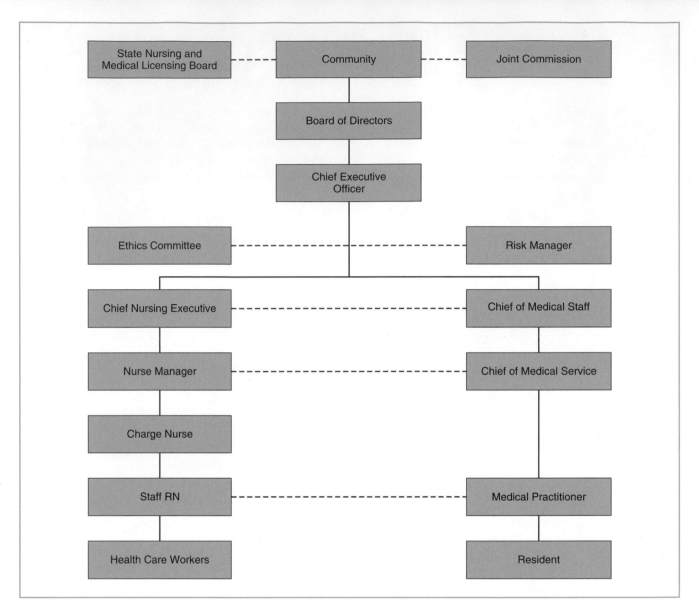

Figure 16-2 Organizational chain of command.

DELEGATION DECISION-MAKING TREE

The National Council of State Boards of Nursing (NCSBN) has developed a Delegation Decision-Making Tree (Figure 16-3).

The steps of the Decision-Making Tree are as follows:

- Assessment and Planning
- Communication
- Surveillance and Supervision
- Evaluation and Feedback

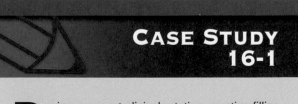

CASE STUDY 16-1

During your next clinical rotation, practice filling out the NCSBN Delegation Decision-Making Tree in Figure 16-3 for one of your patients. Identify the patients' needs, and identify what an RN could safely delegate. What did you note?

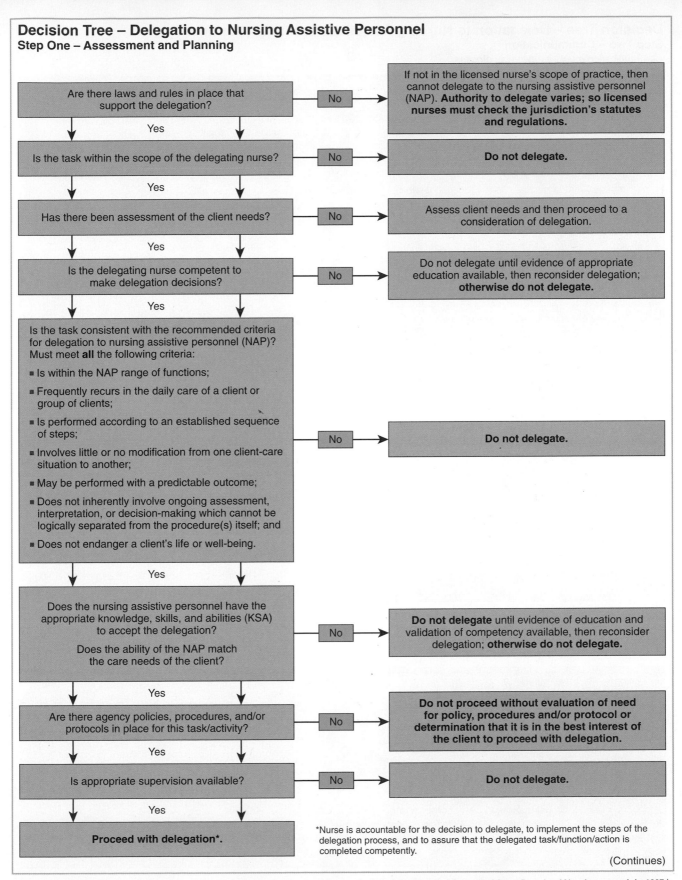

Decision Tree – Delegation to Nursing Assistive Personnel
Step One – Assessment and Planning

Are there laws and rules in place that support the delegation?

→ No → If not in the licensed nurse's scope of practice, then cannot delegate to the nursing assistive personnel (NAP). **Authority to delegate varies; so licensed nurses must check the jurisdiction's statutes and regulations.**

↓ Yes

Is the task within the scope of the delegating nurse?

→ No → **Do not delegate.**

↓ Yes

Has there been assessment of the client needs?

→ No → Assess client needs and then proceed to a consideration of delegation.

↓ Yes

Is the delegating nurse competent to make delegation decisions?

→ No → Do not delegate until evidence of appropriate education available, then reconsider delegation; **otherwise do not delegate.**

↓ Yes

Is the task consistent with the recommended criteria for delegation to nursing assistive personnel (NAP)? Must meet **all** the following criteria:

- Is within the NAP range of functions;
- Frequently recurs in the daily care of a client or group of clients;
- Is performed according to an established sequence of steps;
- Involves little or no modification from one client-care situation to another;
- May be performed with a predictable outcome;
- Does not inherently involve ongoing assessment, interpretation, or decision-making which cannot be logically separated from the procedure(s) itself; and
- Does not endanger a client's life or well-being.

→ No → **Do not delegate.**

↓ Yes

Does the nursing assistive personnel have the appropriate knowledge, skills, and abilities (KSA) to accept the delegation?

Does the ability of the NAP match the care needs of the client?

→ No → **Do not delegate** until evidence of education and validation of competency available, then reconsider delegation; **otherwise do not delegate.**

↓ Yes

Are there agency policies, procedures, and/or protocols in place for this task/activity?

→ No → **Do not proceed without evaluation of need for policy, procedures and/or protocol or determination that it is in the best interest of the client to proceed with delegation.**

↓ Yes

Is appropriate supervision available?

→ No → **Do not delegate.**

↓ Yes

Proceed with delegation*.

*Nurse is accountable for the decision to delegate, to implement the steps of the delegation process, and to assure that the delegated task/function/action is completed competently.

(Continues)

Figure 16-3 NCSBN delegation decision-making tree. (Reprinted and used by permission of the National Council of State Boards of Nursing, copyright 1997.)

Decision Tree – Delegation to Nursing Assistive Personnel (Continued)
Step Two – Communication
Communication must be a two-way process

The nurse:	The nursing assistive personnel:	Documentation:

▪ Assesses the assistant's understanding of:
 ▪ How the task is to be accomplished
 ▪ When and what information is to be reported, including:
  ▪ Expected observations to report and record
  ▪ Specific client concerns that would require prompt reporting.
▪ Individualizes for the nursing assistive personnel and client situation
▪ Addresses any unique client requirements and characteristics, and expectations
▪ Assesses the assistant's understanding of expectations, providing clarification if needed
▪ Communicates his or her willingness and availability to guide and support assistant
▪ Assures appropriate accountability by verifying that the receiving person accepts the delegation and accompanying responsibility.
	▪ Asks questions regarding the delegation and seek clarification of expectations if needed
	▪ Informs the nurse if the assistant has not done a task/function/activity before, or has only done infrequently
	▪ Asks for additional training or supervision
	▪ Affirms understanding of expectations
	▪ Determines the communication method between the nurse and the assistive personnel
	▪ Determines the communication and plan of action in emergency situations.
		Timely, complete, and accurate documentation of provided care
		▪ Facilitates communication with other members of the health care team
		▪ Records the nursing care provided.

Step Three – Surveillance and Supervision
The purpose of surveillance and monitoring is related to nurse's responsibility for client care within the context of a client population. The nurse supervises the delegation by monitoring the performance of the task or function and assures compliance with standards of practice, policies and procedures. Frequency, level, and nature of monitoring vary with needs of client and experience of assistant.

The nurse considers the:	The nurse determines:	The nurse is responsible for:
▪ Client's health care status and stability of condition ▪ Predictability of responses and risks ▪ Setting where care occurs ▪ Availability of resources and support infrastructure. ▪ Complexity of the task being performed.	▪ The frequency of onsite supervision and assessment based on: ▪ Needs of the client ▪ Complexity of the delegated function/task/activity ▪ Proximity of nurse's location.	▪ Timely intervening and follow-up on problems and concerns. Examples of the need for intervening include: ▪ Alertness to subtle signs and symptoms (which allows nurse and assistant to be proactive, before a client's condition deteriorates significantly) ▪ Awareness of assistant's difficulties in completing delegated activities ▪ Providing adequate follow-up to problems and/or changing situations is a critical aspect of delegation.

Step Four – Evaluation and Feedback
Evaluation is often the forgotten step in delegation.

In considering the effectiveness of delegation, the nurse addresses the following questions:
▪ Was the delegation successful? ▪ Was the task/function/activity performed correctly? ▪ Was the client's desired and/or expected outcome achieved? ▪ Was the outcome optimal, satisfactory, or unsatisfactory? ▪ Was communication timely and effective? ▪ What went well; what was challenging? ▪ Were there any problems or concerns; if so, how were they addressed? ▪ Is there a better way to meet the client need? ▪ Is there a need to adjust the overall plan of care, or should this approach be continued? ▪ Were there any "learning moments" for the assistant and/or the nurse? ▪ Was appropriate feedback provided to the assistant regarding the performance of the delegation? ▪ Was the assistant acknowledged for accomplishing the task/activity/function?

Figure 16-3 NCSBN delegation decision-making tree (Continued)

STATE BOARDS OF NURSING

Many states specify nursing tasks that may be delegated in their rules and regulations. Although the excerpts in the example in Table 16-6 are similar to those of some other states, there is variation in rules and regulations from state to state. Check state requirements with your state board of nursing at www.ncsbn.org.

DELEGATION SUGGESTIONS FOR RNs

RNs concerned with appropriate delegation find it helpful to use the delegation suggestions in Table 16-7.

TABLE 16-6	DELEGATION TASK EXAMPLES

Nursing Tasks That May Not Be Delegated

- Assessment (physical, psychological, and social assessment, which requires professional nursing judgment, intervention, referral, or followup). Data collection without interpretation is not assessment
- Planning of nursing care

Evaluation of the patient's response

- Implementation that requires judgment
- Health teaching and health counseling
- Medication administration

Tasks Most Commonly Delegated

- Noninvasive and nonsterile treatments
- Collecting, reporting, and documenting data, such as the following:
  - Vital signs, height, weight, intake and output, urine test for glucose
  - Ambulation, positioning, and turning
  - Transportation of the patient within the facility
  - Personal hygiene and elimination, including cleansing enemas
  - Feeding, cutting up food, or placing meal trays
  - Socialization activities
  - Activities of daily living

Nursing Tasks Not Routinely Delegated

Note that these may sometimes be delegated if the LPN has received special credentialing, for example, education and competency testing.

- Sterile procedures
- Invasive procedures, such as inserting tubes in a body cavity or instilling or inserting substances into an indwelling tube
- Care of broken skin other than minor abrasions or cuts generally classified as requiring only first aid treatment
- Intravenous therapy

TABLE 16-7   ADDITIONAL DELEGATION SUGGESTIONS FOR RN

- Consider prior to delegating
  - ☐ Who has the time to complete the delegated project?
  - ☐ Who is the best person for the project?
  - ☐ What is the urgency of the project?
  - ☐ Are there any deadlines?
  - ☐ Who do you want to develop their skills?
  - ☐ Who is the best person to meet the patients needs?
  - ☐ Who would enjoy the project?
- Be clear on the qualifications of the delegate, that is, education, experience, and competency. Require documentation or demonstration of current competence by the delegate for each task. Clarify patient care concerns or delegation problems. Click on ANA position statements at www.nursingworld.org and at your state board of nursing, as necessary.
- Speak to your delegates as you would like to be spoken to. There is no need to apologize for your delegation. Remember that you are carrying out your professional responsibility.
- Communicate the patient's name, room number, and duty to be performed and identify the time frame for completion. Discuss any changes from the usual procedures that might be needed to meet special patient needs and any potential patient abnormalities that should be reported to the RN. The expectations for personnel before, during, and after duty performance should be stated in a clear, pleasant, direct, and concise manner.
- Identify the expected patient outcome and the limits of the delegate's authority.
- Verify the delegate's understanding of delegated tasks and have the delegate repeat instructions, as needed. Verify that the delegate accepts responsibility and accountability for carrying out the task correctly. Require regular, frequent mini reports about patients from staff.
- Avoid removing duties once assigned. This should be considered only when the duty is above the level of the personnel such as when the patient's care is in jeopardy because the patient's status has changed.
- Monitor task completion according to standards. Make frequent walking rounds to assess patient outcomes. Intervene as needed.
- Accept minor variations in the style in which the duties are performed. Individual styles are acceptable as long as the patient standards are met and good outcomes are achieved. Use opportunities to teach less experienced staff.
- Try to meet staff needs for learning opportunities, and consider any health problems and work preferences of the staff as long as it doesn't interfere with meeting patient needs.
- If a delegate doesn't meet the standards, talk with them to identify the problem. If this is not successful, inform the delegate that you will be discussing the problem with your supervisor. Document your concerns, as appropriate. Follow up with your supervisor according to your organization's policy.
- Avoid high risk delegation. The RN may be at risk if the delegated task can be performed only by the RN according to law, organizational policies and procedures, or professional standards of nursing practice; or if the delegated task could involve substantial risk or harm to a patient: or if the RN knowingly delegates a task to a person who has not had the appropriate training or orientation; or if the RN fails to adequately supervise the delegated activity and does not evaluate the delegated action by reassessing the patient (ANA, 1996).

Source: Adapted from Boucher (1998), and Zimmermann (1996).

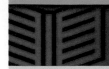

EVIDENCE FROM THE LITERATURE

Citation: Johnson, S. H. (1996). Teaching Nursing Delegation: Analyzing Nurse Practice Acts. *The Journal of Continuing Education in Nursing, 27*(2), 52–58.

Discussion: This author notes policies common to many state Nurse Practice Acts. These policies include the following:

- Only nursing tasks can be delegated, not nursing practices.
- The RN must perform patient assessment to determine what can be delegated.
- UAP do not practice professional nursing.
- The RN can delegate only what is in the scope of nursing practice.
- The LPN works under the direction/supervision of the RN.
- The RN delegates care based on the knowledge and skill of the person selected to perform the task.
- The RN determines competency of the person to whom the nurse delegates.
- The RN cannot delegate activity that requires RN professional skill and knowledge.
- The RN is accountable and responsible for delegated tasks.
- The RN must evaluate patient outcomes resulting from delegated activity.
- Health care facilities can develop special delegation protocols provided they meet state board of nursing delegation guidelines.
- Delegation requires critical thinking by the RN.

You should review your own state Nurse Practice Act and look for the following items to better understand delegation:

- Definition of delegation
- Items that cannot be delegated
- Items that cannot be routinely delegated
- Guidelines for the RN on what can be delegated
- Description of professional nursing practice
- Description of LPN/LVN and unlicensed nursing assistant roles
- Degree of supervision required
- Guidelines for lowering risk of delegation
- Warning about inappropriate delegation
- Restricted use of the word "nurse" to licensed nurses

Implications for Practice: Reviewing your own state's Nurse Practice Act can increase your knowledge and skill in using delegation appropriately. Note that many state nursing boards' contact information as well as information about model Nurse Practice Acts can be accessed at www.ncsbn.org. Search this site for Model Nursing Practice Acts and then state boards of nursing.

TRANSCULTURAL DELEGATION

Nurses and patients come from diverse cultural backgrounds. Transcultural delegation requires that personnel perform duties with this cultural diversity taken into consideration. Poole, Davidhizar, and Giger (1995) suggest there are six cultural phenomena to be considered when delegating to a culturally diverse staff: communication, space, social organization, time, environmental control, and biological variations.

COMMUNICATION

Communication, the first cultural phenomenon, is greatly affected by cultural diversity in the workforce. Elements of communication, including dialect; volume; use of touch; context of speech; and kinesics, such as gestures, stance, and eye behavior, all influence how messages are sent and received (Poole, Davidhizar, & Giger, 1995). For example, if a nurse were talking to UAP in a loud voice, it could be interpreted as anger. However, the nurse may be from a cultural background whose members always speak loudly—she may not be angry at all. Alternately, a nurse,

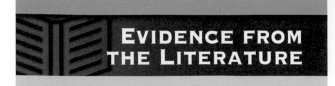

EVIDENCE FROM THE LITERATURE

Citation: Quallich, S. A. (2005). A bond of trust: Delegation. *Urological Nursing, 25*(2), 120–123.

Discussion: The article discusses a realistic approach to delegation of tasks that addresses real-life issues. Combining the five rights of delegation with concepts of establishing a trusting relationship is the premise of the article. Obstacles related to delegation encompass topics often avoided, including tasks that are time consuming and unpleasant. An updated list of tasks that can be delegated is included.

Implications for Practice: It is important for health care staff to address delegation from various points of view. Reviewing the updated list of tasks that can be delegated is useful.

because of cultural upbringing, may view people from other cultures differently (Table 16-8).

SPACE

Cultural background influences the space that individuals maintain between themselves. Some cultures prefer physical closeness, whereas other cultures prefer more distance to be maintained between people. Ineffective delegation can take place when an individual's space is violated. Some delegators stand too close when speaking.

Conversely, some members of a group may feel left out if they are not sitting close to the delegator. They may not feel included or important.

SOCIAL ORGANIZATION

In different cultures, the social support in a person's life varies from support in one's own family to support from collegial relationships with the staff. If staff look to other staff for social support, those staff may have difficulty fulfilling any tasks delegated to them that could threaten their social organization.

TIME

Another cultural phenomenon affecting delegation is the concept of time. How often have you heard people say, "They are on their own time schedule"? Some people tend to move slowly and are often late, whereas other people move quickly and are prompt in meeting deadlines.

Poole, Davidhizar, and Giger (1995) describe different cultural groups as being either past-, present-, or future oriented. Past-oriented cultures focus on their tradition and its maintenance. For example, these cultures invest time into preparation of food that is traditional even though the food can be bought prepared in a store. Present-oriented cultures focus on day-to-day activities. For example, our present-oriented culture works hard for today's wages and does not plan for the future. Future-oriented cultures worry about what might happen in the future and prepare diligently for a potential problem, perhaps financial or health related. A nurse delegator should always be aware of duties to be completed and their deadline so that appropriate personnel can achieve their responsibilities in a timely fashion. Otherwise, people who meet deadlines in a timely fashion may be frustrated by those who do not.

TABLE 16-8	CULTURAL VIEWS

- What is your cultural stereotype of Hispanics? Africans? Chinese? Filipinos? Germans? Irish? Others?
- How do your grandparents, parents, family, and close friends view people from these cultures?
- Have your interactions with these cultural groups been positive? Negative? Neutral?
- How do you feel about going into a neighborhood or into the home of a person from one of these cultural groups?
- Does your cultural stereotype allow for socioeconomic differences?
- What culturally based health practices do you think characterize people from these cultures? How are these practices different from your own culturally based health practices?

Source: Compiled with information from Swanson, J., & Nies, M. (1997). *Community health nursing: Promoting the health of aggregates.* (2nd ed.). Philadelphia: WB Saunders.

CASE STUDY 16-2

A new nursing graduate, Jamilla, has been assigned to work with Abdul, a UAP, and five patients. Jamilla introduces herself to Abdul and asks him what types of patient care he usually performs. He tells Jamilla that he gives baths and takes vital signs. Jamilla asks Abdul to get all of the vital signs and give them to her written on a piece of paper. She asks Abdul if he documents them. He states that he does document them.

Later that morning, Dr. Kent is making rounds on his patients, two of whom are Jamilla's patients. He asks Jamilla for the most recent vital signs. She then asks Abdul for the vital signs on all the patients. Abdul tells her he has not taken them yet. Dr. Kent then asks Jamilla to get the vitals herself. By the time Jamilla returns with the vital signs, Dr. Kent has gone and has written orders she cannot read.

There are several factors in this delegation situation that should have been handled differently. Can you name any?

Do you think the new graduate was ready to delegate to the UAP? Why?

Were the duties delegated appropriate for the UAP?

Would review of the job description for each health care personnel identified in this case study help solve this problem in the future?

ENVIRONMENTAL CONTROL

Poole, Davidhizar, and Giger (1995) define environmental control as people's perception of their control over their environment. This is also called internal locus of control. Some cultures place a heavier weight on fate, luck, or chance, believing, for example, that a patient is cured from cancer based on chance. They may think the health care treatment had something to do with the cure but was not the sole cause of it. How personnel perceive their control of the environment may affect how they delegate and perform duties. Personnel with an internal locus of control are geared toward taking more personal initiative and not requiring assistance in decision making. They believe in taking action and not relying on fate. Personnel with an external locus of control may wait for fate and luck to determine their actions.

BIOLOGICAL VARIATIONS

The sixth and final cultural phenomenon is biological variations. Biological variations are the biopsychological differences between racial and ethnic groups. These biopsychological variations include physiological differences, physical stamina, and susceptibility to disease. Such factors need to be considered. For example, it would be problematic if the care of a comatose patient who weighs more than 300 pounds and needs frequent turning were delegated to a small nurse who cannot physically handle the patient. Hospital policy must address how to meet all patient and staff needs safely. Perhaps this patient can be assigned to two nurses. A nurse who is pregnant

CRITICAL THINKING 16-6

The Luck Factor (Wiseman, 2004) discusses research that illustrates luck as something that can be learned if one pays attention to four principles.

- Lucky people create, notice, and act on the chance opportunities in their life.
- Lucky people make successful decisions by using their intuition and gut feeling.
- Lucky people's expectations about the future help them fulfill their dreams and ambitions.
- Lucky people are able to transform their bad luck into good fortune.

Do you agree with Wiseman's findings? Can you use your "luck" to improve your nursing career? Your ability to delegate? Your life?

may not be assigned to this patient because of the potential injury to the baby and nurse. Likewise, a pregnant nurse would not be assigned to a patient with radium implants because of the risks that the radium poses to the baby and mother. Biological variations must be considered, for the sake of both the health care providers and the patient.

CRITICAL THINKING 16-7

Note the following selected list of values:

Mainstream American Values	Other Cultural Values
Make your own luck.	Fate and luck determine your life.
Like change.	Like tradition.
Arrive on time.	Frequently arrive late.
Value the individual.	Value the group.
Value competition.	Value cooperation.
Set goals for the future.	Enjoy life and just let it happen.
Value directness.	Value being subtle.
Believe that all have a fairly equal chance to achieve status.	Believe that some people will always have higher status.

Which of these values do you hold? Which do members of your staff hold? How can you work to improve communication around these values and improve your working relationships?

KEY CONCEPTS

- Delegation is a practiced and learned behavior.

- The RN must have a clear definition of what constitutes the scope of practice of all personnel.

- The five rights of delegation are the right task, the right circumstance, the right person, the right direction and communication, and the right supervision and evaluation.

- Accountability is being responsible and answerable for actions or inactions of self or others.

- Responsibility involves reliability, dependability, and the obligation to accomplish work when one accepts an assignment. Responsibility also includes each person's obligation to perform at an acceptable level.

- Authority occurs when a person who has been given the right to delegate based on the state Nurse Practice Act also has the official power from an agency to delegate.

- The RN is accountable for the delegation and performance of all nursing duties.

- There are several potential barriers to good delegation.

- Transcultural delegation is encouraged to provide a patient with optimal care.

- Supervision is the provision of guidance or direction, evaluation, and followup by the licensed nurse for accomplishment of a nursing task delegated to UAP.

- Assignment is the downward or lateral transfer of both the responsibility and accountability of an activity from one individual to another.

- Key elements must be in place in an organization for efficient nursing delegation to occur.

- Professional judgment is the intellectual (educated, informed, and experienced) process that a nurse exercises in forming an opinion and reaching a clinical decision based upon an analysis of the available evidence.

- Organizations interested in quality patient care provide staff with guidelines on how to use the chain of command.

- The NCSBN Delegation Decision-Making Tree is a useful tool when developing skill in delegating patient care.

- All members of the health care team must fulfill their delegated responsibilities.

- Nursing staff provide direct and indirect patient care.

KEY TERMS

accountability   indirect patient care activities
authority   responsibility
delegation   supervision
direct patient care activities

REVIEW QUESTIONS

1. What types of information are often discussed with new nurse employees during hospital orientation? Select all that apply.
   _____ A. Nurse Practice Act
   _____ B. UAP job description
   _____ C. Hospital policy for delegation of duties
   _____ D. LPN job descriptions

2. If a patient being discharged requires teaching reinforced, the most appropriate caregiver to perform this would be a(n)
   A. unit secretary.
   B. LPN/LVN.
   C. nurse technician.
   D. UAP.

3. When a nurse asks another nurse to observe his or her group of patients while at lunch, and one patient falls out of bed, which nurse is responsible?
   A. The nurse originally assigned to the patient who went to lunch is responsible.
   B. The nurse who was observing the group of patients is responsible.
   C. Neither nurse is responsible.
   D. The action of both nurses will be reviewed.

4. After a patient's blood transfusion is completed, which health care personnel can obtain the vital signs? Select all that apply.
   _____ A. RN
   _____ B. LPN
   _____ C. UAP
   _____ D. New graduate nurse

5. A new graduate nurse is assigned a patient who is a two-day postoperative who has had a colostomy. The patient has an order to have a nasogastric tube inserted immediately. The new graduate has never inserted this type of tube in a patient. How should the new graduate nurse proceed in this situation?
   A. Delegate the task to a UAP.
   B. Read over the procedure, and then insert the tube.
   C. Notify the practitioner of the new graduate's inexperience.
   D. Ask an experienced RN for assistance with the procedure.

6. Which patient is most appropriate to assign to the UAP for basic care on a general medical unit?
   A. Patient with acute peritonitis
   B. Patient with stable congestive heart failure
   C. New postop acute appendectomy patient
   D. Recent head injury patient

7. If a nurse has difficulty completing nursing duties on schedule, a transcultural phenomenon to be considered is
   A. biological variations.
   B. time.
   C. space.
   D. social organization.

8. The charge nurse working with an RN, an LPN, and a UAP is very busy with the group of patients on the unit. One patient's intravenous line has just infiltrated, a practitioner is on the phone waiting for a nurse's response, a patient wants to be discharged, and the UAP has just reported an elevated temperature on a new surgical patient. Who should be assigned to restart the intravenous line?
   A. LPN
   B. UAP
   C. RN
   D. Charge nurse

9. Which patient will you delegate to the LPN?
   A. The patient who has a fleet enema ordered.
   B. The patient who needs to be started on a twenty-four-hour urine collection.
   C. The patient who is elderly and needs help with frequent ambulation.
   D. The patient who is two days post-op and needs an abdominal wound irrigation and dressing change every shift.

REVIEW ACTIVITIES

1. Have you had any clinical opportunities to delegate duties? Identify to whom and what you delegated. Discuss how it affected the patient and your work. What would you do differently next time?

2. Observe delegation procedures at your institution. Is transcultural delegation considered? If so, which phenomena have you observed?

3. You are caring for a new patient in Room 2510. You are trying to decide whether to delegate his care to UAP Jill or to UAP Penny. Use the Decision Grid below to decide.

Decision Grid

	Certified	Easy to work with?	Do their fair share?	Other?
Jill				
Penny				

4. Review the job descriptions of UAP and RNs in the institution in which you are having your clinical rotation. Compare the job descriptions. Do the job descriptions identify what the UAP can do? What the RN can do?

5. Discuss with a UAP and an RN regarding their preparation in regard to delegation. How much education or training has each of them received? How long ago did they receive it? What type of education or training did they receive? Is the RN familiar with the five rights of delegation and the delegation tree? How is the education of the RN and the training of the UAP different?

EXPLORING THE WEB

■ Log on to *www.aacn.org*
Click on Public Policy and find the advisory team member of your state. Note what policies, if any, consider delegation of care to UAP and LPNs.

■ Log on to *www.nursingworld.org*,
the American Nurses Association (ANA) site, to view safety and quality of care issues.

■ Visit *www.njssna.org*
to read about how school nurses in the state of New Jersey delegate patient care.

■ Visit the *www.aasa.dshs.wa.gov*
Website for delegation classes offered by the Aging and Disability Service Administration of the state of Washington.

REFERENCES

American Association of Critical Care Nurses (AACN). (2004). *AACN Delegation Handbook*. Aliso Viejo, CA: Author.

American Nurses Association (ANA). (1996). *Registered professional nurses and unlicensed assistive personnel*. (2nd ed.). Washington, DC: Author.

ANA. (2005). *Principles for Delegation*. Silver Spring, MD: Author.

Benner, P., Tanner, C. A., & Chesla, C. A. (1996). *Expertise in nursing practice: Caring clinical judgement and ethics*. New York City, NY: Springer Publishing Company.

Boucher, M. A. (1998). Delegation alert. *American Journal of Nursing, 98*(2), 26–32.

Franck, P., & Price, M. (1980). *Nursing Management* (2nd ed.). NCSBN: New York.

Hansten, R. I., & Washburn, M. J. (2004). *Clinical Delegation Skills*. (3rd ed.). Boston: Jones and Bartlett.

Johnson, S. H. (1996). Teaching Nursing Delegation: Analyzing Nurse Practice Acts. *The Journal of Continuing Education in Nursing, 27*(2), 52–58.

Kelly-Heidenthal, P., & Marthaler, M. (2005). Delegation of Nursing Care. In P. Kelly-Heidenthal, *Nursing Leadership and Management*. Clifton Park, NY: Thomson Delmar Learning.

National Council of State Boards of Nursing (NCSBN). (1995). *Delegation: Concepts and decision making process*. Chicago: Author.

NCSBN. (1997). Five rights of delegation. Retrieved from http://www.ncsbn.org/fiverights.pdf.

NCSBN. (2004). Working with others: *NCLEX-RN Test Plan*. A Position paper. Chicago: Author.

Nightingale, F. (1859). *Notes on nursing: What it is and what it is not.* London: Harrison & Sons.

Parkman, C. A. (1996). Delegation: Are you doing it right? *American Journal of Nursing, 96*(9), 46–48.

Poole, V., Davidhizar, R., & Giger, J. (1995). Delegating to a transcultural team. *Nursing-Management, 26*(8), 33–34.

Quallich, S. A. (2005). A bond of trust: Delegation. *Urological Nursing, 25*(2), 120–123.

Timm, S. E. (2003). Effectively delegating nursing activities in home care. *Home Healthcare Nurse, 21*(4), 260–265.

Westfall, P. (1998). Nurse attorney organization makes UAP recommendation. *Insight, 7*(2).

Wiseman, R. (2004). *The Luck factor: Changing your luck, changing your life—The four essential principles*. Orlands, FL: Miramax Books.

Zimmermann, P. G. (1996, June). Delegating to assistive personnel. *Journal of Emergency Nursing, 22*(3), 206–212.

SUGGESTED READINGS

ANA. (2004). *Nursing: Scope and standards of practice*. Washington, DC: Author.

Ballard, K. A. (2003). Patient Safety: A shared responsibility. *Online Journal of Issues in Nursing, 8*(3), 105–118.

Burns, H. (2004). Patient safety: Developing policies for engagement in the prevention of harm to patients. *Journal of Professional Nursing, 20*(1), 4, 75.

Cohen, S. (2004). Delegating vs. dumping: Teach the difference. *Nursing Management, 35*(10), 14–15.

Crawford, L. (2004). Nurses educated in other countries: Coming to America. *Journal of Nursing Administration Healthcare Law, Ethics, and Regulation, 6*(3), 66–68.

Dumpel, H. (2005). Contemporary issues facing international nurses. *California Nurse, 18–22.*

Hansten, R., & Washburn (1992). Delegation: How to deliver care through others. *American Journal of Nursing, 92*(8), 87–88, 90.

Hanston, R. I. (2005), Relationship and results-oriented health care. *Journal of Nursing Administration, 35*(12), 522–524.

Ireland, A. M., DePalma, J. A., Arneson, L., Stark, L., & Williamson, J. (2004). The oncology nursing society ambulatory office nurse survey. *Oncology Nursing Forum, 31*(6), 147–156.

Jones, A. (2003). Changes in practice at the nurse-doctor interface. Using focus groups to explore the perceptions of first level nurses working in an acute care setting. *Journal of Clinical Nursing, 12,* 124–131.

Kleinman, C. (2004). Leadership strategies in reducing staff nurse role conflict. *Journal of Nursing Administration, 34*(7/8), 322–324.

McIntosh, J. (2003). Questions we should ask about community nursing practice. *Primary Health Care Research and Development, 4,* 137–145.

Mikos, C. A. (2004). Beware the consequences of license relinquishment. *Nursing Management, 35*(10), 16–17.

Nurses Board of South Australia. (2004). *Standards: Delegation by a registered nurse or midwife to an unregulated healthcare worker.* Unpublished manuscript (available at www.ncsbn.org).

O'Keefe, C. (Jan/Feb, 2005). State laws and regulations for dialysis: An overview. *Nephrology Nursing Journal, 32*(1), 31–37.

O'Rourke, M. W. (2003). Rebuilding a professional practice model: The return of role-based practice accountability. *Nursing Administration Quarterly, 27*(2), 95.

Potter, P., & Grant, E. (2004). Understanding RN and unlicensed assistive personnel working relationships in designing care delivery strategies. *Journal of Nursing Administration, 34*(1), 19–25.

Rowe, A. R., Savigny, D., Lanata, C., & Victora, C. G. (2005). How can we achieve and maintain high-quality performance of health workers in low-resource settings? *Lancet, 366,* 1026–1035.

Stiehl, R. (2004). Quality Assurance requirements for contract/agency nurses. *Journal of Nursing Administration Healthcare Law, Ethics, and Regulation, 6*(3), 69–74.

Ulrich, B. (1992). *Leadership and management according to Florence Nightingale.* Norwalk, CT: Appleton & Lange.

Whitman, M. (2005). Return and Report. *American Journal of Nursing, 105*(3), 97.

Williams, J. K. & Cooksey, M. M. (2004). Navigating the difficulties of delegation. *Nursing, 34*(9), 12.

CHAPTER 17

Organization of Patient Care

Kathleen F. Sellers, PhD, RN

The object of shared governance is to build a structure that supports the point of care delivery, and the patient, and sustains ownership and accountability there (Tim Porter-O'Grady, 1995).

OBJECTIVES

Upon completion of this chapter, the reader should be able to:

1. Relate the organization of patient care.
2. Identify elements of strategic planning—philosophy, mission, vision.
3. Distinguish a model of nursing shared governance.
4. Differentiate among Benner's concepts of novice, advanced beginner, competent, proficient, and expert nursing practice.
5. Illustrate accountability-based nursing practice.
6. Identify measures of a unit's performance.

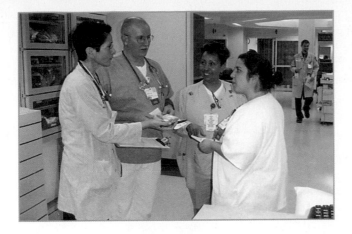

The patient care manager of an acute care surgical unit has been informed that there are plans to merge that unit with an ambulatory surgery unit that currently cares for patients requiring 24-hour observation. As a visionary with a great depth of experience, the patient care manager has been recommended to oversee the development of the new work unit. The institution believes the creation of this new unit will enhance revenue, staff productivity, and continuity of patient care. Therefore, resources are available to design and staff the new work unit in a manner that is congruent with the institution's mission with the understanding that the investment will bring added value to the organization.

What are your reactions as a new nurse on this unit?

What unit structures and patient care processes need to be put in place?

What committees and/or work teams would you get involved with so that you will have a voice in creating this new work environment?

What care delivery system would you like to practice within?

How will you ensure your competency and continued professional growth on this new unit?

Organization of patient care is the coordination of resources and clinical processes that promote patient care delivery. Coordination of resources, clinical processes, and, therefore, care delivery occurs through senior, middle, and front-line staff nurse-management levels. Regardless of the level, organization of patient care management utilizes the nursing process to assess, plan, implement, and evaluate the outcomes of care for populations of patients. The organization of patient care management is akin to conducting a large orchestra. Like the conductor, the patient care manager's primary function is to lead or coordinate a team of diverse individuals with varied talents and expertise toward a common goal (MacGregor–Burns, 1979). The orchestra creates beautiful music. The patient care team provides an outcome of quality, cost-effective patient care.

Successful organization of patient care management requires governance structures, patient care delivery processes, and measures of the outcomes of care delivery. These must be consistent with the mission and vision of the organization and are built on a philosophy of professional practice. The organization of patient care management is built on the tenets of professional nursing practice and requires a structure of shared decision making or shared governance between nursing management and clinical nursing staff. Such a framework creates an environment in which the processes of patient care delivery demand an accountability-based system where staff are able to report, explain, and justify their actions. In such an environment, the outcomes of care delivery, clinical quality, access, service, and cost can regularly be evaluated and staff can continue to grow.

UNIT STRATEGIC PLANNING

Strategic planning is a process designed to achieve goals in dynamic, competitive environments through the allocation of resources.

ASSESSMENT OF EXTERNAL AND INTERNAL ENVIRONMENT

As outlined in Figure 17-1, strategic planning involves clarifying the organization's philosophical values or what is important to the organization; identifying the mission of why the organization exists; articulating a vision statement of what the organization wants to be; and then conducting an environmental assessment, or SWOT analysis, which examines the Strengths, Weaknesses, Opportunities, and Threats of the organization. This information provides data that then drive the development of three- to five-year strategies for the organization. Tactics are then created and prioritized. Finally, goals and objectives are concretized into annual operating work plans for the organization, which can be measured. This same process is used for unit or departmental strategic planning. In developing a strategic plan, unit staff must also examine their organization's mission, vision, strategic plan, and annual operating plans. Unit strategic plans should be congruent with and support the mission and vision of the organizational system of which they are a part. Therefore, communication with the nurse executive who is responsible for the unit is a key step.

DEVELOPMENT OF A PHILOSOPHY

A **philosophy** is a statement of beliefs based on core values—inner forces that give us purpose (Raphael,

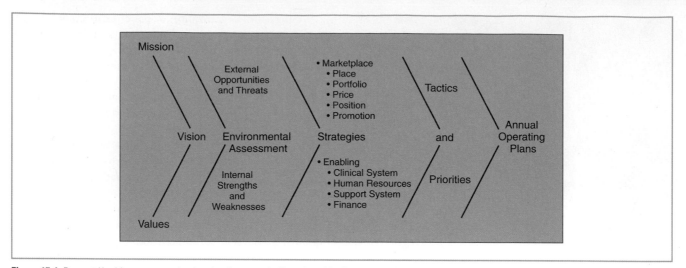

Figure 17-1 Bassett Healthcare strategic planning framework. (Developed by Gennaro J. Vasile, PhD, FACHE.)

REAL WORLD INTERVIEW

At our academic health science center, leaders in the organization, board members who represent the community, and customer stakeholders develop the strategic plan. After the strategic plan is developed, it is published and reviewed at a centerwide management meeting. It is then reviewed in divisional meetings and presented to staff through unit staff meetings. This is where the voice of the chief nursing officer has the most impact. I essentially interpret the rationale for the corporate strategic plan to my staff and glean their reactions. I then communicate the staff's feedback to the corporate level.

Articles are also published in our organizational newsletter for all staff describing the plan and addressing points of clarification. Each division and department then undertakes the process of developing divisional and department plans that support the strategic plan. For example, in the strategic plan a few years ago, it was articulated that our academic center would become a major cardiac center with a state-of-the-art cardiac catheterization laboratory. The department of cardiac services then included development of a state-of-the-art cardiac catheterization laboratory into its plan.

Anne L. Bernat, RN, MSN, CNAA
Chief Nursing Officer
Arlington, Virginia

1994). A unit's mission and vision are most authentic if they are developed based on the philosophy or core beliefs of the staff work team (Wesorick, Shiparski, Troseth, & Wyngarden, 1998). Core beliefs may be complex as those expressed in Table 17-1. Or they can be short statements developed from a staff brainstorming session, such as "patient centered," "partnering," "healing environment," and the like. A unit's core beliefs or values are then incorporated into the unit's mission and vision statements.

MISSION STATEMENT

A **mission** is a call to live out something that matters or is meaningful (Wesorick et al., 1998). An organization's mission reflects the purpose and direction of the health care agency or a department within it, that is, why the agency exists.

Covey (1997) states, "An organizational mission statement—one that truly reflects the shared vision and values of everyone within that organization—creates a unity and tremendous commitment" (p. 139). For the

TABLE 17-1	**CORE BELIEFS**

- Quality exists where shared purpose, vision, values, and partnerships are lived.

- Each person has the right to health care, which promotes wholeness in body, mind, and spirit.

- Each person is accountable to communicate and integrate his or her contribution to health care.

- Partnerships are essential to plan, coordinate, integrate, and deliver health care across the continuum.

- Continuing to learn and think in different ways is essential to improve health.

- A healthy culture begins with each person and is enhanced through self-work, partnerships, and systems supports.

Source: From "Mission and Core Beliefs," by B. Wesorick, *CPMRC Connections . . . for Continuous Learning,* December 2000, 3, p. 3.

The Bassett Nursing Association is a diverse group of autonomous, professional nurses committed to patients, their families, the Bassett and larger community, and each other. We strive for nursing and patient care excellence based on a solid foundation of professional standards, multidisciplinary teamwork, ongoing education, and evidence.

Figure 17-2 The Bassett Nursing Association's mission. (Courtesy of Connie Jastremski, MS, RN, VP Nursing and Patient Care Services, Bassett Healthcare.)

unit mission statement to have the greatest effect, all members of the unit staff should participate in its development.

Questions to be answered by the group charged with development of the unit mission include the following:

- What do we stand for?
- What principles or values are we willing to defend?
- Who are we here to help?

A mission statement reflects why the unit exists. It provides a clear view of what it is trying to accomplish. It indicates what is unique about the care that is provided (www.csuchico.edu).

Mission statements are often so broad that many nursing units adopt the nursing department's mission statement shown in Figure 17-2, which is based on the overall organization mission statement.

VISION STATEMENT

The unit vision statement reflects the organization's vision of what the organization wants to be.

Following are four elements of a vision:

1. It is written down.
2. It is written in present tense, using action words, as though it were already accomplished.
3. It covers a variety of activities and spans broad time frames.
4. It balances the needs of providers, patients, and the environment. This balance anchors the vision to reality (Wesorick et al., 1998).

An environmental assessment of strengths, weaknesses, opportunities and threats (SWOT) to the organization is useful.

GOALS AND OBJECTIVES

The next step in the strategic planning process is to develop broad strategies that span the next three to five years and then develop annual goals and objectives to meet each of these strategies. A **goal** is a specific aim or target that the unit wishes to attain within the time span of one year. An **objective** is the measurable step to be taken to reach a goal. Performance measures of the goals and objectives can be included in a performance improvement plan like the plan illustrated later in this chapter.

THE STRUCTURE OF PROFESSIONAL PRACTICE

In an organization in which professional nursing practice is valued, strategic initiatives are developed and implemented most effectively through a structure of shared

REAL WORLD INTERVIEW

We plan every year, but I'd say we look at our unit philosophy based on our core values and reevaluate the strategic plan every two to three years. We had three core values that guided us, and then this year, with all the external pressures, we added a fourth. We keep these core values in the forefront when we do our annual planning. The process we used to develop and reevaluate the core values was really very powerful and staff driven.

SPAN—Staff Planning Action Network—is our unit-based shared governance organization. SPAN met and developed draft mission and vision statements from our philosophy, which is based on our current core values—patient centered, partnering, and healing environment. They then transcribed these draft statements onto three flip charts, and for 15 minutes per shift, circulated these terms throughout the unit and got staff's reaction and feedback to the statements. Revisions were made from the feedback received. These were then presented at a staff meeting. What was emerging from the feedback was a focus on the need for continuing education and training related to the rapidly changing environment. So we added a fourth value—knowledge.

Pat Roesch, BSN, RN
Patient Care Manager
Cooperstown, New York

governance and shared decision-making between management and clinicians.

SHARED GOVERNANCE

Shared governance is an organizational framework grounded in a philosophy of decentralized leadership that fosters autonomous decision making and professional nursing practice (Porter-O'Grady, Hawkins, & Parker, 1997). Shared governance, by its name, implies the allocation of control, power, or authority (governance) among mutually (shared) interested vested parties (Stichler, 1992).

In most health care settings, the vested parties in nursing fall into two distinct categories: (1) nurses practicing direct patient care such as staff nurses and (2) nurses managing or administering the provision of that care such as managers. In shared governance, a nursing organization's management assumes the responsibility for organizational structure and resources. Management relinquishes control over issues related to clinical practice. In return, staff nurses accept the responsibility and accountability for their professional practice.

Unit-based shared governance structures are most successful if there is an organization-wide structure of nursing shared governance in place that unit-based functions can articulate with. The nursing shared governance structure is most effective if the entire health care system is supported by whole-systems shared governance. In most health care organizations, nursing

shared governance was adopted first as nursing is the largest professional workgroup and practices closest to the point of service delivery, the patient (Porter-O'-Grady, Hawkins, & Parker, 1997). However, the principles of **whole-systems shared governance**, that is, partnership, equity, accountability, and ownership, apply to all professionals practicing in the organization. The principle of partnership connotes horizontal linkages with nursing and other staff roles that are clearly negotiated. With the principle of equity, individual staff roles are based on relationships, not titles. The contributions stemming from staff roles are understood and valued. The principle of accountability comes from within. Individuals are encouraged to report, explain, and justify their actions. This leads to the principle of ownership for the work performed.

Nursing shared governance structures are usually council models that have evolved from preexisting nursing or institutional committees. In a council structure, clearly defined accountabilities for specific elements of professional practice have been delegated to five main arenas: clinical practice, quality, education, research, and management of resources (Porter O'Grady et al., 1997). Figure 17-3 illustrates a shared governance model.

CLINICAL PRACTICE COUNCIL

The purpose of the clinical practice council is to establish the practice standards for the workgroup. Often this

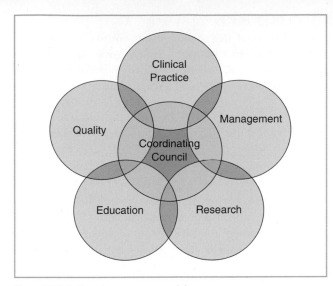

Figure 17-3 A shared governance model.

QUALITY COUNCIL

The purpose of the quality council is twofold: (1) to credential staff and (2) to oversee the unit quality management initiatives. In the role of credentialing staff, this committee is responsible for interviewing potential staff and reviewing their qualifications, or credentials. It then makes recommendations regarding hiring. The quality committee also serves as the body that reviews staff credentials on an ongoing basis and makes recommendations regarding promotion.

Quality management initiatives for which the council is responsible can include review of indicators of the unit's overall clinical performance, such as medication errors, patient falls, family satisfaction, and response time in answering call lights. At times, a unit will also participate in an organizational disease-management study looking at the care of a specific patient population such as patients with diabetes.

council or committee is a unit-level committee that works in conjunction with the organizational committee accountable for determining policy and procedures related to clinical practice. Evidence-based practice fostered by research utilization initiatives ensures that practice standards are developed based on the state of the science of clinical practice and not merely on tradition.

EDUCATION COUNCIL

The purpose of the education council is to assess the learning needs of the unit staff and develop and implement programs to meet these needs. According to Peter Senge (1990), **learning organizations** promote professional practice through the encouragement of personal mastery, an awareness of our mental models, and team

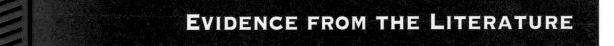

EVIDENCE FROM THE LITERATURE

Citation: Parsons, M. L. (Oct–Dec 2004). Capacity building for magnetism at multiple levels: A healthy workplace intervention, part 1; An emergency department's health workplace process and outcomes part 2. *Topics in Emergency Medicine, 26*(4), 296–304; 287–295.

Discussion: Parsons outlines a theoretical model that guides an intervention to build capacity for magnetism to create healthy workplaces. The theoretical model and intervention address an existing gap. The gap existed between the hospital-wide shared governance organizational level and the nursing unit level. A unit-based capacity-building intervention promoted collaboration and communication, enhancing patient care and workplace empowerment through staff organization and clinical decision making. The intervention was implemented using principles of participatory action research with infrastructure support.

Staff called the phases of the intervention "The Creating Our Future Program." Tangible practice and process improvements resulted from four action planning teams focused on (1) organized patient care, (2) rapid patient disposition, (3) diagnostics, and (4) initiation of care. Outcomes included the elimination of RN vacancies and agency use and improvements in patient and employee satisfaction, including interaction between staff and practitioners. Staff reported feeling empowered to continuously improve the emergency department.

Implications for Practice: A culture of shared governance on a nursing unit facilitates process improvements with outcomes of increased patient and staff satisfaction resulting in enhanced staff retention.

learning. Personal mastery goes beyond competence and skills to include continually clarifying and deepening our personal vision and focusing our energies and developing patience to see reality objectively. Mental models are deeply ingrained assumptions, generalizations, and biases that influence how we understand the world. Mental models influence how we take action. Therefore, the more insight we have into what our mental models are, the more effective we will be at team learning. Team learning is a workgroup's ability to align and develop their collective talents for the purpose of attaining a shared vision (Smith, 2001).

The education council usually works closely with organizational education and training departments. Unit orientation programs and training programs related to new clinical techniques and new equipment are examples of programs sponsored by the education council.

RESEARCH COUNCIL

At the unit level, the research council advances evidence-based practice with the intent of staff incorporating research-based findings into the clinical standards of unit practice. Evidence-based practice involves staff critiquing the available research literature and then making recommendations to the practice council so that clinical policies and procedures can be based on evidence-based research findings. The research council may also coordinate research projects if advanced practice nurses are employed at the institution.

MANAGEMENT COUNCIL

The purpose of the management council is to ensure that the standards of practice and governance agreed upon by unit staff are upheld and that there are adequate resources to deliver patient care. The first-line patient care manager is a standing member of this council. Other members include the assistant nurse managers and the charge or resource nurses from each shift.

COORDINATING COUNCIL

Shared governance structures also include a coordinating council. The purpose of the coordinating council is to facilitate and integrate the activities of the other councils. This council is usually composed of the first-line patient care manager and the chairpeople of the other councils. This council usually facilitates the annual review of the unit mission and vision and develops the annual operational plan (Sellers, 1996).

Unit-based shared governance structures may be less diverse. Often some of the councils are combined into one council, for example, education and research. Or a council may contain subcommittees whose purposes are to perform very specific tasks, for example, credential and promote staff or recruit and retain staff. Unit-based structures are varied, with the primary purpose being to empower staff by fostering professional practice while meeting the needs of the work unit. A shared governance structure and shared decision making among disciplines integrates various functions and thus fosters the organization's patient care management of services (Porter-O'Grady et al., 1997).

CRITICAL THINKING 17-1

As a nurse practicing in a shared governance organization, you remember a decade ago when the organization decentralized, made a commitment to nursing professional practice, and implemented shared governance. Everywhere you went, people were talking about it and displaying posters and other signs of nursing's importance to the organization. That was six years ago, before managed care and all the changes and before this latest nursing shortage. Now you do not hear people talking about it so much. You wonder, does professional practice still exist? How can you tell? How does your organization compare with other organizations that do not have shared governance? Is this an organization that you can be proud to work in? Are you a magnet organization?

ENSURING COMPETENCY AND PROFESSIONAL STAFF DEVELOPMENT

Professional practice through the vehicle of shared governance requires competent staff. Competency is defined as possession of the required skill, knowledge, qualification, or capacity (*Merriam-Webster*, 2005) and is best determined in practice by a group of one's peers. Alspach (1984) defines competency as a determination of an individual's capability to perform to defined expectations (p. 656). Competency of professional staff can be ensured through credentialing processes developed around a clinical or career ladder staff promotion framework. A **clinical ladder** acknowledges that staff members have varying skill sets based on their education and experience. As such, depending on skills and experience, staff members may be rewarded differently and carry differing responsibilities for patient care and the governance and professional practice of the work unit.

BENNER'S NOVICE TO EXPERT

Benner's (1984) **Novice to Expert Model** provides a framework that, when developed into a clinical or career promotion ladder, facilitates professional staff development by building on the skill sets and experience of each practitioner. Benner's model acknowledges that there are tasks, competencies, and outcomes that practitioners can be expected to have acquired based on five levels of experience. Note that the Ten Year Rule states that it takes a decade of heavy labor to master any field (Ross, 2006).

Benner's Novice to Expert model is based on the Dreyfus and Dreyfus (1980) model of skill acquisition applied to nursing. There are five stages of Benner's model: novice, advanced beginner, competent, proficient, and expert. Table 17-2 discusses Benner's model and shows the appropriate application to nursing practice

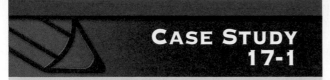

CASE STUDY 17-1

You are a staff nurse who is a member of the credentialing committee of the quality council. A fellow peer has presented his credentials for review in hopes of being promoted to the next level on the clinical ladder. You review the packet and make the recommendation that he be promoted. However, at the credentialing committee meeting, it is revealed that the patient care manager and the individual's preceptor, another member of the committee, have not recommended promotion.

You wonder if your colleague is aware that there were concerns about his performance.

Are there guidelines and standards that you are not aware of that have not been met?

What is the next course of action for the committee?

What should your response be at this meeting?

REAL WORLD INTERVIEW

I'm a new graduate nurse. I understand how tough it is adjusting straight out of school into a "real" job. My fellow new graduates and I did some brainstorming and came up with a couple of things to help make your transition at Bassett an easier one. Here goes!

- Ever wonder where all the Carpujets are? Just when you need to flush an IV, you can't find one anywhere. Guess what, Carpujets are located at the pharmacy! Just give them a call, and they will send you a bunch.
- How about all those tabs on the edge of the charts? It took me two months to find out what they mean on surgery! Red is for STAT orders. Blue is for medicine orders. Yellow alerts the unit clerk. Green alerts the RN.
- How to make your shift run smoother. It's always a good idea to round with the doctors. They know all kinds of information you need to know, and it's a great time to give your input. Collaboration!
- Know what team your patient is on and what doctor is on that specific team and who is coming onto the shift and who is leaving. Nothing is worse than trying to page a doctor before you realize they aren't there! That can be a little embarrassing, not to mention time consuming.
- Words of Wisdom: Write things down, it helps you remember.
- Just one more tidbit. Always bring any documentation and vital information with you to the phone before you page the doctor. Then, you'll have the answers for questions.

I hope that this information will be useful to you.

Christina Denton, RN, Surgery Unit
Bassett Healthcare
Cooperstown, New York

TABLE 17-2	BENNER'S MODEL OF NOVICE TO EXPERT

Stage of Model	Application to Nursing Practice
Novice nurses are recognized as being task oriented and focused on the rules. They need a directing, telling style from a mentor. They tend to see nursing as a list of tasks to do rather than seeing the big picture of patient care needed to meet patient care goals. After novices have mastered most tasks required to perform their ascribed roles, they move on to the phase of advanced beginner.	The novice nurse is educated in techniques associated with delegation. A nurse new to the direct patient care setting may have been educated in principles of delegation, but she has not used them in the clinical setting. These nurses are very task oriented and focused and are often still in orientation. They may delegate tasks clearly outlined by the hospitals, for example, they may ask the unlicensed assistive personnel (UAP) to pass water. They often cannot decide what to delegate. Novices often tend to do all tasks themselves and need a directing, telling style from mentors.
Advanced beginner nurses demonstrate marginally acceptable independent performance. This nurse still focuses on the rules but is more experienced and just needs some coaching. This nurse still needs help identifying priorities.	This nurse is out of orientation, has worked for a short while on the unit, and is able to perform most nursing tasks that are required for patient care. This nurse is becoming more comfortable independently delegating simple tasks to UAP, that is, errands, assisting in positioning of patients, bathing, and taking vital signs. The nurse is often reluctant to delegate to staff whose personality is resistant to delegation. This nurse still needs coaching from a mentor.
Competent nurses have developed the ability to see their actions as part of the long-range goals set for their patients. They lack the speed of the proficient nurse, but they are able to manage most aspects of clinical care.	One to three years in the same role has allowed these nurses to develop the ability to delegate to UAPs and LPNs. They have developed a higher-level of ability to apply the nursing process and use nursing skills. The competent nurse is more able to assess the UAP's abilities, communicate expectations effectively, and gather clinical information from the UAP. The competent nurse is more comfortable communicating and delegating to staff, even in the presence of personality conflicts. This nurse expects that all staff must work to meet the requirements of their job description.
Proficient nurses characteristically perceive the whole situation rather than a series of tasks. They have often been on the job several years and have been delegated total responsibility for their patient's care. They develop a plan of care and then guide the patient from point A to point B. This nurse needs minimal guidance and control and only occasional support from a mentor. They draw on their past experiences and know that in a typical situation, a patient must exhibit specific behaviors to meet specific goals. They realize that if those behaviors are not demonstrated within a certain time frame, then the plan needs to change.	These nurses are often charge nurses developing plans of care for the whole unit. They can see delegation of tasks as an important part of guiding patients from point A to point B. They are able to use past experiences with patients and UAPs to guide the delegation process. They may need a little occasional support from their mentors.
Expert nurses intuitively know what is going on with their patients. Their expertise is so embedded in their practice that they have been heard to say, "There is something wrong with this patient. I'm not sure what is going on, but you had better come and evaluate them." Not heeding the call derived from the intuitive sense of an expert nurse can result in a patient's condition deteriorating with subsequent development of the nurse-sensitive outcome, cardiac arrest. These expert nurses usually seek continuing education.	This nurse intuitively knows what is going on with patients and their needs. They can quickly assess what needs to be delegated. They evaluate the situation continuously.

Source: Developed with information from Benner (1984), Hersey and Blanchard (1993), and Kelly-Heidenthal (2005).

CRITICAL THINKING 17-2

Review the interview from Christina Denton. This was published in the newsletter of Bassett Healthcare's Nursing Association. Christina is functioning as an excellent patient care manager as a new graduate by sharing what she has learned with her peers in a public forum, the newsletter.

How might you contribute to the management and leadership of your organization as a new graduate?

REAL WORLD INTERVIEW

There are five levels of our clinical ladder, which is similar to Benner's Novice to Expert model. The RN novices are the new graduates and people in orientation. The experts are the clinical specialists. A lot of them have also become nurse practitioners so that the organization can receive some reimbursement for their patient care services. This is a good thing because otherwise I'm afraid we wouldn't have these expert nurses anymore. They are the true mentors for nursing staff, especially when you are working with a very complex or difficult patient situation.

Staff nurses also mentor each other. During orientation, your preceptor guides you along the path from RN I to RN II. When you decide you'd like to advance to RN III, you can choose another mentor. RN IIIs provide much more clinical leadership for staff and for the overall unit. I decided I was ready to be promoted to that level when other staff consistently were coming to me for clinical guidance and with patient care questions. Now, as an RN III, I am the chairperson of our unit-credentialing committee, which is part of the quality council of our shared governance model.

Our clinical ladder uses a portfolio as the main tool to evaluate the nurse's readiness to advance. When you are an RN I in orientation, you are first introduced to the idea of a portfolio and how to put it together. It is difficult at first, as people do not know what is expected. However, after that first time when you are promoted from an RN I to an RN II, it becomes easier. You just build on what is already in the portfolio.

A portfolio should include the following:

Licenses
Your resume
Letters of reference
Evaluations
Clinical documentation of patient care
Validations for competencies related to technical skills
　(medication administration, IV therapy)

Examples of participation in development of the team
　plan of care
Exemplars
CEU certificates
Presentations
Publications

The portfolio tells the story of your practice. When a group of people are ready for promotion, the members of the credentialing committee meet. We review the portfolios and make recommendations related to advancement. The nurse manager is a member of this committee. She always reviews the portfolio and gives us her feedback even if she is unable to attend the credentialing meeting. I enjoy reading the exemplars the best. Exemplars are mini stories that paint the pictures of each nurse's practice, and they are all so different.

Stacey Conley, RN, BS
Staff Nurse
Cooperstown, New York

Colorado Differentiated Practice Model

The Colorado Differentiated Practice Model for Nursing has a separate clinical ladder for the six preparatory backgrounds depicted on the conceptual model (Diagram 1). A nurse selects the education clinical ladder according to the nursing credential she or he has attained.

The framework for each educational ladder has four distinct stages. These stages allow nurses to self-pace their advancement. A nurse is placed in a stage according to his or her own competency and experience.

Each nursing ladder has four weighted components as follows:
• Competency Statements 60%   • Institutional Goals 15%
• Skills 10%   • Professional Activities 15%

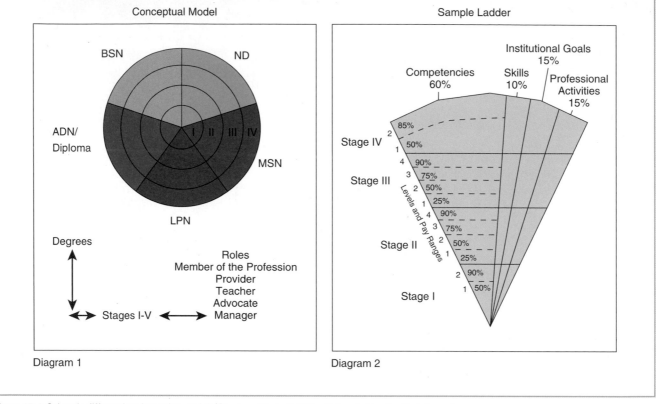

Figure 17-4 Colorado differentiated practice model. (Courtesy Marie E. Miller, Colorado Nursing Task Force.)

that a professional nurse would be expected to perform at each level. Proficiency in completion of these tasks contributes to readiness for promotion along a career ladder. Note that all nurses who care for patients must meet basic criteria for safe care.

The Colorado Differentiated Practice Model (Figure 17-4) builds on the work of Benner (1984) regarding career ladder stages. Stage I is characterized as the entry/learning stage. Stage II is characterized by the individual who competently demonstrates acceptable performance adapting to time and resource constraints. Stage III is characterized by the individual who is proficient. And stage IV is characterized by the individual who is an expert. The stages in this model are specifically defined by behaviors that are consistently exhibited or practiced over a defined period of time.

THE PROCESS OF PROFESSIONAL PRACTICE

Ongoing professional staff development is part of the regular performance feedback that staff can expect to receive from the patient care manager or the credentialing committee. However all patient care managers provide ongoing professional development of staff in their daily

REAL WORLD INTERVIEW

I have a particularly touching story to tell you. D.T. was a 44 year-old man who was admitted from our ear, nose, and throat clinic with a large mass at the base of his tongue. Upon arrival on the unit, the patient appeared very anxious, not knowing what he would face in the next few days. The patient and his wife had been told that he would end up having a tracheostomy placed. This was quite a shock to their systems. They were both feeling overwhelmed with the situation.

As it happened, I was present for every major event that occurred with this family during that admission. I can recall the day when the patient was told that the mass was cancerous. He and his family were devastated. I went in to talk with the family and proceeded to tell them I could not begin to imagine what they must be going through, but that if they needed to talk, I was a good listener. I could tell that they very much appreciated that.

During the next few days, the family began to accept what was going on, and we began working together to teach them all they needed to know about tracheostomies and how to care for them. D.T. and his wife learned quickly how to be independent with tracheostomy care. In the coming days, the patient underwent a feeding tube placement so that he could get some nutrition. I taught him and his wife how to care for the feeding tube and how to hang tube feedings. They learned so quickly that toward the end of the hospital stay, they were doing all his care independently. The patient was informed that he would need to undergo radiation and chemotherapy. In preparation for the treatment, the patient needed to have a complete dental extraction. Considering all that D.T. and his wife went through in such a short amount of time, they both responded quite well to the situation.

Upon discharge, I set the patient up with Lifeline (an emergency response service), nursing services, and equipment for the tracheostomy and tube feedings. This was no easy task because they did not have much money and their insurance company was quite difficult to deal with. As their primary nurse, I literally spent days on the phone in preparation for their discharge. It was quite challenging but rewarding when all was accomplished. It was both a happy and a sad day when the patient and his wife were discharged. Since the patient has left, I have kept in touch through writing, and in person when he has been readmitted to the medical floor for his chemotherapy treatment. I am glad to report that thus far D.T. is doing well.

This was a particularly touching experience for me. This family was very special to me, and I am glad for the opportunity I had to get to know them and be a special part of their lives. As an unknown author says, in the end, we will not remember the years we spent nursing, we will only remember the moments.

Stacey Conley, RN, BS
Staff Nurse
Cooperstown, New York

interactions on the unit by identifying projects and activities that meet a staff member's readiness for leadership development and advancement.

SITUATIONAL LEADERSHIP

The leadership framework developed by Hersey and Blanchard (1993), when combined with an individual's position on a clinical/career ladder, is useful to a patient care manager in discerning the best approach to take in developing the potential of staff members. **Situational leadership** maintains that there is no one best leadership style, but rather that effective leadership lies in matching the appropriate leadership style to the individual's or group's level of task-relevant readiness. Readiness is how able and motivated an individual is to perform a particular task. A basic assumption of situational leadership is the idea that a leader should help followers grow in their readiness to perform new tasks as far as they are able and willing to go. This development of followers is accomplished by adjusting leadership behavior through four styles along the leadership continuum: directing, coaching, supporting, and delegating (Figure 17-5).

According to Hersey and Blanchard's (1993) leadership framework, individuals with low leadership readiness, such as novice nurses, require a directing, telling style on the part of the mentor initially. They need strong direction if they are to be successful and productive. For example, if a patient requires a new IV line to be started,

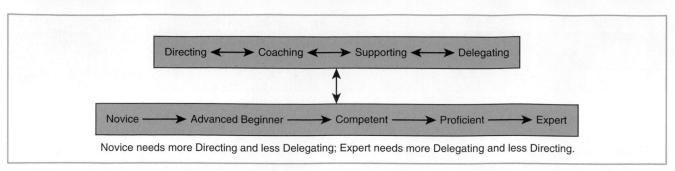

Figure 17-5 Leadership continuum. (Compiled with information from Hersey and Blanchard (1993) and Benner (1984).

REAL WORLD INTERVIEW

I am an acute care inpatient case manager. I'm a member of an interdisciplinary patient care team. My role is multifaceted, with three broad areas of responsibility: utilization management, variance tracking, and complex discharge planning. Utilization management is the process of monitoring the usage of inpatient resources. The hospital purchases nationally developed criteria. These criteria set the standards for admission and continued inpatient stays. Many of the insurance companies use the same or similar criteria. Every admission is reviewed to determine whether or not the patient met the criteria to be admitted. Concurrent reviews are done to determine if the continued stay criteria is being met. I also meet daily with the team to review each patient. We discuss the patient's current health care status, the plans for the day, and attempt to project tentative discharge dates. After three years, many of the doctors have learned the value of these meetings. By taking 15 to 20 minutes each morning to meet and discuss our patients, we have decreased the length of stay and have developed a forum to discuss potential utilization concerns. Many of the insurance companies call daily to get clinical information on their clients. I spend much of my day talking with them, attempting to justify why the patient requires inpatient care. Some of the companies can be nitpicky and cost driven.

The reviews and daily rounds are important to the variance tracking I do. I attempt to identify delays in service, unnecessary usage of inpatient resources, and ways to improve outcomes. The variance data will help the hospital identify ways to improve how they do business.

In the hospital where I work, the primary or staff nurse is responsible for the development of the patients' discharge plan. They will develop this plan with the patient and arrange for equipment, transportation, and home care services. During the patient's stay, if it is determined that the patient has more complex needs, I will become involved in the discharge arrangements. Sometimes my involvement will be to get needed equipment or services approved by the third-party payer. I have spent hours on the phone with the insurers, advocating for patients with complex needs, then spent time convincing the patient's physician to write letters of justification for the care that they deem necessary. Once I successfully got approval for a bariatric lift for a 600-pound woman who was bed bound. This lift enabled her to go home with her family and avoid nursing home placement.

In addition to assisting with complex home discharges, I also work with patients that have needs such as posthospital rehabilitation or skilled nursing facility placement. With the help of the other members of the team, I am able to present the options to the patient and their family. Together we discuss the options, how these options are paid for, and arrange for their placement in a rehabilitation or a skilled nursing facility.

I enjoy my role as case manager. It has evolved a great deal in the three years I've been in this position. I look forward to its continued development.

Cynthia Whispell, BSN, RN
Nursing Case Manager
Cooperstown, New York

the mentor should inform the novice that this needs to be done and then review the steps required to start the new line using the evidenced-based clinical practice standard followed on that unit. This allows the novice to ask questions and obtain guidance. This enhances the likelihood that the task will be performed correctly the first time, improving patient satisfaction and self-confidence in the novice.

As the professional nurse grows in leadership readiness, the mentor should shift to a coaching style where staff are rewarded with increased relationship behavior, that is, positive reinforcement and socioemotional support. Then, when individuals reach higher levels of leadership readiness, as a proficient or expert nurse, the mentor should respond by decreasing control. The mentor moves first to a participatory, supportive style characterized by a high-quality working relationship with the proficient staff and a lower need to give task direction. The mentor then moves to a style of more complete delegation, communicating a sense of confidence and trust. Highly competent individuals respond best to this greater freedom.

Individuals' readiness to learn and accept new tasks may change for a variety of reasons. When patient care managers discern a change, they must readjust their style of interaction with the nurse—moving forward or backward through the leadership continuum from directing to coaching to supporting to delegating, and provide the appropriate level of support and direction to facilitate that individual's continued development, productivity, and success as a member of the patient care team. Development of professional staff based on their innate readiness to accept new tasks and responsibilities facilitates their promotion along a continuum of novice to expert and ensures a patient care team that is able to consistently deliver accountability-based patient care.

ACCOUNTABILITY-BASED CARE DELIVERY

Accountability-based care delivery is essential in today's value-driven workplace. Accountability-based care delivery systems focus on roles, their relationship to the work to be

CASE STUDY 17-2

You are a staff nurse working as part of the interdisciplinary orthopedic team. You notice that there are an increasing number of diabetic patients being admitted for elective total hip surgery. Because the length of stay is so short and your team has such a surgical focus in caring for patients, their underlying chronic diseases have not been a focus on the unit. However, you are aware that the larger organization is beginning to evaluate how different populations of patients, such as diabetics, are cared for across the continuum of care.

What should you do to improve care for your patients?

done, and the outcomes they are intended to achieve. In a professional context, accountability includes the exercise of activities inherent to a role that cannot and are not legitimately controlled outside the role. Competence, in accountability-based approaches to work, is evidenced not by what a person brings to the work, but instead by the results of the application of the person's skills to the work (Porter-O'Grady, 1995). Individuals who are accountable, by definition, are able to report, explain, or justify their actions (*Merriam-Webster*, 2005) (Table 17-3).

MEASURABLE QUALITY OUTCOMES

An important component of organizational patient care management is regular evaluation of a work unit's performance to ensure that the outcomes of care delivery are meeting the objectives of professional practice as outlined in the unit's annual operational plan. The development

TABLE 17-3	**ELEMENTS OF ACCOUNTABILITY-BASED CARE DELIVERY**
■ Accountability is about outcomes, not processes. ■ Accountability is individually defined.	■ Accountability is inherent in the role, not delegated. ■ Accountability is the foundation for evaluation. (Porter-O'Grady, 1995)

2005 PERFORMANCE IMPROVEMENT PLAN

As part of Bassett's commitment to quality, the Surgical Unit will strive to improve performance through a cycle of planning, process design, performance measurement, assessment and improvement. There will be ongoing assessment of important aspects of care and service and correction of identified problems. Problem identification and solution will be carried out using a systematic intra- and interdepartmental approach organized around patient flow or other key functions, and in concert with the approved visions and strategies of the organization. Priorities for improvement will include high risk, high volume and problem-prone procedures.

The Surgical Unit will:

- Promote the Plan-Do-Check-Act methodology for all performance improvement activities
- Provide staff education and training on integrated quality and cost improvement
- Collect data to support objective assessment of processes and contribute to problem resolution

In identifying important aspects of care and service, the Surgical Unit will select performance measures in the following operational categories:

A. Clinical Quality
1. Patient safety

- Patient falls
- Indicator: # of patient falls per month/# of patient days with upper control limits set by the research department based on statistical deviation

- Medication and IV errors
- Indicator: # of patient IV/medication errors per month/# of patient days with upper control limits set by the research department based on statistical deviation

- Restraint use
- Indicator: % of compliance with policy for use of restraints and overall rate of restraint use

2. Pressure ulcer prevention
- Indicator: Rates of occurrence-quarterly tracking report

3. Surveillance, prevention and control of infection
- Indicator: Infection control statistical report of wound and catheter associated infections
- Indicator: Quarterly monitoring of compliance with standards for Acid Fast Bacilli (AFB) room use; evidence of staff validation in AFB practice

4. Employee safety
- Injuries resulting from
- Back and lifting-related injuries
- Morbidly obese patients
- Orthopedic patients
- Indicators: # of injuries sustained by employees and any resultant workmen's compensation (Human Resources quarterly report)
- 100% competency validation in lifting techniques and back injury prevention
- Respiratory fit testing
- Indicator: competency record of each employee

5. Documentation by exception
Indicators:
- 100% validation of RN/LPN staff
- Monthly chart audit (10% average daily census or 20 charts) meeting compliance with established standards

B. Access:
- Maintenance of the 30 minute standard for bed assignment of ED admissions
- Indicator: Quarterly review of ED tracking record

C. Service:
Patient Satisfaction
Indicator: Patient Satisfaction Survey: 90% or above response to, "Would return", and "Would recommend"

D. Cost:
- Nursing staff productivity will remain at 110% of target of 8.5 worked hours per adjusted patient day within a maximum variance range of 10%

For each of the above performance measures, this performance improvement plan will:

- Address the highest priority improvement issues
- Require data collection according to the structure, procedure and frequency defined
- Document a baseline for performance
- Demonstrate internal comparisons trended over time
- Demonstrate external benchmark comparisons trended over time
- Document areas identified for improvement
- Demonstrate that changes have been made to address improvement
- Demonstrate evaluation of these changes; document that improvement has occurred or, if not, that a different approach has been taken to address the issue

The Inpatient Surgical Unit will submit biannual status reports to the Bassett Improvement Council (BIC) through the Medical Surgical Quality Improvement Council (MSQIC).

Approved by:_____ Date:_____

(Chief or Vice President)

Figure 17-6 Inpatient surgical unit, 2005 Performance Improvement Plan. (Courtesy Patricia Roesch, BS, RN, Bassett Healthcare.)

of process improvement measures in today's health care organizations is driven by the multiple domains of quality required by the Joint Commission (JC), formerly known as the Joint Commission on Accreditation of Healthcare Organizations (JCAHO), (www.jointcommission.org) and the National Council for Quality Assurance (NCQA) (www.ncqa.org), the credentialing organization that certifies managed care organizations.

UNIT-BASED PERFORMANCE IMPROVEMENT

To develop a comprehensive unit-based quality improvement program to meet the requirements of today's competitive, value-driven health care system, outcomes should be tracked from four domains: access, service, cost, and clinical quality. These outcomes reflect the unit's goals and objectives. See Figure 17-6 for the inpatient surgical unit 2005 performance improvement plan.

Outcomes of unit quality improvement programs can be succinctly displayed using the Quality Compass (Nelson, Mohr, Batalden, & Plume, 1996). The Bassett Quality Compass in Figure 17-7 measures quality from four domains: functional status, clinical outcomes, cost and utilization, and patient satisfaction. This Quality Compass depicts the outcomes of an organization-wide disease management asthma study prior to an asthma disease management intervention. The Compass tells us that functionally 30% of the population has moderately severe asthma and that the majority of asthmatics have little documented teaching in use of a peak flow meter or metered-dose inhalers (MDIs), which is the current standard of care. More than 30% of the patient visits for asthma are urgent visits, indicating that a large portion of the asthma population will benefit from the disease management intervention of increased patient teaching and development of individual specific asthma care plans.

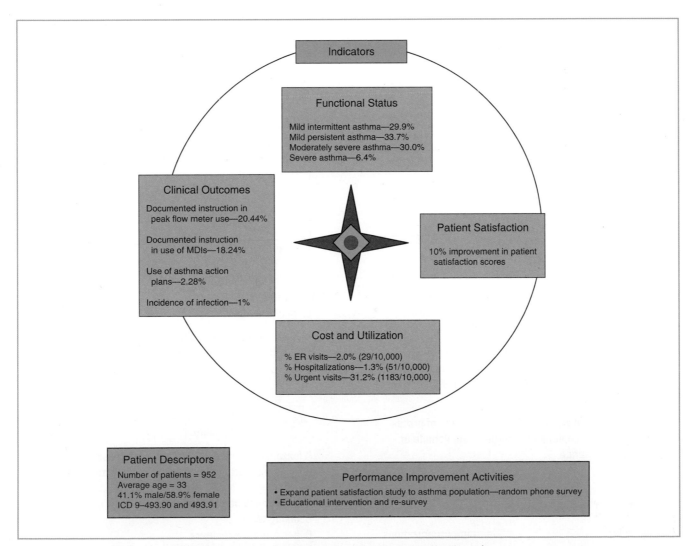

Figure 17-7 Bassett Healthcare quality compass. (Courtesy Kathleen F. Sellers, PhD, RN, Bassett Healthcare.)

The Quality Compass provides a framework to guide the development of a unit-based quality improvement program and provides a tool with which to present the outcomes of quality improvement in the succinct visual format of an executive summary.

Patient care managers are the fundamental operations people in the health care system. Successful orchestration of a patient care area in today's health care system is achieved through vision-driven professional practice. Implementing this vision is achieved through a governance structure of shared decision making, an accountability-based patient care delivery system, and regular evaluation of performance based on the tenets of performance improvement.

KEY CONCEPTS

- Successful orchestration of patient care in today's health care environment is achieved through vision-driven professional practice.

- Strategic planning is a process that is designed to achieve goals in dynamic, competitive environments through the allocation of resources.

- Shared governance is an organizational framework grounded in a philosophy of decentralized leadership that fosters autonomous decision making and professional nursing practice.

- Benner's model of novice to expert provides a framework that facilitates professional staff development.

- Situational leadership maintains that there is no one best leadership style but rather that effective leadership lies in matching the appropriate leadership style to the individual's or group's level of task-relevant readiness.

- Individuals who are accountable are, by definition, able to report, explain, or justify their actions.

- Accountability-based care delivery systems include primary nursing, patient-focused care, and case management.

- A comprehensive unit-based quality improvement program should include outcomes that are tracked from four domains: access, service, cost, and clinical quality.

- Organization of patient care management is the coordination of resources and clinical processes that promote service delivery.

- A learning organization supports the tenets of professional practice implemented through the vehicle of shared governance.

KEY TERMS

clinical ladder
goal

learning organizations
mission

novice to expert model
objective
philosophy
shared governance

situational leadership
strategic planning
whole-systems shared
  governance

REVIEW QUESTIONS

1. Shared governance is
   A. an accountability-based care delivery system.
   B. a tested framework of organizational development.
   C. a competency-based career promotion system.
   D. an allocation of control, power, or authority among mutually interested vested parties.

2. The five levels of a clinical promotion ladder built on Benner's theoretical framework include all of the following except:
   A. Proficient
   B. Competent
   C. Orientee
   D. Expert

3. The principles of whole-systems shared governance include
   A. partnership.
   B. equity.
   C. accountability.
   D. ownership.
   E. all of the above.

4. In developing a unit-based performance improvement plan, which of the following areas should be considered? Select all that apply.
   _____ A. Service
   _____ B. Cost
   _____ C. Access
   _____ D. Clinical quality

5. A learning organization promotes professional practice through encouragement of personal mastery, team learning, and
   A. awareness of our mental models.
   B. taking tests.
   C. performance reviews.
   D. mandatory education.

REVIEW ACTIVITIES

1. You have been asked by your organization to participate on a performance improvement team looking at care of the diabetic patient. What areas other than clinical quality will you evaluate? Identify indicators for each area to measure.

2. You have been practicing now for three years. This summer, you have been precepting a new graduate. He is having difficulty mastering changing a sterile dressing. You must give him feedback. You are uncertain on how to do this most effectively and wonder if you are part of the reason he is having difficulty. Review situational leadership. At what level of readiness is this new graduate? Has your leadership style been appropriate for that level of experience and motivation?

3. You have been practicing as a new graduate for a little over a year. You are feeling more confident about your clinical practice and think you might want to expand your leadership experience. Your unit governance framework is shared governance. Review the common councils of shared governance. Given your education and experience, which council would you like to join?

EXPLORING THE WEB

■ You have been asked by your nurse manager and members of the credentialing committee to revamp the current clinical promotion ladder so that it more clearly differentiates and rewards nurses for their education level as well as expertise. Go to *www.uchsc.edu*

Note what the University of Colorado's Clinical Ladder incorporates.

■ Go to the Magnet Hospitals site, and see if there is information that would help your organization foster professional nursing practice. Striving for magnet hospital designation increases an organization's capability to recruit and retain nurses.
www.ana.org

■ Go to *www.nursingsociety.org*
This site provides weekly literature updates from Sigma Theta Tau International, the nursing profession's honor society. What new books and periodicals are available that may be helpful to you in your practice?

■ Go to *www.vitalsmarts.com*
Access your style under stress. Enhanced insight allows for improved personal mastery and effectiveness as a patient care manager, whether you are leading others or communicating with peers.

REFERENCES

Alspach, J. (1984). Designing a competency-based orientation for critical care nurses. *Heart and Lung, 13,* 655–662.

Benner, P. (1984). *From novice to expert.* Menlo Park, CA: Addison-Wesley.

California State University School of Management. (2006). *Developing a Vision & Mission.* Retrieved August 23, 2006, from http://www.csuchico.edu/mgmt/strategy/module1/sld008.htm

Covey, S. R. (1997). *The seven habits of highly effective people.* New York: Simon & Schuster.

Denton, C. (September, 2002). TIPS from TINA. *Nursing Matters, 9*(3), 4.

Dreyfus, S. E., & Dreyfus, H. L. (1980). *A five stage model of the mental activities involved in directed skill acquisition.* Unpublished report supported by the Air Force Office of Scientific Research (AFSC), USAF (Contract F49620-79-C-0063), University of California at Berkeley.

Hersey, R. E., & Blanchard, T. (1993). *Management of organizational behavior.* Riverside, NJ: Simon & Schuster.

Joint Commission (2007). Comprehensive accreditation manual for hospitals. Chicago: Joint Commission. The Official Handbook. Retrieved from http://www.jointcommission.org

Kelly-Heidenthal, P. (2005). Essentials of Nursing Leadership and Management. Clifton Park, NY: Thomson Delmar Learning.

MacGregor–Burns, J. (1979). *Leadership.* New York: Harper & Row.

Merriam-Webster. (2005). Merriam-Webster's online dictionary. Retrieved March 26, 2006, from http://www.m-w.com

Nelson, E., Mohr, J. J., Batalden, P. B., & Plume, S. K. (1996, April). Improving health care, part 1: The clinical value compass. *Joint Commission Journal on Quality Improvement, 22*(4), 243–258.

Parsons, M. L. (2004, Oct.–Dec.). Capacity building for magnetism at multiple levels: A healthy workplace intervention, part 1. *Topics in Emergency Medicine, 26*(4), 296–304; 287–295.

Parsons, M. L., Cornett, P. A., Sewell, S., & Wilson, R. W. (2004, Oct–Dec). Capacity building for magnetism at multiple levels: A healthy workplace intervention; An emergency department's health workplace process and outcomes part 2. *Topics in Emergency Medicine, 26*(4), 296–304; 287–295.

Porter-O'Grady, T. (1992). *Implementing shared governance creating a professional organization.* St. Louis, MO: Mosby-Year Book, Inc.

Porter-O'Grady, T. (1995). *The leadership revolution in health care.* Gaithersburg, MD: Aspen Publishers, Inc.

Porter-O'Grady, T., Hawkins, M. A., & Parker, M. L. (1997). Whole-systems shared governance. Gaithersburg, MD: Aspen Publishers, Inc.

Raphael, D. D. (1994). Moral philosophy (2nd ed.). New York: Oxford University Press.

Roesch, P. (2000, Oct.). Surgical unit practice. *Nursing Matters, 7*(3), 1. Bassett Healthcare, Cooperstown, New York.

Ross, P. E. (2006, August). The expert mind. *The Scientific American, 8,* 64–71.

Sellers, K. F. (1996). The meaning of autonomous nursing practice to staff nurses in a shared governance organization: A hermeneutical analysis. Unpublished doctoral dissertation, Adelphi University, Garden City, New York.

Senge, P. (1990). *The fifth discipline.* New York: Doubleday.

Smith, M. K. (2001). Peter Senge and the learning organization: The encyclopedia of informal educaton. Retrieved March 26, 2006, from http://www.infed.org/thinkers/senge.htm

Stichler, J. F. (1992). A conceptual basis for shared governance. In N. D. Como & B. Pocta (Eds.), *Implementing shared governance: Creating a professional oranization* (pp. 1–24). St. Louis, MO: Mosby.

Wesorick, B. (2006). The way of respect in the workplace. Retrieved August 22, 2006, from http://www.cpmnc.com

Wesorick, B. (2000, Dec). Mission and core beliefs. *CPMRC connections . . . for continuous learning, 3,* 3.

Wesorick, B., Shiparski, L., Troseth, M., & Wyngarden, K. (1998). *Partnership council field book.* Grandville, MI: Practice Field Publishing.

Zander, K. (1995). *Managing outcomes through collaborative care: The application of care mapping and case management.* Chicago: American Hospital.

SUGGESTED READINGS

Bradford, R. J. (2003). From survival to success: It takes more than theory. *Nursing Administration Quarterly, 27*(2), 106–119.

Doyle, V., & Turkie, W. (2006). Transforming the organization of care. *Nursing Management—UK, 13*(2), 18–21.

Institute of Medicine. (2006). *Keeping patients safe: Transforming the work environment of nurses.* Retrieved August 21, 2006, from http://www.iom.edu/Default.aspx?id=16173

Personality Pathways. (2006). *Introduction to type.* Retrieved August 22, 2006, from http://www.personalitypathways.com/MBTI_intro

Porter-O'Grady, T. (2003). A different age for leadership part 2: New rules, new roles. *Journal of Nursing Administration, 33*(3), 173–178.

Scott, L., & Caress, A. (2005). Shared governance and shared leadership: Meeting the challenges of implementation. *Journal of Nursing Management, 13*(1), 4–12.

Thompson, P., Navarra, M., & Anderson, N. (2005). Patient safety: The four domains of nursing leadership. *Nursing Economics, 23*(6), 331–333.

Tracey, C., & Nicholl, H. (2006). Mentoring and networking. *Nursing Management—UK, 12*(10), 28–32.

Turkel, M. (2004). Magnet status: Assessing, pursuing, and achieving nursing excellence. *Journal of Nursing Administration, 29*(2), 14–20.

Wesorick, B. (2006). *Clinical practice model resource center.* Retrieved August 22, 2006, from http://www.cpmrc.com

Wheeler-Harbaugh, J. (2003). Strategic planning: Drafting your roadmap to success. *Gastroenterology Nursing, 26*(3), 93–95.

Wolf, G. (2003). Coming of age in health care: Changes, challenges, choices. *Reflections on Nursing Leadership, 29*(4), 32–34.

Zemke, R., et al. (2000). Generations at work: Managing the clash of veterans, boomers, xers, and nexters in the workplace. New York: AMA.COM.

CHAPTER
18

Time Management and Setting Patient Care Priorities

Patsy Maloney, RN, BC, EdD, MSN, MA, CNAA

Time is the coin of your life. It is the only coin you have, and only you can determine how it will be spent (Carl Sandberg).

OBJECTIVES

Upon completion of this chapter, the reader should be able to:

1. Apply principles of priority setting to patient care situations.
2. Apply time management strategies to the reality of delivering effective nursing care.
3. Relate time management strategies to enhance personal productivity.

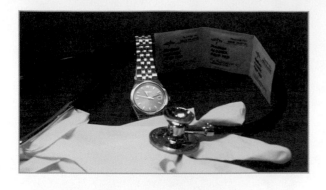

Inez has just completed her medical-surgical orientation as a new graduate registered nurse. This evening is her first solo shift, but she is frightened and feels like she is holding up the world on her new graduate shoulders. Although she feels that all rests on her, she is not really alone. Inez and Carole, the other RN, are responsible for 12 possible patients on this section of the unit along with one certified nursing assistant. Currently, there are 10 patients in this section, but a new admission is on the way, another patient is returning from surgery, the dinner trays are arriving, and Inez has medications to pass. Just as the dinner trays arrive, a patient's family member runs out to Inez and states that her mom is confused and incontinent, and has pulled out her IV.

What would you do if you were Inez?

What would you do first?

Many nurses become nurses out of idealism. They want to help people by meeting all their needs. Unfortunately, most new graduates find it impossible to meet all or even most of their patients' needs. Needs tend to be unlimited, whereas time is limited. In addition to the direct patient care responsibilities, there are shift responsibilities, charting, practitioner's orders to be transcribed or checked, medication supplies to be restocked, and reports to be given.

New graduates often go home feeling totally inadequate. They wake up remembering what they did not accomplish. One young nurse shared with tears in her eyes that once, when she answered a call bell late in her shift, the patient requested a pain medication. She went to the narcotics cabinet to get the medication but was interrupted by an emergent situation. When she arrived home, she was so exhausted that she fell asleep rapidly, only to awaken with the realization that she had not returned with her patient's medication. Her guilt was tremendous. She had gone into nursing to relieve pain, not to ignore it.

Time management allows the novice nurse to prioritize care, decide on outcomes, and perform the most important interventions first. Time management skills are important not just for nurses on the job but for nurses in their personal lives as well. They allow nurses to make time for fun, friends, exercise, and professional development.

GENERAL TIME MANAGEMENT CONCEPTS

Time management has been defined as "a set of related common-sense skills that helps you use your time in the most effective and productive way possible" (Mind Tools, 2006a, p. 1). Another way to say this is that time management allows us to achieve more with available time. Three valuable time management concepts to master are the relative effectiveness of effort (the Pareto Principle), the importance of outcome versus process orientation, and the value of analyzing how time is currently being used. It is important to analyze and manage time to achieve key outcomes effectively and efficiently.

THE PARETO PRINCIPLE

Time management requires a shift from wasting time on the process of being busy to organizing time to achieve desired outcomes and get things done. Often times, a busy frenzy of activity is reinforced with sympathy and assistance. Too often, this frenzied behavior is accomplishing very little because it is not directed at the right outcome. The **Pareto Principle** states that 20% of focused effort results in 80% of outcome results, or conversely that 80% of unfocused effort results in 20% of outcome results (Figure 18-1).

Pareto's Principle, named after Vilfredo Pareto, was invoked by the Total Quality Management (TQM) movement and now is reemerging as a strategy for balancing life and work through prioritization of effort (Reh, 2002). Effective time management requires that a shift is made from doing unfocused activities that require 80% of time for achieving 20% of desired results to doing planned and focused activities that use only 20% of time or input to achieve 80% of desired outcomes. It is important to analyze how your time is being used to manage time and achieve desired outcomes.

If time management achieves more outcomes, why do so many people continue at a crazy, hurried pace? There are several possible explanations for this. They do not know about time management, they think they do not have time to plan, they do not want to stop to plan, or they love crises (Mind Tools, 2006a).

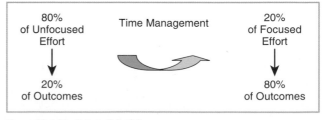

Figure 18-1 The Pareto Principle.

OUTCOME ORIENTATION

With the Pareto Principle in mind, it is important to recognize that more is achieved through an outcome orientation than through an emphasis on the process of task completion. Long-term goals must be determined. It is best to break long-term goals down into achievable outcomes that are the steps toward long-term goals. Long-term goals cannot be achieved overnight. Long-term goals and outcomes should be written down in a planner or in a personal data assistant (PDA). Even though these goals are written, they should remain flexible. Flexibility should be built into any outcome orientation. There may come a time when the outcome may no longer be realistic or should be shifted to a more realistic goal as circumstance changes (Reed & Pettigrew, 2006).

TIME ANALYSIS

Another time management concept is analysis of time to effectively use it. Nurses cannot possibly know how to better plan time without knowing how they currently use it. When keeping track of time, it is important to consider the value of a nurse's time as well as the use of the time.

VALUING NURSING TIME

Nurses often undervalue their time. Consider salary and benefits. Benefits are frequently forgotten, but they raise employer costs by 15% to 30% of salary. If a nurse is making $26.00 an hour, benefits add $3.90 to $7.25 to the hourly cost of a nurse's time. The value of nursing time in this example, excluding what the organization is paying in workman's compensation and payroll taxes, is $29.90 to $33.25 an hour. The organization has also invested in nurse recruitment, orientation, and development, which easily can exceed $20,000 per nurse. Nursing time is an expensive commodity. Keeping this in mind when considering what tasks can be delegated to personnel who receive less compensation, or when considering what tasks are busy work and do not support achieving an outcome, is invaluable.

USE OF TIME

Numerous studies have shown how nurses use their time. Most studies have been done on acute care nurses because they comprise the majority of nurses. Only 30% to 35% of nursing time is spent on direct patient care (Scharf, 1997). Twenty-five percent of a nurse's time is spent on charting and reporting, and the remainder of time is spent on admission and discharge procedures, professional communication, personal time, and providing care that could be provided by unlicensed personnel, such as transportation and housekeeping (Upenieks, 1998). Urden and Roode (1997) summarized various work sampling studies to show that RNs spend 28% to 33% of time on direct patient care, defined as activities performed in the presence of the patient or family;

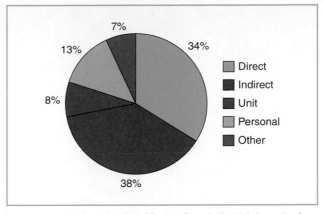

Figure 18-2 Use of nursing time. (*Source:* Compiled with information from "Patterns of nursing: A review of nursing in a large metropolitan hospital" by M. Fitzgerald, A. Pearson, K. Walsh, L. Long, and N. Heinrich, 2003, *Journal of Clinical Nursing, 12*(3), 326–332.)

42% to 45% of time on indirect care activities, which include all activities done for an individual patient but not in the patient's presence; 15% on unit-related activities, which include all unit general maintenance activities; and 13% to 20% on personal activities, which include activities that are not related to patient care or unit maintenance. Fitzgerald, Pearson, Walsh, Long, and Heinrich (2003) found a similar distribution to previous studies—34% of nursing time was spent giving direct care; 38% in indirect support activities to include documentation, obtaining supplies, and professional communication; 8% on unit activities—cleaning and tidying; 7% on other activities such as looking for other personnel, equipment, and professional reading; and 13% personal time for breaks, personal conversations, and reading (Figure 18-2).

Given such a distribution of nurses' time, shifting the use of time could have a major impact on outcomes. If nonnursing activities could be performed by nonnursing personnel instead of nurses, more time could be redirected toward essential nursing responsibilities.

How do you use your time? Memory and self-reporting of time have been found to be unreliable. Nurses are often unaware of the time spent socializing with colleagues, making and drinking coffee, snacking, and other nonproductive time. Self-reporting of time is not recommended for estimating the total number of activities or the average time an activity takes to complete (Pelletier & Duffield, 2003).

An **activity log** is a time management tool that can assist the nurse in determining how time is used. The activity log (Table 18-1) should be used for several days. Behavior should not be modified while keeping the log. The nurse should record every activity, from the beginning of the shift until the end, as well as periodically note feelings while doing the activities—alert, energetic, tired, bored, and so on. Review of this log will illuminate time use as well as time wasted. Analysis of the log will allow

TABLE 18-1   WORK ACTIVITY LOG

Time	Name of Activity (Medication administration, vital signs, bed-making, patient transport, and so on)	Time Required and Feelings (Energetic, bored, and so on)	Could be better done by someone else? Who? (LPN, nursing assistant, housekeeper, and so on)	Toward what outcome achievement? (Increase in patient's functional status, prevention of complication, and so on)
0500				
0530				
0600				
0630				
0700				
0730				
0800				
0830				
0900				
0930				
1000				
1030				
1100				
1130				
1200				
1230				
1300				
1330				
1400				
1430				
1500				
1530				
1600				
1630				
1700				
1730				
1800				
1830				
1900				
1930				
2000				
2030				
2100				
2130				
2200				

the separation of essential professional activities from activities that can be performed by someone else (Grohar-Murray & DiCroce, 2003; Sullivan & Decker, 2004).

PRIORITIZING USE OF TIME

To plan effective use of time, nurses must understand the big picture, decide on desired outcomes, and do first things first.

UNDERSTAND THE BIG PICTURE

Before priorities are set, the big picture must be examined. No nurse works in isolation. Nurses should know what is expected of their coworkers, what is happening on the other shifts, and what is happening beyond the unit. If nurses know what is expected of their coworkers, they can offer assistance during coworkers' busy times and in turn receive assistance during their own busy times. If the previous shift was stressed by a crisis, a shift may not get started as smoothly (Hansten & Jackson, 2004). If areas outside of the unit are overwhelmed, someone might be moved from one unit to assist on the overwhelmed unit elsewhere in the hospital. When nurses take the big picture into consideration, they are less likely to be frustrated when asked to assist others on their unit or others on other units in the hospital. They can also build into their time management plan the possibility of giving and receiving assistance.

DECIDE ON OPTIMAL DESIRED OUTCOMES

When nurses begin their shifts, they need to decide what outcomes can be achieved. **Desired optimal outcomes** are the best possible objectives to be achieved given the resources at hand.

As nurses decide on desired optimal outcomes, they must consider what can and should be achieved given less-than-optimal circumstances and limited resources. These circumstances could include a rough start to a busy shift; personnel late, absent, or uncooperative; and a patient crisis. It is hard for nurses to give themselves permission to do less-than-optimal work, but sometimes achievement of these outcomes is the best that can be expected. These outcomes should be achieved given less-than-optimal circumstances and limited resources.

DO FIRST THINGS FIRST

To decide what is reasonable to accomplish, a nurse has to come to terms with the resources that are available and the outcomes that must be achieved. If someone has called in sick and no replacement is available, it might be unreasonable for a nurse to plan to reinforce teaching or discuss the home environment with a patient scheduled to leave the next day. However, there would be no question that interventions that prevent life-threatening emergencies or save a life when a life-threatening event occurs are priorities. They must be done no matter how short the staffing. It is imperative that nurses protect their patients and maintain both patient and staff safety as well as perform the activities essential to the nursing and medical care plans (Hansten & Jackson, 2004).

FIRST PRIORITY: LIFE-THREATENING OR POTENTIALLY LIFE-THREATENING CONDITIONS

Life-threatening conditions include patients at risk to themselves or others and patients whose vital signs and level of consciousness indicates potential for respiratory or circulatory collapse (Hansten & Jackson, 2004). A patient whose condition is life threatening is the highest priority and requires monitoring until transfer or stabilization. Life-threatening conditions can occur at any time during the shift and may or may not be anticipated.

A quick guide to assessing life-threatening emergencies is as simple as ABC. A stands for Airway. Is the airway open and patent or in danger of closing? This is the highest priority of care. B stands for Breathing. Is there respiratory distress? C stands for circulation. Is there any circulatory compromise? This is a way of prioritizing actions. Although there is clearly an order of importance, ABC is often assessed simultaneously while observing the patient's general appearance and level of consciousness (Figure 18-3 and Table 18-2). Patients with life-threatening conditions usually have an IV access line and receive continuous monitoring of their cardiac rhythm, blood pressure, pulse, respiration, and oxygen saturation level. Their temperature and urinary output is monitored closely as well.

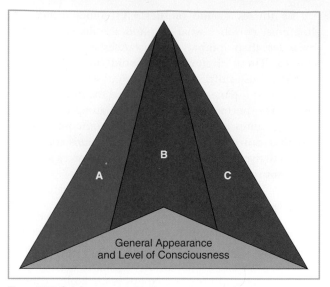

General Appearance
and Level of Consciousness

Figure 18-3 Quick assessment tool.

SECOND PRIORITY: ACTIVITIES ESSENTIAL TO SAFETY

Activities that are essential to safety are very important and include those responsibilities that ensure the availability of life-saving monitoring, medications, and equipment, and that protect patients from infections and falls. They include asking for assistance or providing assistance during two-people transfers, or turning and movement of heavy patients (Hansten & Jackson, 2004). They also include monitoring the patient for the prevention of nurse-sensitive outcomes.

THIRD PRIORITY: ACTIVITIES ESSENTIAL TO THE PLAN OF CARE

Activities that are essential to the plan of care lead to the outcomes that relieve symptoms and/or lead to healing. They are the activities that, if omitted, will hinder the patient's recovery. These essential activities include those

TABLE 18-2	TOP PRIORITY PATIENTS WITH POTENTIAL THREATS TO THEIR ABCs
Respiratory Patients	■ Airway compromise
	■ Choking
	■ Asthma
	■ Chest trauma
Cardiovascular Patients	■ Cardiac arrest
	■ Shock
	■ Hemorrhage
Neurological Patients	■ Major head injury
	■ Unconscious
	■ Unresponsive
	■ Seizures
Other Patients	■ Major trauma
	■ Traumatic amputation
	■ Major burn, especially if airway involvement
	■ Abdominal trauma
	■ Vaginal bleeding
	■ Anaphylaxis
	■ Diabetic with altered consciousness
	■ Septic shock
	■ Child or elder abuse

Source: Compiled with information from the *Canadian Pediatric Triage and Acuity Scale: Implementation Guidelines for Emergency Departments.* Retrieved October 20, 2003, from www.caep.ca.

that relieve symptoms—pain, nausea, and so on, and those that promote healing, such as nutrition, ambulation, positioning, and medication administration (Figure 18-4).

Covey, Merrill, and Merrill (1994) developed another way of setting priorities. Activities are classified as urgent or not urgent, as important or not important. If an activity is neither important nor urgent, then it becomes the lowest priority (Figure 18-5).

Some activities that are often thought of as important may not be. Sometimes laboratory data, vital signs, and intake and outputs are ordered to be monitored more frequently than the status of the patient indicates. Frequent monitoring of these parameters may make no significant difference in patient outcomes. When nurses begin their shifts, they should question the activities that make no difference in outcomes (Hansten & Jackson, 2004). If a practitioner orders these activities, a nurse should work to get the order changed. If there is a nursing order that does not make a difference, the nurse should change it. Nurses should give priority to the activities that they know are going to make a difference in patient outcomes.

APPLICATION OF TIME MANAGEMENT STRATEGIES TO THE DELIVERY OF CARE

After priorities are set, nurses know which are the most important activities to accomplish first. Time management strategies can be used in all areas of care delivery to maximize the effectiveness of the nurse's time and minimize lost time and efforts.

ESTIMATE ACTIVITY TIME CONSUMPTION

Nurses need to estimate how much time each activity will take and plan accordingly. The previously discussed activity log may help estimate how much time many activities will take. Perhaps a patient tends to need more time for medication administration than other patients do, so the wise nurse will save the patients medication administration until last. By estimating the time of activities, nurses can schedule the best time to perform activities. Nurses may notice when passing 6 P.M. medications that water pitchers are empty and juice cups dry. Scheduling the nursing assistant to fill water pitchers and pass refreshments prior to medication administration will be a prudent response to such an observation.

CREATE AN ENVIRONMENT SUPPORTIVE OF TIME MANAGEMENT AND PATIENT CARE

Often in the frenzy of giving care, nurses forget the obvious. Where are the linens, supplies, medications, and so on located? Are there optimal locations? Is stocking things a priority in order to make them available? Do nurses really stop and think before going to a patient's room with pain medications or for a treatment?

How many trips does one treatment take? It should take only one trip, but if a nurse hurries in and leaves something at the nurse's station, then the nurse will have to return to retrieve it. How many times do nurses count

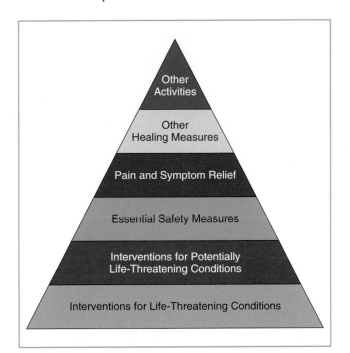

Figure 18-4 Prioritization triangle.

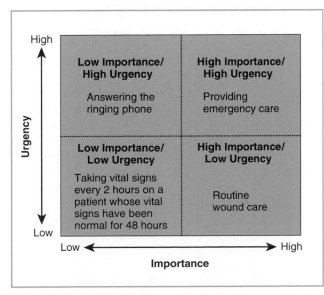

Figure 18-5 Determining priorities.

EVIDENCE FROM THE LITERATURE

Citation: Benner, P. (1984). *From novice to expert: Excellence and power in clinical nursing practice* (pp. 151–161). Menlo Park, CA: Addison-Wesley.

Discussion: Patricia Benner's work is a classic. It addresses issues faced by beginning nurses who struggle with time management issues and explains how expert nurses deal with time management using contingency planning.

Benner's study of how nurses cope with staffing shortages found that nurses who continuously respond to the challenge of each situation frequently end up feeling that they fail to meet their patients' needs in a timely manner. They lack two important sources of job satisfaction—interpersonal connection and a sense of accomplishment and competency that comes from meeting patients' needs when they need it. Nurses who work successfully and who consistently deal with a heavy workload develop a system of contingency planning that allows them to meet their patients' needs in a timely manner. This contingency planning includes rapidly assessing patient needs and setting and shifting priorities. They continuously evaluate routine standards and procedures. Standard priorities include attending to radically abnormal vital signs, signs and symptoms of respiratory or circulatory compromise, intravenous medications running dry, and intravenous medication administration. But even these priorities can be shifted when a patient on the unit actually is in a crisis. Expert nurses learn to anticipate and prevent periods of extreme workload within a shift.

Implications for Practice: This study emphasizes the importance of new nursing graduates learning to prioritize care and finding the human connection and a sense of competency and accomplishment in their work. Benner quotes a nurse who left nursing because of the lack of time to truly care for his patients. Often nurses leave practice before they develop time management skills that allow them to prioritize care and develop shift contingency plans.

narcotics that have not been used in months? These are simple things that take time. The nurse should give consideration to all aspects of the unit environment and get together with coworkers to make a difference. Are specialty carts such as those for intravenous infusion, isolation, laboratory collections, wound care, and so on needed to become more efficient and effective?

UTILIZE SHIFT HANDOFF REPORT

Prior to making a plan for the shift of duty, the end of shift handoff report at best can lead to an efficient, effective, and safe start to the shift. At worst, it can leave the oncoming shift with inadequate or old data on which to base their plan. The Joint Commission (JC) included a standardized approach to shift handoff communication as one of its patient safety goals for 2006 (Kirkpatrick, 2006). So the day of haphazard shift handoff reporting will soon end. There are several ways to conduct an end of shift handoff report—a face-to-face meeting, audiotaping, and walking rounds (Table 18-3).

Whether the report is conducted face to face, via audiotape, or through walking rounds, information has to be transmitted and time must be provided for questions and answers. A procedure that allows time for both transmission of information and for questions and answers

facilitates safe, effective, and efficient care. If the outgoing nurse fails to cover all pertinent points, the oncoming shift must ask for the appropriate information. See Table 18-4 for a tool for taking and giving shift handoff reports.

FORMULATE THE SHIFT ACTION PLAN

Having received pertinent information from the shift report, nurses can consider the big picture; decide on optimal and reasonable outcomes; and set priorities based on life-threatening conditions, safety considerations, and activities essential to safety and the plan of care. The nurse can then formulate a **shift action plan**, a written plan that sets the priorities for the accomplishment of shift outcomes that are both optimal and reasonable (Table 18-5).

This plan needs to be written so that all team members are aware of it. Such a plan works for a variety of patient populations and allows professional nurses to do the real work of nursing instead of concentrating on tasks (Hansten & Jackson, 2004).

The shift action plan must be clearly based on priorities set at the beginning of the shift with built-in flexibility

TABLE 18-3	METHODS OF END-OF-SHIFT HANDOFF REPORT: ADVANTAGES AND DISADVANTAGES

Method	Advantages	Disadvantages
Face-to-face report	■ Nurses get clarification and can ask questions. ■ Nurse giving report has actual audience and tends to be less mechanical. ■ Nurses are more likely to give pertinent information than they would give to a tape recorder.	■ It is time consuming. ■ It is easy to get sidetracked and gossip or discuss nonpatient-related business. ■ Both oncoming and departing nurses are in report. ■ Patients are not included in planning.
Audiotaped report	■ Report is brief due to lack of interruptions by questions and comments. ■ Departing shift tapes report for oncoming shift prior to arrival of new shift workers. ■ Previous shift can provide care while oncoming shift gets report.	■ Variables in the taping process such as the quality of tape and machine, the clarity and diction of the nurse who is recording, and the hearing of the oncoming shift can interfere with the communication. ■ It is difficult to get questions answered. The nurse must find the caregiver after report to ask questions. ■ Information is taped earlier in the shift and may no longer be accurate. ■ There is sometimes not enough information given due to the tendency of the person talking into the tape recorder to read from kardex instead of explaining about patient.
Walking rounds	■ Provides the prior shift and incoming shift staff the opportunity to observe the patient while receiving report. Staff can address any assessment or treatment questions. ■ Information is accurate and timely. ■ Patient is included in the planning and evaluation of care. ■ Accountability of outgoing care provider is promoted. ■ Patient views the continuity of care. ■ Incoming shift makes initial nursing rounds. ■ Departing nurse can show assessment and treatment data directly to oncoming nurse.	■ It is time consuming. ■ There is a lack of privacy in discussing patient information.

TABLE 18-4	TOOL FOR END-OF-SHIFT HANDOFF REPORT

		Notes
Demographics	■ Room number ■ Patient Name ■ Sex ■ Age ■ Practitioner	
Diagnoses	■ Primary ■ Secondary ■ Nursing ■ Medical ■ Surgery Date	
Patient status	■ Do Not Resuscitate (DNR) status ■ Current vital signs ■ Problem with ABCs, level of consciousness, or safety ■ Oxygen saturation ■ Pain score ■ Skin condition ■ Ambulation ■ Fall risk ■ Suicide risk ■ Presence/absence of signs & symptoms of potential complications ■ New orders/changes in treatment plan	
Fluids/tubes/ oxygen Laboratory tests and treatments	■ IV fluid, rate, site ■ Tube feedings—type of tube, solution, rate, and toleration ■ Oxygen rate, route, other tubes, e.g., chest tube, NG tube, foley, and so on, type and drainage ■ Abnormal lab and test values ■ Labs and tests to be done on oncoming shift ■ Treatments done on your shift, include dressing changes (times, wound description) and procedures ■ Identify treatments to be done during next shift	
Expected shift outcomes	■ Priority outcomes for one or two nursing diagnoses ■ Patient learning outcomes	

(Continues)

TABLE 18-4	TOOL FOR END-OF-SHIFT HANDOFF REPORT (CONTINUED)

		Notes
Plans for discharge	■ Expected date of discharge ■ Referrals needed ■ Progress toward self-care and readiness for home	
Care support	■ Availability of family or friends to assist in ADL/IADL (activities of daily living/instrumental activities of daily living)	
Priority interventions	■ Interventions that must be done this shift	

TABLE 18-5	SHIFT ACTION PLAN

Concern	**Considerations**
Plan: What is the big picture?	How many patients? Any staffing issues? Any environmental concerns?
What are the desired outcomes?	If everything goes well and as expected, what does the nurse hope to accomplish? If unexpected setbacks occur, what can the nurse, staff, and patients really accomplish?
What are the priorities?	Who is at greatest risk for potential life-threatening complications? Has all emergency equipment been checked? Are patients who are at a high risk for falls or suicide identified and measures taken? Who are the patients suffering from significant symptoms—airway, breathing, circulation?
Intervene: What are the parts to be accomplished?	Monitoring? Medication administration? Treatments? Teaching? Counseling? Physical and functional care? Unit support, e.g., stocking, maintenance?
Who is available to do the work, and what skills and attributes do the personnel have?	RN? LPN? UAP?
What can the RN do? What about the LPN? What can the UAP do?	RN teaches, counsels, supervises all nursing care. LPN can do medication administration and treatments. UAP can complete physical care such as bathing, performing oral care, and obtaining vital signs. Assign and delegate accordingly.

(Continues)

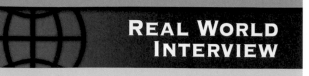

calls to make while driving can be a dangerous practice unless the car is equipped with a hands-free phone.

Sometimes it is important just to sit back and enjoy the scenery or the company. Time management princi-ples aim at creating more enjoyable time, not filling every moment with chores.

CONTROL UNWANTED DISTRACTIONS

Personal life is not immune from distractions that get in the way of accomplishing personal goals. These may include such distractions as visitors, unplanned phone calls, low priority tasks, and requests for assistance (Table 18-7 and Table 18-8).

FIND PERSONAL TIME FOR LIFELONG LEARNING

Finding time for lifelong learning is a struggle for recent graduates and even more-seasoned nurses.

There are ways to achieve your dreams and work, and have a personal life. Flaherty (1998) offers tips for balancing school, family, and work in Table 18-9.

Returning to school is certainly a challenge, but with time management skills, the return to school can result in the accomplishment of personal outcomes, a degree, and new knowledge.

TABLE 18-7	**STRATEGIES FOR AVOIDING PERSONAL TIME DISTRACTIONS**
Distraction	**Strategies**
Casual visitors	Make your environment less inviting. Remain standing. Remove your visitor chair. Keep a pen in your hand.
Unplanned phone calls	Use an answering machine or voice mail. Consider a humorous message. Set a time to return calls.
Unwanted/ low-priority jobs	Say no to jobs that have little value or in which you have little interest. Leave low-priority tasks undone.
	If an unwanted job must be done, pay or ask for assistance.
Requests for assistance	Encourage others to be more independent.
	Give them encouragement but send them back to complete the job. Decisions to help should be conscious decisions, not drop-in distractions.
Clutter	Clear your work area of clutter, and keep it clean. Organize your work area, and take a few minutes at the end of your shift to prepare your area for the next shift.
Interruptions	Open your mail over the garbage can. Respond, delegate, or throw it out. Organize your papers. Keep your notebooks, calendar, and phone lists in one three ring binder, so you have your essentials together.
Procrastination	Break a task down into manageable segments, and return to it again and again until it is complete.
Perfectionism	Become a pursuer of excellence, not a perfectionist as you pursue your goals (Table 18-8).

TABLE 18-8	BEHAVIORS OF PERFECTIONISTS VS. PURSUERS OF EXCELLENCE

Perfectionists

- Hate criticism
- Are devastated by failure
- Get depressed and give up
- Reach for impossible goals
- Value themselves for what they do
- Have to win to maintain high self-esteem
- Can only live with being number one
- Remember mistakes and dwell on them

Pursuers of Excellence

- Welcome criticism
- Learn from failure
- Experience disappointment but keep going
- Enjoy meeting high standards within reach
- Value themselves for who they are
- Do not have to win to maintain high self-esteem
- Are pleased with knowing they did their best
- Correct mistakes, and then learn from them

Source: Courtesy of White L. (2000). *Critical Thinking in Practical/Vocational Nursing.* Clifton Park, NY: Thomson Delmar Learning.

TABLE 18-9	PERSONAL TIME MANAGEMENT WHEN RETURNING TO SCHOOL

- Let your employer know that you are interested in returning to school. Most employers are supportive of additional education and will be flexible with your schedule. But they will continue to expect a competent, dedicated employee.
- Develop computer skills. By using a computer, you can e-mail professors and classmates at any time. You can do online research. You can easily incorporate constructive criticisms into papers and build on previous work. Technology is the working student's friend.
- Discover a flexible, educational program. Many programs offer several classes in a row on a single day, offer weekend and night classes, or offer immersion classes for a week at a time. Some programs offer distance-learning opportunities.
- Do not be surprised by the demands of school. Courses will be difficult and demanding of time. Remember that you have faced difficult demands and challenges before. Use the same techniques that helped you in the past, and develop some new ones.
- Solicit support from family and friends. They may offer emotional support, financial assistance, household assistance, child care, and so forth.
- Use all available resources at the school and at work. Develop mentors and role models. Establish relationships with faculty. Discover and use academic support services such as writing centers and tutors. Read syllabi and course instructions carefully.
- Focus on the outcome. Keep the end in sight and do not give up. Take it one course at a time. Reward yourself along the way. When a course is completed, celebrate.
- Be careful of the sacrifices. You may replace some hobbies with school. But save some time for the things that are really meaningful to you and your family.
- Manage time. Ten minutes spent on planning saves time and energy later. Keep your sense of humor.
- Take care of yourself and your responsibilities. Set aside a day to take care of personal chores and errands.
- If you need a break, take one. Take time to reflect on what you are accomplishing. If you are feeling overwhelmed, take only one course or take a semester off.
- Study on the run. Taping lectures and listening to them as you commute is a great way to study on the run.

Source: Developed with information from Flaherty, M. (1998). "The juggling act: Ten tips for balancing work, school, and family." *Nurseweek.* Retrieved on March 5, 2006, from http://www.nurseweek.com/features/98-5/juggle.html.

KEY CONCEPTS

- General time management strategies include an outcome orientation, analysis of time cost and use, focus on priorities, and visualizing the big picture.

- Shift planning begins with developing both optimal and reasonable outcomes.

- Priority setting takes into account what is life threatening or potentially life threatening, what is essential to safety, and what is essential to the plan of care.

- The shift action plan assigns activities aimed at outcome achievement within a time frame.

- There are three alternative methods for end-of-shift handoff report: face-to-face meeting, audiotaped report, and walking rounds.

- The shift action plan is evaluated at the end of the shift by asking if optimal or reasonable outcomes have been achieved.

- Time wasters that might interfere with outcome achievement include procrastination, inability to delegate, inability to say no, management by crisis, haste, indecisiveness, interruptions, socialization, complaining, perfectionism, and disorganization.

- Time management applies to personal life as well as the job.

- Quality time can be achieved by analyzing time use and energy patterns.

- Delegation and getting up one hour earlier can create time.

- Additional time can be found by productive use of travel time and waiting time.

- Distractions can be controlled by making your environment less inviting, by using voice mail or an answering machine, by saying no, and by encouraging others to be independent.

- It is possible to balance work, family, and school.

KEY TERMS

activity log	shift action plan
desired optimal outcomes	time management
Pareto Principle	

REVIEW QUESTIONS

1. The nurse has just finished the change of shift report. Which patient should the nurse assess first?
   A. A postoperative cholecystectomy patient who is complaining of pain but received an IM injection of Morphine five minutes ago

   B. A postoperative appendectomy patient who will be discharged in the next few hours
   C. A patient with asthma who had difficulty breathing the prior shift
   D. An elderly patient with diabetes who is on the bedpan

2. The staff RN's assignment on the 7 A.M. to 3 P.M. shift includes a newly admitted patient with pneumonia who has arrived on the unit, a new postoperative surgical patient requesting pain medication, and a patient diagnosed with nephrolithiasis who is complaining of nausea. What should the nurse do first after shift report?
   A. Assess the newly admitted pneumonia patient.
   B. Give morphine to the new postoperative patient.
   C. Set up the 9 A.M. medications.
   D. Administer Zofran (Ondansetron hydrochloride) to the patient complaining of nausea.

3. The nurse has been assigned to a medical-surgical unit on a stormy day. Three of the staff can't make it in to work, and no other staff is available. How will the nurse proceed?
   A. Prioritize care so that all patients get safe care.
   B. Provide nursing care only to those patients to whom the nurse is regularly assigned.
   C. Have the patient's family and ambulatory patients take care of the other patients.
   D. Refuse the nursing assignment as the increased number of patients makes it unsafe.

4. The nurse has just completed listening to morning report. Which patient will the nurse see first?
   A. The patient who has a leaking colostomy bag
   B. The patient who is going for a bronchoscopy in two hours
   C. The patient with a sickle cell crisis and an infiltrated IV
   D. The patient who has been receiving a blood transfusion for the past two hours and had a recent hemoglobin of 7.2 grams/dL

5. A new graduate RN organizing her assignment asks the charge nurse "Of the list of patients assigned to me, who do you think I should assess first?" What is the best response the charge nurse could make?
   A. "Check the policy and procedure manual for whom to assess first."
   B. "Assess the patients in order of their room number to stay organized."
   C. "I would assess the patient who is having respiratory distress first."
   D. "See the patient who takes the most time last."

6. Of the following new patients, who should be assessed first by the nurse?
   A. A patient with a diagnosis of alcohol abuse with impending delirium tremens (DTs)

B. A patient with a newly casted fractured fibula complaining of pain

C. A patient admitted two hours ago who is scheduled for a nephrectomy in the morning.

D. A patient diagnosed with appendicitis that has a temperature of 37.8°C (100.2°F) orally

7. The nurse has just come on duty and finished hearing morning report. Which patient will the nurse see first?
   A. The patient who is being discharged in a few hours
   B. The patient who requires daily dressing changes
   C. The patient who is receiving continuous IV Heparin per pump
   D. The patient who is scheduled for an IV Pyelogram this shift

8. A nurse can enhance personal productivity by
   A. analyzing time, getting up an hour early and delegating unwanted tasks.
   B. getting up an hour early, answering the phone, and inviting a friend in to talk.
   C. analyzing use of time, getting up early, and waiting patiently.
   D. avoiding working and going to school at the same time.

9. You received report on the following patients, who would you make patient care rounds on first?
   A. Patient who is concerned that he had no bowel movement for two days
   B. Patient who has suffered several acute asthmatic attacks within the last 24 hours.
   C. Patient who is now comfortable but has had several episodes of breakthrough pain since yesterday
   D. Patient who is severely allergic to peanuts who just ate potato chips fried in peanut oil

10. Who would you make rounds on second?
    A. Patient who is concerned that he had no bowel movement for two days
    B. Patient who has suffered several acute asthmatic attacks within the last 24 hours
    C. Patient who is now comfortable but has had several episodes of breakthrough pain since yesterday
    D. Patient who is severely allergic to peanuts who just ate potato chips fried in peanut oil

REVIEW ACTIVITIES

1. For the next three days, complete an activity log (Table 18-1) for both your personal time and your work time. On what activities are you spending the majority of time? When is your energy level the highest? Is your energy level related to food intake?

2. Compare your use of nursing time to work to Figure 18-2. Are there any distractions that you can eliminate? What

time management concepts might assist you in improving your time management?

3. You go to work one day and there are too many staff members on the unit. Several patients have been discharged. The nursing supervisor asks you to float to another medical-surgical unit. Note the example of the use of priority setting in caring for a group of three patients on this unit (see box).

PRIORITY ASSESSMENTS, GROUP I

Patient	Priority Nursing Assignments
Ms. JD is a 68-year-old who is post-op day one after a total shoulder replacement following a traumatic fall. She is confused and on multiple medications with a history of hypertension and multiple falls. She is anxious and frightened by the "visiting spirits." Her daughter stays with her at all times.	Vital signs, safety, distal pulse, incision/dressing check, and breath sounds. See this patient third during rounds. Safety is a prime concern with this confused patient as well as watching for any postoperative concerns.
Mr. DB is a 55-year-old with insulin-dependent diabetes mellitus, juvenile onset at age 12. He is post-op day two after a right below-the-knee amputation. He complains of severe right leg pain and is restless. Mr. DB has a history of noncompliance with diet and is on sliding scale insulin administration.	Vital signs, Glucoscan at 4 P.M. and 9 P.M., safety, incision/dressing check, pain, DB teaching. See this patient second during rounds. He has pain, restlessness, and a relatively new amputation. He is a diabetic and could have a postoperative complication or an insulin reaction. If in doubt, check Glucoscan.
Mr. JK is a 35-year-old patient with a history of alcohol abuse admitted for severe abdominal pain. He is throwing up coffee-ground-like emesis.	Level of consciousness, seizure and shock potential, hematemesis, DTs, safety, vital signs, CBS, hematocrit, type and cross-match, 16 gauge IV line, pulse oximeter, cardiac monitor. See this patient first during rounds. He is a candidate for the development of shock.

Now, identify the priority nursing assessments for this next group of patients back on your regular unit.

PRIORITY ASSESSMENTS, GROUP II

Patient	Priority Nursing Assignments
Mrs. Hohman, a 61-year-old with a hypertensive crisis three days ago, blood pressure decreasing daily, now 180/102. She periodically complains of headache.	
Mrs. Glusak, a 67-year-old transferred two hours ago from ICU with a recent Brain Attack/CVA, responsive to painful stimuli, and has right-sided paralysis. Family at bedside.	
Mrs. Zurich, a 78-year-old with cellulitis of the right toe and a history of diabetes mellitus, needs teaching.	

4. What are your distractions from outcome achievement? Develop a plan to minimize your distractions.

5. Use Table 18-4, Tool for End-of-Shift Handoff Report, to organize your patient care report.

EXPLORING THE WEB

- If you would like to find a system for managing your time, the following Websites offer electronic organizers:
  www.casio.com
  www.sharp-usa.com
  www.palm.com

- If you prefer a less technological time management system, the following Websites offer nonelectronic organizers and systems for time management:
  www.daytimer.com
  www.covey.com
  www.franklin.com

- Find a free online calendar that you can access from anywhere at
  http://calendar.yahoo.com

- Look at all the hints and free tools on time management at the Mind Tools Website. Can you put any of the ideas to use?
  www.mindtools.com

- If you find time management an impossible challenge, you can find professional assistance at the Professional Organizers Website.
  www.organizerswebring.com

- Check out this University of Michigan site for time management tips as part of their stress management strategies.
  www.umich.edu

- Take a look at the personal time management guide at
  www.time-management-guide.com

- Enjoy the Pickle Jar Theory
  www.alistapart.com

- Check out the myths on time management
  www.couns.uiuc.edu

REFERENCES

Benner, P. (1984). *From novice to expert: Excellence and power in clinical nursing practice.* Menlo Park, CA: Addison-Wesley Publishing.

Covey, S. R., Merrill, A. R., & Merrill, R. R. (1994). *First things first: to love, to learn, to leave a legacy.* New York: Simon & Schuster.

del Bueno, D. (2005). A crisis in critical thinking. *Nursing Education Perspectives, 2*(5) 6, 278–282.

Fitzgerald, M., Pearson, A., Walsh, K., Long, L., & Heinrich, N. (2003). Patterns of nursing: A review of nursing in a large metropolitan hospital. *Journal of Clinical Nursing, 12*(3), 326–332.

Flaherty, M. (1998). The juggling act: Ten tips for balancing work, school, and family. *Nurseweek.* Retrieved on March 5, 2006, from http://www.nurseweek.com/features/98-5/juggle.html

Grohar-Murray, M. E., & DiCroce, H. R. (2003). Managing resources. In *Leadership and management in nursing* (3rd ed., pp. 291–315). Stanford, CT: Appleton & Lange.

Hansten, R. I., & Jackson, M. (2004). *Clinical delegation skills: A handbook for professional practice* (3rd ed.). Sudbury, MA: Jones and Bartlett Publications.

Kirkpatrick, C. (2006). *Safety first: JC's patient safety goals for 2006.* Nursing Spectrum. Retrieved on March 5, 2006, from http://www2.nursingspectrum.com/CE/Self-Study_modules/syllabus.html?ID=331

Marquis, B. L., & Huston, C. J. (2005). *Leadership roles and management functions in nursing: Theory and application.* Hagerstown, MD: Lippincott, Williams & Wilkins.

Mind Tools. (1999–2006a). *How to achieve more with your time.* Retrieved February 27, 2006, from http://www.mindtools.com/tmintro.html

Mind Tools. (1999–2006b). *How to achieve more with your time.* Retrieved February 27, 2006, from http://www.mindtools.com/tmgetup.html

Pelletier, D., & Duffield, C. (2003). Work sampling: Valuable methodology to define nursing practice patterns. *Nursing and Health Sciences, 5,* 31–38.

Reed, F. C., & Pettigrew, A. C. (2006). Self-management: stress and time. In P. S. Yoder-Wise (ed.), *Leading and managing in nursing* (4th ed., pp. 413–430). St. Louis: Mosby.

Reh, F. J. (2002). *Pareto's principle—The 80-20 rule.* Retrieved February 25, 2006, from http://management. about.com/cs/generalmanagement/a/Pareto081202.htm

Scharf, L. (1997). Revising nursing documentation to meet patient outcomes. *Nursing Management, 28*(4), 38–39.

Sullivan, E. J., & Decker, P. J. (2004). *Effective leadership and management in nursing.* Lebanon, IN: Pearson.

Upenieks, V. B. (1998). Work sampling: Assessing nursing efficiency. *Nursing Management, 49*(4), 27–29.

Urden, L., & Roode, J. (1997). Work sampling: A decision-making tool for determining resources and work redesign. *Journal of Nursing Administration, 27*(9), 34–41.

Vacarro, P. J. (2001, April). Five priority-setting traps. *Family Practice Management, 8*(4), 60.

SUGGESTED READINGS

Barker, A. M., Sullivan, D. T., & Emery, M. J. (2006). *Leadership competencies for clinical managers.* Sudbury, MA: Jones and Bartlett Publishers.

Cohen, S. (2005). Reclaim your lost time with better organization. *Nursing Management, 36*(10), 11.

Denton, K. D. (2003). Using the intranet to get rid of work. *Canadian Manager, 28*(4), 11–14.

Hendry, C., & Walker, A. (2004). Priority setting in clinical practice: Literature review. *Journal of Advanced Nursing, 47*(4), 427–436.

Jackson, M., Ignatavicius. D. D., & Case, B. (2006). *Conversations in critical thinking and clinical judgment.* Sudbury, MA: Jones and Bartlett Publishers.

Patterson, E. S., Roth, E. M., Woods, D. D., Chow, R., & Gomes, J. O. (2004). Handoff strategies in settings with high consequences for failure: Lessons for health care operations. *International Journal for Quality in Health Care, 16*(2), 125–132.

Robinson, J., & Godbey, G. (2005). Time in our hands. *The Futurist, 39*(5), 18–22.

Walls, H. (2003). Pareto people. *Industrial Engineer, 35*(7), 22.

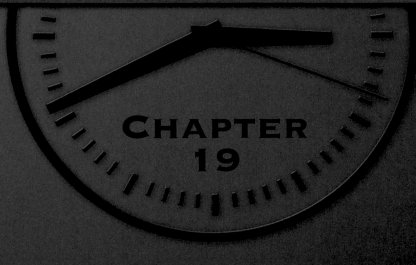

CHAPTER 19

Patient and Health Care Education

Paul Heidenthal, MS ✪ Nancy Braaten, RN, MS ✪ Martha Desmond, RN, MS, Post Masters Certificate in Nursing Education ✪ Susan Abaffy Shah, RN, MS

Education takes place when the learner's, not the teacher's, objectives have been achieved (Florence Nightingale).

OBJECTIVES

Upon completion of this chapter, the reader should be able to:

1. Identify five major steps of a teaching methodology.
2. Relate the major learning domains.
3. Differentiate the four components of a behavioral objective.
4. Summarize the relationship between terminal and enabling objectives.
5. Construct behavioral objectives for a teaching session.
6. Create a lesson plan for a teaching session.

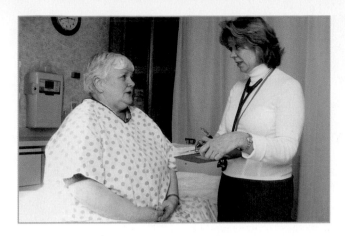

Your patient, Mrs. Melendez, age 72, has been diagnosed with heart failure. She is anxious about this diagnosis and is concerned about her treatment plan.

What resources will you provide to Mrs. Melendez?

What teaching strategies will you use to implement a treatment plan?

Patient and staff health care education is the communication of facts, ideas, and skills to change knowledge, attitudes, values, behaviors, and skills of patients, families, and fellow health care workers. Education is an inherent part of nursing. Teaching is a tool through which nurses bolster patients' self-care abilities by providing patients with information about specific disease processes, treatment methods, and health-promoting behaviors.

Patient education is also a legal component of the nursing process. In most states, patient education is a required function of nurses. Patient education is also mandated by several accrediting bodies, such as the Joint Commission (JC), formerly known as the Joint Commission on Accreditation of Healthcare Organizations (2006). The American Hospital Association's *Patient's Bill of Rights* (1992) also calls for the patient's understanding of health status and treatment approaches.

The goal of staff education is to increase staff proficiency to function at the highest level of competency. Staff education is incorporated at all levels of nursing practice, including informally mentoring a patient care technician in how to utilize safe transfer techniques in assisting a patient with a new amputation. Staff education includes distributing an evidence-based practice article or sharing an overview of a conference attended. It also includes formal ongoing education of nurses and other disciplines regarding health care issues facing nurses, patients, and their families.

INFORMAL AND FORMAL PATIENT EDUCATION

Patient education occurs informally and formally in combination with almost all nursing interventions. Informal education can be as basic as exchanging information during a conversation with the patient, such as explaining a medication, procedure, or laboratory result. Formal education is planned, structured, and directed toward specific topics and goals. Formal education also contains evaluation, which measures the patient's success in retaining and applying information.

INDIVIDUAL AND GROUP EDUCATION

The nurse provides education in an individual or group setting. Individual patient education frequently occurs in a clinical environment, often when an individual is facing the immediate impact of a specific health care situation. The term *patient education* may also be a misnomer in many of these situations because the nurse may be teaching the patient's family members or health care providers along with or instead of the patient. Even when others are involved, however, the focus of the education usually remains on the needs of an individual patient.

Although most patient and staff education occurs on an individual basis, nurses are increasingly becoming involved in teaching on a group level. As hospitals and other health care organizations adopt a proactive approach to health care, they are increasingly reaching out to the community, providing informational seminars and wellness classes that address common health care situations or emphasize preventive behavior.

METHODOLOGY

Whether conducted in an individual or group setting, the educational process is more effective when it follows a structured, standardized approach. Such an approach is called a **methodology**. The methodology presented in Table 19-1 contains five major steps in the development and delivery of formal education.

ANALYSIS

The first step in developing any educational program is to perform an analysis, to define the type of education needed. The nurse should analyze three major elements:

- Context
- Learner
- Content

TABLE 19-1   EDUCATIONAL DEVELOPMENT METHODOLOGY

Analysis	Design	Development	Implementation	Evaluation
■ Context	■ Objectives	■ Format	■ Environment	■ Learner
■ Learner	■ Sequence Content	■ Strategies	■ Learner	■ Teaching
■ Content		■ Media	■ Presentation	
		■ Lesson Plan	■ Content	

REAL WORLD INTERVIEW

I had severe pain in my right foot, around the middle toe area. The diagnosis was Morton's neuroma. The nurse explained how it developed, how the doctor would remove it, and, most importantly, what the after effects would be. I've never had the aftereffects explained to me; I never even thought to ask!

To me this represents quality care. The nurse told me what to expect. The majority of my nonhealth care friends and myself don't even know enough to think of the questions. I really appreciated this information.

Tessie Dybel
Patient
Schererville, Indiana

CONTEXT ANALYSIS

The context consists of the situational context in which the educational need arose and the instructional context in which the education will occur.

The situational context is the situation that creates the need for education. For example, is the patient facing a particular health care procedure such as a heart operation? Has the patient expressed concerns over an existing or potential health care condition such as diabetes? Is the patient receiving a new chemotherapy agent, or is there a practitioner initiating a new neurosurgery procedure, requiring staff education?

The instructional context refers to the conditions under which education will occur. In what environment will the education be presented? Is it a health care facility, a home, a community environment, or some other setting? How will this affect the ability to provide and access resources? How will it affect the nurse's ability to effectively control the education environment? How will it affect the learner's attention and motivation?

The instructional context also includes the time for education: When will the education occur and how long will the nurse have? Is the amount of time planned for education adequate? Is the amount of time flexible or is it fixed such as one hour allotted at a community center for giving a course on diabetes management?

LEARNER ANALYSIS

The nurse should also conduct a learner analysis (Figure 19-1). **Learner analysis** is the process of identifying the learner's unique characteristics and needs and the ways in which these can influence the education process. Understanding the learner's particular needs and characteristics is an important consideration when developing an individualized education plan that is relevant and effective.

Although at one level people can be said to be similar, at another level they are all unique. Even though education is based on a standard methodology, it is also a human interaction, and its success is influenced by the individual personalities of the people involved. Understanding the patient's unique characteristics may not guarantee success in education, but it can contribute to its effectiveness. The patient-centered and empathetic traits inherent in the nursing process can help nurses develop personal understanding and awareness of their patients.

The first question facing the nurse is: Who is the learner? Is it the patient, family, nursing staff, ancillary staff, other?

In most cases, the learner will be the patient. However, in some cases, the patient may be unable or unwilling to participate in the learning process. In other instances, there may be other learners in addition to the patient, such as family members, legal guardians, or others, who may make health care decisions for the patient. Learners may be caregivers who, whether related or not,

Education topic _____

Target Audience (check all that apply)

_____ Patient   _____ Professional staff   _____ Nonprofessional staff

_____ Individual   _____ Group

_____ Adult   _____ Elderly   _____ Adolescent   _____ Child

Relationship of group

(staff of same unit, multiple units, multidisciplinary team, family members)

_____

Purpose of Education

_____ Informational   _____ Skill, procedure, technique

_____ Professional development   _____ Infection control issue

_____ Introduction of new equipment   _____ Quality improvement

Gender _____

Learner's primary language _____   Translation assistance needed _____

Limitations and barriers to patient/staff learning? Describe.

Cognitive _____

Physical _____

Emotional _____

Cultural/religious/lifestyle _____

Motivational _____

Other _____

Literacy—education material at the appropriate reading level?

_____

Previous health care experience with this topic?

_____

Learning style assessment _____

_____

Figure 19-1 Learner analysis for patient or staff education.

CRITICAL THINKING 19-1

You work on a nursing unit that cares for cancer patients. Many of these patients are in constant pain. How can you educate patients who are in pain? How can you reduce the stress of these patients and increase the likelihood of their retaining your education? Is it possible to educate these patients? Who else can you involve in their patient education?

will be participating in the patient's care. Others may not directly participate in the care, but with the patient's permission, may require or desire information.

DEMOGRAPHICS Various demographic characteristics can influence a learner's response to the health care and learning environments. These factors include the following:

- Cultural background
- Language
- Age
- Education
- Health care background
- Physiological condition

The nurse's major goal is to identify characteristics that may indicate how the patient may respond to education. Some of these are physical, such as pain or physical discomfort, that will affect the patient's concentration. Others may be psychosocial, such as cultural beliefs that influence the patient's ideas about health care—for example, reliance on folk remedies. Cultural factors may also influence how a patient reacts to the nurse during an education session. Culturally influenced suspicion of or deference to health care staff may prevent the patient from effectively communicating with the education. People born in a common generation, may share similar values and attitudes, which they carry with them throughout life. These common traits may have implications for the way they approach learning.

The nurse may not be able to identify all of these characteristics prior to the education session. However, the more the nurse knows about the patient, the more the nurse can develop education that effectively incorporates the patient's unique characteristics and needs.

LEARNING STYLES   A **learning style** is a particular manner in which a learner responds to and processes learning. Traditional education often has expected the learner to adjust to the education style of the instructor rather than vice versa. In recent decades, this attitude has changed, and educational researchers and the educational community have come to agree on a principle that many people have always espoused: People learn differently.

The different ways in which people learn are still being determined and debated. Several theories of learning style exist, although they typically fall into one of three categories: perception, information processing, and personality (Conner & Hodgins, n.d.).

PERCEPTION   Perception theories emphasize the way in which people's senses affect learning. For example, some learners easily retain information when they can see or visualize it. Others retain best when they hear information. Still others learn best through physical action or involvement. Examples of perception theories include the Visual-Auditory-Kinesthetic (VAK) Model (Rose, 1985), shown in Table 19-2, and Gardner's Multiple Intelligences (Gardner, 1993), shown in Table 19-3.

INFORMATION PROCESSING   Information processing theories emphasize different styles of thinking. Does the learner prefer concrete facts or abstract theory, reflective observation or direct experience? An example is the Kolb Experiential Learning Style (Kolb, 1984), shown in Figure 19-2. In Kolb's theory, there are four major thinking styles: sensing and abstracting (which are opposites) and doing and watching (also opposites). An individual's style combines two of these styles, with one dominating. For example, a person whose style combines sensing and watching, with sensing dominant, is described by Kolb as a reflector personality. Such a person is likely to prefer concrete information rather than abstractions, prefers social situations to solitary ones, and judges performance by external measures rather than by personal criteria. Educationally, this person would probably learn best in an interactive group setting in which performance expectations are clearly stated and information is specific and factual.

PERSONALITY   Personality theories emphasize how personality differences affect learning. Traits such as introversion or extroversion, and preference for rational objectivity or instinctive "gut feeling" affect the individual's learning. An example is a theory based on the Myers-Briggs Personality Dichotomies (Figure 19-3), which in turn are based on personality theories of Carl Jung (Briggs Myers, & Myers, 1995).

The Myers-Briggs theory suggests that personality is made up of four complementary sets of traits: extroversion-introversion, sensing-intuition, thinking-feeling, and judging-perceiving. Within each of these sets, there is a sliding scale, so to speak. For example, on the extroversion-introversion scale, 1 might be completely extroverted, 10 completely introverted, and 5 equally both. In most cases, one or the other usually dominates. Through testing, an individual can be identified as one of sixteen possible types, based on the person's score in each of the

TABLE 19-2	ROSE'S VISUAL–AUDITORY–KINESTHETIC (VAK) MODEL OF LEARNING

Style	Design	Description
Visual learner	Learn best when they see; prefer graphic images and written text	■ Use charts, graphs, pictures, diagrams, and so on. ■ Include outlines, handouts, and other material for reading and note taking. ■ Allow plenty of empty space in materials for learner to take notes, draw diagrams, and so on. ■ Preview and review teaching content visually through flip charts, outlines, or other visual means. ■ Include both textual and graphic versions of information within material.
Auditory learner	Learn best when they hear and say	■ Present material verbally. ■ Include verbal preview and review of material. ■ Involve learner through verbal questions and answers, discussion. ■ Include verbal activities, such as brainstorming, discussion, and quiz show activities that require verbal response.
Kinesthetic learner	Learn best when they touch and move	■ Use activities to get learners up and moving. ■ Use music and color during presentation (these stimulate senses). ■ Whenever possible, physically demonstrate learning and have learner physically practice it. ■ Provide frequent breaks during presentation so learners can get up and move around. ■ Provide toys, models, equipment, or other objects learners can touch. ■ For complex tasks, have learners visualize physically performing the task.

Source: Compiled from *Accelerated Learning,* by C. Rose, 1985, New York: Dell.

four areas. The personality type is identified by a four-letter indicator. For example, an INTJ would be an introvert-intuitive-thinking-judging personality. An ESFP would be an extrovert-sensory-feeling-perceiving personality. In the theories of Jung and Myers-Briggs, each personality type has specific characteristics that affect the individual's approach to life experiences, including learning. Extroverts prefer to interact with people; introverts prefer to be alone. Thinking personalities prefer an objective, unwavering approach; feeling personalities are more likely to bend the rules if they think it makes people happy. Sensing people rely on their senses and prefer facts and structure to make decisions, whereas intuitive people are creative and see possibilities. Judging people like to be organized and decisive, whereas perceiving people work well in a spontaneous, flexible atmosphere.

TABLE 19-3	**GARDNER'S MULTIPLE INTELLIGENCES**	
Type	**Characteristics**	**Teaching Considerations**
Verbal—linguistic	Responds to rhythms and patterns of words, whether written or oral	Prefers activities that involve listening, speaking, writing
Logical—mathematical	Responds to reasoning, logic, recognition of patterns and structures	Prefers activities that involve abstract symbols, formulas, numbers, problem solving
Musical	Responds to pitch, melody, rhythm, and tone	Prefers activities that involve audio, musical rhythms, tonal patterns, melodic sound
Spatial	Responds to two- and three-dimensional visual representations	Prefers using or creating graphics and models, "visualizing" abstract information
Bodily—kinesthetic	Responds to physical movement and activity (sports, dancing)	Prefers activities involving physical movement and gestures
Interpersonal	Responds to social interactions and relationships	Prefers group activities or other situations that involve human interaction or collaboration
Intrapersonal	Responds to personal, inner emotions to understand self and others	Prefers activities that use introspection, processing emotions, reflection
Naturalist	Responds to intricacies and subtleties of patterns and relationships in nature	Prefers activities that provide involvement in the natural world (plants, animals, other natural phenomena)

Source: Compiled from *Frames of Mind*, by H. Gardner, 1993, New York: Basic Books.

Such personality differences can affect the way individuals approach and engage in a learning experience. Knowledge of learning styles is essential because it directly influences the nurse's choices when it comes to selecting education strategies and media. For example, if the patient is a visual learner, using graphics and charts is a logical education choice. This choice can significantly affect the teaching process.

Knowledge of learner demographics and learning style is more useful in individual education sessions. Tailoring to specific individuals is usually not possible in group education because members of the group will have a variety of characteristics. Rather than tailor group education to one style or characteristic, the nurse will need to incorporate education methods that address various styles and characteristics.

CONTENT ANALYSIS

After context and learner analysis, the next step in the analysis phase is content analysis.

During content analysis, the nurse begins to identify specific information that education should address. For example, the practitioner has just written an order for a medication you rarely administer on your unit. What specific information would you obtain to educate yourself and your coworkers on this medication? Could you use the same content information to educate the patient? Content information might include the following:

■ Confirmation by pharmacy on the use of the medication for your unit
■ Action of the medication
■ Safe dose

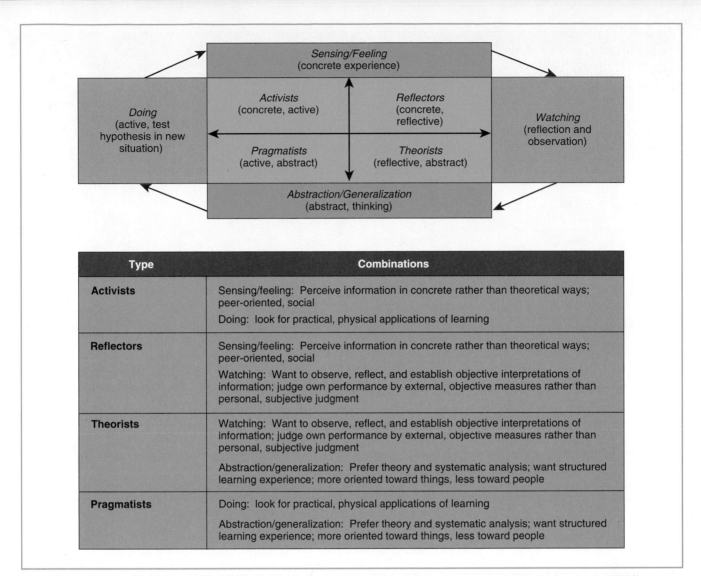

Type	Combinations
Activists	Sensing/feeling: Perceive information in concrete rather than theoretical ways; peer-oriented, social
	Doing: look for practical, physical applications of learning
Reflectors	Sensing/feeling: Perceive information in concrete rather than theoretical ways; peer-oriented, social
	Watching: Want to observe, reflect, and establish objective interpretations of information; judge own performance by external, objective measures rather than personal, subjective judgment
Theorists	Watching: Want to observe, reflect, and establish objective interpretations of information; judge own performance by external, objective measures rather than personal, subjective judgment
	Abstraction/generalization: Prefer theory and systematic analysis; want structured learning experience; more oriented toward things, less toward people
Pragmatists	Doing: look for practical, physical applications of learning
	Abstraction/generalization: Prefer theory and systematic analysis; want structured learning experience; more oriented toward things, less toward people

Figure 19-2 Kolb's experiential learning style. (Compiled from *Experiential Learning,* by D. A. Kolb, 1984, Englewood Cliffs, NJ: Prentice-Hall/TPR.)

- Side effects
- Route of administration
- Interactions with other medications or food

The nurse must also determine what information is essential to the education session. Although there may be a wealth of information available for a topic, all the available information may not be necessary information. Some of it may be irrelevant, redundant, or nonessential.

A typical rule of thumb in choosing content for educating is to distinguish between need to know versus nice to know. Need-to-know information can further be identified as common and critical. Education should address information the learner must commonly use, such as how to obtain and interpret a blood sugar reading, and information the patient must know to address or avoid critical situations, such as how to administer an insulin injection. Any information that does not fall into these categories is considered nonessential and can be classified as nice to know, for example, the history of diabetes management in the United States. Nice-to-know information can be shared with the patient if there is time and the patient has mastered essential information, but it has a lower priority in the education session.

In health care, such information may already be dictated by health care standards. Therefore, nurses will find that many content decisions may have already been made. However, there may still be additional information that can potentially be included. The nurse must analyze such information and determine whether it fits in the education situation.

LEARNING DOMAINS

The goal of education is not just dispensation of knowledge but change in behavior. This is especially true in health care.

Extrovert
Energized around a crowd
Like excitement around a project
Able to multitask
Act before thinking

1 2 3 4 5 6 7 8 9 10

Introvert
Private, energized by working alone
May be anxious in group settings
Think before acting
Prefer one-to-one relationships

Sensing
Take in information through the five senses
Make practical, realistic decisions
Trust facts and focus on details
Recall of past highly detailed

1 2 3 4 5 6 7 8 9 10

Intuitive
Creative
Trust their hunches
Focus on big picture, sees possibilities
Recall of past in patterns, context, connections

Thinking
Logical, objective, analytical
Fair, and stress cause and effect reasoning
Clear goals and objectives
Prefer expectations in clear, concrete terms

1 2 3 4 5 6 7 8 9 10

Feeling
Oriented to human values and needs
Stress empathy and harmony
Like group exercises

Judging
Decisive, organized
Make plan and lists, goal oriented
Value action and planning
Manage life around goals and deadlines

1 2 3 4 5 6 7 8 9 10

Perceiving
Curious, spontaneous, flexible
Process oriented
Continually gathering information
Best with small, frequent tasks
and deadlines

Figure 19-3 Myers-Briggs personality dichotomies. (Compiled from *Gifts Differing,* by I. Briggs Myers and P. B. Myers, 1995, Palo Alto, CA: Davies-Black, and *Patient Teaching* by P. Heidenthal in *Essentials of Nursing Leadership & Management,* by P. Kelly-Heidenthal, 2004, Clifton Park, NY: Thomson Delmar Learning.)

REAL WORLD INTERVIEW

I work in a wound center in a small community hospital. A patient with a peripherally inserted central catheter (PICC) was due to come in for a hyperbaric chamber treatment. I would have to access the PICC prior to the patient's entry into the hyperbaric chamber. We do not usually have patients here with central lines so I was feeling a bit apprehensive about using the PICC. I put in a call to the clinical nurse specialist who specializes in intravenous therapy to see if she could inservice the staff on my unit. She came to the unit with a policy on PICC management as well as a demonstration on how to access the PICC. She demonstrated the correct way to flush the PICC before and after disconnecting the patient from her medication. It was very helpful to have a resource person to be able to go to for this education session.

Sabrina Mosseau, RN, BS
Northeast Health
Albany, New York

Learning theory suggests that learning can be classified into taxonomies, or **learning domains**, each based on the major type of learning involved.

Each taxonomy is organized into a hierarchy that progresses from simple to complex behaviors. These behaviors can be observed and measured. This means that the nurse does not just present information to a patient and hope that the patient has learned and mastered it, but that the nurse can document behavioral changes by measuring the patient's performance at appropriate levels. The nurse can also examine what types of behavior the information represents: acquiring knowledge, gaining skill, or changing attitude.

Educators have identified three domains of learning:

1. Cognitive (Bloom & Krathwohl, 1956)
2. Psychomotor (Simpson, 1971)
3. Affective (Krathwohl, Bloom, & Masia, 1999)

The **cognitive domain** is centered on knowledge, or what the learner knows (Table 19-4).

The **psychomotor domain** is centered on skill, or what the learner does (Table 19-5).

TABLE 19-4	TAXONOMIES OF LEARNING: COGNITIVE DOMAIN	
Level	**Description**	**Actions**
Knowledge	Recalls information	Define, describe, identify, know, label, list, name, recall, recognize, select, state
Comprehension	Understands meaning of information, as demonstrated by the ability to restate the information in the learner's own words	Comprehend, convert, defend, distinguish, estimate, explain, generalize, give example of, interpret, paraphrase, rewrite, summarize, translate
Application	Uses information in a new situation	Apply, change, compute, construct, demonstrate, discover, manipulate, modify, predict, prepare, produce, relate, solve
Analysis	Separates information into component parts to understand the overall structure	Analyze, break down, compare, contrast, diagram, deconstruct, differentiate, discriminate, distinguish, identify, illustrate, outline, relate, select, separate
Synthesis	Puts information together to form a new meaning or structure	Categorize, combine, compile, compose, create, devise, design, generate, modify, organize, plan, rearrange, reconstruct, reorganize, revise, summarize
Evaluation	Makes judgments about the value of ideas	Appraise, compare, conclude, contrast, criticize, critique, defend, evaluate, explain, interpret, justify, support

Source: Compiled from *Taxonomy of Educational Objectives, Handbook 1,* by B. S. Bloom and D. Krathwohl, 1956, Boston: Addison-Wesley.

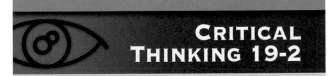

CRITICAL THINKING 19-2

Think about how you learn. How would you describe your own learning style? When you develop educational programs, does your learning style reflect your own learning preferences, or does it reflect the learning style of the patient? Look at a recent education session you observed. What changes would you make so that it addresses a different learning style?

The **affective domain** is centered on attitude, or what the learner feels/believes (Table 19-6).

The emerging pattern of behaviors sets the stage for the design phase of teaching development, in which the nurse translates the behaviors into objectives, develops education topics corresponding to the objectives, and arranges those topics into a structured topic sequence. This provides an organized, structured framework on which to build an effective education session.

DESIGN

The purpose of the design phase is for the nurse to organize and structure the content identified in the analysis phase. The nurse accomplishes this by establishing objectives and by sequencing content.

ESTABLISHING BEHAVIORAL OBJECTIVES

The behaviors identified in content analysis are now translated into behavioral objectives. A **behavioral objective** states a specific and measurable behavior that should

TABLE 19-5	TAXONOMIES OF LEARNING: PSYCHOMOTOR DOMAIN	
Level	**Description**	**Actions**
Perception	Observes behaviors involved in a performance	Choose, describe, detect, differentiate, distinguish, identify, isolate, relate, select
Set	Demonstrates readiness to perform; understands steps in a task, adopts physical posture to perform the task	Begin, display, explain, move, proceed, react, show, state
Guided response	Imitates performance and refines it through trial and error, practice	Copy, trace, follow, react, reproduce, respond
Mechanism	Performs task comfortably	Assemble, calibrate, construct, dismantle, fasten, fix, manipulate, measure, mend, mix, organize
Complex overt response	Performs task skillfully and automatically (increased proficiency, accuracy, and coordination)	Same as for Mechanism, but adverbs/ adjectives indicate increase in speed or accuracy of performance
Adaptation	Alters performance to adapt to new situations	Adapt, alter, change, rearrange, reorganize, revise, vary
Origination	Creates an original skill	Arrange, build, combine, compose, construct, create, design, initiate, make, originate

Source: Compiled from "Educational Objectives in the Psychomotor Domain," by E. Simpson, in *Behavioral Objectives in Curriculum Development,* edited by M. Kapfer, 1971, Boston: Educational Technology.

result from the education session. Behavioral objectives define what the nurse will teach, thereby providing the skeleton of the education session. They also provide the basis for evaluation because the success of learning is gauged by whether the learner achieves these objectives.

The essential component of a behavioral objective is a performance, specifically one that can be observed and measured. For example, the following is a behavioral objective: "List patient injection sites that are used to administer insulin."

However, this statement leaves some elements undefined. Who is doing the listing? The person(s) who performs the behavior is the *audience.*

This objective also does not state how well the person should perform the objective. Is 20% accuracy acceptable, or 50%, or 80%? The *degree* identifies how well the behavior is performed.

When we add audience and degree to the objective, it reads this way: "The patient will list six injection sites that he can use to administer insulin, with 100% accuracy."

These three elements—audience, performance, degree—should always be present in an objective.

A fourth, optional component of an objective is called the condition. The condition indicates any restrictions or specific requirements involved in performing the behavior. For example: Given an outline of the human body and a pencil, the patient will mark six injection sites where he can administer insulin with 100% accuracy. In this example, the condition is the phrase, "given an outline of the human body and a pencil."

One way to remember the components of an objective is to think of the ABCD method: A = Audience, B = Behavior, C = Condition, and D = Degree (Table 19-7).

TABLE 19-6   **TAXONOMIES OF LEARNING: AFFECTIVE DOMAIN**

Level	Description	Actions
Receiving/ attending	Displays attention, willingness to listen	Ask, choose, describe, follow, give, identify, locate, name, select, use
Responding	Displays active participation, willingness, motivation	Answer, assist, aid, comply, conform, discuss, help, label, perform, practice, present, read, recite, report, select, tell, write
Valuing	Shows acceptance, preference, and commitment for the value	Complete, demonstrate, differentiate, explain, follow, form, initiate, invite, join, justify, propose, read, report, select, share, study
Organization	Organizes and prioritizes values through contrasting them, resolving value conflicts, and developing a personal value system	Adhere, alter, arrange, combine, complete, defend, explain, formulate, generalize, identify, integrate, modify, order, organize, propose, relate, synthesize
Characterization (internalizing values)	Exhibits a value system that drives the individual's behavior	Act, discriminate, display, influence, modify, perform, practice, propose, qualify, question, revise, serve, solve, verify

Source: Compiled from *Taxonomy of Educational Objectives, Handbook 2,* by D. Krathwohl, B. S. Bloom, and B. B. Masia, 1999, Boston: Addison-Wesley.

TABLE 19-7   **COMPONENTS OF A BEHAVIORIAL OBJECTIVE**

Audience	Behavior	Condition	Degree
Who will perform the behavior	What the performer will do	What limitations or other conditions will be placed on the performance	What degree of measurement will be used to determine successful performance
The patient	*Will identify the major valves of the heart*	*Using the anatomical heart chart provided by the teacher*	*With an accuracy of 100%*

It is up to the nurse to determine how detailed objectives should be. The important consideration is that they indicate a behavior that is measurable.

TERMINAL AND ENABLING OBJECTIVES   When developing education, the nurse often begins with a primary goal for the session—for example, the patient will demonstrate strategies for stroke management. As the nurse develops objectives, a hierarchy of objectives may evolve, much like an outline or a hierarchical organization chart. Certain primary behaviors, each supporting the session goal, become evident. A **terminal objective** identifies a major behavior that contributes to achievement of the overall session goal. Terminal behaviors

TABLE 19-8	EXAMPLE OF SESSION GOAL, TERMINAL OBJECTIVES, AND ENABLING OBJECTIVES

Session Goal: The patient will be able to demonstrate strategies for stroke prevention and management

Terminal Objective 1: Perform an accurate blood pressure reading	**Terminal Objective 2: Develop a stroke management and prevention plan**	**Terminal Objective 3: Develop a Coumadin management program**
Enabling Objectives:	Enabling Objectives:	Enabling Objectives:
1. Identify equipment for taking blood pressure reading	1. Identify signs and symptoms of a stroke	1. Discuss medication and precautions
2. Demonstrate the procedure for taking blood pressure	2. List modifiable risk factors for stroke	2. Identify food interactions
3. State the acceptable range of blood pressure measurements	3. Discuss a low-salt, low-cholesterol diet plan	3. Demonstrate knowledge of INR/PT laboratory tests
	4. Develop an exercise/rehabilitation plan	

may in turn be achieved through the performance of related, secondary behaviors. An **enabling objective** identifies a secondary behavior that contributes to, or enables, achievement of terminal objectives.

Table 19-8 illustrates this concept of terminal and enabling objectives.

Objectives also dictate the items for learner evaluation. Each evaluation item should correspond to an objective. If the nurse is creating objectives for performances that are not relevant or necessary to evaluate, the nurse should examine those objectives and eliminate them.

SEQUENCING CONTENT

As the nurse analyzes content and develops objectives, the main topics within the education session and the order in which they appear become clearer. The nurse should then choose a specific topic-sequencing structure. In many situations, there will be only one choice, such as when teaching a procedure in the order in which the steps are performed. In other situations, no one sequence is obvious, and the nurse has various options from which to choose.

Table 19-9 describes common sequencing structures.

DEVELOPMENT

In the design phase, the nurse essentially determines what objectives education should accomplish and what information will support those objectives. During the development phase, the nurse clarifies how to teach by determining what strategies and resources to use.

Objectives should support evidenced-based practices. It is important to show how utilizing evidenced-based

CASE STUDY 19-1

Mr. Zel-Awi, a 72-year-old male, was admitted last week with a stroke. He is ready for discharge to home. You are working on his discharge plan. He will be discharged on antihypertensives, anticoagulants, and lipid-lowering medications. What resources will you utilize to develop a teaching plan that will include self-management of medications, diet, and activity? Who else will you involve in the teaching plan?

practice improves the quality of care. Nurses need to identify the learners' needs and target the education to achieve a positive outcome for that patient (Violana, Corjulo, Bozzo, & Diers, 2005).

FORMAT

Modern educators have come up with various formats for teaching. One of the most common is Gagne's nine events of instruction (Gagne, 1985), described in Table 19-10. This provides an effective framework for conducting the education session.

Any education session should incorporate certain effective elements. Sharing knowledge, experiences, and

TABLE 19-9	COMMON SEQUENCING STRUCTURES

Type	Characteristics
Chronological	Information is arranged in time sequence, based on the sequential occurrence of events. Typically used for teaching history.
Procedural (step by step)	Presents the steps in a procedure in the order in which they are performed.
Categorical	Information is organized into categories that are related to the primary topic. Allows the nurse to develop an arbitrary, but logical, structure when the information does not fit any of the other structures described here.
Topical	Patient is immediately placed in the middle of a topical problem or issue. Education may then address how the issue originated and the concerns surrounding its resolution.
Parts to whole; whole to parts	Presents the parts, and then shows how they relate to the whole, or presents the whole, and then talks about each part.
General to specific; specific to general	Similar to the preceding; presents the "big picture" first, and then presents details, or presents details first, and then shows how they fit into the big picture.
Problem to resolution	Presents a problem/situation, and then presents the topics involved in its resolution.
Known to unknown; unknown to known	Known to unknown begins with patient's existing information/experience and uses it as a bridge to new, unknown information. Unknown to known presents unfamiliar information, later showing its connection to what the patient already knows.
Theoretical to practical; practical to theoretical	Presents the theory, and then demonstrates how it is used, or shows practical applications of information, and then presents the theory.
Simple to complex; complex to simple	Begins with information that is easier to present or easier for the patient to learn, and then moves to more difficult information, or presents the most complex material first, and then progresses to easier information.

Source: Based on *Designing Powerful Training,* by M. Milano and D. Ullius, 1998, San Francisco: Jossey-Bass.

resources through the learning process, the education can help to facilitate learning and help to empower the learner (Minnesota Department of Health, 2001).

REPETITION   There is an old adage in adult training: Tell them what you're going to tell them; tell them what you want to tell them; tell them what you just told them.

In other words, preview information, present the information, and then review information. Previewing information allows the patient to understand what is to come and mentally prepare, much like providing a road map of an upcoming trip. It also provides a framework so that when information is presented, the patient knows where he is in the process. Finally, review provides the patient with an opportunity to organize the information and reinforce the learning. Therefore, repetition provides one of the most effective methods of education and should be incorporated into the education as much as possible.

INTERACTION   Learning works best when there is interaction between the learner and teacher, and when the learner is involved, whether it be nurse to patient or nurse to nurse. Interaction is stimulated using constant discussion, incorporating activities, and questioning the learner.

TABLE 19-10	GAGNE'S NINE EVENTS OF INSTRUCTION

Event	Explanation
1. Gain attention.	Engage the learner and stimulate interest and motivation.
2. Inform learner of objective.	Stating objectives establishes the expectations for the learner and provides an opportunity to preview the content of the education event.
3. Stimulate recall of prerequisite learning.	Try to relate the content to previous learning or experience. This provides the learner with a familiar context in which to approach learning.
4. Present stimulus materials.	Present the content.
5. Provide learning guidance.	Perform/demonstrate the learning for the learner or in conjunction with the learner.
6. Elicit performance.	Have the learner practice or demonstrate the learning.
7. Provide feedback.	Help the learner refine learning by providing feedback and suggestions.
8. Assess performance.	Evaluate learner performance in terms of the learning objectives.
9. Enhance retention and transfer.	Review learning and encourage learner to use learning in new situations.

Source: Compiled from *The Conditions of Learning and the Theory of Instruction,* by R. Gagne, 1985, New York: Holt, Rinehart & Winston.

PRESENTATION, PERFORMANCE, PRACTICE   In the case of patient education, the nurse can incorporate repetition, as well as interaction, into education through a format of presentation, performance, and practice. The nurse presents material to the patient, the nurse performs a demonstration either alone or along with the patient, and then the patient practices the performance, either independently or with nurse observation. This format allows the patient to repeat and reinforce learning while also increasing the patient's interaction with the nurse and active involvement in the learning.

VARIETY   A certain amount of variety in education maintains the learner's interest. Using different approaches and media can add variety to the education session. However, when working with patients, too much variety can break continuity and confuse the patient.

STRATEGIES

Although Gagne's events provide a structure for the overall education session, they do not prescribe how education will occur at the topic level. At this level, education can take various forms, commonly called strategies. Examples of education strategy include lecture, group discussion, fact sheets, and role play. The number and types of strategies the nurse chooses depend on several factors such as the type of content being taught, the audience's learning style, the nurse's own comfort level with various strategies, the resources available, the education environment, and so on. The nurse may use a single education strategy throughout the session or may vary strategy from topic to topic. Strategy may also be influenced by the education event; that is, it may be different during presentation and performance.

The nurse has wide latitude in selecting education strategies, but the nurse should choose strategies and be able to adapt the education methods to be effective in meeting the needs and preferences of the learner (Minnesota Department of Health, 2001).

MEDIA

Equally important to consider are the resources to be used during the education session. Resources consist of various media such as written, visual, audio, video, computer-based, or other material, or combinations of these materials. As in selecting an education strategy, a single medium may be used throughout the event, or several may be used, depending on such factors as content type, education strategy, patient learning style, teacher preference, or the limitations of what is available. The nurse has several options but should make decisions based on the idea of what would be best for the patient's learning style.

The nurse must consider two categories of media for patient education—media to be used during education and media to be provided to the patient for reference.

Because the latter is likely to be used outside the presence and supervision of the nurse, it is especially important that it be appropriate for the patient.

MEDIA EVALUATION AND SELECTION When possible, the nurse should use media resources that are already available. This frees the nurse from the task of creating materials and allows for more time to be devoted to developing and managing the education event. However, the nurse must examine available materials and determine whether they are truly suitable for use in education.

The nurse should look at several factors. Is the content presented in the material appropriate for the patient's needs? Is it accurate? Is the material of suitable quality; for example, is the audio understandable, is video of appropriate visual quality, are graphics understandable, is text readable or at the appropriate reading level? Is the source reliable; for example, does information on a Website come from a reputable and verifiable source?

Web-based education has made many advancements, and with the increased computer knowledge of today's patients and nursing staff, this type of education can be ideal. Formal online educational programs allow the nurse to learn about the most recent evidence-based practices, thus allowing them to bring this information to their patient education sessions. Many online educational programs can be accessed from home, making it more convenient for the nurse (Belcher & Vonderhaar, 2005).

MATERIALS DEVELOPMENT The nurse may use existing materials when developing an education session. In many situations, the nurse's organization will have existing materials and encourage their use. In other situations, the nurse may have greater freedom in selecting education materials.

In some situations, the nurse may find that no materials exist, or existing materials are not appropriate for the content to be taught. The nurse may need to create materials, either to augment existing materials or to fill a void. Keep in mind that creating materials can be both a creative and a frustrating endeavor.

Many times, nurses are busy and unable to attend in-services and classes. Fact sheets are a good alternative. Fact sheets provide bedside nurses with up-to-date research. They are usually one page in length with easy to read bullets that bring out the most important aspects nurses need to apply to their practice (Valente, 2003) (see Table 19-11).

LESSON PLAN

So far, the nurse has analyzed education content, designed behavioral objectives, organized the sequence of content, established the overall format of education, and selected appropriate education strategies and materials. All these decisions will be reflected in the lesson plan. A **lesson plan** is a document that provides the blueprint for the education session. See Table 19-12 and Table 19-13 for sample lesson plans. They provide the necessary information for the nurse or other educator to conduct the education session.

IMPLEMENTATION

During the implementation phase, the nurse actually conducts the education. The lesson plan defines the objectives, topics, strategies, and materials needed for the session. Using this plan, the nurse begins the education session.

When the nurse begins the education session, various factors will affect the success of the session. Some of these factors are highly controllable, others less so. Some of the more influential factors are environment, patient condition, the nurse's education and communication skills.

ENVIRONMENT

The environment in which the education will occur can have a major impact on the effectiveness of education. Before beginning to educate, the nurse should evaluate physical environment factors such as lighting, temperature, and sound quality. Also consider the learner's privacy needs, interior or exterior distractions, and the environment's ability to support the education session. The nurse may have to quickly adapt the education session in the case of unexpected situations.

LEARNER

The nurse must also assess the learner's condition at the time of the education session and be prepared to adapt accordingly. The learner's condition can be affected by physical factors, such as discomfort or pain, and by psychological factors, such as depression or learner anxiety. Any of these factors can seriously affect the learner's ability to learn. The nurse must decide how to address these factors or whether to postpone education until a more appropriate time.

PRESENTATION AND CONTENT

An effective educator must bring certain qualities to the education event. Although every individual will have varying degrees of talent in each area, nurse educators must constantly be aware of these qualities and strive to exhibit them in the education session. These qualities include the following:

- *Content knowledge:* The nurse may not be an expert on a topic but must be able to demonstrate reasonable knowledge to the patient.
- *Education experience:* The nurse must demonstrate experience and professionalism.
- *Communication:* The nurse must be able to communicate clearly and at a professional level.

TABLE 19-11   SAMPLE FACT SHEET

Preventing Ventilator-Associated Pneumonia (VAP)

Ventilator-Associated Pneumonia

- Common complication of patients in the Intensive Care Unit (ICU)
- Risk for developing VAP increases from 1% to 3% for each day a patient is intubated and on a ventilator

Definition

- Inflammation of lung parenchyma, caused by infectious agents

Symptoms

- Fever > 100.4°F
- Chest pain
- Crackles
- Mental status changes
- Purulent tracheobronchial secretions
- Decreased gas exchange
- Hypoxemia

Diagnosis Determined

- Chest X-ray showing infiltrate
- Leukocytosis
- Positive gram stain in sputum

Interventions to Prevent VAP

- Hand washing—after removal of gloves and between patient contacts
- Semi-recumbent positioning—head of bed elevation to 35–45 degrees decreases gastrointestinal reflux and aspiration
- Sedation and neuromuscular-blocking agents (NBAs)—oversedation and use of NBAs may prolong mechanical ventilation
- Adequate oral hygiene—use of Sage Toothette for Oral Care
- Endotracheal (ET) tubes with subglottic suctioning—Hi-Lo Evac ET tube helps to prevent aspiration of colonized bacteria
- Lateral rotation therapy/continuous oscillation beds—should be started within 24 hours of intubation
- Ventilator suctioning—catheters should be changed and suctioning done only when necessary
- Stress ulcer prophylaxis—some agents reduce acidity causing an environment for growth of bacteria; use is recommended when high risk of bleeding present
- Oral vs. nasal intubation—nasal intubation should be avoided whenever possible due to risk of sinusitis
- Nasogastric/enteric tubes—tube provides route for bacteria to travel from stomach to orophyranx
- Noninvasive positive pressure ventilation—eliminates need for ET tube

Source: Prepared by Susan Shah RN, MS. Compiled with information from Grap M, Munro C. L. (2004). Oral Health and Care in the Intensive Care Unit: State of the Science. *American Journal of Critical Care, 13,* 25–34; and Schleder, B. J. (2003). Taking Charge of Ventilator-associated Pneumonia. *Nursing Management, 34,* 29–32.

TABLE 19-12	SAMPLE STAFF LESSON PLAN FOR STROKE MANAGEMENT

Setting: 4th Floor Stroke Unit

Learner: 4th Floor Unit Staff

Overall Goal: The staff on the 4th floor will verbalize knowledge of Stroke Management

Objectives: After completion of this session, the staff will:

1. Verbalize a definition of a stroke.
2. Identify the signs and symptoms of stroke.
3. Discuss prevention and treatment of stroke.

Topic: In this lesson, the staff will receive the following information:

Definition of stroke: A decrease in the blood supply of the brain due to bleeding or a blood clot. This results in loss of function of the affected parts of the body.

Signs and symptoms of stroke: Loss of muscle tone, headaches, dizziness, tingling in the arms and legs, numbness, vision disturbances or temporary blindness in one eye, confusion, faintness, loss of consciousness, slurred speech or inability to talk.

Causes: Stroke is caused by bleeding or a blood clot that causes decreased blood flow to the brain.

Prevention: Exercise daily, do not smoke, check blood pressure regularly, follow a recommended diet, daily aspirin may help.

Treatment: Thrombolytics, anticoagulants, and/or aspirin, physical therapy, speech therapy, and so on.

Strategy: PowerPoint presentation

Medium: Handouts—Stroke Management

Evaluation: Provide a five question True or False quiz to each staff member; they must obtain a score of 80% or better.

Evaluation Tool for Stroke Management: Mark the correct answer.

____T____ F 1. A stroke is a temporary increase in blood supply to the brain.

____T____ F 2. Numbness and tingling is a symptom of a stroke.

____T____ F 3. A stroke can be caused by full blockage of a small artery in the brain.

____T____ F 4. One way to avoid a stroke is to avoid smoking.

____T____ F 5. Two medications which may be prescribed for a stroke patient are aspirin and Coumadin.

Source: Compiled from www.americanheart.org (Accessed in February, 2006).

TABLE 19-13   SAMPLE LESSON PLAN

Lesson Plan Title: Diabetic Self-Management

Patient	Juan Abado
Presenter	John Reilley, RN
Setting	Patient's hospital room
Brief patient/learner summary	Patient is a 50-year-old English-speaking Hispanic male, college graduate, newly diagnosed with diabetes and unfamiliar with the self-injection process. No other learners involved. No physical limitations to learning. Mild anxiety about self-injection, but high motivation. Initial interview suggests preference for learning through visual means.
Overall goal	The patient will understand and demonstrate diabetic self-care.
Objectives	After completing the session, the patient will be able to do the following:

- Perform an accurate blood sugar reading
  - □ Identify equipment for taking blood sugar reading
  - □ Demonstrate the procedure for taking a blood sugar reading
  - □ State the acceptable range of blood sugar level

- Develop a diabetic behavior management plan
  - □ Identify symptoms of hypoglycemia and hyperglycemia
  - □ List foods that can raise blood sugar levels
  - □ Discuss the ADA diet plan
  - □ Develop a regular exercise plan

- Administer insulin self-injection
  - □ Identify equipment necessary for insulin self-injection
  - □ Discuss insulin and method for self-injection
  - □ Demonstrate correct procedure for insulin self-injection

Topic outline (excerpt)

Time: 1 minute	Preview In this session, we will learn about diabetes and three major elements of diabetic self-care:

- Monitoring blood sugar
- Developing appropriate diet and exercise
- Insulin self-injection

Time: 3 minutes	Objective: Identify equipment for taking a blood sugar reading

Topics:

1. Importance of taking a blood sugar reading
2. When/how often to take a blood sugar reading
3. Equipment for taking a blood sugar reading
   a. Accu-Check and similar machines
   b. Interpretation strips

Strategy: Lecture and demonstration/return demonstration

Medium: Handout—*Monitoring Blood Sugar*

(Continues)

TABLE 19-13	**SAMPLE LESSON PLAN (CONTINUED)**

Time: 10 minutes

Objective: Demonstrate the procedure for taking a blood sugar reading

Topics:

1. How to put the interpretation strip in the machine
2. How to disinfect the finger
3. How to stick the finger
4. How to apply the blood to the interpretation strip
5. How to interpret the results

Strategy: Presentation of video and discussion with patient; nurse demonstration followed by patient demonstration

Medium: Equipment—Accu-Check machine and interpretation strips; video segment—*Taking a Blood Sugar Reading;* handout—*Monitoring Blood Sugar*

(Continue with this format for each objective in the session. Each segment lists the objective, the related topics to be covered, the teaching strategy used, and the presentation medium. It is also helpful to indicate the estimated amount of time needed to conduct each segment.)

Time: 3 minutes

Review

(In this segment, the nurse reviews the major objectives and topics covered in the session. This is also a useful time for asking the patient whether there are any topics he is unsure of or has further questions about.)

Strategies for retention/transfer

(In this segment, the nurse indicates any methods for helping the patient apply the teaching to future situations.)

Have patient perform own blood sugar tests four times daily during remaining time in hospital.

Evaluation

(This segment can take the form of a behavioral checklist, in which the nurse checks off that the patient has acceptably performed the behavior, or specific evaluation items, such as questions or other forms of evaluation. The example below contains samples of each.)

Identifies equipment for taking blood sugar reading   ☐ Yes   ☐ No

Demonstrates the procedure for taking a blood sugar reading   ☐ Yes   ☐ No

Blood sugar readings are taken using an Accu-Check machine and _____.

Before sticking the finger, you should:

A. Put the blood on the strip.
B. Read the blood sugar results.
C. Disinfect the finger.
D. Close your eyes.

EVIDENCE FROM THE LITERATURE

Citation: Valente, S. M. (2003). Research dissemination and utilization. *Journal of Nursing Care Quality, 18*(2), 114–121.

Discussion: This article discusses the need to disseminate research on evidence-based practice in an efficient manner to clinicians. The article provides the reader with the steps to develop a fact sheet. The fact sheet is a one-page research based sheet that is concise and can be posted on nursing units for all staff members to read.

Implications for Practice: Knowledge of research dissemination and utilization is helpful to nurses in clinical practice. A fact sheet is a quick and easy tool to accomplish this.

CRITICAL THINKING 19-3

You are caring for a patient with lung cancer. Smoking cessation has been difficult for her. Your preceptor would like you to identify key elements that would assist the patient and staff in the plan of care for this patient. Can you identify one topic that you could use to educate the patient using a fact sheet? What research literature will you use to develop your information? How can you make the fact sheet appealing to the eyes and draw the attention of the staff and patient?

- *Intelligence:* The nurse must be intelligent and able to grasp the complexities of the content.
- *Adaptability:* The nurse must be able to adapt to changes in the education content and format and be able to adapt to unforeseen changes in the education session.
- *Patience:* The nurse must be patient and caring with learners.
- *Self-confidence:* The nurse must maintain a poised and professional manner when interacting with learners.
- *Self-direction:* The nurse must be able to assume initiative, identify needs, and solve problems. The nurse must be able to work independently without supervision.
- *Interactive:* The nurse must enjoy people and interacting with them and be able to work with difficult people.

- *Organization:* The nurse must be able to organize and prioritize tasks and information to work efficiently.

COMMUNICATION SKILLS

Although communication can be viewed as another education skill, it is more significant than all others in producing successful education. Both verbal and nonverbal communication skills are essential to effective education.

As much as possible, the nurse should maintain a professional speaking voice:

- Tone should be calm and reassuring yet authoritative.
- Volume should be appropriate enough that the patient can hear.
- Pace should be appropriate enough for the patient to hear and process information.
- Avoid the use of fillers, such as "um," "you know," and so on.
- Speak clearly and with correct grammar.
- Speak in an active voice.

The nurse should also be careful about use of health care terminology. The patient is not likely to have the same familiarity with health care concepts and terms. Avoid using technical terminology if possible or take the time to explain terms to the patient. If using such terminology, use terms consistently to avoid confusing the patient. However, do not talk to the patient in condescending terms.

Listening skills are critical for effective education. The nurse must constantly watch and listen to the patient, looking for cues as to the patient's reaction to the education. The nurse must involve the patient in learning and look for opportunities to clarify, support, encourage, and incorporate patient responses. This further involves the patient in the learning process and increases patient motivation.

Body language says a lot about the nurse's level of interest and motivation. The nurse should maintain a professional appearance during the education event. Eye contact, use of hands, movement, and distance between nurse and patient all send messages about the nurse's attitude toward the education event.

EVALUATION

Evaluation is the process of determining the effectiveness of education. The two major components of evaluation are learner evaluation and education evaluation:

- *Learner evaluation:* Did the learners learn what they were supposed to learn?
- *Education evaluation:* Was the education presented in an effective manner?

LEARNER EVALUATION

What to evaluate is determined by the objectives. There should be a direct correlation between the objectives established for the education and the learner evaluation that occurs during the education.

TABLE 19-14	EDUCATION EVALUATION

Possible Areas for Education Evaluation

Patient learning	Did the patient learn the appropriate content, as indicated by such tools as learner evaluation results and follow-up observations? Were learner evaluation items appropriate and reliable?
Patient satisfaction/ comfort	Was the patient satisfied with the content presented? With the effectiveness of the presenter? Did the patient feel that questions were addressed appropriately?
Environment	Was the environment conducive to learning? Were there distractions from inside or outside the room? Was lighting appropriate? Room temperature?
Design	Were the objectives appropriate? The topics? The order of sequence?
Knowledge	Did the materials and/or teacher reflect adequate knowledge of the content?
Organization	Was the information well organized?
Accuracy	Was the information presented accurate?
Relevance	Was information presented not relevant to the patient's situation? Or was relevant information missing?
Delivery	Were education strategies effective? Materials?
Pacing	Did education move too fast or too slow? Were demonstrations at a pace the patient could follow? Was the patient given enough time for practice?
Variety	Was there too much of one type of activity? Not enough variety in education methods or presentations? Too much variety, creating a sense of confusion?
Involvement	Was there enough patient involvement? Was there a lack or shortage of activities and/or practice time?
Communication	Did the nurse communicate clearly and effectively with the patient?
Focus	Did the materials and/or educator stay on the topics?
Assistance	Did the educator provide enough assistance? Did the materials provide cues or explanations to assist the user in completing activities?

The following demonstrates an objective and the related evaluation item:

- *Objective:* Identify three medications for the treatment of diabetes.
- *Evaluation item:* List three medications for the treatment of diabetes.

Learner evaluation can take many forms. Asking the learner to recall information, answer questions, perform procedures, solve relevant problems, analyze a situation, or construct a plan of action are all forms of learner evaluation. The nurse should choose evaluation events based on how effectively they reflect the associated learning objective, how realistically the learner can be expected to perform the evaluation, and how practically the nurse can observe and measure successful performance. If possible, the nurse may also want to consider the learner's learning style when planning learner evaluation. For example, if the patient is more of an auditory learner, questions can be posed verbally rather than in written form.

The nurse must also remember that the purpose of evaluation is to validate that the patient and staff have effectively processed and adopted the information. Many learners feel anxious at any event that has the slightest hint of "testing." The nurse can reduce learner anxiety by presenting evaluation in the context of a review of the education. If the learner is having trouble with certain topics, the nurse can revisit those topics or, if conditions make that approach impractical, provide additional resources or referrals to the learner.

EDUCATION EVALUATION

Education evaluation is concerned with whether the education event itself was effectively constructed and presented. It is useful for the nurse to examine the education session and identify areas for improvement as well as areas to reinforce the effective elements.

Education evaluation can involve feedback from the nurse-educator, the patient, and/or third-party observers. Measurement can be formal or informal and can involve verbal or written feedback.

Table 19-14 (on previous page) identifies some of the elements that can be examined in education evaluation.

Patient and staff education is an important component of clinical practice. The staff needs to be kept up-to-date on the latest nursing and health care research. Evidence-based nursing care is of the utmost importance to the bedside clinical nurse.

Patient and staff education is a rewarding experience for the nurse. The nurse can provide a professional and gratifying learning situation through application of a structured approach to the design, development, and delivery of education.

KEY CONCEPTS

- A standard education methodology contains five major phases: analysis, design, development, implementation, and evaluation.
- Analysis consists of context analysis, learner analysis, and content analysis.
- The design phase of education consists of establishing objectives and sequencing content into an organized, structured framework.
- The development phase of education consists of establishing format, selecting strategies and media, and finalizing the lesson plan.
- The implementation phase of education consists of conducting education based on the lesson plan.
- The evaluation phase of education consists of learner evaluation, which measures how well the learner learned, and the education evaluation, which measures how well the education was conducted.
- Learners have individual learning styles and respond to specific educational methods.

- Gagne's nine events of instruction provide structure for education.
- All learning can be classified under three domains: cognitive, psychomotor, and affective. Each contains a hierarchy of behaviors.
- Behavioral objectives specify the audience, behavior, condition, and degree of measurement of the education session.
- Terminal and enabling objectives clarify learning.
- The lesson plan documents the objectives, content, sequence, format, strategies, media, and evaluation methods of the teaching session.
- A lesson plan is developed for educating patients and staff.

KEY TERMS

affective domain
behavioral objective
cognitive domain
enabling objective
evaluation
learner analysis

learning domains
learning style
lesson plan
methodology
psychomotor domain
terminal objective

REVIEW QUESTIONS

1. You are a new graduate on the unit, and your preceptor has asked you to demonstrate an insulin injection to your patient. The primary learning style you will utilize when the patient does his return demonstration is which of the following?
   A. Visual learning
   B. Auditory learning
   C. Kinesthetic learning
   D. Logical learning

2. Referring to Gagne's nine events of instruction (Table 19-10), a nurse has just instructed her asthmatic patient on the use of an inhaler. One event the nurse can utilize to evaluate the patient's skill is which of the following?
   A. Ask the patient to watch the nurse demonstrate the skill again
   B. Have the patient demonstrate the use of the inhaler
   C. Document the education session on the patient's chart
   D. Provide the patient with a lecture on asthma

3. The nurse has just instructed the patient on stroke management as part of discharge planning for home. The patient states "I don't feel I am ready to go home so soon. I am scared." What should the nurse say next?
   A. Tell the patient to call the rehabilitation nurse every hour for reassurance
   B. Ask the patient in a calm reassuring voice to verbalize his/her concerns
   C. Review the stroke education information again in a loud emphatic voice
   D. Stand over the patient without eye contact and ask the patient to verbalize his concerns

4. The major goal of education is to spread and share knowledge as well as which of the following?
   A. Utilize group learning
   B. Change behavior
   C. Enable student learning
   D. Learn new behavior

5. Utilizing a fact sheet such as the one on VAP (ventilator associated pneumonia), the nurse's instruction should include which of the following?
   A. A loved one should be flat in bed at all times.
   B. VAP is not a common occurrence in the ICU.
   C. Hand washing is a measure to prevent VAP.
   D. VAP is an inflammation of the lining of the heart.

6. Evaluating the effectiveness of an education event can be done by which of the following?
   A. Asking the patient if all questions have been answered
   B. Being sure that all information is repeated at least four times
   C. Noting a change in the learner's behavior
   D. Noting a decrease in patient stress

7. The nurse is an important component in patient education because of which of the following?
   A. Caring attitude
   B. Knowledge and expertise
   C. Ability to comfort others
   D. Professional appearance

8. Which learning domain involves changes in learner's feelings and beliefs?
   A. Cognitive domain
   B. Psychomotor domain
   C. Affective domain
   D. Reflective domain

9. Which of the following forms of analysis is concerned with the situation that created the need for education and with the conditions under which education will occur?
   A. Context learning
   B. Learner analysis
   C. Content learning
   D. Design analysis

REVIEW ACTIVITIES

1. Identify a patient education project that you can develop for one of your patients. Develop a lesson plan for this patient. Are your objectives in one, two, or three domains of learning?

2. Identify a patient in a clinical unit who needs education. Are there any learner characteristics that would affect the education for this patient? How would you adjust the education to address these characteristics?

3. You have developed a lesson plan for nursing staff on a new computer order-entry system that is to take effect on all the clinical units in your institution. Look at Table 19-14, which lists areas for education evaluation. How would you develop an evaluation tool for your lesson plan by using all or some of these areas? Are there other areas you would want to include in the evaluation?

4. Develop a staff education plan for staff on a unit where you have your clinical rotation. Use Table 19-12 to do this.

EXPLORING THE WEB

■ Go to the Keirsey Website: *www.keirsey.com* Take the Keirsey temperament Sorter-II test. This test describes temperament and character types. Does it seem to fit your temperament? Would it help to know your coworkers' temperament types to understand how they respond to efforts at teamwork and education?

- The following sites provide online health information for consumers:

  www.medlineplus.org
  Search for MedlinePlus Guide to Healthy Web Surfing.

  www.mayoclinic.com

  www.webmd.com

  www.patients.uptodate.com

  http://healthline.com

  How useful are these sites?

  How accurate is the information they provide?

  Who developed and maintains the Websites?

  Search for the same information on each site. What is the reading level of the information?

  Determine which type of patient would benefit from each site. Would you give the Website address to patients to look up their own information?

  Could you use the Website for professional information?

  Would you encourage your coworker to use the Website for information?

- These sites provide information on evaluating health Websites:

  www.nlm.nih.gov

  www.hon.ch

  Use the preceding criteria and evaluate some of the sites listed here.

- This site is a tutorial from the National Library of Medicine on evaluating Internet health information: *www.nlm.nih.gov*

- The following sites represent major health organizations in the United States. What kind of information do these sites contain that would be useful in patient education? What information would be useful for sharing with coworkers for professional development? How would you evaluate these sites in comparison to the consumer sites listed previously?

  American Dietetic Association: *www.eatright.org*

  American Diabetes Association: *www.diabetes.org*

  American Heart Association: *www.americanheart.org*

  American Cancer Society: *www.cancer.org*

  National Institute of Health: *www.nih.org.gov*

- The following Websites are for international health information. What kind of information do they provide? When are they useful?

  Canada: *www.canadian-health-network.ca*

  United Kingdom: *www.nhsdirect.nhs.uk*

  Australia: *www.healthinsite.org*

REFERENCES

American Hospital Association. (1992). *A Patient's bill of rights.* Retrieved August 23, 2006, from http://www.patienttalk.info/AHA-Patient-Bill-of-Rights.htm

Belcher, J. V., & Vonderhaar, K. J. (2005). Web-delivered research-based nursing staff education for seeking magnet status. *Journal of Nursing Administration, 35*(9), 382–386.

Bloom, B. S., & Krathwohl, D. (1956). *Taxonomy of educational objectives: Handbook I: Cognitive domain.* Boston: Addison-Wesley.

Briggs Myers, I., & Myers, P. B. (1995). *Gifts differing.* Palo Alto, CA: Davies-Black.

Conner, M., & Hodgins, W. (n.d.). *Learning styles.* Retrieved November, 2005, from http://www.learnativity.com/learningstyles.html

Gagne, R. M. (1985). *The conditions of learning and the theory of instruction* (4th ed.). New York: Holt, Rhinehart, & Winston.

Gardner, H. (1993). *Frames of mind: The theory of multiple intelligences* (10th anniversary ed.). New York: Basic Books.

Grap, M., & Munro, C. L. (2004). Oral health and care in the intensive care unit: State of the science. *American Journal of Critical Care, 13,* 25–34.

Joint Commission. (2006). *Comprehensive accreditation manual for hospitals: The official handbook.* Chicago: Author.

Kolb, D. A. (1984). *Experimental learning: Experience as the source of learning and development.* Englewood Cliffs, NJ: Prentice-Hall/TPR.

Krathwohl, D. R., Bloom, B. S., & Masia, B. B. (1999). *Taxonomy of educational objectives: Handbook 2: Affective domain.* Boston: Addison-Wesley.

Milano, M., & Ullius, D. (1998). *Designing powerful training.* San Francisco: Jossey-Bass.

Minnesota Department of Health. (2001, March). *Public health interventions: Applications for public health nursing practice. Health teaching.* Retrieved February 2, 2006, from http://www.health.state.mn.us/divs/chs/phn/interventions.html

Rose, C. (1985). *Accelerated learning.* New York: Dell.

Schleder, B. J. (2003). Taking Charge of ventilator-associated pneumonia. *Nursing Management, 34,* 29–32.

Simpson, E. (1971). Educational objectives in the psychomotor domain. In M. Kapfer (Ed.), *Behavioral objectives in curriculum development.* Englewood Cliffs, NJ: Educational Technology.

Valente, S. M. (2003). Research dissemination and utilization. *Journal of Nursing Care Quality, 18*(2), 114–121.

Violano, P., Corjulo, M., Bozzo, J., & Diers, D. (2005). Targeting Educational Initiatives. *Nursing Economics, 23*(5), 248–252.

SUGGESTED READINGS

Bastable, Susan, B. (2003). *Nurse as Educator* (2nd ed.). Boston: Jones and Bartlett Publishers.

Bastable, Susan, B. (2006). *Essentials of Patient Education.* Boston: Jones and Bartlett Publishers.

Cutilli, C. C. (2006). Do your patients understand? How to write effective healthcare information. *Orthopaedic Nursing, 25*(1), 39–50.

Falvo, D. (2004). *Effective Patient Education: a Guide to Increased Compliance* (3rd ed.). Boston: Jones and Bartlett Publishers.

Hamilton, S. (2005). Clinical consultation. How do we assess the learning style of our patients? *Rehabilitation Nursing, 30*(4), 129–131.

Lau-Walker, M. (2004). Cardiac rehabilitation: The importance of patient expectations—a practitioner survey. *Journal of Clinical Nursing, 13*(2), 177–184.

Rankin, S. R., Stallings, K. D., & London, F. (2005). *Patient Education in Health and Illness* (5th ed.). Philadelphia: Lippincott Williams & Wilkins.

Ridge, R. (2005). A dynamic duo: Staff development. *Nursing Management, 36*(7), 28–35.

Sewchuk, D. H. (2005). Experiential learning: A theoretical framework for perioperative education. *Association of Operating Room Nurses Journal, 81*(6), 1311–1316.

Sparlnig, L. A. (2001). Enhancing the learning in self-directed learning modules. *Journal for Nurses in Staff Development, 17*(4), 199–205.

CHAPTER 20

Managing Outcomes Using an Organizational Quality Improvement Model

Mary McLaughlin, RN, MBA ⊕ Karen Houston, RN, MS

Go the extra mile, It's never crowded (Executive Speech Writer Newsletter).

OBJECTIVES

Upon completion of this chapter, the reader should be able to:

1. Relate major principles of quality and quality improvement (QI), including customer identification; the need for participation at all levels; and a focus on improving the process, not criticizing individual performance.

2. Explain how quality improvement affects the patient and the organization.

3. Compare the Plan Do Study Act Cycle, the FOCUS methodology, and other methods for quality improvement.

4. Identify how data are utilized for QI (time series data, Pareto charts).

5. Outline the difference between risk management and QI.

6. Relate how the principles of QI are implemented in the organization.

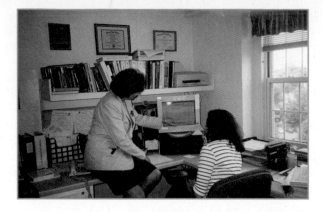

University HealthSystem Consortium (UHC), a group of about 110 academic health science centers, did a benchmark study on total hip arthroplasty. Albany Medical Center, an organization that participated in that study, noted that compared to other organizations, its average length of stay (LOS) was long (the Albany Medical Center LOS was 7.07 days; the average LOS for UHC was 5.78 days). It also noticed that the percentage of patients that used a pneumatic compression device (a device to decrease the postoperative rate of deep vein thrombosis) was 85% for UHC but only 53% for Albany Medical Center. The percentage use of indwelling catheters in total hip arthroplasty patients at Albany Medical Center (indwelling catheters are associated with an increase in postoperative urinary tract infections, or UTIs) was 53%. Although this catheter use was lower than the UHC average, the team believed it could decrease the rate further. Albany Medical Center also delivered an average of three physical therapy (PT) visits postoperatively per patient, whereas UHC's average was five visits per patient. There was also an increased cost at Albany Medical Center versus the average cost at UHC.

Albany Medical Center decided to assign an interdisciplinary team the responsibility of identifying opportunities for improvement. The team began by developing a clinical pathway based on the most recent research in this area. Using data and research, the team looked for ways to improve the patient care process. The team incorporated the best practices that they found: this meant designing into the clinical pathway increased use of the pneumatic compression device, more physical therapy, earlier catheter removal, and an earlier discharge date. To prepare the patient properly for the earlier discharge, the team added preoperative home visits to the clinical pathway. The Visiting Nurses Association would make the home visit and then make a recommendation for discharge planning prior to the patient's admission. This process expedited initiation of referrals to an acute rehabilitation facility or home care following discharge, if needed. If the family home had to be rearranged to accommodate limited ambulation or stair use, these recommendations were made early in an effort to allow the family to prepare ahead of time.

The higher costs at Albany Medical Center seemed to be related to the number of prosthetic vendors. When fewer vendors are used, the volume with each vendor is higher, allowing more competitive price negotiation among vendors. The organization

worked with the surgeons on the team to decrease the number of vendors to a ratio of 0.25 vendors to surgeons.

How does attention to cost and quality improve patient care?

Continuous quality improvement has been shown to be a powerful tool to help make health care organizations more effective. Ransom, Joshi, and Nash (2005) stress the importance of management and leadership commitment to the success of quality improvement. Organizational leadership often has a significant say in activities in which staff are involved. Organizational leadership can designate required resources and remove obstacles to making change and improving care. The improvement philosophies of quality experts such as Deming (1986) and Crosby (1989) also emphasize the commitment of management, and without that commitment, successful quality improvement is jeopardized.

Quality improvement is described as both a science and an art. The science of improvement is the development of new ideas, the testing of those ideas, and the implementation of change. As Carey and Lloyd (2001) describe, W. Edwards Deming, Joseph M. Juran, and Philip B. Crosby have been the gurus of continuous quality improvement and have provided important contributions to the science

CRITICAL THINKING 20-1

Refer back to the chapter's opening scenario. If you were a staff nurse on the orthopedic unit at Albany Medical Center, what could you do to improve the quality of care? How would you encourage the decreased use of indwelling catheters? How would you encourage the use of a pneumatic compression device?

How could you bring your ideas to other staff members without making them feel that the quality of their care was being criticized? For example, many staff members feel that catheter use is better for the patient's skin and reduces the need for assistance in ambulating the patient to the bathroom. You know that research shows indwelling catheters and decreased ambulation increase risk of complications. How do you deal with these competing positions?

What measures would you use to ensure that while you were improving some aspects of care, you were not decreasing other critical outcome measures? For example, as you decrease catheter use, what is happening to UTI and fall rates?

of improvement. Deming's components of appreciating a system, understanding variation, and applying knowledge and psychology are fundamental improvement principles. Quality improvement is also described as an art that taps into creative, "out of the box" ideas. It is about systematically testing new ideas to improve customer care. Health care customers are patients, families, practitioners, nurses, staff, and so forth. If the change is planned and measured, there are limitless boundaries to what can be achieved.

Adapting the concepts of science and art in improving health care can create an enthusiasm for change and a passion for results. This chapter will discuss and provide examples of the application and implementation of quality improvement principles in a health care setting.

HISTORY OF QUALITY ASSURANCE

Consider Berwick and Plsek's red bead example (1992):

> In a group of beads in a bag, there are 90 blue beads and 10 red beads. There are four workers whose job it is to take blue beads out of a bag. They cannot see what color bead they are taking. The supervisor watches to see how many red beads are pulled out of the bag. The first day, worker A has 1 red bead, worker B has 4 red beads, worker C has 3 red beads, and worker D has 2 red beads. The supervisor states that worker A has done a great job and worker B has done a terrible job. He tells them they have to improve. The beads go back in the bag, and they start over the next day. This day, worker A has 4 red beads, worker B has 0 red beads, worker C has 2 red beads, and worker D has 4 red beads. The supervisor praises worker B for the improvement and yells at workers A and D for not doing a good job. The truth is these workers do not have any ability to change the number of red beads that they pull out of the bag.

This example demonstrates random variation. Using inspection in systems to reward or punish random variation results in tampering with the system rather than quality improvement. Instead of improving the process, the tampering encourages staff to look for someone to blame rather than to change the process to improve outcomes. So the question is, how much variability do we expect? This can be calculated on a time series chart and will be discussed in more detail later in the chapter.

Prior to the 1980s, focus was on **quality assurance** (QA), rather than on quality improvement (QI). QA began as an inspection approach to ensure that health care institutions—mainly hospitals—maintained minimum standards of patient care quality. The use of QA

grew over time, as did federal and state regulatory controls. QA departments became the organizational mechanism for measuring performance against standards and reporting incidents and errors, such as mortality and morbidity rates. This approach was reactive and fixed the errors after a problem was noted. QA's methods consisted primarily of retrospective chart audits of various patient diagnoses and procedures. The method was thought to be punitive, with its emphasis on "doing it right," and did little to sustain change or proactively identify problems before they occurred. It did, however, accomplish the task of monitoring minimum standards of performance.

TOTAL QUALITY MANAGEMENT

Total quality management (TQM), also referred to as quality improvement (QI) and performance improvement (PI), began in the manufacturing industry with W. Edwards Deming and Joseph Juran in the 1950s. TQM, QI, and PI are terms that are frequently interchanged. For the purposes of this chapter, **quality improvement (QI)** will be referred to as a systematic process of organization-wide participation and partnership in planning and implementing continuous improvement methods to understand, meet, or exceed customer needs and expectations and improve patient outcomes. This proactive approach emphasizes "doing the right thing" for customers. It was integrated into the health care industry in the 1980s when purchasers of care and accrediting bodies began to push providers to document quality (Carey & Lloyd, 2001). Movement into QI is thought to be more of an overall management approach than a single program. Integrating concepts of quality into daily organizational operations is key to successful outcomes. Table 20-1 notes the difference in focus between QA and QI.

GENERAL PRINCIPLES OF QUALITY IMPROVEMENT

Quality improvement principles include the following:

1. The priority is to benefit patients and all other internal and external customers.
2. Quality is achieved through the participation of everyone in the organization.
3. Improvement opportunities are developed by focusing on the work process.
4. Decisions to change or improve a system or process are made based on data.
5. Improvement of the quality of service is a continuous process.

TABLE 20-1	DIFFERENCE IN FOCUS BETWEEN QUALITY ASSURANCE AND QUALITY IMPROVEMENT

Focus of Quality Assurance (doing it right)

- Assessing or measuring performance retrospectively
- Reviewing chart audits and incident reports
- Determining whether performance conforms to standards
- Improving performance when standards are not met

Focus of Quality Improvement (doing the right thing)

- Meeting the needs of the customer proactively
- Building quality performance into the work process
- Assessing the work process to identify opportunities for improved performance
- Employing a scientific approach and using data for assessment and problem solving
- Improving health care performance and changing the health care system continuously as a management strategy, not just when standards are not met

Early QA literature focused on fixing problems, "doing it right," and having zero defects. Over time, a gap was found between theory and practice. It was determined that quality is not about being perfect. First, it is about being better, doing the right thing the first time, and being better than the competition. This increases an organization's chances of survival during highly turbulent and competitive times. Second, quality is about health care professionals seeing themselves as having customers. The notion of "customer" requires major shifts in mindset for the health care professional. The term *customer* is frequently used in business, and calling a patient a "customer" was initially thought by some to undermine the professional care provided to patients. Designing health care processes from the customer's point of view versus the professional's point of view is a challenge and requires changes in thinking and redesign of health care processes. Health care involves work processes in which one step leads to the next step. Improving these steps in the work process is an important part of improving care and customer satisfaction. Customer satisfaction is rooted in the way health professionals treat their patients/customers and in the quality of their outcomes. Having the goal of astounding patients with quality in every interaction is key to achieving satisfaction and loyalty. Third, quality directs health professionals to give their customers more than the basics so that customers will recommend and demand these services. This is achieved by proactively seizing opportunities to perform better, driving for quality consistently and continuously, and not waiting for a problem to be pointed out or for pressure from a competitor to improve. Improvements are sustained over time when interdisciplinary teams collaborate and decisions about change are supported by data.

The primary benefits of adopting quality improvement concepts and principles include discovering performance issues more quickly and efficiently by looking at every problem as an opportunity for improvement. QI involves staff in how the work is designed and carried out. This improves staff satisfaction and empowers staff to identify and implement improvement in the health care system and results in improved patient outcomes. Increasing the customer's perception that you care by designing health care work processes to meet the customer's needs, rather than the health care provider's, and decreasing unnecessary costs from waste and rework, lost business, and not meeting regulations are also quality concepts. These quality improvement concepts should be emphasized until they become work habits and part of an organization's daily operations.

CUSTOMERS IN HEALTH CARE

A customer is anyone who receives the output of your efforts. There are internal and external customers. An internal customer is anyone who works within the organization and receives the output of another employee. Internal customers include health care staff such as practitioners, nurses, pharmacists, physical therapists, respiratory therapists, occupational therapists, pastoral caregivers, and so on. An external customer is anyone who is outside the organization and receives the output of the organization. The patients are external customers, but they are not the only external customers. Other external customers include private practitioners, insurance payers, regulators such as the Department of Health, the Joint Commission (JC), formerly known as the Joint Commission on Accreditation of Healthcare Organizations (JCAHO), and the community you serve.

PARTICIPATION OF EVERYONE IN THE ORGANIZATION

QI is achieved through the participation of everyone in the organization at all levels. A participation and empowerment initiative must be built by first offering employees the opportunity for appropriate involvement. An organization that encourages empowerment promotes a culture of employee ownership. In this type of culture, employees do the following:

- Take responsibility for the success or failure of an organization
- Take an active part in developing new ways of doing business and securing new customers
- Trust that their efforts are valued

A new staff member can participate in the design and improvement of daily work practices and processes on an individual, unit, or organizational level. For example, as an individual, a nurse could change the organization of the day to spend more time with patients' families. On a unit level, a nurse could work with others on the unit to change the way patient report is given to be more time efficient. On an organizational level, a nurse could suggest that the process for notifying pharmacy about a missing medication could be improved. The nurse could participate on a team to find a solution.

All members of the staff are encouraged to participate in quality improvement processes. These include the nursing and medical practitioners, physical therapist, occupational therapist, speech therapist, pharmacist, case management worker, social worker, medical technologists, and any member of the health care team who cares for the patient or contributes to the care of the patient. The goal of QI efforts, as well as the process being worked on, determines who participates on the team. For example, if you were trying to decrease the time a patient waits outside the radiology suite for a test, you would need to include the patient transportation staff, unit clerks, unit RNs, and radiology staff in your QI efforts. If you were trying to ensure that patients with congestive heart failure are discharged understanding the importance of weighing themselves daily, you would need the cardiac unit's RN, clinical dietician, Visiting Nurses Association staff, primary care practitioner, cardiologist, pharmacist, the patient, and the patient's family. The key in determining who participates is including the point-of-service staff: the

workers on the front line who do the direct care involved in the work process you are trying to change. They are the people who have the most knowledge of the work process so they can look for potential areas of improvement. There should be a clearly identified way for staff to suggest improvement opportunities that they see in their day-to-day work. For example, an x-ray technologist may note steps in the process of scheduling and transporting patients that create a long wait time for x-ray testing. If a mechanism for suggesting improvement exists in the radiology department, the technologist could suggest and test ideas for change.

FOCUS ON IMPROVEMENT OF THE HEALTH CARE WORK PROCESS

Improvement opportunities are focused on the process of work that the health care team delivers. A **process** is a set of causes and conditions that repeatedly come together in a series of steps to transfer inputs into outcomes (Langley, Nolan, Norman, Provost, & Nolan, 1996). All work processes have inputs, steps, and outputs. Deming (2000) points out that "Every activity, every job is part of a process." A process in health care includes the work process or activities that constitute health care (i.e., diagnosis, treatment, rehabilitation, prevention, and patient education) and also other work processes or activities that help make the care happen (i.e., food preparation, transportation, technical support) (Donabedian, 2003). The people involved in these health care activities or work processes include all types of health care workers, such as, nursing and medical practitioners, technicians, housekeeping and so on. An example of a health care work process is illustrated by a patient who presents in the emergency department with chest pain. When it is determined that the patient has had a Myocardial

Infarction (MI), several work processes should occur. These work processes include an appropriate set of interventions for the patient with an MI such as pertinent blood work, the right diet, the right medication in the right time frame, and patient assessments done on a regular interval to identify complications early or before they happen. All the steps of the work process can be measured. These measurements are then reviewed, applying evidence-based principles, as appropriate to improve patient care. Steps of the work process may be eliminated or changed and then standardized so that all staff use the improved work process. For instance, in the example of the patient with the MI, health care evidence shows that all patients with an MI should receive aspirin within a specific time frame. In an organization with a focus on quality improvement, the steps of aspirin administration to the patient are reviewed and changed until the measurement data shows that all patients with an MI receive aspirin in the appropriate time frame. This would mean a review of when the practitioner ordered the drug, when the order was transcribed, when the pharmacy got the aspirin to the staff, when the staff gave it to the patient, and so on. A decrease in variability of the work process leads to improved care. The care is standardized to assure the best result.

IMPROVEMENT OF THE SYSTEM

A **system** is an interdependent group of items, people, or processes with a common purpose (Langley et al., 1996). In a system, the work processes as well as the relationships among the work processes lead to the outcome. You can improve the outcome by examining these work processes and relationships. In a system, every step of a work process affects the following step. For example, if the x-ray staff members place the patient who has had a chest x-ray in the hall and call transportation to take the patient back to his room but do not monitor and consider the transportation

process, they may decrease the total time a patient is in radiology but increase the patient's time in the hall waiting for transportation. You cannot improve care unless you review all the steps in the system's work process.

A CONTINUOUS PROCESS

Improvement of quality of service is a continuous process. Walter Shewhart, the director of Bell Laboratories in the mid-1920s, is credited with the concept of the cycle of continuous improvement. This concept suggests that products or services are designed and made based on knowledge about the customer. Those products or services are marketed to and judged by the customer. These judgments lead to improved products and services. Hence, the process of QI is continuous, because it is linked to changing customer needs and judgments.

In addition to being a continuous process, as we discussed earlier in the example of the patient with an MI, quality improvement focuses on standardization of a work process. Variation in a work process increases complexity and the risk of error (Ransom et al., 2005). Technology increasingly offers tools for standardization of work processes, however, there are challenges with technology. Ransom et al. explain it like this: "Imagine how difficult it would be to drive a rental car if every manufacturer placed gas pedals, brake pedals, and shifts in completely different locations with varying designs." As we increase the use of technology to assist in the standardization of work processes, we need to bear in mind the need to standardize the technology itself.

IMPROVEMENT BASED ON DATA

Decisions to change or improve a work system or work process are made based on data. When someone says, "The patients are waiting too long to return from radiology," it is time to look at the data. Review the waiting

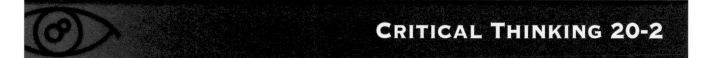

CRITICAL THINKING 20-2

In the opening scenario at the start of this chapter, when the original length of stay data by nursing unit was examined, one unit had a much shorter length of stay than the other. At first there was discussion about this variance, and the idea emerged of just going to the floor with the longer length of stay and fixing things there. The group members decided that rather than approach the task from this limited perspective, they would study the work process as a whole and determine whether there were steps they could take to improve the work process. Several excellent opportunities for improvement were identified, as noted previously—for example, preoperative home evaluation, increased physical therapy involvement, and shorter Foley catheter use. All these areas contributed to the work process improvement, and the outcome was that both units ended up reducing their lengths of stay. These opportunities would have been lost had the group members used the data only to say that one unit was doing a bad job. They needed to review the work process as a whole to improve the length of stay on both units.

How could you improve care in a patient care unit that you are familiar with? What patient care work process could be improved? Who would you ask to work on the improvements with you?

time data to see whether waiting times are increasing. The data clarify these issues. Using data correctly is important. Data should be used for learning, not for judging. It is critical to look at work processes rather than people for improvement opportunities. In the radiology example, if we jumped to the conclusion that someone was not doing the job correctly, we might criticize the transportation staff person who returned the patient from radiology. This would not foster improvement ideas. By not analyzing the process (patient has chest x-ray, is put in hall, clerk at desk calls transportation, transportation clerk pages transportation aide, and so on) and the relationships among the processes (waiting times between calls, transportation phone process, page system, and so on), we could miss finding where the real improvement opportunity lies. Perhaps it has nothing to do with the transportation person who returned the patient to the room. It may be that the actual root cause of the problem is a long delay in the paging system. Reviewing the wait time data is an example of examining the work process, not the people carrying out the work process.

IMPLICATIONS FOR PATIENT CARE

The implications of quality improvement for patient care can be measured by the overall value of care. Value is a function of both quality outcomes and cost. Outcomes can be a patient's clinical or functional outcomes. For example, did the patient live; can the patient go back to work? Outcomes can also be measured by patient satisfaction. For example, would the patient recommend this health care facility to someone else? Cost is the cost of both direct and indirect patient care needs. Direct cost is the cost of the care of the patient, for example, cost of medications, operating room equipment, and direct patient caregiver salaries. Indirect costs are the costs of nondirect care activities, including electricity and salaries of nondirect patient caregivers such as secretaries or human resource staff.

$$Value = \frac{Quality\ of\ outcomes}{Cost}$$

In most QI efforts, as quality is improved by standardizing care delivery work processes and applying evidence-based principles, the cost of care decreases. The example in the opening scenario illustrated this. The length of stay decreased as the team found ways to standardize care and evaluate the patient prior to admission to plan for discharge and prepare the family. A decrease in length of stay generally translates into a decrease in costs.

CRITICAL THINKING 20-3

The third-party payer system in the United States is complex and constantly changing. Third-party payers are the organizations that pay patients' hospital bills. They include government payers, such as Medicaid and Medicare and private payers such as health insurance companies. For example, to some payers, decreasing lengths of stay may mean decreasing payments. Other payers will pay for a patient admission using a **diagnosis-related group** (DRG) payment reimbursement schedule with preset fees, regardless of the length of stay. DRG payment schedules are based on groups of patients that are medically related with respect to diagnosis or condition, presence of a surgical procedure, age, and presence or absence of comorbidities or complications. So under this type of payment, if the patient is discharged in a short time, generally the facility will make money. If patients stay a long time, hospitals will lose money.

What do you think of these types of cost reimbursement? What can you do to keep health care costs down for your patient? Is there a benefit to the hospital if length of stay is decreased in the DRG system? What can an RN do to prevent delay in discharge of a patient?

METHODOLOGIES FOR QUALITY IMPROVEMENT

There are several models that outline methodologies for quality improvement. Two are reviewed here: the Plan Do Study Act (PDSA) Cycle and the FOCUS methodology. Improvement comes from the application of knowledge (Langley et al., 1996). Thus, any approach to improvement must be based on building and applying knowledge.

THE PLAN DO STUDY ACT CYCLE

The PDSA Cycle starts with the following three questions (Ransom et al., 2005):

1. What are we trying to accomplish?
2. How will we know that a change is an improvement?
3. What changes can we make that will result in improvement?

REAL WORLD INTERVIEW

I n my job, I review a patient's chart and compare it to evidence-based guidelines from research and the literature to see if the patient's health care is being performed in the appropriate setting. I will review if the patient's care is medically necessary. If it is not, I assist the hospital case managers or physicians to move the patient to the appropriate level of care. For example, IV antibiotics can sometimes be administered at home or in another facility. When the situation at home is such that the family cannot manage it, the patient could move to a subacute facility, if available, or the patient could stay in the hospital with the hospital paid at a different rate. Documentation is critical in this type of review. An accurate clinical picture of the patient needs to be reflected in the documentation.

Marguerite Montysko, RN
Case Manager, Albany Medical Center
Albany, New York

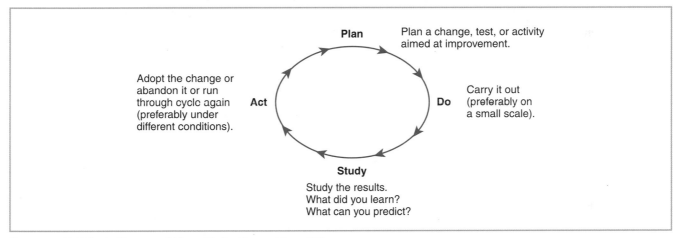

Figure 20-1 PDSA Cycle. (Courtesy of Albany Medical Center, Albany, NY.)

As these questions are being answered, testing needs to be done to evaluate any proposed changes. Testing is done to evaluate the effect of a proposed change and to learn about different alternatives (Figure 20-1). The goal is to increase the ability to predict the effect that one or more changes would have if they were implemented (Langley et al., 1996). The plan for testing should cover who will do what, when they will do it, and where they will do it. Using the PDSA Cycle encourages ongoing quality improvement.

THE FOCUS METHODOLOGY

The FOCUS methodology describes in a stepwise process how to move through the improvement process (Figure 20-2).

F: Focus on an improvement idea. This step asks, "What is the problem?" "What is the opportunity?" During this phase, an improvement opportunity is articulated

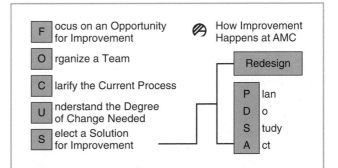

Figure 20-2 FOCUS Method. (Courtesy of Albany Medical Center, Albany, NY.)

and data are obtained to support the hypothesis that an opportunity for improvement exists.

O: Organize a team that knows the work process. This means identifying a group of staff members who are

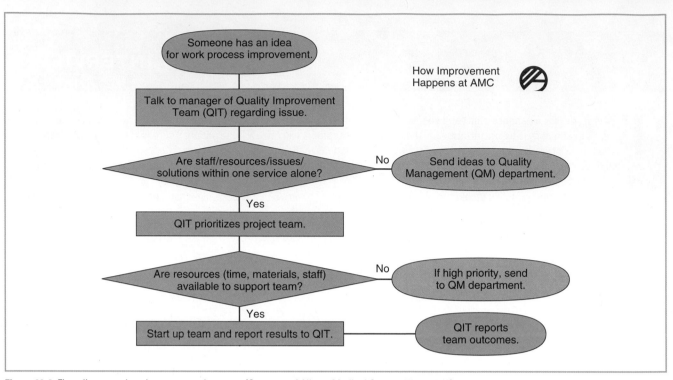

Figure 20-3 Flow diagram—how improvement happens. (Courtesy of Albany Medical Center, Albany, NY.)

direct participants in the work process to be examined—the point-of-service staff. A team leader is identified who will appoint team members.

C: Clarify what is happening in the current work process. A flow diagram (Figure 20-3) is very helpful for this. A detailed flowchart can be analyzed in two ways to uncover possible problems—at a macro level and at the micro level.

At the macro level, scan the flowchart for any indication that the work process is broken. Red flags include the following:

- Many steps that represent quality checks or inspections for errors. When you notice too many boxes in your flow diagram describing similar steps, this could indicate rework or lack of clarity in roles.
- Areas in the work process that are not well understood or cannot be defined. If the work process cannot be defined well, you can be certain it is not being performed efficiently, with maximized outcomes.
- Many wait times between work processes. Wait times should always be minimized to improve efficiency of the process.
- Multiple paths that show lots of people involved in the activity or delivering the service to the customer. Too many staff involved is wasteful and confusing to the patient.

If the existing work process seems reasonable, with one or two areas needing improvement, then a micro-level analysis of your flow diagram is needed.

- Examine decision symbols (diamonds) that represent quality inspection activities. For example, in the flow diagram in Figure 20-3, the "Are resources available . . . ?" diamond is a decision point. Either the resources are available or they are not. Can material, etc., be eliminated? Do some errors go undetected? Is the issue high priority? This examination will ensure limited rework and maximum clarity.
- Examine each work process in the diagram for redundancy and value. If a step in the work process is repeated or does not have any value for the customer, it should be eliminated.
- Examine work processes for waiting time areas. The work process should be changed to eliminate these wait times.
- Examine all work processes for rework loops. A step should not be repeated. Resources are always limited, especially in hospitals today.
- Check that handoffs are smooth and necessary. Handoffs are times when a work process is handed from one staff person or department to another. Handoffs always leave room for error. During this phase, cause-and-effect diagrams and Pareto charts can be helpful. These tools will be illustrated later.

U: Understand the degree of change needed. In this stage, the team reviews what it knows and enhances its knowledge by reviewing the literature, available data,

Bed Access Improvement Team
Phase 2 Work Plan: Transition to Daily Management and Evaluation

Activity	Responsible Party	8/98	9/98	10/98	11/98	12/98
1.0 Modify the Team						
1.1 Identify Phase 2 Tasks to Be Completed	Team	▓				
1.2 Review & Modify Team Composition/Membership	Team	▓				
1.3 Develop Work Plan	Planning Team	▓				
1.4 Review Work Plan with Team	Myers/Nolan		▓			
2.0 Review/Modify Ideal Design						
2.1 Identify Modifications/Opportunities for Additional Change	Team				▓	
2.2 Revise Ideal Flow Chart	Team					
3.0 Modify Structure & Supports: People/Forms Needed						
3.1 Revise Process Management Structure • Modify Job Descriptions—Triage Manager and Admitting Coordinator	Triage Management Subgroup				▓	
3.2 Assess Communication Needed with Nursing Units	Team					
4.0 Draft/Standardize Tasks						
4.1 Draft/Standardize Tasks					▓	
5.0 Transition to Daily Operations, Develop Data Collection Process, Evaluate, Monitor						
5.1 Evaluate Bed Access Simulation • Review ED & PACU Data • Identify Accomplishments and Opportunities of Structure and Ideal Process	Team					▓
5.2 Develop Plan to Transition Process and Structure to Daily Operations	Planning Team					▓
5.3 Develop Data Collection Process	Planning Team					▓
5.4 Evaluate Process & Structure (Milestone Meeting)	Team					▓
5.5 Identify Subgroup of Pt Care Delivery System QIT to Monitor Progress	Team					▓

Figure 20-4 Gantt chart/workplan. (Courtesy of Albany Medical Center, Albany, NY.)

REAL WORLD INTERVIEW

I felt that benchmarking was useful because it allowed us to compare ourselves to other organizations. It allowed us to network with other similar facilities to share ideas and strategies. It allowed us to test our strategies to see if we were making any improvements.

Karen Petronis, RN, MS
Orthopedic Clinical Nurse Specialist
Albany, New York

and competitive benchmarks. How are other health care organizations doing the process?

S: Solution: Select a solution for improvement. The team can brainstorm and then choose the best solution. It can then use the PDSA Cycle to test this solution.

An implementation plan should be used to track progress and the steps required. This implementation plan can be in the form of a work plan or Gantt chart. This is a chart in the form of a table that identifies what activity is to be completed, who is responsible for it, and when is it going to be done (Figure 20-4). It outlines the steps needed to implement the change.

OTHER IMPROVEMENT STRATEGIES

Improvement strategies identified at the organizational level involve benchmarking, meeting regulatory requirements, identifying opportunities for system changes following sentinel event review, using visual measurements, and using a storyboard.

BENCHMARKING

Benchmarking is the continual and collaborative discipline of measuring and comparing the results of key work processes with those of the best performers. It is learning how to adapt these best practices to achieve breakthrough process improvement and build healthier communities (Gift & Mosel, 1994). Benchmarking focuses on key services or work processes, for example, length of time from the patient entering the emergency department until the time of a treatment PCI procedure. A benchmark study will identify gaps in performance and provide options for selection of processes to improve, ideas for redesign of care delivery, and ideas for better ways of meeting customer expectation. There are various types of benchmarking studies, such as clinical, financial, and operational. A clinical benchmark study will review outcomes of patient care, for example, reviewing standards of managing the outcomes of care of patients with diabetes or a stroke. Financial benchmarking studies examine cost/case charges and length of stay. Operational benchmarking studies review systems that support care, for example, the case management system in an organization. It is key for benchmarking studies to be linked to organizational improvement priorities to ensure that change and system redesign are supported by senior administration. The outcomes of clinical, financial, and operational studies are compared or benchmarked with another high-quality organization's outcomes.

REGULATORY REQUIREMENTS

The Joint Commission (JC) has developed standards to guide critical activities performed by health care organizations. Preparation for an accreditation survey and the survey results will provide a wealth of information and data, which can be utilized as ideas for improvement strategies. In January 2003, the first six National Patient Safety Goals (NPSG) were approved by the JC. Each year, the JC publishes new goals that organizations must have in place to promote specific improvements in care related to patient safety. Recognizing that system design is intrinsic to the delivery of safe, high-quality health care, the goals focus on systemwide solutions wherever possible. The NPSG goals focus on Communication, Patient Identification, Medication Safety, Falls, Surgical Fines, and Medication Reconciliation. Specific information regarding the history and ongoing requirements can be found at the JC Website. (www.jointcommission.org). JC requires that specific data be collected and reported during a survey (ORYX measures). In addition, the Center for Medicare (CMS) requires reporting on key quality measures, some linked to pay for performance. Reporting on quality measures is required in clinical areas such as Acute Myocardial Infarction, Congestive Heart Failure, Pneumonia, and Surgical Infection Prevention.

SENTINEL EVENT REVIEW

An adverse **sentinel event** is an unexpected occurrence involving death or serious physical or psychological injury to a patient. Events are called sentinel because they require immediate investigation. During analysis of these sentinel events, opportunities for improving the system will arise and should be taken advantage of. Linkage of sentinel event review to the organization's quality improvement system will identify strategies for prevention of future sentinel events. An example of a sentinel event is surgery performed on the wrong side of a patient. Reviewing the surgical process and developing a system to mark the appropriate site is a change in the work process to prevent future harmful occurrences.

MEASUREMENTS

To assess and monitor outcomes, heath care organizations collect and report measures at various levels in the organization. The terms dashboard, balanced scorecard, report cards, and clinical value compass are often used to describe the concept of measuring performance at both a strategic and operational level in the organization. Indicators may be patient clinical or functional status, patient satisfaction measures, cost measures, or organizational performance measures. Figure 20-5 illustrates these in the form of a clinical value compass (Caldwell, 1998).

Such an approach allows those reviewing data to examine all aspects of care. For example, patient outcomes are reflected in a patient's functional status and clinical status. Patient satisfaction and cost balance this to ensure value. Data can be arranged to create a balanced scorecard, in an approach that uses the organization's priorities as categories for indicators. For example, three priorities might be customer service, cost-effectiveness, and positive clinical outcomes. These priorities help sort out what should be measured to give a balanced view of whether a strategy is working. Indicators are selected based on what they have in common, so that if a change occurs in the cost-effectiveness category, it will affect the data in another category. For example, if we decrease cost for orthopedic surgery, does that affect the customer's satisfaction positively or negatively? If we decrease the length of stay for these patients, does it increase or decrease complication rates? After indicators are selected, data are tracked over time at regular intervals (every month or every quarter, for example). Figure 20-6 shows how the balanced scorecard was used on an orthopedic unit. From the control charts, you can see that the total hip pathway length of stay increased and then decreased. The satisfaction scores remained at around 90%, so even though the length of stay decreased, the satisfaction did not deteriorate. The ratio of complications went down; the average number of physical therapy visits varied and then went up. This reporting mechanism offers a balanced view. Kaplan and Norton (1996) describe a Balanced Scorecard approach used strategically to align customer service cost-effectiveness and clinical outcome measures. These measures are utilized to monitor organizations' priorities. The goal is to assess that changing a strategy in one area does not negatively impact another indicator. For

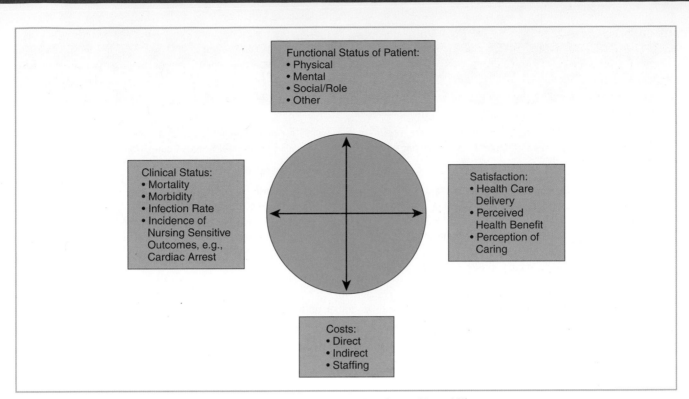

Figure 20-5 Clinical value compass. (Developed with information from Albany Medical Center, Albany, NY.)

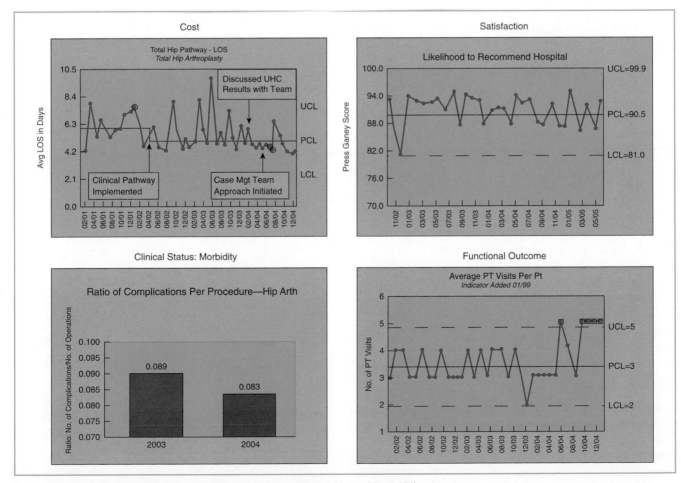

Figure 20-6 Orthopedic Balanced Scorecard. (Courtesy of Albany Medical Center, Albany, NY.)

EVIDENCE FROM THE LITERATURE

Citation: Cossette, S., Cote, J. K., Pepin, J., Ricard, N., Di'Aoust, L. (2006). A dimensional structure of nurse-patient interactions from a caring perspective: Refinement of the Caring Nurse-Patient Interaction Scale (CNPI-Short Scale). *Journal of Advanced Nursing, 55*(2), 198–214.

Discussion: The development of a short version of the Caring Nurse-Patient Interaction Scale is discussed in this article. Measuring caring to assess its effect on patient health outcomes is a priority for nursing. The short version of the 70-item scale was developed based on both inductive and deductive process to assess attitudes and behaviors associated with Watson's ten carative factors. Evidence of validity and reliability of the Short Scale is presented. The Short Scale comprises 23 items, reflecting four caring domains: Humanistic Care (four items), Relational Care (seven items), Clinical Care (nine items), and Comforting Care (three items). The items of the CNPI-Short Scale are identified in the article.

Implications for Practice: The CNPI-Short Scale has potential for use in clinical research settings, particularly when questionnaire length is an issue. It is a useful tool for research aimed at demonstrating that caring is indeed fundamental to nursing.

TABLE 20-2   BALANCED SCORECARD

Mission—Why We Exist	Balanced Scorecard Measures
Values—What's Important To Us	■ Clinical and functional
Vision—What We Want To Be	■ Financial
Strategy—Our Game Plan	■ Organizational
	■ Satisfaction

Source: Compiled with information from Kaplan, R. S., and Norton, D. P. (2004). *Strategy maps.* Boston: Harvard Business School Publishing.

example, as an organization increases patient volume and reduces length of stay, is there any change noted in the patient readmission rate or patient satisfaction? The Balanced Scorecard reflects the organization's mission, vision, and values (Table 20-2).

STORYBOARD: HOW TO SHARE YOUR STORY

Quality improvement teams share their work with others using a storyboard. The storyboard usually takes the major steps in the improvement methodology and visually outlines the progress in each step. The storyboard can be displayed in a high-traffic area of the organization to inform

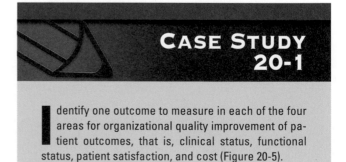

CASE STUDY 20-1

Identify one outcome to measure in each of the four areas for organizational quality improvement of patient outcomes, that is, clinical status, functional status, patient satisfaction, and cost (Figure 20-5).

other staff of the QI efforts under way. Storyboarding can be done when a QI process is complete, or used during the QI process to communicate information.

PATIENT SATISFACTION DATA

Health care facilities get feedback from patients by having them fill out a questionnaire that asks how they felt about their health care encounter. It is most helpful if this data can be compared or benchmarked with other organizations' data. This requires that several organizations use the same data collection tools. All patient responses are put into a database so the results can be compared. Another method of patient data collection is via a phone call. One method of doing this is as a follow-up phone call after patient discharge. Another method to obtain patient satisfaction information is via a focus group or postcare interview or phone call. This means talking with one or more patients after their discharge and getting feedback on their perceptions of their stay.

USING DATA

Several different types of charts are used to examine data in QI efforts. These include time series charts, Pareto charts, histograms, flowcharts, fishbone diagrams, pie charts, and check sheets.

TIME SERIES DATA

Time series data (Figure 20-7) allow a QI team to see change in quality over time. A time series chart allows the user to determine whether a process is in control, meaning that the process has normal variation rather than dramatic changes that are not predictable. Although bar charts are useful, there are times in process improvement efforts when time series data display the process more clearly.

In the bar graph at the top of Figure 20-7, you can see that from year one to year two the percentage of the time that Foley catheters were in for greater than two days decreased dramatically. However, if you look at the time series chart of the same data for two different units,

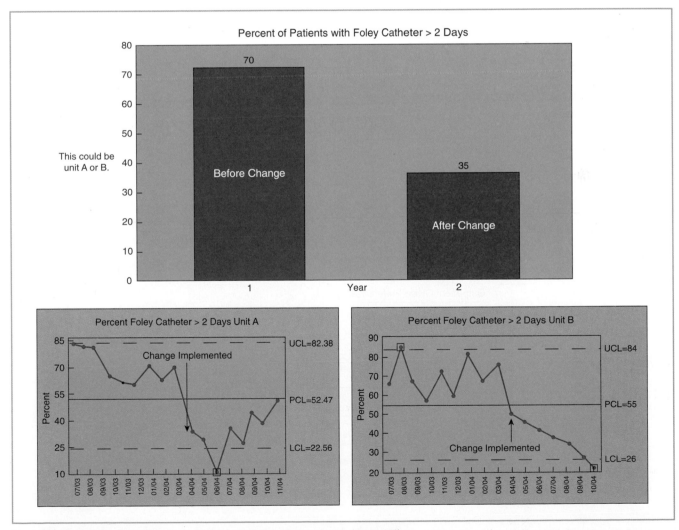

Figure 20-7 Time series versus bar charts. (Courtesy of Albany Medical Center, Albany, NY.)

the actual process for each unit is quite different. Unit A had a good initial decrease after the change was implemented. However, it could not hold the gains, and the rate of Foley use has begun to creep back up. Unit B, however, made progress and has continued to decrease its rate over time. Determining next steps for these two units in this process improvement initiative would require very different strategies.

Tracking data over time allows you to see how a process is behaving. A time series graph is used for this. Graphs or charts—rather than tables of numbers—are used to display data because graphs are faster to interpret. As you can see from the graph of the total hip arthroplasty pathway length of stay in Figure 20-6, a time series data graph contains data points at particular intervals, every two months for example. The process centerline (PCL) represents the average, and the upper control limit (UCL) and lower control limit (LCL) represent acceptable boundaries for expected performance (Wheeler, 1993). If the process were changed in some way, you would expect to see the data change at that time. The time series chart is used to look for trends, shifts, and unusual data.

CHARTS: PARETO, HISTOGRAM, FLOWCHARTS, FISHBONE DIAGRAMS, PIE CHARTS, AND CHECK SHEETS

In addition to time series data graphs, information can be displayed in several different ways to enhance decision making. These include Pareto diagrams, pie charts, flowcharts, and histograms. Figure 20-8 is an example of a fishbone diagram. (Fishbone diagrams are also referred to as root cause diagrams, cause-and-effect diagrams, or Ishikawa diagrams.) Note that many factors contribute to a problem. Review of a cause-and-effect chart encourages staff to look for all the causes of a problem, not just one cause. Figures 20-9 and 20-10 show a flowchart, a check sheet, a Pareto chart, and a control chart. A full discussion of these tools is outside the scope of this chapter.

PRINCIPLES IN ACTION IN AN ORGANIZATION

How are these principles and tools of quality management actually used on a day-to-day basis in a health care facility? This is done through setting up a structure for the organization, using a process for quality, and monitoring outcomes.

ORGANIZATIONAL STRUCTURE

Most organizations today are structured to maximize QI efforts. This allows an organization to be flexible and nimble in a very turbulent health care environment. An organization accomplishes this through an organizational structure that encourages accountability and communication and by focusing all staff on the priorities of the organization.

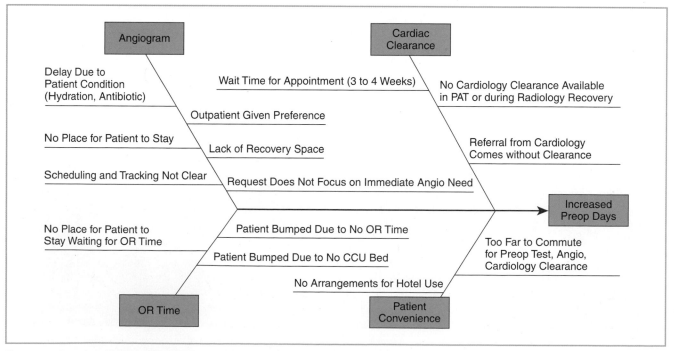

Figure 20-8 Root cause/fishbone diagram. (Courtesy of Albany Medical Center, Albany, NY.)

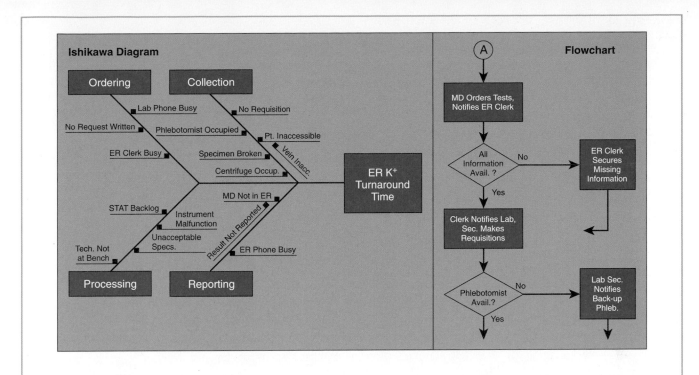

Figure 20-9 Ishikawa Diagram, Flowchart, and Check Sheet. (Reprinted with permission from *Total quality and the management of laboratories* by K. N. Simpson, A. D. Kaluzny, and C. P. McLaughlin, 1991, *Clinical Laboratory Management Review, 5*(6), 448–449, 452–453, 456–458 PASSIM. ©Clinical Laboratory Management Association, Inc. All rights reserved.)

Figure 20-11 is an organizational chart that shows a structure for quality improvement. Note that it includes staff from the board level to staff on individual quality improvement teams (QITs). Within an organizational structure, it is vital that nursing leadership is represented at all levels. In the structure represented in Figure 20-11, the Chief Nursing Officer participates at Board/Hospital Affairs, Executive Management Council, and Center Quality Council. The CNO and the Nursing Directors co-lead the Service Quality Improvement Teams (QITs). Nursing and other health care staff are represented on the QITs and are vital to promoting input and ideas for change in

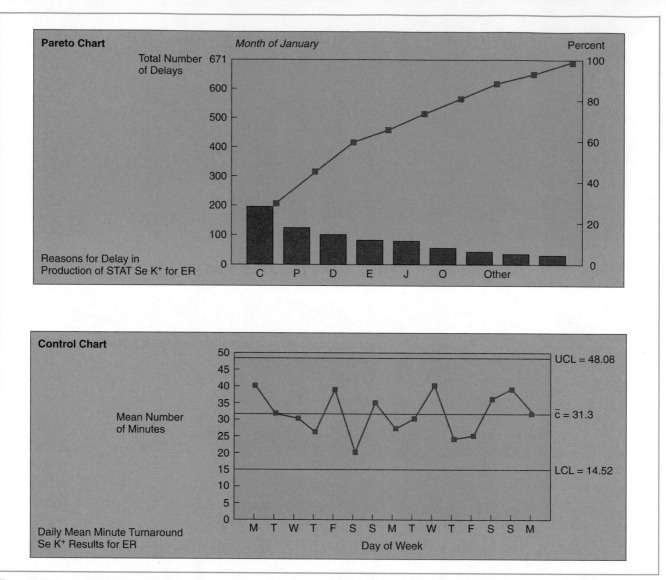

Figure 20-10 Pareto Chart and Control Chart. (Reprinted with permission from Total quality and the management of laboratories by K. N. Simpson, A. D. Kaluzny, and C. P. McLaughlin, 1991, *Clinical Laboratory Management Review, 5*(6), 448–449, 452–453, 456–458 PASSIM. ©Clinical Laboratory Management Association, Inc. All rights reserved.)

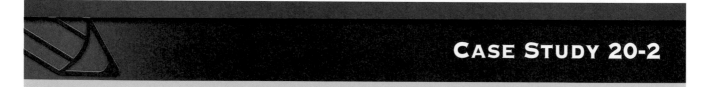

CASE STUDY 20-2

You have been caring for groups of patients following myocardial infarctions. You have also developed a good working relationship with the other nursing and medical staff on your unit. You believe that the care delivery on your unit could improve, thus improving patient satisfaction and clinical outcomes and decreasing the length of stay. How would you proceed? Whose support would you enlist first? Who should be involved? What quality indicators could be measured?

workflow and work processes to improve patient care. Communicating priorities at all levels in the organization is key. Staff members must realize how their day-to-day work influences the accomplishment of strategic goals.

Mission, vision, and value statements help accomplish this clarity of focus. This is discussed more in Chapter 10. These statements guide the quality improvement teams, and the outcomes can be measured.

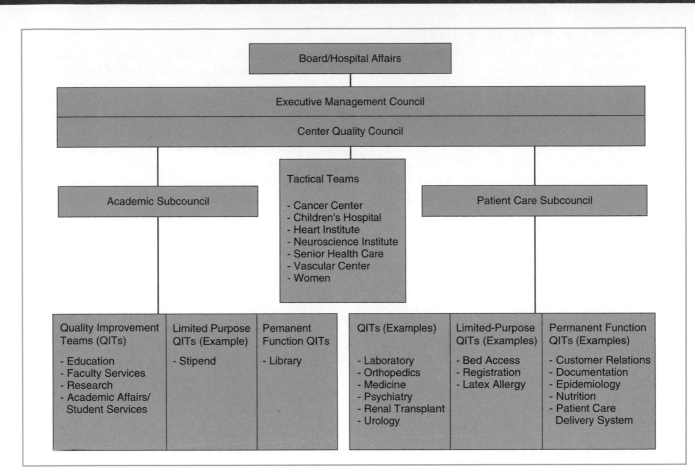

Figure 20-11 Structure for quality improvement. (Courtesy of Albany Medical Center, Albany, NY.)

CRITICAL THINKING 20-4

There are times when some care practitioners see clinical pathways and other standardized guidelines as cookie-cutter medicine. All health care providers like to think they give their patients the best care possible. Standardization and evidence-based clinical guidelines are meant to communicate the latest evidence as to the best practice for a given patient problem. In the absence of evidence-based practices, consensus of the team should be used to develop the clinical pathway.

A group that was developing a clinical pathway for the care of patients with acute myocardial infarction noted evidence showing that these patients should receive acetylsalicylic acid (ASA) on admission. The research in this area was very clear, and most providers believed this was being done. When a chart audit was performed to determine whether this was, in fact, the practice on the unit, it was discovered that only 48% of the patients were receiving ASA within eight hours of admission. The team added this to the clinical pathway. After this was implemented, 85% of the patients received ASA within the first eight hours of admission.

What clinical practices do you see on your clinical unit that are based on an evidence-based clinical pathway? How can you participate in improving the care of more patients using evidence-based clinical pathways?

OUTCOMES MONITORING

Outcomes are a measurement of the patient response to structure and process. Outcomes measure actual clinical progress. Outcomes can be short term, such as the average length of stay for a patient population, or long term, such as a measure of patients' progress over time (e.g., survival rate for a transplant patient one, two, and three years after treatment). Outcomes are studied to identify potential areas of concern. This may lead to an investigation of structure and process to determine any root causes of a negative outcome. For example, when a postoperative infection rate was used as an outcome measure, an increase in the number of infections per month was noted. This led the team to review the patient care process being used. It was discovered that, often, preoperative prophylactic antibiotics were not given to the patient because the order was not written. The team added this order to the initial order set, and all patients received prophylactic antibiotics. The number of postoperative infections decreased. Outcome monitoring is critical to quality improvement.

KEY CONCEPTS

- Quality improvement is a continuous process focused on maintaining regulatory compliance and improving patient care processes and outcomes.

- Patient care needs should drive improvement opportunities.

- Decisions should be driven by data.

- Improvement initiatives should be linked to the organization's mission, vision, and values.

- Organizational goals and objectives should be communicated up and down the organization.

- There should be a balance in improvement goals focused on patient clinical and functional status, cost, and patient satisfaction outcomes.

- Customers of health care are patients, nurses, doctors, the community, and so on.

- A clinical value compass identifies key outcomes that are monitored for quality improvement.

- The PDSA Cycle and FOCUS Method are used to improve quality in organizations.

- Everyone in an organization is part of quality improvement efforts.

- Systems for quality improvement will work to improve care in an organization.

- Benchmarks are used to monitor quality.

- Organizations are structured to improve quality.

KEY TERMS

benchmarking
diagnosis-related group
process
quality assurance (QA)

quality improvement (QI)
sentinel event
system

REVIEW QUESTIONS

1. Which of the following describes the benchmarking process?
   A. Reviewing your own unit's data for opportunities
   B. Collecting data on an individual patient
   C. Reviewing data in the literature
   D. Comparing your data to that of other organizations to identify improvement opportunities

2. Identifying QI opportunities in the health care arena is the responsibility of which group?
   A. Administration
   B. Practitioners
   C. Patients
   D. All health care personnel

3. Following a sentinel event, which step would be initiated first?
   A. No action
   B. Corrective action of personnel
   C. Reporting to health department/root cause analysis
   D. Immediate investigation

4. What document defines the purpose of an organization?
   A. Mission
   B. Fishbone diagram
   C. Balanced scorecard
   D. Process flowchart

5. What tool could be used to track a change in a process over time?
   A. Flowchart
   B. Histogram
   C. Time series chart
   D. Pie chart

6. Standardizing a process has which of the following effects? It:
   A. removes all chance of error.
   B. removes unwanted variation from a work process, decreasing risk for error.

C. increases complexity because it is hard to communicate the standard to everyone.

D. makes care delivery too "cookie cutter" in nature.

REVIEW ACTIVITIES

1. Risk management, infection control practitioners, and a benchmark study have revealed that your unit's utilization of Foley catheters is above average. Brainstorm reasons why this may be occurring. Creating a fishbone (root cause) diagram may help.

2. After you have identified the root causes for the overuse of Foley catheters, use the PDSA Cycle to identify improvement strategies.

3. Think about your last clinical rotation experience. Identify one work process that you believe could be improved and describe how you would begin improving the process. Use the FOCUS Method in Figure 20-2.

EXPLORING THE WEB

■ Use these sites for potential benchmark data: University HealthSystem Consortium (UHC): *www.uhc.edu*

Institute for Healthcare Improvement (IHI): *www.ihi.org*

■ These sites are recommended for a team that is looking for evidence-based guidelines or research studies for a particular diagnosis:

National Guideline Clearinghouse: *www.guideline.gov*

Cochrane Library: *www.cochrane.org*

PubMed's Clinical Queries: *www.ncbi.nlm.nih.gov/entrez/query.fcgi*

Evidence-Based Practice Internet Resources: *http://hsl.mcmaster.ca/ebm* *www.zynxhealth.com*

■ The Joint Commission: *www.jointcommission.org*

■ Note this AACN Website for nursing staffing levels: *www.aacn.nche.edu*

Health grades: *www.healthgrades.com*

REFERENCES

Berwick, D., & Plsek, P. (1992). *Managing medical quality videotape series.* Woodbridge, NJ: Quality Visions.

Caldwell, C. (1998). *Handbook for managing change in health care.* Milwaukee, WI: ASQ Quality Press.

Carey, R. G., & Lloyd, R. C. (2001). *Measuring quality improvement in healthcare: A guide to statistical process control applications.* Milwaukee, WI: Quality Press.

Cossette, S., Cote, J. K., Pepin, J., Ricard, N., D'Aoust, L. (2006). A dimensional structure of nurse-patient interactions from a caring perspective: Refinement of the Caring Nurse-Patient Interaction Scale (CNPI-Short Scale). *Journal of Advanced Nursing, 55*(2), 198–214.

Crosby, P. B. (1989). *Let's talk quality.* New York: McGraw-Hill.

Deming, W. E. (1986). *Out of the crisis.* Cambridge, MA: Center for Advanced Engineering Study.

Deming, W. E. (2000). *Out of Crisis.* Cambridge, MA: The MIT Press.

Donabedian, A. R. (2003). *An introduction to quality assurance in health care.* New York: Oxford University Press.

Gift, R. G., & Mosel, D. (1994). *Benchmarking in health care: A collaborative approach.* Chicago: American Hospital Publishing.

Institute of Medicine. (1999). *To err is human.* Washington, DC: National Academy Press.

Kaplan, R. S., & Norton, D. P. (1996). *Balanced scorecard: Translating strategy into action.* Boston: Harvard Business School Publishing.

Kaplan, R. S., & Norton, D. P. (2004). *Strategy maps.* Boston: Harvard Business School Publishing.

Langley, G. J., Nolan, K. M., Norman, C. L., Provost, L. P., & Nolan, T. W. (1996). *The improvement guide.* San Francisco: Jossey-Bass.

Ransom, S. B., Joshi, M. S., & Nash, D. B. (2005). *The healthcare quality book: Vision, strategy, and tools.* Chicago: Health Administration Press.

Simpson, K. N., Kaluzny, A. D., & McLaughlin, C. P. (1991). Total quality and the management of laboratories. *Clinical Laboratory Management Review, 5*(6), 448–449, 452–453, 456–458.

Wheeler, D. J. (1993). *Understanding variation: The key to managing chaos.* Knoxville, TN: SPC Press.

SUGGESTED READINGS

Albert, N. M. (2006). Evidence-based nursing care for patients with heart failure. *AACN Advanced Critical Care, 17*(2), 170–185.

Beyea, S. C. (2006). Surgical Care Improvement Project: An important initiative. *Association of Operating Room Nurses Journal, 83*(6), 1371–1373.

Institute of Medicine. (2001). *Crossing the quality chasm: A new health system for the 21st century.* Washington, DC: National Academy Press.

Joint Commission (2007). *Comprehensive accreditation manual for hospitals.* Oakbrook, IL: Joint Commission.

Ring, N., Coull, A., Howie, C., Murphy-Black, T., & Watterson, A. (2006). Analysis of the impact of a national initiative to promote evidence-based nursing practice. *International Journal of Nursing Practice, 12*(4), 232–240.

Sanfilippo, J. S., & Robinson, C. L. (2002). *The risk management handbook for healthcare professionals.* New York: The Parthenon Publishing Group.

Shortell, S. M., & Kaluzny, A. D. (2006). *Health care management organization design and behavior* (6th ed.). Clifton Park, NY: Thomson Delmar Learning.

Stubblefield, A. (2005). *The Baptist health care journey to excellence: Creating a culture that wows!* Hoboken, NJ: John Wiley & Sons, Inc.

Wheeler, D. J. (2000). *Understanding variation: The key to managing chaos* (2nd ed.). Knoxville, TN: SPC Press.

Evidence-Based Strategies to Improve Patient Care Outcomes

Mary Anne Jadlos, MS, APRN, BC, CWOCN ✛ Glenda B. Kelman, PhD, APRN, BC

The best outcomes evaluation is likely to come from partnerships of technically proficient analysts and clinicians, each of whom is sensitive to and respectful of the contributions the other can bring (Robert L. Kane, Professor of Public Health, University of Minnesota, 1997).

OBJECTIVES

Upon completion of this chapter, the reader should be able to:

1. Discuss the use of outcomes research in evidence-based practice.
2. Describe selected evidence-based models.
3. Apply the Model for Improvement to implement evidence-based practice in specific patient care situations.
4. Identify resources available to generate outcomes/benchmarks in clinical practice.

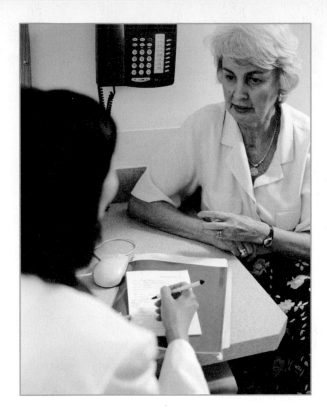

During report, the staff nurse tells you about a 60-year-old woman, Miss Kelly, who was admitted to the unit today with shortness of breath and left hip and sciatic pain after a recent fall at home. The nurse also tells you that Miss Kelly has lymphedema of her right hand and arm and a very large right breast mass that is foul-smelling and bleeds intermittently. Miss Kelly presented to her practitioner with a problem about two weeks ago, and she has been diagnosed with breast cancer.

You immediately begin to suspect she has a pathologic hip fracture. The staff nurse interrupts your thoughts and says, "Wait, there is more. Miss Kelly has also developed a pleural effusion, which necessitated the insertion of a chest tube this morning. Her dyspnea has improved and her pulse oximetry is 99% on two liters of oxygen via nasal cannula. She appears anxious, and has indicated that she is uncomfortable and afraid to move. Miss Kelly rates her pain as 8 on a scale of 0 to 10. She has Tylenol with codeine ordered orally every four hours as needed for pain but has been very reluctant to use the medication because she is afraid that she may become confused. Results of a bone scan and CT scan of the abdomen and pelvis indicate that she has metastatic involvement of the left acetabulum. This also could be the cause of her left hip pain with tumor replacing the bone."

Miss Kelly is single, has no children, and lives with her brother and five cats. She does not smoke or drink. She is a retired clerk for the state Department of Labor. She has been followed by a cardiologist for hypertension for several years. Prior to this illness, she had not actually seen a doctor for almost two years. She would call for prescription refills but then cancel her appointments because she feared what the doctor would find or say.

What are your thoughts about how you will approach this patient?

What additional data do you need to develop a protocol of care to improve Miss Kelly's outcomes?

What priorities should be addressed to manage Miss Kelly's care?

This chapter will identify evidence-based strategies used to improve patient care outcomes. Information from nursing theory and an evidence-based practice model for improvement will be applied to a selected patient case study. By asking the simple question "Why?" you are beginning the journey of gathering data and evidence either to support your current practice or to change how you provide care and interact with patients and families to improve patient care outcomes. The focus is the patient.

EVIDENCE-BASED PRACTICE

Evidence-based practice (EBP) is defined as the conscientious, explicit, and judicious use of current best evidence in making decisions about the care of individual patients (Sackett, Rosenberg, Gray, Haynes, & Richardson, 1996). EBP uses outcomes research and other current research findings to guide the development of appropriate strategies to deliver quality, cost-effective care. Outcomes research provides evidence about benefits, risks, and results of treatments so individuals can make informed decisions and choices to improve their quality of life. Research seeks to understand the end results of particular health care practices and interventions. End results may include changes in a person's ability to function and carry out routine activities of daily living. Outcomes research can also identify potentially effective strategies that can be implemented to improve the quality and value of care.

Evidence-based practice is a total process that begins with knowing what clinical questions to ask, how to find the best practice, and how to critically appraise the evidence for validity and applicability to the particular care situation. The best evidence is then applied by a clinician with expertise based on the patient's unique values and needs. The final aspect of the process includes evaluation of the effectiveness of care and continual process improvement. Responsibilities related to achieving quality outcomes will be addressed in this chapter. They include: (1) provide evidence-based, clinically competent care; (2) demonstrate critical thinking, reflection, and problem-solving skills; (3) take responsibility for quality of care and health outcomes at all levels; and (4) contribute to continuous improvement of the health care system.

Historically, health care providers have relied primarily on biomedical parameters or measures such as laboratory and diagnostic tests to determine whether a health intervention is necessary and whether it is successful. However, these measures often do not fully reflect the multidimensional outcomes that matter most to the patients, such as quality of life, family, work, and overall level of functioning. Traditionally, outcome measures have included physical measures, such as blood pressure to assess the effectiveness of antihypertensive medications. They have also sometimes included patient satisfaction measures to assess patient satisfaction with the care or services provided.

The Institute of Medicine (IOM) released two landmark reports on health care safety and quality, *To Err is Human* (1999) and *Crossing the Quality Chasm* (2001). These studies provided a broad agenda for the nation in addressing quality improvement in health care.

The Institute for Healthcare Improvement (IHI) in December 2004 decided to launch a national initiative, the 100,000 Lives Campaign, with a goal of saving 100,000 lives among patients in hospitals through improvements in safety and the effectiveness of care. Six areas for evidence-based interventions were identified:

1. Deploy Rapid Response Teams
2. Deliver Reliable Evidence-Based Care for Acute Myocardial Infarction
3. Prevent Adverse Drug Events through Medication Reconciliation
4. Prevent Central Line Infections
5. Prevent Surgical Site Infections
6. Prevent Ventilator-Associated Pneumonia

All of the nation's 5,759 hospitals were invited to join and share their progress in reducing mortality. Other organizations that joined the IHI to support the campaign interventions included the Agency for Healthcare Research and Quality (AHRQ), Centers for Medicare & Medicaid Services (CMS), Surgical Care Improvement Project, Joint Commission (JC), formerly the Joint Commission on Accreditation of Healthcare Organizations (JCAHO), and the Leapfrog group. The organizations and examples of their target goals are included in Table 21-1.

ROLE OF THE ANA

The American Nurses Association (ANA) was an active advocate of outcomes evaluation as early as 1976. Outcomes were emphasized as a measure of quality care. The 1980 ANA *Social Policy Statement* stated that one of the four defining characteristics of nursing is the evaluation of the effects of actions in relation to phenomena. In 1986, the ANA approved policies related to the development of a classification system, including outcomes. In 1995, the ANA developed a *Nursing Report Card for Acute Care Settings,* which lists indicators for patient-focused

CRITICAL THINKING 21-1

You have attended a conference to implement one of the initiatives of the 100,000 Lives Campaign. After returning from the conference, a committee is formed to develop a Rapid Response Team. The committee meets to identify sources of information to review current best practice to prevent cardiac arrest or facilitate transfer to intensive care.

What other guidelines should the committee review that support the 100,000 Lives Campaign interventions?

outcomes, structures of care, and care processes. In 2003, the ANA revised the *Social Policy Statement* and included "Nurses use their theoretical and evidence-based knowledge of these phenomena in collaborating with patients to assess, plan, implement, and evaluate care. Nursing interventions are intended to produce beneficial effects and contribute to quality outcomes. Nurses evaluate the effectiveness of their care in relation to identified outcomes and use evidence to improve care (p. 7)."

EVOLUTION OF EBP

Evidence-based practice has evolved from a nice-to-know perspective to a need-to-know essential strategy in health care. Patients, health care providers, and payers recognize the significance of collecting data and analyzing outcomes to achieve safe, quality, cost-effective care. Outcome strategies used in EBP by nurses and members of the health care team include the creation of clinical protocols, guidelines, pathways, algorithms, and so on, which become the tools for health care interventions. A **practice guideline** is a descriptive tool or a standardized specification for care of the typical patient in the typical situation. These guidelines are developed by a formal process that incorporates the best scientific evidence of effectiveness and expert opinions. Synonyms or near synonyms include *practice parameter, preferred practice pattern, algorithm, protocol,* and *clinical standard.*

Evidence-based practice is used to guide practice interventions and is most successful when the entire organization and interdisciplinary team buy into EBP and participate and support the process. By linking the care that people receive to the outcomes they experience, EBP or outcomes research has become key to identifying and developing better strategies to monitor and improve the quality of care.

EBP is not a cookbook approach to patient care, however. The nurse and members of the health care team

TABLE 21-1	EXAMPLES OF ORGANIZATIONS SUPPORTING IHI'S 100,000 LIVES CAMPAIGN AND SELECTED EXAMPLES OF SPECIFIC GOALS/INITIATIVES

Organization	Selected Examples of Initiatives
Agency for Healthcare Research and Quality www.ahrq.gov	Patient safety practices ■ Appropriate prophylaxis to prevent venous thromboembolism ■ Semirecumbent positioning to prevent ventilator-associated pneumonia
Centers for Medicare and Medicaid Services www.cms.hhs.gov	Conditions targeted by the Hospital Quality Initiative ■ Improved care for patients with acute myocardial infarction ■ Prevention of surgical site infection
Institute of Medicine www.iom.edu	Priority areas for transforming health care ■ Ischemic heart disease—prevention and reduction of recurring events ■ Medication management—preventing medication errors ■ Nosocomial infections—prevention and surveillance
Joint Commission www.jointcommission.org	National Patient Safety Goals for Hospitals 2007 ■ Reduce the risk of health care-associated infections ■ Improve the safety of using medications ■ Improve the effectiveness of communication among caregivers
Surgical Care Involvement Project www.cfmc.org	Target Areas ■ Surgical site infections ■ Deep vein thrombosis ■ Postoperative, ventilator-associated pneumonia
The Leapfrog Group www.leapfroggroup.org	Practices endorsed by the National Quality Forum and The Leapfrog Group ■ Create a heath care culture of safety ■ Adhere to effective methods of preventing central venous catheter-associated bloodstream infections

assess each patient and determine whether a guideline is appropriate. Many nursing theorists such as Nightingale, Peplau, Benner, and others have identified that the uniqueness of nursing is based upon the relational and integrative nature of healing, involving the person and environments. Nursing is the only discipline that views the whole person within the context of the person's environment. Nurses must not mimic medical practitioners but must focus on the art and science of nursing that comforts, cares, nurtures, heals, and builds on nursing theory to guide practice. There is a difference between evidence-based practice and evidence-based nursing practice.

Ingersoll has defined **evidence-based nursing practice (EBNP)** as the conscientious, explicit, and judicious use of theory-derived, research-based information in making decisions about nursing care delivery to individuals or groups of individuals and in consideration of individual needs and preferences (2000). Evidence-based practice has a medical focus, whereas evidence-based nursing practice considers the individual's needs and preferences based on nursing theory and research.

The role of the nurse is to participate in developing a comprehensive, interdisciplinary evidence-based plan of care in conjunction with the patient and members of

CRITICAL THINKING 21-2

Two nurses on the oncology unit are having coffee. They are discussing the new clinical findings related to Miss Kelly. An x-ray of the left femur has confirmed a pathologic fracture. They are wondering how they can incorporate the pain management protocol to meet her total comfort care needs, including the left hip pain, discomfort from the open draining breast mass, and her anxiety related to the situation.

How can they adapt or modify the pain management protocol to accommodate all of Miss Kelly's needs?

CRITICAL THINKING 21-3

An elderly patient is admitted with CHF and venous stasis ulcers on her legs. The doctor orders normal saline gauze dressings to be changed twice a day. The evening staff RN is giving report to the night nurse. She states that the dressings are always wet, and they are saturating the bed linens. The RN wonders whether the prescribed dressing regime is the best choice for this patient.

Where do you find answers to your clinical questions?

What health care personnel are available as resources to you?

the health care team. This plan of care integrates the art and science of caring, not merely the medical model of the absence or presence of disease. Nurses must use innovation, creativity, and technology to plan care.

Benner, Hooper-Kyriakidis, Hooper, Stannard, & Eoyang (1998) identify aspects of what they refer to as the skilled know-how of managing a crisis. They state that some of this knowledge is assumed based on training, skill, and experience. Other nursing responsibilities are accepted or imposed based on necessity or a sense of moral obligation. These responsibilities might include stocking equipment at the bedside, prioritizing interventions and

procedures, organizing the team and orchestrating their actions in a way that enhances their ability to function, recognizing the effect of therapies, and asking for help as appropriate. These skills are all relatively invisible in daily nursing practice. They become more visible in crisis situations. Mastery of and comfort with these skills come only with practice, practice, practice.

Nurses are expected to manage the care of acutely ill patients. Beginning nurses should be encouraged to thoughtfully acknowledge their personal abilities and limitations. There must be a blend between knowing and

REAL WORLD INTERVIEW

The pain documentation sheet helps the nursing staff advocate for patients to effectively manage their pain. Having all pain information on one sheet helps us to see at a glance what medications the patient is receiving, how much, and how well the pain is being managed. If a patient's pain is not controlled, I use the sheet to talk with doctors and pharmacists about making adjustments in pain medications. For example, if a patient's pain rating is 6 or above, and he is getting around-the-clock prn Morphine, we can see quickly how much medication is being given within a 24-hour period and also side effects of the medication. Based on this information, we can change the medication to a longer acting medication or increase the dosage to help improve control of the patient's pain while alleviating the side effects. We can also individualize the care by documenting any measures that have helped patients previously when they are in pain. As a preceptor for nursing students and new graduates, I find the protocol and flow sheet especially helpful. Pain management can be complicated. The new graduates like the protocol and flow sheet because all pain-related information is organized in one place and makes pain management easier to understand. It is a great education and communication tool.

Beth Woods, RN
Albany, New York

EVIDENCE FROM THE LITERATURE

Citation: Persson, E., & Larsson, B. W. (2005). Quality of care after ostomy surgery: A perspective study of patients. *Ostomy Wound Management, 51,* 40–48.

Discussion: This study examined ostomy patients' perceptions of quality of care in terms of their evaluation of actual care conditions, as well as the subjective importance they ascribe to those conditions, using an internationally documented instrument to measure quality of care. 49 patients from nine Swedish hospitals completed a postoperative, Quality of Care from the Patient's Perspective (QPP) questionnaire modified to include stoma care variables. The questionnaire is an internationally documented instrument to measure quality of care and consists of items addressing patient perceptions of medical-technical competence of the caregivers, degree of identity-orientation in the attitudes and actions of the caregivers, physical-technical conditions of the care organization, and sociocultural atmosphere of the care organization. The questionnaire was modified to contain an additional thirteen items designed to assess ostomy-specific aspects of care. Medical care, personal necessities, being personal, and physical caring items on the questionnaire received the highest perceived reality scores. Interest in view-of-life, care-room characteristics, and participation items on the questionnaire received the lowest scores. On the subjective importance questions, medical care, physical caring, and care equipment received highest ratings, whereas interest in view-of-life and care-room characteristics scored lowest. On the stoma-specific portion, where to get advice and support regarding the ostomy received the highest perceived reality and subjective importance scores. Satisfactory information regarding the stoma appliance and the possibility to practice handling my stoma in private also received high perceived reality scores. Satisfactory dialogue with Enterostomal Therapy (ET) nurse about sexuality received the lowest scores on perceived reality and subjective importance items. Most items in the QPP questionnaire, including the ostomy-related questions, received high scores on subjective importance, and so reflected the patients' point of view. Patients regarded most aspects of care as important and perceived quality of care received was high. High scores for medical care were thought to be due to the fact that patients with a serious diagnosis had successfully undergone an operation. Enterostomal Therapy (ET) nurses were regarded as experts in stoma care. This finding supports other study findings. Patients may not have desired to talk with ET nurses about sexual concerns due to the questionnaire being completed at the hospital, soon after surgery. Most people did not place high value on caregiver interest in their view-of-life with regard to the quality of their health care. Of note, patients did not feel they were informed about what was happening. Nor did they feel they had the opportunity to voice their feelings regarding their situation. The authors encourage more quality of care research to improve care of ostomy patients in all care settings. In particular, they suggest that interesting and useful results might be derived through diagnosis-related analysis of the quality of care of ostomy patients. Discussion did not indicate whether all hospitals had an ET nurse on staff. It would be interesting to do a research study on patient satisfaction for ostomy care in institutions with and without ET nursing.

Implications for Practice: Patients with ostomies benefit from quality health care in the preoperative, perioperative, and postoperative period. Patient satisfaction is likely to be higher if the hospital has the benefit of ET nursing care. Medical and nursing staff should be encouraged to utilize ET nurses skill in all phases of the patient's care. Periodic outpatient followup, not only with the medical practitioner but with the ET nurse, would most likely enhance patient satisfaction.

doing. It is important that the beginning nurse realize that gaining knowledge and skill is a gradual process. As the beginning nurse develops aspects of skilled know-how, the nurse will become aware of the ability to deliver safe patient care, minimize patient discomfort, decrease stress and anxiety, and assist in optimizing team performance. Guidelines based on EBP can help to direct care but cannot replace learning by hands-on delivery of patient care. As beginning nurses gain clinical experience and learn new theoretical knowledge, they will be able to contribute to the development and revision of EBP guidelines. Remember, EBP guidelines outline practice parameters based on evidence or research, but they do not outline how to deliver individualized patient care.

EVIDENCE-BASED MULTIDISCIPLINARY PRACTICE MODELS

Several models are used in EBP. They include the University of Colorado Hospital model and the Model for Improvement.

THE UNIVERSITY OF COLORADO HOSPITAL MODEL

The University of Colorado Hospital model (Figure 21-1) is an example of an evidence-based multidisciplinary practice model (Goode et al., 2000; Goode & Piedalue, 1999). This model presents a framework for thinking about how you use different sources of information to change or support your practice. The health care team or team member uses valid and current research from sources such as journals, conferences, and clinical experts as the basis for clinical decision making. The model depicts nine sources of evidence that are linked to the research core. This model provides a way for the nurse to organize information and data needed not only to care for a patient but also to evaluate the care provided. In other words, did this patient receive the best possible care not only that this institution can offer, but that is available in this world?

The elements of the University of Colorado's practice model can be applied to the case of Miss Kelly in the Opening Scenario of this chapter (Table 21-2). For example, to assess Miss Kelly's progress related to her diagnosis of breast cancer, it would be important to review evidence using institutional and national benchmarks comparing length of stay for Miss Kelly with other breast cancer patients' length of stay. **Benchmarking** is defined as the continuous process of measuring products, service, and practices against the toughest competitors or those customers recognized as industry leaders (Camp, 1994). The wound care regime related to nursing time and product use could be analyzed

for cost-effectiveness. How much time does it take for a nurse to complete a dressing? How much do the dressings, tape, and other supplies used for the dressing cost?

Pathophysiology would be analyzed by reviewing Miss Kelly's biopsy results, bone scan results, and CT scan results to rule out metastatic disease. These results could be discussed with the practitioner regarding implications related to the prognosis, treatment, and survival rates for breast cancer. A concurrent or ongoing review could be conducted using the Braden Scale for Predicting Pressure Sore Risk (Bergstrom, Braden, Laguzza, & Holman, 1987) and documenting the assessment score daily.

Data collected for quality improvement purposes could include information on the incidence and management of infection, bleeding, pressure ulcers, and pain. The pain and pressure ulcer guidelines from the Agency for Healthcare Research and Quality (AHRQ; formerly the Agency for Health Care Policy and Research) are examples of national evidence-based standards that could be used to benchmark and manage cancer pain (AHCPR, 1994a), prevention of pressure ulcers (1992b), and treatment of pressure ulcers (1994b) for Miss Kelly. In addition, the National Pressure Ulcer Advisory Panel (NPUAP) published a monograph related to the prevalence, incidence and implications of pressure ulcers in America (2001). Other evidence would be continually sought in the literature. Infection control data could include a review of wound culture results and the use of appropriate institutional wound precautions. The nurse could discuss with Miss Kelly, document, and then implement Miss Kelly's wishes regarding advance directives. Utilization of clinical expertise could include consulting the acute care nurse practitioners (ACNPs) and other health care practitioners for input regarding wound, skin, and pain management initially and on an ongoing basis.

THE MODEL FOR IMPROVEMENT

Another model for using EBP is the Model for Improvement (Langley, Nolan, Nolan, Norman, & Provost, 1996). Some elements of this model (Figure 21-2) were discussed in another chapter. The model begins with these questions:

1. What are we trying to accomplish?
2. How will we know that a change is an improvement?
3. What change can we make that will result in improvement?

These three questions provide the foundation for the Model for Improvement and will help focus the use of the Plan, Do, Study, Act (PDSA) Cycle (Figure 21-3) to complete the Model for Improvement. (Note that the PDSA Cycle may also be referred to as Plan-Do-Check-Act [PDCA] Cycle.) We will apply the Model for Improvement to the Opening Scenario presented at the beginning of this chapter in relation to pain, pressure ulcers, and wound management.

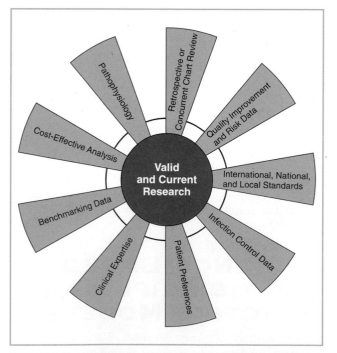

Figure 21-1 University of Colorado Hospital evidence-based multidisciplinary practice model. (By permission of University of Colorado Hospital Research Council, Denver, CO.)

TABLE 21-2	PRACTICE APPLICATION TO ELEMENTS OF THE UNIVERSITY OF COLORADO HOSPITAL MODEL

Model Element	Application
Benchmarking data	Compare length of stay for Miss Kelly with that of other breast cancer patients in this hospital and other hospitals nationally. Review the literature.
Cost-effective analysis	Analyze cost-effectiveness of wound care regimens, including nursing time and use of actual products (for example, hydrogel vs. normal saline dressings).
Pathophysiology	Review biopsy results/findings of testing for metastatic disease and implications.
Retrospective/ concurrent chart review	Assess changes in condition related to pressure ulcer development using the Braden Pressure Ulcer Risk Assessment Scale.
Quality improvement and risk data	Review and analyze documentation regarding patient progress and risk assessment (for example, infection, bleeding, pressure ulcer development); outcomes assessment (for example, pain rating, dosage of narcotic administration, and falls).
International, national, and local standards	Assess effectiveness of care related to AHRQ guidelines and other evidence-based literature for cancer pain and pressure ulcers.
Infection control data	Review wound culture results and institute appropriate precautions and treatment.
Patient preferences	Discuss, document, and implement patient's wishes regarding advance directives, pain management, and so on.
Clinical expertise	Consult acute care nurse practitioner and other practitioners for wound, skin, and pain management.

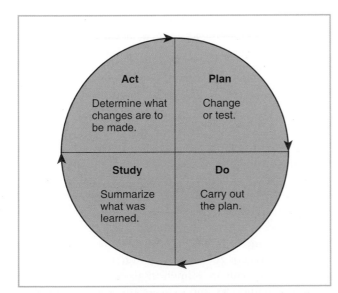

Figure 21-2 The Model for Improvement. (From *A Practical Approach to Enhancing Organizational Performance* [p. 7], by G. J. Langley, K. M. Nolan, T. W. Nolan, C. L. Norman, and L. P. Provost, 1996, San Francisco: Jossey-Bass. Reprinted by permission of Jossey-Bass, Inc., a subsidiary of John Wiley & Sons, Inc.)

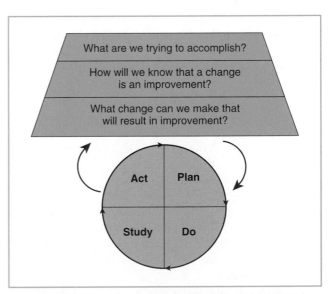

Figure 21-3 The PDSA Cycle. (From *A Practical Approach to Enhancing Organizational Performance* [p. 3], by G. J. Langley, K. M. Nolan, T. W. Nolan, C. L. Norman, and L. P. Provost, 1996, San Francisco: Jossey-Bass. Reprinted by permission of Jossey-Bass, Inc., a subsidiary of John Wiley & Sons, Inc.)

PAIN MANAGEMENT

Unrelieved pain remains a major health problem, and 50% to 80% of individuals with cancer do not receive adequate pain relief (American Pain Society, 1995; SUPPORT Study Principle Investigators, 1995). In August 1997, a collaborative project was initiated with the Robert Wood Johnson Foundation and the Joint Commission (JC) to integrate pain assessment and management into the standards that the JC uses to accredit health care facilities. The pain management standards received approval of the JC board of commissioners in May 1999 and are published in the 2006 Comprehensive Accreditation Manual for Hospitals: The Official Handbook (CAMH). The pain management standards emphasize respect for patient values, beliefs, preferences and dignity, pain assessment in all patients, data collection to monitor effectiveness of pain management, and patient rights to pain management.

APPLICATION OF THE MODEL FOR IMPROVEMENT TO PAIN MANAGEMENT

Let's revisit the scenario related to Miss Kelly described at the beginning of this chapter and apply the Model for Improvement.

1. *What are we trying to accomplish?* The overall objective is to reduce or alleviate Miss Kelly's pain, which may be related to a variety of physiological, psychosocial, and spiritual issues. Cancer pain may be related to the breast cancer compression of tissue and nerves, pressure from a pleural effusion, discomfort related to a chest tube, fear of diagnosis and prognosis, social isolation, and perceived lack of opportunity to participate in spiritual activities.

   The nurse can begin by asking Miss Kelly where her pain is and asking her to describe the quality and characteristics of her pain. Miss Kelly may express a range of sensations related to the different sources of her pain. The nurse will ask her to rate her pain on a scale from 0 to 10, with 0 meaning no pain, and 10 meaning the highest pain possible. The nurse will then document the pain rating and the degree of relief that medications or other pain relief strategies provide and will also identify any alleviating or aggravating factors. The nurses in conjunction with the other members of the health care team will identify, implement, and document the best strategies that reduce, minimize, or alleviate her pain.

2. *How will we know that a change is an improvement?* Miss Kelly will state that her pain is decreased or relieved. Behaviors that may indicate decreased pain include her verbal or nonverbal expression of pain relief or improved comfort, her ability to

reposition herself, and statements such as "I feel more rested," along with an improved mood.

3. *What change can we make that will result in improvement?* To standardize pain management for patients like Miss Kelly, the nursing staff created a protocol that includes implementation of a pain management flow sheet (Figure 21-4). Note that this flow sheet documents the patient's pain status as reported by the patient and pain interventions at various points in time.

IMPLEMENTATION OF THE PDSA CYCLE

The PDSA Cycle can be individual or system focused. It can be used to solve a specific patient problem or to structure strategies to manage groups of patients with common problems. Based on our answers to the three questions, we will apply the PDSA Cycle as follows.

PLANNING PHASE   Once the three Model for Improvement questions have helped staff identify what should be improved, the interdisciplinary staff (nursing and medical practitioners, pharmacists, and so on) would develop a plan for improvement. The plan would include using the pain management flow sheet and implementing unit standards for assessing and monitoring patient comfort.

DOING PHASE   Nursing staff decided to trial the pain management flow sheet to collect data on Miss Kelly during her hospital stay. All nurses assigned to care for Miss Kelly were asked to complete the documentation tool. Data to be collected would include the patient's pain rating, her nonverbal behaviors, level of consciousness, respiratory rate, side effects, activity, nonpharmacological therapies, pharmacological interventions, and patient teaching.

STUDYING PHASE   Data was collected for a period of two weeks. The nurses on the unit met and reviewed the documentation. Several improvements and issues were identified. Documentation of pain assessment and pain parameters had been completed 66% of the time during the two-week period. Staff nurses reported that they referred to the pain management flow sheet when giving report to the doctor about Miss Kelly's pain status, and also to the nurses at the change of shifts. As a result, Miss Kelly's pain management was central in discussions regarding her care, and decisions about changes in her pain medication regimen were made in a timely manner. The nursing and medical practitioners, and pharmacists verbalized satisfaction with the flow sheet in terms of being able to see at a glance the amount and type of medication she was getting, how often, and her rating of pain. Within one week, Miss Kelly was reporting her pain level improved at 2 to 3

PAIN MANAGEMENT FLOW SHEET - DIRECTIONS

1. X PREDOMINANT site of pain on the figures below.
2. Ask patient to rate pain using the Pain Intensity Scale.
3. For VERBAL patients, enter "●" on the flow chart and connect ●----●
   For NON-VERBAL patients, document in the space provided using the key.
4. Document teaching / analgesia / intervention(s).

ASSESSMENT

DATE						
TIME						
INITIALS						
WORST PAIN 10						
9						
8						
7						
6						
5						
4						
3						
2						
1						
NO PAIN 0						
NON-VERBAL BEHAVIOR						
LOC						
RESPIRATORY RATE						
SIDE EFFECTS						
ACTIVITY						
ALTERNATE THERAPY						
MEDICATION REGIME						

INTERVENTION

PCA / EPIDURAL / INTRATHECAL / IV DRIP (Circle) Medication _____

Concentration _____ / cc

RATE (cc/hr)						
BOLUS DOSE (mg)						
TOTAL cc INFUSED						
PT / FAMILY TEACHING						

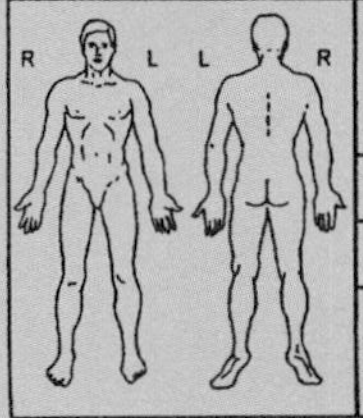

NON-VERBAL BEHAVIORS
G = Grimacing   R = Restless
M = Moaning   — = Not Applicable
Patient-Specific:
1.
2.

0-10 NUMERIC PAIN INTENSITY SCALE
0 1 2 3 4 5 6 7 8 9 10
No Pain — Pain as bad as you can imagine

LEVEL OF CONSCIOUSNESS (LOC)
0 = Normal Sleep
1 = Awake
2 = Occasionally Drowsy; Easy to arouse
3 = Frequently Drowsy; Easy to arouse
4 = Somnolent; Difficult to arouse

SIDE EFFECTS
N = Nausea
V = Vomiting
CNF = Confusion
C = Constipation
R = Urinary Retention
MSD = Motor / Sensory Deficit
HA = Headache
O = Itching
O = Other
— = Not Applicable

ACTIVITY
B = Bed Rest
C = Chair
A = Ambulation
AA = Anticipated Activity
PT = Physical Therapy

ALTERNATE THERAPY
RP = Reposition
H = Heat
C = Ice Pack
M = Massage
TENS = Tens Unit
D = Distraction
— = Not Applicable

MEDICATION REGIME (Drug Name/Dose/Route)
1.
2.
3.
4.

PT / FAMILY TEACHING
P = Per Protocol
R = Reinforced
NN = Narrative Note
RSE = Reinforce Side Effects

Figure 21-4 Pain management flow sheet. Courtesy M.A. Jadlos, G.B. Kelman, K. Marra, and A. Lanoue. (1996). *Oncology Nursing Forum 23*, 1451-1454.

on a scale of 0 to 10. She was receiving around-the-clock medication and bolus dosing three to four times a day as necessary. She remained alert and oriented and had no problems with constipation, urinary retention, or other medication side effects. Radiation therapy was started to her left leg in an effort to control her pain.

ACTING PHASE After a meeting with the nurse manager, clinical nurse specialist, practitioners, pharmacist, staff nurse, and other health care staff to discuss the findings, the staff agreed to continue to trial the pain management flow sheet for four months on all patients admitted to the oncology unit. This next step in the improvement process reflects the use of additional multiple PDSA cycles (Figure 21-5) to improve not only Miss Kelly's individual care but also to improve the total care delivery system.

MULTIPLE USES OF THE PDSA CYCLE

Multiple PDSA cycles were used to improve care, not just for Miss Kelly but for all patients.

PLANNING PHASE The inpatient oncology staff agreed to collect data for four months using the pain management flow sheet on Miss Kelly and all new patients admitted to the oncology unit. A start date and stop date for the pilot study were identified. The pilot study also included a plan to orient the staff to the purpose, development, and procedures for using the tool. A plan was also developed to orient the pharmacist and all practitioners.

DOING PHASE All nursing staff working on the inpatient oncology unit attended an inservice reviewing the purpose, development, and procedures for using the pain management flow sheet. After all the staff had completed the orientation, the data collection period was implemented. The pharmacist and practitioners were oriented individually by the clinical nurse specialists and provided with an opportunity to ask questions. Data was collected by the nurses for a period of four months on all patients admitted to the oncology unit.

STUDYING PHASE Documentation practices and clinical outcomes were reviewed after four months. Documentation of pain assessment was completed on 78% of all patients' charts on admission to the inpatient unit, 67% were completed 24 hours after admission, and 50% were completed 48 hours after admission. The majority of the unit's nurses agreed that they were using the pain management flow sheet as a basis for their report to the practitioner regarding the patient's pain status. The pharmacist and the practitioner reported that they did review the pain management flow sheet approximately 50% of the time, but they most often relied on the staff to verbally share with them the information to improve the patient's pain status.

ACTING PHASE A protocol for pain assessment, management, and documentation was developed and integrated with the pain management flow sheet (Figure 21-6). Eventually, this process was published in the oncology literature (Jadlos, Kelman, Marra, & Lanoue, 1996).

This example using the Model for Improvement provides a framework to think about how to apply knowledge and increase the ability to make changes in individual patient care, ultimately resulting in improvement for many patients. The next two applications of the Model for Improvement are still related to the Opening Scenario but focus on other aspects of comfort care, including pressure ulcer and wound management. Benner et al.'s research with critical care nurses provided a description of clinical judgment and thinking-in-action referred to as clinical grasp and clinical forethought. In addition, they identified nine domains of practice common to complex

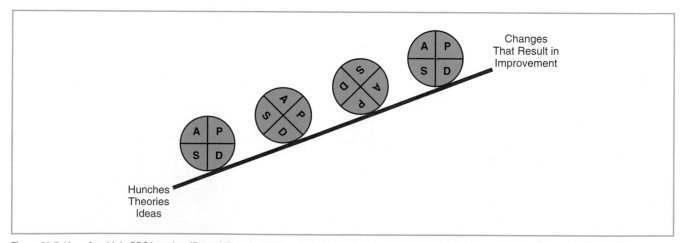

Figure 21-5 Use of multiple PDSA cycles. (From *A Practical Approach to Enhancing Organizational Performance* [p. 5], by G. J. Langley, K. M. Nolan, T. W. Nolan, C. L. Norman, and L. P. Provost, 1996, San Francisco: Jossey-Bass. Reprinted by permission of Jossey-Bass, Inc., a subsidiary of John Wiley & Sons, Inc.)

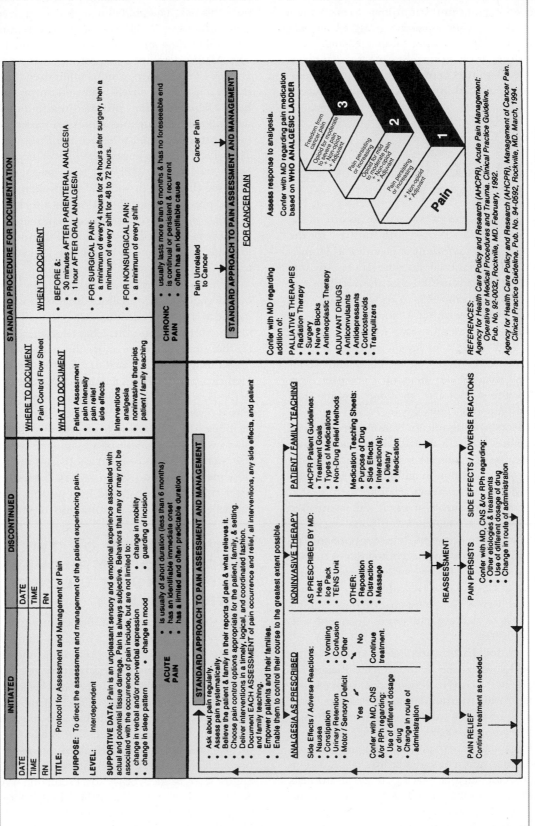

Figure 21-6 Protocol for assessment and management of pain. Courtesy M.A. Jadlos, G.B. Kelman, K. Marra, and A. Lanoue. (1996). *Oncology Nursing Forum* 23, 1451-1454.

patient care situations. One domain includes providing comfort measures. Benner et al. explain that skin is a point of connection and central or primary to many nursing interventions. Touching a patient; giving a back rub; assessing a wound for erythema, drainage, and odor; changing an ostomy appliance; and caring for an incontinent patient are all points of connection with the patient. One of the most essential aspects of nursing practice is comfort care.

PRESSURE ULCER MANAGEMENT

Reducing the prevalence of pressure ulcers is one of the major goals of the Healthy People 2010 Initiative for the nation's health (U.S. Department of Health and Human Services, 2000). The National Pressure Ulcer Advisory Panel (NPUAP) (2001) reported that the incidence of pressure ulcers varies from 0.4% to 38% in acute care, 2.2% to 23.9% in long-term care, and 0% to 17% in home care. Prevalence rates also vary from 10% to 18% in acute care, 2.3% to 28% in long-term care, and 0% to 29% in home care. Research by Zhan and Miller (2003) reported that development of a pressure ulcer adds $10,845 to the cost of care, prolongs hospital stays by 3.98 days, and increases mortality by 7.23%.

Pressure ulcers are a significant health concern for all patients with limited mobility and activity levels. Pressure ulcers occur because of a complex interaction among a variety of risk factors in addition to mobility and activity levels. These include environmental factors, such as skin moisture and cutaneous shear forces, as well as intrinsic biological factors, such as a patient's nutritional status and sensory perception. The economic impact of pressure ulcers is significant. The cost in the United States to heal one pressure ulcer has been reported to range from $5,000 to $40,000. Cost analyses reveal that prevention is cost-effective. However, few cost-effectiveness studies measure the cost to achieve measured treatment outcomes (Phillips, 1997).

The Agency for Healthcare Policy and Research (AHCPR), now known as the Agency for Healthcare Research and Quality (AHRQ), developed evidence-based guidelines that provide the foundation for evidence-based pressure ulcer prevention and management. *Pressure Ulcers in Adults: Prediction and Prevention* (1992b), based on research findings and expert multidisciplinary opinion, recommends identification of at-risk individuals and identification of specific factors placing those individuals at risk. The guidelines recommend use of a validated instrument such as the Braden Scale (Bergstrom, Braden, Laguzza, & Holman, 1987; Bergstrom, Braden, Kemp, Champagne, & Ruby, 1998) (Figure 21-7) to identify

patients at risk for development of pressure ulcers. A protocol should then be initiated for these patients to minimize this risk. The guideline includes three categories of preventive care: 1) skin care and early treatment, 2) mechanical loading and support surfaces, and 3) education. The AHRQ developed a second guideline, *Treatment of Pressure Ulcers* (1994b), which emphasized that underlying causes must be effectively managed for pressure ulcers to heal. These guidelines provided the foundation for tool development to document pressure ulcer healing. The two most widely used tools are the Pressure Sore Status Tool (PSST) (Bates-Jensen, 1998) and the Pressure Ulcer Scale for Healing (PUSH) (Berlowitz et al., 2005). Whereas the PSST provides a comprehensive assessment of the pressure ulcer, the PUSH tool seeks to select the minimal number of assessment parameters needed to monitor healing or deterioration of the ulcer. The PUSH tool has been found to be reliable and easy to use and teach to others (Berlowitz et al., 2005).

Prevention of pressure ulcers is imperative when the overall goal is to cure an illness, to rehabilitate the individual, or to help the individual live optimally with a chronic illness. More recently, there has been increased attention on the prevention of pressure ulcers in the elderly residing in long-term care facilities. In 2004, the Centers for Medicare and Medicaid Services (CMS), formerly known as the Health Care Financing Administration (HCFA), released revised guidelines on pressure ulcers for long-term facilities. The CMS considers a pressure ulcer to be a sentinel event in a resident of a long-term care facility who has been assessed as being at low risk for the development of a pressure ulcer (Ayello, 2002). Therefore, pressure ulcer risk assessment should be a priority of patient care regardless of age, physical condition, or setting.

APPLICATION OF THE MODEL FOR IMPROVEMENT TO PRESSURE ULCER MANAGEMENT

In the scenario presented at the beginning of the chapter, we identified a patient with a need for pain management, and we will now focus on prevention and treatment of pressure ulcers in this same patient. Since admission, Miss Kelly's mobility was limited to bed rest because of multiple factors, including presence of a chest tube, shortness of breath, right arm lymphedema, and metastatic left leg pain from her breast cancer. The Braden Scale for Predicting Pressure Sore Risk demonstrated she was at high risk, with a score of 12 initially and daily for two weeks. See Figure 21-7 Braden Scale for Predicting Pressure Sore Risk, with documentation of Miss Kelly's score. The preventive interventions from the Skin Care Protocol and Flow Sheet were implemented upon admission (see Figure 21-8). A dynamic alternating air mattress was placed

PATIENT *Miss Kelly – Room 6006-1*

The Braden Scale for Predicting Pressure Sore Risk

SENSORY PERCEPTION ability to respond meaningfully to pressure-related discomfort.	**1 Completely Limited** Unresponsive (does not moan, flinch, or grasp) to painful stimuli, due to diminished level of consciousness or sedation OR limited ability to feel pain over most of body surface.	**2 Very Limited** Responds only to painful stimuli. Cannot communicate discomfort except by moaning or restlessness OR has a sensory impairment which limits the ability to feel pain or discomfort over half of body.	**3 Slightly Limited** Responds to verbal commands but cannot always communicate discomfort or need to be turned OR has some sensory impairment which limits ability to feel pain or discomfort in 1 or 2 extremities.	**4 No Impairment** Responds to verbal commands. Has no sensory deficit which would limit ability to feel or voice pain or discomfort.	*3*
MOISTURE degree to which skin is exposed to moisture	**1 Completely Moist** Skin is kept moist almost constantly by perspiration, urine, etc. Dampness is detected every time patient is moved or turned.	**2 Very Moist** Skin is often but not always moist. Linen must be changed at least once a shift.	**3 Occasionally Moist** Skin is occasionally moist, requiring an extra linen change approximately once a day.	**4 Rarely Moist** Skin is usually dry, linen only requires changing at routine intervals.	*3*
ACTIVITY degree of physical activity	**1 Bedfast** Confined to bed.	**2 Chairfast** Ability to walk severely limited or nonexistent. Cannot bear own weight and/or must be assisted into chair or wheelchair.	**3 Walks Occasionally** Walks occasionally during day but for very short distances with or without assistance. Spends majority of each shift in bed or chair.	**4 Walks Frequently** Walks outside the room at least twice a day and inside room at least once every 2 hours during waking hours.	*2*
MOBILITY ability to change and control body position	**1 Completely Immobile** Does not make even slight changes in body or extremity position without assistance.	**2 Very Limited** Makes occasional slight changes in body or extremity position but unable to make frequent or significant changes independently.	**3 Slightly Limited** Makes frequent though slight changes in body or extremity position independently.	**4 No Limitations** Makes major and frequent changes in position without assistance.	*2*
NUTRITION *usual* food intake pattern	**1 Very Poor** Never eats a complete meal. Rarely eats more than one third of any food offered. Eats 2 servings or less of protein (meat or dairy products) per day. Takes fluids poorly. Does not take a liquid dietary supplement OR is NPO and/or maintained on clear liquid or IVs for more than 5 days.	**2 Probably Inadequate** Rarely eats a complete meal and generally eats only about half of any food offered. Protein intake includes only 3 servings of meat or dairy products per day. Occasionally will take a dietary supplement OR receives less than optimum amount of liquid diet or tube feeding.	**3 Adequate** Eats over half of most meals. Eats a total of 4 servings of protein (meat, dairy products) each day. Occasionally will refuse a meal, but will usually take a supplement if offered OR is on a tube feeding or TPN regimen, which probably meets most of nutritional needs.	**4 Excellent** Eats most of every meal. Never refuses a meal. Usually eats a total of 4 or more servings of meat and dairy products. Occasionally eats between meals. Does not require supplementation.	*1*
FRICTION & SHEAR	**1 Problem** Requires moderate to maximum assistance in moving. Complete lifting without sliding against sheets is impossible. Frequently slides down in bed or chair, requiring frequent repositioning with maximum assistance. Spasticity, contractures or agitation leads to almost constant friction.	**2 Potential Problem** Moves feebly or requires minimum assistance. During a move, skin probably slides to some extent against sheets, chair, restraints, or other devices. Maintains relatively good position in chair or bed most of the time but occasionally slides down.	**3 No Apparent Problem** Moves in bed and in chair independently and has sufficient muscle strength to lift up completely during move. Maintains good position in bed or chair at all times.		*1*

TOTAL SCORE: *12*

9 or less = very high risk   10–12 = high risk   13–14 = moderate risk   15–18 = at risk   19–23 = not at risk

**If other major risk factors are present, advance to the next level of risk
(*advanced age, fever, poor dietary intake of protein, diastolic pressure below 60, hemodynamic instability*)

**Total Braden Score of 18 or below is considered predictive for
the development of a pressure ulcer unless preventive measures are taken.**

Figure 21-7 Braden Scale for Predicting Pressure Sore Risk. (Copyright Barbara Braden and Nancy Bergstrom, 1988. Reprinted with permission, documentation added.)

Albany Memorial Hospital
Samaritan Hospital
Northeast Health

Room: 6006-1

Patient: Miss Kelly

SKIN CARE PROTOCOL & FLOW SHEET

Initiate if Braden Score for Pressure Ulcer Risk = 18 or less

PREVENTIVE MEASURES—Documentation Directions:

Enter *START* date, your initials, & indicate selected preventive skin care measures by placing a check mark (✔) in the spaces provided. *Refer to the regimen daily & implement!* Re-document ONLY if regimen *changes!*

		START/ CHANGE DATE	1/2	1/10					COMMENTS
		INITIAL		BF					
MOISTURE RELIEF		Keep CLEAN and DRY	✔	✔					
		Barrier Lotions *routinely*	✔	✔					
		NO DIAPER USE							
PRESSURE RELIEF	**Bedrest**	Air Mattress **S**tatic **D**ynamic **R**otational	D	D					
		Turning Schedule (30 degree angle)	✔	✔					
		Elevate heels off surfaces	✔	✔					
		ICU/CCU Prone Positioner Precautions							
	Chair	Air Cushion **R**egular **B**ariatric		B					
		Limit sitting *based on pt's needs/goals*		✔					
		Remind pt to shift own weight *frequently*							
		Foot Waffle (✔) ❑ R ❑ L							
SHEAR/ FRICTION RELIEF		HOB lower than 30 degrees	✔	*					* tube feeding started
		Barrier Lotions to skin folds/bony prominences *routinely*	✔	✔					
		Assistive Device to reposition/transfer pt	✔	✔					
NUTRITION		Nutrition Consult	✔	✔					
		Assist/Set up pt for meals/feeding	✔						
		Feed pt/Administer tube feeding		✔					

FORM# VN3000(9/06)

Figure 21-8 Skin Care Protocol and Flow Sheet. (Courtesy of Northeast Health, Samaritan and Albany Memorial Hospitals, Acute Care Division, Troy and Albany, NY, with documentation.)

on Miss Kelly's bed. Miss Kelly's appetite was poor, and her serum albumin was low at 1.8 gram/dL. When she was repositioned, Miss Kelly continued to complain of a pulling, stretching, sharp pain radiating from the thigh to the lower leg. She rated the pain as an 8 on a scale of 0 to 10. She had started to take oral Tylenol with codeine as needed every three to four hours. The radiation oncologist initiated a course of radiation therapy to the left leg to help control the leg pain. Her limited mobility necessitated the use of a bedpan for urination and defecation. As a result of her limited mobility and repeated use of the bedpan, Miss Kelly developed a sacral decubitus ulcer and open painful superficial skin breakdown between the buttocks. She tended to lie on her back in bed continuously. When asked why she laid on her back all the time, she stated that her left leg hurt when she moved and that she was afraid her leg would break if she moved the wrong way.

We apply the Model for Improvement and start with the three questions:

1. *What are we trying to accomplish?* The overall goal is to treat and heal the sacral decubitus ulcer, treat and heal the open excoriated skin between the buttocks, and prevent further skin breakdown. The primary risk factors for pressure ulcers are immobility and limited activity levels, so an additional overall goal in managing this patient for pressure ulcer

treatment would include improvement in her mobility and activity level.

2. *How will we know that a change is an improvement?* Miss Kelly's sacral decubitus ulcer and the open skin between her buttocks will show signs of healing. Miss Kelly will verbalize less discomfort related to the open skin between her buttocks. Miss Kelly will demonstrate increased mobility in bed and increased activity such as getting out of bed with assistance and sitting in a chair.

3. *What change can we make that will result in improvement?* We will initiate the Skin Care Protocol and Flow Sheet (Figure 21-8). We will consult the acute care nurse practitioner for additional recommendations regarding treatment of the open skin. We will consult other members of the health care team such as nursing and medical practitioners, physical therapists, a nutritionist, and so on. We will conduct a multidisciplinary patient care conference to coordinate strategies for pressure relief, skin care, mobility, and nutrition. Finally, we will involve Miss Kelly and decide on her goals and care recommendations together.

IMPLEMENTATION OF THE PDSA CYCLE

Based on our answers to the three Model for Improvement questions, we will begin the PDSA Cycle as follows.

PLANNING PHASE   A multidisciplinary patient care conference including the patient and her brother, nursing staff, the ACNP, the medical practitioners, the physical therapists, the nutritionist, and the clinical resource manager was held. All conference members agreed that a change in Miss Kelly's skin care regimen and activity and mobility was necessary in addition to pain and anxiety relief measures. The nurse practitioner wrote orders for pressure relief and management of the sacral ulcer and the open skin on Miss Kelly's buttocks. A dynamic alternating air mattress overlay and air cushion for chair sitting was ordered. A physical therapy consultation was ordered for strengthening exercises and nonweight-bearing instruction for the left leg when out of bed. The Skin Care Protocol (Figure 21-9) was continued to guide interventions and the Skin Care Flow Sheet (Figure 21-10) was used to document the skin care treatment plan for the sacral and buttock ulcers. The Wound and Skin Care Instructions in Figure 21-11 were followed.

DOING PHASE   The staff nurses implemented the agreed-upon plan of care. The Braden Scale for Pressure Sore Risk was assessed daily (Figure 21-7). Preventive interventions that were implemented included a two-hour turning schedule and adherence to limiting chair sitting to a maximum of two hours daily (Figure 21-8). The chest

REAL WORLD INTERVIEW

Miss Kelly had a lot of different worries and concerns that she did not tell us about at first. We were able to see her almost every day, and she grew to trust us. We got to know her and were able to engage her in planning and delivering her care. Miss Kelly said she was afraid about her condition and its treatment. Her physical care was complicated. If her nursing care was not coordinated and monitored closely, she would not have progressed as well as she did and would have developed unnecessary problems. I think that the continuity in care provided by the nurse practitioners helped the entire staff to provide quality care for Miss Kelly, from nursing to physical therapy to medicine to discharge planning.

Mary Anne Jadlos, APRN, BC
Nurse Practitioner
Wound, Skin, Ostomy Service
Albany, New York

TITLE: SKIN CARE PROTOCOL

PURPOSE: To optimize conditions for maintenance of skin integrity and the treatment of open skin for acutely ill patients with Braden Risk Assessment Score of 18 or less.

LEVEL: Independent

Supportive Data: Signs of infection include pus, periwound erythema/edema/pain, change in color of exudate, foul odor, elevated body temperature, and elevated WBC count.

STANDARD PROCEDURE FOR DOCUMENTATION
1. Data Collection Record/Assessment Flow Sheet
2. Skin Care Flow Sheet
3. PPR: evaluative statement (i.e. Improvement or worsening)
4. MEDEX/KARDEX: Treatment/Dressing with frequency

PATIENT/FAMILY EDUCATION
■ Wound & Skin Care Instructions

U N S T A G E A B L E

Deep Tissue Injury (DTI)—A pressure-related injury to subcutaneous tissues under intact skin. Initially, these lesions have the appearance of a deep bruise, and are unstageable. These lesions may herald the subsequent development of a Stage 3 or 4 pressure ulcer even with optimal management.

Eschar—Pressure ulcer covered with necrotic black leathery tissue. Until the eschar is removed, the ulcer can't be accurately visualized and so is unstageable.

U N S T A G E A B L E

Stage 1 Pressure Ulcer (PU)

An observable pressure-related alteration of intact skin whose indicators, as compared with the adjacent or opposite area on the body, may include changes in one or more of the following: skin temperature (warmth or coolness), tissue consistency (firm or boggy feel), & / or sensations (pain, itching). The ulcer appears as a defined area of persistent redness in lightly pigmented skin, whereas, in darker skin tones, the ulcer may appear with persistent red, blue, or purple hues.

STANDARD PROCEDURES FOR SKIN BREAKDOWN

Complete Braden Scale for Predicting Pressure Sore Risk DAILY

Nutrition Consult if Braden Score 18 or less.

Moisture Relief
■ Keep clean and dry
■ Apply Barrier Cream/Lotion/Ointment
■ Consult MD re: condom or indwelling catheter
■ Fecal Incontinence Collector for watery stools.

Pressure Relief—Bed
■ Air Mattress (static, dynamic, rotational)
■ Turning schedule (30 degree angle)
■ Keep heels of mattress

Pressure Relief—Chair
■ Air Cushion (regular, bariatric)
■ Limit time in chair based on patient needs/goals
■ Remind patient to shift own weight, if able
■ Foot Waffle Boot(s)

Shear Relief
■ Head Of Bed lower than 30 degrees

Friction Relief
■ Apply Barrier Cream to skin folds & bony prominences
■ Use assistive devices to reposition/transfer patient

ICU/CCU Prone Positioner Precautions
■ Off-load pressure over the chin, jaw, breasts, anterior ribs, pelvic bones, male genitalia, anterior knees, and toes
■ Place hydrocolloid dressing (ie. Duoderm) over sternum to prevent friction effects on skin
■ Assess facial edema & adjust devices to relieve pressure (hourly)
■ Administer oral care to avoid skin maceration from saliva

PARTIAL THICKNESS WOUNDS

Abrasion   Skin Tear   Superficial Burn   Friction Injury
Radiation Injury   Denudation due to Moisture

Stage 2 Pressure Ulcer (PU)

Pressure-induced injury located over a body prominence & characterized by epidermal sloughing & changes in skin temperature, tissue consistency, & / or sensation.

FULL THICKNESS WOUNDS

Deep Burn   Tumor   Surgical Wound
Venous Insufficiency   Arterial Insufficiency

Stage 3 Pressure Ulcer (PU)

Skin loss involving damage or necrosis of subcutaneous tissue, which may extend down to but not through underlying fascia. The ulcer presents clinically as a deep crater, with or without undermining of adjacent tissue.

Stage 4 Pressure Ulcer (PU)

Skin loss with extensive destruction, tissue necrosis, or damage to muscle, bone or supporting structures (such as tendon, joint capsule).

PRESSURE RELIEF SURFACE SELECTION—For pts with Stage 3/4 PUs OR suspected DTI OR at-risk pts without ulcers.
For specialty products/consults, call Purchasing. Order static air products from Storeroom.

For pts with COMPLEX care needs, check Braden Subscale scores: Sensory Perception, Activity, Mobility & Moisture
***If two or more of these scores = 2 or less obtain alternating low air loss (LAL) mattress (eg. Size-Wise PULSATE)

For BARIATRIC pts AT RISK for pressure ulcers, obtain a Specialty Surface Consult (eg. Size-Wise)
re: necessary bed frame, pressure relief surface & other bedside equipment.

DRESSING SELECTION—Consider:

Condition of wound bed   Amount/Type of wound drainage   Location of wound   Pain related to the wound
Goal of Care (healing, prevention of wound deterioration, comfort)

If signs of infection are present, notify M.D.

Antimicrobial (topical or within dressing)

Granular Wound Bed

Partial & Full Thickness / Stage 2
Nondraining   →   Draining
Transparent   Foam
Hydrocolloid   Calcium alginate
Hydrogel   Hydrofiber
Use Gauze as a secondary dressing, if needed.

Necrotic Wound Bed

Full Thickness / Stage 3 or 4
Nondraining   →   Draining
Transparent   Foam
Hydrogel   Calcium alginate
Hydrocolloid   Hydrofiber
Gauze (moist)   Gauze (moist or dry)

Debridement

Surgical / Mechanical / Autolytic / Enzymatic

Excoriated Skin—Consult with MD/NP re:
Petrolatum (eg. Aquaphor) Ointment
+ / − Anesthetic (eg. Lidocaine) Gel if pain

┌─────────────────────────────┐
│ CONSULT WOUND & SKIN CARE   │
│ NURSE PRACTITIONER for: │
│ Stage 3 or 4 Pressure Ulcers or │
│ suspected Deep Tissue Injury │
└─────────────────────────────┘

Original: 8/8/89
REVIEW:
REVISION: 11/11/92   1/14/98
            6/9/93   9/2/02
            5/10/95   9/21/04
            8/9/95   9/19/06

APPROVAL:

COO & CNO,
Albany Memorial & Samaritan Hospitals

Figure 21-9 Skin Care Protocol. (Courtesy of Northeast Health, Samaritan and Albany Memorial Hospitals, Acute Care Division, Troy and Albany, NY.)

SKIN CARE FLOW SHEET

DIRECTIONS:

1. Mark wound/skin site(s) on body figure, number and circle.
2. For each site, identify wound/skin condition and place ✔.
3. Document assessment(s) and treatment(s) daily in acute care, and at least weekly in home and long-term care, using the:

Assessment Key:

- ❖ **I** = intact   **P** = pink   **R** = red   **S** = slough   **Y** = yellow   **G** = green   **W** = white   **E** = eschar
- ❖❖ **S** = superficial or record in **cm.**
- ❖❖❖ **S** = serosanguinous   **B** = bloody   **Y** = yellow   **G** = green   **0** = none

Treatment Key: **DSD** = Dry Sterile Dsg   **NS** = Normal Saline Dsg   **DD** = Duoderm   **A** = Aquacel   **Aag** = Aquacel Ag   **F** = Flexzan   **GEL** = Hydrogel   **CS** = Collagenase Santyl
AP = Aquaphor   **B** = Barrier Cream/Ointment   **BS** = Barrier Spray   **T** = Tegaderm   **OTA** = Open to air   ***Other:** _____

☐ Abrasion   ☐ Ecchymosis   ☐ Skin Tear   ☐ Tumor   ☐ Burn   ☐ Radiation   ☐ Surgical Wound   ☐ Chest Wall
☐ Pressure Ulcer—Stage 1   2A   2B   3   4   (Circle one)   ☑ Other   _Tumor_

SITE # 1

DATE	10/3	10/4	10/5	10/6	10/7	10/8	10/9	10/10	10/11	10/12			
INITIALS	DT	MAJ	BW	DT	DT	DT	MAJ	BW	DT	MAJ			
Wound bed appearance ❖	RYS	RYS	RYS	RYS	RYS	RY	RY	RY	R	R			
Wound edge appearance ❖	P	P	P	P	P	P	P	P	P	P			
Size (cm.)	15.0	15.0	15.0	15.0	15.0	15.0	15.0	14.5	14.5	14.5			
Depth ❖❖	0.125	0.125	0.125	0.125	0.125	0.125	0.125	0.125	0.125	0.125			
Drainage ❖❖❖	BY	BY	BY	BY	BY	BY	BY	S	S	S			
Odor (Y/N)	Y	Y	Y	N	N	N	N	N	N	N			
Maceration (Y/N)	N	N	N	N	N	N	N	N	N	N			
Inflammation (Y/N)	N	N	N	N	N	N	N	N	N	N			
Undermining (Y/N)	N	N	N	N	N	N	N	N	N	N			
TREATMENT	GEL	GEL	GEL	GEL	GEL	GEL	GEL	GEL	GEL	GEL			

(Continues)

Figure 21-10 Skin Care Flow Sheet. (Courtesy of Northeast Health, Samaritan and Albany Memorial Hospitals, Acute Care Division, Troy and Albany, NY, with documentation.)

SITE #2

□ Abrasion   □ Ecchymosis   □ Skin Tear   □ Tumor   □ Burn   □ Radiation   □ Surgical Wound   □ Sacral Ulcer
☑ Pressure Ulcer—Stage 1   2A   ②A ②B   3   4   (Circle one)   □ Other

DATE	10/9	10/10	10/11	10/12
INITIALS	MAJ	BW	DT	MAJ
Wound bed appearance ❖	R	R	R	R
Wound edge appearance ❖	P	P	P	P
Size (cm.)	3.0	3.0	3.0	2.5
Depth ❖	S	S	S	S
Drainage ❖❖❖	S	S	O	O
Odor (Y/N)	N	N	N	N
Maceration (Y/N)	N	N	N	N
Inflammation (Y/N)	N	N	N	N
Undermining (Y/N)	N	N	N	N
TREATMENT	AP	AP	AP	AP

SITE #3

□ Abrasion   □ Ecchymosis   □ Skin Tear   □ Tumor   □ Burn   □ Radiation   □ Surgical Wound   □ Buttocks
☑ Pressure Ulcer—Stage 1   ②A   2B   3   4   (Circle one)   □ Other

DATE	10/9	10/10	10/11	10/12
INITIALS	MAJ	BW	DT	MAJ
Wound bed appearance ❖	R	R	R	R
Wound edge appearance ❖	R	R	R	R
Size (cm.)	10.0	10.0	10.0	10.0
Depth ❖	S	S	S	S
Drainage ❖❖❖	O	O	O	O
Odor (Y/N)	N	N	N	N
Maceration (Y/N)	N	N	N	N
Inflammation (Y/N)	N	N	N	N
Undermining (Y/N)	N	N	N	N
TREATMENT	B OTA	B OTA	B OTA	B OTA

cm   1   2   3   4   5   6   7   8   9   10

Figure 21-10 Skin Care Flow Sheet (Continued).

Wound & Skin Care Instructions

PRODUCT	GOAL	APPLICATION PROCEDURE
Calcium Alginate *Sorbsan/Calcicare/Tegagen*	Absorb drainage and promote granulation	Change once a day/prn if drainage strikes through outer dressing: ■ Place dressing into wound filling all "dead space." ■ Cover with 4 × 4 gauze dressing and secure with tape.
Foam *Flexzan/Lyofoam*	Absorb drainage and facilitate wound closure	Change every 5 to 7 days/prn if nonadherent: ■ Wipe periwound skin with "skin prep" and allow to dry. ■ Place dressing. ■ Wipe edges with "skin prep" or frame with tape.
Hydrocolloid *Duoderm/Restore/Tegasorb*	Autolytically debride necrotic tissue and facilitate wound closure	Change every 2 to 3 days/prn if nonadherent: ■ Remove paper backing, and then apply dressing. ■ Frame edges with tape.
Hydrofiber *Aquacel/Aquacel Ag* *(with silver)*	Absorb drainage, promote granulation, and decrease bacterial load	Change once a day/prn if drainage strikes through outer dressing: ■ Place dressing into wound filling all "dead space." ■ Cover with 4 × 4 gauze dressing a secure with tape.
Hydrogel *Saf-Gel/Solosite/Tegagel*	Hydrate dry wound bed and facilitate wound closure	Change 1 to 2 times a day: ■ Apply coat of barrier ointment onto periwound skin. ■ Apply hydrogel to wound bed. ■ Cover with 4 × 4 gauze dressing and secure with tape.
Debridement Gel *Collagenase Santy/Accuzyme*	Enzymatically debride devitalized tissue	Change once a day: ■ Apply coat of barrier ointment onto periwound skin. ■ Apply debridement gel to wound bed. ■ Cover with 4 × 4 gauze dressing and secure with tape.
Wet-to-Dry Gauze *Normal Saline*	Mechanically debride necrotic tissue	Change 2 to 3 times a day/prn if soiled: ■ Moisten gauze and wring out. ■ Unfold gauze and place into wound bed, with all surfaces in contact with the gauze. ■ Cover with dry gauze/ABD pad dressing and secure with tape.
Hemostatic *Surgicel*	Stop bleeding	Do not remove. Allow the dressing to fall off: ■ Place the dressing onto the site of persistent bleeding. ■ Cover with a dry ABD pad dressing as desired by the patient. ■ DO NOT TAPE. Mesh netting may be used to secure.
Topical Antibiotic *Cleocin Spray/Flagyl Spray*	Decrease bacterial load and eliminate foul odor	Apply to secondary dressing when changed and prn: ■ Spray antibiotic solution onto a dry gauze dressing. ■ Place moist side of dressing over the wound bed. ■ Cover with dry gauze/ABD pad dressing and secure with tape.
Topical Antimicrobial *Bactroban/SilvaSorb/Silvadene*	Treat local signs of infection	Apply as prescribed by MD or NP: ■ Apply prescribed agent onto wound bed. ■ Cover with 4 × 4 gauze/ABD pad dressing and secure with tape.
Transparent Film *Tegaderm/OpSite*	Autolytically debride devitalized tissue	Change once a day: ■ Remove paper backing carefully from the dressing. ■ Place over wound bed/periwound skin.

Figure 21-11 Wound and skin care instructions. (Courtesy of Northeast Health, Samaritan and Albany Memorial Hospitals, Acute Care Division, Troy and Albany, NY.)

wall tumor (Site # 1) was treated with Hydrogel dressings three times a day. The sacral ulcer (Site # 2) was treated with Aquaphor ointment applied every shift and prn. The buttocks excoriation (Site # 3) was treated with Dimethicone-based barrier lotions every shift and as needed. Both sacral ulcer and buttocks sites were left open to air. The staff nurses documented the status of Miss Kelly's skin breakdown and worked with the nurse practitioners to assess the progress of the patient's wounds. Physical therapists worked with the patient every day on range of motion, transfer techniques, and nonweight-bearing measures. The dietician also was consulted to assess Miss Kelly's nutritional status and made dietary recommendations, which were implemented. Discharge planning was initiated by the clinical resource manager with input from the multidisciplinary team.

STUDYING PHASE Five days after the proposed plan of care was implemented, the open skin between Miss Kelly's buttocks was completely healed. The sacral ulcer, however, looked the same regarding size, depth, appearance of the wound bed, inflammation, and drainage. The patient had received three cycles of chemotherapy and had completed a course of radiation therapy to the left leg. Miss Kelly's left leg pain was minimal, with the patient giving the pain a score of 3 at its worst level. Miss Kelly was making every effort to get out of bed into the chair. In fact, she tried to get out of bed to the chair on her own at first. She thought the doctor wanted her to do this. After this unsuccessful attempt, the nursing staff and practitioner reinforced to Miss Kelly that she ask for assistance for all transfers. She did this. She did not change her position much when in bed, however. She stated that she wanted to sit up in bed most of the time and be on her back so she could look out the doorway.

ACTING PHASE The nursing staff decided to continue the same care regime for the skin of Miss Kelly's buttocks. The ACNP continued to monitor the sacral ulcer with the staff. A revised local wound care regimen was implemented. The staff agreed to continue the PDSA Cycle until there was evidence of improvement in the condition of the sacral ulcer. Miss Kelly's level of mobility and activity would continue to be monitored and would progress as tolerated.

EVIDENCE FROM THE LITERATURE

Citation: Siegel, T. (2006). Do registered nurses perceive the anchoring of indwelling urinary catheters as a necessary aspect of nursing care? *Journal of Wound, Ostomy, and Continence Nursing, 33,* 140–144.

Discussion: This study was done to determine if RNs employed at an acute care facility perceived the anchoring of indwelling urinary catheters (IUC) as a necessary aspect of care. Anchoring was defined as taping the catheter to the patient's inner thigh or using a catheter holder leg strap. A descriptive exploratory pilot study was conducted utilizing the investigator's Catheter Anchoring Survey (CAS) (Siegel, 2003). The CAS was developed based on the responses from the WOCN continence forum, a review of the literature, and discussion with colleagues. The CAS consisted of six questions, and nurses were asked to indicate a response from Strongly Agree to Strongly Disagree. Content validity was established by a panel of eight certified continence nurses who reviewed and made some modifications to the tool. A convenience sample of 82 medical-surgical and critical care nurses completed the survey. Approximately 61% of the sample had more than 10 years of nursing experience, more than 50% had baccalaureate degrees in nursing, and 30% were certified by specialty nursing organizations. Ninety-eight percent of the nurses agreed that securing indwelling urinary catheters was a necessary aspect of care. Their response did not match the prevalence data that was obtained prior to the survey. The prevalence rate found only three catheters were stabilized in 68 patients (4.4%).

Implications for Practice: Nurses may want to consider including the assessment of catheter stabilization as part of their daily routine patient assessment. Further studies are needed to determine the benefits of anchoring IUCs.

WOUND MANAGEMENT

Patients with cancer may experience disruptions in skin integrity related to the disease or its treatment. Alteration in skin integrity may be caused by breast cancer with chest wall involvement as in the case of Miss Kelly. Breast tumors are often very vascular and, if superficially eroded, may bleed easily. Chemotherapy-related lowering of the blood counts, particularly white blood cells and platelets, may result in complications such as bleeding or infection. Tumors also are frequently necrotic and have varying amounts of foul-smelling drainage. Therefore, local wound care needs to incorporate measures to maintain a moist environment, aid debridement, promote epithelialization, and increase comfort. Care must be taken to control exudate and odor, minimize frequency of dressing changes, and remove dressings without trauma.

APPLICATION OF THE MODEL FOR IMPROVEMENT TO WOUND MANAGEMENT

Miss Kelly, as noted previously, has metastatic breast cancer with a large right breast tumor and right arm lymphedema. The right breast tissue was essentially replaced by tumor and the superficial skin had eroded, producing a draining, bloody, malodorous, necrotic wound. The medical oncologist recommended systemic chemotherapy to decrease the size of the breast tumor and treat the metastatic spread of the disease. Potential side effects of this chemotherapy included lowering of the blood counts with risk of infection and bleeding, hair loss, nausea, vomiting, neuropathy, cardiotoxicity, and muscle and joint aches. These side effects were reviewed with Miss Kelly and her brother. An Infusaport was placed for intravenous access, and the chemotherapy treatments were started. Lowered blood counts related to her chemotherapy did occur and resulted in intermittent bleeding from the breast wound. This complicated Miss Kelly's care.

We start with the three questions:

1. *What are we trying to accomplish?* Our goals are to prevent wound infection and bleeding and control odor and exudate. We will work to facilitate epithelialization, if possible, and promote comfort and preserve Miss Kelly's sense of body image.
2. *How will we know that a change is an improvement?* The size of the wound bed will decrease. There will be minimal or no bleeding from the wound bed. There will be no signs of wound infection.
3. *What change can we make that will result in improvement?* We will consult the acute care nurse practitioner for wound care recommendations. We will conduct a multidisciplinary care conference to

coordinate the wound care strategies. Wound care of Miss Kelly's right breast wound can be coordinated with selected members of the nursing staff who are familiar with the patient. The ACNP may initially change the dressing on a regular basis to ensure consistency, optimize wound healing, and prevent complications.

IMPLEMENTATION OF THE PDSA CYCLE

Based on our answers to the three questions, we will begin the PDSA Cycle as follows.

PLANNING PHASE   The nursing staff and the ACNP examined the right breast wound. Based on this examination, the ACNP recommended a regimen of hydrogel gauze dressing changes twice daily. The ACNP explained to the staff and the patient that the use of a hydrogel dressing would maintain a moist environment, conform easily to the wound, and reduce pain. Removal of the secondary dressing would be easier because of the moist, nonadherent wound surface. Hydrogel also provides some autolytic debridement through softening of necrotic tissue (Bates-Jensen, 1998). If there was a significant amount of loosened necrotic tissue, consideration would be given to removal of the tissue by debridement. Any debridement would be performed by the ACNP or medical practitioner. In addition, an antibiotic spray solution for application onto the gauze was prescribed to help decrease the foul odor. The dressing was to be stabilized using mesh netting around the patient's trunk to alleviate the need for taping onto the patient's skin.

DOING PHASE   The staff nurses implemented the agreed-upon plan of care. The ACNPs assisted by changing the dressing two to three times a week and communicating with the staff. Miss Kelly's platelet levels were monitored closely and debridement of the wound bed was not performed on the days that the platelet counts were low. If bleeding occurred during the dressing change, the nursing staff was instructed not to apply pressure directly on the wound area but to hold a dry gauze next to the site until the bleeding stopped.

STUDYING PHASE   Eight weeks after the implementation of the proposed plan of care, the patient had received three cycles of chemotherapy. During this time, the patient received antibiotic therapy and colony-stimulating factors (CSFs) to maintain her white blood count and reduce the risk of infection. The topical

---

CASE STUDY 21-1

Mr. Albert is a 52-year-old male diagnosed with metastatic rectal cancer. He is admitted with intractable abdominal pain and has a colostomy. He has developed chemotherapy-related peripheral neuropathy and has a limited ability to feel pain in his legs. Other pertinent assessment information includes the following:

- Alert and oriented.
- Height = 5'10" and weight = 165 lbs.
- Bedbound; makes occasional slight changes in body or extremity position but unable to make frequent or significant changes independently; refuses to be turned due to pain.
- Frequently slides down in bed requiring frequent repositioning with maximum assistance.
- Incontinent of urine at least four times a day; colostomy.
- Rarely eats more than one-third of any food offered; takes fluids poorly; refuses liquid dietary supplements.
- Hgb = 7.2; serum albumin = 1.7; pulse oximetry = 90% on room air.
- Admitting orders include Morphine Sulfate 4 mg IV every three to four hours as necessary for pain.

Calculate a Braden Score using the Braden Scale for Pressure Sore Risk.

---

antibiotic spray was effective in eliminating wound odor. The breast wound had dramatically decreased in size, with 90% of the original wound bed covered by epithelial tissue. The remainder of the wound bed was clean with minimal serous drainage. The patient was much more comfortable as a result.

ACTING PHASE   As the breast wound continued to heal, the hydrogel was discontinued. The ACNP continued to monitor the breast wound in conjunction with the nursing staff. A revised regimen was implemented using different types of dressings. The staff agreed to continue using the PDSA Cycle until the wound was healed.

KEY CONCEPTS

■ Evidence-based practice (EBP) represents a multidisciplinary approach to the utilization of current research findings to guide the development of appropriate strategies to deliver quality, cost-effective care.

■ Outcomes research provides evidence about benefits, risks, and results of treatment so individuals can make informed decisions and choices to improve their quality of life.

■ The American Nurses Association (ANA) has been an active advocate of outcomes evaluation.

■ EBP provides a "static" snapshot of a conclusion based on previous clinical trials about a condition or situation, but the clinician still must make a clinical judgment about an individual considering his or her unique characteristics (such as, gender, age, clinical history, socioeconomic status, support system, ethical concerns, and the illness experience).

■ The University of Colorado Hospital model is an example of a multidisciplinary EBP model for using different sources of information to change or support your practice.

■ The Model for Improvement (PDSA) can be applied to a system or an individual.

KEY TERMS

benchmarking

evidence-based nursing practice (EBNP)

evidence-based practice (EBP)

practice guideline

REVIEW QUESTIONS

1. To participate effectively in the use of EBNP, nurses must
   A. participate in the development, use, and evaluation of practice guidelines.
   B. read and analyze outcomes of research studies.
   C. involve themselves in everyday patient care and nursing practice.
   D. do all of the above.

2. Why is it important for nurses to recognize and value patient-focused outcome indicators?
   A. To achieve safe, quality, cost-effective care for patients in daily practice
   B. To realize that individual nursing practice styles directly affect the rates at which patients recover
   C. To prevent development of unnecessary complications and injury
   D. All of the above

3. Which of the following are examples of national evidence-based practice guidelines?
   A. Hospital policy on how to staff a nursing unit
   B. AHRQ pressure ulcer treatment guidelines
   C. Hospital procedure on how to insert a catheter
   D. JCAHO accreditation standards

4. What was the primary focus of The Institute for Healthcare Improvement's initial 100,000 Lives Campaign?
   A. Enroll 100,000 patients in Safety Prevention Programs.
   B. Save 100,000 lives in U.S. hospitals by June 2006.
   C. Enroll 100,000 hospitals worldwide to improve health care.
   D. Save $100,000 annually in U.S. hospitals to promote cost-effective care.

5. Which organization released two landmark reports on health care safety and quality entitled *To Err Is Human* and *Crossing the Quality Chasm?*
   A. The Leapfrog Group
   B. Institute of Medicine
   C. Agency for Healthcare Research and Quality
   D. The Joint Commission

6. Which of the following is true about the Model for Improvement (PDSA Cycle)?
   A. It provides a framework to think about how to apply evidence-based knowledge, facilitating ability to make changes in individual patient care.
   B. It is a process that can be applied to a system or an individual.
   C. It is a process that can be used to test hunches, theories, and ideas about patient care resulting in actual changes that result in improvement.
   D. All of the above

7. Which of the following is an example of a component of the planning phase of the PDSA Cycle?
   A. Revision of a current pain documentation flow sheet
   B. Implementation of a skin care protocol for bariatric patients
   C. Initiation of a multidisciplinary conference to discuss reduction in patient falls
   D. Evaluation of patient progress after implementation of a new pressure relief device

8. A source of data used to modify or adapt patient care may include which of the following?
   A. A patient's concerns, preferences, and changing clinical condition
   B. Study results of pressure ulcer prevalence survey
   C. The Website for the Institute for Healthcare Improvement (IHI)
   D. All of the above

9. Which organization revised its Social Policy Statement to include statements about the evaluation of the effectiveness of care in relation to identified outcomes and the use of evidence to improve care?
   A. JC
   B. IHI
   C. ANA
   D. AHRQ

10. The continuous process of measuring products, service, and practices against the toughest competitors or those customers recognized as industry leaders is referred to as which of the following?
    A. Process Evaluation
    B. Benchmarking
    C. Quality Improvement
    D. Cost Analysis

11. The Model for Improvement by Langley, et al., utilizes the PDSA Cycle and begins with what question?
    A. How will we know that change is an improvement?
    B. What change can we make that will result in an improvement?
    C. What have we learned from this process up to this point?
    D. What are we trying to accomplish?

REVIEW ACTIVITIES

1. Review the IHI initiative in Table 21-1. Select one of the initiatives, and review a relevant research study or clinical practice article that discusses the use of evidence-based practice to improve patient outcomes related to this initiative.

2. The University of Colorado Hospital model is one example of an evidence-based multidisciplinary practice model. This model presents a framework for thinking about how you use different sources of information to change or support your practice. Select a situation from your clinical practice and apply the model. For example, if you were caring for an elderly patient, admitted with a hip fracture sustained during a fall at home, what benchmarking data would you review to compare the patient's length of stay with that of other patients with fractured hips? What standards of care would be used? Are these institutional specific or do they also incorporate any specific outside organizations' guidelines?

3. Another model for achieving improvement is the Model for Improvement. Based on what you have read, consider the three questions:
   A. What are we trying to accomplish?
   B. How will we know that a change is an improvement?
   C. What changes can we make that will result in an improvement?

Apply the PDSA Cycle to a situation that involves patient safety.

4. Imagine you want to initiate a pain-management team in your setting. Search one of the Websites listed in the chapter that addresses evidence-based practice related to pain management. *HINT:* Start with the IHI to review what other organizations are doing related to pain management and reducing adverse drug events. See "Exploring the Web."

EXPLORING THE WEB

- Thirteen AHRQ Evidence-Based Practice Centers: *www.ahrq.gov*

- Best Evidence: *www.acponline.org*

- Best Practices Network: *www.best4health.org*

- Centre for Health Evidence: *www.cche.net*

- Clinical Information Systems Database for Nursing & Allied Health Literature (1982 to present): *www.cinahl.com*

- Education Resources Information Center (for bibliographies and abstracts): *www.eric.ed.gov*

- Institute for Healthcare Improvement: *www.ihi.org*

- The Cochrane Library (regularly updated evidence-based health care databases): *www.cochrane.org*

- The Joint Commission: *www.jointcommission.org*

- Medline—National Library of Medicine & National Institutes of Health Database: *http://medlineplus.gov*

- Medscape (Free to access. Allows you to access other Websites and databases, download, and print.): *www.medscape.com*

- National Institute for Clinical Excellence (NICE): *www.nice.org.uk*

- National Center for Biotechnology Information (National Library of Medicine and National Institutes of Health): *www.ncbi.nlm.nih.gov*

Pain Web Resources

- American Pain Society: *http://ampainsoc.org*

- City of Hope Provider Education: *www.cityofhope.org*

- International Association for the Study of Pain (Desirable Characteristics For Pain Treatment Facilities): *www.iasp-pain.org*

■ National Pain Data Bank and VA Chronic Pain Management Website: *www.vachronicpain.org*

■ Partners Against Pain: *www.partnersagainstpain.com* accessed March 30, 2007

Wound/Skin Web Resources

■ Agency for Healthcare Research and Quality 1994 pressure ulcer guidelines: *www.ahcpr.gov* Click on Clinical information: Clinical practice guidelines.

■ American Academy of Wound Management: *www.aawm.org*

■ Braden Risk Assessment Scale: *www.webmedtechnology.com/public/ BradenScale-skin.pdf*

■ The European Wound Management Association: *www.ewma.org*

■ National Pressure Ulcer Advisory Panel: *www.npuap.org*

■ American Nurses Association Nursing Information and Data Set Evaluation Center (ANA Recognized Classification Systems listed): *www.nursingworld.org*

■ World Council of Enterostomal Therapists: *www.wcetn.org*

■ Wound Ostomy and Continence Nurses Society: *www.wocn.org*

■ Wound Ostomy and Continence Nurses Certification Board: *www.wocncb.org*

REFERENCES

Agency for Health Care Policy and Research. (1992a). *Acute pain management: Operative or medical procedures and trauma* (Clinical Practice Guideline, Pub. No. 92-0032). Rockville, MD: Author.

Agency for Health Care Policy and Research. (1992b). *Pressure ulcers in adults: Prediction and prevention* (Clinical Practice Guideline, Pub. No. 92-0047). Rockville, MD: Author.

Agency for Health Care Policy and Research. (1994a). *Management of cancer pain* (Clinical Practice Guideline Pub. No. 94-0592). Rockville, MD: Author.

Agency for Health Care Policy and Research. (1994b). *Treatment of pressure ulcers* (Clinical Practice Guideline, Pub. No. 95-0652). Rockville, MD: Author.

American Pain Society, Quality of Care Committee. (1995). Quality improvement guidelines for the treatment of acute pain and cancer pain. *Journal of the American Medical Association 23,* 1874–1880.

Ayello, E. A., & Braden, B. (2002). How and why to do pressure ulcer risk assessment. *Advances in Skin & Wound Care, 15*(3), 125–131.

Bates-Jensen, B. M. (1998). Management of necrotic tissue. In C. Sussman & B. M. Bates-Jensen (Eds.), *Wound care: A collaborative practice manual for physical therapists and nurses* (pp. 139–158). Gaithersburg, MD: Aspen.

Benner, P. E., Hooper-Kyriakidis, P., Hooper, P. L., Stannard, D., & Eoyang, T., (1998). *Clinical wisdom and interventions in critical care: A thinking-in-action approach.* Philadelphia: Saunders.

Bergstrom, N., Braden, B. J., Kemp, M., Champagne, M., & Ruby, E. (1998). Predicting pressure ulcer risk: A multisite study of the predictive validity of the Braden Scale. *Nursing Research, 47,* 261–269.

Bergstrom, N., Braden, B. J., Laguzza, A., & Holman, V. (1987). The Braden Scale for Predicting Pressure Sore Risk. *Nursing Research, 36*(4), 205–210.

Camp, R. (1994). Benchmarking applied to healthcare. *The Joint Commission on Quality Improvement, 20,* 229–238.

Goode, C. J., & Piedalue, F. (1999). Evidence-based clinical practice. *Journal of Nursing Administration, 29,* 15–21.

Goode, C. J., Tanaka, D. J., Krugman, M., O'Connor, P. A., Bailey, C., Deutchman, M., et al. (2000). Outcomes from use of an evidence-based practice guideline. *Nursing Economic$, 18,* 202–207.

Ingersoll, G. L. (2000). Evidence-based nursing: What it is and what it isn't. *Nursing Outlook, 48,* 151–152.

Institute of Medicine (IOM). (2001). *Crossing the quality chasm: A new health system for the 21st century.* Washington, DC: National Academies Press.

Jadlos, M. A., Kelman, G. B., Marra, K., & Lanoue, A. (1996). A pain management documentation tool. *Oncology Nursing Forum, 23,* 1451–1454.

Joint Commission on Accreditation of Healthcare Organizations. (2006). *Comprehensive accreditation manual for hospitals: The official handbook (CAMH).* Oakbrook Terrace, IL.

Kane, R. L. (1997). *Understanding health care outcomes research.* (1st ed.). Gaithersburg, MD: Aspen.

Kohn, K. T., Corrigan, J. M., & Donaldson, M. S. (1999). *To err is human: Building a safer health system.* Washington, DC: National Academies Press.

Krasner, D. (1998). Painful venous ulcers: Themes and stories about living with the pain and suffering. *Journal of Wound, Ostomy, and Continence Nursing, 25*(3), 158–168.

Langley, G. J., Nolan, K. M., Nolan, T. W., Norman, C. L., & Provost, L. P. (1996). *The improvement guide: A practical approach to enhancing organizational performance.* San Francisco: Jossey-Bass.

NPUAP. (2000). *NPUAP position statement on reverse staging: The facts about reverse staging in 2000.* Retrieved February 12, 2006, from http://www.npuap.org

Persson, E., & Larsson, B. W. (2005). Quality of care after ostomy surgery: A perspective study of patients. *Ostomy Wound Management, 51,* 40–48.

Phillips, T. J. (1997). Cost effectiveness in wound care. In D. Krasner & D. Kane, (Eds.), *Chronic wound care: A clinical source book for healthcare professionals* (pp. 369–372). Wayne, PA: Health Management Publications.

Sackett, D. L., Rosenberg, W. M., Gray, J. A., Haynes, R. B., & Richardson, W. S. (1996). Evidence based medicine: What it is and what it isn't. *British Medical Journal, 312*(7023), 71–72.

Siegel, T. (2006). Do registered nurses perceive the anchoring of indwelling urinary catheters as a necessary aspect of nursing care? *Journal of Wound, Ostomy, and Continence Nursing, 33,* 140–144.

SUPPORT Study Principle Investigators. (1995). A controlled trial to improve care for seriously ill hospitalized patients: A study to understand prognoses and preferences for outcomes and risks of treatments (SUPPORT). *Journal of the American Medical Association, 274,* 1591–1598.

U.S. Department of Health and Human Services. (2000, Nov.). *Healthy people 2010: Understanding and improving health* (2nd ed). Washington, DC: U.S. Government Printing Office.

Zhan, C. & Miller, M. R. (2003). Excess length of stay, charges, and mortality attributable to medical injuries during hospitalization. *Journal of the American Medical Association (JAMA), 290,* 1868–1874.

SUGGESTED READINGS

Agency for Health Care Policy and Research. (1999, July 13). *Clinical information: Clinical practice guidelines online.* Retrieved January 30, 2002, from http://www.ahcpr.gov/clinic

American Nurses Association. (2004). *Nursing: Scope and standards of practice.* Washington, DC: Author.

Ayello, E. A., Baranoski, S., Lyder, C. H., & Cuddigan, J. (2004). Pressure ulcers. In S. Baranoski & E.A. Ayello (Eds.), *Wound care essentials: Practice principles.* Philadelphia, PA: Lippincott, Williams & Wilkins.

Ayello, E. A., Baranoski, S., & Salati, D. S. (2005). Wound care survey report. *Nursing 2005, 35*(6), 36–47.

Ayello, E. A. (2006). 20 years of wound care: Where we have been, where we are going. *Advances in Skin & Wound Care, 19*(1), 28–33.

Baranoski, S., & Ayello, E. A. (2004). *Wound care essentials: Practice principles.* Springhouse, PA: Lippincott Williams & Wilkins.

Bates-Jensen, B. M. (1997). The pressure sore status tool a few thousand assessments later. *Advances in Wound Care, 10*(5), 65–73.

Bergstrom, N., Bennett, M. A., Carlson, C. G., et al. (1994). Treatment of pressure ulcers in adults. Clinical practice guideline, Number 15. Rockville, MD: Public Health Service, U.S. Dept. of Health and Human Services; Agency for Health Care Policy and Research publication 95-0652.

Berlowitz, D. R., Ratliff, C., Cuddigan, J., Rodeheaver, G. T., & the National Pressure Ulcer Advisory Panel. (2005). The PUSH tool: A survey to determine its perceived usefulness. *Advances in Skin & Wound Care, 18*(9), 480–483.

Berwick, D. M., Calkins, D. R., McCannon, B. A., & Hackbarth, A. D. (2006). The 100,000 Lives Campaign: Setting a goal and a deadline for improving health care quality. *Journal of the American Medical Association, 295*(3), 324–327.

Hess, C. T. (1998). *Nurse's clinical guide: Wound care.* Springhouse, PA: Springhouse.

Hiser, B., Rochette, J., Philbin, S., Lowerhouse, N., TerBurgh, C., & Pietsch, C. (2006). Implementing a pressure ulcer prevention program and enhancing the role of the CWOCN: Impact on outcomes. *Ostomy Wound Management, 52*(2), 48–59.

Krasner, D., & Kane, D. (Eds.). (1997). *Chronic wound care: A clinical source book for healthcare professionals.* Wayne, PA: Health Management Publications.

Maklebust, J., Sieggreen, M. Y., Sidor, D., Gerlach, M.A., Bauer, C., & Anderson, C. (2005). Computer-based testing of the Braden Scale for Predicting Pressure Sore Risk. *Ostomy Wound Management, 51*(4), 40–52.

Morison, M., Moffatt, C., Bridel-Nixon, J., & Bale, S. (1997). *Nursing management of chronic wounds.* London: Mosby.

National Pressure Ulcer Advisory Panel Board of Directors, Cuddigan, J., Berlowitz, D. R., & Ayello, E. A. (Eds). (2001). Pressure ulcers in America: Prevalence, incidence, and implications for the future. An executive summary of the National Pressure Ulcer Advisory Panel Monograph. *Advances in Skin and Wound Care, 14*(4), 208–215.

National Pressure Ulcer Advisory Panel (2003a). Frequently asked questions. Retrieved February 12, 2006, from http://www.npuap.org/npuap-faq.htm

NPUAP PUSH Task Force. (1997). Pressure ulcer scale for healing: Derivation and validation of the PUSH tool. *Advances in Wound Care, 10*(5), 96.

Pompeo, M. (2003). Implementing the PUSH tool in clinical practice: Revisions and results. *Ostomy Wound Management, 49*(8), 32–46.

Sussman, C., & Bates-Jensen, B. M. (Eds.). (1998). *Wound care: A collaborative practice manual for physical therapists and nurses.* Gaithersburg, MD: Aspen.

Wound, Ostomy, Continence Nurses Society (WOCN). (2003). *Guideline for prevention and management of pressure ulcers.* WOCN Clinical Practice Guideline Series. Glenview, IL: WOCN.

CHAPTER 22

Decision Making and Critical Thinking

Sharon Little-Stoetzel, RN, MS

When you have to make a choice and don't make it, that is in itself a choice (William James).

OBJECTIVES

Upon completion of this chapter, the reader should be able to:

1. Apply decision making to clinical situations.
2. Explain how problem solving, critical thinking, reflective thinking, and intuitive thinking relate to decision making.
3. Apply decision-making tools and technology to nursing care.
4. Facilitate group decision making using various techniques.
5. Examine limitations to effective decision making.
6. Apply strategies to strengthen the nurses role in decision making for patients.

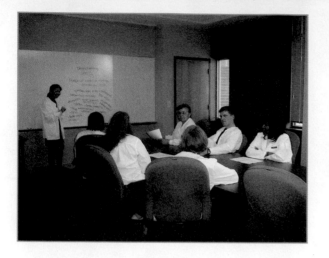

You are a staff nurse in the Medical Intensive Care Unit in your hospital. The nurse manager has requested that you be a task force committee member to determine a new method of scheduling to be implemented in the unit. Currently, the manager writes the schedule after staff members have submitted their requests for days off for that time period. The manager has received consistent feedback that the staff would like to try a new method of scheduling, but the staff has been unable to come to a decision as to what new method they should try. The task force consists of three RNs from the unit in addition to you. There are two nurses from night shift and two nurses from day shift. One day shift nurse has been on the unit for five years and is the chairperson of the committee.

What should be the first step of the task force?

Can the decision-making process help the group solve the situation?

Rapid changes in the health care environment have expanded the decision-making role of the nurse. Because the health care market is more competitive, decision making and critical thinking by nurses tend to be necessary for the agency's survival. Additionally, stringent budgets require that nurse managers and staff alike do more with less. Patient care is more complex as acuity rises. With patients being discharged from acute care institutions earlier, effective decisions regarding treatment must be made in a timely manner.

Critical thinking is essential when making decisions and solving problems. This chapter explores the decision-making process and how it relates to critical thinking, reflective thinking, intuitive thinking, and problem solving. Application of decision-making models to clinical nursing decisions is presented. The chapter examines advantages and limitations to group decision making as well as the use of technology in decision making. Finally, it discusses limitations to effective decision making and strategies for improving the nurses role in decision making for patients.

DECISION MAKING

In everyday practice, nurses make decisions about patient care. As the nurse gains experience in clinical practice, decision making will become somewhat automatic in certain circumstances, but other decisions will remain complex. DeLaune and Ladner (2006) define **decision making** as "considering and selecting interventions from a repertoire of actions that facilitate the achievement of a desired outcome" (p. 89). Critical, reflective, and intuitive thinking may be used during the decision-making process as illustrated in Figure 22-1.

Although decisions are unique to different situations, the same decision-making process can be applied to most all situations. The decision-making process consists of five steps (Table 22-1):

Step 1: Identify the need for a decision.
Step 2: Determine the goal or outcome.
Step 3: Identify alternatives or actions along with the benefits and consequences of each action.
Step 4: Decide which action to implement.
Step 5: Evaluate the decision.

In the following clinical application, the decision-making process is applied to a clinical situation.

CLINICAL APPLICATION

You are the night shift nurse caring for Mr. Cintas. In the morning, Mr. Cintas is scheduled for a permanent pacemaker insertion to replace his temporary pacemaker, which is still functioning. Hospital policy states that no visitor may stay all night with a patient unless that patient is very critically ill. Mr. and Mrs. Cintas are both requesting that Mrs. Cintas stay in a chair beside Mr. Cintas's bed because both are anxious about his upcoming

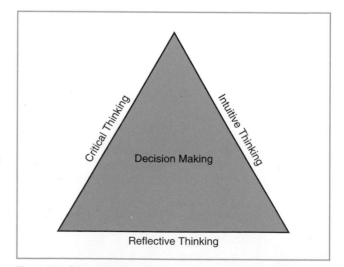

Figure 22-1 Critical thinking, intuitive thinking, and reflective thinking are incorporated throughout the decision-making process.

TABLE 22-1   THE DECISION-MAKING PROCESS

1. Identify the need for a decision.

2. Determine the goal or outcome desired.

3. Identify alternatives.

    a. Identify consequences of each alternative.

    b. Identify benefits of each alternative.

4. Make the decision.

5. Evaluate the decision.

procedure. Use your decision-making skills to help you decide what to do.

Step 1: Identify the need for a decision. Should you let Mrs. Cintas spend the night? Consider all the information (hospital policy, the patient's wishes, anxiety level, and so on).

Step 2: Determine the outcome. What is the goal? Questions to consider include the following: Can an exception to hospital policy be made? Is the goal to alleviate Mr. and Mrs. Cintas's anxiety? Will Mr. Cintas's level of anxiety affect the outcome of the surgery? Will Mr. and Mrs. Cintas be satisfied customers?

Step 3: Identify all alternative actions and the benefits and consequences of each. If you enforce hospital policy, the benefits are that all patients are treated equally, and the written policy supports the decision. The consequences are that Mr. and Mrs. Cintas's anxiety level increases, perhaps adversely affecting the outcome of his surgery, and they will not be advocates for the health center. The other alternative is to allow Mrs. Cintas to stay all night. The benefits are that Mr. and Mrs. Cintas's level of anxiety will decrease, and they will be satisfied customers. The consequence is that a precedent is set that may make it difficult to enforce the existing hospital policy.

Step 4: Make the decision. Consider the two alternatives and the benefits and consequences of each, and then implement the decision. The decision was made to let Mrs. Cintas spend the night with her husband. The nurse determined that the couple's anxiety level in relation to the outcome of the surgery was the most important consideration and the goal in this scenario.

Step 5: Evaluate the decision. Was the goal achieved? The nurse must evaluate the decision that was implemented. The decision to allow Mrs. Cintas to spend the night was a good decision. It allowed Mr. Cintas to get a good night's rest as well as decreased his overall anxiety. Decreasing a patient's anxiety prior to a surgery is an important nursing intervention. This decision might lead to a change in the current policy, allowing for more customer satisfaction.

From the beginning of their careers, new graduate nurses are faced with the responsibility of making decisions regarding patient care. For the beginning nurse, it is common to have more questions than answers. When nurses are faced with a difficult clinical decision, they should get others close to the situation involved. These may include other RNs on the unit or house supervisors. Experienced nurses have a wealth of information regarding clinical decision making. New nurses should tap into that valuable resource. Depending on the situation, recognize that you also have knowledge and intuition that are valuable. With more experience comes greater trust in your decision making.

CRITICAL THINKING

What does it mean to be a critical thinker? Paul (1992) defines **critical thinking** as "thinking about your thinking while you're thinking in order to make your thinking better" (p. 7). Paul points out that there are many accurate definitions of critical thinking, and most are consistent with each other. From a nursing perspective, Ignatavicius (2001) defines critical thinking as "purposeful, outcome-directed thinking that is based on a body of scientific knowledge derived from research and other courses of evidence" (p. 31). A good critical thinker is able to examine decisions from all sides and takes into account varying points of view. A good critical thinker does not say "We've always done it this way," and refuse to consider alternate ways. The critical thinker generates new ideas

TABLE 22-2	THE SPECTRUM OF UNIVERSAL INTELLECTUAL STANDARDS

Clear	_____	Unclear
Precise	_____	Imprecise
Specific	_____	Vague
Accurate	_____	Inaccurate
Relevant	_____	Irrelevant
Consistent	_____	Inconsistent
Logical	_____	Illogical
Deep	_____	Superficial
Complete	_____	Incomplete
Significant	_____	Insignificant
Adequate	_____	Inadequate
Fair	_____	Unfair

Source: Adapted from The Foundation for Critical Thinking, Dillon, CA. Retrieved April 25, 2003 from www.criticalthinking.org.

and alternatives when making decisions. The critical thinker asks "why" questions about a situation to arrive at the best decision. Critical thinking skills should be used all through the decision-making process. Four basic skills—critical reading, critical listening, critical writing, and critical speaking—are necessary for the development of critical thinking skills. These skills are part of the process of developing and using thinking for decision making. Ability in these four areas can be measured by the extent to which one achieves the universal intellectuals standards provided in Table 22-2.

As you begin to apply critical thinking to nursing, use these universal intellectual standards when you are reading material from a textbook, listening to an oral presentation, writing a paper, answering test questions, or presenting ideas in oral form. Ask yourself whether the ideas are clear or unclear, precise or imprecise, specific or vague, accurate or inaccurate. Are they relevant or irrelevant, consistent or inconsistent, logical or illogical, deep or superficial, complete or incomplete, significant or insignificant, adequate or inadequate, or fair or unfair. You will improve your critical thinking skills over time and with practice.

REFLECTIVE THINKING

Pesut and Herman (1999) describe **reflective thinking** as watching or observing ourselves as we perform a task or make a decision about a particular situation. We have two

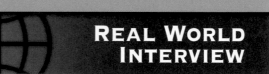

REAL WORLD INTERVIEW

Journaling has helped me reflect on how I interacted with a patient on a particular day and helped teach me how I would interact with a future patient in a similar situation. Analyzing the situation after it has occurred helps to put perspective on the tasks that were carried out during that clinical experience. During one particular clinical day, I cared for a patient who needed basic nursing care. It was challenging in the sense that she wasn't easy to care for even though the needs she had were simple. I learned the importance of the therapeutic relationship, and reflecting on this in my journal helped me to realize the true meaning of nursing.

Tabetha Carson
Student Nurse
Independence, Missouri

selves, the active self and the reflective self. The reflective self watches the active self as it engages in activities. The reflective self acts as observer and offers suggestions about the activities. To be a good critical thinker, you must practice reflective thinking. Reflection upon a situation or problem after a decision is made allows you to evaluate the decision. Nurse educators assist students to become better reflective thinkers through the use of clinical journals. Using journals helps students reflect on clinical activities and improve their clinical decision-making abilities.

For example, when a new nurse performs an abdominal sterile dressing change on a surgical patient, the reflective self will watch the process. The reflective self will then make suggestions as to how to make the process more efficient the next time. The reflective self might make suggestions such as having all the supplies in the room prior to the process, including an extra pair of sterile gloves, or having an extra table in the room. Reflection upon a situation or problem after a decision is made allows the individual to evaluate the decision. New nurses should continue to use reflective thinking throughout their practice to build their confidence in the clinical decisions they make.

INTUITIVE THINKING

Intuition and **intuitive thinking** is described as an innate feeling that nurses develop that helps them to act in certain situations (Gardner, 2003). It has also been described as a gut feeling that something is wrong. Intuitive thinking may result from unconscious assessment and analysis of data based on an individual's past experience. Nurses may make decisions about patient care based, in part, on intuitive thinking. This may seem contrary to using the logical, evidenced-based reasoning that is so prevalent in nursing literature. Alfaro-LeFevre (2003) contends that expert thinking is usually the result of using intuition and drawing on evidence at the same time to make well-reasoned decisions. The following Real World Interview represents an example of a new nurse using intuitive thinking.

PROBLEM SOLVING

Problem solving is an active process that starts with a problem and ends with a solution. Nurses address multiple needs and problems of patients on a daily basis. Some problems are uncomplicated and require one simple solution. Other problems may be complex and require more analysis by the nurse. The problem-solving process consists of the following five steps: identify the problem, gather and analyze data, generate alternatives and select an action, implement the selected action, and evaluate the action. Note the similarities to the decision-making process and to the nursing process steps of assessment, diagnosis, outcome identification, planning, implementation, and evaluation. The nursing process is applied to patient situations or problems, whereas the problem-solving process and decision-making process may be applied to a problem of any type (Table 22-3).

TABLE 22-3	**REVIEW OF TERMS**
Decision making	Behavior exhibited when making a selection and implementing a course of action from alternatives. It may or may not involve an immediate problem.
Critical thinking	Thinking about your thinking while you're thinking in order to make your thinking better (Paul, 1992).
Reflective thinking	Watching or observing ourselves as we perform a task or make a decision about a particular situation (Pesut & Herman, 1999).
Intuitive thinking	An innate feeling that nurses develop that helps them to act in certain situations (Gardner, 2003).
Problem solving	An active process that starts with a problem and ends with a solution.

DECISION-MAKING TOOLS AND TECHNOLOGY

Nurse managers are faced with complex decisions at times. Decisions related to budget are common in our current health care environment with its emphasis on cost containment and quality maintenance. Disciplining an employee also creates a complex situation in which managers must make decisions regarding the employee's future. A decision-making grid may help to separate the multiple factors that surround a situation. Figure 22-2 illustrates use of a decision-making grid by nurses who were told they had to reduce their workforce by two full-time equivalents (FTEs). This grid is useful in this example to visually separate the factors of cost savings, effect on job satisfaction of remaining staff, and effect on patient satisfaction. The nurse needs to determine the priorities when developing a grid.

A decision-making grid is also useful when a nurse is trying to decide between two choices. Figure 22-3 is an

Methods of Reduction	Cost Savings	Effect on Job Satisfaction	Effect on Patient Satisfaction
Lay off the Two Most Senior Full-Time Employees	$93,500	Significant Reduction	Significant Reduction
Lay off the Two Most Recently Hired Full-Time Employees	$63,200	Significant Reduction	Moderate Reduction
Reduce by Staff Attrition	$78,000	Minor Reduction	Minor Reduction

Figure 22-2 Sample decision-making grid.

Elements	Importance Score (Out of 10)	Likelihood Score (Out of 10)	Risk (Multiply Scores)
If I Work at Hospital A			
Learning Experience	10	10	100
Good Mentor Support	8	8	64
Financial Reward	6	6	36
Growth Potential	8	8	64
Good Location	10	10	100
Total			364
If I Work at Hospital B			
Learning Experience	8	8	64
Good Mentor Support	7	7	49
Financial Reward	8	8	64
Growth Potential	9	9	81
Good Location	6	6	36
Total			294

Figure 22-3 Sample decision-making grid for weighing options.

example of a decision grid used by a nurse deciding between working at hospital A or hospital B.

The Program Evaluation and Review Technique (PERT) is useful in determining timing of decisions. The flowchart provides a visual picture depicting the sequence of tasks that must take place to complete a project. Jones and Beck (1996) provide an example of a PERT flow diagram depicting a case management project (Figure 22-4).

The vice president for nursing plans to change all units to include case managers. She believes that this can be accomplished within a year and a half. For this to be achieved, the following activities and events have to occur:

Activity Symbol	Activity Descriptions
A	Form a multidisciplinary advisory group
B	Agree upon definitions
C	Notify members of subcommittees
D	Write job descriptions
E	Advertise for candidates for case manager
F	Review qualifications of candidates
G	Select candidates for case manager
H	Review patient charts
I	Write patient care maps
J	Meet with case managers
K	Orient case managers
L	Orient unit and hospital staff
M	Utilize case management process

	Events
1.	Project begins
2.	Meeting of multidisciplinary committee
3.	Formation of subcommittees
4.	Subcommittee for job description meets
5.	Subcommittee for patient care maps meets
6.	Candidates for case managers are interviewed
7.	Candidates are hired
8.	Subcommittee for patient care maps meets to finalize maps
9.	Orientation begins
10.	Implementation begins
11.	Project is evaluated

Expected   **Time Calculations**

Activity	Duration
A	0.5 month
B	1 month
C	0.5 month
D	1 month
E	1 month
F	2 months
G	1 month
H	1 month
I	2 months
J	1 month
K&L	1 month
M	3 months

Figure 22-4 PERT diagram with critical path for implementation of case management.

CRITICAL THINKING 22-1

Yˉou have just received report from the night shift nurse in the surgical ICU. Your patient had a hip replacement the previous day and was in the ICU due to respiratory complications in the PACU. The night shift nurse reported that the patient's heart rate was starting to rise slightly during the last hour of her shift. You have been on duty for 45 minutes, and the patient's heart rate has gone from 100 beats per minute to 112 beats per minute. The patient is currently sleeping, and his blood pressure is 116/76. Use your nursing knowledge and critical thinking skills to determine possible causes of the elevation in heart rate.

EVIDENCE FROM THE LITERATURE

Citation: White, A., Allen, P., Goodwin, L., Breckinridge, D., Dowell, J., & Garvy, R. (2005). Infusing PDA technology into nursing education. *Nurse Educator, 30*(4), 153–154.

Discussion: Article discusses the Nursing Education program at Duke University, where students use PDAs and software to access current drug and infectious disease information, calculations, growth charts, immunization guidelines, and Spanish and English language translations to improve clinical decision making. Information about this can be accessed at www.pepidedu.com.

Implications for Practice: Use of the PDA can improve clinical decision making.

The chart shows the amount of time taken to complete the project and the sequence of events to complete the project. An advantage of the PERT diagram is that participants can visualize a complete picture of the project, including the timing of decisions from beginning to end.

DECISION TREE

A decision tree can be useful in making the alternatives visible. Figure 22-5 is a decision tree for choosing whether to go back to school.

Figure 22-6 identifies a decision analysis tree for a patient who smokes.

GANTT CHART

A Gantt chart can be useful for decision makers to illustrate a project from beginning to end. Figure 22-7 illustrates a Gantt chart used to show the progression of a nursing unit's pilot project.

USE OF TECHNOLOGY

Nurses use technology as a support for decision making. The best source of clinical decision making and judgment is still the professional practitioner. However, computer technology has many uses to support information

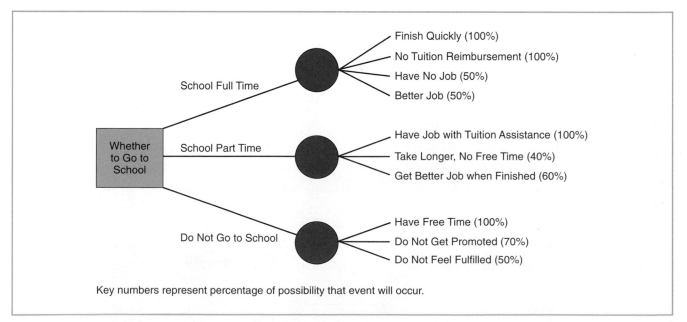

Figure 22-5 Decision tree for deciding whether to go back to school.

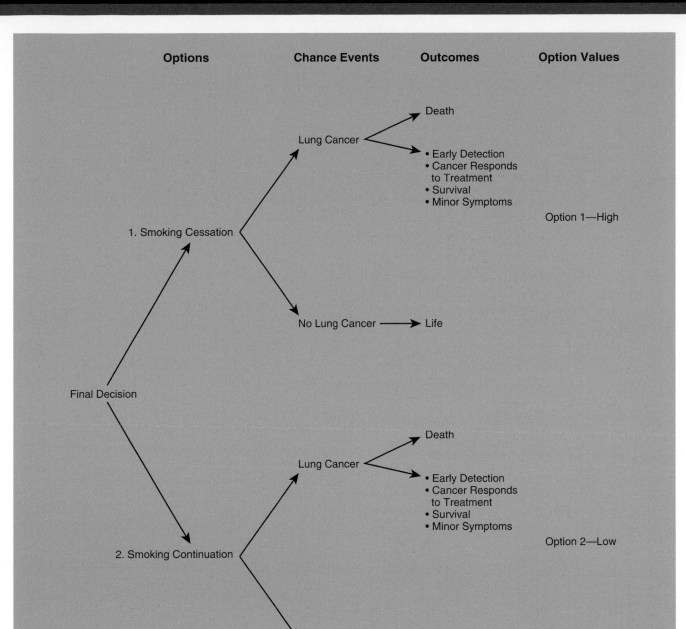

Figure 22-6 Decision analysis tree for a patient who smokes.

systems for nurses. Patient classification systems, inventory control, scheduling staff, and changes in policies and procedures are but a few examples of how computers can assist nurses with tracking the information needed for patient care. Many nurses today are using PDAs (see Figure 22-8) to improve patient care. PDAs are used for medication administration and accessing the literature, information on pathophysiology, nursing care plans, and nursing diagnosis. NCLEX questions are also available on PDAs.

GROUP DECISION MAKING

Certain situations call for group decision making. Vroom and Yetton (1973) identified certain questions managers should ask themselves before making a decision alone. There are occasions when it is more appropriate for a group to make the decision rather than the individual manager. Each situation is different, and an effective

A nurse is working on a unit that will pilot a new care delivery system within six months. The Gantt chart can be used to plan the progression of the project.

Activities	Sept	Oct	Nov	Dec	Jan	Feb	Mar	Apr	May
Discuss Project with Staff	─ X								
Form an Ad Hoc Planning Committee	─	X							
Receive Report from Committee			X	─					
Discuss Report with Staff			─	─ X					
Educate All Staff to the Plan				─	─ X				
Implement New System						─	───		
Evaluate System and Make Changes							─	─	X

Key
─── Proposed Time
___ Actual Time
X   Complete

Figure 22-7 Gantt chart: Implementation of care delivery system.

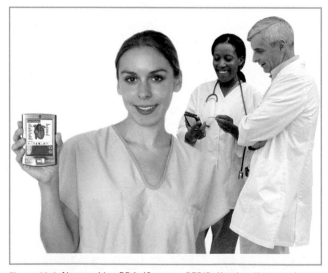

Figure 22-8 Nurse with a PDA. (Courtesy PEPID, Heather Hautman.)

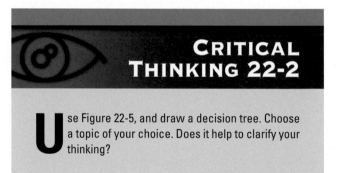

CRITICAL THINKING 22-2

Use Figure 22-5, and draw a decision tree. Choose a topic of your choice. Does it help to clarify your thinking?

manager adopts the appropriate mode of decision making—group or individual. The eight questions in Table 22-4 may assist the manager in determining which mode to use.

Today's leadership and management styles include people in the decision-making process who will be most affected by the decision. Decisions affecting patient care should be made by those groups implementing the decisions.

The effectiveness of groups depends greatly on the group's members. The size of the group and the personalities of group members are important considerations when choosing participants. More ideas can be generated with groups, thus allowing for more choices. This increases the likelihood of higher-quality outcomes. Another advantage of groups is that when followers participate in the decision-making process, acceptance of the decision is more likely to occur. Additionally, groups may be used as a medium for communication.

TABLE 22-4   INDIVIDUAL VS. GROUP DECISION-MAKING QUESTIONS

1. Does the individual nurse have all the information needed?

2. Does the group have supplementary information needed to make the best decision?

3. Does the individual nurse have all the resources available to obtain sufficient information to make the best decision?

4. Is it absolutely critical that the group accept the decision prior to implementation?

5. Will the group accept the decision I make by myself?

6. Does the course of action chosen make a difference to the organization?

7. Does the group have the best interest of the organization or patient foremost when considering the decision?

8. Will the decision cause undue conflict among the group?

Source: Adapted from *Leadership and Decision-Making* (pp. 21–30), by V. Vroom and P. Yetton, 1973, Pittsburgh, PA: University of Pittsburgh Press.

TABLE 22-5   ADVANTAGES AND DISADVANTAGES OF GROUPS

Advantages	Disadvantages
■ Easy and inexpensive way to share information	■ Individual opinions influenced by others
■ Opportunities for face-to-face communication	■ Individual identity obscured
■ Opportunity to become connected with a social unit	■ Formal and informal role and status positions evolve—hierarchies
■ Promotion of cohesiveness and loyalty	■ Dependency fostered
■ Access to a larger resource base	■ Time consuming
■ Forum for constructive problem solving	■ Inequity of time given to share individual information
■ Support group	■ Existence of nonfunctional roles
■ Facilitation of esprit de corps	■ Personality conflicts
■ Promotion of ownership of problems and solutions	

A major disadvantage of group decision making is the time involved. Without effective leadership, groups can waste time and be nonproductive. Group decision making can be more costly and can also lead to conflict. Groups can be dominated by one person or become the battleground for a power struggle among assertive members. See Table 22-5 for a listing of the advantages and disadvantages of groups.

TECHNIQUES OF GROUP DECISION MAKING

There are various techniques of group decision making. Nominal group technique, Delphi technique, and consensus building are different methods to facilitate group decision making.

NOMINAL GROUP TECHNIQUE

The nominal group technique was developed by Delbecq Van de Ven and Gustafson in 1971. The word *nominal* refers to the nonverbal aspect of this approach (Cawthorpe & Harris, 1999). In the first step, there is no discussion; group members write out their ideas or responses to the identified issue or question posed by the group leader. The second step involves presentation of the ideas to the group members along with the advantages and disadvantages of each. These ideas are presented on a flip board or chart. The third phase offers an opportunity for discussion to clarify and evaluate the ideas. The fourth phase includes private voting on the ideas. The ideas receiving the highest number of votes are the solutions implemented.

EVIDENCE FROM THE LITERATURE

Citation: Bucknall, T. (2003). The clinical landscape of critical care: Nurses' decision making. *Journal of Advanced Nursing, 43*(3), 310–319.

Discussion: The purpose of this study was to investigate and describe influences that the critical care setting has on nurses' decision making. The researchers observed eighteen critical care nurses in a variety of hospital settings. The nurses were interviewed within twenty-four hours after observation regarding the clinical situations. Three key environmental influences were recognized: the complexity of the patient; resource availability, including staffing; and interpersonal relationships. The complexity of the patient contributed to the amount and speed of the decisions. A more stable patient required less assessment, whereas an unstable patient required more monitoring and intervention. Resource availability included the layout of the unit, available equipment, and staffing. Interpersonal relationships included the amount of nursing teamwork, relationships with practitioners, and the relationships among patients, families, and nurses. These three main influences directly affect the decision making of the critical care nurse.

Implications for Practice: Practicing nurses need to be aware of how external influences contribute to their decision-making processes. Reflection on past decisions and the influences on these decisions will help the nurse develop this awareness. Nurse educators should include an examination of external influences on decision making for students in the clinical setting.

CRITICAL THINKING 22-3

You are working for a home health agency that employs seventeen registered nurses. There have been concerns about staffing and scheduling as the agency's census has increased. The manager has said that until more staff can be hired, there will be an increased need for on-call and overtime scheduling. The manager has given the responsibility to the entire group to figure out the best way to cover the patient assignments.

What would be the best group decision-making strategy to use? What should the group do first?

DELPHI GROUP TECHNIQUE

Delphi technique differs from nominal technique in that group members are not meeting face to face. Questionnaires are distributed to group members for their opinions, and these are then summarized and disseminated with the summaries to the group members. This process continues for as many times as necessary for the group members to reach consensus. An advantage of this technique is that it can involve a large number of participants and thus a greater number of ideas.

CONSENSUS BUILDING

Consensus is defined by the Merriam-Webster's Collegiate Dictionary (2003) as "a general agreement; the judgment arrived at by most of those concerned; group solidarity in sentiment and belief" (p. 265). A common misconception is that consensus means everyone agrees with the decision 100%. Contrary to this misunderstanding, **consensus** means that all group members can live with and fully support the decision regardless of whether they totally agree. Building consensus is useful with groups because all group members participate and can realize the contributions each member makes to the decision. A disadvantage to the consensus strategy is that decision making requires more time. This strategy should be reserved for important decisions that require strong support from the participants who will implement them. Consensus decision making works well when the decisions are made under the following conditions: all members of the team are affected by the decision; implementation of the solution requires coordination among team members; and the decision is critical, requiring full commitment by team members. Although consensus can be the most time-consuming strategy, it can also be the most gratifying.

GROUPTHINK

Groupthink and consensus building are different. In consensus, the group members work to support the final decision, and individual ideas and opinions are valued. In groupthink, the goal is for everyone to be in 100% agreement. Groupthink discourages questioning and

EVIDENCE FROM THE LITERATURE

Citation: Ruth-Sahd, L., & Hendy, H. (2005). Predictors of novice nurses' use of intuition to guide patient care decisions. *Journal of Nursing Education, 44*(10), 450–458.

Discussion: One of the purposes of the study was to openly discuss the use of intuition in novice nurses as they are likely to use intuition at the bedside to guide their decisions about patient care. The authors surveyed 323 novice nurses over a total of 151 nursing programs. The researchers measured the nurses' use of intuition with Miller's Willingness to Act on Intuition scale. They also questioned the nurses' personal experiences (age, gender, number of hospitalizations, self-esteem, and religiosity), interpersonal experiences (number of children and relationships with others), and professional experiences (learning methods in school, GPA, and number of months experience) as these factors may influence the use of intuition. The results of the study suggested that older novice nurses, those with more social support and those with more hospitalizations use intuition more often in making decisions about patient care. Additionally, the use of intuition was affected by personal and interpersonal experience as opposed to professional experience in these subjects.

Implications for Practice: Intuition needs to be acknowledged in nursing education and clinical practice more openly. Students should be able to discuss intuition with nurse educators to better develop the use of their own intuition. As age was a factor associated with more frequent use of intuition, nurse educators should ensure that age groups are mixed in learning groups. Strong mentoring or support systems are also important for the new nurse to help in guiding their decision making and use of intuition.

divergent thinking. It hinders creativity and usually leads to inferior decisions (Jarvis, 1997). The potential for groupthink increases as the cohesiveness of the group increases. An important responsibility of the group leader is to recognize symptoms of groupthink. Janis (as cited in Jarvis, 1997) described examples of these symptoms. One symptom is that group members develop an illusion of invulnerability, believing they can do no wrong. This problem has the greatest potential to develop when the group is powerful and group members view themselves as invincible. The second symptom of groupthink is stereotyping outsiders. This occurs when the group members rely on shared stereotypes—such as, all Democrats are liberal or all Republicans are conservative—to justify their positions. People who challenge or disagree with the decisions are also stereotyped. A third symptom is that group members reassure one another that their interpretation of data and their perspective on matters are correct regardless of the evidence showing otherwise. Old assumptions are never challenged, and members ignore what they do not know or what they do not want to know.

Numerous problems can arise when groupthink is present. Groups may come to one solution to a problem early in the course of problem solving without considering all available options (Shortell & Kaluzny, 2006). Groups may not be willing to seek expertise or be open to new information when groupthink is present. Groups may believe so strongly in their decisions that they may not develop contingency plans in case the decision is wrong (Shortell & Kaluzny, 2006). Clearly, these problems would be detrimental to any group decision-making process.

Strategies to avoid groupthink include appointing group members to roles that evaluate how group decision-making occurs. Group leaders should encourage all group members to think independently and verbalize their individual ideas. The leader should allow the group time to gather further data and reflect on data already collected. A primary responsibility of the managers or the group leader is to prevent groupthink from developing.

LIMITATIONS TO EFFECTIVE DECISION MAKING

What are obstacles to effective decision making? Past experiences, values, personal biases, and preconceived ideas affect the way people view problems and situations. Incorporating critical thinking into the decision-making process helps to prevent these factors from distorting the process. Delaune and Ladner (2006) have identified

EVIDENCE FROM THE LITERATURE

Citation: Bakalis, N. A., & Watson, R. (2005). Nurses' decision making in clinical practice. *Nursing Standard, 19*(23), 33–39.

Discussion: This exploratory study was carried out to determine types of clinical decisions that medical-, surgical-, and critical care nurses make. The investigators also wanted to know if the clinical setting made a difference in nurses' clinical decision making. Sixty nurses were given a questionnaire related to direct patient care, supervision and management decisions, and decisions related to nurses' extended roles. In all three specialties investigated, nurses regularly made decisions related to direct patient care. Critical care nurses made more decisions related to emergency situations than did medical nurses or surgical nurses. The more senior nurses made more decisions related to management and supervision. Investigators did not note the educational preparation of the nurses.

Implications for Practice: The researcher identified three implications for practice: student nurses should have multiple opportunities to participate in clinical decision making during their educational program, postgraduate nurses should be encouraged to participate in clinical decision making, and nurses should also be encouraged to participate in research that will increase their knowledge about clinical decisions. Nurses should also realize that some of the decision making they encounter in practice is particular to their specialty area.

actions that may negatively affect the decision-making or problem-solving processes:

- Jumping to conclusions without examining the situation thoroughly
- Failing to obtain all of the necessary information
- Choosing decisions that are too broad, too complicated, or lack definition
- Failing to choose and communicate a rational solution
- Failing to intervene and evaluate the decision or solution appropriately

STRATEGIES TO STRENGTHEN THE NURSES' ROLE IN DECISION MAKING FOR PATIENT CARE

In today's world, patients are taking a more active role in treatment decisions. The consumers of health care are more knowledgeable and cost conscious and have more options than in previous years. Nurses must be aware of patients' rights in making decisions about their treatments, and they must assist patients in their decision making. When patients are active participants, compliance with

CASE STUDY 22-1

The nurse has identified a problem for the nursing unit: low patient satisfaction. Patients are dissatisfied with the long waiting periods, lack of information, and impersonal attitude of staff. Apply the decision making process to this problem. How would you assess the problem? How would you gather information? Who would you involve to solve the problem?

prescribed treatments is more likely to follow. Empowering the patient in this manner ultimately promotes a more positive outcome.

Comfort with decision making improves with experience. Early in the nurse's career, the nurse is commonly indecisive or uncomfortable with decisions. Alfaro-LeFevre (2003) has identified several strategies that help to improve critical thinking, which, in turn, will also help to improve decision making. Do you have all the information needed to make a decision? At times, delaying a decision until more information is obtained may be the best approach. Asking "why," "what else," and "what if" questions will help you arrive at the best decision. When

TABLE 22-6	**DOS AND DON'TS OF DECISION MAKING**

Do

Make only those decisions that are yours to make.

Write notes and keep ideas visible about decisions to utilize all relevant information.

Write down pros and cons of an issue to help clarify your thinking.

Make decisions as you go along rather than letting them accumulate.

Consider those affected by your decision.

Trust yourself.

Don't

Make snap decisions.

Waste your time making decisions that do not have to be made.

Consider decisions a choice between right and wrong; decisions are a choice among alternatives.

Prolong deliberation about decisions.

Regret a decision; it was the right thing to do at the time.

Always base decisions on the "way things have always been done."

Source: Adapted from *The Small Business Knowledge Base,* 1999. Retrieved February 19, 2002, from http://www.bizmove.com.

more information becomes available, decisions can be revised. Very few decisions are set in stone. Another helpful strategy for improving decision making is to anticipate questions and outcomes. For example, when calling a practitioner to report a patient's change in condition, the nurse will want to have pertinent information about the patient's vital signs and current medications readily available.

Nurses who practice strategies to promote their own critical thinking will, in turn, be good decision makers. A foundation for good decision making comes with experience and learning from those experiences. Table 22-6 gives the nurse some additional tips to consider when making decisions. By turning decisions with poor outcomes into learning experiences, nurses will enhance their decision-making ability in the future.

KEY CONCEPTS

- The ever-changing health care system calls for nurses to be effective decision makers.

- In the decision-making process, there are five steps: Step 1—identify the need for a decision; Step 2—determine the goal or outcome; Step 3—identify alternatives or actions, along with their benefits and consequences; Step 4—decide the action and implement; Step 5—evaluate the decision.

- Critical thinking involves examining situations from every viewpoint when faced with any problem or situation. Use of the universal intellectual standards will improve a nurse's critical thinking.

- Practicing reflective thinking helps individuals become better critical thinkers.

- Nurses should recognize the importance of intuitive thinking. Recognizing their own use of intuition will help nurses develop their intuitive thinking skills.

- Problem solving involves five steps: (1) identify the problem, (2) gather and analyze data, (3) generate alternatives and select action, (4) implement the selected action, and (5) evaluate the selected action.

- Decision-making grids may be helpful when the nurse needs to separate multiple factors surrounding a situation during the decision-making process.

- There are situations in which a nurse needs to make individual decisions. Other decisions call for group decision making.

- Consensus building is a strategy utilized when working with a group to make a decision.

- Groupthink occurs when individuals are not allowed to express creativity, question methods, or engage in divergent thinking.

- The nurse must recognize the importance of empowering patients in making their own treatment decisions. The nurse needs to provide the patient with information and assist the patient in exploring all possible options.

- There are many strategies to improve decision making. Obtaining all the information, asking "why" and "what if" questions, and developing good habits of inquiry are a few of the strategies that will help nurses improve decision making.

KEY TERMS

consensus	intuitive thinking
critical thinking	problem solving
decision making	reflective thinking

REVIEW QUESTIONS

1. A nurse needs to assist a patient in walking down the hall twice daily as part of the patient's postoperative activities. It is the middle of the afternoon, and the patient is asleep. The nurse would like to allow the patient to sleep because the patient was awake a majority of the night. However, if the nurse does not ambulate the patient now, it is possible that the rest of the nurse's afternoon activities will prevent her from returning to the patient to ambulate before the end of her shift. The nurse must decide whether to ambulate the patient now. What is the next step of the decision-making process?
   A. Determine the outcome or goal that is desired.
   B. Generate alternatives and determine benefits and consequences of each.
   C. Evaluate the decision.
   D. Make the decision.

2. A nurse is asked to participate on a committee to interview and assist in making selections of staff in conjunction with the nurse manager. An applicant is interviewed, and the committee is discussing her qualifications. A committee member states, "If we hire her, then we will have all of our positions filled, then no one will get any overtime." A discussion ensues about the consequences of no overtime, and the committee determines that they shouldn't hire the nurse. What dysfunctional characteristic of group decision making may be going on in this group?
   A. Consensus
   B. Groupthink
   C. Stereotyping outsiders
   D. Group believes it is invincible

3. A nursing assistant approaches the RN to tell her that her patient care assignment is too difficult of a patient load. She will be unable to complete all of her work, which is unusual for this assistant. She asks the RN if she will review the assignments to see if a more equitable assignment can be made. The RN makes rounds on the patients and reviews patient acuities as well as other nursing assistant assignments. Which step of the problem-solving process is the RN performing?
   A. Identifying the problem
   B. Selecting an action
   C. Gathering and analyzing data
   D. Generating alternatives

4. A nurse manager decides to form a task force to identify reasons and solutions for patient dissatisfaction on your unit. What are the advantages of forming this task force? Select all that apply
   _____A. The decisions will be made more quickly.
   _____B. Higher quality decisions due to more solutions being generated.
   _____C. Acceptance of the decision is more likely.
   _____D. There is access to a larger resource base.
   _____E. There is less likely to be conflict during the decision-making process.
   _____F. This will help to promote ownership of the problem.

5. A new nurse is trying to set her goals for the next five years. She plans to eventually become an acute care nurse practitioner in the ICU setting. She knows she needs to become more experienced, obtain appropriate certification, go back to school, and take the practitioner exam. She would like to see a visual of the time it will take her to realistically accomplish those goals. She should use which of the following?
   A. Decision tree
   B. Gantt chart
   C. Decision grid
   D. Problem-solving process

6. A task force designed to examine solutions for low patient satisfaction in an emergency has decided to write their ideas down, present their ideas to the task force, discuss the ideas, and then, vote on the ideas. This is an example of which group process?
   A. Consensus building
   B. Delphi technique
   C. Problem-solving process
   D. Nominal group technique

7. Your friend tells you that the nurse manager over the Pediatrics unit, where you wanted to work, is a "terrible" nurse manager. Because of this information, you decide to pursue employment elsewhere. Making this decision might have involved which of the following?

A. Making a decision based upon the first available information

B. Being comfortable with the status quo

C. Assigning inaccurate probabilities to alternatives

D. Making a decision to justify a previous decision

8. A nurse needs to determine whether she should work overtime next week for two shifts. The nurse is having difficulty deciding because she will miss her child's program if she works, but feels the extra income might be worth it. She also believes it will be beneficial to work because the manager might give her preference for time off in the next pay period, but the nurse will miss a continuing education program she has been wanting to attend if she works overtime. The nurse could make the best decision by using which of the following?

A. PERT diagram

B. Gantt chart

C. Group consensus

D. Decision-making grid

9. A nurse has finished her shift and is on her way home from her job. She is mulling over the activities of the day and thinks about the teaching she completed on a patient with diabetes. The nurse decides that the patient had some difficulty understanding the insulin injections because she (the nurse) did not explain the differences in the two types of insulin in terms the patient could understand. The nurse decides that next time she will use more nonmedical terms in her explanations. This is an example of which of the following?

A. Critical thinking

B. Intuitive thinking

C. Reflective thinking

D. Decision making

REVIEW ACTIVITIES

1. You are a nurse on a surgical unit that consists of twelve beds. Your supervisor informs you that twelve more beds will be opened for neurosurgical patients. Draw a PERT diagram to depict the sequence of tasks necessary for the completion of the project.

2. The education forms are not being filled out correctly or in a timely manner on new admissions in your medical-surgical unit. Decide on your own the best action to take in this situation. Then, get into a group and attempt to reach consensus on the best action to take. Compare the differences between individual and group decision making. What did you learn about developing consensus?

3. Identify a problem that you have been considering. Using the decision-making grid at the bottom of the page, rate the alternative solutions to the problem that you have been considering on a scale of 1 to 3 on the elements of cost, quality, importance, location, and any other elements that are important to you.

  Did this exercise help you in thinking through your decision?

4. Identify a current problem in health care. Use the decision making process in a group to find a solution. Employ the nominal group technique or the Delphi technique.

EXPLORING THE WEB

- Visit these critical thinking sites:
  www.criticalthinking.org

  www.insightassessment.com

- Note the following site for clinical decision making, which includes software for clinical decision making: *www.apache-msi.com*

- Review these sites for extra information on intuitive thinking: *www.typelogic.com*

  www.intuitivethinking.com

- Review this site on applying artificial intelligence to clinical situations: *www.medg.lcs.mit.edu*

REFERENCES

Alfaro-LeFevre, R. (2003). *Critical thinking and clinical judgment: A practical approach* (3rd ed.). Philadelphia, PA: W. B. Saunders.

Bakalis, N. A., & Watson, R. (2005). Nurses' decision making in clinical practice. *Nursing Standard, 19*(23), 33–39.

Bucknall, T. (2003). The clinical landscape of critical care: Nurses' decision making. *Journal of Advanced Nursing, 43*(3), 310–319.

Cawthorpe, D., & Harris, D. (1999). Nominal group technique: Assessing staff concerns. *Journal of Nursing Administration, 29*(7/8), 11, 18, 37, 42.

	Cost	Quality	Importance	Location	Other
Alternative A					
Alternative B					
Alternative C					

Delaune, S., & Ladner, P. (2006). *Fundamentals of nursing, standards and practice* (3rd ed.). Clifton Park, NY: Thomson Delmar Learning.

Gardner, P. (2003). *Nursing process in action.* Clifton Park, NY: Thomson Delmar Learning.

Ignatavicius, D. (2001). Six critical thinking skills for at-the-bedside success. *Dimensions Of Critical Care Nursing, 20*(2), 30–33.

Jarvis, C. (1997). *Groupthink.* Retrieved June 2, 1999, from Brunel University Website: http://sol.brunel.ac.uk/~jarvis/bola/communications/groupthink.html

Jones, R. A. P., & Beck, S. E. (1996). *Decision making in nursing.* Clifton Park, NY: Thomson Delmar Learning.

Merriam-Webster. (2003). *Merriam-Webster's Collegiate Dictionary* (11th ed.). Springfield, MA: Author.

Paul, R. (1992). *Critical thinking: What every person needs to survive in a rapidly changing world.* Santa Rosa, CA: Foundation for Critical Thinking.

Pesut, D. J., & Herman, J. (1999). *Clinical reasoning: The art & science of critical & creative thinking.* Clifton Park, NY: Thomson Delmar Learning.

Ruth-Sahd, L., & Hendy, H. (2005). Predictors of novice nurses' use of intuition to guide patient care decisions. *Journal of Nursing Education, 44*(10), 450–458.

Shortell, S., & Kaluzny, A. (2006). *Health care management* (5th ed.). Clifton Park, NY: Thomson Delmar Learning.

The Small Business Knowledge Base. (1999). Retrieved January 19, 2002, from http://www.bizmove.com

Sullivan, E., & Decker, P. (2001). *Effective leadership and management in nursing.* Menlo Park, CA: Addison Wesley Longman.

Vroom, V. H., & Yetton, P. W. (1973). *Leadership and decision-making.* Pittsburgh, PA: University of Pittsburgh Press.

White, A., Allen, P., Goodwin, L., Breckinridge, D., Dowell, J., & Garvy, R. (2005). Infusing PDA technology into nursing education. *Nurse Educator, 30*(4), 153–154.

SUGGESTED READINGS

Carr, S. (2004). A framework for understanding clinical reasoning in community nursing. *Journal of Clinical Nursing, 13,* 850–857.

Evans, C. (2005). Clinical decision-making theories: Patient assessment in autonomy and extended roles. *Emergency Nurse, 13*(5), 16–20.

Hamilton, S. (2004). Clinical decision making: Thinking outside the box. *Emergency Nurse, 12*(6), 18–20.

Harbison, J. (2001). Clinical decision making in nursing: Theoretical perspectives and relevance to practice. *Journal of Advanced Nursing, 35*(1), 126–133.

Hendry, C. (2004). Priority setting in clinical nursing practice: Literature review. *Journal of Advanced Nursing, 47*(4), 427–436.

Higuchi, K. (2002). Thinking processes used by nurses in clinical decision making. *Journal of Nursing Education, 41*(4), 145–153.

Manias, E. (2004). Decision-making models used by "graduate nurses" managing patients' medications. *Journal of Advanced Nursing, 47*(3), 270–278.

Murphy, J. (2004). Using focused reflection and articulation to promote clinical reasoning: An evidence-based teaching strategy. *Nursing Education Perspectives, 25*(5), 226–231.

O'Callaghan, N. (2005). The use of expert practice to explore reflection. *Nursing Standard, 19*(39), 41–47.

Potter, P. (2005). Understanding the cognitive work of nursing in the acute care environment. *Journal of Nursing Administration, 35*(7/8), 327–335.

CHAPTER 23

Legal Aspects of Health Care

Judith W. Martin, RN, JD ✛ Sister Kathleen Cain, OSF, JD ✛
Chad S. Priest, RN, BSN, JD

A nurse who concludes that an attending physician has misdiagnosed a condition or has not prescribed the appropriate course of treatment may not modify the course set by the physician simply because the nurse holds a different view . . . However, the nurse is not prohibited from calling on or consulting with nurse supervisors or with other physicians . . . concerning those matters, and when the patient's condition reasonably requires it the nurse has a duty to do those tasks . . . (Berdyck v. Shinde, 613 N.E.2d 1014, 1024 [Ohio, 1993]).

OBJECTIVES

Upon completion of this chapter, the reader should be able to:

1. Identify the sources and types of laws and regulations, and recognize their impact on nursing practice.

2. Analyze common areas of nursing practice that lead to malpractice actions, and outline actions a nurse can take to minimize these risks.

3. Relate legal protections for nursing practice.

4. Explain privacy laws related to nursing actions.

5. Analyze the nurse's role as patient advocate and the duty to follow another practitioner's orders.

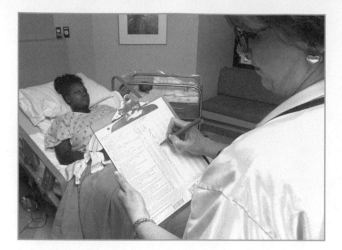

You are working on a postsurgical unit and have been given an order to discharge a 72-year-old male who has just had a total hip replacement. Per hospital policy, you obtain a set of vital signs before discharging him home and note his temperature to be 100.9°F (38.3°C). Upon assessing the patient, he tells you that he feels a bit "chilled." You notify the practitioner of the elevated temperature and the patient's comments, but you are told to continue with the discharge.

> *After notifying the practitioner about the elevated temperature, do you need to gather additional information about the patient's condition before you discharge him?*

> *What do you do if the patient appears to be too ill for discharge? Is there anyone else you can contact?*

> *If you discharge the patient and he develops sepsis or a serious illness, are you responsible or is the practitioner responsible?*

Law that affects the relationship between individuals is called civil law. Law that specifies the relationship between citizens and the state is called public law. This chapter reviews how laws are enacted and implemented and how the various types of law affect nursing practice.

SOURCES OF LAW

The authority to make, implement, and interpret laws is generally granted in a constitution. A **constitution** is a set of basic laws that specifies the powers of the various segments of the government and how these segments relate to each other.

Generally, it is the role of a legislative body, both on the federal and state levels, to enact laws. Agencies under the authority of the administrative branch of the government draft the rules that implement the law. Finally, the judicial branch interprets the law as it rules in court cases. Table 23-1 gives examples of these relationships.

Also, a judicial decision may set a precedent that is used by other courts and, over time, has the force of law. This type of law is referred to as common law.

PUBLIC LAW

Public law consists of constitutional law, criminal law, and administrative law and defines a citizen's relationship with government.

CONSTITUTIONAL LAW

Several categories of public law affect the practice of nursing. For example, the nurse accommodates patients' constitutional right to practice their religion every time the nurse calls a patient's clergy as requested, follows a specific religious custom for preparation of meals, or prepares a deceased person's remains for burial.

Controversial constitutional rights that may affect the nurse's practice include the recognized constitutional rights of a woman to have an abortion and an individual's right to die (see *Roe v. Wade* [1973] and *Cruzan v. Director* [1990]). Nurses may not believe in either of these rights personally and may refuse to work in areas in which they would have to assist a patient in exercising these rights. Nurses may not, however, interfere with another person's right to have an abortion or to forgo life-saving measures.

CRIMINAL LAW

Criminal law focuses on the actions of individuals that can intentionally do harm to others. Often the victims of such abusive actions are the very young or the very old. These two categories of people generally cannot defend themselves against physical or emotional abuse. The nurse, in caring for patients, may notice that a vulnerable patient has unexplained bruises, fractures, or other injuries. Most states have mandatory statutes that require the nurse to report unexplained or suspicious injuries to the appropriate child or elderly protective agency. Generally, the institution in which the nurse is employed will have clear guidelines to follow in such a situation. Failure of the nurse to report the problem as required by law can result in criminal penalties.

Another aspect of criminal law affecting nursing practice is the state and federal requirement that criminal background checks be performed on specified categories of prospective employees who will work with the very young or the elderly in institutions such as schools and nursing homes. Again, this is an attempt to protect the most vulnerable citizens from mistreatment or abuse. Failure to conduct the mandated background checks can result in the institution having to defend itself for any harm done by an employee with a past criminal conviction.

	Legislative Branch	**Administrative Branch**	**Judicial Branch**
TABLE 23-1		**THE THREE BRANCHES OF GOVERNMENT**	
Example at federal level	Americans with Disabilities Act (ADA) (1990)	The Equal Employment Opportunity Commission (EEOC) publishes rules specifying what employers must do to help a disabled employee.	In 1999, the U.S. Supreme Court interpreted the law to require that to be protected by this law, the individual must have an impairment that limits a major life activity and that is not corrected by medicine or appliances (glasses, blood pressure medicine). *Sutton v. United Airlines* (1999); *Murphy v. United Parcel Service, Inc.* (1999)
Example at state level	Nurse Practice Act	The state board of nursing develops rules specifying the duties of a registered nurse in that state.	Courts and juries determine whether a nurse's actions comply with the law governing the practice of nursing in a state.

A third area in which criminal law concerns affect nursing practice is the prohibition against substance abuse. Both federal and state law requires health care agencies to keep a strict accounting of the use and distribution of regulated drugs. Nurses routinely are expected to keep narcotic records accurate and current.

Nurses' behavior when off duty can also affect their employment status. Abusing alcohol or drugs on one's own time, if discovered, can result in nurses being terminated from employment and their license to practice nursing restricted or revoked (Mantel, 1999). Frequently, boards of nursing have programs for the nurse with a drug problem, and completion of such a program may be required before the nurse can resume practice. Additionally, health care facilities may require nurse employees to submit to random drug screens to identify those who may be using illegal substances.

ADMINISTRATIVE LAW

Both the federal government and state governments have administrative laws that affect nursing practice. The laws pertaining to Social Security and, more specifically, Medicare, are interpreted in the *Code of Federal Regulations*, which contains the administrative rules for the federal government. These rules have specific requirements that hospitals, nursing homes, and other health care providers must adhere to if they are to qualify for payment from federal funds. Likewise, state laws are interpreted in

administrative rules that specify licensing requirements for health care providers in the state.

FEDERAL

Administrative law deals with protection of the rights of citizens. It extends some rights and protections beyond those granted in the federal and state constitutions. An example of this type of law, at the federal level, is the Civil Rights Act of 1964, which prohibits many forms of discrimination in the workplace. This law may necessitate that the nurse manager make some scheduling accommodations for such things as an employee's religious practices.

Another federal law that affects nursing practice is the Health Insurance Portability and Accountability Act (HIPAA), which was enacted to, among other things, safeguard certain private medical information. Under the law, disclosure of certain protected health information, such as a patient's medical diagnosis or plan of care, can result in criminal penalties. HIPAA is implicated anytime that a patient's private medical information may be shared with another, whether intentional or accidental (Frank-Stromborg, 2004).

Nurses in all practice areas, and of all experience levels, face HIPAA issues each day. For example, wipe-erase boards were once common features in hospital emergency rooms and inpatient units and were displayed in highly visible areas. On these boards, nurses used to list the names of all the patients on the unit,

CRITICAL THINKING 23-1

You are a new nurse working on the OB unit of your local hospital. Your close friend George Nurse also got a job on this unit. George has a reputation as a smart, likeable, and hard-working nurse, who also knows how to let loose and have a good time when work is out. However, lately George has been coming to work late and appears "out of it." You spoke with George, who told you that he was having a difficult time at home, and had not been as focused at work as he needed to be. He promised that he would try to leave his personal life at home.

For a month after your discussion with George, everything seemed fine. However, in the past two weeks, you have noticed that George has had bloodshot eyes, and his speech seems slurred at times. He looks unkempt and unclean, and the narcotic count for Vicodin was off for three separate shifts that he worked. You are concerned that George may be using drugs or alcohol and that it may be impacting his nursing care.

What action do you take? Who can you go to for help in this situation?

---

their practitioners, and perhaps their diagnoses. Today, such a practice might be a violation of HIPAA, as it would disclose the private health information of individual patients. Another example is the chart that many nurses, especially new nurses, use to organize their patient care tasks. Typically these charts identify the patients the nurse is responsible for, their diagnoses, and what medications and treatments they will need. Although these forms are invaluable tools for new nurses learning to organize their clinical practice, they contain sensitive protected health information that, if disclosed, may violate HIPAA. As such, nurses must be on guard to carefully destroy these forms when they are no longer needed (Adams, 2004).

As with most federal laws, the agency responsible for implementing the law has a great deal of power to draft specific rules and regulations. For example, the Occupational Safety & Health Administration, an administrative agency, works to establish a safe workplace for employees. This includes enacting regulations concerning storage of hazardous substances, protection of employees from infection, and protection of employees from violence in the workplace. Hospitals are subject to numerous OSHA regulations designed to protect the health and safety of nurses and other health care workers. From the minute the new nurse joins the hospital staff, he or she is likely to come into contact with OSHA-mandated products or programs every day. For example, any unvaccinated nurse joining the staff of a hospital will be offered Hepatitis B vaccination pursuant to OSHA regulations. Additionally, nurses working with patients who may have tuberculosis will be issued special OSHA-approved respirators to prevent the nurse from becoming infected. Every day, nurses will utilize OSHA mandated and approved "sharps" containers

that hold used needles, and personal protective equipment such as gloves, gowns, and surgical face-masks. New nurses should review hospital policies and procedures to ensure they are using these safety devices properly.

STATE

An example of a state's administrative law is its Nurse Practice Act. Under Nurse Practice Acts, state boards of nursing are given the authority to define the practice of nursing within certain broad parameters specified by the legislature, mandate the requisite preparation for the practice of nursing, and discipline members of the profession who deviate from the rules governing the practice of nursing. Other professions such as medicine and dentistry have similar practice acts established in state law.

An important issue to nurses is the transferability of their nursing license from one state to another. A license to practice nursing is generally valid only in the state where it is issued. In most cases, a nurse wanting to practice in a state other than where his or her license was issued must apply for a license in that state. For nurses who frequently move from one state to another, this can be a burdensome process. There is an ongoing movement to allow nurses licensed in one state to automatically receive licensure to practice in another state. The Nurse Licensure Compact, a project of the National Council of State Boards of Nursing, is an agreement among states to allow nurses licensed in other states who are parties to the agreement to practice without applying for a new license (Hellquist & Spector, 2004). As of the date of this writing, only nineteen states had joined this agreement, meaning that most states still require nurses to apply for a license in the state where they want to practice. You may check the Web to determine if your state is a member of the compact by pointing your browser to www.ncsbn.org. Of course, nurses should always contact the board of nursing in any state where they intend to practice to determine eligibility and licensure requirements.

CIVIL LAW

Civil law governs how individuals relate to each other in everyday matters. It encompasses both contract and tort law.

CONTRACT LAW

Contract law regulates certain transactions between individuals and/or legal entities such as businesses. It also governs transactions between businesses. An agreement must contain the following elements to be recognized as a legal contract:

- Agreement between two or more legally competent individuals or parties stating what each must or must not do
- Mutual understanding of the terms and obligations that the contract imposes on each party to the contract
- Payment or consideration given for actions taken or not taken pursuant to the agreement

The terms of the contract may be oral or written; however, a written contract may not be legally modified by an oral agreement. Another way this is often expressed is by the phrase "all of the terms of the contract are contained within the four corners of the document," that is, if it is not written, it is not part of the agreement or contract. A contract may be express or implied. In an express contract, the terms of the contract are specified, usually in writing. In an implied contract, a relationship between parties is recognized, although the terms of the agreement are not clearly defined, such as the expectations one has for services from the dry cleaner or the grocer.

CRITICAL THINKING 23-2

You are assigned to a medical-surgical unit, working the night shift. Your supervisor calls and says that one of the RNs assigned to the critical care unit has called in sick, and you must work that unit instead of your usual assignment. You have never worked in the critical care setting before and have received no orientation to this unit. You are now asked to work there when it is short of staff.

What should you do?

The nurse is usually a party to an employment contract. The employed nurse agrees to do the following:

- Adhere to the policies and procedures of the employing entity
- Fulfill the agreed-upon duties of the employer
- Respect the rights and responsibilities of other health care providers in the workplace

In return, the employer agrees to provide the nurse with the following:

- A specified amount of pay for services rendered
- Adequate assistance in providing care
- The supplies and equipment needed to fulfill his responsibilities
- A safe environment in which to work
- Reasonable treatment and behavior from the other health care providers with whom he must interact

This contract may be express or implied, depending on the practices of the employing entity. Sometimes, what is determined to be "reasonable" by the employer is not considered "reasonable" by the nurse. For instance, after twenty years of working as a nurse on the orthopedic unit, a nurse may not view it as reasonable to be pulled to the labor and delivery unit for duty as a nurse there. It would be prudent to express any misgivings to the supervisor and to take assignments that are in keeping with the experience one has on an orthopedic unit.

TORT LAW

Black's Law Dictionary (2000) defines **tort** as a civil wrong for which remedy may be obtained. A tort can be any of the following:

- The denial of a person's legal right
- The failure to comply with a public duty
- The failure to perform a private duty that results in harm to another

A tort can be unintentional, as occurs in malpractice or neglect, or it can be the intentional infliction of harm such as assault and battery. In a tort suit, the nurse can be named as a defendant because of something she did incorrectly or because she failed to do something that was required. In either case, the suit is usually classified as a tort suit (Fiesta, 1999a). Other tort charges that a nurse may face include assault and battery, false imprisonment, invasion of privacy, defamation, and fraud (see Table 23-2).

NEGLIGENCE AND MALPRACTICE

If a nurse fails to meet the legal expectations for care, usually defined by the state's Nurse Practice Act, the patient, if harmed by this failure, can initiate an action against the

TABLE 23-2	SELECTED TORTS	
Tort	**Definition**	**Example**
Assault	Threat to touch another person in an offensive manner without that person's permission.	Nurse who threatens to give a patient a treatment against his will.
Battery	Touching of another person without that person's consent.	Nurse who forces a treatment against a patient's will.
Invasion of privacy	All patients have the right to privacy and may bring charges against any person who violates this right.	Nurse who discloses confidential information about a patient or photographs a patient without consent.
False imprisonment	This occurs when individuals are physically prevented, or incorrectly led to believe they are prevented, from leaving a place.	Nurse who restrains a patient who is of sound mind and is not in danger of injuring himself or others.
Defamation, including libel and slander	Intentionally false communication or publication, including written (libel) or verbal (slander) remarks that may cause the loss of a person's reputation.	Nurse who makes a statement that could either ruin the patient's reputation or cause the patient to lose his job.

nurse for damages. The term **malpractice** refers to a professional's wrongful conduct in the discharge of his or her professional duties or failure to meet standards of care for the profession, which results in harm to another individual entrusted to the professional's care. **Negligence** is the failure to provide the care a reasonable person would ordinarily provide in a similar situation.

Simply proving malpractice or negligence is not sufficient to recover damages. Proof of liability or fault requires the proof of the following four elements:

1. A duty or obligation created by law, contract, or standard practice that is owed to the complainant by the professional
2. A breach of this duty, either by omission or commission
3. Harm, which can be physical, emotional, or financial, to the complainant (patient)
4. Proof that the breach of duty caused the complained of harm

A Louisiana appellate court described the plaintiff's (patient's) specific burden of proof in a negligence or malpractice case against a nurse as follows:

[T]he three requirements which a plaintiff must satisfy to meet its burden of proving the negligence

of a nurse are: (1) the nurse must exercise the degree of skill ordinarily employed, under similar circumstances, by the members of the nursing or health care profession in good standing in the same community or locality; (2) the nurse either lacked this degree of knowledge or skill or failed to use reasonable care and diligence, along with her best judgment in the application of that skill; and (3) as a proximate result of this lack of knowledge or skill or the failure to exercise this degree of care, the plaintiff suffered injuries that would not otherwise have occurred (*Odom v. State Dept. of Health & Hospitals*, [1999]).

After a plaintiff presents his case, the defendant nurse must refute the claims either by showing that if a duty was owed, it was fulfilled, or by demonstrating that the breach of that duty was not the cause of the plaintiff's harm.

Proving that a duty was owed is not difficult. The person need only show that the nurse was working on the day in question and was responsible for the plaintiff's care. This can usually be accomplished by producing staffing schedules and assignment sheets.

To demonstrate a breach of duty, the courts employ a *reasonable man* standard by asking what a reasonable nurse would do in a like situation. This is accomplished

TABLE 23-3	SELECTED SOURCES OF EVIDENCE REGARDING THE STANDARD OF CARE

- Evidence-based health care literature
- Nursing and medical textbooks, articles, and research
- State professional practice acts, such as Nurse Practice Act, Physician Practice Act
- Standards of professional association, for example, American Nurses' Association Standards
- Equipment manufacturers manuals, for example, cardiac monitoring equipment manuals
- Written policies and procedures of a facility, such as Foley catheter insertion procedures
- Nurse, practitioner, or other health care professional expert testimony
- Professional health care accreditation agency criteria, for example, JC (Joint Commission) criteria
- Medication books, such as *Physician's Desk Reference, American Society of Health System Pharmacists Drug Information Book*, and so on

Note: Not all sources are used in all states.

by reviewing the employing institution's policies and procedures and other evidence, including the state's Nurse Practice Act and hearing testimony from nurses who are accepted as expert witnesses to the standard of nursing practice in the community (Table 23-3).

The defendant nurse would employ the same methodology to refute the plaintiff's charges. The nurse would present evidence that the institution's policies and procedures were followed and that the care rendered adhered to accepted nursing standards. To present the nurse's case, the nurse's attorney would also use expert witnesses to document that the care given fulfilled the duty owed, was the kind that would be given by a reasonable nurse in such a circumstance, and that it was not the cause of the plaintiff's harm.

It is not sufficient for a patient plaintiff to show a breach of duty to prevail in a tort suit. He must also show that the breach of the duty caused him harm. Even if it is proved that a nurse made a medication error, if the error was not the cause of the plaintiff's harm, he will not win in recovering damages from the nurse. In a recent malpractice case, a patient with sickle cell anemia died after suffering a cardiopulmonary arrest, attributed to an aspiration that was witnessed by a visitor. The visitor immediately called for and obtained help. Although revived, the patient never regained consciousness and was eventually taken off of life support. At trial, the plaintiff was able to prove that the nurse assigned to this patient did not follow the institution's policy of documenting frequent observations, which were mandated because the patient was receiving a blood transfusion at the time of the cardiac arrest. In reviewing the case on appeal, the appellate court noted the following:

> [T]he record contains no evidence which suggests what could have been done even if the nurse had been seated at his bedside prior to the arrest. Plaintiff has failed to offer any proof that more immediate assistance would have prevented the catastrophic results of his aspiration. Based on the evidence in this record, we conclude that more frequent monitoring would have made no difference (*Webb v. Tulane Medical Center Hospital,* [1997]).

Thus, even though the plaintiff successfully proved a breach of a duty, the breach was not found to be the cause of the patient's death, and the nurse was not found to be guilty of negligence.

Table 23-4 represents the results of a study examining the types and frequency of nursing malpractice actions throughout the United States.

When a nurse is listed as a party in a malpractice lawsuit, the nurse's liability is determined by state laws, such as the Nurse Practice Act, the standards for the practice of nursing, and the institution's policies and procedures. Thus, if state laws mandate that a nurse must have a practitioner's order before doing something, then a practitioner's order must be present. Problems arise when the orders are verbal, and later it is claimed that the nurse misunderstood and acted in error. Another pitfall is illegible writing, which is then misinterpreted, and the result causes harm to the patient.

TABLE 23-4   NURSING MALPRACTICE CASES*

Treatment

- Failed to prevent and treat pressure ulcers and malnutrition, resulting in death
- Mishandled shoulder dystocia during delivery, resulting in brachial plexus injury
- Failed to perform intrauterine resuscitation, leading to infant's brain damage
- Failed to properly handle telephone triage calls, resulting in death
- Failed to incorporate patient's emergency room records into patient's hospital chart, resulting in death
- Failed to properly treat pediatric glaucoma, resulting in vision loss
- Burned patient with hair dryer, resulting in third-degree burns
- Failed to accurately count sponges after operation, resulting in retained sponge
- Failed to provide adequate nutrition and implement nursing plan of care, resulting in death
- Injected patient with used needle, leading to emotional distress from possible hepatitis infection
- Failed to properly treat patient's jaundice, resulting in infant's brain damage
- Failed to treat dehydration and pressure ulcers, resulting in death
- Removed internal pacemaker wires improperly, resulting in infection
- Administered suction tube improperly, leading to aspiration and death by suffocation
- Failed to detect arterial blockage after surgery, leading to leg amputation
- Failed to adequately hydrate patient prior to Cesarean delivery, resulting in maternal hypotension and infant's brain damage
- Failed to administer supplemental oxygen, resulting in vision loss and brain damage

Communication

- Failed to notify physician of:
  - Patient burns
  - Bleeding gastric ulcer, resulting in death
  - Increased heart rate, resulting in death
  - Fetal distress, resulting in fetal death or brain damage
  - Newborn jaundice, resulting in brain damage
  - Prothrombin time level
  - Pain and numbness after spinal surgery, resulting in cauda equina syndrome
  - Vision problems, resulting in vision loss
- Failed to report sexual abuse of patient/resident to police and/or state department of human resources
- Failed to institute chain of command when practitioner refused to come to the hospital promptly

Medication

- Administered insufficient Heparin, leading to death by pulmonary embolism
- Administered doses of Dilantin and insulin to a patient in excess of practitioner's order, leading to patient's disorientation and burns by bedside heater
- Administered excessive dose of IV antibiotics (Nafcillin), leading to chemical burn

TABLE 23-4   NURSING MALPRACTICE CASES* (CONTINUED)

Medication (cont.)

- Failed to send antibiotics home with patient with meningitis, leading to cerebral palsy
- Failed to recognize dosage error in doctor's order and thereby administered excessive dose of Dilaudid, leading to brain damage

Monitoring/Observing/Supervising

- Failed to monitor premature newborn, leading to death by cardiac arrest
- Failed to detect fetal distress, resulting in fetal death or brain damage
- Failed to monitor patient, leading to third-degree burns
- Failed to timely call a "code blue" in response to patient's respiratory arrest, resulting in death
- Failed to seek timely medical intervention, leading to death from bleeding ulcer
- Failed to properly monitor heart rate after surgery, resulting in death
- Misidentified and mixed up newborns in nursery
- Failed to monitor respiratory rate after surgery, resulting in death
- Failed to take vital signs of patient in waiting room, resulting in brain damage
- Failed to restrain demented patient, resulting in death
- Failed to properly insert Foley catheter during delivery, resulting in urinary sphincter trauma and incontinence
- Failed to monitor cornea in facial palsy, leading to corneal scarring and vision loss
- Failed to reattach cardiac monitor after x-rays, resulting in death
- Failed to detect brain swelling, resulting in vision loss and diminished I.Q.

*Reported in *Professional Negligence Law Reporter,* July 2001 through July 2002 (Courtesy, Pozza, R., Unpublished manuscript, 2003).

The institution's policies and procedures describe the performance expected of nurses in its employ, and a nurse deviating from them can be liable for negligence or malpractice. Occasionally, such failure to adhere to institutional protocol can result in the employer denying the nurse a defense in a lawsuit.

Practicing nurses must also adhere to the standards of practice for the nursing profession in the community. These standards include such things as checking the six "rights" in medication administration or repositioning the bed-bound patient at regular intervals.

NEGLIGENCE AND NURSING ADVOCACY

The American Nurses Association Code of Ethics and many state Nursing Practice Acts require nurses to serve as patient advocates (ANA Code, 2001). A patient's illness, combined with the institutional nature of hospitals, often results in patients becoming passive recipients of health care instead of active partners. Nurses are often called

upon to help patients communicate their desires and needs to the health care team and to be vigilant in protecting the patient's safety and even legal rights. For example, occasionally a provider's order may appear suspect or clearly contrary to accepted medical practice. In such situations, the nurse must exercise professional judgment and refuse to carry out the order if it would put the patient in danger. Most hospitals have policies and procedures to assist the nurse in carrying out this advocacy function. These procedures often require the nurse to take the issue up the "chain of command," from the nursing manager up through the medical staff if necessary. Nurses are increasingly being held liable for negligence in failing to question potentially improper provider orders.

Nurses also serve as advocates by safeguarding patient legal interests, such as the right to make informed health care decisions. In this role, nurses frequently collaborate with other members of the health care team and provide patient education to ensure that patients understand the risks and benefits of procedures, medication

REAL WORLD INTERVIEW

Nursing practice in today's health care environment is multifaceted and complex. Our patients and our communities expect quality care from nurses at all levels of practice. Responsibility to keep abreast of current practices is an integral component of a nurse's licensure requirements. Nursing professionals must understand their scope of practice and the legal requirements necessary to maintain their license in good standing. As a former member of a State Board of Nursing, I can assure you that this is important for all nurses, novice or experienced.

Increased emphasis is being placed on patient safety through regulatory agencies, JC, and other national initiatives. Commitments to reducing medication errors and surgical infections, and improving patient outcomes are just a few of the ongoing issues that have become a fundamental component of nursing practice.

As a sustained focus is placed on improvement of care and patient safety, evidence-based practice must be integrated into the daily practice patterns of patient care. Proven methods and research-based policies and procedures need to dictate how patient care is administered, rather than "this is how we have always done it." Failure to adhere to best practices within your scope of practice can result in negative patient outcomes and ultimately lead to licensure problems or legal action.

Above all, staying current in skills, knowledge, and education helps nurses to meet the practice standards that are expected in today's health care environment.

Marsha King RN, MS, MBA, CNAA
Chief Nursing Officer, Past President of the Indiana State Board of Nursing
Indianapolis, Indiana

regimens, or laboratory tests. Additionally, nurses may help patients express their desires regarding end-of-life decisions to the medical team. Both of these issues are discussed in detail later in this chapter.

It is not uncommon for a nurse to find conflicts between an employer's expectations and the nursing standard of care. A nurse working in a medical-surgical ward, for example, may be asked to take care of an unsafe number of patients, or a surgical nurse with no experience working in the ER may be asked to "float" to this unit. In these situations, nurses must advocate on behalf of their patients and their profession, and consider whether it is appropriate to take on such an assignment. If the nurse determines that he or she cannot safely carry out the hospital's order, the nurse must not do so. A nurse in this situation would be wise to offer to help hospital staff and patients and notify the supervisor of the patient safety concerns.

ASSAULT AND BATTERY

Assault is a threat to touch another in an offensive manner without that person's permission. **Battery** is the touching of another person without that person's consent. In the health care arena, complaints of this nature usually pertain to whether the individual consented to the treatment administered by the health care professional. Most states have laws that require patients to make informed decisions about their treatment.

CRITICAL THINKING 23-3

Review the malpractice cases in Table 23-4. Have you ever seen a similar case or one that might result in a malpractice charge? How would you handle it if you saw it?

Informed consent laws protect the patient's right to practice self-determination (Aveyard, 2001). The patient has the right to receive sufficient information to make an informed decision about whether to consent or to refuse a procedure. The individual performing the procedure has the responsibility of explaining to the patient the nature of the procedure, benefits, alternatives, and the risks and complications. The signed consent form is used to document that this was done, and it creates a presumption that the patient had been advised of the appropriate risks.

Often the nurse is asked to witness a patient signing a consent form for treatment. When you witness a patient's signature, you are vouching for two things: that the patient signed the paper and that the patient knows he is signing a consent form (Olsen-Chavarriaga, 2000). For a consent form to be legal, a patient, in most states, must be at least eighteen-years-old; be mentally competent; have the procedures, with their risks and benefits, explained in a manner he can understand; be aware of the available alternatives to the proposed treatment; and consent voluntarily. The nurse must also be familiar with which other people are allowed by state law to consent to medical treatment for another when that person cannot consent for himself. Frequently, these include the person possessing medical power of attorney; a spouse; adult children; or other relatives, if no one is available in one of the other categories listed.

A nurse may also face a charge of battery for failing to honor an advance directive, such as a medical power of attorney, durable power of attorney, or living will. Federal law requires that a hospital ask the patient, upon admission, whether she has a living will; if she does not, the hospital must ask the patient whether she would like to enact one. A **living will** is a written advance directive voluntarily signed by the patient that specifies the type of care she desires if and when she is in a terminal state and cannot sign a consent form or convey this information verbally. It can be a general statement such as "no life sustaining measures" or specific such as "no tube feedings or respirator." Often, the patient's family has difficulty allowing health care personnel to follow the wishes expressed by the patient in a living will, and conflicts arise. These should be communicated to the hospital ethics committee, pastoral care department, risk management, or whichever hospital department is responsible for handling such issues. If the patient verbalizes her wishes regarding end-of-life care to the family, such difficult situations can sometimes be avoided, and the patient should be encouraged to do this, if possible.

The nurse should be familiar with the requirements for the implementation of a living will in the state where the nurse practices.

Do Not Resuscitate (DNR) Orders

The attending medical practitioner may write a do not resuscitate (DNR) order on an inpatient, which directs the staff not to perform the usual cardiopulmonary resuscitation (CPR) in the event of a sudden cardiopulmonary arrest. The practitioner may write such an order without evidence of a living will on the medical record, and the nurse should be familiar with the institution's policies and state law regarding when and how a practitioner can write such an order in the absence of a living will. Often, a DNR order is considered a medical decision that the practitioner can make, preferably in consultation with the family, even without a living will executed by the patient. If the nurse feels such a DNR order is contrary to

the patient's or family's wishes, the nurse should consult the policies and procedures of the institution. These may include going up the chain of command until the nurse is satisfied with the course of action. This may entail notifying the nursing supervisor, the medical director, the institution's chief operating officer, state regulators, or the Joint Commission (JC). Often an institution has an ethics committee that examines such issues and makes a determination of the appropriateness of the order.

False Imprisonment

False imprisonment occurs when individuals are incorrectly led to believe they cannot leave a place. This often occurs because the nurse misinterprets the rights granted to others by legal documents such as powers of attorney and does not allow a patient to leave a facility because the person with the power of attorney (agent) says the patient cannot leave. A **power of attorney** is a legal document executed by an individual (principal) granting another person (agent) the right to perform certain activities in the principal's name. It can be specific, such as "sell my house," or general, such as "make all decisions for me, including health care decisions." In most states, a power of attorney is voluntarily granted by the individual and does not take away the individual's right to exercise his own choices. Thus, if the principal (patient) disagrees with his agent's decisions, the patient's wishes are the ones that prevail. If a situation occurs in which an agent, acting on a power of attorney, disagrees with your patient regarding discharge plans, contact your supervisor for further assistance in deciding an action consistent with your patient's wishes and best interests.

The authority to make medical decisions for another may be granted in a general power of attorney document or in a specific document limited to medical decisions only, such as a medical power of attorney. The requirements for a medical power of attorney vary from state to state, as do most legal documents.

A claim of false imprisonment may be based on the inappropriate use of physical or chemical restraints. Federal law mandates that health care institutions employ the least restrictive method of ensuring patient safety. Physical or chemical restraints are to be used only if necessary to protect the patient from harm when all other methods have failed. If the nurse uses restraints on a competent person who is refusing to follow the practitioner's orders, the nurse can be charged with false imprisonment or battery. If restraints are used in an emergency situation, the nurse is to contact the practitioner immediately after application to secure an order for the restraints. Also, the nurse must check the institution's policies regarding the type and frequency of assessments required for a patient in restraints and how often it is necessary to secure a reorder for the restraints. These policies ensure the patient's safety and must be consistent with state law.

CASE STUDY
23-1

Y ou are working the night shift. One of your patient's practitioners has ordered a dose of a medication to be given to a patient that you know is too high for this patient. You are unable to locate the practitioner to check the order. What would you do to ensure safe care for your patient?

INVASION OF PRIVACY

The nurse is required to respect the privacy of all patients. The nurse may be privy to very personal information and must make every effort to keep it confidential. This often necessitates policing conversations with coworkers that have the potential for being overheard by others so that no patient information is accidentally revealed. Sometimes the protection of a patient's privacy conflicts with the state's mandatory reporting laws for the occurrence of specified infectious diseases such as syphilis or human immunodeficiency virus (HIV). The need to protect an individual's privacy may also conflict with the state's mandatory reporting laws on suspected patient abuse, discussed previously. Other information that state or federal law may require to be revealed include a patient's blood alcohol level, incidences of rape, gunshot wounds, and adverse reactions to certain drugs. Failing to strictly follow reporting laws could lead to criminal-, civil-, or disciplinary action, termination of employment, or all of these; nurses must consult the institution's policies and confer with its risk management department to ascertain their responsibilities and course of action. The ANA Code for Nurses states that nurses must protect the patient and the public when incompetence or unethical or illegal practice compromise health care and safety. Many states have adopted this concept in their Nurse Practice Acts, thereby creating a legal obligation to report. Nurses who observe unethical behavior in a hospital should report this as directed in the institution's policies and procedures manual or by the laws of the state.

LEGAL PROTECTIONS IN NURSING PRACTICE

As discussed earlier in this chapter, nursing practice is guided by state Nurse Practice Acts and agency policies and procedures. Other resources for the nurse include Good Samaritan laws, skillful communication, and risk management programs.

GOOD SAMARITAN LAWS

Good Samaritan laws have been enacted to protect the health care professional from legal liability. The essential

EVIDENCE FROM THE LITERATURE

Citation: Croke, E. M. (2003). Nurses, negligence, and malpractice. *American Journal of Nursing, 103*(9), 54–64.

Discussion: This article discusses the actions that prompted charges of negligence that led to malpractice lawsuits against nurses from 1995 to 2001. It identifies several factors that have contributed to the increase in malpractice cases against nurses. According to the National Practitioner Data Bank (NPDB), 2,311 nonspecialized nurses made malpractice payments in cases reported to NPDB from 1990 to 2001. Annual Reports of the NPDB are available at www.npdb-hipdb.com. Author states that the majority of payments by nonspecialized nurses in malpractice suits resulted from problems relating to monitoring, treatment, medication, obstetrics, and surgery. Negligence areas discussed include failure to act as a patient advocate; failure to communicate adequate information to the practitioner or patient; inadequate patient assessment, nursing interventions, or nursing care; medication errors; inadequate infection control; failure to document; and unsafe or improper use of equipment. Monetary awards were paid either directly by independent practitioners or by employers according to the doctrine of respondeat superior. The author also discusses strategies for reducing potential liability.

Implications for Practice: Knowledge of the legal implications of nursing practice is necessary to assure that you are taking action to reduce your liability.

elements of commonly enacted Good Samaritan law are as follows:

- The care is rendered in an emergency situation.
- The health care worker is rendering care without pay.
- The care provided did not recklessly or intentionally cause injury or harm to the injured party.

Note that these laws are intended to protect the volunteer who stops to render care at the scene of an accident. They would not protect an emergency medical technician (EMT) or other health care professionals rendering care at the scene of an accident as part of their assigned duties and for which they receive pay. In doing their duties, these paid emergency personnel would be evaluated according to the standards of their professions.

SKILLFUL COMMUNICATION

The nurse must communicate accurately and completely both verbally and in writing. In the cases detailed earlier in Table 23-4, many cited a lack of communication by the nurse. Either the nurse failed to monitor the patient and notify the practitioner of a change in the patient's status, or the nurse failed to document the assessments performed. It is essential that the nurse chart accurately and completely. Often a case involving patient care takes several years to come to trial; by that time, the nurse may have no memory of the incident in question and must rely on the written record done at the time of the incident. This record is frequently in the courtroom, blown up to billboard size for all to see. All errors are apparent and omissions stand out by their absence, especially if it is data that should have been recorded per institutional policy. The old adage that "if it isn't written, it wasn't done" will be repeated to the jury numerous times. To protect themselves when charting, nurses should use the FLAT charting acronym: F—factual, L—legible, A—accurate, T—timely:

F: Charting should be *factual*—what you see, not what you think happened.
L: Charting should be *legible,* with no erasures. Corrections should be made as you have been taught, with a single line drawn through the error and initialed.
A: Charting should be *accurate* and complete. What color was the drainage and how much was present? How many times, and at what times, was the practitioner notified of changes? Was the supervisor notified?
T: Charting should be *timely,* completed as soon after the occurrence as possible. "Late entries" should be avoided or kept to a minimum.

Patient safety and risk management are synonymous terms. Health care delivery processes are inherently complex, high risk, and problem prone. In order to create an environment that promotes optimal patient outcomes, basic nursing and patient care processes and procedures must be well designed. Well-designed nursing care processes possess the following characteristics:

- Staff-level nursing policies and procedures should be designed with input and participation by those closest to the process, that is, staff level nurses.
- Nursing care policies, processes, and procedures should be simple, practical, and written in universally understandable terms.

During a shadowing experience, I was once asked by a BSN student, "What can bedside nurses do to protect themselves and the organization from liability?" My answer was multifaceted. The single most important risk-management tool is well-documented nursing care. It is a challenge in today's nursing environment to assure that an accurate reflection of all patient care details is made. Many hospitals utilize "charting by exception," which is designed for efficiency and to capture the essence of nursing care delivery under "normal" circumstances without variation. However, in-depth narrative must be documented with changes in patient condition or care needs along with the patients' response to our interventions.

The medical record is the only document we will have several years out if a patient care incident results in litigation. For this reason, it must tell a vivid story in complete detail about what the patient looked like, smelled like, felt like, and sounded like at accurate points in time during our care as well as everything we did for the patient and how they responded to what we did. It is the nurse's responsibility to supplement any standard form to provide this type of information.

Communication between nurses, physicians, and other health care team members is another critical element of safe patient care and effective risk management.

Patient safety and risk management is every individual's responsibility, and everyone has a role to play.

Tamara L. Awald, RN, BSN, MS
Vice-President of Patient Care Services/Risk Manager
Plymouth, Indiana

RISK-MANAGEMENT PROGRAMS

Risk-management programs in health care organizations are designed to identify and correct system problems that contribute to errors in patient care or to employee injury. The emphasis in risk management is on quality improvement and protection of the institution from financial liability. Institutions usually have reporting and tracking forms that record incidents that may lead to financial liability for the institution. Risk management will assist in identifying and correcting the underlying problem that may have led to an incident, such as faulty equipment, staffing concerns, or the need for better orientation for employees. After a system problem is identified, the risk-management department may develop educational programs to address the problem.

The risk-management department may also investigate and record information surrounding a patient or employee incident that may result in a lawsuit. This helps personnel remember critical factors if called to testify at a later time. The nurse should notify the risk-management department of all reportable incidents and complete all risk-management and/or incident report forms as mandated by institutional policies and procedures. Note also that employee complaints of harassment or discrimination can expose the institution to significant liability and should promptly be reported to supervisors and the risk-management department, human resources, or whichever department is specified in the institution's policies. See Table 23-5 for a checklist of actions to decrease the risk of nursing liability.

TABLE 23-5	**ACTIONS TO DECREASE THE RISK OF LIABILITY**

- Communicate with your clients by keeping them informed and listening to what they say. Treat clients and their family with kindness and respect.

- Acknowledge unfortunate incidents and express concern about these events without either taking the blame, blaming others, or reacting defensively.

- Chart and time your observations immediately, while facts are still fresh in your mind.

- Take appropriate actions to meet the client's nursing needs. Be assertive and professional.

- Acknowledge and document the reason for any omission or deviation from agency policy, procedure, or standard.

- Maintain clinical competency and professional certifications; Acknowledge your limitations. If you do not know how to do something, ask for help.

- Promptly report any concern regarding the quality of care, including the lack of resources with which to provide care, to a nursing administration representative.

- Delegate patient care based on the documented skills of licensed and unlicensed personnel.

- Communicate the patient's name, room number, and expectations for staff before, during, and after duty performance in a pleasant, direct, and concise manner when delegating patient care.

- Identify realistic, attainable outcome standards to use to identify completion of any task that is delegated. Make frequent walking rounds to assure quality patient outcomes after delegation.

- Follow evidence-based standards of care and the facility's policy and procedure for administering care and reporting incidents. Document the reason for any omission or deviation from agency policy, procedure, or standard.

- Avoid taking telephone and verbal orders. If needed, repeat the order back to the practitioner to assure clarity. Document that you did this with Verbal Order Repeated Back (VORB).

- Encourage the development of clearly written and/or computerized orders from all practitioners.

- Document the time of nursing actions and changes in conditions requiring notification of the practitioner. Include the response of the practitioner. Use the chain of command at your agency to report any concerns.

- Complete incident reports immediately after they occur. Discuss critical factors with the risk manager to increase your retention of the facts.

- Follow professional guidelines for safe transfer of all patients both inside and outside the agency.

CRITICAL THINKING 23-4

You are the only licensed nurse assigned to give 9 A.M. medications on a 52-bed nursing home unit. To avoid being classified as a drug error according to the institution's policy and usual nursing practice, administration of the medications must occur within 45 minutes of the ordered time. Also, nursing practice mandates you verify the "six rights": the right drug, the right dose, the right patient, the right time, the right route, and the right documentation.

What problems are there with this assignment? What would you do?

REAL WORLD INTERVIEW

Most nurses are familiar with the phrase, "If it was not documented, it was not done." Insofar as this phrase is used to encourage thorough documentation, it reflects good nursing practice. Timely, accurate, and complete documentation is an excellent way to protect oneself from litigation. However, lawyers who represent plaintiffs in medical malpractice cases are aware of this "rule" and often attempt to use it against nurses in health care liability claims.

Imagine the following scenario: A patient is admitted to the hospital, and Nurse A performs an initial assessment of the patient. Nurse A notes in the patient's chart that the patient has good capillary refill. Nurse A proceeds to take the patient's vital signs, including capillary refill, hourly throughout Nurse A's eight-hour shift. The patient's capillary refill remains good, and the nurse makes no further documentation in the chart relating to the patient's capillary refill. After Nurse A's shift, Nurse B takes over the patient's care. One hour into Nurse B's shift, the patient codes and expires. The patient's family sues Nurse A. The plaintiffs' lawyer is cross-examining Nurse A.

Lawyer: "Nurse A, are you familiar with the phrase, 'If it wasn't charted, it wasn't done'?"

Nurse A: "Yes."

Lawyer: "That's a common rule in nursing practice, isn't it?"

Nurse A: "Yes."

Lawyer: "You were taught that in nursing school, weren't you?"

Nurse A: "Yes, I was."

Lawyer: "And after you documented that the patient had good capillary refill upon admission, you did not document anything relating to the patient's capillary refill for the next eight hours, did you?"

Nurse A: "Well, no."

Lawyer: "So if we use your rule, 'If it wasn't documented, it wasn't done,' we can assume you never checked the patient's capillary refills during your shift after the initial assessment, right?"

Nurse A: "No. I checked, but it hadn't changed, so I didn't chart anything . . ."

Do you see what just happened? Nurse A provided competent nursing care, but the lawyer made it appear as if Nurse A was negligent. A nurse involved in litigation should not blanketly agree with this documentation rule. You simply cannot document everything noted in an assessment of a patient. Moreover, most nurses would agree that patient care takes priority over charting. This rule ignores that. Bad charting looks bad. Good charting protects you. Even lapses in charting do not correlate with bad nursing care. Nurses should not lose sight of that when faced with litigation.

Robyn D. Pozza Dollar, JD
Austin, Texas

MALPRACTICE/ PROFESSIONAL LIABILITY INSURANCE

Nurses may need to carry their own malpractice insurance. Nurses often think their actions are adequately covered by the employer's liability insurance, but this is not necessarily so. If, in giving care, the nurse fails to comply with the institution's policies and procedures, the institution may deny the nurse a defense, claiming that because of the nurse's failure to follow institutional policy, or because of the nurse working outside the scope of employment, the nurse was not acting as an employee at that time. Also, nurses are being named individually as defendants in malpractice suits more frequently than in the past. Consequently, it is advantageous for the nurse to be assured of a defense independent of that of his employer. Professional liability insurance provides that assurance and pays for an attorney to defend the nurse in a malpractice lawsuit.

NURSE/ATTORNEY RELATIONSHIP

Despite the nurse's best intentions, a nurse may be named as a defendant in a lawsuit and need to retain the services of an attorney. LaDuke (2000) made the following suggestions for consulting and collaborating with an attorney:

1. Retain a specialist. Generalists are competent to handle many matters, but professional malpractice, professional disciplinary proceedings, and employment disputes are best handled by specialists in those areas.
2. Be attentive. Read the documents the attorney produces and travel to court proceedings to observe the attorney's performance.
3. Notify your insurance carrier as soon as you are aware of any real or potential liability issue. Inform your agent about the status of your case every few months, even if it is unchanged.
4. Keep costs sensible. Your attorney should explain initially how the fee will be computed and how you will be billed. The attorney may require you to pay a retainer fee.
5. Keep informed. The attorney should address your questions and concerns promptly. You are entitled to be kept informed about the status of your case. You are entitled to copies of all correspondence, legal briefs, and other documents.
6. Weed through writing. Your attorney needs to explain all facts and options. Examine all relevant documents and do not hesitate to make corrections in the same way you would correct a medical record by drawing a line through the incorrect or misleading information, writing in the correction, and signing your initials after it.
7. Set your own course. Insist on a collaborative relationship with your attorney for the duration of your case.

KEY CONCEPTS

- Nursing practice is governed by civil, public, and administrative laws.

- Nurses are legally responsible for their actions and can be held liable for negligent care.

- Nurses have an ethical and legal obligation to advocate for patients.

- Every institution has its own policies and procedures designed to help nurses carry out their professional responsibilities.

- Nurses need to be familiar with their institution's policies and procedures in giving care and in reporting variances, illegal activities, or unexpected events.

- HIPPA legislation was enacted to safeguard private health care information.

- Many sources of evidence are used to identify the standard of care.

- Nursing malpractice examples include treatment problems, communication problems, medication problems, and monitoring/observing/supervising problems.

- The ANA Code of Ethics requires nurses to serve as a patient advocate.

- Legal protections in nursing practice include Good Samaritan laws, skillful communication, and risk-management programs.

- Common torts include negligence and malpractice, assault and battery, false imprisonment, invasion of privacy, and defamation.

- Nurses need to be familiar with their state Nurse Practice Act.

- Good Samaritan laws exist in many states.

- Risk-management programs improve the quality of care and protect the financial integrity of institutions.

KEY TERMS

administrative law	Good Samaritan laws
assault	living will
battery	malpractice
civil law	negligence
constitution	power of attorney
contract law	public law
false imprisonment	tort

REVIEW QUESTIONS

1. You are given a written order by a provider to administer an unusually large dose of pain medicine to your patient. In this situation, which of the following is an appropriate nursing action?
   A. Administer the medication because it was ordered by a provider.
   B. Refuse to administer the medication, and move on to another patient.
   C. Speak with the provider about your concerns, and clarify whether the medication dose is accurate.
   D. Select a dose that you feel comfortable with, and administer that dose.

2. A practitioner has ordered you to discharge Mr. Jones from the hospital, despite a new temperature of 102.0°F (38.8°C). The practitioner refuses to talk with you about the patient. In this situation, which of the following is an appropriate nursing action?
   A. Administer an antipyretic medication, and discharge the patient.
   B. Discharge the patient with instructions to call 911 if he has any problems.
   C. Do not discharge the patient until you have discussed the matter with your nursing manager and are satisfied regarding patient safety.
   D. Discharge the patient, and tell the patient to take Tylenol when he gets home.

3. A practitioner has issued a Do Not Resuscitate (DNR) order for your patient, a fifty-five-year-old man with cancer. You spoke with the patient this morning, and he clearly wishes to be resuscitated in the event that he stops breathing. What is the most appropriate course of action?
   A. Ignore the patient's wishes because the practitioner ordered the DNR.
   B. Consult your hospital's policies and procedures, speak to the practitioner, and discuss the matter with your nurse manager.
   C. Attempt to talk the patient into agreeing to the DNR.
   D. Contact the medical licensing board to complain about the practitioner.

4. The Health Insurance Portability and Accountability Act (HIPAA) protects which of the following?
   A. A patient's right to be insured, regardless of employment status or ability to pay
   B. The confidentiality of certain protected health information
   C. The nurse's right to health insurance
   D. The hospital's right to disclose protected health information

5. Which of the following elements is not necessary for a nurse to be found negligent in a court of law?
   A. A duty or obligation for the nurse to act in a particular way
   B. A breach of that duty or obligation
   C. The nurse's intention to be negligent
   D. Physical, emotional, or financial harm to the patient

6. Which type of law authorizes state boards to enact rules that govern the practice of nursing?
   A. State law
   B. Federal law
   C. Common law
   D. Criminal law

7. You are a new nurse working on a medical-surgical unit. One of your patients, an elderly woman, has an advanced directive that requests that no CPR be done in the event that she stops breathing. One day she stops breathing, and someone on your unit calls a "code" and begins resuscitative efforts. You go along with the team and help to resuscitate the patient. She regains a pulse but never regains consciousness. She is now ventilator dependent and her family is very angry with you and the staff. Which of the following is a potential legal action you will face?
   A. Violation of patient privacy
   B. Battery
   C. Criminal recklessness
   D. Revoked nursing license

8. Which of the following is not an essential element of a Good Samaritan law?
   A. The care is rendered in an emergency situation.
   B. The health care worker is rendering care without pay.
   C. The health care worker is concerned about the safety of the victims.
   D. The care provided did not recklessly or intentionally cause injury or harm to the injured party.

REVIEW ACTIVITIES

1. Talk to the risk manager at a hospital in which you have your clinical assignments. Ask the risk manager how she handles an incident report. Is it used for improving the hospital's care in the future? How?

2. Identify the various ways in which nurses you observe in your clinical rotations discuss orders and treatments with practitioners and other nurses. How do nurses address incorrect or dangerous medication orders? Talk with nurses you encounter about how they handle these situations.

3. Research the various companies that offer nursing malpractice insurance, and determine the cost and coverage associated with a nursing malpractice policy. Go to an Internet search engine, such as www.google.com. Search for Nursing Malpractice Insurance. What did you find? Note the Nursing Service Organization (NSO) Website at www.nso.com. Recent legal cases are reported there.

EXPLORING THE WEB

- Go to this site to find malpractice information for your state: *www.mcandl.com*

- Where can you find state and federal laws regulating hospitals? *www.findlaw.com*

- You have a patient who is to be transferred to a nursing home for recuperation. Where can you tell the family to look to evaluate the local nursing homes regarding their adherence to the federal regulations for nursing homes? *www.medicare.gov*

- Where can you find a copy of the ANA Code of Ethics? *www.ana.org*

- Note the Medical Liability Monitor at *www.medicalliabilitymonitor.com*
  Also check this site
  http://aspe.hhs.gov/daltcp/reports/mlupd1.htm
  What did you find there?

- Go to *www.google.com,* and type in "living wills" and "power of attorney."
  What did you find there?

REFERENCES

Adams, S. (2004). HIPAA patient confidentiality requirements. *Journal of Emergency Nursing, 30*(1), 70.

American Nurses Association. (2001). Code of Ethics. Silver Springs, MD: Author.

Aveyard, H. (2001). The requirement for informed consent prior to nursing care procedures. *Journal of Advanced Nursing, 37*(3), 243–249.

Croke, E. M. (2003). Nurses, negligence, and malpractice. *American Journal of Nursing, 103*(9), 54–64.

Cruzan v. Director, Missouri Department of Health, 110 S.Ct. 2841 (1990).

Fiesta, J. (1999a). Do no harm: When caregivers violate our golden rule, part 1. *Nursing Management, 30*(8), 10–11.

Frank-Stromborg, M. (2004). They're real and they're here: The new federally regulated privacy rules under HIPAA. *Dermatology Nursing, 16*(1), 13–24.

Garner, B., & Black, H. C. (2000). *Black's Law Dictionary* (7th ed.). St Paul, MN: West.

Hellquist, K., & Spector, N. (2004). A primer: The national council of state boards of nursing nurse licensure compact. *Journal of*

Nursing Administration's Healthcare Law, Ethics, and Regulation, 6(4), 86–89.

Hughes, N. (2006). Respiratory protection, part 1. *American Journal of Nursing, 106*(1), 96.

LaDuke, S. (2000). What should you expect from your attorney? *Nursing Management, 31*(1), 10.

Mantel, D. L. (1999). Legally speaking: Off-duty doesn't mean off the hook. *Registered Nurse, 62*(10), 71–74.

Murphy v. United Parcel Service, 527 U.S. 516 (1999).

Odom v. State Department of Health & Hospitals, 322 So. 2d 91 (La. 1999).

Olson-Chavarriaga, D. (2000). Informed consent: Do you know your role? *Nursing 2000, 30*(5), 60–61.

Roe v. Wade, 410 U.S. 133 (1973).

Sheehan, J. P. (2000). Protect your staff from workplace violence. *Nursing Management, 31*(3), 24–45.

Sutton v. United Airlines, 527 U.S. 471 (1999).

Webb v. Tulane Medical Center Hospital, 7000 So. 2d 1142 (La. 1997).

SUGGESTED READINGS

Brensilver, P. (2002). E-formed consent: Evaluating the interplay between interactive technology and informed consent. *The George Washington University Law Review, 70*(613).

Clark, A., & Gerhardt, S. (2003). HIPAA is here: Did you hear what that nurse just said? *Clinical Nurse Specialist, 17*(4), 188–190.

Erlen, J. (2004). HIPAA: Clinical and ethical considerations for nurses. *Orthopaedic Nursing, 23*(6), 410–413.

Hewitt, J. (2001). A critical review of the arguments debating the role of the nurse advocate. *Journal of Advanced Nursing, 37*(5), 439–445.

Kay Hall, J. (2004). After Schiavo: Next issue for nursing ethics. *Journal of Nursing Administration's Healthcare Law, Ethics, and Regulation, 7*(3), 94–98.

Kroll, M. (2003). What were you thinking: Charting rules to keep you legally safe. *Journal of Gerentological Nursing, 29*(3), 15–16.

LaDuke, S., & Biondo, T. (2003). Protect your future with personal liability insurance. *Nursing, 33*(2), 52–53.

Murphy, E. (2003). Charting by exception. *Association of Operating Room Nurses Journal, 78*(5), 821–823.

Priest, C. (2005). Held liable. *Reflections on nursing leadership, 31*(1), 20–22, 36.

Ziel, S. (2004). Guard against HIPAA violations. *Nursing Management, 35*(4), 26–27.

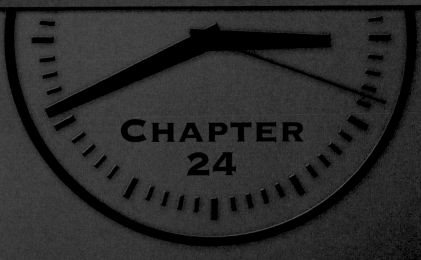

CHAPTER 24

Ethical Aspects of Health Care

Camille B. Little, MS, RN, BSN ✛ Joan Dorman, RN, MS, CEN

Moral excellence comes about as a result of habit, we become just by doing just acts, temperate by doing temperate acts, brave by doing brave acts (Aristotle).

OBJECTIVES

Upon completion of this chapter, the reader should be able to:

1. Relate ethics and morality.
2. Identify historical and philosophical influences on nursing practice.
3. Devise a personal philosophy of professional nursing.
4. Analyze ethical theories, virtues, principles, and values as the basis for professional nursing practice.
5. Support participation on ethics committees in hospitals.
6. Explain values clarification.
7. Apply a guide for ethical decision making to an ethical dilemma.
8. Evaluate ethical issues encountered in practice, including cost containment, use of technology, and patients' rights.
9. Support ethical leadership and responsibility in professional practice and organizations.

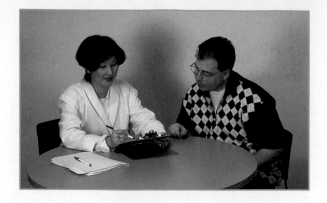

In a large teaching hospital, a patient you are caring for says he does not want to go on living. He has had cancer for several years and states he is tired of being sick. When you ask him whether he has shared these feelings with his family, he says that he does not want them to think he is giving up. You report the patient's statements to the next shift and explain how you encouraged him to talk with his family and his practitioner. That evening, the patient suddenly arrests, and a code is called. The patient ends up on a ventilator, receives five units of blood, and is comatose. The patient did not have advance directives, and Do Not Resuscitate (DNR) orders had not been signed.

> *What are your thoughts about maintaining the patient's life in this situation?*
>
> *Who should make the decision about the patient's situation since he is comatose?*
>
> *Does the nurse who spoke with the patient have the right to share that conversation with the patient's family?*

Throughout its history, nursing has relied on ethical principles to serve as a guideline in determining care. Nurses are confronted with ethical dilemmas in all types of practice settings. This chapter provides an overview of the nursing profession's ethics and the increased ethical challenges faced by nurses in today's health care environment.

DEFINITION OF ETHICS AND MORALITY

Ethics is the branch of philosophy that concerns the distinction of right from wrong on the basis of a body of knowledge, not just on the basis of opinions. **Morality** is behavior in accordance with custom or tradition and usually reflects personal or religious beliefs (DeLaune & Ladner, 2006). Ethics governs professional groups and provides a framework for determining the right course of action in a particular situation. For nurses, the actions they take in practice are primarily governed by the ethical principles of the profession. These principles influence practice, conduct, and relationships that nurses are held accountable for in the delivery of care. Health care ethics, also called **bioethics**, are ethics specific to health care and serve as a framework to guide behavior in **ethical dilemmas**. An ethical dilemma occurs when there is a conflict between two or more ethical principles; there is no "correct" decision.

Laws, in contrast, are state and federal government rules that govern all of society. Laws mandate behavior. In some situations in health care, the distinctions between law and ethics are not clear. There are cases in which ethics and law are similar; there are others where ethics and law differ.

HISTORICAL AND PHILOSOPHICAL INFLUENCES ON NURSING PRACTICE

Nursing practice evolved from the needs of society and has been strongly influenced by religions and women. Society created the profession of nursing for the purpose of meeting specific, perceived health needs (Burkhardt & Nathaniel, 2002). Nursing fulfilled the need to care for people with illnesses. Likewise, a strong instinct for preservation of humanity gave people the motivation to help one another. The concern for health of the community was evident in antiquity and continued as civilizations developed (Donahue, 1996). A complementary relationship evolved as social needs and individual motivation to care for others developed.

RELIGIOUS INFLUENCES

Workers who were engaged in nursing, usually women, were often trained in the doctrines of the church, including unquestioning obedience, humility, and sacrificing one's self for the good of others. An individual nurse did not make independent decisions but followed instructions given by a priest or practitioner.

WOMEN'S INFLUENCES

Donahue states that nursing has its origin in the mother-care of helpless infants and must have coexisted with this type of care from earliest times (Donahue, 1996). Mothers cared for family members when they were helpless and sick. During the Christian era, women were selected by Jesus because of the compassion they showed as they ministered to the poor and sick. Thus, Christianity greatly enhanced women's opportunities for useful social service (Donahue, 1996).

PHILOSOPHY

Philosophy is the rational investigation of the truths and principles of knowledge, reality, and human conduct. Personal philosophies stem from an individual's beliefs and values. These beliefs and values, in turn, develop based upon a person's experiences in life, cultural influences, and education.

PHILOSOPHY OF NURSING

A professional nurse's personal philosophy affects that nurse's philosophy of nursing. Throughout the nursing educational process, students begin forming their philosophy of nursing. This philosophy is influenced significantly by a student's personal philosophy and experiences. One's personal philosophy should be compatible with the philosophy of the nursing department where the nurse works. This helps the nurse to be an effective leader and practitioner. See Figure 24-1 for a nursing department's philosophy statement. An example of a personal nursing philosophy is the following:

> I believe professional nursing care promotes an optimal level of wellness in body, mind, and spirit to those being served. I believe professional nurses must hold themselves to the highest standards of the profession and honor the profession's code of ethics in all aspects of practice.

Many health care centers have addressed ethical concerns by developing professional practice models. These

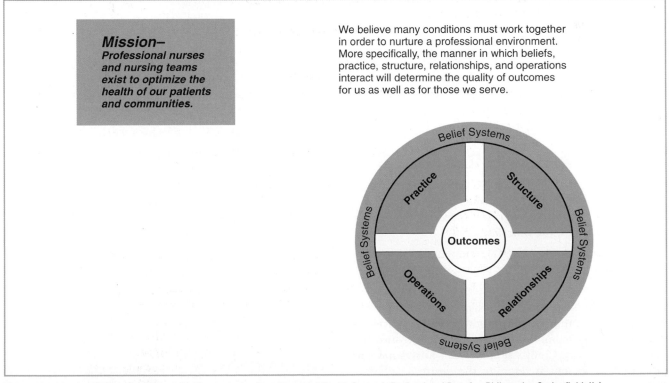

Figure 24-1 Nursing philosophy. (Adapted with permission from Memorial Health System's Professional Practice Philosophy, Springfield, IL.)

TABLE 24-1	SELECTED ETHICAL THEORIES

Ethical Theory	Interpretation
Deontology	Actions are based on moral rules and unchanging principles, such as, "do unto others as you would have them do to you." An ethical person must always follow the rules, even if doing so causes a less desirable outcome. Theory states that the motives of the actor determine the goodness or value of the act. Thus, a bad outcome is acceptable as long as the intent was good.
Teleology	A person must take those actions that lead to good outcomes. The theory states that the outcome of an act determines whether the act is good or of value and that achievement of a good outcome justifies using a less desirable means to attain the end.
Virtue ethics	Virtues such as truthfulness and trustworthiness are developed over time. A person's character must be developed so that by nature and habit, the person will be predisposed to behave virtuously. Living a virtuous life contributes both to one's own well-being and to the well-being of society.
Justice and equity	A "veil of ignorance" regarding who is affected by a decision should be used by decision makers because it allows for unbiased decision making. An ethical person chooses the action that is fair to all, including those persons who are most disadvantaged.
Relativism	There are no universal ethical standards, such as "murder is always wrong." Ethical standards are relative to person, place, time, and culture. Whatever a person thinks is right, is right. Theory has been largely rejected.

models illustrate how a code of ethics is essential to all other aspects of patient care. These practice models are shared with employees and consumers to illustrate the institution's commitment to excellence.

ETHICAL THEORIES

The study of ethical behavior has resulted in different theories that may apply to nursing practice and form a framework for ethical decision making. Table 24-1 describes some of these theories.

VIRTUES

Burkhardt and Nathaniel (2002) list four virtues that are more significant than others and that are illustrative of a virtuous person: compassion, discernment, trustworthiness, and integrity. Compassion is a trait nurses have, as perceived by society. It refers to the desire to alleviate suffering. Discernment is possession of acuteness of

CRITICAL THINKING 24-2

New graduates should formulate a philosophy of nursing based on personal beliefs and on values. Reflections on the following questions can assist in the development of a philosophy:

What do I believe about nursing practice?

Should nurses be patient advocates?

How should professionals conduct themselves?

How can I influence patient care based on my nursing philosophy?

Are the virtues of compassion, discernment, trustworthiness, and integrity essential both personally and professionally?

CRITICAL THINKING 24-3

Mr. Johanssen smokes three packs of ciga-rettes a day and is seen in a free clinic for chronic obstructive pulmonary disease. All attempts at getting him to stop smoking have failed. Mr. Johanssen tells you that smoking is the one pleas-ure he has in life, and he does not want to give it up.

Do you respect Mr. Johanssen's wishes? Does he still have a right to the free treatment and medications? Are limits to Mr. Johanssen's treatments justified?

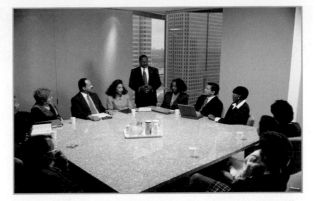

Figure 24-2 Ethics committee at work. (Photo courtesy of Photodisc.)

CRITICAL THINKING 24-4

You are caring for Mr. Trout, who has been labeled a malingerer. He is in and out of the hospital frequently and always has some type of pain requiring parenteral medications. The order is to give a placebo when he asks for pain medication. When you take the placebo in, Mr. Trout asks you what the medication is.

What principles can guide your actions regarding Mr. Trout? What theories can guide your actions in rela-tion to this patient? Is a nurse ethically required to disclose placebo medication?

judgment. Trustworthiness is present when trust is well-founded or deserving. Integrity may be considered firm adherence to a code of conduct or an ethical value. Trust-worthiness and integrity are traits expected in all people but are especially necessary for professional nurses. These traits form the foundation for an ethically princi-pled discipline and have been endorsed throughout the profession's history (Burkhardt & Nathaniel, 2002).

ETHICAL PRINCIPLES AND VALUES

In addition to the theories, ethical principles and values provide a basis for nurses to determine the appropriate action when faced with an ethical dilemma in the prac-tice setting. See Table 24-2 for a summary of the major ethical principles.

ETHICS COMMITTEES

The complexities found in health care today have pre-sented numerous ethical dilemmas to nurses in patient care, management, and administrative situations. To assist with decision making in these situations, many health care organizations are looking to an organizational ethics com-mittee for assistance. These committees are interdiscipli-nary in their membership and include representatives from clinical nursing and administration, medicine, clergy, clinical social service, nutritional service, pharmacy, and the legal profession. Additional participants may be invited on an as-needed basis (Figure 24-2).

Anyone on the health care team has the opportunity to refer a situation that has an ethical dilemma associ-ated with it to the ethics committee. Cases, such as the one described in the opening scenario of this chapter,

may be referred to the committee for direction. The role of the ethics committee is to provide guidance that assists with decisions involving ethical dilemmas. The ethics committee uses guidelines and criteria developed at the time of its inception to assist with the resolution. In the case in the opening scenario, the ethics commit-tee may invite family members of the patient and other nurses and practitioners to assist the ethics committee with the review.

VALUES AND VALUES CLARIFICATION

Values are personal beliefs about the truth of ideals, standards, principles, objects, and behaviors that give meaning and direction to life. If you were told that you must pack a bag for a special trip but you may bring only three items from your belongings, what items would you choose? The ones selected are what you value. Suppose

TABLE 24-2   ETHICAL PRINCIPLES

Ethical Principle	Definition	Example
Beneficence	The duty to do good to others and to maintain a balance between benefits and harms	■ Provide all patients, including the terminally ill, with caring attention. ■ Become familiar with your state laws regarding organ donations. ■ Treat every patient with respect and courtesy.
Nonmaleficence	The principle of doing no harm	■ Always work within your scope of practice. ■ Never give information or perform duties you are not qualified to do. ■ Observe all safety rules and precautions. ■ Keep areas safe from hazards. ■ Perform procedures according to facility protocols. Never take shortcuts. ■ Ask an appropriate person about anything you are unsure of. ■ Keep your skills up to date.
Justice	The principle of fairness that is served when an individual is given that which he or she is due, owed, deserves, or can legitimately claim	■ Treat all patients equally, regardless of economic or social background. ■ Learn the state laws and your facility's policies and procedures for handling and reporting suspected abuse.
Autonomy	Respect for an individual's right to self-determination; respect for individual liberty	■ Be sure that patients have consented to all treatments and procedures. ■ Become familiar with state laws and facility policies dealing with advance directives. ■ Never release patient information of any kind unless there is a signed release. ■ Do not discuss patients with anyone who is not professionally involved in their care. ■ Protect the physical privacy of patients.
Fidelity	The principle of promise keeping; the duty to keep one's promise or word	■ Be sure that necessary contracts have been completed. ■ Be very careful about what you say to patients. They may only hear the "good news."
Respect for others	The right of people to make their own decision	■ Provide all persons with information for decision making. ■ Avoid making paternalistic decisions for others.
Veracity	The obligation to tell the truth	■ Admit mistakes promptly. Offer to do whatever is necessary to correct them. ■ Refuse to participate in any form of fraud. ■ Give an "honest day's work" every day.

EVIDENCE FROM THE LITERATURE

Citation: Kopala, B., & Burkhart, L. (2005, Jan.–Mar.). Ethical dilemma and moral distress: Proposed new NANDA diagnoses. *International Journal of Nursing Terminologies and Classifications, 16*(1), 3–13.

Discussion: Nurses experience ethical dilemmas and the resulting moral distress on a regular basis. Nurses need to have the ability to diagnose ethical or moral situations in health care. Two NANDA diagnoses, moral distress and ethical dilemma, have been proposed to fill the void in the current terminology. This will enable nurses to recognize and track nursing care related to ethical and moral situations.

Implications for Practice: Ethical and moral issues faced by the nurse are often unspoken and not identified as problems. Because problem-oriented nursing is the norm, these additional diagnoses add validity to the problem and will point toward its resolution.

CRITICAL THINKING 24-5

Administration announces that the nurse manager must decrease full-time staff by two people. What are the nurse manager's choices? How will the rest of the personnel on the unit view having to work with fewer staff? As one of the staff nurses on this unit, or as a new nurse accepting a position as a staff RN, the nurse-to-patient ratio will be high on your list of priorities. You may be faced with the choice of looking elsewhere for employment. Often, the decisions of management force subsequent decisions among employees. Will patient care be compromised if staffing is too low? To what extent can the nurse manager compromise personal and unit values?

the staff, in Critical Thinking 24-5 concerning a proposed workforce reduction, refused to work under the circumstances they would face if the numbers were reduced as directed? What could be said about the staff's values? What could be said about the administration's values?

VALUES CLARIFICATION

Values clarification is the process of analyzing one's own values to better understand what is truly important. In their classic work *Values and Teaching*, Raths, Harmin, and Simon (1978, p. 47) formulated a theory of values clarification and proposed a three-step process of valuing, as follows:

1. *Choosing:* Beliefs are chosen freely (that is, without coercion) from among alternatives. The choosing

step involves analysis of the consequences of various alternatives.
2. *Prizing:* The beliefs that are selected are cherished (that is, prized).
3. *Acting:* The selected beliefs are demonstrated consistently through behavior.

Nurses must understand that values are individual rather than universal; therefore, nurses should not try to impose their own values on patients.

A GUIDE FOR ETHICAL DECISION MAKING

Burkhardt and Nathaniel (2002) developed a guide for decision making, which new nurses may find useful when confronted with an ethical decision. The main points are noted in Figure 24-3.

AN ETHICS TEST

A practical way of improving ethical decision making is to run decisions that you are considering through an ethics test when any doubt exists. The ethics test presented here was used at the Center for Business Ethics at Bentley College (Bowditch & Buono, 1997) as part of ethical corporate training programs. Decision makers are taught to ask themselves:

- Is it right?
- Is it fair?
- Who gets hurt?
- Would you be comfortable if the details of your decision were reported on the front page of your local newspaper or through your hospital's e-mail system?
- Would you tell your child or young relative to do it?
- How does it smell? This question is based on a person's intuition and common sense.

Gather Data and Identify Conflicting Moral Claims

- What makes this situation an ethical problem? Are there conflicting obligations, duties, principles, rights, loyalties, values, or beliefs?
- What are the issues?
- What facts seem most important?
- What emotions have an impact?
- What are the gaps in information at this time?

Identify Key Participants

- Who is legitimately empowered to make this decision?
- Who is affected and how?
- What is the level of competence of the person most affected in relation to the decision to be made?
- What are the rights, duties, authority, context, and capabilities of participants?

Determine Moral Perspective and Phase of Moral Development of Key Participants

- Do participants think in terms of duties or rights?
- Do the parties involved exhibit similar or different moral perspectives?
- Where is the common ground? The differences?
- What principles are important to each person involved?
- What emotions are evident within the interaction and with each person involved?
- What is the level of moral development of the participants?

Determine Desired Outcomes

- How does each party describe the circumstances of the outcome?
- What are the consequences of the desired outcomes?
- What outcomes are unacceptable to one or all involved?

Identify Options

- What options emerge through the assessment process?
- How do the alternatives fit the lifestyle and values of the person(s) affected?
- What are the legal considerations of the various options?
- What alternatives are unacceptable to one or all involved?
- How are alternatives weighed, ranked, and prioritized?

Act on the Choice

- Be empowered to make a difficult decision.
- Give yourself permission to set aside less acceptable alternatives.
- Be attentive to the emotions involved in the process.

Evaluate Outcomes of Action

- Has the ethical dilemma been resolved?
- Have other dilemmas emerged related to the action?
- How has the process affected those involved?
- Are further actions required?

Figure 24-3 Guide for decision making. (From *Ethics and Issues in Contemporary Nursing* (2nd ed.) by M. A. Burkhardt and A. K. Nathaniel, 2002, Clifton Park, NY: Thomson Delmar Learning.)

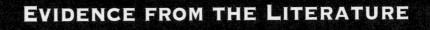

EVIDENCE FROM THE LITERATURE

Citation: Gutierrez, K. M. (2005). Critical care nurses' perceptions of and responses to moral distress. *Dimensions of Critical Care Nursing, 24*(5), 229–241.

Discussion: In an effort to describe and analyze the nursing phenomena of moral distress, a qualitative, descriptive methodology was implemented in a study of critical care nurses working in a surgical ICU at a large teaching hospital in a Midwestern region of the United States.

Main themes identified in the study centered around lack of collaboration between nurses and medical practitioners regarding patient care decisions resulting in nurses' perceptions of powerlessness; ineffective communication between nurse, patient, and practitioner; and nurses' inability to find meaning in patient and family suffering or influence the situation. Suggestions for clinical application were delineated, including promoting ethical discourse between patients, families, nurses, and medical practitioners and integrating palliative care principles into the plan of care for all patients by addressing and treating all aspects of suffering and promoting care based on patient goals rather than diagnosis.

Implications for Practice: Nurses frequently experience conflict regarding health care decisions, yet are expected to implement actions that they may perceive to be morally wrong. Research has described the deleterious effects of this moral incongruency, coined moral distress, on nurses' well being and has identified it as a causative agent in nursing turnover, burnout, and nurses leaving the profession. Moral distress may also affect nurses' provision of care.

CRITICAL THINKING 24-6

To better relate the study of ethics to yourself, take the following self quiz. Do you agree or disagree with the following statements?

1. I would report a nursing coworker's drug abuse.
2. I would tell the truth to a patient who asked if he was dying.
3. I see no harm in giving ordered drugs on a temporary basis to a drug-addicted patient who presents to the emergency department.
4. When applying for a nursing position, I would cover up the fact that I had been fired from a recent job.
5. If I received $100 for doing some odd jobs, I would not report it on my income tax returns.
6. I see no harm in taking home a few nursing supplies.
7. It is unacceptable to call in sick to take a day off, even if only done once or twice a year.
8. I would accept a permanent, full-time job even if I knew I wanted the job for only six months.

C.S. Faircloth, RN, personal communication, March 13, 2003.

ETHICAL ISSUES ENCOUNTERED IN PRACTICE

Numerous events contribute to ethical issues that professional nurses encounter in today's practice. Cost containment, technology, and patient rights have all influenced the increased numbers of ethical dilemmas nurses face.

COST CONTAINMENT AND ISSUES RELATED TO TECHNOLOGY

Cost containment and the sophisticated technology available in health care today are related. The more technology that is developed and used, the more costly health care becomes. There are several factors that contribute to the high costs of receiving treatment in our system. ICUs are full of expensive equipment designed to breathe for patients, monitor vital signs automatically, and communicate if the heart is failing in some way. Scores of devices all have the same purpose—to let us know what needs to be done to sustain life.

Although the use of technology has brought many benefits, two significant questions arise about its use. When do we refrain from the use of technology? When do we stop using it once we have started? Who is entitled to it in our society?

PATIENT RIGHTS

The American Hospital Association developed a Patient's Bill of Rights (Table 24-3) with the expectation that when patients and families participate in treatment decisions, the outcome will be more effective care. See the "Exploring the Web" section at the end of this chapter to view this document online.

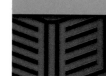

REAL WORLD INTERVIEW

One of my most difficult cases involved a man in his early forties who was in a coma, ventilator dependent, and declared brain dead. The patient was from a different culture, and when the family arrived six weeks later from the country abroad, they refused to allow him to be removed from the ventilator. His parents said they were told by the gods that their son would be well several months in the future. After two months in the hospital, the administration began to put pressure on the family to transfer the patient.

Emily Davison, RN
Case Manager
Pleasant Hill, Missouri

ETHICAL LEADERSHIP AND MANAGEMENT

Nurse leaders are in the position to assure that the setting in which they practice is ethically principled and that it accepts accountability for the Code of Ethics set by the profession of nursing. The professional environment can empower nurses and can foster autonomy and an appreciation of the diversity of persons and opinions. Treating others with fairness, dignity, and respect, nurse leaders can influence the decisions made by the organization.

ORGANIZATIONAL BENEFITS DERIVED FROM ETHICS

Highly ethical behavior and socially responsible acts are not always free. Investing in work/life programs, granting social leaves of absence, and telling patients the absolute truth about potential problems may not have an immediate return (DuBrin, 2000). Nevertheless, recent evidence suggests that high ethics and social responsibility are related to good financial performance (Positive Leadership, 1998). Profits and social responsibility seem to work two ways. More profitable firms seem more able to afford to invest in social responsibility initiatives, and these initiatives in turn seem to lead to more profits. Being ethical also helps avoid the costs of paying huge fines for being unethical, and a big payoff from socially responsible acts is that they often attract and retain socially responsible employees and customers (DuBrin, 2000).

EVIDENCE FROM THE LITERATURE

Citation: Candela, L., Michael, S. R., & Mitchell, S. (2003). Ethical debates. *Nurse Educator, 28*(1), 37–39.

Discussion: This article discusses a format for classroom debate on ethical issues. A portion of the format is as follows:

Select an ethical issue and phrase as a question starting with the word, "Should."

Select a moderator for the group. The moderator will introduce the issue and be responsible for debate flow and adhering to time requirements.

Divide the group into two subgroups. One subgroup will argue for the question, one subgroup will argue against the question.

Be sure to consider all pertinent ethical principles, any conflict between principles, relationship to ethical codes, legal implications, people involved and impacted, and any relevant sociocultural, political, or religious aspects that may influence this ethical issue. All major points must be grounded in the literature.

Each group member must articulate a position. Be sure to credit your sources as you speak. Be familiar with your part so you can "talk it" versus "read it."

Implications for Practice: Nurses can use this format to clarify their own thinking on various ethical issues.

TABLE 24-3	**A PATIENT'S BILL OF RIGHTS**

Introduction

Effective health care requires collaboration between patients and physicians and other health care professionals. Open and honest communication, respect for personal and professional values, and sensitivity to differences are integral to optimal patient care. As the setting for the provision of health services, hospitals must provide a foundation for understanding and respecting the rights and responsibilities of patients, their families, physicians, and other caregivers. Hospitals must ensure a health care ethic that respects the role of patients in decision making about treatment choices and other aspects of their care. Hospitals must be sensitive to cultural, racial, linguistic, religious, age, gender, and other differences as well as the needs of persons with disabilities.

The American Hospital Association presents *A Patient's Bill of Rights* with the expectation that it will contribute to more effective patient care and be supported by the hospital on behalf of the institution, its medical staff, employees, and patients. The American Hospital Association encourages health care institutions to tailor this bill of rights to their patient community by translating and/or simplifying the language of this bill of rights as may be necessary to ensure that patients and their families understand their rights and responsibilities.

Bill of Rights*

1. The patient has the right to considerate and respectful care.

2. The patient has the right to and is encouraged to obtain from physicians and other direct caregivers relevant, current, and understandable information concerning diagnosis, treatment, and prognosis. Except in emergencies when the patient lacks decision-making capacity and the need for treatment is urgent, the patient is entitled to the opportunity to discuss and request information related to the specific procedures and/or treatments, the risks involved, the possible length of recuperation, and the medically reasonable alternatives and their accompanying risks and benefits. Patients have the right to know the identity of physicians, nurses, and others involved in their care, when those involved are students, residents, or other trainees. The patient also has the right to know the immediate and long-term financial implications of treatment choices, insofar as they are known.

3. The patient has the right to make decisions about the plan of care prior to and during the course of treatment and to refuse a recommended treatment or plan of care to the extent permitted by law and hospital policy and to be informed of the medical consequences of this action. In case of such refusal, the patient is entitled to other appropriate care and services that the hospital provides or transfer to another hospital. The hospital should notify patients of any policy that might affect patient choice within the institution.

4. The patient has the right to have an advance directive (such as a living will, health care proxy, or durable power of attorney for health care) concerning treatment or designating a surrogate decision maker with the expectation that the hospital will honor the intent of that directive to the extent permitted by law and hospital policy. Health care institutions must advise patients of their rights under state law and hospital policy to make informed medical choices, ask if the patient has an advance directive, and include that information in patient records. The patient has the right to timely information about hospital policy that may limit its ability to implement fully a legally valid advance directive.

5. The patient has the right to every consideration of privacy. Case discussion, consultation, examination, and treatment should be conducted so as to protect each patient's privacy.

6. The patient has the right to expect that all communications and records pertaining to his/her care will be treated as confidential by the hospital, except in cases such as suspected abuse and public health hazards when reporting is permitted or required by law. The patient has the right to expect that the hospital will emphasize the confidentiality of this information when it releases it to any other parties entitled to review information in these records.

7. The patient has the right to review the records pertaining to his/her medical care and to have the information explained or interpreted as necessary, except when restricted by law.

(Continues)

TABLE 24-3	A PATIENT'S BILL OF RIGHTS (CONTINUED)

8. The patient has the right to expect that, within its capacity and policies, a hospital will make reasonable response to the request of a patient for appropriate and medically indicated care and services. The hospital must provide evaluation, service, and/or referral as indicated by the urgency of the case. When medically appropriate and legally permissible, or when a patient has so requested, a patient may be transferred to another facility. The institution to which the patient is to be transferred must first have accepted the patient for transfer. The patient must also have the benefit of complete information and explanation concerning the need for, risks, benefits, and alternatives to such a transfer.

9. The patient has the right to ask and be informed of the existence of business relationships among the hospital, educational institutions, other health care providers, or payers that may influence the patient's treatment and care.

10. The patient has the right to consent to or decline to participate in proposed research studies or human experimentation affecting care and treatment or requiring direct patient involvement, and to have those studies fully explained prior to consent. A patient who declines to participate in research or experimentation is entitled to the most effective care that the hospital can otherwise provide.

11. The patient has the right to expect reasonable continuity of care when appropriate and to be informed by physicians and other caregivers of available and realistic patient care options when hospital care is no longer appropriate.

12. The patient has the right to be informed of hospital policies and practices that relate to patient care, treatment, and responsibilities. The patient has the right to be informed of available resources for resolving disputes, grievances, and conflicts, such as ethics committees, patient representatives, or other mechanisms available in the institution. The patient has the right to be informed of the hospital's charges for services and available payment methods.

The collaborative nature of health care requires that patients, or their families/surrogates, participate in their care. The effectiveness of care and patient satisfaction with the course of treatment depend, in part, on the patient fulfilling certain responsibilities. Patients are responsible for providing information about past illnesses, hospitalizations, medications, and other matters related to health status. To participate effectively in decision making, patients must be encouraged to take responsibility for requesting additional information or clarification about their health status or treatment when they do not fully understand information and instructions. Patients are also responsible for ensuring that the health care institution has a copy of their written advance directive if they have one. Patients are responsible for informing their physicians and other caregivers if they anticipate problems in following prescribed treatment.

Patients should also be aware of the hospital's obligation to be reasonably efficient and equitable in providing care to other patients and the community. The hospital's rules and regulations are designed to help the hospital meet this obligation. Patients and their families are responsible for making reasonable accommodations to the needs of the hospital, other patients, medical staff, and hospital employees. Patients are responsible for providing necessary information for insurance claims and for working with the hospital to make payment arrangements, when necessary.

A person's health depends on much more than health care services. Patients are responsible for recognizing the impact of their life-style on their personal health.

Conclusion

Hospitals have many functions to perform, including the enhancement of health status, health promotion, and the prevention and treatment of injury and disease; the immediate and ongoing care and rehabilitation of patients; the education of health professionals, patients, and the community; and research. All these activities must be conducted with an overriding concern for the values and dignity of patients.

---

* These rights can be exercised on the patient's behalf by a designated surrogate or proxy decision maker if the patient lacks decision-making capacity, is legally incompetent, or is a minor.

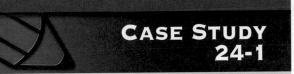

CASE STUDY 24-1

S elect an ethical issue of your choice in class, for example, should patients be given placebo medications?

Ask for one volunteer to give the reasons why patients should be given placebos and one volunteer to give the reasons why patients should not be given placebos.

Instruct your volunteers to consider all pertinent ethical theories and principles, any conflict between them, any relationship to ethical codes, legal implications, people involved and impacted, and any relevant sociocultural, political, or religious aspects that may influence this ethical issue.

Each volunteer must state his or her position and references.

What were the pros identified? What were the cons? Did any of the comments alter your own position on this question? Is a nurse ethically required to disclose placebo medication?

Developed with information from Candela, L., Michael, S. R., & Mitchell, S. (2003). Ethical debates. *Nurse Educator, 28*(1), 37–39.

CREATING AN ETHICAL WORKPLACE

Establishing an ethical and socially responsible workplace is not simply a matter of luck and common sense. Nurse managers can develop strategies and programs to enhance ethical and socially responsible attitudes. These may include the following:

1. Formal mechanisms for monitoring ethics, such as an ethics program or ethics hotline.
2. Written organizational codes of conduct (Table 24-4).
3. Widespread communication in the hospital to reinforce ethical and socially responsible behavior.
4. Leadership by example: If people throughout the firm believe that behaving ethically is "in" and behaving unethically is "out," ethical behavior will prevail.
5. Encouraging confrontation about ethical deviations: Unethical behavior may be minimized if every employee confronts anyone seen behaving unethically.
6. Training programs in ethics and social responsibility, including messages about ethics from managers, classes on ethics at colleges, and exercises in ethics (DuBrin, 2000).

NURSE-PHYSICIAN RELATIONSHIPS

Nurses working in organizations often confront ethical dilemmas in working with patients and their families. To resolve these dilemmas, the nurse must often work

EVIDENCE FROM THE LITERATURE

Citation: Greene, J. (2002, Mar.). No abuse zone. *Hospitals and Health Networks, 26*, 28.

Discussion: An astounding number of health care workers, 62% to 96%, say that they experienced or witnessed abusive behavior in the past year from a supervisor, a medical practitioner, or even a patient. For example, a nurse working the night shift gets a medication order she can't read and calls the medical practitioner at 2 A.M. for clarification. He yells at her and hangs up without answering the question. The nurse is afraid to call back and gives a fatal dose of the wrong drug.

This article discusses guidelines for a five-stage process to rid health care workplaces of abusive behavior. Deborah Anderson, president of Respond 2, Inc., St. Paul, Minnesota, is developing the guidelines in conjunction with the Hennepin Medical Society, Minneapolis, Minnesota. The Respond 2 five-stage process includes building a team that meets monthly, surveying employees with an assessment tool about their experiences with workplace abuse, devising a plan to deal with workplace abuse, evaluating outcomes with a resurvey, and infusing the workplace with an atmosphere of collegiality by changing policies and procedures that affect culture, hiring, employee orientation, training, reporting processes, performance evaluation, and appropriate patient safety- and quality-related initiatives. In developing this five-stage process, it is imperative that strong support be in place from the leaders of the organization.

Implications for Practice: This five-stage process can be very useful in developing a no-abuse workplace.

TABLE 24-4	ORGANIZATIONAL ELEMENTS TO SUPPORT AN ETHICAL WORKPLACE

- Follow professional standards for education, licensure, and competency in all hiring decisions, orientation, and ongoing continuing education programs.

- Have clear job descriptions and ongoing licensing and credentialing policies for nursing and medical practitioners LPN/LVNs, unlicensed assistive personnel (UAP), and other health care staff. The organization must ensure that all staff are safe, competent practitioners before assigning them to patient care. Orient all staff to each other's roles and job descriptions.

- Facilitate clinical and educational specialty certification and credentialing of all practitioners and staff.

- Provide standards for ongoing supervision and periodic licensure/competency verification and evaluation of all staff.

- Provide access to professional health care standards, policies, procedures, library, and medication information with unit availability and efficient Internet access.

- Facilitate regular evidence-based review of critical standards, policies, and procedures.

- Have clear policies and procedures for delegation and chain of command reporting lines for all staff from RN to charge nurse to nurse manager to nurse executive and, as appropriate, to risk management, the hospital ethics committee, the hospital administrator, medical practitioners, the chief of the medical staff, the board of directors, the State Licensing Board for Nursing and Medicine, and the Joint Commission (JC).

- Provide administrative support for supervisors and staff who delegate, assign, monitor, and evaluate patient care.

- Clarify nursing and medical practitioner accountability, for example, if the medical practitioner delegates a nursing task to UAP, the medical practitioner is responsible for monitoring that care delivery. This must be spelled out in hospital policy. If the RN notes that the UAP is doing something incorrectly, the RN has a duty to intervene and to notify the ordering practitioner of the incident. The RN always has an independent responsibility to protect patient safety. Blindly relying on another nursing or medical practitioner is not permissible for the RN.

- Provide standards for regular RN evaluation of UAP and LPN/LVN and reinforce need for UAP and LPN/LVN accountability to RN. RNs must delegate and supervise. They cannot abdicate this professional responsibility.

- Develop physical, mental, and verbal, "No Abuse" policy to be followed by all professional and nonprofessional health care staff.

- Consider applying for magnet status for your facility. This status is awarded by the American Nurses Credentialing Center to nursing departments that have worked to improve nursing care, including the empowering of nursing decision making and delegation in clinical practice.

- Consider a shared governance model of nursing practice to empower nursing decision making and delegation in clinical practice.

- Monitor patient outcomes, including nurse-sensitive outcomes, staffing ratios, and other clinical, financial, and organizational quality indicators, as well as developing ongoing clinical quality improvement practices.

- Maintain ongoing monitoring of incident reports, sentinel events, and other elements of risk management and performance improvement of the process and outcome of patient care.

- Develop systematic, error-proof systems for medication administration that ensure the six rights of medication administration, that is, the right patient, right medication, right dose, right time, right route, and right documentation. Include computerized order entry.

- Provide documentation of routine maintenance for all patient care equipment.

- Attain JC Patient Safety Goals, 2007.

- Develop safe intra hospital and intra agency transfer policies.

closely with the medical practitioner. The nurse often finds that medical practitioners hold different beliefs about values, communication, trust and integrity, role responsibilities, and organizational politics and economics. These beliefs affect their ethical beliefs, which, in turn, affect their decisions about treatment, which may lead to conflicts between nurses and practitioners. These conflicts can be limited with clear ethical guidelines and policies, established by interdisciplinary teams and overseen by an ethical administration. When an ethical issue arises, resolution might be tedious and possibly riddled with resentment without guidelines and policies.

The Gallup Organization's 2005 annual poll on professional honesty and ethical standards ranked nurses number one. Of the 21 professions tested, six have high ethical ratings: nurses (82%), pharmacists (67%), medical practitioners (65%), high school teachers (64%), policemen (61%), and clergy (54%). For more information, see http://poll.gallup.com.

ETHICAL CODES

One mark of a profession is the determination of ethical behavior for its members. Several nursing organizations have developed codes for ethical behavior. The International Council of Nurses Code for Nurses appears in Table 24-5.

The ANA has also developed a Code for Nurses. See the "Exploring the Web" section at the end of this chapter for a site to view this document online.

CRITICAL THINKING 24-7

A nurse administered the wrong medication to a patient. The patient then had to be transferred to the intensive care unit and required a longer stay in the hospital. The nurse freely admitted the mistake to her nurse manager. The manager recommended that the two of them go talk with the patient and explain what happened. Then the administration heard about the incident and advised the manager against telling the patient immediately about the error. The situation was also referred to the hospital ethics committee. How can the nurse make the right decision? Who is the nurse manager an advocate for? Where does loyalty belong when the patient, the staff nurse, the organization, and the nurse manager are all involved? Use the guide for decision making and the ethics test to help you decide.

TABLE 24-5   INTERNATIONAL COUNCIL OF NURSES CODE OF ETHICS FOR NURSES

An international code of ethics for nurses was first adopted by the International Council of Nurses (ICN) in 1953. It has been revised and reaffirmed at various times since, most recently with this review and revision completed in 2005.

Preamble

Nurses have four fundamental responsibilities: to promote health, to prevent illness, to restore health, and to alleviate suffering. The need for nursing is universal.

Inherent in nursing is respect for human rights, including cultural rights, the right to life and choice, to dignity and to be treated with respect. Nursing care is respectful of and unrestricted by considerations of age, colour, creed, culture, disability or illness, gender, sexual orientation, nationality, politics, race or social status.

Nurses render health services to the individual, the family and the community and co-ordinate their services with those of related groups.

(Continues)

TABLE 24-5	INTERNATIONAL COUNCIL OF NURSES CODE OF ETHICS FOR NURSES (CONTINUED)

The ICN Code

The *ICN Code of Ethics for Nurses* has four principal elements that outline the standards of ethical conduct.

Elements of the Code

1. Nurses and people

The nurse's primary professional responsibility is to people requiring nursing care.

In providing care, the nurse promotes an environment in which the human rights, values, customs and spiritual beliefs of the individual, family and community are respected.

The nurse ensures that the individual receives sufficient information on which to base consent for care and related treatment.

The nurse holds in confidence personal information and uses judgement in sharing this information.

The nurse shares with society the responsibility for initiating and supporting action to meet the health and social needs of the public, in particular those of vulnerable populations.

The nurse also shares responsibility to sustain and protect the natural environment from depletion, pollution, degradation and destruction.

2. Nurses and practice

The nurse carries personal responsibility and accountability for nursing practice, and for maintaining competence by continual learning.

The nurse maintains a standard of personal health such that the ability to provide care is not compromised.

The nurse uses judgement regarding individual competence when accepting and delegating responsibility.

The nurse at all times maintains standards of personal conduct which reflect well on the profession and enhance public confidence.

The nurse, in providing care, ensures that use of technology and scientific advances are compatible with the safety, dignity and rights of people.

3. Nurses and the profession

The nurse assumes the major role in determining and implementing acceptable standards of clinical nursing practice, management, research and education.

The nurse is active in developing a core of research-based professional knowledge.

The nurse, acting through the professional organization, participates in creating and maintaining safe, equitable social and economic working conditions in nursing.

4. Nurses and co-workers

The nurse sustains a co-operative relationship with co-workers in nursing and other fields.

The nurse takes appropriate action to safeguard individuals, families and communities when their health is endangered by a co-worker or any other person.

Source: Reproduced with permission from the International Council of Nurses. (2000). *Code for nurses.* Geneva: Author.

CASE STUDY 24-2

A patient is brought to the hospital in an extremely critical state. The family has supporting documentation that the patient wanted a DNR order at a time such as this. The medical practitioner delays writing the order.

How do the nurses caring for the patient deal with this situation if the patient arrests? Who does the nurse advocate for in a situation of this type?

THE FUTURE

Ethical issues in the future that will challenge nursing practice include the allocation of resources, advanced technologies, an aging population, and an increase in behavior-related health problems. These issues all magnify the importance of professional nurses providing leadership that emphasizes ethical behavior in all practice settings.

KEY CONCEPTS

- Ethics is a branch of philosophy that concerns the distinction of right from wrong.
- Society created the profession of nursing for the purpose of meeting specific health needs.
- A person's beliefs and values will influence his or her philosophy of nursing.
- Teleology, deontology, virtue ethics, justice and equity, and relativism are examples of ethical theories.
- Ethical principles and rules include beneficence, non-maleficence, fidelity, justice, autonomy, respect for others, and veracity.
- Ethics committees provide guidance for decision making in ethical dilemmas in the health care setting.
- Values clarification is an important step in decision making.
- The Burkhardt and Nathaniel guide for decision making is a helpful tool.
- Numerous ethical issues face today's nurses.
- Patients' rights is an area in which nurses are held accountable.
- Nurses have the obligation to uphold the trust society places in the nursing profession.
- Nurse leaders who are dedicated to ethical principles can influence organizational ethics.

KEY TERMS

autonomy
beneficence
bioethics
ethical dilemma
ethics
fidelity
justice

morality
nonmaleficence
philosophy
respect for others
values
veracity

REVIEW QUESTIONS

1. When the nurse is obtaining the patient's consent, the patient states that the surgeon did not inform the patient of the risks of surgery. The nurse should
   A. tell the patient the risks.
   B. report the surgeon to the ethics committee.
   C. report the surgeon to the unit manager.
   D. inform the surgeon that the patient is unaware of the risks.

2. The nurse notices a coworker has been drinking and is not able to practice safely. The nurse should
   A. inform the manager or shift director immediately.
   B. warn the coworker that black coffee is in order.
   C. discuss the situation with the other nurses working.
   D. do nothing, but keep an eye on the nurse.

3. The nurse demonstrates nonmaleficence by doing which of the following? Select all that apply.
   ____ Observing the six rights of medication administration.

_____ Reviewing practitioner orders for accuracy and completeness.

_____ Keeping knowledge and skill up-to-date.

_____ Dressing professionally with name badge clearly visible.

4. The nurse manager has an ethical responsibility to
   A. the patient.
   B. the organization.
   C. the profession.
   D. the patient, the organization, the profession, and society.

5. The primary role of an ethics committee is to
   A. decide what should be done when ethical dilemmas arise.
   B. prevent the practitioner from making the wrong decision.
   C. provide guidance for the health care team and family of the patient.
   D. prevent ethical dilemmas from occurring.

6. Ethical dilemmas may be referred to the ethics committee by
   A. medical practitioners only.
   B. nursing and medical practitioners, lawyers, all health care team members, and families of patients.
   C. lawyers only.
   D. hospital administration only.

7. Mrs. Jones rides the elevator to the fifth floor where her husband is a patient. While on the elevator, Mrs. Jones hears two nurses talking about Mr. Jones. They are discussing the potential prognosis and whether Mr. Jones should be told. The nurses are violating which of the following ethical principles?
   A. Autonomy
   B. Confidentiality
   C. Beneficence
   D. Nonmaleficence

8. The nurse realizes that neglecting to inform the patient about the plan of care is a violation of
   A. the Patient's Bill of Rights.
   B. the patient's right to privacy.
   C. the patient's right to confidentiality.
   D. the fifth amendment of the constitution.

9. During morning report, the night nurse tells you that Mr. P, who is admitted for pancreatitis, is a drug addict and an alcoholic and caused all his own problems. You realize this nurse is exhibiting a lack of
   A. autonomy.
   B. compassion.
   C. discernment.
   D. trustworthiness.

REVIEW ACTIVITIES

1. An elderly woman, age 88, is admitted to the Emergency department in acute respiratory distress. She does not have a living will, but her daughter has power of attorney (POA) for health care and is a health care professional. The patient has end-stage renal disease, end-stage Alzheimer's disease, and congestive heart failure. Her condition is grave. The doctors want to intubate her and place her on a ventilator. The sons agree. The daughter states that their mother would not want to be on a machine just to prolong her life.

   Divide into groups and discuss the ethical theories that can be applied to this situation. Use the theories and principles discussed in this chapter to help you.

2. As a hospice nurse, you are involved with pain control on a regular basis. Many of the medications prescribed for the management of pain also depress respirations.

   Determine a protocol for the use of these medications, keeping in mind that the purpose of hospice is to promote comfort. Support your decisions with ethical theories and principles.

EXPLORING THE WEB

■ See what this Website says about nursing competencies and ethics.
   www.nursingworld.org

■ What Website could you recommend to nursing managers who need to clarify values of the staff? How else can this Website be used?
   www.ana.org

■ Go to the following site to view the American Hospital Association's "Patient's Bill of Rights":
   www.aha.org

■ View the American Nurses Association _Code for Nurses with Interpretive Statements_ (2001) at:
   www.nursingworld.org

■ Use the International Council of Nurses Website to find the ICN Code for Nurses:
   www.icn.ch

REFERENCES

American Hospital Association. (1992). _A patient's bill of rights._ Chicago: Author.

Bowditch, J. L., & Buono, A. F. (1997). A primer on organizational behavior (4th ed.). New York: Wiley.

Burkhardt, M. A., & Nathaniel, A. K. (2002). _Ethics & issues in contemporary nursing_ (2nd ed.). Clifton Park, NY: Thomson Delmar Learning.

Candela, L., Michael, S. R., & Mitchell, S. (2003). Ethical debates: Enhancing critical thinking in nursing students. *Nurse Educator, 28*(1), 37–39.

Corley, M. (1998). Ethical dimensions of nurse physician relations in critical care. *Nursing Clinics of North America, 33,* 325–337.

DeLaune, S. C., & Ladner, P. K. (2006). *Fundamentals of nursing* (3rd ed.). Clifton Park, NY: Thomson Delmar Learning.

Donahue, M. P. (1996). *Nursing, the finest art* (2nd ed.). St. Louis, MO: Mosby.

DuBrin, A. J. (2000). *The Active Manager.* Clifton Park, NY: Southwestern College Publishing.

Greene, J. (2002, Mar.). No abuse zone. *Hospitals and Health Networks, 26,* 28.

Gutierrez, K. M. (2005). Critical care nurses' perceptions of and responses to moral distress. *Dimensions of Critical Care Nursing, 24*(5), 229–241.

International Council of Nurses. (2000). *Code for nurses.* Geneva: Author.

Kopala, B., & Burkhart, L. (2005). Ethical dilemma and moral distress: Proposed new NANDA diagnoses. *International Journal of Nursing Terminologies and Classifications, 16*(1), 3–13.

Positive Leadership. (1998). Research reported in sample issue. *Positive Leadership, 5.*

Raths, L., Harmin, M., & Simon, S. (1978). *Values and teaching* (2nd ed.). Columbus, OH: Merrill.

Schroeder, S. A. (1995). Cost containment in U.S. health care. *Academic Medicine, 70*(10), 861–866.

Sullivan, E., & Decker, P. (2001). *Effective leadership and management in nursing* (5th ed.). Upper Saddle River, NJ: Prentice-Hall.

SUGGESTED READINGS

American Nurses Association. (2002). *Code of ethics for nurses with interpretive statements.* Washington, DC: American Nurses Publishing.

Arries, E. (2005). Virtue ethics: An approach to moral dilemmas in nursing. *Curationis, 28*(3), 64–72.

Beidler, S. M. (2005). Ethical considerations for nurse-managed health centers. *Nursing Clinics of North America, 40*(4), 759–770.

Corley, M. C., Minick, P., Elswick, R. K., & Jacobs, M. (2005). Nurse moral distress and the ethical work environment. *Nursing Ethics, 12*(4), 381–390.

Crigger, N. J. (2004). Always having to say you're sorry: An ethical response to making mistakes in professional practice. *Nursing Ethics, 11*(6), 568–576.

Dreezen, I., & Nys, H. (2003). Human rights: Implications for patients and staff. *EDTNA ERCA J., 29*(2), 93–95.

Faithful, S., & Hunt, G. (2005). Exploring nursing values in the development of a nurse-led service. *Nursing Ethics, 12*(5), 440–452.

Falk-Rafael, A. (2005). Speaking truth to power: Nursing's legacy and moral imperative. *Advanced Nursing Science, 28*(3), 212–223.

Ferrell, B. (2005). Ethical perspectives on pain and suffering. *Pain Management Nursing, 6*(3), 83–90.

Gallagher, A., & Wainwright, P. (2005). The ethical divide. *Nursing Standards, 20*(7), 22–25.

Gutierrez, K. M. (2005). Critical care nurses' perceptions of and responses to moral distress. *Dimensions of Critical Care Nursing, 24*(5), 229–241.

Jacobson, J. (2005). When providing care is a moral issue. *American Journal of Nursing, 105*(12), 16.

Johnstone, M. J. (2003). Moral activism and the nursing profession: Meeting the challenge to be involved. *International Nursing Review, 50*(4), 193–194.

Kennedy, W. (2004). Beneficence and autonomy in nursing. A moral dilemma. *British Journal of Perioperative Nursing, 14*(11), 500–506.

Milton, C. L. (2005). The Metaphor of nurse as guest with ethical implications for nursing and healthcare. *Nursing Science Quarterly, 18*(4), 301–303.

Randers, I., & Mattiasson, A. C. (2004). Autonomy and integrity: Upholding older adult patients' dignity. *Journal of Advanced Nursing, 45*(1), 63–71.

Sorlie, V., Kihlgren, A., & Kihlgren, M. (2005). Meeting ethical challenges in acute nursing care as narrated by registered nurses. *Nursing Ethics, 12*(2), 133–142.

Tschudin, V. (2006). How nursing ethics as a subject changes: An analysis of the first eleven years of publication of the journal Nursing Ethics. *Nursing Ethics, 13*(1), 65–85.

CHAPTER 25

Culture, Generational Differences, and Spirituality

Karen Luther Wikoff, RN, PhD

If we are to achieve a richer culture, rich in contrasting values, we must recognize the whole gamut of human potentialities, and so weave a less arbitrary social fabric, one in which each diverse human gift will find a fitting place (Margaret Mead, 1935).

OBJECTIVES

Upon completion of this chapter, the reader should be able to:

1. Apply cultural considerations to the role of a nurse leader.
2. Compare and contrast the demographics of the U.S. population and U.S. nurses.
3. Describe how organizational culture can influence leading a team.
4. Describe the current generations and their behaviors that influence leading and delivering patient care.
5. Identify methods of assessment and meeting spiritual needs of patients.
6. Apply knowledge of spirituality to problem solving in the nurse leader role.

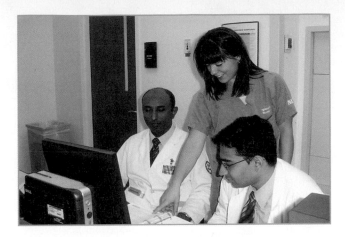

Mr. Hernandez, a recent Mexican immigrant who came over the border without any documentation, arrived in the Emergency Room bleeding profusely from his right arm following an accident with a chain saw. A pressure dressing is applied while he keeps repeating in Spanish that he is in pain. As you try to do his assessment, he grimaces in pain but refuses to answer any questions or cooperate with the nurse. You have asked another nurse to translate your questions and plans for care to Mr. Hernandez, but he keeps attempting to leave.

Considering his status as an undocumented worker, how will you convince him to be treated?

How does his undocumented status affect his access to health care?

We live in a global society rich with ever-changing different cultures, traditions, religions, spiritual beliefs, and generations, all of which influence the delivery of health care. New immigrants arrive daily. Consideration of all of these differences and sensitivity to patient and health care staff diversity is necessary in all nursing roles as situations arise that call for evaluating patient and staff behavior. Though each person is first and foremost an individual, each is also a member of a cultural group. Clues to people's behaviors come from understanding the cultural, generational, and spiritual focus of the individual or group. This chapter will enable the nurse to begin the process of preparing for cultural, generational, and spiritual aspects of leadership and management with patients and health care staff. These concepts are also discussed further in Chapter 8 on Personal and Interdisciplinary Communication and Chapter 11 on Effective Team Building.

CULTURE

Culture refers to the integrated patterns of human behavior that include the language, thoughts, communication, actions, customs, beliefs, values, and institutions of racial, ethnic, religious, or social groups (Munoz &

Luckmann, 2005). Although people from all cultures share most human characteristics, the study of culture highlights the way individuals differ and are similar to individuals in other cultures. Individuals from different cultures may think, solve problems, and perceive and structure the world differently from individuals of another culture. Cultural beliefs serve as a conscious and unconscious point of reference that guides the outlook and decisions of people. Culture incorporates the experience of the past and influences the present. It transmits traditions to future members of a culture. Culture influences what we eat, the language we speak, the values we believe in, and the actions we take. Values serve important functions:

- They provide people with a set of rules by which to govern their lives.
- They serve as a basis for attitudes, beliefs, and behaviors.
- They help to guide actions and decisions.
- They give direction to people's lives and help them solve common problems.
- They influence how individuals perceive and react to other individuals.
- They help determine basic attitudes regarding personal, social, and philosophical issues.
- They reflect a person's identity and provide a basis for self-evaluation (Munoz & Luckmann, 2005).

When interacting with members from your own culture, an awareness of the rules that guide behavior is usually a known truth. However, when interacting with members of other cultures, these rules may be unknown or not well understood.

Culture is learned and then shared. People learn about their culture from parents, teachers, religious and political leaders, and respected peers. As children grow up, they gradually internalize the values and beliefs of their culture and they, in turn, share these values and beliefs with their children.

Normally, children learn about their culture while growing up. However, when people emigrate from their native cultures into a new culture, they often experience culture shock. Culture shock develops when the values and beliefs upheld by this new culture are radically different from the person's native culture. For successful assimilation into a new culture, immigrants must learn and internalize that culture's important values.

In addition to belonging to a major cultural group, people also belong to a variety of subcultures, or smaller groups within a culture. Each culture has its own value system and related expectations. Subcultures may be based on the following:

- Professional and occupational affiliations (RNs)
- Nationality or race (a shared historical and political past)

- Age groups (adolescents, senior citizens)
- Gender (feminists, men's groups)
- Socioeconomic factors (working class, middle class, upper class)
- Political viewpoints (Democrat, Republican)
- Sexual orientation (gay and lesbian groups)

For example, when you studied to be a nurse, you entered a nursing subculture, and initially you probably suffered from some degree of culture shock. You had to learn a whole new value system. During your years of study, you gradually internalized the values taught by your instructors. Eventually you became comfortable with the values and behaviors you learned in your school of nursing, and, by the time you graduate, you will be assimilated into the professional nursing subculture.

Upon admission to a hospital, patients also become members of a culture. In this world filled with strange sights, unfamiliar sounds, and strangers, many patients experience culture shock. This shock intensifies for patients who are recent immigrants or who do not speak English (Cohen & Luckmann, 2005).

RACE AND ETHNICITY

Race describes a geographical or global human population distinguished by genetic traits and physical characteristics such as skin color or facial features. Major U.S. Census classification of race are American Indian, Asian, Black African, Pacific Islander/Hawaiian, or White, as shown in Figure 25-1 (www.census.gov). Cultural ethnicity identifies a person or group based on a racial, tribal, linguistic, religious, national, or cultural group, for example, Jewish, Irish. In years past, when new immigrants

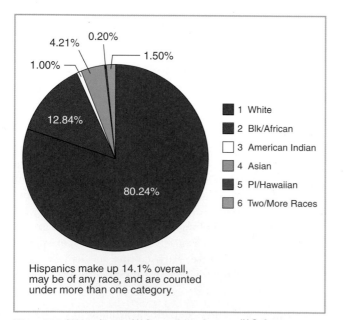

4.21%   0.20%

1.00%

1.50%

12.84%

80.24%

- 1 White
- 2 Blk/African
- 3 American Indian
- 4 Asian
- 5 PI/Hawaiian
- 6 Two/More Races

Hispanics make up 14.1% overall, may be of any race, and are counted under more than one category.

Figure 25-1 2004 estimate of U.S. population by race. (U.S. Census Bureau, Census 2000 [www.census.gov].)

CRITICAL THINKING 25-1

E xamine the community in which you live. What cultures are represented there? How does your community compare to other surrounding communities? Do any cultural differences in these communities affect health care?

arrived in the United States, they sought to become acculturated to their new country by adopting the conditions, language, and customs of the United States. Acculturation has taken a generation or two in the past and often resulted in the loss of a separate cultural identify. Today's immigrant population is more likely to maintain a strong tradition of valuing their historical cultural customs and identity.

INCREASING DIVERSITY

The ethnic and racial composition of the population of the United States has changed dramatically since the 1990s. There is increasing diversity in languages, beliefs, lifestyles, and practices among residents in rural and urban areas throughout the country. The percent of the U.S. population that is White has decreased since the 1970s. The reduction in percentage is due in part to increasing immigration from Asian and Latin American nations and in part to a higher population growth rate among Blacks (Munoz & Luckmann, 2005).

POPULATION GROUPS

It is important to recognize that within each of the broad, statistical categories, there are numerous cultural groups. These groups are characterized by variations in lifestyles, values and beliefs, health-related and illness-related practices, preferences for care, and family member patterns of interaction. For example, many cultural groups are included in the category of White (sometimes also referred to as Anglo-American or Caucasian). Individuals in these groups may trace their heritage to a European nation, Australia, North America, or many other nations and regions. Among individuals who are White, the largest group of 58 million people has a German ancestry. Another 39 million Americans trace their roots to Ireland, and more than 32.6 million Americans have an English ancestry (U.S. Census Bureau, 2001). The prevailing value system for many mainstream White Americans is based on the White, Anglo-Saxon, Protestant (WASP) ethics of Northern Europe over 2 centuries ago (Munoz & Luckmann, 2005).

There is also great diversity among the individuals who are included in the Hispanic population category. There are differences in their countries of origin, in the dialects spoken, and in customs and beliefs, including practices related to health and illness. Hispanics may include people from the Caribbean, Cuba, El Salvador, Guatemala, Puerto Rico, Mexico, Central and South America, and Spain (Munoz & Luckmann, 2005).

The term Black is similarly very inclusive and may refer to individuals who are refugees or immigrants from the African nations, such as Eritrea, Kenya, and the Caribbean, Haiti, the Dominican Republic, or individuals who can trace their heritage through multiple generations of residency in the United States. Furthermore, the term Native American too often blurs distinctions among members of more than 500 Native American groups who reside in North America, for example, Cherokees, Navajo, Chippewa, Sioux, Choctaw, American Indian/Athapaskan, Aleuts, and Eskimos. Likewise, the term Asian refers to the Japanese, Chinese, Indochinese, Filipino, Korean, Vietnamese, Cambodian, Laotian, Thai, Indonesian, Pakistani, Hmong, and Indian populations, each of which contains numerous, diverse subcultures. Religions practiced by this group include Buddhism, Taoism, Christianity, Confucianism, Zen Buddhism, Shintoism, and Hinduism (Munoz & Luckmann, 2005).

REAL WORLD INTERVIEW

The U.S. population is becoming more diverse while access to care for racial and ethnic minority populations has not improved. The challenge for nursing leadership is to attract a workforce that will mirror the diversity of the population and promote culturally competent clinical care. Nursing leadership in any health care work environment must recognize the uniqueness of each person and respect, protect, and advocate for the individual's right to self-determination, self-expression, confidentiality, and dignity. Nurses must embrace the belief that the relationships established while caring for the patient and family have the inherent capacity to promote health, healing, and wholeness. Caring and compassionate behaviors are the essence of nursing and therefore essential in today's work environment.

Carol Robinson, RN, MPA, CNAA, FAAN
Senior Associate Director, Patient Care Services
University of California Davis Health System
Sacramento, California

HEALTH CARE DISPARITY

Because of differences in cultural beliefs, there is often the **marginalization** or separation of some cultural groups away from the mainstream. Marginalized groups often suffer from higher rates of morbidity, mortality, and the burden of disease (Keltner, Kelley, & Smith, 2004). These increased rates may be due to a lack of health care access, inadequate financial resources, immigrant resident status, or a lack of knowledge on how to seek help.

According to the U.S. Census Bureau, 30% of Native Americans live below the poverty line compared with 29.5% of Blacks, 25.3% of Hispanics, 14.1% of Asian/Pacific Islanders, and 9.8% of Whites. Also, Native Americans have the lowest life expectancy of any ethnic group in the United States. Native Americans can expect to live only two-thirds as long as other people in the United States.

As nurse leaders understand problems in their local community, they can facilitate problem-solving activities, including seeking health care access, securing grants for health care, and increasing the health care knowledge of the community. For example, in one Southern California community, there is a relatively high percentage of Hispanic people, yet there is little Hispanic representation in the licensed health care staff. As a result of this cultural disparity, there is often a lack of knowledge and understanding of what to expect from health care. Nursing leaders have been actively involved in breaking down barriers and ensuring access to education and care. Participating in community outreach and education, serving as a role model for an ethnic group, and serving as a community activist for universal access to health care are several methods of reaching out to the marginalized in a community.

RACISM AND PREJUDICE

Some authors have suggested that racism exists in American nursing as a formidable barrier that severely undermines patient care. According to Barbee (1993), certain attributes of nursing prevent nurses from openly confronting the racism that exists in their profession.

- *An emphasis on empathy:* Nurses perceive themselves as caring individuals who see all people as the same rather than different. Nurses are taught that illness has no color and that their vocation is to help sick people, regardless of their color, creed, or race. This perception of themselves as caring makes it very difficult for nurses to acknowledge that they are capable of racism.
- *An individual orientation:* The major concepts that nurses learn in school are individualistic rather than group oriented. Although nursing theory seems to emphasize families, groups, and communities, nursing practice is geared to the needs of

REAL WORLD INTERVIEW

In the southern part of California, we have an underrepresentation of Hispanic nurses in our hospitals. To encourage and promote nursing enrollment, we have brought Hispanic nurses from Mexico to experience our health care system. They are provided with a hospital orientation of key programs in their areas of interest. They also spend time in the clinical area.

At the high school level, we have brought a group of about thirty high school students, the majority Hispanics, to the hospital. We talk to them about health care, nursing opportunities, and the need for Hispanic nursing staff.

As a nursing executive, I feel that it is important to be a role model for minority students. Recently, I participated in mock interviews for high school students. The majority of these students were Hispanic, Black, and Asian. We wanted to mentor and coach them on how to successfully interview for jobs. These are students without role models in their lives. Just by seeing that other people have done it creates a high sense of inspiration and desire to do better because they see that it is possible.

Pablo Velez, PhD, RN
Chief Nursing Officer
Sharp Chula Vista Medical Center
Chula Vista, California

individuals. Also, schools of nursing require students to study the hard sciences such as chemistry and physics, whereas social sciences such as sociology and anthropology are usually electives. As a consequence, nurses fail to learn enough about cultural diversity and the multicultural milieu in which they will be working.

- *A preference for homogeneity and a need to avoid conflict:* According to Brink (1990), selection committees on nursing faculties prefer a homogeneous student body because it tends to be more efficient, less challenging, and less threatening than a heterogeneous one.

Such characteristics reduce conflict and promote solidarity within the nursing ranks (Munoz & Luckmann, 2005).

These attributes have allowed the following three types of racism to flourish in American nursing (Barbee, 1993):

- *Denial:* There are several ways nurses can deny racism. Nurses, Black and White, may simply refuse to use the terms, *race* or *racism.* Black nurses may believe that their humanitarian work makes them immune to racism, and thus for them, racism does not exist. White nurses may substitute the more benign terms of ethnocentrism, cultural bias, and cultural diversity for the politically incorrect term of racism, thereby denying its existence.
- *Color-blind perspective:* Nurses who adhere to the color-blind perspective believe that race is a social

category that has no relevance to an individual's behavior, and thus "individuals should not notice each other's racial group membership" (Barbee, 1993). For those who adopt the color-blind perspective, race is a taboo topic, and they view social relationships as interpersonal rather than intergroup relationships. The color-blind perspective helps nurses to (a) avoid overt conflict with people of other races, (b) minimize the discomfort and embarrassment that is associated with discussions of race or racism, (c) ignore or distort the fact that cultural differences exist, and (d) protect themselves from charges of discrimination in the workplace.

- *Aversive racism:* According to Barbee (1993), "aversive racism is characterized by ambivalence: feelings and beliefs associated with an egalitarian value system conflict with unacknowledged negative feelings and beliefs concerning Blacks." This form of racism is subtle because aversive racists do not see themselves as prejudiced or discriminatory in any way.

Although racism distorts communication, prejudices between the nationalities, social classes, and sexes within a culture can also cause communication problems. For example, prejudices within the Hispanic culture may make professionals from the Dominican Republic reluctant to work with Puerto Ricans. Second-generation Mexican-American nurses may not want to take orders from Central American nurses or practitioners. Some Black men object to working for Black women. Some Latin men refuse to take directions from Latin or Black women (Burner, Cunningham, & Hattar, 1990).

CULTURAL COMPETENCE

Nurses providing care need to ensure that the cultural needs of their patients are considered. **Culturally competent care** is a complex integration of knowledge, attitudes, and skills that enhance cross-cultural communication and appropriate and effective interactions (American Academy of Nursing, 1992). Cultural competence has also been defined as a process that includes components of cultural awareness, cultural knowledge, cultural skills, cultural encounters, and cultural desire (Campinha-Bacote & Munoz, 2001). A baseline for delivering culturally competent care can be developed by completing an assessment of your beliefs, your organization, and your community. Table 25-1 provides a list of items to consider when preparing to provide culturally competent care. This preparation should include education regarding cultural groups specific to your local community as well as education on methods of obtaining sensitive personal information from patients.

Many nursing schools added curricula in the 1990s to ensure that nurses have adequate preparation for cultural competence. In addition, all nurses need to commit themselves to enhancing their knowledge of different cultures by reading about cultures, seeing films about different cultures, talking with patients and coworkers about their cultural backgrounds, or acting as a participant observer in a cultural setting such as an ethnic neighborhood. You can develop cultural competence by assessing your level of skill, practicing various techniques to improve your skills, evaluating your new skills, and deciding what improvements you still need to make. Note that every new person you meet who is

> ## CRITICAL THINKING 25-2
>
> You discovered what seems to be the perfect job, based on your family scheduling needs, as a clinic nurse for a nearby Native American tribe. What research will you do about this tribe? How do you prepare for the interview? What questions will you ask to enhance your understanding of their culture?

from another culture will help to broaden your appreciation of different cultures and improve your cultural competence.

A new nurse leader is often asked to work with people who are different because of their ethnicity, race, culture, religion, or age. This can result in workplace difficulties with communication and the development of problems. To manage and understand these potential difficulties, cultural nursing theories and conceptual models offer some direction. Table 25-2 reviews several of these: Leininger's Transcultural Nursing (1978, 1997), Purnell's Model for Cultural Competence (2005), Campinha-Bacote's Process of Cultural Competence in the Delivery of Health Care Service (2003), and Giger and Davidhizar's Transcultural Assessment Model (2004). Each of these models offers the nurse insight into examining the cultural beliefs and needs of culturally diverse patients. Choosing a model to direct your practice offers a path for implementation of the nursing process. In lieu of choosing a model, the nurse must be aware of his or her personal cultural values, be sensitive

TABLE 25-1	**PREPARATION FOR PROVIDING CULTURALLY COMPETENT CARE**

- Identify cultural groups in your community.
- Assess your own feelings about working with different cultural groups.
- Compare your community analysis with the patient population.
- Review common cultural barriers often encountered in working with various cultural groups.
- Review any challenges you have had working with patients and families from diverse cultures.
- Develop culturally competent approaches to these challenges.
- Review organizational polices and procedures regarding cultural diversity.
- Attend community and organizational educational offerings to improve your knowledge.

TABLE 25-2   **CULTURAL NURSING THEORIES AND MODELS**

Theorist	Characteristics	Basic Tenets	Implications for Nursing Practice
Leininger (1978, 1997) Transcultural Nursing	Formal approach to the study and practice of comparative holistic cultural care and health and illness patterns while respecting differences.	All cultures have caring behaviors that may vary from culture to culture. Each culture identifies what it values for care. An understanding of each culture is important to providing care and meeting patient needs. Need to evaluate world view, social structure, language, ethno-history, environmental context, and folk and professional systems.	Initial theory was created in the 1960s and is frequently updated and edited. Seeks to provide culturally congruent nursing care that is meaningful to the recipient.
Purnell (2005) Model for Cultural Competence	An organizing framework for assessing culture across disciplines. States that cultural competence is a process, not an endpoint.	The model is represented by a circle with rims moving from the global society to the community, to the family, and to the individual. The inner circle has twelve pie slices representing twelve domains of culture, that is, overview/heritage, communication, family roles and organization, workforce issues, biocultural ecology, high-risk behaviors, nutrition, pregnancy, death rituals, spirituality, health care practices, and health care practitioners.	This grand theory offers direction for practice. Analyzing the patient belief system in each of the twelve domains gives direction to the nursing process.
Campinha-Bacote (2003) The Process of Cultural Competence in the Delivery of Health Care Service	Cultural competence is a process where the nurse works to effectively meet needs within a cultural context.	Cultural Desire leads the nurse to engage in developing cultural competence. Cultural Awareness is a self-examination and exploration of one's own cultural background. Cultural Knowledge is learning about diverse groups and understanding beliefs and values specific to the patient. Cultural Skill is the ability to collect data and complete a cultural assessment. Cultural Encounters occur when the nurse is engaged in interactions with diverse patients meeting their needs in a culturally sensitive manner.	This process reflects the need for the nurse to have an awareness of patient needs and then to actively seek to meet those needs. The model serves as a guide for becoming culturally competent.
Giger and Davidhizar (2004) Transcultural Assessment Model	Method for completing and evaluating the outcomes of cultural assessment.	Has five concepts that focus on transcultural nursing and the provision of culturally diverse nursing care, provision of culturally competent care, identification of the cultural uniqueness of individuals, development of culturally sensitive environments, and development of culturally specific illness and wellness behaviors.	Consider communication, space, social organization, time, environmental control, and biological variations when assessing culture.

CASE STUDY 25-1

Following are different levels of response you might have toward a person.

Levels of Response:

- *Greet:* I feel I can greet this person warmly and welcome him or her sincerely.
- *Accept:* I feel I can honestly accept this person as he or she is and be comfortable enough to listen to his or her problems.
- *Help:* I feel I would genuinely try to help this person with his or her problems as they might be related to or arise from the label or stereotype given to him or her.
- *Background:* I feel I have the background of knowledge and experience to be able to help this person.
- *Advocate:* I feel I could honestly be an advocate for this person.

The following is a list of individuals. Read down the list and place a check mark by anyone you would not Greet or would hesitate to Greet. Then move to response level 2, Accept, and follow the same procedure for all five response levels. Try to respond honestly, not as you think might be socially or professional desirable. Your answers are only for your personal use in clarifying your initial reactions to different people. How did you do?

Individual	1 Greet	2 Accept	3 Help	4 Background	5 Advocate
1. White Anglo-Saxon American (WASP)					
2. Child Abuser					
3. Jewish American					
4. Iranian American					
5 Hispanic American					
6. IV drug user					
7. Catholic American					
8. Senile elderly American					
9. Native American					
10. Prostitute					
11. Jehovah's Witness American					
12. Cerebral palsied person					
13. Asian American					
14. Gay/Lesbian American					
15. Muslim American					
16. American with AIDS					
17. Chinese American					
18. Black African American					
19. Unmarried expectant teen					
20. Protestant					
21. Amputee					
22. Pacific Islander American					
23. Filipino American					
24. Alcoholic					
25. Amish American					

Source: Compiled with information from Munoz & Luckmann, 2005.

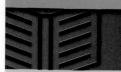

EVIDENCE FROM THE LITERATURE

Citation: DeRosa, N., & Kochurka, K. (2006, Oct.). Implement culturally competent healthcare in your workplace. *Nursing Management,* 18–26.

Discussion: This article discusses selected verbal and nonverbal communication patterns of culture. Even when two people speak the same language, communication may be hindered by different values or beliefs. Nonverbal differences or ethnic dialects can also block mutual understanding. Communication differences include the following:

- *Conversational style:* Silence may show respect or acknowledgement. In some cultures, a direct "no" is considered rude, and silence may mean "no." A loud voice or repeating a statement may mean anger or simply emphasis, enthusiasm, or a request for help.
- *Personal space:* Beliefs about personal space vary. Someone may be viewed as aggressive for standing "too close" or as "distant" for backing off when approached.
- *Eye contact:* In some cultures, direct eye contact may be a sign of respect. In other cultures, direct eye contact may be seen as a sign of disrespect.
- *Subject matter and conversation length:* Even appropriate subject matter, when it's appropriate to discuss, and how long the discussion should last vary from culture to culture. Some cultures value communication that's subtle and circumspect; forthright discussion is considered rude. In some cultures, it's acceptable to discuss topics such as sexuality and death, whereas in other cultures, these topics are taboo.

The article also discusses elements of a cultural assessment, including nutrition, medications, pain, and psychological and primary language assessment. It also explores how to approach the patient with educational needs.

Implications for Practice: Be aware of these cultural differences when working with patients and staff from other cultures. Remember that not everyone sees things the way that you do.

to and accepting of the influence of culture, have a commitment to continual learning about different cultures, and provide care that is in harmony with the cultural beliefs and lifestyle of patients.

Although it is not possible to learn every nuance of every culture, it is essential to learn as much as possible about the cultures represented in your community. Table 25-3 provides an overview of cultural norms, health care beliefs and religious beliefs seen in America. The content in this table provides information to begin a dialogue between the nurse and the patient. Note that the norms and beliefs may not be valid for all individuals within a cultural group.

ORGANIZATIONAL CULTURE

Before leaving the concept of culture, it is important to discuss organizational culture. In an organizational culture, the norms of behavior and beliefs influence the outcomes for the organization. **Organizational culture** is the system of shared values and beliefs that actively influences

the behavior of organization members. The term, *shared values,* is important because it implies that many people are guided by the same values and that they interpret them in the same way. Values develop over time and reflect an organization's history and traditions. Culture consists of the culture of an organization, such as being helpful and supportive toward new members.

Five dimensions of organizational culture are of major significance in influencing organizational culture (Ott, 1989):

- *Values:* Values are the foundation of any organizational culture. The organization's philosophy is expressed through values, and values guide behavior on a day-to-day basis.
- *Relative diversity:* The existence of an organizational culture assumes some degree of similarity. Nevertheless, organizations differ in how much deviation can be tolerated.
- *Resource allocation and reward:* The allocation of money and other resources has a critical influence on culture. The investment of resources sends a message to people about what is valued in the organization.

TABLE 25-3	CULTURAL NORMS, HEALTH CARE BELIEFS, AND RELIGIOUS BELIEFS*		
Cultural Group	**Cultural Norms**	**Health Care Beliefs**	**Religious Beliefs**
Hispanic	■ Maintaining eye contact is valued. ■ A pat on the back or arm is considered friendly. ■ Treating others with respect is valued. ■ Cakes and sweets may be a regular part of the diet. ■ Children are highly valued and loved. ■ May have different perception of time, for example, may have a problem in being late for appointments.	■ Fatalistic and may view illness as a punishment from God. ■ View health as the ability to rise in the morning and go to work. ■ May or may not follow medical advice. ■ May consult a folk healer, for example, curandero. ■ Will use Western medications but will stop when feels can no longer afford it.	■ Are often Roman Catholic but may be member of other Christian group, may light candles, attend mass, pray to God, Jesus, the Virgin Mary, and saints. ■ Traditional men view religion as a preoccupation of women. ■ May have statues of saints at home.
White Anglo-Saxon Protestant (WASP)	■ Value independence, individuality, youth, wealth, comfort, cleanliness, achievement, punctuality, work, aggression, and assertiveness; rational and oriented to the future; and value mastery of their own fate. ■ Set long-term goals.	■ May not feel comfortable answering personal questions. ■ May feel a visit to practitioner is incomplete without a prescription. ■ May be resistant to authority.	■ May be Episcopalians, Presbyterians, or members of United Church of Christ. Others may be methodists, Lutherans, Baptist, Unitarian, Congregationalist, Disciples of Christ, and so forth.
Black African	■ Have tradition of involving many in raising children. ■ Many households are headed by women. ■ May be frank and direct in speech. ■ Unrelated persons often live in the home. ■ High incidence of poverty. ■ Oriented to the present.	■ Often distrust or have discomfort with majority group and health care system. ■ May be private about their health and may not want family members present during care or treatment. ■ May try self care first and use all forms of pharmacological and some nonpharmacological, alternative and complimentary medicines prior to seeking care. ■ View health as being in harmony with nature, and view illness as disharmony. ■ Some have fatalistic attitude about illness.	■ Are heavily involved in key religious groups, such as, churches or mosques. ■ Black minister is strong influence in community. ■ May use faith healers or herbalists. ■ Are active in singing, praying, and reading the Bible. ■ Illness is between the individual and God; illness may be viewed as punishment from God. ■ May see illness as the will of God.

(Continues)

TABLE 25-3	CULTURAL NORMS, HEALTH CARE BELIEFS, AND RELIGIOUS BELIEFS (CONTINUED)		
Cultural Group	**Cultural Norms**	**Health Care Beliefs**	**Religious Beliefs**
Asians	■ Work hard, have respect for elders and nature, have esteem for self control and loyalty to all family and extended family. ■ Are traditionally patriarchal. ■ Have respect for elders. ■ May not consider shaking hands to be polite. ■ Submissive to authority. ■ Pride and honor are extremely important.	■ Prefer a same sex health care practitioner. ■ Expect health care to include an injection or prescription. ■ May not make important decisions without checking with an astrologer or almanac for a lucky day.	■ Have broad group of practices from Christianity to Buddhism, Taoism, ancestor worship, Muslim, and many others, depending on the geographic area. ■ Prayer and offerings are dominant in many groups. ■ May use faith healers or herbalists.
Pacific Islanders	■ May ascribe to a holistic world view—interconnectedness of family, environment, self, and spiritual world. ■ Family and community play an important role and often live in close proximity or tightly knit communities. ■ Interpersonal and social behavior is based on mutual respect and sharing.	■ Often distrust Western style of health care. Rarely respond positively to health education and treatment based on scare tactics. ■ Stoic; do not complain. ■ May use Western medication but choose over-the-counter drugs for minor ailments. ■ Massage is a method to achieve harmony.	■ Have deeply rooted spiritual connections. ■ Hold belief in unity, balance, and harmony. ■ Use traditional healers. ■ Some may be Christian.
Native Americans	■ Family and tribal affiliations are part of daily life. ■ May have extended family structure living with relatives from both sides of the family. ■ Have a holistic view of life and health. ■ Often suffer from poverty, poor nutrition, and inadequate access to health care. ■ Avoid eye contact. ■ Elders often assume leadership role. ■ Share goods with others. ■ Cooperate with others. ■ Work for good of the group.	■ Physical illness may be due to violation of a taboo or being out of harmony. ■ Skeptical regarding the benefit and habit-forming properties of medications. ■ Holistic orientation to health. ■ May wait to see Western practitioner until seen by a healer. ■ Oriented to the present. ■ Accept nature rather than try to control nature.	■ Religion or spiritual affiliation is based on personal choice. ■ May have Christian beliefs and traditional beliefs. ■ Have spiritual orientation. ■ May fear witchcraft as cause of illness and use a medicine bag received from a healer, which should be kept with the patient at all times. ■ May carry object at all times to guard against witchcraft.

*The information presented is from multiple sources and is meant to serve as a starting point to understanding. All people are individuals and these norms and beliefs may not be valid for all within a cultural group identified in the table.

Source: Compiled with information from *The providers guide to quality and culture.* Retrieved April 2, 2007, from http://erc.msh.org/ mainpage.cfm?file=1.0htm&module=provider&language=English; and Lipson, J. G. & Dibble, S. L. (2005). *Culture and clinical care.* San Francisco: UCSF Nursing Press; and Munoz, C., & Luckmann, J. (2005). *Transcultural Communication in Nursing.* Clifton Park, NY: Thomson Delmar Learning.

TABLE 25-4	QUESTIONS TO ASK WHEN ASSESSING ORGANIZATIONAL CULTURE

- Are the organization's values consistent with your values?
- Is the organization or the department centralized or decentralized?
- What is the formal chain of command?
- What is the informal chain of command?
- Do individuals participate in changing policies or procedures?
- What are the rules about how things should be done?
- Where does one take new ideas or suggestions?
- Are risk and change encouraged?
- How are individuals rewarded for quality improvement, or are all rewards oriented toward the group?
- How does the team work together?

- *Degree of change:* A fast-paced, dynamic organization has a culture different from that of a slow-paced, stable one. Top-level managers, by the energy or lethargy of their stance, send messages about how much they welcome innovation.
- *Strength of the culture:* The strength of a culture, or how much influence it exerts, is partially a byproduct of the other dimensions. A strong culture guides employees in many everyday actions. It determines, for example, whether employees will inconvenience themselves to satisfy a patient. If the culture is not so strong, employees are more likely to follow their own whims, that is, they may decide to please patients only when convenient for them.

Each organization will have embedded in its environment the dos and don'ts that are specific to its workplace. When beginning in a new organization, observe and ask questions to learn about the organization and culture and how decisions are made (Table 25-4).

ORGANIZATIONAL SOCIALIZATION

As a new member of a team or workgroup, it is important to be socialized into the organization. In most organizations, this socialization begins as part of the new employee's orientation process. This allows the organization to promote the organization's values to the new employee from the beginning. The individual responsible for a new hire's orientation is often also responsible for enhancing the socialization process. When there is a good fit of ethics, values, and behaviors between the preceptor and a new individual, the socialization process goes smoothly and often occurs rapidly. To ensure socialization that meets the organizational goals, it is important to monitor the orientation process. Frequent evaluation by both the preceptor and the new hire are critical to the success of the new employee and the organization.

Socialization is beneficial to the organization when employees are a good fit, that is, the employee has a high commitment to the organization, little intention to leave, high levels of job satisfaction, and little work-related stress. Things to consider when entering a new work environment in any culture are the organizational behavior style for greetings, titles, punctuality, body language, and dress (Table 25-5).

These organizational styles are important to the workplace milieu. Additionally, it is important for employees to avoid assumptions about how other individuals think, act, or speak. New employees should consider these organizational behavioral styles and work to ensure organizational cohesiveness (Table 25-6).

Most organizations have a workplace culture that has a strong mission and vision, and its members work tirelessly to ensure its success. However, there will be organizations that can only be described as toxic. In these organizations, the staff and/or leadership is dysfunctional. Instead of problem solving, the goal of these organizations is faultfinding and placing blame. Staff may observe excessive control on the part of the leader or a unit or worker in a constant state of crisis. This dysfunctional toxic environment may be a unit within a hospital or the entire organization. Choosing your workplace environment wisely will make your work life more satisfying.

TABLE 25-5	UNITED STATES ORGANIZATIONAL BEHAVIORAL STYLES

Concepts	Things to Consider
Greetings	■ Americans usually acknowledge each other with a smile, nod of the head, and/or verbal greeting, such as "Hello," or "Hi." ■ When greeting someone in a business situation, a firm handshake is appropriate, such as when greeting a manager of nursing or human resources.
Titles	■ When introducing yourself or others, give your first name followed by your last name. ■ Use the appropriate title the first time you address an individual, such as Mrs., Dr., Ms., or Mr. Wait to be directed to call them by their first name.
Time	■ Punctuality is highly respected in nursing, so be on time to interview appointments and work. ■ Know where you are going and plan to be on time.
Body language	■ Use of direct eye contact is expected in all work situations and when working with patients. However, some patients may not respond to direct eye contact, depending on their culture. ■ In conversation, it is important to keep approximately one arm length's distance from the speaker; closer proximity is often considered rude.
Dress	■ When in doubt, use business attire, that is, a professional suit with white blouse or shirt for meetings and interviews. ■ For your work environment, ask what traditional dress is in a particular work area or nursing unit before starting a new job or purchasing new uniforms. ■ Even in areas where daily dress is casual, business situations should be considered formal.

TABLE 25-6	WORKPLACE BEHAVIOR GUIDELINES

■ To be successful in health care, work to adapt to your organization's culture.

■ People from other cultures often may not think and behave the way that you do. What might be normal behavior in your culture may be inappropriate in another culture and vice versa.

■ Communication requires listening and clarifying meaning to ensure understanding. It is often a good idea to rephrase what you heard to test your understanding.

■ When seeking clarification, go to the source of the communication. Do not ask other coworkers to clarify work requests that originated from a third party or from your leadership personnel.

■ Observe for cultural differences in the workplace, and attempt to understand and accommodate those differences.

■ In health care, holidays and weekends are considered part of the work requirements for nurses. If you need time off to celebrate a cultural or religious holiday, make arrangements early with your manager. Also, realize that health care is a 24/7 business.

CRITICAL THINKING 25-3

In today's diverse workplace, you will work closely with RNs, nursing students, medical practitioners, and ancillary personnel who are from different cultures and who speak English as a second language. How do you feel about working with practitioners who are from foreign countries, or from different racial or ethnic groups? Take a minute to answer the following questions. You do not need to share your answers with anyone, so be honest with yourself.

	Agree	Neutral	Disagree
I would rather work with an American nurse than a foreign nurse.			
I find it frustrating to work with medical and nursing practitioners who are not proficient in English.			
If I thought that a medical or nursing practitioner was not fulfilling duties because of cultural or language problems, I would hesitate to report the person for fear that I would be considered prejudiced.			
I enjoy working with a skilled foreign nurse. I feel that I can learn a lot from this person.			
I like to attend classes and informal meetings where I can learn more about how nurses from other countries are educated.			
I do not feel prepared to work with or supervise an unlicensed assistive worker who has some problems with understanding English.			

Source: Compiled with information from Munoz & Luckmann, 2005.

CRITICAL THINKING 25-4

You are hired to work on a ten-bed nursing unit. During your orientation, you discover that you are the only individual of your cultural group. What actions will you take to enhance your socialization into the group? What actions should the group take?

WORKING WITH STAFF FROM DIFFERENT CULTURES

Staff nurses from different cultures may have different perceptions of staff responsibilities to each other, different perceptions of the nurse's role in patient care, a different locus of control, different time orientation, and a different language.

DIFFERENT PERCEPTIONS OF STAFF RESPONSIBILITIES

Cultural values deeply influence what a person feels is most important, that is, the welfare of the individual or the welfare of the group. Individualism emphasizes the importance of individual rights and rewards. Collectivism emphasizes the importance of group decisions and places the rights of the group as a whole above the rights of any individual in the group. For example, some nurses tend to accept difficult assignments without complaint. They also may be more willing to do what other nurses might consider demeaning, for example, cleaning cabinets. Because nurses from some cultures value the group, they believe that a nurse's individual duties have less value than the combined work of all of the nurses on the unit. Also, when assigned to difficult or menial tasks, nurses from some cultures may feel it is inappropriate to confront a supervisor or demand a change of assignment. Maintaining face and ensuring harmony are Eastern cultural values that may be more important to some nurses than upsetting a supervisor to get an easier assignment. An emphasis on minimizing

CRITICAL THINKING 25-5

When you are asked to work with people from a different culture, it is natural to have some concerns. How do you feel about this? Are you worried that you will not be able to communicate clearly with people from other cultures? Try to respond as honestly as possible to the following statements. The answers are for your use only.

	Agree	Neutral	Disagree
People are the same. I don't behave any differently toward people from a cultural background that differs from mine.			
I always know what to say to someone from a different cultural background.			
I look forward to working with people from a different cultural background.			
I can learn something when I work with people from diverse cultural backgrounds.			
I always introduce myself to new people who I work with.			
I prefer to work with staff from my own cultural group because it is easier.			
Responsible adults prepare for the future and strive to influence events in their lives.			
Intelligent, efficient people use their time well and are always punctual.			
It is disrespectful to address people by their first name unless they give you permission to do so.			
It is rude and intrusive to obtain information by asking direct questions.			

Source: Compiled with information from Munoz & Luckmann, 2005.

conflict, and maintaining harmony, teamwork, and commitment to group loyalty typify most Asian cultures.

In contrast, nurses educated in Western culture generally place more value on individualism and independence. Thus, Western nurses may complain to the supervisor if they feel assignments are unfair or involve menial work. This assertive behavior is consistent with ingrained values of equitable work distribution and the respect for education and professionalism that define the American work style.

Western nurses also want to be individually recognized for their work; for instance, they may want a promotion, or they may dream of being publicly honored for giving outstanding patient care or other accomplishments (Munoz & Luckmann, 2005).

DIFFERENT PERCEPTIONS OF THE NURSE'S ROLE

Nurses from different cultures have different perceptions of the nurse's role and nursing care values, which American nurses may not appreciate. For example, in a study of Philippine American nurses, the most important finding was the theme of obligation to care that prevailed in all aspects of their work (Spangler, 1992). This theme, which epitomized the Philippine American nurses' values, was expressed in three important ways: an expressed dedication to work, an attentiveness to the patient's physical comfort needs, and through the respect and patience that the nurses carried into their relationships with patients.

The theme of an obligation to care reflected the Philippine American nurses' strong belief that bedside nursing is truly the core of nursing. This value conflicted with the attitude of some American nurses that the physical care of patients is devalued work with low prestige and should therefore be delegated to ancillary personnel (Spangler, 1992).

DIFFERENCES IN LOCUS OF CONTROL

Locus of control refers to the degree of control that individuals feel that they have over events. People who feel in control of their environment have an internal locus of control. People who believe that luck, fate, or chance controls their lives have an external locus of control.

Health care providers who are trained in the United States typically have an internal locus of control. American medical and nursing practitioners and nurses feel that it is their duty to diagnose disorders, plan interventions, carry out procedures, and do everything possible to save the patient's life.

Conversely, health care providers from cultures that promote an external locus of control (some Mexican Americans, Appalachians, and Puerto Ricans) may have a more fatalistic attitude toward their patients and thus feel that they cannot control matters of life and death. For example, when a patient who is expected to die does die on the operating room table, care providers with an external locus of control may be puzzled when hospital administration asks for a quality review of the case (Giger & Davidhizar, 1996). Finally, some American Indians, Chinese Americans, and Japanese Americans believe themselves to be in harmony with nature rather than being controlled by nature or in control of nature (Giger & Davidhizar, 1996).

DIFFERENCES IN TIME ORIENTATION

Cultural groups are either past-, present-, or future oriented. Americans generally value the future over the present. Southern Blacks and Puerto Ricans value the present over the future. Southern Appalachians, traditional Chinese Americans, and Mexican Americans value the present (Munoz & Luckmann, 2005).

The ways in which different cultural groups value time can create challenges in the health care workplace. For example, people who work in the OR must be both future- and presented oriented. To plan and adhere to the OR schedule, the person must be future oriented and abide by the calendar and clock. However, after the surgical procedure begins, the surgeon and nurses must now switch to a present orientation (Giger & Davidhizar, 1996).

Staff meetings also are influenced by the time orientation of staff members. For instance, staff members who are meeting to plan for the future may become annoyed with members who want to spend all of the time on present-day problems and issues.

EDUCATIONAL DIFFERENCES

Foreign nurses are educated differently from American nurses. Generally, nursing education outside of the United States is less theory oriented, focusing primarily on the development of clinical skills. Also, there is less emphasis on meeting the psychosocial needs of patients.

Another cultural difference in the education of nurses revolves around who provides the majority of care—the nurse, the patient's family, or the patient. Some nurses may feel it's the nurse's duty to give patients complete physical care. Other nurses, educated outside of the United States, may have been taught that it is the family's duty to bathe the patient and provide personal care. In contrast, nurses educated in the United States are taught that patients should perform self-care whenever possible. In keeping with the American values of independence and self-reliance, American nurses encourage patients to be ambulatory, active, and self-sufficient as soon as possible.

Even when nurses are from other English-speaking countries, they are educated differently from American nurses. English nurses, taught under the system of socialized medicine, may find it difficult to adjust to the concept that health care in the United States is a business, and practitioners are in private practice. These nurses may not be familiar with practitioner referral services, charging patients for supplies, or the use of extreme measures to prolong the lives of terminally ill patients.

LANGUAGE DIFFERENCES

Language differences, perhaps more than any other barrier, raise the potential for serious miscommunications between health care providers and patients. Today, large medical centers in the United States may be primarily staffed by nurses and practitioners for whom English is a second language. For example, in urban medical centers on the East Coast, it is not unusual to hear a Filipino nurse and a Haitian nurse attempting to communicate with a resident practitioner who has been educated in India. Unless these caregivers take the time to clarify their communications, serious errors may result. The potential for miscommunication exists (especially over the telephone), unless words are clarified by a coworker or practitioner (Munoz & Luckmann, 2005).

Nonverbal communication can also create misunderstandings. For example, an Asian nurse may think that it is rude to sustain prolonged eye contact with a patient; the patient, on the other hand, may interpret the lack of eye contact as lack of interest. As a result of this confusion, the patient may request an American nurse, a request that could cause the foreign nurse to feel inadequate and disrespected.

Language differences are also a source of friction between American nurses and foreign nurses. When frictions escalate, foreign nurses may form cliques on a unit. By speaking in their native language and excluding

English-speaking nurses, foreign nurses may feel unified, even though they are alienating themselves even further from the rest of the nursing staff (Burner, Cunningham, & Hattar, 1990). English-speaking nurses may believe that they are being talked about by the foreign nurses and thus demand that personnel speak only English on the unit. Foreign nurses, denied the right to speak their own language at work, can feel even more threatened and angry, a feeling that presents further obstacles to communication (Munoz & Luckmann, 2005).

IMPROVING COMMUNICATION ON THE TEAM

If you are assigned to work with a nurse or staff member who is from a different culture and who speaks English as a second language, try these techniques to facilitate communication:

- Recognize that your coworker probably has an educational background in nursing that is very different from your own.
- Acknowledge that the coworker's value system and perception of what constitutes good patient care may differ from your own.
- Try to assess your coworker's level of understanding of verbal and written communication. For example, ask a coworker to explain a practitioner's order to you in her own words. It also helps to assess a patient with the coworker and note what terms the person uses to describe the patient's signs and symptoms.
- Avoid the use of slang terms and regional expressions. For example, Chinese, Japanese, and Filipino nurses may not understand such terms as piggybacking, doing a double, or rigging something to work.
- Provide your coworker with resources, such as written procedures and protocols, that may help to reinforce your verbal communication.
- Remember to praise your coworker's competency in technical skills. Inspiring self-confidence in a foreign nurse will make it easier for that person to ask for assistance when needed.
- Appreciate the knowledge that you can gain by working alongside a skilled nurse from another culture. Observe how foreign nurses relate to patients who are from their culture. If you have an open mind, working with foreign coworkers can increase your knowledge of other cultures, enrich your work as a nurse, and foster personal growth (Tilki, Papadopoulos, & Alleyne, 1994).
- When offering constructive criticism, try to use *I* statements instead of *you* statements. For example: "I think that it's very important to address the

patient's emotional state when you chart" is better than "You never seem to chart anything about the patient's emotional state."

- If you feel you cannot achieve effective communication with a coworker, request to work with another person. You do not want to be held accountable for the actions of a nurse with whom you cannot communicate.
- Report to your supervisor if you feel that a nurse or a practitioner is endangering patients because of language difficulties or different cultural values. Record any problems that occur, and keep a copy of the notes you provide to your supervisor (Munoz & Luckmann, 2005).

COMMUNICATION WITH OTHERS

Sometimes you may need to work with a foreign practitioner who is difficult to understand because of language differences or a strong accent. In this case, do not take verbal orders, particularly over the telephone. Even when an order is written, take the time to clarify the order with the practitioner. Because patients may also find it difficult to understand a foreign practitioner, you may need to listen carefully and then explain the practitioner's remarks to the patient (Munoz & Luckmann, 2005).

Another group of health care workers who may have difficulty understanding and speaking English are unlicensed assistive personnel (UAP) (Walton & Waszkiewiez, 1997). If you are called upon to supervise an unlicensed worker who speaks English as a second language, follow these cautions:

- Delegate appropriate tasks to an unlicensed worker. Match assignments to the worker's level of understanding and skill.
- Do not stop at just delegating an assignment or giving instructions. Instead, make sure that the worker understands your instructions.
- Restate your instructions in clear, concrete terms, and give a demonstration of a procedure if necessary.
- To reduce miscommunication, check for understanding by asking the worker to repeat instructions or do a return demonstration.
- If you are still not satisfied that the communication between the two of you is accurate and effective, repeat your directions and request a repeat demonstration.
- Establish a time frame for the worker to complete assigned tasks. For example, "I want you to feed Mr. Brown before you get Mr. Black out of bed."
- Observe how the worker communicates with patients and performs duties.
- Give workers clear feedback concerning their communication skills and performance of duties. If the

worker has performed a procedure incorrectly, offer suggestions for improvement. Demonstrate the procedure as it should be done and ask for a return demonstration.

■ If, despite your best efforts, the worker is still unable to perform because of language difficulties, ask your supervisor to work with the person. Again, you do not want to be held responsible for a worker with whom you cannot communicate (Munoz & Luckmann, 2005).

MANAGERIAL RESPONSIBILITY

Jamieson and O'Mara (1991) have laid out a broad, six-step program for nurse managers to follow to actively manage a diverse nursing staff:

1. Determine which cultural groups are represented on staff.
2. Understand the organization's values and goals.
3. Decide on what is best for the future of the organization.
4. Analyze present conditions within the organization.
5. Plan ways to reach the desired future state, and decide how to manage transitions.
6. Evaluate the results.

Nurse managers might consider using the following approaches to diminish tensions between staff members and improve communication:

■ Plan informal meetings for nurses to discuss their cultural values. For example, it may benefit Asian nurses to share with American-born nurses their cultural values concerning respect for authority.

■ Provide cultural workshops, and ask knowledgeable individuals to present information about the values, behaviors, and communication patterns of the different cultural groups that are represented on staff.

■ Provide classes in English as a second language for foreign nurses who do not speak fluent English or who have difficulty pronouncing words.

■ Establish a program for orienting foreign nurses to the hospital or agency (Jein & Harris, 1989). The orientation program should be designed to help newcomers adjust to the new work environment. It is helpful to assign each new nurse to a preceptor who will assist in the orientation process. If possible, the preceptor should be a member of the nurse's cultural group. For maximum benefits, the nurse manager needs to interview each new nurse every week to find out how that person is adapting to the new hospital culture (Williams & Rodgers, 1993).

■ Plan potluck events at which nurses, practitioners, and other staff members can socialize and discuss cultural differences informally, in a relaxed environment. For example, each unit in the hospital might plan one potluck event for each shift on a monthly basis. Potluck meals could be planned around a cultural theme, for instance, a traditional Vietnamese dinner one month and a traditional Costa Rican meal the next month (Burner, Cunningham, & Hattar, 1990).

■ Confer with specialists in transcultural communication; also hire experts to identify potential areas of conflict and resolve conflicts peacefully before they erupt into legal battles (Munoz & Luckmann, 2005).

GENERATIONAL PERCEPTIONS

Generational perceptions and different values and beliefs are created as each generation deals with the experiences of their lives as they are altered by the changing times. A **generation** is a group that shares birth years, age, location, and significant life events (Kupperschmidt, 2000). A generation is approximately fifteen to twenty years in length and has a different value system from the preceding generation and later generations. Like culture, we take our generational differences with us into patient care and the work environment. We often assume that those around us are like us and think like us. This is not always true.

Four distinct generations make up the current patient and workforce population. These generations are the Traditional Generation, born before 1940; the Baby Boomers, born between 1940 and 1960; Generation X (Gen Xers), born between 1960 and 1980; and the newest generation to hit the workforce, the Generation Y (Echo Boomers or Millennials), those born after 1980.

The Traditional Generation came of age after the Great Depression and were raised to be disciplined and obey their elders. They feel obligated to conform and believe that work is one's duty. The Traditional Generation was followed by the Baby Boomers, who came of age during a time of much available education and economic expansion. They work for the challenge of work and career advancement (Calhoun & Strasser, 2005). Baby Boomers have been characterized as workaholic, strong-willed individuals who are working for material gain, promotions, recognition, job security, and corner offices. Baby Boomers are the largest generation. They have had a dramatic financial impact on the present and are anticipated to impact the future dramatically as they begin to retire in 2006.

The Gen Xers are often called latch-key kids, as their parents were often away working. They learned to be self-reliant and independent. The Gen Xers are busy looking for career security, not job security. They are willing to change jobs and have little loyalty to their employers. They observed their parents going through multiple changes in their work organizations, such as downsizing and rightsizing. They are not workaholics, and they seek a balance between work and leisure. Gen Xers want a work environment that is technologically current, has competent leadership, and provides a mentor or coach for a boss.

Generation Yers are primarily the children of the Baby Boomers. They grew up with the end of the Cold War, the Internet, and a speak-your-mind philosophy. This generation is just beginning to make its mark on the workforce. What is known is that they are focusing on early retirement. Change is their mantra, and they expect countless options.

In the workplace, these generations all have different goals and needs (Kupperschmidt, 2000). For example, while the Traditional Generation and the Baby Boomers are retiring, many have elected to stay working, and they are now working, alongside the younger generations.

Nursing leadership of this diverse group of workers requires a different management style and increased

flexibility. The ACORN Model discussed by Kupperschmidt (2000) illustrates how a new leader can use opportunities to accommodate employee differences; create workplace choices; operate from a theoretically sound, sophisticated management style; and nourish nursing retention. For example, when creating workplace choices, a nurse leader might devise multiple scheduling options, that is, one size does not fit all. Furthermore, this leader would provide multiple opportunities for cross training and lateral and upward movement through the organization. Each generation has different needs for orientation, training, and opportunities for advancement and benefits. While meeting these different needs, the nurse manager still needs to bring the groups together and begin to form a team (Hu, Herrick, & Hodgin, 2004). Chapter 11 provides more information on effective team building.

SPIRITUALITY

In nearly every culture, spirituality is a component of healing, yet many nurses seldom assess the concept of spirituality or work to help patients meet their spiritual needs. In the workplace, spiritual considerations are often ignored unless an individual pushes the issue.

During the first sixty years of the twentieth century, there was considerable attention paid by nursing to religious issues. Then during the cultural change of the 1960s and 1970s, little was written on religion. In the mid 1980s, interest developed in the holistic component of spirituality. Each succeeding year thereafter, there has been an increasing amount of research and thought on spirituality. For many years, the focus was on defining the term, *spirituality*. The researchers found the term difficult to quantify and finally concluded that spirituality is a

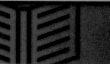

CRITICAL THINKING 25-6

When working on a nursing team, consider the values, goals, and outcomes of the members and generations on the team. Make a list of how your generation is different from the one before it and the generation after your own. How can you improve your ability to work together?

EVIDENCE FROM THE LITERATURE

Citation: Grossman, C. L. (2006, Sept. 12). View of God can reveal your values and politics. *USA Today*, 1A.

Discussion: Article reports on the Baylor University religion survey of 1,721 Americans. The survey found that 91.8% of those surveyed say they believe in God, a higher power, or a cosmic force. The other respondents said they were atheists, did not answer, or weren't sure. Respondents had four distinct views of God's personality, that is, Authoritarian, Benevolent, Critical, and Distant. The article discusses how these four views of God affect politics, such as gay marriage, stem cell research, war, abortion, and federal government involvement in life and world affairs.

Implications for Practice: Many Americans believe in God and may want assistance with their spiritual needs during times of illness and stress. Nurses can play a role in helping patients obtain the assistance they need.

complex and enigmatic concept (Martsolf & Mickley, 1998; McSherry & Draper, 1998). Foley, Wagner, and Waskel (1998) described spirituality as a multifaceted concept specific to the spiritually lived experience of an individual. This description gives the nurse little direction in assessing or intervening when there is evidence of spiritual need or distress.

SPIRITUAL ASSESSMENT

Providing holistic patient care includes assessing the spiritual needs of the patient in addition to the biophysical and psychosocial needs. To provide spiritual care, an understanding of the patient's beliefs can be used to plan appropriate interventions. In contemporary nursing, spirituality has become an important area of assessment during hospitalization. The national health care accrediting body, the Joint Commission, recently focused on the assessment of spirituality, requiring nurses to ask patients some questions regarding their spiritual needs. However, asking the questions, "What is your religion?" or "What religious needs can we meet during your hospitalization?" leaves the nurse with only descriptive labels. To meet the spiritual needs of patients, nurses need to understand more than these labels. Patients may be asked if they would like to see their spiritual leader or advisor, with the understanding that not all patients will want to meet with a clergy member. Nurses need to know and use various resources available for providing spiritual support to patients. Many inpatient facilities have pastoral care departments that conduct formal services, visit and pray with patients and their families, conduct support groups (for example, bereavement), and provide information regarding organ donation, living wills, and other end-of-life services (Duldt, 2002). Kuepfer, as cited in Ray (2004) addresses a shift in the duties of hospital chaplains from focusing mainly on providing religious rites to empowering the hospital staff members to serve the community.

REAL WORLD INTERVIEW

Only when you meet the spiritual needs of your patient can you say that you have treated the patient as a whole. Spiritual realities exist whether one believes in them or not. In fact, nurses consider all world views when directing or providing care.

Celeste Lynn Hagen Proctor, MS, RN
Roseville, California

Several research tools are used for measuring spirituality:

- *Spiritual Well-Being:* This tool measures the psychological dimension of spiritual wellness (Ellison & Paloutzain, 1999).
- *JAREL Spiritual Well-Being Scale:* This tool measures harmony as a function of interconnectedness (Hungelmann, Kenkel-Rossi, Klassen, & Stollenwerk, 1989).
- *Spiritual Perspective Scale:* This tool measures the extent to which one holds spiritual views during spirituality-related interactions (Reed, 1986).

For the nurse looking to understand spirituality in an effort to provide comfort to patients during illness or crisis, these tools provide some guidance.

SPIRITUAL DISTRESS

Spiritual distress is a North American Nursing Diagnosis Association (NANDA) term used to identify when an individual has an impaired ability to integrate meaning and purpose in life through the individual's connectedness with self, others, art, music, literature, nature, or a power greater than oneself (Ackley & Ladwig, 2006). To decrease or eliminate spiritual distress, it is expected that an individual will connect with the elements he or she considers important to arrive at meaning and purpose in life. These elements may include meditation; prayer; participating in religious services or rituals; communing with nature, plants, and animals; sharing of self; and caring for self and others. The Wikoff (2003) Spiritual Focus Questionnaire (Table 25-7) is designed to ascertain what is spiritually important to the individual. It assesses the concepts of relationships with a Higher Power, Self, other Family and Friends, Nature, and Religion. Each question can be scored on a 0-4 scale arriving at a total score for each area of the questionnaire. The tool is not designed to measure the strength or amount of spirituality. The higher score(s) suggest the concepts most important to the patient, thereby allowing the nurse to develop interventions that can assist the individual in finding that meaning and purpose.

Reviewing the Spiritual Focus Questionnaire and knowing a patient's spiritual needs helps a nurse develop interventions to help patients. Nursing interventions for spiritual needs could include the nurse requesting a visit from a patient's spiritual leader or helping a patient obtain spiritual or religious tapes or music. The nurse can offer the patient uninterrupted quiet time to allow the patient time for personal prayer or reading of spiritual and religious material. Most religious groups from Christians to Jews to Muslims to Buddhists communicate spiritually through prayer or meditation.

TABLE 25-7   WIKOFF SPIRITUAL FOCUS QUESTIONNAIRE

Spiritual Focus Questionnaire Instructions: The following questions assess your expressions of spirituality. Please rate each question by checking the box indicating importance to you as 4=very important, 3=somewhat important, 2=not important, 1=very unimportant, 0=neither important or unimportant.

Question	4	3	2	1	0
1. My strongest relationship is with a Higher Power.					
2. The time I spend in connection with a Higher Power is essential.					
3. In my personal life, I feel close to a Higher Power/Supreme Being.					
4. I spend time daily talking to a Higher Power.					
Higher Power Total Score					
5. I count on myself as my spiritual center.					
6. I feel an internal calmness when I am at peace with myself.					
7. My spirituality comes from within me.					
8. To find spiritual peace, I look inside myself.					
Self Total Score					
9. I renew my spirit with my family/friends.					
10. Special people within my life are my spiritual focus.					
11. When spiritually discouraged, I seek help from my family/friends.					
12. Others around me help quiet my spirit.					
Others Total Score					
13. I make an effort to spend time in the quiet solitude of nature.					
14. In nature, I reflect on its magnitude and importance to me.					
15. My connection with natural things helps me find inner peace.					
16. When in nature, I feel thankful for my blessings.					
Nature Total Score					
17. Through my religion, I find inner calmness.					
18 My religion gives my life spiritual focus.					
19. The time I spend in religious activities renews my spirit.					
20. My religion helps me keep my life in perspective.					
Religion Total Score					
Overall Total					

Source: Wikoff, 2003.

REAL WORLD INTERVIEW

I t is extremely important to recognize the problems that caregivers experience as they make decisions and struggle through their loved ones' stages of Alzheimer's Disease. These problems include stress, guilt, religious, spiritual, and emotional turmoil. In northern Indiana, there have been over 36,500 patients diagnosed with Alzheimer's Disease. Seven out of ten patients live at home. Seventy-five percent of them are cared for by family and friends. Those family members and friends need to take care of themselves, also, as they are vital to their loved ones. They must maintain some normalcy in their own lives and stay mentally and physically healthy for their own well-being as well as for the well-being of their loved ones. To assist them, Alzheimer's Services of Northern Indiana (ASNI), a nonprofit organization, shares information, at no cost to the families, about respite home care, adult day care centers, specialized Alzheimer's units in nursing homes, local support groups, and family outreach programs. We offer a 24 hour toll-free HELP line (1-888-303-0180). ASNI's mission statement, which we take quite seriously, is "Bringing hope and help to Alzheimer's families in northern Indiana."

Leona Bachan, Community Relations Coordinator
Alzheimer's Services of Northern Indiana
Munster, Indiana

EVIDENCE FROM THE LITERATURE

Citation: Tzeng, H. M., & Yin, C. Y. (2006). Learning to respect a patient's spiritual needs concerning an unknown infectious disease. *Nursing Ethics, 13*(1), 17–28.

Discussion: While the location of this article is Taiwan, there are parallels for nursing practice anywhere a new disease might develop. The first readily transmissible disease of the twenty-first century was Severe Acute Respiratory Syndrome (SARS). It occurred in twenty-nine countries. In a Taiwanese hospital, there was a substantial outbreak of SARS. All staff and patients were quarantined within the hospital. Despite their medical knowledge in a time of rapid technological development, the Taiwanese community began to see the disease from the framework of a religious concept called a taboo. A taboo in Taiwan acts as a part of folk religion that serves as a cultural and psychological remedy for society. It is thought that this religious concept of the taboo worked to unite the community to overcome the crisis. To illustrate the shift to folk belief by patients during a time of crisis, a diary written by a medical doctor who developed a case of SARS is shared in the article. The story the medical doctor tells is of his own increasing reliance on prayer to the gods, seeking divine advice, and asking others to pray for him during his episode of SARS. While his traditional medical beliefs were important, he also prayed to Jehovah, the Virgin Mary, the Goddess of Mercy, the Buddha, and Bodhisattva. He discusses his sense of powerlessness in the article and his sense of not knowing what he could do to aid his recovery during his illness.

Implications for Practice: In times of crisis, it can be expected that many will return to their cultural religious heritage for reassurance regarding healing and a return to wellness. Nurses need to be willing to respect personal beliefs that may be foreign to them and even against known scientific data. These personal beliefs may help the patient shift toward or away from survival.

BARRIERS TO SPIRITUAL CARE

Barriers to providing spiritual care are often more common for nurses than barriers to providing any other type of care or service. One of the barriers that nurses face (McEwen, 2005) may be those of a personal nature where the nurse believes that spiritual needs are private and not the purview of the nurse, and therefore, not a nursing responsibility. The nurse may be uncomfortable or embarrassed by their own spirituality and find it upsetting to

TABLE 25-8   SPIRITUAL NURSING INTERVENTIONS

- Open a dialogue with the patient regarding the purpose and meaning of life.

- Allow the patient to describe their spiritual life.

- Ask the patient if prayer plays a role in their life. If comfortable, you can offer to pray with the patient.

- Offer to seek the spiritual or religious leader of their choice, such as, pastor, priest, imam, rabbi, and so on.

- Be physically present, and listen to the patient. Seek a quiet, noninterrupted environment.

- Use therapeutic touch by holding the patient's hand or gently touching the patient's arm.

- Seek an answer to how you may provide support to the individual patient.

- Support patient-directed spiritual activities, such as receiving sacraments, anointing meditation, and so on.

- Focus on spiritual relationships and how you might provide support for patients with spiritual needs.

Source: Compiled with information from Ackley, B. J., & Ladwig, G. B. (2006). *Nursing diagnosis handbook: A guide to planning care* (7th Ed.). St. Louis, MO: Mosby.

deal with the issues that bring up spiritual distress, such as death and dying or suffering and grief. A lack of knowledge regarding the specific beliefs of a patient's religion and how to facilitate those spiritual needs are other potential barriers to quality nursing care delivery. Finally, there is often insufficient nursing time or privacy to allow a patient to discuss their spiritual beliefs.

These barriers to spiritual care sometimes form an apparently legitimate reason for nurses to avoid the necessary interaction to determine the patient's spiritual needs. Spiritual needs are often ignored, forgotten, and never dealt with. As a result, patients experience even more distress and suffering. This distress can be avoided by supporting and spending time with the patient. Other nursing interventions to help patients are included in Table 25-8.

CHAMPIONING SPIRITUALITY

The nurse leader who champions spirituality for all staff ensures that this component of holistic nursing is not for-

gotten or marginalized. For example, there may be an employee requesting a Saturday or Sunday every week off to attend religious services. When nurses are needed to work every other weekend, this can pose a problem for the nurse leader. A possible solution is to pair two nurses, where one works every Saturday and the other works every Sunday. Both nurses are then able to meet their spiritual needs without a negative impact on staffing a nursing unit.

There are religious holidays or celebrations that have spiritual and cultural significance. An understanding and empathetic approach to vacation requests will ensure contented staff and minimize turnover. It is also important to consider important markers of life such as weddings, births, and deaths. There are many cultural and spiritual overtones to these life events that need to be respected by nursing leadership practices. Sensitivity to the spiritual practices of the staff will enable the nurse manager to provide a compassionate and caring leadership.

DEVELOPING SPIRITUAL LEADERSHIP

Spiritual leadership involves using values and beliefs as the basis for dealing with all staff and patients within an organization. It is using compassion, caring, and nurturing to create an environment that reflects the values and beliefs of the leaders, patients, and staff. Spiritual leaders develop trust and connect with their staff on both a personal and professional level. This connection is then the basis for change and growth within the organization. The ability to connect and build relationships among staff and leadership, inspire others, and spot problems early results in a cohesive and positive workplace.

CRITICAL THINKING 25-7

How does your own spirituality influence the way you provide nursing care? Are you comfortable with your spirituality?

EVIDENCE FROM THE LITERATURE

Citation: Villagomeza, L. R. (2006). Mending broken hearts: The role of spirituality in cardiac illness: A research synthesis, 1991–2004. *Holistic Nursing Practice, 20*(4), 169–186.

Discussion: This research synthesis analyzed research on spirituality in cardiac illness from 1991 to 2004 to identify progress, gaps, and priorities for research. Articles were retrieved from PubMed and CINAHL. Twenty-six studies met the inclusion criteria. Moody's Research Analysis Tool, Version 2004, was used to analyze studies. Lack of a conceptual model and a universal definition of spirituality are major knowledge gaps identified. A proposed conceptual model is presented.

The proposed conceptual model of spirituality has seven distinct but overlapping constructs: a sense of connectedness, value system, sense of self-transcendence, sense of inner strength and energy, sense of inner peace and harmony, sense of purpose and meaning in life, and faith and a religious belief system.

Implications for Practice: Heart disease has been reported as bringing "one's spiritual side into greater focus." Spirituality, the dimension of human life that been regarded as the central artery that permeates, energizes, and enlivens all other dimensions, may serve as buffer for the stressful physical, emotional, and psychologic events associated with illness. Spirituality is the manner by which human beings make sense of life events and establish the meaning of their existence amid potentially life-threatening illnesses. Nurses concerned with quality patient care can help strengthen this spirituality buffer.

KEY CONCEPTS

- Culture affects both the nursing staff and the patient.

- Cultural competence is an important component of nursing.

- Organizations that nurses work in have distinct cultures.

- Each culture has its own values.

- Five major population groups are counted in the U.S. Census.

- Nurses are moving to increase the number of various population groups in nursing.

- Each generation has different values, goals, and expected outcomes from its work and life experiences.

- Spirituality may include religion and reflects one's values and beliefs.

- Spiritual Assessment is a requisite of holistic nursing.

- Many barriers can interfere with meeting a patient's spiritual needs.

KEY TERMS

culture
culturally competent care
generation
marginalization

organizational culture
race
spiritual distress

REVIEW QUESTIONS

1. Stephanie, the Gen X night shift charge nurse, is requesting more time off than any other charge nurse. What reason for this best represents her generation? She
   A. prefers to work the day shift and is hoping for a schedule change.
   B. believes that there are other nurses just as capable to do her role.
   C. wants to increase her leisure time to balance with work.
   D. seeks to be rewarded for time spent at work.

2. Nurses may fail to meet spiritual needs because of which of the following?
   A. Lack of compassion
   B. Lack of knowledge regarding the patient's illness
   C. Lack of understanding of the patient's spiritual beliefs
   D. Lack of chaplains in the care area

3. During orientation to work on a new unit, the nurse experiences a sense of isolation from his preceptors. Which of the following actions will best increase his socialization into the preceptor group? The nurse should
   A. ask as many questions as he can.
   B. request that his orientation be increased for two more weeks.
   C. study the differences between his values and his preceptor group's values.
   D. arrive late for duty frequently.

4. An organization's workplace culture reflects which of the following?
   A. The cultural affiliations of the staff
   B. The religion practiced by the hospital's leadership group
   C. The culture of its preceptors
   D. The values and beliefs of the organization

5. The Traditional Generation may do which of the following?
   A. Value working as one's duty
   B. Have a speak-your-mind philosophy
   C. Value working primarily for the challenge
   D. Use the Internet daily as a part of their life

REVIEW ACTIVITIES

1. You are called to problem solve a situation between a patient and a staff nurse. The patient is refusing to allow the nurse to take care of him because the nurse is wearing a headscarf. How will you handle the situation?

2. You live in a small community with little diversity. A patient that you are scheduled to take care of is visiting from a large city. This patient is from India and speaks only Hindi, a language unfamiliar to the staff. When you walk in the room, there are no visitors or anyone to translate. How will you approach your care in a culturally competent manner?

3. You are hiring several new graduate nurses to work on a unit that has had little turnover in the past ten years. Many of the current staff are Traditionals and Baby Boomers and have been in this organization for the entire length of their career. How will you go about integrating the Generation Xers and Generation Yers of nurses into this group?

4. You are taking care of a trauma patient in the ER. The patient has 70% burns over his body. The likelihood of the patient's survival is unknown. There is a lot of noise and distraction in the ER as well as many family members within earshot. The patient asks you to pray for him and his family. How will you respond?

5. As the nurse manager, you are asked to intervene with a male patient and his family. The nursing staff are concerned that the adult children of the male patient do not allow the patient to do anything for himself. The patient always has someone at his bedside who does all the care and refuses to allow the father to do anything, including feeding himself. The family's behavior is out of a cultural belief of caring for and respecting their elders. As the patient has had a recent cerebral vascular accident (CVA), you know that self-care is a requisite to healing. How will you intervene in a culturally competent way?

EXPLORING THE WEB

- This Website is devoted to developing cultural awareness and diversity in health care. It includes a list serve. *www.diversityrx.org*

- The International Sigma Theta Tau (nursing honor society) site's position paper on diversity. What does the nursing honor society believe about diversity? *www.nursingsociety.org*

- This site contains information about cultural beliefs and medical issues pertinent to the health care of recent immigrants to the United States. Who are the most recent immigrants and what are their cultural needs? *www.ethnomed.org*

- Access the Center for the Study of Cultural Diversity in Health Care at the University of Wisconsin. Find Webcasts from recent conferences. *http://cdh.med.wisc.edu*

- The U.S. Department of Health and Human Services-Office of Minority Health. *www.omhrc.gov*

- The Provider's Guide to Quality and Culture: *http://erc.msh.org*

- Canadian Nurses Association. *www.can-nurses.ca*

- National Alaska Native American Indiana Nurses (NANAINA): *www.nanainanurses.org*

- National Black Nurses Association, Inc.: *www.nbna.org*

- Transcultural Nursing Society: *www.tcns.org*

- U.S. Census Bureau: *www.census.gov*

- Islamic Information Center of American (IICA): *www.iica.org*

- Islamic Information Office: *www.iio.org*

- U.S. Citizenship and Immigration Services: *www.uscis.gov*

- American-Arab Antidiscrimination Committee: *www.adc.org*

- American Civil Liberties Union (ACLU): *www.aclu.org*

- American Indian Culture Research Center: *www.bluecloud.org*

- American Indian Heritage Foundation: *www.indians.org*

- American Jewish Community: *www.ajc.org*

- Anti-Defamation League: *www.adl.org*

- Asia Society: *www.asiasociety.org*

- Asian and Pacific Islander Partnership for Health: *www.apiph.org*

- National Association for the Advancement of Colored People: *www.naacp.org*
- Urban League: *www.nul.org*
- International Council of Nurses: *www.icn.ch*
- Global Health Council: *www.globalhealth.org*
- World Health Organization: *www.who.org*
- United States Committee for Refugees: *www.irsa.org*

REFERENCES

Ackley, B. J., & Ladwig, G. B. (2006). *Nursing diagnosis handbook: A guide to planning care* (7th ed.). St. Louis, MO: Mosby.

American Academy of Nursing. (1992). AAN expert panel report: Culturally competent health care. *Nursing Outlook, 40*(6), 277–283.

American Association of Colleges of Nursing (AACN). (2002). *Peaceful death: Recommended competencies and curricular guidelines for end-of-life nursing care.* Retrieved July, 2004, from http://www.aacn.nche.edu

Barbee, E. L. (1993). Racism in U.S. nursing. *Medical Anthropology Quarterly, 7*(4), 3436–3462.

Brink, P. J. (1990). Cultural diversity in the nursing profession. In J. C. McCluskey & H. K. Grace (eds.), *Current issues in nursing* (3rd ed.). Boston: Blackwell Scientific.

Burkhart, M. A., & Nagai-Jacobson, M. G. (2002). *Spirituality· Living our connectedness.* Clifton Park, NY: Thomson Delmar Learning.

Burner, O. Y., Cunningham, P., & Hattar, H. S. (1990). Managing a multicultural nurse staff in a multicultural environment. *Journal of Nursing Administration, 20*(6), 30–34.

Calhoun, S. K., & Strasser, P. B. (2005). Generations at work. *AAOHN, 53*(11), 469–471.

Campinha-Bacote, J., & Munoz, C. (2001). A guiding framework for delivering culturally competent services in case management. *The Care Manager, 12,* 48–52.

Campinha-Bacote, J. (2003, Jan. 31). Many faces: Addressing diversity in health care. *Online Journal of Issues in Nursing, 8*(1), manuscript. Retrieved April 18, 2006, from http://nursingworld.org/ojin/topic20/tpc20_2.htm

DeRosa, N., & Kochurka, K. (2006, Oct.). Implement culturally competent healthcare in your workplace. *Nursing Management, 18*–26.

DiJoseph, J., & Cavendish, R. (2005, July/Aug.). Expanding the dialogue on prayer relevant to holistic care. *Holistic Nursing Practice,* 147–155.

Duldt, B. (2002). The spiritual dimension of holistic care. *Journal of Nursing Administration, 32*(1), 20–24.

Ellison, C. W., & Paloutzain, R. F. (1999). *Measures of Religiosity.* Birmingham, AL: Religious Education Press.

Foley, L., Wagner, J., & Waskel. S. (1998). Spirituality in the lives of older women. *Journal of Women and Aging, 10*(2), 85–91.

Giger, N., & Davidhizar, R. J. (1996). When the operating room has a multicultural team. *Today's Surgical Nurse, 18*(5), 26–32.

Giger, J., & Davidhizar, T. (2004). Transcultural nursing: Assessment and intervention (4th ed.). St. Louis, MO: Mosby Year Book.

Grossman, C. L. (2006, Sept. 12). View of God can reveal your values and politics. *USA Today,* 1A.

Hu, J., Herrick, C., & Hodgin, K. A. (2004). Managing the multigenerational nursing team. *The Health Care Manager, 23*(4), 334–340.

Hungelmann, J., Kenkel-Rossi, E., Klassen, L., & Stollenwerk, R. (1989). Development of the JAREL Spiritual Well-Being Scale. In R. M. Carroll-Johnson (Ed.), *Classification of nursing diagnoses proceedings of the eighth conference North American nursing diagnosis association* (393–398). Philadelphia: Lipinncott.

Jamieson, D. & O'Mara, J. (1991). *Managing workforce 2000: Gaining the diversity advantage.* San Francisco: Jossey-Bass.

Jein, R. F., & Harris, B. L. (1989). Cross-cultural conflict: The American nurse manager and a culturally mixed staff. *Journal of the New York State Nurses Association, 20*(2), 16–19.

Joint Commission. (2003). Comprehensive accreditation manual for hospitals. Chicago: Author.

Keltner, B., Kelley, F., & Smith, D. (2004). Leadership to reduce health disparities: A model for nursing leadership in American Indian communities. *Nursing Administration Quarterly, 28*(3), 181–190.

Koenig, H. G., George, L. K., & Titus, P. (2004). Religion, spirituality, and health in medically ill hospitalized old. *Journal of American Geriatric Society, 2*(4), 554–562.

Kupperschmidt, B. R. (2000). Multigeneration employees: Strategies for effective management. *Heath Care Management, 19*(1), 65–76.

Leininger, M. (1978). *Transcultural nursing: Concepts, theories and practice.* New York: Wiley.

Leininger, M. (1997). Transcultural nursing research to nursing education and practice: 40 years. *Image Journal of Nursing Scholarship, 29*(4), 341–347.

Lipson, J. G. & Dibble, S. L. (2005). *Culture and clinical care.* San Francisco: UCSF Nursing Press.

Martsolf, D. S., & Mickley, J. R. (1998). The concept of spirituality in nursing theories: differing world-views and extent of focus. *Journal of Advanced Nursing, 27,* 294–303.

Mazanec, P., & Tyler, M. K. (2004). Cultural considerations in end-of-life care: How ethnicity, age, and spirituality affect decisions when death is imminent. *Home Healthcare Nurse, 22*(5), 317–324.

McCord, G., Gilchrist, V., Grossman, S., King, B., McCormick, K., Oprandi, A., et al. (2004). Discussing spirituality with patients: A rational and ethical approach. *Annals of Family Medicine, 2*(4), 356–361.

McEwen, M. (2005, July–Aug.). Spiritual nursing care. *Holistic Nursing Practice,* 161–168.

McSherry, W., & Draper, P. (1998). The debates emerging from the literature surrounding the concept of spirituality as applied to nursing. *Journal of Advanced Nursing, 27*(4), 683–691.

Mead, M. (2001). *Sex and temperament in three primitive societies.* New York: Harper Collins Publishers.

Molter, N. (2003). Creating a healing environment for critical care. *Critical Care Nursing Clinics of North America, 15*(3), 295–304.

Munoz, C., & Luckmann, J. (2005). *Transcultural communication.* Clifton Park, NY: Thomson Delmar Learning.

Nussbaum, G. (2003). Spirituality in critical care. *Critical Care Nursing Quarterly, 26*(3), 214–220.

Ott, J. (1989). *The organizational culture perspective* (20–48). Chicago: Dorsey Press.

Purnell, L. (2005). The Purnell model for cultural competence. *The Journal of Multicultural Nursing and Health, 11*(2), 7–15.

Ray, R. (2004). The faith connection. *NurseWeek, A Nursing Spectrum Publication, 11*(9), 17–20.

Reed, P. G. (1986). Spirituality and well-being in terminally ill hospitalized adults. *Research in Nursing and Health, 35,* 368–374.

Spangler, A. (1992). Transcultural care values and practices of Philippine-American nurses. *Journal of Transcultural Nursing, 4*(2), 28–31.

Spector, R. E. (2004). *Cultural diversity in health and illness* (6th ed.). Upper Saddle River, NJ: Pearson Prentice Hall.

Taylor, E. J. (2002). *Spiritual care: Nursing theory, research and practice.* Upper Saddle River, NJ: Prentice Hall.

The Providers Guide to Quality & Culture. Retrieved April 2, 2007, from http://erc.msh.org/mainpage.cfm?file=1.0.htm&module=provider&language=English

Tzeng, H. M., & Yin, C. Y. (2006). Learning to respect a patient's spiritual needs concerning an unknown infectious disease. *Nursing Ethics, 13*(1), 17–28.

U.S. Census Bureau. (2001). U.S. Department of Commerce News. Washington, DC. Retrieved March 12, 2001, from *www.census.gov/PressRelease2001*

U.S. Department of Health and Human Services Preliminary Findings: 2004 National Sample Survey of Registered Nurses. (n.d.). Retrieved on May 30, 2006, from http://bhpr.hrsa.gov/healthworkforce/reports/rnpopulation/preliminaryfindings.htm

Villagomeza, L. R. (2006). Mending broken hearts: The role of spirituality in cardiac illness: A research synthesis, 1991–2004. *Holistic Nursing Practice, 20*(4), 169–186.

Walton, J. C., & Waszkiewiez, M. (1997). Managing unlicensed assistive personnel: Tips for improving quality outcomes. *Medsurg Nursing, 6*(1), 124–128.

Wikoff, K. L. (2003). Development and psychometric evaluation of the Wikoff Spiritual Focus Questionnaire. *Dissertation Abstracts International, 64*(04), 1691. (UMI No. AAT 3088678).

Williams, J., & Rodgers, S. (1993). The multicultural workplace: Preparing preceptors. *Journal of Continuing Education in Nursing, 24*(3), 101–104.

SUGGESTED READINGS

Ai, A. L., Peterson, C., Tice, T. N., Bolling, S. F., & Koenig, H. G. (2004). Faith-based and secular pathways to hope and optimism subconstructs in middle-aged and older cardiac patients. *Journal of Health Psychology, 9*(3), 435–450.

Davidhizar, R., & Giger, J. (2004). A review of the literature on care of clients in pain who are culturally diverse. *International Council of Nurses, 51,* 47–55.

Dossey, B. M., Keegan, L., & Guzzetta, G. E. (2003). *Holistic nursing: a handbook for practice* (3rd ed.). Boston: Jones & Bartlett.

Foley, R., & Wurmuser, T. A. (2004). Culture diversity: A mobile workforce command creative leadership, new partnerships, and innovative approaches to innovation. *Nursing Administrative Quarterly, 28*(2), 122–128.

Frankl, V. (1985). *Man's search for meaning.* New York: Washington Square Press.

Kaplan, M. (2005). You are special: Recognizing the gifts you bring to oncology nursing. *Clinical Journal of Oncology Nursing, 9*(3), 313–316.

North Amerian Nursing Diagnosis Association (NANDA). (2007). *Nursing diagnoses: Definitions and classification 2007–2008.* Philadelphia: Author.

Reb, A. M. (2003). Palliative and end-of-life care: Policy analysis. *Oncology Nursing Forum, 30*(4), 551–555.

Salimbene, S. (2005). *What language does your patient hurt in? A practical guide to culturally competent patient care.* Amherst, MA: Diversity Resources, Inc.

Taylor, E. J. (2002). *Spiritual care: Nursing theory, research and practice.* Upper Saddle River, NJ: Prentice Hall.

Ulrich, B. (2004). Keep the faith. *NurseWeek, A Nursing Spectrum Publication, 11*(9), 2.

Villagomeza, L. R. (2005, Nov.–Dec.). Spiritual distress in adult cancer patients. *Holistic Nursing Practice,* 285–294.

Wieck, K. L. (2005, Aug.–Oct.). Generational approaches to current nursing issues. *ISNA (Indiana State Nurses Association) Bulletin,* 27–30.

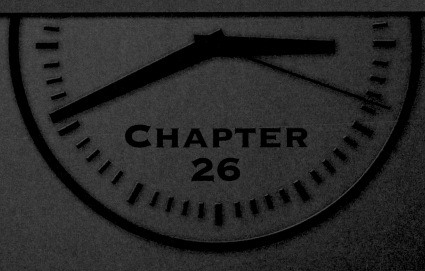

UNIT V
Leadership and Management of Self and the Future

CHAPTER 26

Collective Bargaining

Janice Tazbir, RN, MS, CCRN

You will have much opposition to encounter. But great works do not prosper without great opposition (Florence Nightingale, 1864, cited in Ulrich, 1992).

OBJECTIVES

Upon completion of this chapter, the reader should be able to:

1. Relate the history of collective bargaining and associated legislation.
2. Identify collective action models and associated terminology.
3. Outline the steps of whistle-blowing.
4. Identify the process of unionization.
5. Identify collective bargaining agents.
6. Summarize professionalism and unionization.
7. Relate the process of managing in a union environment.
8. Analyze pros and cons of collective bargaining in the workplace.

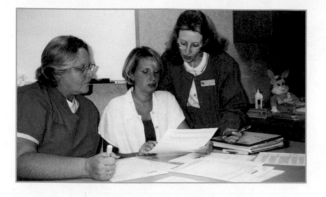

You are a new nurse on an orthopedic unit. You walk into a discussion between two nurses. Juanita, a registered nurse with 10 years of experience, states, "I'm tired of low pay and work assignments that are unsafe." Peggy, a registered nurse with five years of experience, states, "Have you brought your complaints to management?" Juanita replies, "Of course. I point out unsafe situations and the lack of raises, but no one cares." Peggy says, "I bet we would have better success with these issues if we nurses came together as a group."

What are your thoughts about this situation?

What are some of the choices the nurses have?

Historically, nurses have often been perceived as hard-working, submissive staff who do what they are told. The scope of nursing has changed so drastically that today nurses cannot afford to have a submissive image and do only what they are told. Patients, their illnesses, and their families are more complex than ever. Nurses are educated to advocate for their patients and themselves. Clinical situations arise in which nurses must voice their opinions and stand up for what is best for patients. To be effective in today's world, nurses must understand the tools available to deal with problems.

Collective action, or simply acting as a group with a single voice, is one method of dealing with problems. **Collective bargaining** is the practice of employees, as a collective group, bargaining with management in reference to wages, work practices, and other benefits. This chapter discusses different types of collective action models as they may function in the health care environment, and also includes information concerning unionization, as well as professionalism within the context of unionization.

TABLE 26-1	**SUMMARY OF SELECTED LEGISLATION AFFECTING THE WORKPLACE**
Year and Title of Legislation	**Summary**
1898: Erdman Act	Outlawed discrimination by employers against union activities
1935: National Labor Relations Act (Wagner Act)	Gave private employees the right to organize unions to demand better wages and safer work environments
1938: Fair Labor Standards Act	Set minimum wage and maximum hours that can be worked before overtime is paid
1947: Taft-Hartley Act	Returned some rights to management; somewhat equalized balance between unions and management
1962: Kennedy Executive Order 10988	Amended National Labor Relations Act to allow public employees to join unions
1964: Civil Rights Act	Set equal employment standards such as equal pay for equal work
1965: Executive Order 11246	Set affirmative action guidelines
1967: Age Discrimination Act	Protects against forced retirement
1973: Rehabilitation Act	Protects rights of disabled people
1973: Vietnam Veterans Act	Provides reemployment rights
1974: Taft-Hartley Amendments to the Wagner Act	Allows nonprofit organizations to join unions

History of Collective Bargaining and Collective Bargaining Legislation in America

Collective bargaining and unionization have existed in the United States since the 1790s. Traditionally, people who formed and joined unions were highly skilled craftspeople. People found that by working collectively, they could set wages and standards for their trades. The Erdman Act, passed in 1898, was the first federal legislation to deal with collective bargaining. Since then, numerous legislative acts have been passed to ensure the rights of employees (Table 26-1). The rights many workers have today came from the struggles of others with the fortitude to stand up for what they believed was right.

Collective Action Models

One of the main purposes of collective action for nurses is to advance the profession of nursing (Budd, Warino, & Patton, 2004). Many nurses belong to numerous collectives, including specialty nursing organizations, church organizations, special interest clubs, community groups, and so on. The reason most people belong to these organizations is to better themselves and their communities or to promote and support the special interests of a group. Two types of nursing collective action are discussed in this chapter: workplace advocacy and collective bargaining. Shared governance, another type of collective action, is discussed in Chapter 17.

Workplace Advocacy

Workplace advocacy refers to activities nurses undertake to address problems in their everyday workplace setting. This type of collective action is probably the most common in nursing. An activity that falls under workplace advocacy is forming a committee to address problems, devising alternatives to achieve optimal care, and inventing new ways to implement change.

An example of an issue that would be addressed by workplace advocacy is patient advocacy. Patient advocacy is preserving and protecting the wishes of patients (Beyea, 2005). Patients rely on nurses to do this. Often, in the workplace, nurses are too busy to serve as a patient advocate, which causes the nurses and patients distress.

Other Forms of Workplace Advocacy

Nurses in many hospitals serve on professional practice councils. These councils are often part of a shared governance organization within the hospital that works to improve patient care and the environment for staff. Shared governance is discussed in Chapter 17.

Note that a supportive management will view workplace advocacy as a way to strengthen staff and promote teamwork. If the management is authoritative, however, workplace advocacy may not be encouraged because it may be perceived as a threat to management and its policies.

Collective Bargaining

In collective bargaining, the group is bargaining with management for what the group desires. If the group cannot achieve its desires through informal collective bargaining with management, the group may decide to use a collective bargaining agent to form a union.

Factors Influencing Nurses to Unionize

In general, nurses who are content in their workplace do not unionize (Forman & Grimes, 2004). It is when nurses feel powerless that they initiate attempts to unionize. Other motivations to unionize include job stress and physical demands (Budd et al., 2004). Nurses are also motivated to join unions when they feel the need to communicate concerns and complaints to management without fear of losing their jobs. Some nurses believe that they need a collective voice so that management will hear them and changes will be instituted.

Issues that are commonly the subject of collective bargaining include poor wages, unsafe staffing, health and safety issues, mandatory overtime, poor quality of care, job security, and restructuring issues such as cross-training nurses for areas of specialty other than those in which they were hired to practice (United American Nurses, 2006). Many nurse managers believe that it is best to deal quickly and effectively with issues that arise to avoid collective bargaining because of the increase in

EVIDENCE FROM THE LITERATURE

Citation: Cimiotti, J. P., Quinlan, P. M., Larson, E. L., Pastor, D. K., Lin, S. X., & Stone, P. W. (2005, Nov./Dec.). The magnet process and the perceived work environment of nurses. *Nursing Research, 54*(6), 384–390.

Discussion: This study compared the differences between characteristics of hospitals and nurses from three hospital types—magnet hospitals, hospitals in the process of applying for magnet certification, and nonmagnet hospitals—and how nurses from these hospitals perceive their work environment. Data were available from 2,092 nurse surveys. Over a third of the respondents were from magnet-in-process hospitals and almost half were from nonmagnet hospitals. The majority of nurses were female and from large hospitals in the Atlantic region. The mean age of nurses was 39.5 years, and the mean years of work experience in the Intensive Care Unit (ICU) was 10.2 years. Nurses from magnet hospitals had a positive perception of nursing competence in their work environment.

Implications for Practice: A magnet hospital has organizational, leadership, and professional practice characteristics that are consistent with a discrete set of research-based attributes associated with positive nursing and patient outcomes, more so than other hospitals. Nurses seeking employment may want to consider a magnet hospital.

costs to the hospital that results from collective bargaining and the limitations it places on managers.

UNIONS

A **union** is a formal and legal group that works through a collective bargaining agent to present desires to management formally, through the legal context of the National Labor Relations Board (NLRB).

Table 26-2 lists some collective action terminology. This is useful in understanding the collective bargaining process.

WHISTLE-BLOWING

As patient advocates, nurses protect patients from known harm. Nurses are often aware of health care fraud in the form of people violating laws or endangering public health or safety. However, some nurses who are aware of health care fraud do nothing because of fear of retribution. Fraud costs the federal government and ultimately costs the taxpayer.

Whistle-blowing is the act in which an individual discloses information regarding a violation of a law, rule, or regulation, or a substantial and specific danger to public health or safety. The government has recouped more than $2 billion since 1995 from whistle-blowers exposing fraud (Weinberg, 2005). Health care fraud can range from filing false claims to performing unnecessary procedures. As patient advocates, nurses have an ethical and moral duty to protect their patients. In 1986, the False Claims Act was modified to encourage whistle-blowers to come forward.

CRITICAL THINKING 26-2

You are caring for Mr. San Filipe, a 65-year-old man who was admitted for congestive heart failure. He is a retired steelworker from an area steel mill. He states, "I worked in that mill for 30 years, and I am thankful for the union. Because of the union, my medical costs are covered for the rest of my life. The union served me well. Do nurses have unions or groups that help them get what they want?"

How will you respond to Mr. San Filipe? Name two collective groups to which you belong. What are these collective groups able to get done as a whole? Are these collective groups more effective and stronger than you are as an individual in these interest areas? What are the downsides of belonging to a collective group?

Whistle-blowing claims are brought in *qui tam* lawsuits (Weinberg, 2005), which anyone can file on both the government's behalf and their own behalf. If the government believes an individual has a case of fraud, the government will pay all expenses for the lawsuit, and the individual will be entitled to 15% to 25% of the government's recovery. To date, over $199 million has been

TABLE 26-2　　COLLECTIVE BARGAINING TERMINOLOGY

Term	Definition
Agency shop	Synonymous with "open shop." Employees are not required to join the union but may join it.
Arbitration	Last step in a dispute. Indicates a nonpartial third party will be involved and may make the final decision. Arbitration may be voluntary or imposed by the government.
Collective bargaining	The practice of employees, as a collective, bargaining with management in reference to wages, work practices, and other benefits.
Collective bargaining agent	An agent that works with employees to formalize collective bargaining through unionization.
Contract	A set of guidelines and rules voted and agreed upon by union members that guides their work practices, wages, and other benefits.
Dispute	A disagreement between management and the union. A dispute may go through (1) mediation and conciliation, (2) arbitration, and possibly (3) a strike. A dispute may be settled at any stage.
Employee at will	An employee working without a contract. The employee agrees to work under given rules and may be terminated if the employee breaks any rules imposed by management.
Fact finding	Fact finding is used in labor management disputes that involve government-owned companies. It is the process in which claims of labor and management are reviewed. In the private sector, fact finding is usually performed by a board of inquiry.
Grievance	A grievance occurs when a union member believes that management has failed to meet the terms of the contract or labor agreement and communicates this to management.
Grievance proceedings	A formal process in which a union member believes that management has failed to meet the terms of the contract. The steps usually include (1) communication of the grievance to management, (2) mediation with a union representative and a member of management, and possibly (3) arbitration. The dispute may be settled at any step.
Lockout	Closing a place of business by management in the course of a labor dispute to attempt to force employees to accept management terms.
Mediation and conciliation	A step in the grievance process in which a nonpartial third party meets with management and the union to assist them in reaching an agreement. In this step, the third party has no actual power in decision making.
National Labor Relations Board (NLRB)	The National Labor Relations Board was formed to implement the Wagner Act. The two major functions of the board include (1) determining and implementing the free democratic choice of employees as to whether they choose to be or choose not to be in a union and (2) preventing and remedying unfair labor practices by employers or unions.
Professional	A person who has knowledge from formal studies and has autonomy.

(Continues)

TABLE 26-2   COLLECTIVE BARGAINING TERMINOLOGY (CONTINUED)

Term	Definition
Self-expression	"The expressing of any views, argument, or opinion, or the dissemination thereof, whether in written, printed, graphic or visual form[,] if such expression contains no threat or reprisal or force or promise of benefit" (National Labor Relations Act, 1994).
Strike	An act in which union members withhold the supply of labor for the purpose of forcing management to accept union terms.
Supervisor	A person with the authority to (1) impart corrective action and (2) delegate to an employee.
Union	A formal and legal group that brings forth desires to management through a collective bargaining agent and within the context of the National Labor Relations Board.
Union dues	Money required of all union employees to support the union and its functions.
Union shop	A place of employment in which all employees are required to join the union and pay dues. *Union shop* is synonymous with the term *closed shop*.
Whistle-blowing	Whistle-blowing is the act in which an individual discloses information regarding a violation of a law, rule, or regulation, or a substantial and specific danger to public health or safety.

CRITICAL THINKING 26-3

You are a nurse working at an institution in which there is limited flexibility in the scheduling. You want to institute self-scheduling, with the staff nurses responsible for making and maintaining the schedule. Make a plan to present this idea to the manager. How will you elicit the support of other nurses? Now put yourself in the role of the manager. How would you respond to this request?

received by whistle-blowers (Weinberg, 2005). The name of the person filing the suit will not be divulged if the government does not consider the matter to involve health care fraud, thereby protecting the person from any retribution from the employer. The employer will not know who attempted to "blow the whistle." If nurses are aware of

fraud in their practice setting, the proper steps for them to take include the following:

- File a *qui tam* lawsuit in secret with the court.
- Do not let the agency or hospital know you filed a lawsuit.
- Serve a copy of the complaint to the Department of Justice with a written disclosure of all the information you have concerning the fraud.
- If the government decides to go forward with the lawsuit, the government will bear responsibility for litigating the lawsuit, and the government will pay for it.

PROCESS OF UNIONIZATION

The process of choosing a collective bargaining unit and negotiating a contract may take three months to three years. There are formal steps to follow to legally form a union. A **collective bargaining agent** is an agent that works with employees to formalize collective bargaining through unionization. The American Nurses Association (ANA) outlines the steps in organizing a collective bargaining unit through a state nurses association in Table 26–3.

MANAGERS' ROLE

RNs have the legal authority to participate in collective bargaining in the majority of health care facilities in the country. Over the years, there has been debate over the composition of collective bargaining units in the health care industry. In 1989, the NLRB deemed eight collective bargaining units, including one for RNs, appropriate in the hospital setting. Some other collective bargaining units in the hospital include licensed practical nurses (LPNs), secretaries, and housekeepers. Managers who

---

CASE STUDY 26-1

You are a nurse working in a cardiac catheterization unit. You notice that a certain practitioner routinely performs cardiac catheterizations on patients who are in their early forties, have no risk factors for cardiac history, and are on Medicaid. The catheterizations are always negative for disease. You love your job but are troubled by this practice. You are fearful that patients will have complications. You ask the practitioner why these procedures are performed on patients who do not appear to need this testing. The response is, "You don't worry about what I do; these procedures keep us all employed with healthy paychecks." You discuss this with your nursing manager and the chief nursing executive, who both say, "Just do your job and let the practitioner decide what is best for your patients."

You decide that whistle-blowing is your next action. What is your first step? Should you notify management of your whistle-blowing? What policies exist in your agency to guide the nurse when the nurse finds unprofessional activities?

TABLE 26-3	**STEPS IN ORGANIZING A COLLECTIVE BARGAINING UNIT**

- Bring together a group of nurses supportive of collective bargaining.
- Arrange a meeting with a representative of the state nurses association to discuss organizing.
- Assess the feasibility of an organizing campaign at your facility.
- Conduct the necessary research, such as what are the needs and/or complaints of the employees, to develop a plan of action.
- Establish an organizing committee and subcommittees to facilitate organizing.
- Begin the process of obtaining union authorization cards from the National Labor Relations Board to legally vote on a collective bargaining agent.
- Schedule an informal meeting for nurses eligible for the collective bargaining unit.
- Keep the lines of communication open with nurses.
- Seek voluntary recognition from the employer.
- Move toward formal organization of the unit.
- Seek certification by the NLRB as the exclusive bargaining agent of the unit.
- Initiate contract negotiations.

Source: Compiled with information from "Nurses Organize" by the United American Nurses, 2006.

EVIDENCE FROM THE LITERATURE

Citation: Ellis, B., & Gates, J. (2006). Achieving magnet status. *Nursing Administration Quarterly, 29*(3), 241–244.

Discussion: Many hospitals are trying to acquire Magnet Service Recognition by the ANA. Magnet status essentially designates hospitals that attract and retain professional nurses and support, value, recognize, and reward the professional nurse. Some hospitals feel that unions are a barrier to achieving magnet status. In union institutions that have attained magnet status, they viewed respectful collective bargaining relationships as vital to maintaining a safe and fair work environment.

Implications for Practice: Nurses and institutions should not view unionization as deleterious in becoming a place that retains and values the nursing profession. In many instances, nurses unionize in an effort to attain many of the same goals that are achieved with magnet status. When hospitals attempt to obtain magnet status, it may be considered a first step in bringing nurses and hospitals together.

unionization is not professional and that the ANA cannot truly support nursing as a profession if it is also a collective bargaining agent. Because nurse managers are excluded from union membership, many nurse managers believe they have been left outside the organization that is supposed to represent all of nursing. Other nurse managers do not feel this separation (Fitzpatrick, 2001).

The ANA represents the interests of nurses in collective bargaining and in many other areas as well. The ANA advances the nursing profession by fostering high standards for nursing practice and lobbies Congress and regulatory agencies on health care issues affecting nurses and the general public. The ANA initiates many policies involving health care reform. It also publishes its position on issues ranging from whistle-blowing to patients' rights. The ANA recently launched a major campaign to mobilize nurses to address the staffing crisis, to educate and gain support from the public, and to develop and implement initiatives designed to resolve the crisis (United American Nurses, 2006). American Nurses Credentialing Center, a subsidiary of the ANA, created the Magnet Recognition Program to recognize health care organizations that provide the very best in nursing care. Since 1994, more than 168 institutions have received this award.

REAL WORLD INTERVIEW

I believe it is professional to be in a union because you have more opportunities to stand up for your patients and your own nursing practice. Having worked in both a union and a nonunion environment, I think being in a union allows you to speak your mind without fear of losing job security. They can't dismiss you for just any reason. There are grievance proceedings. In a nonunion environment, if they don't like you or what you say, they can punish you. But I've also seen the downside of unions. An example is when a contract comes out. The more-senior union nursing staff wants to hold out from agreeing on a contract that does not address all of our concerns while the junior union nursing staff wants to agree on the first contract that is presented. Holding out for what you want is why there is arbitration. The junior nurses don't realize the power of the bargaining unit in nursing. I think most nurses don't realize what we as nurses can accomplish if we stick together.

Susan Zielinski, RN
Staff Nurse
Chicago, Illinois

PROFESSIONALISM AND UNIONIZATION

Requirements for a vocation to be considered a profession include: (1) a long period of specialized education, (2) a service orientation, and (3) the ability to be autonomous (Jacox, 1980). Jacox (1980) defines autonomy as a characteristic of a profession in which the members of that profession are self-regulating and have control of their functions in the work situation. Nurses agree that specialized education and a service orientation are necessary to become a nurse, but many nurses disagree on the concept of autonomy. This disagreement is the central argument that divides nurses with regard to whether it is professional to be part of a union.

Many nurses believe that for nursing to be considered a profession, nurses must exercise autonomy, and like most professionals, work out issues themselves. Many argue that this cannot be done without unionization. The debate about whether it is professional to be a part of a nurse's union has plagued nursing since the inception of nursing unions.

DEFINITION OF SUPERVISOR

Much discussion in nursing unions has revolved around the definition of a supervisor. The National Labor Relations Act (1994), in Title 29 of the United States Code, defines a supervisor as "any individual having authority, in the interest of the employer, to hire, transfer, suspend, lay off, recall, promote, discharge, assign, reward, or discipline other employees, or the responsibility to direct them, or to adjust their grievances, or effectively, to recommend such action, if in connection with the foregoing, the exercise of such authority is not of a merely routine or clerical nature, but requires the use of independent judgment."

Using this definition, conceivably every nurse may be considered a supervisor—if not to another RN, then of LPNs, nurse's aides, and unlicensed personnel. The larger issue for discussion is, if all nurses are supervisors by definition, can they legally be in a union? Nursing unions do not allow nursing managers or supervisors to unionize. Only nurses defined as employees can unionize. The ambiguity of the terms *employees* and *supervisors* has caused legal disputes (Fine, 2006). Dependent on clarification from the legal system, nurses may not always have the privilege to unionize. This very definition of supervisor has not allowed many other professionals to join unions because, by definition of their roles, they are supervisors.

PHYSICIAN UNIONIZATION

As health maintenance organizations (HMOs) and other health care groups change the face of health care, they are changing the role of medical practitioners. These practitioners are considered employees in some settings instead of supervisors and now, like nurses, have the ability to join unions. The recent loss of medical practitioner autonomy and lowered wages have prompted many medical practitioners to join unions (Fine, 2006). Similar to what occurred in nursing, medical practitioners discontent leads to unionization. Approximately 50,000 medical practitioners in the country are already unionized (Fine, 2006). The Service Employees International Union is the largest collective bargaining agent for medical practitioners. The American Medical Association (AMA) supports medical practitioners engaging in collective action with employers but does not favor them formally joining unions (Fine, 2006).

REAL WORLD INTERVIEW

I don't think it's any less professional for a physician to be in a union than any other health care provider. Doctors agree to try to help people. In return, physicians should be able to charge for that service and provide the best care they know how to deliver. Doctors should be able to bargain for better conditions and autonomy like the rest of society. More and more, the governing decision is not so much the patient care as what's cost-effective. Doctors are not making those decisions and that's inherently wrong. As more and more of the medical structure becomes corporate, the workers, which doctors have become, need a means of negotiating with their employers.

Jonathan Fisher, MD
Surgical Resident
Chicago, Illinois

UNIONIZATION OF UNIVERSITY PROFESSORS

The unionization of kindergarten through twelfth-grade teachers is established in this country. Now, though, the number of professors at higher education institutions who are choosing to unionize is increasing. Again, wages and work environment have been reasons stimulating university professors to join unions. As the average age of university faculty increases and fewer people show interest in teaching, unions may be able to protect professors from becoming overburdened and financially reward those who enter teaching at the university level.

MANAGING IN A UNION ENVIRONMENT

Managers must work with the union to manage within the rules and context of contract agreements. In some ways, managing after a union is in place is less difficult because of the explicit language in most union contracts. Corrective actions, rules concerning allowed absences, and so on are agreed upon, voted on, and written in the contract.

GRIEVANCE

When a union member believes that management has failed to meet the terms of the contract or labor agreement and communicates this to management, this process is called a **grievance**. All union contracts specify grievance proceedings for union members. Grievance proceedings usually start with an employee who believes there has been wrongdoing on the part of management. Next, the member talks with a union representative, who helps the employee judge whether the act or condition actually justifies a complaint. The union representative uses knowledge of the contract, knowledge of the NLRB, and judgment to assist the employee. Next, the union member and the union representative meet with the manager to voice the grievance. At this step, the conflict may be resolved. If the conflict is not resolved, the next step may be to appeal management's decision and mediate with a higher-level manager. Grievance proceedings may differ from union to union.

PROS AND CONS OF COLLECTIVE BARGAINING

The decision to support or not to support collective bargaining in the form of a union is a personal one. Table 26-6 summarizes a number of pros and cons of collective bargaining.

Nurses practicing in the United States have the luxury of many laws to protect individuals in the workplace. If nurses prefer a particular collective action model, they can find that model in action in numerous work settings. Nurses have the ability to choose where they practice and under which model they practice.

TABLE 26-6	PROS AND CONS OF UNIONIZATION
Pros	**Cons**
The contract guides standards.	There is reduced allowance for individuality.
Members are able to be a part of the decision-making process.	Other union members may outvote your decisions.
All union members and management must conform to the terms of the contract without exception.	All union members and management must conform to the terms of the contract without exception.
A process can be instituted to question a manager's authority if a member feels something was done unjustly. More people are involved in the process.	Disputes are not handled with an individual and management only; there is less room for personal judgment.
Union dues are required to make the union work for you.	Union dues must be paid even if individuals do not support unionization.
Unions give a collective voice to employees.	Employee may not agree with the collective voice.
Employees are able to voice concerns to management without fear of job security.	Unions may be perceived by some as not professional.

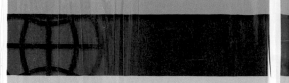

REAL WORLD INTERVIEW

The union affects my role as manager in many ways. There are so many pros and cons with it. I get frustrated as a manager when I feel like I cannot use my judgment because it may contradict the contract. An example is I had an employee that lost a grandparent that I know was essentially their parent, but I couldn't give them time off because it was not technically their parent. The contract also doesn't allow me to really commend employees that really work hard and do their best every day. The hard-working person's pay and benefits are exactly the same as a mediocre employee. My hands are tied.

If you violate the contract, it becomes a time-consuming project for me as the manager. An example of this is if I chose to give the person time off for the grandparent that died. I would have grievances from other people that I did not give time off for their grandparent's death. I would have to document what I did and why and would ultimately lose the grievance and have to find a way to compensate the other people for not giving them time off. I come from a pro-union family, and I understand how unions can protect employees. In general, it is good for employees to have somebody who is on their side and who treats all as equals. It's hard for me to imagine that there are managers who mistreat their employees in other institutions.

Ann Marie O'Connor, RN
Patient Care Manager
Hammond, Indiana

KEY CONCEPTS

- Collective bargaining has existed in the United States since 1790.

- The Wagner Act of 1935 gave private employees the legal right to form unions. Since then, numerous legislative acts have been passed to protect employees from unfair work practices.

- Workplace advocacy is a collective action model that is more informal and encompasses the everyday creativity and problem solving that occurs in nursing.

- Collective bargaining through unionization is a collective action model that is formal and legally based. It uses a written contract to guide nursing and workplace issues.

- Nurses may be aware of fraud and be fearful to report it. *Qui tam* lawsuits allow people to discreetly expose health care fraud.

- Nurses who are unhappy in the workplace because of issues such as wages and unsafe staffing often attempt to unionize to rectify workplace problems. Nurses who are not managers have the legal right to unionize. There are specific steps that can be taken to unionize. Employees and managers must be aware of what steps to take during the initiation of unionization.

- The American Nurses Association is a full-service professional organization that represents the nation's entire registered nurse population. The ANA has a dual role of being a professional organization and a collective bargaining agent. The ANA is politically active and lobbies on issues affecting nursing and the general public.

- Other professionals who do not have a tradition of unionization are opting to unionize. Medical practitioners and university professors are joining unions for the same reasons that some nurses have chosen to join unions.

KEY TERMS

American Nurses
  Association (ANA)
collective action
collective bargaining
collective bargaining agent

grievance
union
whistle-blowing
workplace advocacy

REVIEW QUESTIONS

1. Which statements concerning unions are true? Select all that apply.
   _____ A. Unions work through a collective bargaining agent.
   _____ B. Unions represent only hourly employees.
   _____ C. Unions represent only salaried employees.
   _____ D. Unions formally present a group's desires to management.

2. A manager observes a paper on the unit that states there will be a meeting in the hospital cafeteria to discuss the nurses' rights to organize and choose a collective bargaining agent. Which response by the nurse manager is most appropriate?
   A. Explain to the nurses that the meeting should take place off hospital property.
   B. Tell them they will be fired if they attend the meeting.
   C. Ask if you could join them in the cafeteria.
   D. Explain that nurses cannot join unions because they are supervisors.

3. A staff nurse tells a coworker, "I don't want any part of a union. Unions restrict your individuality, other union members may outvote what I want, they cost too much, and management can still fire you for no reason." Which of those comments by the nurse is not true of a union environment?
   A. Other union members may outvote what you want.
   B. Unions restrict individuality.
   C. Some feel they cost too much.
   D. Management can still fire you for no reason.

4. Which are the correct steps when nurses feel they have witnessed health care fraud? Put these steps in order.
   _____ A. Serve a copy of the complaint to the Department of Justice.
   _____ B. Do not tell your employer you have filed a suit.
   _____ C. File a *qui tam* lawsuit in secret.
   _____ D. Verify to the best of your knowledge that the action witnessed is health care fraud.

5. In which situation does the employee have the right to grieve an action by the manager?
   A. Making the employee work their scheduled weekend
   B. Talking to the nurse in private to discuss a comment made by a patient about them
   C. Changing scheduled work days after the schedule has been put out without consent or knowledge of the nurse
   D. Refusing to grant the vacation request of a nurse with one year seniority in order to grant the request of a nurse that has 15 years seniority

6. Which is correct concerning collective bargaining? Select all that apply.
   _____ A. Collective bargaining is formal and only occurs through unionization.
   _____ B. Collective bargaining agents represent the interests of the nurses.
   _____ C. Collective bargaining is done by a group acting with a single voice.
   _____ D. Workplace advocacy is a type of collective action.

7. Workplace advocacy is best defined as
   A. a management-defined solution for the workplace.
   B. holding managers and nurses accountable.
   C. a formal structure that is voted on.
   D. activities nurses undertake to address problems in the workplace.

8. Common reasons nurses unionize include all of the following EXCEPT
   A. patient care issues.
   B. wages.
   C. staffing issues.
   D. being content in the workplace.

9. Which legislation gave unions the right to organize?
   A. National Labor Relations Act (1935)
   B. Fair Labor Standards Act (1938)
   C. Taft-Hartley Act (1947)
   D. Executive Order 11246 (1965)

REVIEW ACTIVITIES

1. You are a new graduate nurse and have begun working on a medical unit. The nurse manager explains to you that the unit uses workplace advocacy. What is workplace advocacy? How will it affect your functioning as an RN on the unit?

2. You are hired in a hospital that is a union shop. How does unionization differ from other collective action models such as workplace advocacy? Give three examples of how unionization differs from workplace advocacy.

3. You are a graduate nurse, and you found out you passed the NCLEX examination. As an RN, you are represented by the ANA. What is the mission of the ANA? What is meant when it is said that the ANA has a dual role in nursing? Is the ANA active in politics?

EXPLORING THE WEB

- What site would you recommend to someone inquiring about collective bargaining?
  www.nursingworld.org
  Search for collective bargaining.

- Go to the site for the American Nurses Association and find your state nurses association. What did you learn about your state nurses association?
  www.nursingworld.org

- What site would you access to find out the history of collective bargaining?
  www.nlrb.gov

- Visit the American Nurses Credentialing Center Website and see what magnet status is all about. Would magnet status have an impact on your decision of where to be employed?
  www.nursingworld.org/ancc

REFERENCES

American Nurses Association. (2006). Who we are: ANA's statement of purpose. Retrieved on February 25, 2007, from http://www.nursingworld.org/about/mission.htm

Beyea, S. (2005). Patient advocacy-nurses keeping the patients safe. *Association of Operating Room Nurses Journal, 82*(3).

Budd, K., Warino, L., & Patton, M. (2004). Traditional and non-traditional collective bargaining strategies to improve the patient care environment. *Online Journal of Issues in Nursing,* (9). Retrieved February 25, 2007, from www.nursingworld.org/ojin/topic23/ tpc23_5.htm

Cimiotti, J. P., Quinlan, P. M., Larson, E. L., Pastor, D. K., Lin, S. X., & Stone, P. W. (2005, Nov./Dec.). The magnet process and the perceived work environment of nurses. *Nursing Research, 54*(6), 384–390.

Ellis, B., & Gates, J. (2006). Achieving magnet status. *Nursing Administration Quarterly, 29*(3), 241–244.

Fine, S. (2006). Emergence of Unionization a threat or salvation for physicians? *The Osteopathic Family Physician News.* Retrieved January, 2007, from www.acofp.org/member_publications/print/busmar_02.html

Fitzpatrick, M. (2001). Collective bargaining: A vulnerability assessment. *Nursing Management, 32*(2), 40–42.

Forman, H., & Davis, G. (2002). The rising tide of healthcare labor unions in nursing. *Journal of Nursing Administration, 32*(7/8), 376–378.

Forman, H., & Grimes, T. C. (2004). The "new age" of union organizing. *Journal of Nursing Administration, 34*(3), 120–124.

Jacox, A. (1980). Collective action: The basis for professionalism. *Supervisor Nurse, 11*(9), 22–24.

National Labor Relations Act. (1935). Retrieved January, 2007, from www.nlrb.gov

Scheck, T. (2002). The nurses' strike—one year later. Minnesota Public Radio. Retrieved February 25, 2007, from http://news.minnesota.publicradio.org/features/20020626_scheckt_nurseupdate

Ulrich, B. (1992). *Leadership and management according to Florence Nightingale.* Norwalk, CT: Appleton & Lange.

United American Nurses. (2006). Nurses organize! Retrieved February 25, 2007, from www.uannurse.org/organizeindex.html

Weinberg, N. (2005, March). The Dark Side of Whistleblowing. *Forbes,* 90–96.

SUGGESTED READINGS

Armalegos, J., & Berney, J. (2005). 30 years of collective bargaining autonomy, voice in practice. *Michigan Nurse, 78*(2), 6–8.

Mason, D. (2004). Declaration of independence: The UAN adopts a constitution. *American Journal of Nursing, 104*(9), 26.

Polston, D. (1999). Whistleblowing: Does the law protect you? *American Journal of Nursing, 99*(1), 26–32.

Robinson, C. (2001). Magnet nursing services recognition: Transforming the critical care environment. *AACN Clinical Issues, 12*(3), 411–423.

TABLE 27-1	CAREER PLANNING SCENARIOS

Apply the concepts of Career Planning to each of these three graduate nursing student situations as directed later in this chapter.

Student A

Julie, age 21, finished high school with a B average. She had changed her mind frequently during high school regarding a career goal and had finally applied to nursing. Julie was pleasantly surprised by how much she enjoyed nursing. Her decision as to what to do after graduation is now looming. She had very little difficulty with the academics of the nursing program, and at times found her social life interfering with being at the top of her class. The possibility of going on to study at the Masters level led her to review her priorities this year.

Student B

James, age 39, entered nursing following a nine-year career as an emergency ambulance first responder with the Fire and Ambulance Services. He is married and has two children, ages seven and nine. Although emergency work is interesting, he recognizes that life goes on for patients and their families after an emergency. He wants to be part of helping patients with their care after the emergency. To allow time for his studies, he works evening and night shifts during the weekend. This means sacrificing that study time, and he recognizes that this is a necessary tradeoff. His wife works as a legal assistant, which often means long and uncertain hours. James is pulling a B average, and, at times, this is helped by his experience in the ambulance.

Student C

Jane is 28 and comes from a poor family. Her immediate family is supportive of her aspirations to become a nurse. Jane has worked for ten years as a nursing assistant on a pediatric unit. She enjoys working with the pediatric patients but doesn't feel fulfilled in her work.

Jane did not complete high school initially. She returned to school to complete the nursing entrance requirements. She found science courses were particularly challenging. Her family is very proud of the effort she is making to upgrade her education. Jane continues to apply herself in nursing school. Despite feeling overwhelmed at times by the amount of reading demanded by her nursing courses, she maintains an A average.

Some of these changes include such things as dealing with significant diseases such as Severe Adult Respiratory Syndrome (SARS), and dealing with a changing male and female, multigenerational, multicultural nursing workforce in times of nursing shortages. The Registered Nurses Association of Ontario (RNAO) submitted a report on the nursing experience with SARS in Ontario, Canada, to an independent commission. This report illustrates the value of the nursing workforce during a challenging time. The report honored nurses for their resilience while exposing their vulnerability in challenging nursing situations (RNAO, 2003).

Many changes have occurred in the nursing workforce, testing the resilience of nurses. Fifty years ago, nursing was primarily a female occupation with the students entering following completion of high school. Childrearing frequently prevented continuation of nursing employment while the children were at home. At that time, nurses who were returning to their nursing careers after their children were older returned with a goal of lifelong employment and retirement pensions. Nurses today are both female and male. Nurses are often raising a family and working simultaneously. Current research is indicating that many nurses are now leaving nursing in five years or less (Hodges, Keeley, & Grier, 2005). These changing values are shaping the future of nursing and affecting career planning.

Within the current nursing workforce, several generations of nurses working together may have different values. The older nurse may view the recently graduated nurse as placing his or her own interests before that of the organization, thereby seemingly lacking commitment. For example, working overtime may be seen by the older, long-term nurse as an expectation, whereas the younger, newly graduated nurse may resist working overtime and do so only if the remuneration is acceptable or time is given for some

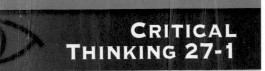

CRITICAL THINKING 27-1

Consider the values that may be significant for our new nurses, Julie, James, and Jane from Table 27-1.

What values may be significant for each?

Do you envision that their values may change over time?

What situations may cause a conflict in values between each of the new nurses and their employer?

other desired activity. With all these changes, it is important to clarify your values and seek employment that is a good fit between you and a health care agency and that prepares you for your vision of the future.

DETERMINING YOUR GOALS

Determining your goals using a common SMART acronym for goal setting is useful. SMART stands for Specific (S), Measurable (M), Achievable (A), Realistic (R), and Timely (T) goal setting. Being SMART will help you describe specifically what you want to accomplish with your strategic planning for your career. For example, when you are planning your career, you may want to work in a specialty patient care unit after graduation. Your SMART career planning goals may be as follows in Table 27-2.

The shortage of nurses has also created the need for unprecedented migration of nurses from other countries resulting in a multicultural workforce. The face of nursing has changed and will continue to change (Callister, 2006). Increasingly, these internationally educated nurses mirror the patient population. Generic nursing programs are

CRITICAL THINKING 27-2

Note the analysis of the components of SMART in Julie's goals listed here. Develop short-term, intermediate, and long-term SMART goals for James and Jane.

- *Short-term goal:* Work as a nurse full-time on an acute medical unit of a community hospital for one year.
- *Intermediate goal:* Work as a nurse for three years part-time in a community health center in a First Nation's Community while studying part-time in a masters program in community health nursing.
- *Long-term goal:* Teach in a baccalaureate nursing program and study at the doctorate level focusing on the interdisciplinary contribution to community health within six years.

Set your own short-term, intermediate, and long-term goals. Did this process help you clarify your strategic career planning goals?

also witnessing an increase in their culturally diverse student populations.

Setting strategic planning goals sounds like it is part of a business plan or venture. Although you may resist this approach at first, consider that your career is your business, and your business is nursing care. Putting your goals in writing permits you to analyze the current situation and make the necessary changes to achieve your goals. Career planners suggest setting short-term goals for one to three years, intermediate goals for three to five years, and long-term goals for six to twenty years.

TABLE 27-2	SMART CAREER PLANNING GOALS
Specific	Employment as an RN in an Emergency Department (ED)
Measurable	Function independently full-time
Achievable	Employment at hospital that allows recently graduated RNs to work in ED
Realistic	Presence of other new graduates that were able to achieve goal
Timely	Achieve goal within two years

PLANNING AND IMPLEMENTING A JOB SEARCH

You can use several methods to search for a job. The first method is networking through family, friends, and your acquaintances. These persons may be able to identify job opportunities you have not noticed. Do you want to work in a large city teaching hospital? A smaller private community hospital?

The next method is to look at positions advertised in the newspaper, bulletin board, or online job listings. It may be helpful to apply for a position that is not advertised in a health care agency that is of interest to you. This may be very effective because the health care agency you would like to work for may have many hidden job opportunities. Your skills and aptitudes may be just what they are looking for. Even if you do not receive a positive response immediately, it is common for prospective employers to keep desirable resumes on file for future reference.

Another method of searching for a job is attending a job fair. This allows you to be exposed to many opportunities in various health care agencies in a limited time. Always review any organizations carefully that you are considering for employment. Is it a magnet hospital? Is it a hospital that you would be proud to be associated with? In 1993, the American Nurses Credentialing Center (ANCC) established the Magnet Services Recognition Program. The ANCC Magnet Program has certified many hospitals in the United States and is expanding internationally (see Chapter 3). Review the Hallmarks of the Professional Nursing Practice Environment, available at www.aacn.nche.edu.

Consider looking for a one-year nursing residency program like the one implemented through a partnership between the American Association of Colleges of Nursing (AACN) and the University HealthSystem Consortium (UHC). In addition to developing clinical judgment and leadership skills for new nurses at the point of care, the goal of the residency program is to strengthen the new nurse's commitment to practice in the inpatient setting by making the first critical year a positive working and learning experience. See Website, www.rwjf.org.

Determine if there is a multistate licensure compact in place in any states where you are interested in working. The multistate licensure compact allows a nurse to have one license (in his or her state of residency) and to practice in other states (both physically and electronically), subject to each state's practice law and regulation. Under this mutual state recognition, a nurse may practice across participating state lines unless otherwise restricted. View guidelines of the multistate licensure compact at www.ncsbn.org. Find the nurse licensure compact map and click on it.

Finally, make an appointment with the nurse recruiter to learn about the mission and services of the organization. When contacted for an interview, displaying knowledge about the organization tells the interviewer that you have done your homework and your interest is serious. It is often helpful to begin a job tracking file (Figure 27-1).

PREPARATION OF A COVER LETTER AND RESUME

Your cover letter and resume are a form of marketing strategy. You are marketing and advertising yourself to a potential employer. Develop your opening sentences carefully. Consider your cover letter to be a brief commercial about yourself. It is a short opportunity to catch the attention of the nurse recruiter. Address your cover letter to a person rather than to a company. It should fit on one page and use dynamic language. Limit repeating information contained in your resume. Do not indent paragraphs. Sign your name in blue or black ink. See Figure 27-2 for an example.

Remember that your first opportunity to market yourself is a well-written cover letter and resume. It gives

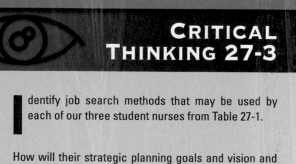

CRITICAL THINKING 27-3

Identify job search methods that may be used by each of our three student nurses from Table 27-1.

How will their strategic planning goals and vision and values focus their job search?

Where should they begin their job search?

Agency and Referral Source	Telephone Number	Contact Name	Resume Sent/ Date	Thank-You Letter	Followup

Figure 27-1 Tracker for job leads. (Courtesy of Karen Polifko-Harris, 2003.)

James Mattern
214 Christie Avenue
Gladstone, OH 43523
(604) 775-3424

April 11, 2007

Ms. Eileen Carter, BSN, RN
Director of Human Resources
Concordia Hospital
100 Seaside Drive
Austin, NJ 12356

Dear Ms. Carter:

I am requesting the opportunity to discuss my career plans with you. I will be graduating on June 30, 2007 from the University of Ohio with a Baccalaureate of Science Degree in Nursing. I will take my NCLEX-RN on July 30, 2007.

I have served as an ambulance attendant for 9 years. This service provided me with the skills to handle emergency calls, including mass disasters such as airline crashes and hotel and apartment fires. I also performed many tasks of varying priorities within many Fire and Police Departments. I feel that these skills, combined with my newly acquired nursing skills, are an asset to your Emergency Department.

I would appreciate the opportunity to discuss my career plans with you. I will call you next week to schedule an appointment to discuss employment possibilities. In the meantime, I can be contacted at (604) 775-3424 or at James123@school.edu.

Thank you for your time and consideration of my resume.

Sincerely,

James Mattern

James Mattern

Figure 27-2 Cover letter.

TABLE 27-3   ACTION VERBS

Communication	Time and Resource Management	Team Support and Leadership	Organizational Skills	Analytical and Technical Skills
address	adapt	demonstrate	arrange	analyze
arrange	advocate	design	classify	apply
clarify	collaborate	eliminate	compile	assess
debate	conceive	explore	distribute	critique
develop	coordinate	generate	generate	detect
document	delegate	innovate	incorporate	examine
illustrate	encourage	institute	order	exercise
introduce	expedite	manage	organize	identify
present	facilitate	master	process	implement
read	modify	motivate	revise	inspect
relate	prevent	negotiate	schedule	investigate
report	refer	oversee	select	perform
summarize	resolve	promote	supply	practice
teach	simplify	respect	update	research
translate	support		verify	solve
write	volunteer			utilize
				validate

the nurse manager or human resources personnel the opportunity to see an example of your work. Both your cover letter and your resume highlight your credentials and skills. Keep it brief and specific. Double-check all spelling and grammar; proofreading is essential. Be sure all dates are accurate. Have someone else read your cover letter and resume, and do not rely only on spell check to pick up a word that is spelled incorrectly or is an error in grammar. Use white, off-white, or ivory, top quality 8.5″ × 11″ paper with matching envelopes. Print only with a laser printer and if sending the same resume to more than one potential employer, print multiple originals instead of making photocopies. Any sloppiness in your cover letter and resume indicates a lack of attention to detail. A prospective employer may question whether your performance in nursing would also be sloppy. Use action verbs in your documents (Table 27-3). Action verbs are powerful. Highlight your skills of communication, time, and resource management, team support and leadership, as well as your organizational, analytical, and technical skills. Never bad-mouth a former employer, and avoid any humor or sarcasm in your documents. Your nursing curricula, both the academic and clinical components, has prepared you to meet the employment needs (Ervin, Bickes, & Schim, 2006).

CRITICAL THINKING 27-4

You are helping some of the new nurses in Table 27-1 prepare their cover letters and resumes.

What job application method is illustrated in James' cover letter?

How would you position Jane so that the nurse recruiter would want to continue reading her cover letter? What strengths may be considered in marketing Jane?

How would you strengthen Julie's position?

RESUME   It is customary to write resumes in either a chronological or a functional style. The choice of resume is dependent upon the message you want to convey. The chronological style lists jobs in reverse chronological order. It illustrates your employment history and is good for those with little or no gaps in work history in the same field in which they are seeking employment. It may also serve to highlight a progression of your work experiences from a position of lesser to greater responsibility. A functional style of resume gives the applicant the opportunity to illustrate experience in multiple careers or dramatically change a career focus. It emphasizes skills and abilities rather than a sequence of job experiences. A resume contains educational status, including any certifications, clinical rotations, personal attributes, societal contributions, and related work experience. In the body of your resume, double-space between sections. See Figure 27-3 for an example of a functional resume. Figure 27-4 is an example of a chronological resume. Note elements of the two resume styles may be combined in one resume.

Itemize your educational qualifications on your resume, including the name of your academic institution, as well as any certifications (such as cardiopulmonary resuscitation [CPR]), and dates obtained. List additional education you have taken to enhance your knowledge base, such as online courses or skills training. Demonstration of a strong knowledge of drug therapy is significant, including knowledge of commonly used drugs. Include a list of your clinical rotations with specific competencies that you have achieved. If your college has a senior clinical practicum experience, highlight the skills you have mastered. For example, note such items as administered intravenous medications using a patient-controlled analgesic pump for three patients, gave antibiotic medications via the burretrol, identified normal and abnormal laboratory results, notified the practitioner of health care problems, and contributed significant data in an interdisciplinary team conference.

Nursing employers are looking for staff with employability skills just as any employer. Include personal attributes on your resume that position you as a continuous learner, effective team player, and consistent performer such as the following:

- Paying attention to detail
- Taking responsibility for own learning
- Seeking out learning opportunities
- Providing a safe and comfortable environment for patients experiencing dementia
- Demonstrating resilience in resolving conflict
- Demonstrating reliability in attendance and punctuality
- Performing therapeutic nursing interventions.

For applicants with limited formal work experience, recruiters may consider societal and professional contributions as significant for the entry-level nurse. It can suggest that the individual is motivated and self-directed. Employers are looking for workers with employability skills that can be transferred between settings. For example, participating in the organization of a health fair for seniors and conducting a session on the need for regular foot care for the diabetic patient demonstrates your interest in the promotion of wellness as you also apply to an illness-oriented setting.

Employability skills are commonly recognized as communication, problem-solving, positive attitudes and behaviors, adaptability, and teamwork. These skills are required whether you choose to work on your own or as part of a team. Within the nursing profession, there are many opportunities within the workplace that may promote your marketability and advance your career.

INTERNET CORRESPONDENCE

Sending cover letters and resumes via the Internet is an acceptable practice. It does require some additional considerations in terms of both safeguards and catching the attention of the reader. It is safest to initially send the e-mail to yourself or to a mentor to determine how it will appear to the reader. Send the resume as an attachment to your cover letter. The human resources personnel or nurse manager can reproduce it readily to circulate it to other managers or members of the interviewing committee.

Catching the attention of human resources personnel is vital. For example, instead of entering *Resume* in the subject line of your e-mail, enter *Resume for nursing position with 9 years EMT experience,* or *Resume for entry-level RN seeking pediatric nursing position,* as appropriate. Human resources personnel are more likely to read this resume quickly.

PREPARATION FOR THE INTERVIEW

Congratulations for securing an interview! Several factors contribute to a productive interview. The employer-applicant interview includes preparation, an introductory phase, a working phase, and a termination phase.

CRITICAL THINKING 27-5

Prepare a cover letter and resume for Jane from Table 27-1.

How can Jane capture the attention of a human resource person who has had an extremely busy day and is reading his or her e-mail subject lines at the end of a workday?

How should Jane develop her cover letter and resume so that she is interviewed for a job on a pediatric patient care unit?

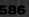

Julie Martin
111 Norberry Place
Maryland, NY 06701
(609) 323-4562
ljm@uscotia.net

Objective

An entry-level staff nurse position on a medical surgical patient care unit.

Education

Bachelor of Nursing (June 2007)   2003–present
University of Scotia
- GPA 3.7
- Dean's list, 2006

Certifications

- CPR, June 2005
- Diabetic Monitoring Devices, June 2006

Clinical Rotations

Senior Practicum   Winter Session, 2006
Calgary Mayo Care Center
- Determined patient need priorities and provided nursing interventions
- Engaged in self-evaluation of clinical performance
- Identified hospital and community resources available to patients

Maternal Child Nursing   Winter Session, 2006
Nightingale Health Center
- Conducted a physical assessment of an infant at 4 hours of age and daily until discharge
- Assessed postpartum mothers, including breast, fundal, lochia discharge, and perineum at one hour, four hours, and daily

Community Health   Winter Session, 2005
Riverdale Community Health Center
- Conducted well baby clinics, including physical assessment using the Rourke assessment form
- Offered contraceptive information
- Provided vaccinations for children under the supervision of the community health nurse
- Participated in a Diabetic Clinic focusing on accurate blood glucose monitoring

Societal/Professional Contributions   1999–present
- Taught swimming to children ages 6–10 at YMCA
- Organized a health fair for seniors in an assisted living complex
- Provided regular reading opportunities to a child experiencing developmental delays
- Tutored first year nursing students in anatomy and physiology
- Seek additional learning opportunities
- Take responsibility for personal learning needs
- Demonstrate conflict resolution skills

Figure 27-3 Functional resume.

Caitlin O'Malley
2424 Sailing Avenue
Cherry Hill, NJ 08080
(609) 444-2212 (home)
Cat24@excite.net

Objective

An entry-level position as a pediatric registered nurse

Education

Bachelor of Science in Nursing, May 2007
University of Pennsylvania, Philadelphia, PA
- Maintained 3.66 GPA, Dean's list
- Senior class president, junior class advocate
- 220-hour preceptorship on the Oncology Unit at the Children's Hospital of Philadelphia

Experience

Patient Care Assistant, Labor and Delivery
St. Mary's Medical Center, Philadelphia, PA
(August 2002–present)
- Assist in preparation of the operating room
- Provide basic patient care monitoring, including vital signs, phlebotomy, glucose screening
- Prepare and stock patient rooms

Life Guard and Camp Counselor
Camp Perry, Point Pleasant, NJ
(Summers 1998–2001)
- Supervise waterfront for 150 campers along with three additional lifeguards
- Perform basic camp counselor duties, including direct supervision of campers ages 9 to 14

Certification

Certified as a Basic Life Support Provider, 1998–present

Professional Organizations

Nursing Student Association, University of Pennsylvania Chapter
National Student Nurses Association
American Red Cross, Blood Drive Volunteer
Philadelphia Free Clinic, Registration Volunteer

Figure 27-4 Resume—Chronological. (Courtesy of Karen Polifko-Harris, 2003.)

In preparation for the interview, learn more about the agency and the possible questions they may ask you or that you should ask (Hart, 2006). You will be wise to ask for a copy of the job description beforehand. Familiarize yourself with it, as this will demonstrate your interest in the position. It will also give you an opportunity to prepare appropriate interview questions. For example, if the job description requires the nurse to demonstrate the use of medical equipment, you can clarify what type of medical equipment is used in the unit. Go online and find the agency's Website. Review what you find there. Search for the agency by name and location by using a search engine, for example, www.google.com.

Arrive shortly before the interview to demonstrate your time-management skills. The interviewer will note this. Prepare a folder that contains a description of the organization and its services, extra copies of your resume, questions you have researched and are prepared to ask, and blank paper as well as a pen and any other documents that may be helpful. Note that various person's perspectives will be assessed as part of the interview process. The nurse manager or representatives of the Human Resources department will verify your license, assess your competency, review your employment references, and complete background and criminal checks, as appropriate. They will assess your ability to meet any health requirements or any other job requirements of a nursing position. Your ability to fit in with the agency's culture as well as the patient care unit's culture will be assessed. Your communication skills, maturity, dependability, learning and nursing skills, as well as your ability to delegate, use initiative, use judgment, and be loyal and dedicated to your work are all items that may be assessed. The nursing representatives and the human resources representatives will usually try to offer you a competitive salary or hourly rate within approved budget guidelines, and they will assure the completion of any required organizational and governmental paperwork. Some organizations may require a group interview with multiple persons interviewing you for some positions to assess such things as your ability to work on a team, and so on. For entry-level position interviews, it is customary to have only the nursing manager or the nurse manager and a nurse recruiter or human resources person present during the interview. In some situations, other staff nurses are included in interviews for new unit staff.

You will also want to assess such items as whether the organization offers a nurse internship program for new graduates, what the program consists of, who serves as preceptors for the program, what are their backgrounds, and what is the salary during the internship. Note that internship programs may vary from organization to organization in content, length of program, preceptor requirements, salary during internship, and so on.

Rehearse an interview scenario with a trusted colleague or by video. Types of interviews can vary from one-to-one interviews, panel interviews, telephone interviews, and followup interviews with varying types of questions involving hypothetical case scenarios. You are applying for an entry-level position, and therefore the questions will be directed at your nursing care knowledge. For example, if you are applying for a nursing position on a general medical unit, be ready to give the nursing interventions for a patient experiencing chest pain or hypoglycemia. You may also be asked to recall a difficult nursing situation and describe your behavior in that situation. For example, you may be asked, "If you are faced with a demanding patient who has been waiting for a long time to have his dressing changed, what would you do?" To respond, use the STAR acronym and include each component. Describe Specifically (S) what happened; the Task (T), problem, or issue; the Action (A) you took; and the Result (R) of the action. What the interviewer is looking for is what you learned from the situation and how you would handle a similar situation in the future (Table 27-4).

Interviews that ask about your behavior are designed to provide the employer with information about how you have handled both negative and positive experiences in the past. Employers are seeking employees who are able to reflect on their past performance and learn from the experience. In this information age, nursing employers are recognizing the need to transform worksites into learning sites (Holden, 2006).

During the introductory phase of the interview, the employer should outline the job and the conditions of employment. If the job and conditions do not reflect your understanding of the position, be sure to clarify by asking questions at this time.

TABLE 27-4	**STAR INTERVIEWS**
Specifics	A patient was overdue for his dressing change. He became angry and demanded that I come now to change his dressing.
Task	I was busy with other high-priority patients. I was having trouble getting to this dressing change.
Action	I called my charge nurse and asked for help. The charge nurse was able to change the patient's dressing, talk with him, and help him to relax. I stopped in to tell the patient I was sorry for the delay.
Result	I asked the charge nurse to review assignments for future care of this type of patient who has extensive dressing change needs. I also resolved to examine the way I prioritize my patients at the beginning of a shift to determine the best way to meet patient care needs. I resolved to change my future patient's dressings early in the shift before it gets busy.

The working phase of the interview will begin with the employer asking you questions that reflect your cover letter and resume. All the questions during the interview will reflect the job description. Familiarize yourself with the legal and illegal questions that may be asked. See Website www.hospitalsoup.com. Legally acceptable questions include your reason for applying, your career goals, any problems you foresee, and your strengths and weaknesses. Illegal questions include asking if you are a citizen of the country, your age, cultural heritage, membership in social organizations, family characteristics, and medical history (Tetterton, 2006).

Rather than refusing to answer an illegal question, which may be seen as being uncooperative or confrontational, respond as if it is a legally acceptable question. For example, should the interviewer ask how many children you are caring for at home, respond by indicating that you are able to handle the demands and hours of the job for which you are applying. Responding in this manner may signal to the interviewer your ability to serve as a team player without compromising the legal or ethical issues of the job requirements.

Highlight specific personal and professional accomplishments as these reflect your ability; however, be careful not to inflate them as this can raise doubts concerning your truthfulness and accuracy. If you give the interviewers reason to question your veracity, you may lose the job opportunity. Respond in a calm, problem-solving fashion to all questions. See Table 27-5 for interview questions you may be asked.

Avoid any discussion of how bad your last employer or faculty was or how incompetent you think that your coworkers or classmates are. Keep the entire interview process as positive as possible. Avoid any discussions of any personal problems. If an employer has a choice between you and the person who lost their last job because they kept calling in sick over child care or personal problems, they're going to pick you every time.

DRESSING FOR THE INTERVIEW Dress appropriately for the position by wearing professionally acceptable, comfortable, and neatly pressed clothing. For women, this may be a solid-color conservative suit with a coordinated blouse, medium-heeled polished shoes, limited jewelry, neat professional hairstyle, and neutral hosiery. Skirt length should be long enough so you can sit down comfortably. Choose a soft color that complements your skin tone and hair color such as brown, tan, beige, black, blue, navy, or gray. Use light makeup and perfume and have neat, manicured nails.

For men, appropriate dress may be a solid-color dark blue, gray, muted pinstripe, or very muted brown conservative suit with a white long-sleeve shirt and conservative tie. Use a conservative stripe or paisley tie that complement your suit, silk or good quality blends only. Wear dark socks with professional polished leather dress shoes, brown, cordovan, or black only. Wear limited or no jewelry and have a neat professional hairstyle. Limit aftershave and have neatly trimmed nails. Both women and men should avoid body piercing jewelry and cover tattoos. Avoid food and don't chew gum or use a cell phone or iPod during the interview. Use a breath mint before you enter the building for the interview.

TERMINATION PHASE OF THE INTERVIEW

Terminating an interview is important. The employer will close an interview by asking if you have any questions (Table 27-6).

Expect to be quite exhausted by the end of the interview. However, take time to review your notes, seek clarification for any concerns, and conclude the interview by asking when you can expect to hear from the employer. Asking when you can expect to hear from the employer indicates that you are actively seeking employment and suggests that if they are serious about hiring you, they may want to offer a position. Many sources recommend waiting to ask questions such as the following until after a position has been offered: What is the salary? When do raises occur? Is there a shift differential? Is there a differential for advanced nursing degrees? What type of health, dental, retirement, vacation, holiday time, sick time, continuing education, and educational reimbursement benefits are offered? Note the regular salary surveys done by many nursing journals, for example, RN (October 2005), Nursing (October 2006), AORN (December 2005), and so on.

OBTAINING REFERENCES Seek permission to use your references prior to your interview to avoid delay and illustrate that you are not hesitant to provide references. Seeking permission to submit a person's name for

---

CRITICAL THINKING 27-6

For many nurse applicants, the most anxiety-producing aspect of searching for a job is the interview. Assume you are seeking employment. Practice answering the questions in Table 27-5. What questions would represent your level of knowledge and skill? What characteristics would you emphasize when you respond to the questions?

TABLE 27-5   **INTERVIEW QUESTIONS**

Question	Potential Response
Tell me about yourself.	Do not go into a long list, but have two to three traits that are solid (for example, "I am a positive person and look for new learning experiences.").
Why do you want to work here?	Describe several attributes of the work environment, the staff, or the patients (for example, "I enjoyed my rotation on 5 West—the staff worked as a team and I am looking for that type of support in my first position."). Comment on any attractive organizational strengths you saw on the organization's Website.
What do you want to be doing in five years?	Identify a long-term goal and your plans to achieve it with progressive responsibilities and achievements.
What are your qualifications?	Discuss experiences that you have had that qualify you for the new position.
What are your strengths?	This is a favorite question. Look at the job description. What qualities do you have that are required? Are you able to work under stress, are you organized, are you eager to learn new skills, do you enjoy new challenges?
What would your references say?	You may want to ask your references this question. Would they say you are easily distracted or focused? A team player or solo player? A problem solver or one who ignores problems?
Are you interested in more schooling?	Most who have just graduated may want to say no, but an employer wants someone who is interested in lifelong learning, especially in the nursing profession.
What has been your biggest success?	Think of a success ahead of time that may fit with the organization. It does not have to be in nursing.
What has been your greatest failure?	Again, think ahead, but this time, make sure you can state what you learned from the negative experience. After all, to fail is to learn, so state what you would do differently next time and why.
Why do you want to leave your current job?	For an RN, you can say that you are seeking new responsibilities, experiences, and challenges. Give an example of a new experience you are looking for.

Source: Compiled with information from Polifko-Harris, 2003.

---

a reference alerts that individual that he can expect a call and from whom. This will prevent any hesitancy in agreeing to provide the reference to the employer while trying to recall who you are, especially if there has been a delay since you had contact with him.

Your past employment history will guide you as to whom to list as references. If you have had past health care employers, like Jane and James, in Table 27-1, you will be wise to list those employers and your manager. You should also include any character references, and at least one nursing professor. For graduates who have not had many work-life experiences, references from volunteer service and high school contributions are also helpful.

TABLE 27-6	**SAMPLE QUESTIONS TO ASK DURING AN INTERVIEW**

- How can I prepare myself to work on this unit and do a good job?
- May I have a copy of the job description and performance appraisal form? How often will I be evaluated?
- Is there a clinical ladder program?
- Who is my preceptor?
- What shift will I be scheduled to work? Will I rotate shifts? Are special requests for time off honored?
- What holidays and weekends am I scheduled to work?
- What type of orientation or internship will I receive? How long is it? Does it address how to work well with other practitioners?
- Is this a magnet hospital? Do you monitor nurse-sensitive outcomes?

Source: Compiled with information from Polifko-Harris, 2003, and Kelly-Heidenthal, 2004.

FOLLOWING UP YOUR INTERVIEW Within twenty-four hours, follow up your interview with a simple thank you note for the interview (Figure 27-5).

If you sensed that the interview did not go well, reflect objectively upon the event with a colleague or friend, avoiding excessive negative talk about yourself or the interviewers. Recognize the confidentiality of the interview for both the employer and yourself. Consider it a good learning experience. If you are not the successful applicant, ask what areas were weak and how you might address them. For example, you may not be considered for a community health nursing position as employers may require you to have two to three years of previous acute medical and surgical nursing experience. By asking for this information, you are demonstrating your interest in addressing your weaknesses and learning from the interview. If the employer is reluctant to spend time with you as an entry-level nurse answering these questions, this employer may not have been the best fit for you. If you have not heard back from the employer in the time indicated at the interview, follow up with a phone call. This will demonstrate your continued interest in the position and your willingness to learn about your weaknesses for future interviews.

If the job is offered to you, suggest a followup meeting to clarify any questions that need further explanations, such as salary. Even within unionized health care agencies, there is negotiation room for where the employer may want to place you on the pay scale. It is important to know your value, know the average salary paid for similar positions with other agencies, and to clearly communicate your expectations.

Should you find the job offer unacceptable, clearly state the reason. You will leave the door open should the employer return with a counter offer. In addition, be sure

CRITICAL THINKING 27-7

Congratulations to Julie, James, and Jane for being selected as the successful candidates! Now anticipate an interview with Julie, James and Jane after two and five years.

1. What were the experiences that provided the greatest learning for them? Were the experiences positive or negative or both?
2. What would they have done differently?
3. Have their initial career plans changed?

to thank them for the opportunity to discuss your career goals and plans.

EVALUATION

Your academic and clinical preparation has placed you in an admirable position to apply the standards of practice expected of the entry-level nurse in accordance with the licensing and professional associations. Carry out every step in your strategic planning for your career with a view toward marketing yourself even if you are rejected. You will leave the impression with the interviewers that you may meet their employment needs in the future. Career planning means thriving rather than surviving.

In today's nursing world, nursing management is seeking nurses who are willing to enter into partnerships

James Mattern
214 Christie Avenue
Gladstone, OH 43523
(604) 555-1212

April 26, 2007

Ms. Eileen Carter, BSN, RN
Director of Human Resources
Concordia Hospital
100 Seaside Drive
Austin, NJ 12356

Dear Ms. Carter:

Thank you for the time you spent with me as I interviewed for a position as a registered nurse at Concordia Hospital. I enjoyed meeting the Emergency Department nurse manager and several of the staff nurses yesterday and was especially impressed with the sense of professionalism among the staff.

I have requested that my transcripts be sent directly to your office, and I will have three of my instructors complete the reference forms you gave me. I look forward to hearing from you soon about my second interview and will contact you in two weeks as directed.

Sincerely,

James Mattern

James Mattern

Figure 27-5 Interview followup letter. (Compiled with information from Polifko-Harris, 2003.)

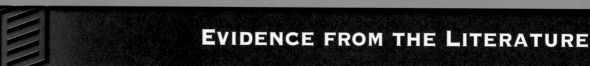

EVIDENCE FROM THE LITERATURE

Citation: Holden, J. (2006). How can we improve the nursing work environment? *The American Journal of Maternal/Child Nursing, 31*(1), 34–38.

Discussion: The mother of our profession, Florence Nightingale, was the first to set the most important patient care goal, which was to do the sick no harm. The article highlights the need for organizations to transform the environment of nurses into learning organizations. When using the framework of a learning organization, health care organizations achieve their goals just as business and industry have done. The article articulates the principles of a learning organization to include systems thinking, personal mastery, team learning, mental models, and shared vision.

Through systems thinking, the processes that exist within an organization are viewed as interrelated. Activities or work processes done in one part of an organization affect the entire organization. Personal mastery relates to developing the person as an evolving growing individual and professional. This can best be realized in an environment where not only individual learning but also team learning is actively promoted. Having a mental model suggests that individuals develop a shared mental vision of a healing environment where individuals are given permission and freedom to address health care deficiencies and promote quality improvement. Having a shared vision of such environments promotes a common goal with a stronger sense of commitment by the entire team. The author relates making a successful and integrated change to a new work environment to the well-known steps of the nursing process: assessment, planning, implementation, and evaluation.

Implications for Practice: When planning your career in nursing, consideration of a potential employer's working environment is important when selecting with whom and for whom you want to work. Before accepting a nursing position, determine the congruence between your values and goals and the operation of the organization. As personal mastery over your own destination is important, select a learning organization that will promote your ultimate success.

with them. The health care industry recognizes that nurses have a unique capacity to influence the health status of its patients as well as improve the nursing work environment (Holden, 2006). Forging respectful partnerships between the employer and employee promotes quality health care for all our citizens. Sharing the mutual goal of providing safe and competent care will be satisfying for both you and your employer. Your consistent application of employability skills will result in a highly marketable reference for any future endeavor.

KEY CONCEPTS

- Career planning for the professional nurse necessitates taking control of the strategic planning, vision, and goal setting process.

- Marketing strategies designed to demonstrate your academic preparation and the critical thinking skills that you honed during your education are key features in your success.

- Values clarification enhances organizational fit and success for both employer and employee.

- Establishing short-term, intermediate, and long-term goals will shape your job search.

- Consider your cover letter and resume as a commercial for marketing yourself.

- Preparation for a job interview requires knowledge of the agency, the job description, and standards of nursing practice.

- Practice your job interview with a trusted colleague.

- Do a job search on the Internet to locate positions that you are interested in.

- Recognizing personal strengths and weaknesses is helpful when working collaboratively as a member of the interdisciplinary health team.

- Follow up your interview with a thank you note.

KEY TERM

career planning

REVIEW QUESTIONS

1. You are being considered for an entry-level nursing position on a busy medical nursing unit. During the interview, the nursing manager poses the following case scenario: During the night shift, one of the patients on the unit becomes unstable. It is difficult to care for him and all the patients in your assignment. How should you handle the situation to provide a safe practice environment?
   A. Ask the UAP to watch the unstable patient while you care for the other patients.
   B. Inform the nursing supervisor of the patient's condition and the patient assignment and request assistance.
   C. Prepare a detailed documentation report to give to the nursing manager in the morning.
   D. Place the patient near the desk so that anyone passing by can check on the patient.

2. During an interview for a position in the Emergency Department, James was asked how he would handle the following situation: The ED is very busy, and a patient arrives with his wife. Some of the nurses refer to him as a "frequent flyer" and tell you to put him in the end room until you have time to care for him. What would be your initial response?
   A. After smelling alcohol on his breath, you realize that he may be intoxicated and comply with the nurses' direction.
   B. You place him on a stretcher and tell his wife to watch him so that he doesn't fall off.
   C. You assess him more thoroughly and take the appropriate nursing action.
   D. You ask the nurse what she means by the term "frequent flyer" because you had never heard it before.

3. During a job interview, the nurse recruiter presents the following hypothetical question: You are working the evening shift and receive a sick call for the night shift. The unit has been very busy on the evening shift. How would you handle the situation?
   A. After an hour, call the nurse back to determine if her health has improved.
   B. Fill out a heavy workload form, and submit it to the union representative.
   C. Assess the unit's patients conditions, and notify the nursing supervisor of the sick call.
   D. Inform the nursing manager that you think the nurse is abusing her sick time.

4. The employer is requesting applicants to undertake an assessment test that includes the following case scenario: You are making early morning rounds and discover that a patient was restrained to the siderails of the bed. What is your initial response?
   A. Assess the patient's condition.
   B. Check the policy of the hospital with respect to the use of restraints.
   C. Contact the nursing manager to witness the presence of the restraint.
   D. Check the practitioner's order for the use of restraints.

5. You are engaged in an employment interview. One of the interview panel members questions you about whether you could handle the hours of the job. Which of the following responses would help you get the job?
    A. Since the hours are in the evening, my partner can look after the children.
    B. I can meet the expectations of the work schedule that this job requires.
    C. I will look for daycare arrangements once I know I have the job.
    D. I would not be available to pick up extra shifts if that is what you are asking.

REVIEW ACTIVITIES

1. Using the acronym SMART, develop short-term, intermediate, and long-term strategic planning vision and goals for James and Jane.

2. You have been hired as a career planner by James and Jane. Your services require you to prepare a cover letter and resume for them.

    What method of job application is illustrated in James' cover letter?

    How would you position Jane so that the human resource person would want to continue reading her cover letter or return to it?

3. Send an e-mail for Julie and Jane to a human resource manager.

    How would you begin to capture the attention of a human resource person who has had an extremely busy day and is reading his or her e-mail at the end of the workday for Julie?

    How would you position Jane so that the human resource personnel would consider reading her e-mail?

    What employment skills does Jane bring to the job?

EXPLORING THE WEB

- For U.S. statistics, review this reference from the U.S. Department of Labor, Bureau of Labor Statistics: *www.bls.gov*

- For the Canadian labor market, review this reference from Statistics Canada: *www.statcan.ca*

- Review these generalized Websites for nursing issues:
  www.nursingworld.org
  www.nursingcenter.com
  www.nurseweek.com
  www.medsearch.com
  www.medzilla.com

- Note great interview questions at these sites:
  http://content.monster.com
  www.hospitalsoup.com

- Review this excellent Website for career information:
  www.ucalgary
  Use these sites for job searching:
  Dogpile: *www.dogpile.com*
  Excite: *www.excite.com*
  WebCrawler: *www.webcrawler.com*
  Go.com: *http://go.com*
  Google: *www.google.com*

- Some examples of job boards specific to health care include the following:
  www.healthcareerweb.com
  www.medjobs.com
  www.monster.com
  www.aone.org (This site requires membership to use.)

- A few examples of other sites with job openings include the following:
  www.rn.com
  www.careercity.com

- There are many Websites specific to nursing employment opportunities. Try some of these:
  www.americanmobile.com
  www.rnwanted.com
  www.healthopps.com
  www.healthcareers-online.com
  www.healthcaretraveler.com

- Look up several of these nursing sites:
  Association of Pediatric Hematology Oncology Nurses: *www.apon.org*
  Association of Rehabilitation Nurses: *www.rehabnurse.org*
  Association of Women's Health, Obstetric and Neonatal Nurses: *www.awhonn.org*
  Trauma Nursing: *www.emergency.com*

- Review these good examples of letters of application in a variety of situations:
  www.career.vt.edu

- For library references by e-mail: *www.ci.austin.tx.us* (type in *library reference*)

- For online journal articles:
  www.medscape.com

- For nursing articles: *www.nursingcenter.com* (click on library of nursing journals)
  www.nursingmanagment.com

- For a magnet listing of hospitals: *www.nursingworld.org* (type in the word *magnet*)

- Check this guide to education and careers in nursing, which includes the most comprehensive directory of nursing schools with full school profiles and detailed nursing Q & As: *www.allnursingschools.com*

REFERENCES

Callister, L. C. (2006). Global health and nursing: It's a small, small world. *The American Journal of Maternal/Child Nursing, 31*(1), 63–63.

Ervin, E. E., Bickes, J. T., & Schim, S. M. (2006). Environments of care: A curriculum model for preparing a new generation of nurses. *Journal of Nursing Education, 45*(2), 75–80.

Harris, K. (2002). *Center of the storm, practicing principled leadership in times of crisis.* Nashville, TN: Thomas Nelson, Inc.

Hart, K. (2006). Student extra: The employment interview: Tips for success selecting an employer for the perfect fit. *American Journal of Nursing, 106*(4), 72AAA–72CCC.

Hodges, H. F., Keeley, A. C., & Grier, E. C. (2005). Professional resilience, practice longevity, and Parse's theory for baccalaureate education. *Journal of Nursing Education, 44*(12), 548–554.

Holden, J. (2006). How can we improve the nursing work environment? *The American Journal of Maternal/Child Nursing, 31*(1), 34–38.

Kelly–Heidenthal, P. (2004). *Essentials of nursing leadership and management.* Clifton Park, NY: Thomson Delmar Learning.

Leiter, M. P., & Laschinger, H. K. S. (2006). Relationships of work and practice environment to professional burnout. *Nursing Research, 55*(2).

Nogueras, D. J. (2006). Occupational commitment, education, and experience as a predictor of intent to leave the nursing profession. *Nursing Economic$, 24*(2), 86–93.

Polifko-Harris, K. (2003). Career Planning. In P. Kelly-Heidenthal *Nursing Leadership and Management.* Clifton Park, NY: Thomson Delmar Learning.

Registered Nurses Association of Ontario. (2003). Report on the nursing experience with SARS in Ontario. RNAO: Public Hearing, September 29. Retrieved March 31, 2006, from http://www.rnao.org/html/PDF/SARS_Unmasked.pdf

Tetterton, S. K. (2006). Interviewing potential staff. Retrieved January 4, 2006, from http://www.libsci.sc.edu/bob/class/clis724/Special LibrariesHandbook/tetterton.htm

SUGGESTED READINGS

Bagnardi, M., & Perkel, L. K. (2005). The learning achievement program, fostering student cultural diversity. *Nurse Educator, 30*(1), 17–20.

Brewer, C. S., Zayas, L. E., Kahn, L. S., & Sienkiewicz, M. J. (2006). Nursing recruitment and retention in New York State: A qualitative workforce needs assessment. *Policy, Politics & Nursing Practice, 7*(1), 54–63.

Hankin, H. (2005). *The new workforce.* New York: AMACOM.

Hill, S. (2006). Inspiring the next generation. *Nursing Times, 102*(21), 18–19.

Johnson, S. A., & Romanello, M. L. (2005). Generational diversity, teaching and learning approaches. *Nurse Educator, 30*(5), 212–215.

Kenworthy, N., & Redfern, L. (2004). *The Churchill Livingstone professional portfolio* (3rd ed.). New York: Churchill Livingstone, Inc.

Kidder, M., & Cornelius, P. B. (2006). Licensure is not synonymous with professionalism: It's time to stop the hypocrisy. *Nurse Educator, 31*(1), 15–19.

Lake, E. T., & Friese, C. R. (2006). Variations in nursing practice environments, relation to staffing and hospital characteristics. *Nursing Research, 55*(1), 1–9.

Langford, B. (2005). *The etiquette edge, the unspoken rules for business success.* New York: AMACOM.

Laschinger, H. K. S., Purdy, N., Cho, J., & Almost, J. (2006). Antecedents and consequences of nurse managers' perceptions of organizational support. *Nursing Economic$, 24*(1), 1–29.

Manion, J. (1990). *Change from within, nurse intrapreneur as health care innovators.* Kansas City, MO: American Nurses Association.

Maxwell, M. (2005). It's not just black and white: How diverse is your workplace? *Nursing Economics, 23*(3), 139–140.

McIntyre, M., Thomlinson, E., & McDonald, C. (2005). *Realities of Canadian nursing: professional, practice, and power issues* (2nd ed.). New York: Lippincott Williams & Wilkins.

Morath, J. M., & Turnbull, J. E. (2005). *To do no harm.* San Francisco: Jossey-Bass, A Wiley Imprint.

Nicklin, P. J., Kenworthy, N., & De Witt, R. (2002). *Teaching and assessing in nursing practice.* Toronto: Bailliere Tindall.

Poster, E., Adams, P., Clay, C., Garcia, B. R., Hallman, A., Jackson, B., et al. (2005). The Texas model of differentiated entry-level competencies of graduates of nursing programs. *Nursing Education Perspectives, 26*(1), 18–23.

Thrasher, C., & Staples, E. (2005). Expanding community health nursing practice, primary health care nurse practitioners. In L. L. Stamler & L. Yiu (Eds.), *Community health nursing, a Canadian perspective* (pp. 333–336). Toronto: Pearson Prentice Hall.

Wagner, S. E. (2006). Staff retention: From "satisfied" to "engaged." *Nursing Management, 37*(3), 25–29.

White, K. M. (2005). Policy highlight: Staffing plans and ratios. What is the latest U.S. perspective? *Nursing Management, 37*(4), 18–24.

Xu, Y., & Kwak, C. (2005). Characteristics of internationally educated nurses in the United States. *Economic$, 23*(5), 233–238.

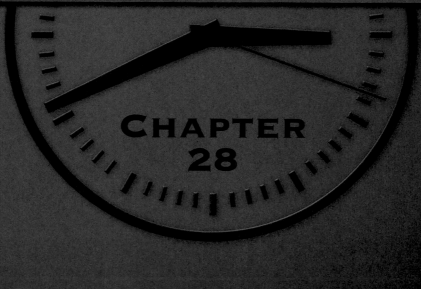

CHAPTER 28

Emerging Opportunities

Stephen Jones, MS, RNC, PNP, ET

Luck is a matter of preparation meeting opportunity (Oprah Winfrey).

OBJECTIVES

Upon completion of this chapter, the reader should be able to:

1. Relate the many nursing opportunities available upon graduation.
2. Identify advanced nursing practice and other nontraditional nursing roles.
3. Identify various opportunities for certification.
4. Relate hospital-based and nonhospital-based nursing practice.
5. Identify directions for the future of nursing.

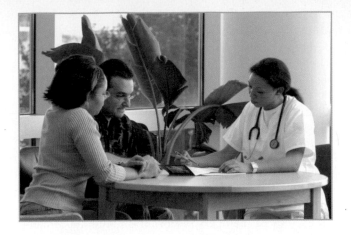

You are within four months of graduation. Your thoughts are focused on moving to a nice city and getting a good job in a health care setting that will stimulate and educate you. You also know individuals who have been nurses for a while. They are doing seemingly incredible activities and interventions. Many are able to write prescriptions, and some even have flexible hours. There are numerous questions that you, the graduating nurse, need to consider:

What do you see yourself doing one year, five years, and ten years from now?

What are your real-life situations and circumstances regarding family, ability to relocate, hours to work?

Do you have financial constraints?

What are your strengths and weaknesses?

Health care facilities have been experiencing nursing shortages since the mid-1980s. In the early 1990s, there was a temporary ease in the nursing shortage. This easing, however, was short-lived; at the turn of the twenty-first century, the nursing demand far exceeded the supply of registered professional nurses. As of 2005, one in ten nursing jobs were unfilled, and according to the Bureau of Labor and Statistics, the nursing shortage will reach one million by 2012 (Erickson et al., 2005). Nurses apply their holistic knowledge to help individuals manage the changes brought on by illness or disease, educate them about preventive health care, and, in general, attempt to improve the quality of health care. Many factors have contributed to the nursing shortages, especially since the mid-1980s. In particular, the number of chronically ill and frail elderly patients has increased, and the demand for nurses who can care for them far exceeds the supply. In addition, the various restructuring efforts in our nation's health care system have made nursing jobs less attractive. This nursing shortage is expected to not only continue but worsen by the year 2015, as mentioned. This shortage is different from those of the past in several ways. Factors contributing to the most recent shortage

include an aging nursing population, a declining number of nursing students in the academic pipeline, and the need for more accommodating working conditions for nurses.

Statistical data from 2004 showed that the average age of nurses was 46.8 years; the average age at graduation for recent RN graduates was 29.6 years; and the number of RNs who are advanced practice nurses is 240,461 or 8.3% of the total RN population. In December 2005, the NLN (National League for Nursing) released statistics indicating that while there was a significant increase of almost 20% enrollment for all types of nursing programs, the number of qualified instructors/professors continued to decline (www.nln.org). Nursing programs rejected 32,617 qualified applicants due to lack of qualified nurse educators available to teach these future generations of RNs, according to preliminary survey data released by the American Association of Colleges of Nursing (AACN) (www.aacn.nche.edu).

Throughout its history, nursing has always responded to changes in society's health care needs. From the days of Florence Nightingale and her service in the mid-1800s to Lillian Wald and public health nursing in the early 1900s to Martha Rogers in the 1930s and 1940s suggesting that nurses prepare themselves to handle the health issues that arise from space travel, nursing has met society's changing health care needs by expanding the roles of nurses. For decades, nurses in acute care settings have been taking on advanced and expanded roles on evening, night, and weekend shifts.

Many of the changes in nursing have evolved naturally and logically. Positions such as staff nurse, nurse manager, director of nursing, and case manager, and organizations such as visiting nurse associations and public health organizations are a direct reflection of these evolutions. Nursing has established itself in hospitals, ambulatory clinics, practitioners' offices, and community and school settings. An issue confronting nursing, however, has been identifying what the appropriate entry-level educational degree should be, and what a nurse really is because of the many levels of educational preparation. In December 1965, the American Nurses Association (ANA) House of Delegates (HOD) adopted a motion that the ANA continue to work toward baccalaureate education as the educational foundation for professional nursing practice. By 1985, the ANA HOD agreed to urge State Nursing Associations to establish the BS degree with a major in nursing as the minimum educational requirement for licensure and to retain the title of registered nurse (RN) (American Nurses Association [ANA], 2000). To date, there are still a variety of paths an individual can take to become an RN. These include a two-year associate degree, a three-year diploma, and a four-year baccalaureate degree. Many four-year baccalaureate schools of nursing have changed the traditional four-year pathway

EVIDENCE FROM THE LITERATURE

Citation: Khomeiran, R., Yekta, Z. P., Kiger, A. M., & Ahmadi, F. (2006, March). Professional competence: Factors described by nurses as influencing their development. *International Nursing Review, 53*(1), 66–72.

Discussion: This study was done to explore and define factors that may influence competence development. This oftentimes controversial issue in health care settings affects many aspects of the nursing profession, including education, practice, and management. This study was a qualitative study with data obtained via tape-recorded semistructured interviews. These interviews were then transcribed verbatim and analyzed according to the qualitative methodology of content analysis. Six descriptive categories were identified from the data: experience, opportunities, environment, personal characteristics, motivation, and theoretical knowledge.

Implications for Practice: These findings suggest that the six identified factors influencing the process of developing professional competence in nursing extend across both personal and extrapersonal domains. Further understanding and research into these areas may enhance the ability of nursing leaders, including educators, to enable student and qualified nurses to pursue effective competency development pathways to prepare themselves for a higher standard of care delivery.

national group in 1955. Clinical nurse specialists (CNSs), which began in psychiatric nursing in the early 1940s, developed specialties and certification by the mid-1970s. The newest, and perhaps most visible role due to its significant presence in primary care, is the nurse practitioner (NP), with its inaugural program beginning in 1965. Currently, there are a variety of patient populations served by the CNS and NP roles. Nurses within these roles assume expanded functions and additional responsibilities, often crossing over into what had been viewed as the role of medicine. The twentieth century was a unique time in nursing's history. The profession struggled to assume its rightful role in the health care arena with its members performing traditional nursing roles, yet it significantly upgraded its educational, clinical, research, and managerial focus. This chapter will examine emerging opportunities for both new graduates who would prefer not to assume advanced or expanded nursing roles and those who are contemplating advanced or expanded roles. The first section will discuss nursing roles that do not require graduate-level preparation. The remaining section of the chapter will discuss advanced practice nursing roles that do require a graduate degree.

EVIDENCE FROM THE LITERATURE

Citation: Schwarz, T. (2006, January). What is past is prologue. *American Journal of Nursing, 106*(1), 13.

Discussion: "... But if you'd asked me on that hot afternoon thirty-five years ago what my future would hold, I would have gazed into a pretty hazy crystal ball. Few of us know from an early age what career path we will follow, and those who think they know are sometimes surprised at the results. It shouldn't have surprised me, therefore, that when I asked a handful of nurse colleagues to describe their goals and aspirations, most wrote about the past rather than the present. With the exception of those whose paths are marked by sheer luck or some controlling obsession, most of us look to the patterns of our past steps to get a fix on our future course."

Implications for Practice: Nursing educators must reach out and help nursing students plan for the future at an early stage in their career. Those who don't plan for the future have no opportunity for control over it.

to a degree and are admitting students who already have a nonnursing baccalaureate degree or an associate's degree. In deciding which education option to pursue, students should consider their future, that is, where they want to be in five to ten years. If advanced practice is a desired goal, then a baccalaureate education is the required first step toward that goal.

A major advancement within nursing has been the emergence of several areas of advanced nursing practice: the certified registered nurse anesthetist (CRNA), the clinical nurse specialist (CNS), the nurse practitioner (NP), and the certified nurse-midwife (CNM). Historically, the oldest American advanced nursing practice role is the nurse anesthetist, which began in the mid 1800s, with a professional nursing association later established in 1931 (Murphy-Ende, 2002). Nurse midwives were the next role to develop, incorporating as a

EMERGING OPPORTUNITIES

Within the traditional hospital setting, the levels of nursing hierarchy are established: vice president/director of nursing, nurse managers, and staff nurses. This hierarchy allow for promotion and advancement. Since the mid-1980s, however, the trend has been to flatten the levels of nursing management; that is, have fewer managers and additional clinical nurses including bedside nurses, nurses with expanded roles, and advanced practice nurses.

CERTIFICATION

Professional certification in nursing is a measure of distinctive nursing practice. The rise in consumerism in the face of a compelling nursing shortage and the profession's movement to elevate nursing as a career option have given prominence to the value of certification in nursing (Shirey, 2005). Certification in nursing represents an example of professional credentialing and is a voluntary process undertaken by practicing nurses. It is a marker of the knowledge and experience of a professional RN and is more than just a symbolic title. The American Board of Nursing Specialists (ABNS) defines the certification process as the formal recognition of the specialized knowledge, skills, and experience demonstrated by the achievement of standards identified by a nursing specialty to promote optimal health outcomes (Stromberg et al., 2005).

Basic eligibility requirements for specialty nursing certification are available at www.nursecredentialing.org. They can also be seen in Table 28-1. The requirements often include the following:

- Hold a currently active RN licensure in the United States or its territories.
- Have practiced the equivalent of two years full-time as an RN in the United States or its territories.
- Hold a baccalaureate or higher degree in nursing. Note that candidates with an associate degree/diploma may apply for certification in several areas of nursing practice.
- Have a minimum of 2,000 hours of clinical practice within the past three years.
- Have had 30 contact hours within the past three years.

Professional certification, through a wide variety of organizations, is also monitored by the American Board of Nursing Specialties (www.abns.org), and includes both the clinical component of nursing (bedside nurses, advance practice nurses, and so on) as well as nursing administration. Several of the larger certifying organizations include the ANA; American Association of Nurse Anesthetists (AANA); National Association of Pediatric Nurse Associates and Practitioners (NAPNAP); Association of Women's Health, Obstetric and Neonatal Nurses (AWHONN); and The Association of Critical Care Nurses (ACCN).

TRAVELING NURSE

As the demand for nursing has increased, the supply has often been very low, and hospitals are frequently

CRITICAL THINKING 28-1

Many nurses are certified in their area of specialty. You are thinking about taking the certification examination but are not sure you really want to spend the time required to prepare for it. Some reflections on what certification might do for you are useful:

What is the reason you want to take this examination? Will becoming certified make a difference in your job? Will becoming certified allow you to further progress in your position? Is certification required for licensure?

EVIDENCE FROM THE LITERATURE

Citation: Marrelli, T. (2006, January). Nursing in flux. *American Journal of Nursing, 106*(1), 19–20.

Discussion: Author states, "When I compare career trajectories with nurses in various fields, I realize that my many shifts in roles and interests are not unusual. The sheer range of opportunity for nurses often beckons us toward change, whether to a new workplace, a new specialty, or another area within the current system. Nursing today offers complex variations on all the old pros and cons. There are more opportunities than ever, more work setting choices, more specialties and certification areas, and a wide range of geographic locations limited only by time and the availability of flights."

Implications for Practice: Nurses must share information about nursing opportunities with potential nurse candidates. This will help nurses in the future prepare for careers they are interested in.

TABLE 28-1	**CERTIFICATIONS AVAILABLE FROM AMERICAN NURSES ASSOCIATION**

Advanced Practice

Nurse Practitioners

- Acute Care
- Adult
- Adult Psychiatric/Mental Health
- Advanced Diabetes Management
- Family
- Family Psychiatric/Mental Health
- Gerontological
- Pediatric

Clinical Nurse Specialists

- Advanced Diabetes Management
- Adult Health
  (formerly known as Medical-Surgical)
- Adult Psychiatric/Mental Health
- Child/Adolescent Psychiatric/Mental Health
- Gerontological
- Pediatric
- Public/Community Health

Other Advanced-Level Exams

- Advanced Diabetes Management—Dietician
- Advanced Diabetes Management—Pharmacist
- Nursing Administration, Advanced

BS in Nursing or Higher Degree

- Cardiac/Vascular Nurse
- Gerontological Nurse
- Informatics Nurse
- Medical-Surgical Nurse
- Nursing Administration
- Nursing Professional Development
- Pediatric Nurse
- Perinatal Nurse
- Psychiatric/Mental Health Nurse
- Public/Community Health Nurse

Associate Degree or Diploma in Nursing

- Cardiac/Vascular Nurse
- Gerontological Nurse
- Medical-Surgical Nurse
- Pediatric Nurse
- Perinatal Nurse
- Psychiatric Mental Health Nurse

Diploma, Associate, Baccalaureate or higher degree in Nursing

- Ambulatory Care Nurse
- Nursing Case Management
- Pain Management

Source: www.nursingworld.org/ancc/cert/index.html.

understaffed. One option to fill the nursing shortage is the traveling nurse. These nurses usually work in three-month assignments on the same unit. They travel to various locations throughout the United States. The financial charge by the traveling nurse company to the employing hospital for a traveler is usually very high. The traveling nurse's salary however, is not as high and is similar to that of fellow employees.

The benefits to the health care institution of using traveling nurses include having a nurse with a variety of experiences providing continuity of care for a three-month period. These traveling nurses often need only the basic hospital and unit orientation because they come with skills applicable to their area of practice. Traveling nurses need to be aware of differing nursing methodologies and licensure requirements from state to state and will require a license for each state in which they practice unless there is a multistate compact for licensure in the new state in which they want to practice. Traveling nurses should also ensure that their contract stipulates clearly what their assignment is and what the institution and agency expect of them. Check this carefully before signing a contact. Most travelers exhibit flexibility, adaptability, assertiveness, strong organizational and interpersonal skills, confidence, independence, and the ability to learn new skills and techniques.

If traveling is in your blood, adventure also lies outside of the United States, as many foreign countries actively recruit American nurses, especially Middle East countries such as Saudi Arabia and Kuwait. This is an opportunity to see other areas of the world, work with different cultures, and learn other interventions. Many of the traveling nurse companies advertise in nursing journals as well as over the Internet.

FLIGHT NURSING

In numerous tertiary care centers, nurses are functioning in the role of flight nurse for both helicopter and fixed-wing transports. Over the years, numerous television shows and movies have portrayed these nurses, in their jumpsuits and helmets, landing on the helipad on the top of the hospital. Flight nursing actually started in 1933 with the emergency Flight Corps of the Armed Services and was present in both the Korean and Vietnam wars. The concept of an air ambulance was initiated in Denver in 1972. One needs numerous advanced technical skills to practice flight nursing, such as patient intubation, EKG interpretation, intravenous (IV) and chest tube insertion, medication administration, sedation, and central line placement.

The vast majority of flight teams consist of an RN and a respiratory therapist. Although team members follow established health care protocols, they still make many independent decisions regarding crisis intervention. These nurses are truly functioning in an expanded role, providing care to infants, children, and adult patients while performing a variety of therapeutic interventions. Flight nurses also provide education to outlying communities and volunteer in emergency situations.

Although there are no true national standards for becoming a flight nurse, most of the opportunities available nationally require the following:

- Two to three years critical care experience
- Advanced Cardiac Life Support certificate (ACLS)
- Pediatric Advanced Life Support certificate (PALS)
- Neonatal Resuscitation Program (NRP)
- Graduation from a nationally recognized trauma program, such as Prehospital Trauma Life Support (PHTLS), Basic Trauma Life Support (BTLS), Trauma Nurse Core Course (TNCC), and/or Transport Nurse Advanced Trauma Course (TNATC).

Certifications such as Critical Care Registered Nurse (CCRN), Certified Emergency Nurse (CEN), or Certified Flight Registered Nurse (CFRN) may also be required.

Most of these courses and certificates are nationally known and offered by a variety of providers. The certification exams are offered and given by their governing bodies, and most exams are offered online, for example, AACN.

If you are interested in flight nursing, it is important to note that a broad-based background is immensely helpful for this position. Large, busy medical centers will afford you a broad range of experiences, such as adult and pediatric critical care, high risk obstetrics, emergency department, and so on.

Many flight nurses have a baccalaureate degree (BS) and many of the certifications listed previously. Some flight nurses may have additional critical care certifications such as critical care registered nurse (CCRN) or certified emergency nurse (CEN). In addition to the

REAL WORLD INTERVIEW

Becoming a flight nurse after being a pediatric intensive care nurse for 7½ years was a huge role change, especially because of the autonomy I now have. I am responsible for performing an assessment on a patient, and then delivering care based on my findings. The care a flight nurse delivers is based on diagnosis-specific standards of care. Many times the patient diagnosis is known, such as when a patient is being transferred from a hospital, but it is the flight nurse's responsibility to ensure that the previous care initiated is still appropriate for this patient. The physical environment is also very different from my previous role. Many of the patients I encounter are located in a very small community hospital with limited resources. When I have a flight mission at an accident scene, the patient may be in an ambulance, trapped in a vehicle, on the ground, or in their house. Once the patient is initially assessed and stabilized, they are moved to the confined and noisy environment of the helicopter. I think that the biggest change from being a staff nurse to a flight nurse is the limited resources available while on a call. Although physician consult is only a radio or phone call away, I am expected to make autonomous clinical decisions in order to save the patient valuable time in receiving lifesaving therapies. At times, I must rely solely on my own experience and that of my partner.

Allison Goodell, BSN, RN, NREMT-P
Flight Nurse
Albany, New York

advanced certifications, education, and clinical skills, nurses qualifying for flight nursing need a strong critical care/emergency room background, with demonstrated clinical skills in a variety of areas. An extensive training program is also provided by the hospital. These training programs include clinical rotations, ambulance and flight observation/ride time, and classroom training. Upon becoming a flight nurse, it is essential that nurses maintain continuing education and certification credits and attend courses offered by agencies such as the U.S. Department of Transportation, the National Flight Nurses Association, and the Emergency Nurses Association in addition to ASTNA (Air and Surface Transport Nurse Association).

HEALTH CARE SALES/ PHARMACEUTICAL REPRESENTATIVES

Some nurses have left clinical staff nursing and have become representatives for companies that work in conjunction with traditional health care institutions. These include companies involved in pharmaceutical sales, durable medical equipment, home care, and insurance coverage, as well as health maintenance organizations (HMOs). These opportunities afford the nurse a perspective into corporate America and the workings of the world of business. There are frequently many salary enhancements, or perks, given with these positions, including having a company car, going on business trips, attending national and regional meetings and conferences, participating in profit-sharing and stock option plans, and meeting a variety of health care personnel. It can be difficult, however, especially with pharmaceutical sales, to meet sales quotas, provide for your customers, and survive the ups and downs of the business world.

RNs are usually seen as desirable employees for these positions because of their knowledge of pharmacology, technology, and health care systems. They understand how items are supposed to work and are excellent problem solvers when events are not going well.

CASE MANAGER

The Case Management Society of America defines case management as a "collaborative process which assesses, plans, implements, coordinates, and evaluates options and services to meet an individual's health needs through communication and available resources" (Lantz, Keeton, Romano, & Degroff, 2004). The ANA defines the goals of case management as "providing quality health care along a continuum, decreasing fragmentation of care across many settings, enhancing the patient's quality of life, and cost containment" (Yamamoto & Lucey, 2005). In accomplishing these goals, case management integrates both patient and provider satisfaction, taking into consideration cost factors. The hope is that this role will optimize the patient's self-care and decrease length of stay while decreasing fragmentation of care by ensuring seamless and coordinated care. Case management's origins date from the early 1970s, when private insurance companies practiced external case management to monitor and control expensive claims caused by catastrophic illness or accidents and to ensure a high quality of care. In the mid-1980s, when hospitals began to feel the financial impact of a changing reimbursement system, internal types of case management were developed to ensure that hospitals were appropriately reimbursed for their services (Yamamoto & Lucey, 2005). During the 1990s and into the twenty-first century, the growth of managed care has prompted the next level of case managers, where not only discharge planning but also utilization review is incorporated into the role. In performing the role, the nurse case manager should have expert clinical skills and knowledge of the health care system, health care finances, and legal issues, as well as be an effective communicator. Within the case management model, the nurse

REAL WORLD INTERVIEW

After receiving my BSN in nursing and passing the NCLEX, I entered the field of nursing in 1998. My career started on a busy pediatric unit filled with an assortment of medical and surgical patients. As my clinical nursing skills greatly improved, I became interested in participating in many of the unit's committees, such as the quality improvement team. This introduced me to the field of case management. As a pediatric case manager, I work with the quality improvement teams to increase patient care quality. Through collaborating with health care teams, we hope to improve care across the continuum. As a case manager, I advocate for the patient to ensure that appropriate nursing and medical interventions are implemented in a timely manner. A case manager also functions as a resource to families, patients, and staff in facilitating education and assisting with the utilization of community resources. Finally, I screen all pediatric patients for appropriateness of admission and length of stay. By doing so, I identify cases that potentially may not be covered by insurance and work to utilize resources to promote the patient's best outcome.

Jennifer Rivers, BSN, RN
Case Manager
Albany, New York

case manager will utilize various tools, such as practice guidelines, critical pathways, variance analysis, protocols, and outcome measurement tools, to achieve quality and cost-effective outcomes. Nurse case managers must provide care that focuses on outcome achievement and assist in arranging, coordinating, and monitoring patient care services. Patient goals include improving access to health care services, providing services that meet the patient's needs, and facilitating support for informal caregivers. System goals include coordinating the service delivery systems so that services are accessed more easily, preventing unnecessary use of services, and containing costs.

NURSE ENTREPRENEUR

Many nurses are leaving the bedside for the world of entrepreneurship in a variety of consultative, educational, or technical areas (Manthey, 1999). With this risk-taking move, these individuals quickly learn that success is based on high-quality work, patient satisfaction, and establishing and building effective relationships.

The concept of entrepreneurship is not a new one. The term is an interpretation of a French word that means "to undertake" (Simpson, 1998). The Merriam-Webster Collegiate Dictionary describes an entrepreneur as "one who organizes, promotes, and manages risks for an activity" (2003). Nurses have always been independent thinkers and somewhat entrepreneurial. At the start of the twentieth century, many nurses functioned independently and contracted directly with the patient or family to provide care. Bedside hospital nursing, as we know it today, was in its infancy, and it was not until the 1930s that nurses moved into the hospital setting and became employees. Nurse entrepreneurs plan, organize, finance, and operate their own businesses (Leong, 2005). Some of the major characteristics and attributes of nurse entrepreneurs include the following:

- Are visionary, self motivated, and a risk taker
- Have common sense
- Are good decision makers and problem solvers
- Are self confident, assertive, autonomous, and creative
- Are responsive to a perceived need
- Are market driven, with good financial foresight
- Recognize the possibility of success as well as the possibility of failure (Leong, 2005; Faugier, 2005; Manthey, 1999; Simpson, 1998; Wilson, 1998)

For Websites that provide information on nurse entrepreneurship, see Table 28-2.

As with any job, there are benefits and drawbacks to becoming a nurse entrepreneur. The benefits include job satisfaction, flexibility in choosing opportunities, and being able to do exactly what you want to do. Some of the downsides of entrepreneurship include enduring tough competition, riding the highs and lows of the market, finding the right product or service to sell, and providing for your own health insurance. It is important to decide what type of product or service you want to provide and develop a solid business plan. Expect to use your personal savings to cover initial start-up expenses, and plan to develop marketing strategies to spread the word about your business. Table 28-3 and Table 28-4 provide additional information about establishing a business plan. As Manthey indicated in 1999, "The process of deciding how to package my experience in such a way as to sell it was one of my most important learning experiences as a consultant" (p. 82).

TABLE 28-2	WEBSITES WITH INFORMATION AND GUIDANCE ON NURSE ENTREPRENEURSHIP

- www.nurse-entrepreneur-network.com
- www.nurseweek.com
- www.nnba.net (National Nurses in Business Association)
- www.nursingentrepreneurs.com (Nurse Entrepreneur)
- www.nursebiz.com (Travel Nursing)
- www.urmc.rochester.edu (University of Rochester Center for Nursing Entrepreneurship)
- www.independentrncontractor.com
- www.sba.gov/smallbusinessplanner/index.html, accessed May 30, 2007

TABLE 28-3	PROCESS OF ESTABLISHING A BUSINESS PLAN

Nursing Process	Business Process
Assess	■ Develop an idea/concept: short term and long term.
	■ Perform a market survey and feasibility study: determine consumer, clientele, location, and business forecast. *Utilize Websites for information.*
	■ Identify resources available: financial, technology, and business support based on your designed product or service to market.
Plan	■ Develop market strategies and financial plan based on market survey and feasibility studies.
	■ Develop product information: literature, brochures, pamphlets.
	■ Develop advertising/public relation methods and material.
	■ Schedule appropriate time to deliver product information and services.
Implement	■ Implement business concepts: direct and indirect methods with follow-up (mailings, telephone, Internet).
	■ Perform services/deliver products or service.
Evaluate	■ Perform periodic assessment of business plan: monthly, biannually, and annually.
	■ Identify strengths and weaknesses, and implement changes.

TABLE 28-4	**ELEMENTS OF A BUSINESS PLAN**
Resources	■ Financial: required capital, personal savings, loans, investors ■ Technology: computer with encryption capabilities, phone, fax, cell phone, beeper, car, credit card provider (usually coordinated through a bank). ■ Business Support Services: Better Business Bureau, Chamber of Commerce, personal contacts, accountant/financial planner
Expenses	■ Labor: self, employees, benefits, wages, health care, retirement ■ Supplies: office supplies (paper, envelopes, stamps, business cards, and so on), technology (computer, phone, fax, car, telephone, and so on) ■ Fees: professional services, equipment repair/maintenance, purchased services and/or products ■ General and administrative: utilities, leases/rentals/mortgages, phone services, taxes, depreciation, continuing education/tuition, travel, health insurance, post office box
Revenue	■ Direct result of services and/or products provided and sold ■ Fair market value

WOUND, OSTOMY, CONTINENCE NURSE SPECIALIST

The field of enterostomal therapy was initiated in 1958 at the Cleveland Clinic, with the first enterostomal therapists (ETs) being nonnurses. The first nursing training program was started in 1961, and in 1972, new standards for the schools of enterostomal therapy were established. The year 1976 marked a significant change when the governing body of the International Association of Enterostomal Therapists determined that only RNs would be admitted to enterostomal therapy educational programs. After this, the scope of practice was expanded beyond just caring for ostomies to include skin care, management of draining wounds and fistulas, pressure sores, and incontinence. At this point, the entry requirements into an enterostomal therapy nursing education program (ETNEP) changed to be a bachelor's degree with a major in nursing.

Nurses with this training and education practice both in hospitals and community-based settings such as visiting nurse associations, public health, nursing homes, and long-term care facilities. Over the past twenty years, these specialists have truly become the clinical experts in managing patients with ostomies, alterations in skin integrity, and wounds.

REAL WORLD INTERVIEW

This field of practice has grown tremendously over the past twenty years and provides the individual with a myriad of clinical challenges on a daily basis. The Wound, Ostomy, Continence (WOC) nurse functions in the role of an independent advanced nurse clinician and is uniquely prepared to assume the role of a specialist in three scopes of practice: wounds, ostomy, and continence. In caring for patients with these alterations, the WOC nurse's practice component may include clinical practice, consultation, education, research, and administration. In addition, the WOC nurse can function effectively in a variety of health care settings and is skilled in collaborative practice with the interdisciplinary team that is required for comprehensive patient care management.

Jane Carmel, MA, RN, CWOCN
Former ETNEP Director
Former Board of Directors, WOCN
Albany, New York

ADVANCED PRACTICE NURSING

The concept of advanced practice nursing originated in the mid- to late nineteenth century, with the creation of the role of nurse anesthetist. The concept further developed in the twentieth century with nurse-midwifery (1925 with the Frontier Nursing Service in rural Kentucky), clinical nurse specialists (1955 at Rutgers University), and finally, nurse practitioners (1965 at University of Colorado with Loretta Ford).

Why is there a need for advanced practice nurses (APNs)? The last quarter of the twentieth century taught that detection, prevention, promotion, early intervention, and education are not only cost-effective but also rational. APNs are ideally suited to deliver this type of health care. Many Americans have been disenfranchised from advances in the health sciences, namely the poor, minority groups, the uninsured or underinsured, and individuals suffering from chronic poor health. This segment of our society is especially vulnerable and one that APNs can certainly assist.

Definitions of advanced practice nursing have been advanced since the early 1990s. In 1992, the ANA defined APNs as nurses who have a graduate degree in nursing and who "conduct comprehensive health assessments, demonstrate a high level of autonomy, and possess expert skills in the diagnosis and treatment of complex responses of individuals, families, and communities to actual or potential health problems" (Robertson, 2004). The AACN has provided a position statement that describes the APN as "an umbrella term appropriate for a licensed registered nurse prepared at the graduate degree level . . . with specialized knowledge and skills that are applied within a broad range of patient populations in a variety of practice settings (McCabe & Burman, 2006; Walden & Wright, 2005). Advanced practice nursing, builds on the foundation of professional nursing practice and responds to the health care needs of the country. The future for APNs will be built on their ability to be politically astute and savvy and take an active role in their own destiny, giving evidence of and demonstrating their worth.

This evidence can be provided through research studies as well as through the APN's day-to-day contributions. Are the APN's contributions unique and valuable, and can this be shown to others? Consider the following:

- *Clinical nurse specialist (CNS):* In a hospital setting, the CNS must be able to identify how performance contributes to the patient-focused mission and goals of the organization. Does the CNS's practice reduce length of stay, improve patient outcomes, or enhance the efficiency of staff nurses?
- *Certified nurse midwife (CNM):* The CNM's ability to better meet patient needs, or to provide services to groups of patients at a lower cost than services provided by practitioners, should be measureable.
- *Nurse practitioner (NP):* In both inpatient and outpatient settings, the NP needs to document both the quantity and quality of services provided to patients and the NP's ability to reduce hospitalization rates.
- *Certified registered nurse anesthetist (CRNA):* In evaluating anesthesia services in a chronic low back pain clinic, the CRNA should clearly document quality of service and patient outcomes.

CERTIFIED REGISTERED NURSE ANESTHETIST (CRNA)

The first recorded nurse administering anesthesia was Sister Mary Bernard, a Catholic nun, in 1877. Alice Magaw, however, is considered the mother of anesthesia for her outstanding contributions to the field. She was also the first nurse anesthetist to publish articles and perform research on the practice of anesthesia. Between 1909 and 1914, four formal educational programs for nurse anesthetists were established. Currently, there are more than 90 approved programs, which may be viewed at www.aana.com (American Association of Nurse Anesthetists).

The **certified registered nurse anesthetist** (CRNA) is an APN specialty requiring the graduate to obtain a master's degree. This individual takes care of the patient's anesthesia needs before, during, and after surgery or other procedures alone or in conjunction with other health care professionals. Today, CRNAs enjoy a high degree of autonomy and professional respect. CRNAs provide anesthetics to patients in every practice setting and for every type of surgery or procedure. They are the sole anesthesia providers in two-thirds of all rural hospitals, and the main provider of anesthesia to expectant mothers and to men and women serving in the U.S. Armed Forces. CRNA programs require a bachelor's of science in nursing as well as at least one year of acute care nursing for entry into the program.

CERTIFIED NURSE-MIDWIFE (CNM)

Midwifery has existed from the beginning of humankind, and throughout history has played a vital and integral role in a community's growth. In the 1920s, Mary Breckenridge (a British midwife), along with other British midwives, worked with the Frontier Nursing Services in Kentucky to provide services for the rural population. The first American midwifery program was established in 1932, with the curriculum adapted and modified from the British model. In 1955, the American College of Nurse-Midwives (ACNM) was formed, with its main goals focused on setting standards for practice and education.

Currently, there are numerous midwifery educational programs offering the master's degree which may be viewed at www.midwife.org. Since 1980, CNMs have been allowed to practice in a variety of settings, including hospitals, homes, and birthing centers, providing care for women throughout the childbearing cycle as well as postpartum. Nurse-midwives and collaborating practitioners agree upon the protocols and procedures. Health education, as well as delivering newborns, comprises a large part of the clinical activities, including the teaching of self-care skills and preparation for childbirth and child rearing. The ANA asserts that the CNM can provide "services to women and their babies in the areas of prenatal care, labor and delivery management, postpartum care, normal newborn care, well-women gynecology, and family planning (ANA, 2000).

CLINICAL NURSE SPECIALIST (CNS)

By the turn of the twentieth century, the greatest percentage of APNs were the CNSs, whose origins can be traced back to 1938. Reiter first coined the term *nurse clinician* in 1943 to designate a nurse with advanced clinical competence and recommended that such clinicians get their preparation in graduate nursing education programs. Educators first developed the **clinical nurse specialist** (CNS) role because of their concern for improving nursing care. They believed that nursing care improvement was dependent upon increasing expertise at the bedside, giving both direct and indirect care, and incorporating role modeling and consultation. The CNS role has evolved to include many specialties. The first CNS master's program in psychiatry was started by Peplau in 1955 at Rutgers University.

The impressive development of the psychiatric CNS role helped to initiate the other CNS specialty programs. Following the passage and enactment of the Nurse Training Act in 1965, clinical specialization in graduate education increased tremendously. Graduates would provide a high level of specialized nursing care, as well as serve as change agents in hospital settings.

The CNS is a hospital-based APN primarily, serving as a clinical expert in evidence-based nursing practice within a specialty area. In this capacity, the CNS uses clinical expertise to influence patients, nurses, and nursing practice, as well as the organization/system with a focus on providing quality, cost-effective care (Darmody, 2005). The four components included within this role are that of direct patient care provider, educator, consultant, and researcher. The 2004 revision of the CNS practice agreement further developed these roles to integrate their practice rather than partition the roles in the previously mentioned activities. Further literature has identified the roles of the CNS, and in addition to the above, includes leader, change agent, practitioner, and case manager (Darmody, 2005; Stacey, All, & Gresham, 2002). A good portion of time is spent in the hospital, in both staff and patient/family education, as well as developing protocols, standards, and pathways that will guide nursing practice. Within the role, the CNS focus can be broad, encompassing adult, pediatric, and obstetric patients, or narrow, including areas such as oncology, the cardiopulmonary system, the pulmonary system, and so on. A study by Wyers, Grove, and Pastorino in 1985 listed essential CNS competencies; which are still valid today.

- Developing an in-depth knowledge base
- Demonstrating clinical expertise in a selected area of clinical practice
- Serving as a role model
- Serving as a practitioner/teacher, consultant, researcher

NURSE PRACTITIONER (NP)

The last decade of the twentieth century witnessed a large increase in the number of nurse practitioner programs and graduates (Ford, 1997). This was driven partially by the changing health care system, hospital downsizing, an increase in ambulatory care, and constraints on managed care. In addition, the American Medical Association (AMA) called for a decrease in admissions to medical school. Simultaneously, the federal government practically eliminated the graduate medical education (GME) funds given to hospitals with residency programs. Many of these circumstances are not unlike those that existed when Loretta Ford, a doctorally prepared RN, and Henry Silver, a medical practitioner, started the first nurse practitioner (NP) training program at the University of Colorado in 1965 (Hoekelman, 1998).

The NP role has had a tremendous evolution from its humble beginnings. This graduate-level educated RN is still primarily practicing within primary care, however, the role has expanded greatly. These NPs are practicing throughout the continuum of health care in a multitude of settings and patient populations. Within ten years of Dr. Ford's first NP program, sixty-five other NP programs were created. The second NP program was started at Duke in 1966, the birthplace of the first physician's assistant program. By 1999, NPs in all states could be directly reimbursed by Medicare and could write prescriptions (Ventura & Grandinetti, 1999).

Although NPs have become fully integrated into the clinical delivery system, they have often been legally and financially dependent on medical practitioners for their jobs. While some states allow NPs to work independently, most states allow NPs to work collaboratively with a medical practitioner. This differs from the physician assistant, who works under the direct supervision of the physician. NPs are competent in delivering primary care that is

REAL WORLD INTERVIEW

As NPs face the new millennium, it is advisable to listen to the wisdom of the famous author on China, Pearl Buck, who said, "To understand today, you have to search yesterday." Further, to envision the future, think "outside the box" creatively, constructively, and globally. Unfortunately, most people hate change; so do professionals. By their very nature, professionals can become myopic, territorial, and conservative. Some that are so resistant to change become arrogant, self-important, and greedy. Nursing must face the future differently. Tomorrow's practitioners will face globalization, not only of economics but of every field of human endeavor. Demographics, technological advances, transportation, and communication will expand beyond imagination and at lightning speed. Health information will no longer belong exclusively to the health professions. The Internet will see to that. The challenge for NPs is to be proactive rather than reactive in creating a social, cultural, political, and physical environment in which to successfully live, work, and thrive as a responsible member of the new society and as an advocate for our patients and their families. So, thoroughly examine the past, keep the enduring human values of caring, compassion, and courage in nursing, listen to your best teachers—the patients—and create your own future accordingly.

Loretta Ford, EdD, RN, FAAN
Founder, Nurse Practitioner Program
Rochester, New York

satisfactory, acceptable to patients, and cost-effective. The keys to the success of the NP role have been the autonomous yet collaborative nature of the practice; accountability as a direct provider of health care services; emphasis on clinical decision making as a foundational clinical skill; the focus on health and healthy lifestyles as a foundation of practice; and the cost-effective, accessible nature of the practice. These basic attributes of NP practice hold true regardless of setting or specialty focus (Ford, 1997).

Although many NPs have practiced in primary nonhospital, nonacute care settings, the neonatal nurse practitioner (NNP) has been hospital based for many years. Recently, a new role, the acute care nurse practitioner (ACNP), has been created. These positions also have a collaborative rather than subordinate relationship with medical practitioners (Kleinpell, 2005). As with all NPs, the ACNP is blending nursing and medicine by taking a holistic patient-management approach while using collaborative treatment protocols frequently involving procedures previously done only by medical practitioners, such as lumbar punctures, chest tube insertion, writing medication prescriptions, and so on.

Although the performance of such roles bodes well for nursing in general and NPs specifically, there is also some discussion about NPs taking on too much within the health care system; the concern is that "if nurses take on an increasing amount of technical and medical work, then characteristics highly valued in the nursing profession may be threatened. It is clear that while NPs

provide autonomous practice and competent patient management, they also must protect their holistic, caring nursing role (Kleinpell, 2005).

CLINICAL NURSE SPECIALIST/NURSE PRACTITIONER (CNS/NP): A COMBINED ROLE

Since the mid-1980s, there has been frequent discussion and published data on the controversial issue of merging the advance practice CNS and NP roles. There is no doubt that both these APNs are key providers meeting the health care needs of many Americans. There are few practice settings or patient populations that have not been served by an APN in some capacity (Lincoln, 2000). Historically, the major differences between the CNS and NP were the setting and focus of their practice. This has changed and in today's health care arena, CNS and NP roles have evolved in response to the changing needs of patients, as well as the changing health care system. Undoubtedly, many aspects of the roles are similar, and both roles have served their patients and each other well. The CNS role has been credited with creating an advanced level of nursing with an eye toward theory-based practice. NP's have been credited with the movement of nursing beyond traditional roles and increasing the public's awareness of advanced practice nursing (Stacey et al., 2002). In 1990, the ANA Council of Clinical Nurse Specialists and the Council of Primary Health Care Nurse Practitioners merged, which sent a powerful message regarding their positions on the issue. Despite this, at the end of the twentieth century, while there are some dual-role educational programs and individuals functioning as both a CNS and NP, many education programs and clinical practice areas are separate. Following are some factors to consider when examining these two roles (Pinelli, 1997):

- Patient populations
- Future roles for CNS and NP
- Narrower perspective and focus for both the CNS and NP
- "Horizontal violence" within nursing—nurses fighting among themselves

It might be said that the role of the APN is emerging with both depth and breadth. Both the NP and CNS possess the skills and knowledge that promote the application of these roles in a variety of settings, both those settings that currently exist and those yet to be created. Research skills and change agent skills allow these APNs to function at multiple and varied levels within the health care system. Through these roles, nursing can resume its mission to provide health care to all individuals and reshape health care with an eye toward wellness and prevention as described originally in Nursing's Agenda for Health Care Reform (1992), and more recently in the national health promotion and disease prevention initiative available at www.healthypeople.gov, Healthy People 2010 (Stacey et al., 2002).

There are both advantages and disadvantages to merging the roles (Table 28-5). Some predict that eventually the two roles will merge as a result of supply and marketplace demands. Additional educational programs for each, however, could still be available for CNSs not desiring to spend the majority of their time in clinical practice, such as CNS/consultant or CNS/educator.

TABLE 28-5   CNS/NP MERGER: ADVANTAGES AND DISADVANTAGES

Advantages	Disadvantages
■ Many similarities: education, clinical settings	■ Different scopes of practice: CNS primarily in hospital-based tertiary care; NP primarily in ambulatory and primary care
■ Expanding and overlapping practice settings	
■ Increased power in numbers	■ Legal issue of trying to include CNS in existing advanced practice legislation
■ Cost savings to universities and education programs	■ Increased length of graduate education program
■ Increased marketability	■ Continued blurring and role confusion

---

REAL WORLD INTERVIEW

Currently, I am functioning as a CNS/NP. When I made the decision to pursue graduate school in order to become an advanced practice nurse, I carefully examined many different schools of nursing and came to the decision that if I wanted to be a nurse practitioner, then I should go to the school with the individual that started the entire field. For me, that was the University of Rochester, where Dr. Loretta Ford had moved in the mid-1970s from Denver. The knowledge and skills I obtained throughout my graduate education, including clinical rotations, course work, and finally my master's thesis, were supportive of where I wanted to be in the years to come, as I combined the two roles both educationally and clinically. I have also had the wonderful opportunity to practice what I preach in the pediatric clinical setting where I have been working since the 1980s.

Stephen Jones, MS, RNC, PNP, ET
Albany, New York

CASE STUDY 28-1

It is March of your senior year at college. You have been offered a position as a staff nurse at a hospital where you really wanted to work. For the past several weeks during your last clinical rotation, however, you have had the opportunity to work with an APN. You start to think that perhaps this is what you would like to do, and you know of a few colleges that will take graduates right into their master's program. You begin to check educational opportunities.

Is this something you could do? Should do?

In coming to an answer, consider the following:

- Have the clinical rotations you had as a student prepared you for an advanced practice role?
- What resources are available to you that would provide information in guiding your decision?
- Would spending time working as a staff nurse better prepare you to be an APN?

EVIDENCE FROM THE LITERATURE

Citation: Larrabee, J. H., Janney, M. A., Ostrow, C. L., Withrow, M. L., Hobbs, G. R., & Burant, C. (2003). Predicting registered nurse job satisfaction and intent to leave. *Journal of Nursing Administration, 33*(5), 271–283.

Discussion: The purpose of this study was to investigate the relative influence of nurse attitudes, context of care, and structure of care on job satisfaction and intent to leave. A nonexperimental, predictive design evaluated these relationships in a nonrandom sample of ninety registered staff nurses using instruments with known psychometric properties. The major predictor of intent to leave was job dissatisfaction, and the major predictor of job satisfaction was psychological empowerment. Predictors of psychological empowerment were hardiness, transformational leadership style, nurse/practitioner collaboration, and group cohesion. Results supported the influence of nurse attitude on job satisfaction relative to other contributing factors.

Implications for Practice: This study provides support for the theoretical relationships among the nurse outcomes of job satisfaction and intent to leave and nurse attitudes, context of care, and structure of care. This finding reaffirms the importance of nurse leaders routinely monitoring satisfaction and evaluating and implementing strategies to address the dimensions of satisfaction that the data indicate need improvement. Specifically, the findings emphasize the importance of creating and maintaining a work milieu in which participative management thrives.

DIRECTION FOR THE FUTURE

In examining the evolution of nursing and the direction in which it is heading, the ANA believes that more effective utilization of RNs to provide primary health care services is part of the solution to the cost and accessibility problems in health care today.

The twenty-first century holds a great deal of promise, but there are many questions to be answered regarding the cost, accessibility, and quality of the health care system in the United States. Nursing has a wonderful opportunity to be a leader in the changing health care delivery system. Few other professions provide as many options. There is a world of emerging opportunities as you prepare to enter the workforce. Take your time, research the possibilities, organize your plan, and live your dream. As Sophia Palmer said in 1897 at the first convention of the American Society of Superintendents of Training Schools for Nursing, "Organization is the power of the day. Without it, nothing great is accomplished" (ANA, 2001).

KEY CONCEPTS

- Nursing possesses myriad emerging practice opportunities.

- Certification is a process readily available to any RN.

- Case management is a growing subspecialty within the hospital setting.

- Entrepreneurship and other nontraditional positions such as travel nursing have proven very successful for nurses.

- Nursing practice has become increasingly specialized.

- Numerous types of APNs are now practicing in both the hospital and community settings.

- Although the CNS is primarily hospital-based, NPs practice both within the hospital and in community-based settings.

- For any RN, a plan to develop professional opportunities is essential.

KEY TERMS

certified registered nurse anesthetist

clinical nurse specialist

REVIEW QUESTIONS

1. Traveling nurses
   A. need to carry a notarized copy of their home state license.
   B. should become ACLS certified.
   C. need to obtain state licenses for each state in which they will be practicing.
   D. should only work for one company.

2. The hospital-based case manager's primary focus is
   A. providing care and services that focus on outcome.
   B. making sure all the patient's expenses are taken care of.
   C. guiding medical and nursing protocols.
   D. ensuring that each patient has a primary nurse.

3. To be a successful nurse entrepreneur, it is imperative that the individual
   A. be able to attain a sizable loan from a bank to help with start-up costs.
   B. attain credit card approval.
   C. understand how the stock market functions.
   D. develop a solid business plan.

4. Which of the following is the best method of determining the effectiveness of an APN's practice?
   A. Patient satisfaction guide
   B. Fewer hospital admissions
   C. Improved patient outcomes
   D. Number of research studies

5. APNs provide both nursing and health care services. APNs can best fulfill this mission by
   A. performing and then publishing research.
   B. responding to patients' health care needs.
   C. maintaining as many certifications as possible.
   D. managing patients in both the hospital and outpatient settings.

REVIEW ACTIVITIES

1. Finally, you have graduated and moved to the city of your choice and are working at the health care facility of your choice. You are starting to apply all the knowledge and skills that you gained at school. You are around all levels and types of mentors and role models and are witnessing firsthand the activities of new and experienced staff nurses, as well as those of APNs.

   What are some of your initial thoughts on where you will be in one, three, five, or ten years from now? Discuss how you will determine your progress.

2. Review categories such as travel nursing, job hunting, and licensure and certification at *Nursing*'s (the journal) Website, located at www.nursing2007.com (this will change with the specific year this journal is being published). What did you see there?

3. Review nursing issues/programs, information, services and certification at ANA's Website (www.nursingworld.org). What did you see there?

4. Peruse and discover hot topics, various resources, and so on at Modern Healthcare's Website (www.modernhealthcare.com). What did you see there?

5. For information on salaries, practice issues, and so on, log on to NLN's site (www.nln.org). What did you see there?

6. Review the RN salary survey by Hader in *Nursing Management, 36*(7), 18–27. How will this information help you plan your future?

7. Review the medical practitioner's salary survey by Westfall C., in the *Physician Executive,* November/December 2005, 32–37. Note how medical practitioners are compensated.

EXPLORING THE WEB

Which sites should you visit regularly, both for your own personal and professional growth?

General Interest and Nursing Issues:

- Centers for Disease Control and Prevention: *www.cdc.gov*

- National Institutes of Health: *www.nih.gov*

- National League for Nursing: *www.nln.org*
- American Nurses Association (ANA): *www.nursingworld.org*
- ANA certification listing: *www.nursingworld.org*
- Discover Nursing: *www.discovernursing.com*
- Center for Nursing: *www.nursingcenter.com*
- National Council of State Boards of Nursing: *www.ncsbn.org*
- General nursing interest site: *www.allnurses.com*
- Health care information: *www.medscape.com* *www.docguide.com*

Specialty Issues:

- American Association of Nurse Anesthetists: *www.aana.com*
- Flight nursing: *www.flightweb.com*
- Small Business Administration: *www.sbaonline.sba.gov*
- Service Corps of Retired Executives: *www.score.org*
- Traveling nurses: *www.healthcareers-online.com*
- American Academy of Nurse Practitioners: *www.aanp.org*
- Nurse Practitioner Central: *www.npcentral.net*

REFERENCES

American Nurses Association [ANA]. (2000). Press release. Retrieved February 25, 2000, from www.ana.org

ANA. (2001). Where we come from. Retrieved February 28, 2002, from http://www.nursingworld.org/centenn/index.htm

Darmody, J. V. (2005, Sept.–Oct.). Observing the work of the Clinical Nurse Specialist: A pilot study. *Clinical Nurse Specialist, 19*(5), 260–268.

Erickson, J., Holm, L., Chelminiak, L., & Ditomassi, M. (2005). Why not nursing. *Nursing 2005, 35*(7), 46–49.

Faugier, J. (2005). Developing a new generation of nurse entrepreneurs. *Nursing Standard, 19*(30), 49–53.

Ford, L. C. (1997). Advanced practice nursing. A deviant comes of age . . . the NP in acute care. *Heart & Lung: Journal of Acute & Critical Care, 26*(2), 87–91.

Hoekelman, C. R. (1998). A program to increase health care for children: The pediatric nurse practitioner program by Henry K. Silver, MD, Loretta C. Ford, EdD, and Susan G. Stearly, MS, Pediatrics, 1967, 39: 756–760. *Pediatrics, 102*(1 Pt. 2), 245–247.

Kleinpell, R. M. (2005). Acute care nurse practitioner: Results of a 5-year longitudinal study. *American Journal of Critical Care, 14*(3), 211–221.

Khomeiran, R., Yekta, Z. P., Kiger, A. M., & Ahmadi, F. (2006, March). Professional competence: Factors described by nurses as influencing their development. *International Nursing Review. 53*(1), 66–72.

Lantz, P., Keeton, K., Romano, L., & Degroff, A. (2004). Case management in public health screening programs: The experience of the national breast and cervical cancer early detection program. *Journal of Public Health Management Practice, 10*(6), 545–555.

Larrabee, J. H., Janney, M. A., Ostrow, C. L., Withrow, M. L., Hobbs, G. R., & Burant, C. (2003). Predicting registered nurse job satisfaction and intent to leave. *Journal of Nursing Administration, 33*(5), 271–283.

Leong, S. (2005). Clinical nurse specialist entrepreneurship. *Internet Journal of Advanced Nursing Practice, 7*(1).

Lincoln, P. E. (2000). Comparing CNS and NP role activities: A replication. *Clinical Nurse Specialist, 14*(6), 269–277.

Manthey, M. (1999). Financial management for entrepreneurs. *Nursing Administration Quarterly, 23*(4), 81–85.

Marrelli, T. (2006, January). Nursing in flux. *American Journal of Nursing, 106*(1), 19–20.

McCabe, S., & Burman, M. (2006, Jan.–Mar.). A tale of two APNs: Addressing blurred practice boundaries in APN practice. *Perspectives in Psychiatric Care, 42*(1), 3–12.

Merriam Webster's Collegiate Dictionary (2003). 11th Edition. Merriam Webster.

Murphy-Ende, K. (2002). Advanced practice nursing: reflections on the past, issues for the future. *Oncology Nursing Forums, 29*(1), 106–112.

Pinelli, J. M. (1997). The clinical nurse specialist/nurse practitioner: Oxymoron or match made in heaven? *Canadian Journal of Nursing Administration, 10*(1), 85–110.

Robertson, J. (2004). Does advanced community/public health nursing practice have a future? *Public Health Nursing, 21*(5), 495–500.

Schwarz, T. (2006, January). What is past is prologue? *American Journal of Nursing, 106*(1), 13.

Shirey, M. (2005). Celebrating certification in nursing: Forces of magnetism in action. *Nursing Administration Quarterly, 29*(3), 245–253.

Simpson, R. L. (1998). Nursing informatics. From nurse to nursing informatics consultant: A lesson in entrepreneurship. *Nursing Administration Quarterly, 22*(2), 87–90.

Stacey, R., All, A., & Gresham, D. (2002). Role preservation of the clinical nurse specialist and the nurse practitioner. *Internet Journal of Advanced Nursing Practice, 5*(2).

Stromberg, M. F., Niebuhn, B., Prevost, S., Fabrey, L., Muenzen, P., Spence, C., et al. (2005, May). More than a title. *Nursing Management, 36*(5), 36–46.

Ventura, M., & Grandinetti, D. (1999). NP progress report: A survey. *RN, 62*(7), 33–35.

Walden, M., & Wright, K. (2005, Jan.–Feb.). Advanced practice registered nurse update: Issues of evolving complexity . . . stay informed (guest editorial). *Journal of Wound, Ostomy & Continence Nursing, 32*(1), 1–2.

Wilson, C. K. (1998). Mentoring the entrepreneur. *Nursing Administration Quarterly, 22*(2), 1–12.

Wyers, M. E., Grove, S. K., & Pastorino, C. (1985). Clinical nurse specialist: In search of the right role. *Nursing Health Care, 6*(4), 202–207.

Yamamoto, L. & Lucey, C. (2005). Case Management "within the walls". A glimpse into the future. *Critical Care Nursing Quarterly, 28*(2), 162–178.

SUGGESTED READINGS

Adams, M. H., & Crow, C. S. (2005). Development of a nurse case management service: A proposed business plan for rural hospitals. *Lippincott's Case Manager, 19*(30), 148–158.

American Journal of Nursing. (2006, January supp.). Your guide to certification. 106, 50–63.

Bryant-Lukosius, D., & DiCenso, A. (2004). A framework for the introduction and evaluation of advanced practice nursing roles. *Journal of Advanced Nursing, 48*(5), 530–540.

Bryant-Lukosius, D., DiCenso, A., Browne, G., & Pinelli, J. (2004). Advanced practice nursing roles: Development, implementation and evaluation. *Journal of Advanced Nursing, 48*(5), 519–529.

Cummings, G., & McLennan, M. (2005). Advanced practice nursing: Leadership to effect policy change. *Journal of Nursing Administration, 35*(2), 61–69.

Ford, L. C. (1995). Nurse practitioners: Myths and misconceptions. *The Pulse, 32*(4), 9–10.

Fulton, J. S. (2005, Sept.–Oct.). Calling blended role programs to account. *Clinical Nurse Specialist, 19*(5), 221–222.

Grainer, P., & Bolan, C. (2006). Perceptions of nursing as a career choice of students in the baccalaureate nursing program. *Nurse Education Today, 26*(1), 38–44.

Hader R. (2005). Salary survey 2005. *Nursing Management, 36*(7), 18–27.

Kleinpell, R. M., & Hravnak, M. M. (2005). Strategies for success in the acute care nurse practitioner role. *Critical Care Nursing Clinics of North America, 17*(2), 177–181.

Leong, S. (2004, Sept.–Nov.). Nurses choosing entrepreneurship path. *Oklahoma Nurse, 49*(3), 28–29.

Lofmark, A., Smide, B., & Wikbald, K. (2006, March). Competence of newly graduated nurses: A comparison of the perceptions of qualified nurses and students. *Journal of Advanced Nursing, 53*(6), 721–728.

Nelson, R. (2005). AJN reports: Is there a doctor in the house? A new vision for advanced practice nursing. *American Journal of Nursing, 105*(5), 28–29.

Pellico, L. (2006, January). We'll leave the light on for you. *American Journal of Nursing, 106*(1), 32–33.

Robbins, C. L., & Birmingham, J. (2005). Issues and interventions: The social worker and nurse roles in case management. *Lippincott's Case Management, 10*(3), 120–127.

Smolenski, M. C. (2005). Cedentialing, certification and competence: Issues for new and seasoned nurse practitioners (Fellows column). *Journal of the American Academy of Nurse Practitioners, 17*(6), 201–204.

Steefel, L. (2005). New doctoral degree aims to advance nursing practice. *Nursing Spectrum: New York & New Jersey edition, 17*(5), 14–15.

Summer, J. F. (2004). Caring—the foundation of advanced practice nursing. *Topics in Advanced Practice Nursing, 4*(4).

Wilson, G. (2005). The case for advanced practice nurses in the ED. *Internet Australian Nursing Journal, 13*(4).

CHAPTER 29

Your First Job

Lyn LaBarre, MS, RN ✪ Dr. Miki Magnino-Rabig, PhD, RN

*Practice nursing with love,
faith, and passion . . .
(Miki Magnino-Rabig, 2006).*

OBJECTIVES

Upon completion of this chapter, the reader should be able to:

1. Identify key elements to consider in choosing a nursing position.
2. Relate typical components of health care orientation.
3. Explain types of performance feedback.
4. Compare and contrast organizational responses to performance.
5. Relate specific strategies to enhance the beginning nursing manager role.
6. Identify mechanisms to enhance professional growth.

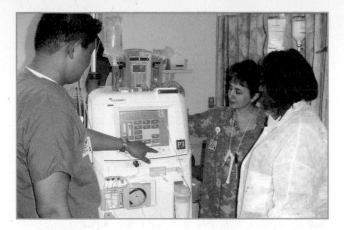

Congratulations! You have just completed your nursing educational requirements, and graduation is one week away. You have decided to stay in this geographic area and have received three job offers: a twelve-hour night position in the surgical intensive care unit of a regional teaching hospital, a rotating shift eight-hour position on a community hospital's medical-surgical floor, and a public health nursing position with your county's health department.

Which position should you accept?

What factors will help you decide which is the best fit for you?

Graduation brings the transition from the role of student to that of RN. A nurse's first job is an opportunity to solidify skills learned in school. It is also the time to establish relationships with mentors and to set down a foundation for future professional growth. This chapter will discuss important considerations regarding your first job.

CHOOSING A POSITION

In the current job market, new nurses are in the enviable position of having broad choices for their first job. Hospitals now recruit new nurses to specialty areas such as obstetrics, psychiatry, and critical care, as well as to the traditional medical-surgical units. Community health organizations are also anxious to hire recent graduates. The federal government has estimated that with the aging population, there will be a 40% increase in the demand for RNs over the next 20 years (Zerweck, 2005).

PATIENT TYPES

One of the most important considerations in selecting a job is choosing the best fit for you in a patient care environment. New nurses who start their career on a general medical or surgical unit typically manage patients with a variety of diagnoses. They learn diverse technical and assessment skills. These nurses develop a working knowledge of many common medications and patient teaching scenarios. In contrast, nurses who choose an entry position on a specialty unit focus on patients with specific diseases, body system disorders, or age groups, such as a cardiology, obstetrics, or neonatology patient. Community health nursing positions can be broad spectrum, sharing the characteristics of a medical or surgical nursing role, or being more specialized, for example, a community neonatal nurse.

WORK ENVIRONMENT

Another facet to consider in choosing a first position is the opportunity to develop organizational skills. In a critical care or specialty area, nurses need to develop the ability to prioritize and plan care for limited numbers of patients, who need highly specialized assessments and technical care. In contrast, the nurse whose first job is on a general floor must organize care for a diverse and much larger group of patients. A new nurse in the community may work alone for most of the day, seeing patients one at a time. Even though each area requires specific skills, the organizational skills for all these nurses include effective time management.

Another consideration in weighing possible positions is the available schedule. Many health care organizations now offer a variety of schedules. Twelve-hour shifts are particularly popular because a full-time nurse can work as few as three shifts per week. For the patient, this means fewer changes in nursing personnel within a day but less continuity throughout the hospital stay. For the new nurse, a twelve-hour shift can be a long work day, but it allows increased flexibility in personal time. Some organizations offer rotations between daytime and other shifts. Others award the more popular day shifts by seniority. When choosing a position, it is important to find out about the process for changing to a different schedule after hiring. Some hospitals restrict new nurses from changing positions for a set period of time. Following are some other questions to ask about your schedule: What will my weekend commitment be? How many holidays will I be expected to work each year? Does the health care organization use a **self-scheduling** system, in which nurses select their own schedule according to unit guidelines, or is time assigned? If time is assigned, how much notice will be required to have a certain day off?

Pay is an obvious element in choosing your first job, but the best-paying job offer is not necessarily the wisest choice, even from a financial point of view. Health care organizations in the same geographic area tend to offer competitive salaries at the start of employment. It is important to ask about an employer's salary policy. Does the hospital you are considering give a raise after you have passed your NCLEX, or would any potential raise be held until your first-year anniversary? Are nurses paid extra for having a BSN degree? What are the differentials, if any, for weekend work or working off shifts? Be sure that nurses are paid for orientation shifts and required courses. When comparing offers between two health care organizations, ask how many hours are paid for a typical workweek. Some employers pay for a full 8- or 12-hour shift by allowing for a 30-minute overlap at change of shifts. Other organizations do not expect staff nurses to overlap, resulting in a shorter shift. Thus at some facilities, a typical pay week includes 40 hours, whereas at others nurses routinely work 37.5 hours per week.

Finally, work environments in health care organizations can vary tremendously. Are you more comfortable in a smaller hospital setting in which it is relatively easy to find your way around and everyone knows each other? Or do you prefer the more complex, perhaps less personal setting of a large teaching facility? Do you enjoy working with resident practitioners in a teaching hospital, or will you be more satisfied interacting with community-based, private attending practitioners?

ORIENTATION CONSIDERATIONS

Different health care organizations also can have very different approaches to new employee orientation and education. Because orientation is a key component of the transition between being a student nurse and becoming a first-time manager of patients, it is important to establish what the organization offers during orientation. Consider the following questions:

- How long should I expect to be in orientation?
- Is it tailored to my learning needs, or is it the same for all incoming nurses?
- Does it all occur at the beginning of my new position, or will it be offered in stages?
- What ongoing education will be available to me?
- Will I be paid for time in education programs?

- In case of short staffing, will I be pulled from orientation?

Many new nurses feel pressured to find just the right setting for their first job, particularly if they have a long-term goal of working in a subspecialty. The focus in the first job needs to be on refining assessment and technical skills and learning to be organized in the delivery of nursing care. These skills, coupled with a positive work record regarding attendance, flexibility, and attitude, will ensure the new nurse of many future opportunities.

ORIENTATION TO YOUR NEW JOB

Orientation fosters a smooth transition from graduate to practicing nurse. At its completion, a new nurse should be able to demonstrate competency in the basic skills needed for safe patient care.

GENERAL ORIENTATION

Many health care organizations divide nursing orientation into general sections and unit-specific sections. General orientation includes information and skills measurement, which all nurses new to the facility need, regardless of their eventual unit assignment. Two examples of information discussed at orientation are validation of CPR competency and an introduction to policies regarding medication administration. General orientation also typically includes explanations of human resource policies and opportunities to hear from representatives of various departments within the organization. Recent concerns about patient safety have expanded orientation to include information about the Joint Commission (JC), formerly the Joint Commission on Accreditation of Health Care Organizations (JCAHO), and National Patient Safety Goals.

REAL WORLD INTERVIEW

When I graduated from nursing school, I had several choices. The community hospital I had worked in as an LPN while I was in nursing school offered to hire me as an RN. I considered taking that position because I was comfortable at that hospital, and it was close to home. I also interviewed at a large academic teaching hospital 40 miles from my home. I decided to take the position at the large teaching hospital as I felt I would learn more at the academic center, and at this stage in my career, the opportunities made the commute worthwhile.

Ken Simek, RN
Recent Graduate
Albany, New York

Some organizations offer sections of general orientation as written materials or on videotape. This allows a more flexible orientation schedule. It is particularly beneficial for new employees who are available to attend orientation only outside daytime hours. Figure 29-1 is a sample schedule for the first week of general orientation at one medical center.

Most facilities offer general orientation first, followed by unit-specific orientation. In this case, new nurses may not actually spend a shift on their unit for two weeks after starting work. Other nurse educators plan orientation so that nurses go to their home unit very early, reserving some of the general content for later in the orientation schedule. The facility works to get information to the new graduates in a meaningful way.

Most organizations tailor their general orientation to individual learners. Thus, an experienced nurse may opt to challenge particular orientation classes by successfully completing the demonstration or written test or demonstrating competency in some fashion.

UNIT-SPECIFIC ORIENTATION

Unit-based orientation, whether it follows the general orientation or is interspersed throughout, focuses on the specific competencies a new nurse needs to care for the diagnoses and ages of patients typical to the assigned unit. These competencies include technical skills as well as beginning mastery of unit-specific processes. Some of the content covered may include topics such as what paperwork is necessary for new admissions and how to get an IV pump for medications.

Most organizations have developed unit-specific competency tools that list those skills orientees need to demonstrate. These lists provide a useful road map with which to plan a learner-specific orientation. Figure 29-2 is an excerpt from an emergency department's unit-based orientation tool.

IDENTIFYING YOUR OWN LEARNING NEEDS

New graduates begin orientation with varied clinical experiences and competencies. Often, beginning nurses are asked to self-rate their level of knowledge or experience with various patient care skills. It is important for new nurses to identify their own learning needs as they become more familiar with their work environment. Orientation is the ideal time for the new nurse to observe coworkers and establish learning priorities. One way to do this is to ask questions of the preceptor or nurse educator. This provides feedback and molds the orientation to the learner's needs.

In addition, plan to do your own self-study to prepare for your new patients. Be sure to review the patient care for the top ten nursing and medical diagnoses seen

---

CRITICAL THINKING 29-1

You are responsible for being the nurse you want to be. To do this, set your goals and monitor and evaluate them regularly. Gather data on the following indicators of being a professional nurse and add to the list, as appropriate:

- Monitor data so that I am up to date on evidence based care for my patients.
- Monitor data that my patients are satisfied, pain free, and feel cared about.
- Monitor data that my patients are complication free and have no nurse-sensitive outcomes.
- Offer professional nursing service to my patients and my community.
- Give and receive professional respect to health care team.
- Speak up about the important role that nurses play in preventing patient complications.
- Network with other professionals.
- Participate in professional committees at work.
- Communicate assertively with the health care team.
- Receive professional salary and benefits.
- Take good care of myself and work for professional and personal balance.
- Continue my education, for example, certification, formal education, continuing education, and so on.
- Join my professional organization.
- Dress like a professional.
- Communicate pride in being a nurse.

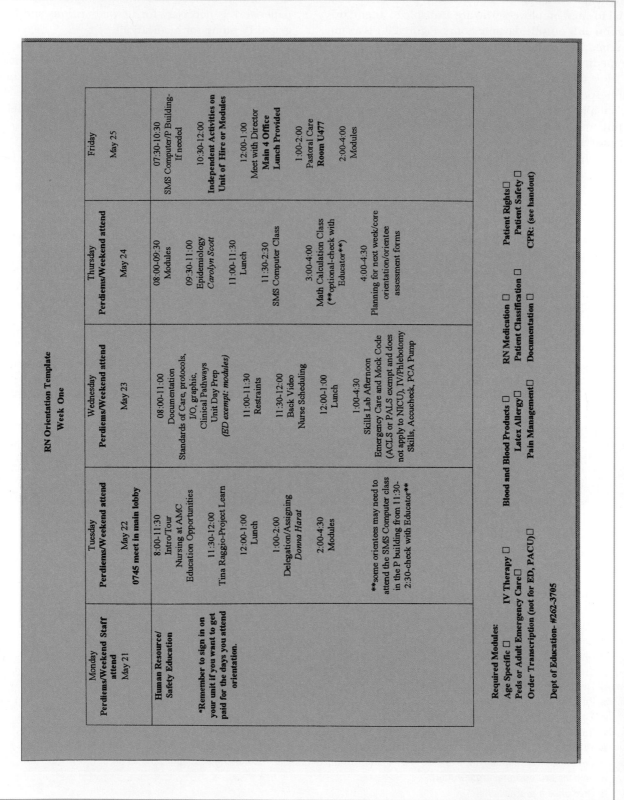

RN Orientation Template Week One

Monday Perdiems/Weekend Staff attend May 21	Tuesday Perdiems/Weekend attend May 22 0745 meet in main lobby	Wednesday Perdiems/Weekend attend May 23	Thursday Perdiems/Weekend attend May 24	Friday Perdiems/Weekend attend May 25
Human Resource/Safety Education	8:00–11:30 Intro/Tour Nursing at AMC Education Opportunities	08:00–11:00 Documentation Standards of Care, protocols, I/O, graphic, Clinical Pathways Unit Day Prep *(ED exempt: modules)*	08:00–09:30 Modules	07:30–10:30 SMS Computer/P Building- If needed
Remember to sign in on your unit if you want to get paid for the days you attend orientation.	11:30–12:00 Tina Raggio-Project Learn		09:30–11:00 Epidemiology *Carolyn Scott*	10:30–12:00 **Independent Activities on Unit of Hire or Modules**
	12:00–1:00 Lunch	11:00–11:30 Restraints	11:00–11:30 Lunch	12:00–1:00 **Meet with Director Main 4 Office Lunch Provided**
	1:00–2:00 Delegation/Assigning *Donna Harat*	11:30–12:00 Back Video Nurse Scheduling	11:30–2:30 SMS Computer Class	1:00–2:00 Pastoral Care **Room U477**
	2:00–4:30 Modules	12:00–1:00 Lunch	3:00–4:00 Math Calculation Class (**optional-check with Educator****)	2:00–4:00 Modules
		1:00–4:30 Skills Lab Afternoon Emergency Care and Mock Code (ACLS or PALS exempt and does not apply to NICU), IV/Phlebotomy Skills, Accucheck, PCA Pump	4:00–4:30 Planning for next week/core orientation/orientee assessment forms	
	some orientees may need to attend the SMS Computer class in the P building from 11:30–2:30–check with Educator*			

Required Modules:

Age Specific ☐	IV Therapy ☐	Blood and Blood Products ☐	RN Medication ☐	Patient Rights ☐
Peds or Adult Emergency Care☐	Latex Allergy☐	Patient Classification ☐	Patient Safety ☐
Order Transcription (not for ED, PACU)☐	Pain Management☐	Documentation ☐	CPR: (see handout)

Dept of Education- #262-3705

Figure 29-1 Registered professional nurse general orientation schedule template—week one. (Courtesy of Albany Medical Center, Albany, NY.)

Name	Preceptor	Unit/Dept.	Emergency Dept	Date:
At the completion of orientation the RPN will perform technical nursing skills specific to the age and characteristics of the patients served consistent with the Standards of Nursing Practice.				
Self Evaluation Scale 1 2 3	RPN Technical Skill Checklist		Method of Validation/ Code	Date Met/ Initials

Self Evaluation Scale 1 2 3	RPN Technical Skill Checklist	Method of Validation/ Code	Date Met/ Initials

	1. Cardiovascular
	  A. Initiate IV therapy
	    1. Adult, non-trauma
	    2. Trauma patient
	    3. Pediatric
	    4. Newborn
	    5. Phlebotomy percutaneous approach
	
	  B. Blood sampling:
	    1. Arterial line,
	    2. Blood sampling: port-a-cath
	    3. Triple lumen/ trauma cath/ central line
	
	  C. Central venous line management: securing/ dressing/ caps/ tubing
	    1. Trauma catheter/ triple lumen
	    2. Implanted device external access (i.e., Hickman)
	    3. PICC line
	    4. Port-a-cath
	
	  D. Infusion pumps
	    1. IV pumps
	    2. Syringe pumps
	    3. Programmable pediatric pump
	    4. Patient Controlled Analgesia
	
	  E. Spacelab bedside and Central monitors
	    1. Cardiac rhythm interpretation
	
	  F. Defibrillator operation
	    1. Zoll
	    2. Physiocontrol 10 and 9
	
	  G. External transcutaneous pacer–Zoll
	
	  H. Transvenous pacer pack: Emergent
	
	  I. Transvenous pacer pack: Urgent
	    1. Pulse generator
	    2. Ushkow's lead
	
	  J. Blood Products administration
	
	  K. Level I blood warmer and rapid infuser
	
	  L. Spun Hct
	
	  M. Utilization of doppler for vascular assessment		

	2. Gastrointestinal
	
	  A. Tubes & Drains
	    1. Salem sump/ Nasogastric tube (age appropriate size)
	      a. Measuring
	      b. Cetacaine administration
	      c. Securing
	    2. Gastric decontamination/ lavage (Code Blue)		

Figure 29-2 Emergency department competency-based orientation tool sample page, excerpt. (Courtesy of Albany Medical Center, Albany, NY.)

on the unit you will work on. Review the common medications, lab tests, diagnostic procedures, and treatments done on your unit. This review will help prepare you for quality patient care delivery and meeting your responsibilities in a professional fashion.

SOCIALIZATION

Socialization to the new workplace is another important part of orientation. Preceptors can play a key role in introducing the new nurse to coworkers and other members of the health team, both on and off the unit. This helps the new nurse identify relationships within the unit and between the unit and the larger health care organization. In practice areas where staff are infrequently together, such as a home health agency, socialization can be difficult. Some nurse managers may arrange a luncheon or coffee hour to introduce new staff members to the workgroup.

WORKING WITH PATIENTS

When you begin to work with patients during your orientation, you soon begin to realize that you are a "real" nurse now. Patients expect you to have the answer. This can be a little intimidating at first. The first time you experience an emergency by yourself, it can be unnerving to realize that you are the nurse in charge of your patient. Your nursing education and hospital orientation should have prepared you for this moment. You can instill confidence by keeping your knowledge base up to date and by looking and acting professional. The more experience you have, the easier this will become.

Work to put your patients at ease and demonstrate a sense of caring to them. Work to become a nursing expert in your patient's eyes and relay to the patient that you possess a body of nursing care knowledge. Demonstrate to your patients that they can trust you, and they will want to continue their relationship with you. Never be afraid to ask other, more experienced nurses for advice or help if you are unsure of a situation; not asking for help is where you can get into trouble.

WORKING WITH DOCTORS

Sometimes, new graduates are intimidated by the practitioners they work with. Cardillo (2001) gives several tips on working with practitioners. She suggests that it is useful to establish rapport and introduce yourself to the practitioners you work with. Do not be intimidated. You and the practitioner are both on the health care team to meet the patient's goals. At least one study has indicated that when nurses and medical practitioners work together, patient death rates or readmission rates decrease (Baggs & Ryan, 1990). Both you and the practitioner are equally important to your patient's welfare; one could not function without the other.

Nurses should be assertive but sincere when calling practitioners. Never fear calling practitioners because they may "yell" at you. If they do so, it's their issue, not yours.

Remember you are the patient's advocate. If you do not understand something, ask questions. Many practitioners love to teach. Be honest and up front. Tell the practitioner if something is new to you.

Give due respect to the practitioners you work with and expect the same from them. If the practitioner is out of line, you might say, "I don't appreciate being spoken to in that way," or "I would appreciate being spoken to in a civil tone of voice, and I promise to do the same with you," or something similar.

Nurses should always seek clarification from the practitioner if an order is unclear and repeat the order and clarify it. If an order is inappropriate or incorrect, rather than saying, "This order does not seem appropriate for this patient," which would likely put the practitioner on the defensive, try, "Teach me something, Dr. Jones; I've never seen a dose of Lopressor that high. Can you explain the therapeutic dynamics to me?" or "Dr. Smith, I can't figure out why you ordered a brain scan on this patient. Can you help me out here?" This approach usually results in the practitioner either reevaluating an order or changing it. If the practitioner does not change an order that you think is inappropriate, let your supervisor know and follow the guidelines of the agency that you work for regarding what to do when an inappropriate order is given. Never give any medication if you have a doubt; clear the doubt first and foremost. Remember, diplomacy works wonders, and it is your license on the line.

LEARNING STYLES

Educators have long realized that people learn in different ways, based in part on their previous experiences. At each stage of the learning process, individuals have different learning styles and need different interventions from their preceptors or leaders. There are more than twenty different learning styles in the literature. New graduates orienting to the clinical area need a preceptor who gives specific directions. They need details and demonstrations of skills. New nurses benefit if the preceptor or educator breaks tasks down into components so that they can readily see the proper order or priority of items. As nurses become more experienced, they do well with a teaching style that emphasizes collaboration and relates the new material to the learner's frame of reference. Taking a learning style inventory can help bring awareness to the orientation process. It can be difficult to match a teaching style to a learning style.

PRECEPTORS

Ideally, the nurse manager assigns each new orientee to a preceptor who understands the need to match the teaching style to the new nurse's learning needs. In many organizations, the learner follows the preceptor's schedule so that orientation is consistent. A successful preceptor is clinically experienced, enjoys teaching, and is committed to

REAL WORLD INTERVIEW

I just finished my unit-based orientation a few weeks ago. Because I'm working in a critical care area, my general orientation included a critical care course, so I wasn't on my unit too much at first. I had two preceptors most of the time—one while I was on the day shift so I could attend classes some days, and the second when I moved to my regular night hours. My preceptors were great—they supported me, taught me new technical skills, and helped me figure out the order to do things. The idea of coming off orientation was scary at first, but I was able to work my schedule so I was on duty the same shifts as my preceptor the first few nights. This gave me the security of knowing I would have a resource available when I needed it.

Jennifer Holscher, RN
Albany, New York

the role. However, if you find it difficult to work with your assigned preceptor, make this known early in the orientation process. The nursing manager or educator should be notified and the situation discussed and resolved. Good preceptors are familiar with the organization's policies and procedures, willing to share knowledge with their orientees, and model behaviors for their orientees.

In some larger organizations, one preceptor is assigned to a group of new nurses. Together, the several orientees work with the preceptor to master core competencies before being assigned to their home unit. For example, several new graduates hired for medical or surgical floors may all be assigned temporarily to one unit, with one preceptor. This has the advantage of providing peer supports to the new nurses and may be more efficient and less expensive than a traditional one-on-one relationship.

In 1974, Kramer described "Reality Shock" and discussed the difficulties some new graduates have in adjusting to the work environment. Kramer identified a conflict between new graduates' expectations and the reality of their first nursing position. A skilled preceptor can assist new nurses through this transition by offering them opportunities to validate their impressions. The support of other new nurses in a similar situation, such as those participating in the same core orientation, is particularly helpful. Note that all nurses may experience reality shock throughout their career whenever they enter a new career area (Brunt, 2005).

PERFORMANCE FEEDBACK

"So, how am I doing?" Everyone wants feedback about their performance, particularly when they are in a new position. Some preceptors and managers recognize new

employees for their progress, but in many cases, the new nurse needs to solicit their feedback. A concrete mechanism to measure your performance is through the objective assessment materials provided by nurse educators. New nurses must successfully pass the written and technical portions of orientation. If the organization has a competency-based orientation tool, the new nurse must meet its performance criteria.

PRECEPTOR ASSESSMENT

New graduates should meet at regular intervals with their preceptor and manager to review progress. This evaluation time is important to make certain that new nurses are being assigned to clinical experiences that match their learning needs. It also provides a chance to ensure a smooth interpersonal relationship between orientee and preceptor. At these meetings, the preceptor, manager, and learner should set goals for the next interval. For example, by the end of next week, the orientee will have progressed to an independent patient assessment, completed a patient admission, and increased the workload to a four-patient assignment.

At each of these sessions, it is important for the new nurse to solicit feedback. Ask, "How do you think I'm doing? Am I at the level you would expect? What should I focus on next?" Answers to questions such as these allow the orientee to measure progress. Many new graduates take negative evaluation personally. It is important that the preceptor identify that it is a skill or behavior that is inappropriate and not the nurse as a person.

FORMAL PERFORMANCE EVALUATION

To maintain accreditation, health care organizations are required to administer performance evaluations for each employee at regular intervals. Individual facilities set

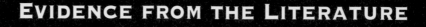

EVIDENCE FROM THE LITERATURE

Citation: Snodgrass, S. G. (2001, June 10). Wish you were a star? Become one! *Chicago Tribune,* D1.

Discussion: The most logical way to predict your future is to create it, so if you want to be a star, start by becoming a top performer now. Companies are drawn to those who use up-to-date skills and leadership to produce measurable results. Organizations seek such people out. Surprisingly, few people understand this. You can begin to position yourself now with exceptional performance.

Start by delivering more than you promise and consistently outperform yourself. Exceed expectations on a regular basis, seek more responsibility, value teamwork and diversity, provide leadership, and always go beyond the call of duty. Communicate effectively and know how to network with others. Be resourceful, comfortable with ambiguity, and open to saying, "I don't know, but I'll find out." In addition, take initiative and persevere until you reach quantifiable results. Finally, assume some personal risk by thinking outside the box and exploring bold, new solutions to challenges. Provide yourself with a margin of confidence through lifelong learning. Be open, flexible, and adapt to new ideas. Spend time with those who challenge your thinking.

You should also be creative, seek innovative solutions, and supplement your past experience with a fresh perspective. Learn how to put your ideas into action and be persistent because achieving results takes time. In addition, do your homework. Understand the business agenda and close any gaps between what you are and what you could be. In other words, define your goals, then create and implement a personal development plan. Finally, demonstrate respect for others, and apply the golden rule. Achieving great results with great behavior enables your star to rise. You can begin the process right now with these specific steps:

- See the big picture. Know why your job was created, how it relates to your organization, and what opportunities it contains. You can positively influence outcomes through performance and achievement.

- Invest in your organization; make decisions as if you owned the company. Determine which actions promise the most significant impact, and then pursue them with zeal.

- Push your comfort zone by seeking challenges, finding the positive in negative situations, taking action, and learning from the past.

- Make time for people; understand the culture, values, and beliefs of the organization; keep things in perspective; and have fun.

- Inspire those around you to exceed expectations; also, convey a sense of urgency, and consistently drive issues to closure.

After you do all this, how do you ensure that you will be noticed? Ask how your company identifies and rewards top performers. Inquire as to whether there is a high-potential category. You should pursue an environment in which the best are recognized and valued. It should be an organization that provides career growth, lifelong learning, and development opportunities.

You also want meaningful work, an opportunity to contribute, and an environment that prizes new ideas and fresh perspectives. In addition, you deserve honest feedback and the opportunity to provide the same in return. Finally, seek an organization that energizes and empowers you, encourages your good health, respects your point of view, and honors your performance. Many such organizations abound.

Implications for Practice: Although a business professional wrote this article, the advice rings true for nurses as well.

their own policies identifying the process and time frames. For many, annual evaluations are the norm.

What should nurses expect from their first formal evaluation? The individual and the nurse manager meet to review progress since either the previous evaluation or date of hiring. The evaluation should be objective, based on the nurse's performance as measured against the job description. See Figure 29-3 for an example of a job description.

Most performance evaluations use some sort of checklist, reflecting whether the individual being evaluated meets standards, exceeds standards, or falls below the organization's standards.

Formal performance evaluation between the manager and staff member serves several purposes. The evaluation is used to ensure competence in the skills required for safe patient care. It is also an opportunity to recognize the nurse's accomplishments in the evaluation

ALBANY MEDICAL CENTER HOSPITAL PATIENT CARE SERVICES
Job Description

JOB TITLE: REGISTERED PROFESSIONAL NURSE

Exempt (Y/N): No	JOB CODE:
SALARY LEVEL: N25.1-4	DOT CODE:
SHIFT:	DIVISION: PATIENT CARE SVC
LOCATION: NURSING UNITS	DEPARTMENT:
EMPLOYEE NAME:	SUPERVISOR: NURSE MANAGER
PREPARED BY: AMY BALUCH	DATE: 03/22/2007
APPROVED BY:	DATE:

SUMMARY: The Registered Professional Nurse utilizes the nursing process to diagnose and treat human responses to actual or potential health problems. The New York State Nurse Practice Act and A.N.A. Code for Nurses with Interpretive Statements guide the practice of the Registered Professional Nurse. The primary responsibilities of the Registered Professional Nurse as leader of the Patient Care Team is coordination of patient care through the continuum, education, and advocacy.

ESSENTIAL DUTIES AND RESPONSIBILITIES include the following. Other duties may be assigned.

— Performs an ongoing and systematic assessment, focusing on physiologic, psychologic, and cognitive status.

— Develops a goal directed plan of care which is standards based. Involves patient and/or significant other (S.O.) and health care team members in patient care planning.

— Implements care through utilization and adherence to established standards which define the structure, process and desired patient outcomes of nursing process.

— Evaluates effectiveness of care in progressing patients toward desired outcomes. Revises plan of care based on evaluation of outcomes.

— Demonstrates competency in knowledge base, skill level and psychomotor skills.

— Demonstrates applied knowledge base in areas of structure standards, standards of care, protocols and patient care resources/references. Practices in compliance with state and federal regulations.

— Demonstrates knowledge of Patient Bill of Rights by incorporating it into their practice.

— Demonstrates ability to identify, plan, implement and evaluate patient/S.O. education needs.

— Participates in development and attainment of unit and service patient care goals.

— Organizes and coordinates delivery of patient care in an efficient and cost effective manner.

— Documents the nursing process in a timely, accurate and complete manner, following established guidelines.

— Utilizes standards in applying the nursing process for the delivery of patient care.

— Participates in unit and service quality management activities.

— Demonstrates self-directed learning and participation in continuing education to meet own professional development.

— Participates in team development activities for unit and service.

(Continues)

Figure 29-3 Albany Medical Center hospital patient care services job description for registered professional nurses. (Courtesy of Albany Medical Center, Albany, NY.)

ESSENTIAL DUTIES AND RESPONSIBILITIES (Cont.)

— Demonstrates responsibility and accountability for professional standards and for own professional practice.

— Supports research and its implications for practice.

— Adheres to unit and human resource policies.

— Establishes and maintains direct, honest and open professional relationships with all health care team members, patients, and significant others.

— Seeks guidance and direction for successful performance of self and team, to meet patient care outcomes.

— Incorporates into practice an awareness of legal and risk management issues and their implications.

QUALIFICATION REQUIREMENTS: To perform this job successfully, an individual must be able to perform each essential duty satisfactorily. The requirements listed below are representative of the knowledge, skill, and/or ability required. Reasonable accommodations may be made to enable individuals with disabilities to perform the essential functions.

EDUCATION and/or EXPERIENCE: Graduate of an approved program in professional nursing. Must hold current New York State registration or possess a limited permit to practice in the State of New York.

LANGUAGE SKILLS: Ability to read and interpret documents such as safety rules and procedure manuals. Ability to document patient care on established forms. Ability to speak effectively to patients, family members, and other employees of organization.

MATHEMATICAL SKILLS: Ability to add, subtract, multiply, and divide in all units of measure, using whole numbers, common fractions, and decimals. Ability to compute rate, ratio, and percent.

REASONING ABILITY: Ability to identify problems, collect data, establish facts, and draw valid conclusions.

PHYSICAL DEMANDS: The physical demands described here are representative of those that must be met by an employee to successfully perform the essential functions of this job. Reasonable accommodations may be made to enable individuals with disabilities to perform the essential functions.

While performing the duties of this job, the employee is regularly required to stand; walk; use hands to probe, handle, or feel objects, tools, or controls; reach with hands and arms; and speak or hear. The employee is occasionally required to sit or stoop, kneel, or crouch.

The employee must regularly lift and/or move up to 100 pounds and frequently lift and/or move more than 100 pounds. Specific vision abilities required by this job include close vision, distance vision, peripheral vision, depth perception, and the ability to adjust focus.

WORK ENVIRONMENT: The work environment characteristics described here are representative of those an employee encounters while performing the essential functions of this job. Reasonable accommodations may be made to enable individuals with disabilities to perform the essential functions.

While performing the duties of this job, the employee is regularly exposed to bloodborne pathogens.

The noise level in the work environment is usually moderate.

Figure 29-3 Albany Medical Center hospital patient care services job description for registered professional nurses. (continued)

period, which can be a real morale boost. This is the ideal time for the manager to enhance future performance by coaching, setting goals, and identifying learning needs. At the end of the performance evaluation, both the manager and the staff member should have a clear understanding of what needs to happen in the next year for that nurse to grow and continue to be successful. Feedback is most useful when it identifies actual examples of good and poor performance with suggestions for change.

360-DEGREE FEEDBACK

Some health care organizations have moved to an evaluation program known as **360-degree feedback**. In this system, an individual is assessed by a variety of people to provide a broader perspective. For example, a nurse may complete a self-assessment and submit a packet detailing the year's progress. This may include documentation of in-services completed in the assessment period, samples of charting, and details related to committee work. The appraisal process also includes peer reviews, evaluation by the nurse's immediate supervisor, and patient interviews.

With 360-degree feedback, the individual can potentially receive a broader, more balanced assessment. To be consistent and objective, nurses who are asked to evaluate their peers need orientation to the process and the specific tool being used. Overall, 360-degree feedback can be time-consuming to complete, yet it provides valuable information.

SETTING GOALS

A key component of any performance appraisal is the opportunity to set goals for the coming year. Goals that are measurable and clearly articulated are more likely to be met. These should be developed jointly by the nurse being evaluated and the nurse's manager.

CRITICAL THINKING 29-2

Seek 360-degree feedback about your professional performance from your supervisor, mentor, coworkers, practitioners, other health care workers, and patients. Think about the feedback, and try not to react before considering it thoughtfully. How well do they think you do on professional behavior, prevention of pain and complications, and prevention of nurse-sensitive outcomes?

A sample performance goals outline might look like the following:

By the next scheduled performance assessment, nurse Joanne Johnson will do the following:

- Successfully complete the advanced pediatric assessment course
- Assume the primary nurse role for patients with an anticipated length of stay of greater than three days
- Become an active participant on a unit-based or hospitalwide committee.

ORGANIZATIONAL RESPONSES TO PERFORMANCE

Many health care organizations have a merit-based compensation structure that is tied to performance evaluations. Employees' pay raises are matched to their performance. But most health care organizations are looking for other ways—in addition to money—to create job satisfaction. Recognition is an important way health care organizations can motivate employee performance.

EMPLOYEE RECOGNITION PROGRAMS

Many health care organizations have developed formal recognition activities. These may take the form of surprising an Employee of the Month with balloons and a plaque, bringing in a national speaker for a celebration of Nurses Day, or presenting recognition pins for years of service. One popular recognition involves selecting an employee from each unit to attend a quarterly luncheon with the organization's administrator. At the luncheon, employees are recognized individually for their contributions to patient care, based on the narratives submitted by the nominating individuals. Figure 29-4 and Figure 29-5 are sample forms used in such a program.

CORRECTIVE ACTION PROGRAMS

Sometimes, appraisal feedback indicates the need for significant performance improvement. Most health care organizations have a prescribed corrective action program. One of the first steps in helping employees improve their performance is identifying whether the poor performance is developmental or related to a failure to follow policies or procedures. For example, a nurse may be having difficulty completing assignments in an appropriate time frame. It is unlikely that the nurse's problem is related to a lack of understanding of the rules. Instead, the manager needs to coach the employee, assisting the

Success Stories Nomination Form

Name: _____

Position: _____ Unit/Dept: _____

Reason for Selection:

_____

_____

_____

_____

_____

_____

_____

_____

_____

_____

_____

Submitted by: Name: _____

Unit/ Ext: _____

Please return complete form to:
Marketing and Retention Committee
M4 Mailbox / MC 73

Figure 29-4 Success stories nomination form. (Courtesy of Albany Medical Center, Albany, NY.)

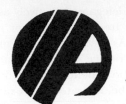

43 New Scotland Avenue, Albany, New York 12208-3478

ALBANY MEDICAL CENTER

October 8, 2007

Dear Managers,

The Marketing and Retention Committee, along with Mary Nolan, has been sponsoring Success Stories luncheons to recognize staff. This December 14, 2007, we will extend this luncheon to include a new staff member, of less than a year on your unit, to accompany the staff member who has been chosen by yourself, another staff member, or the previous Success Story candidate.

Please take this opportunity to submit the name of a staff member who you feel has a positive impact on your department and helps make it a successful one. The individual chosen will receive an invitation to a luncheon with Mary Nolan.

Submissions must be returned to Carole West, Marketing and Retention mailbox on M4, MC73, by November 16, 2007.

Thank you, and we look forward to honoring your "Success Story". If you have any questions, please feel free to call me in the Emergency Department, 262-3131. Your staff member will be honored from noon to 2 PM on December 14, 2007.

Sincerely,

Carole West, RN
Success Luncheon Chairman

Figure 29-5 Invitation to Success Stories luncheon. (Courtesy of Albany Medical Center, Albany, NY.)

nurse with whatever support will help the nurse improve. It may be that the nurse needs remedial work in some particular technical skill or feedback specifically directed to organizing a patient assignment, either of which can affect the nurse's ability to complete the shift on time.

Another category of corrective action is disciplinary corrective action. In this case, an employee receives feedback for failing to follow the organization's policies. Excessive absenteeism is an example. As with the previous example, the goal is to assist the nurse to improve

performance. Most organizations have a series of progressive steps for corrective action in cases in which employee performance does not improve. For example, a manager may begin by providing a verbal warning to an employee whose attendance is minimally acceptable. If the nurse's attendance problem continues, the nurse may receive a written warning. Without improvement, this could proceed to a suspension, final warning, and eventually termination.

In **progressive discipline**, the manager and employee's mutual goal is to take steps to correct performance to bring it back to an acceptable level. In a union environment, the employee may have the right to union representation after a verbal reprimand. It offers a step-wise process with opportunities for continued feedback and clarification of expectations. In any event, the corrective action applied by the manager must be fair. Employees should be forewarned of the consequences of violating an institution's policies so that there are no surprises. The corrective action should be consistent and impartial—each person is treated the same each time the rule is broken. Figure 29-6 is a sample corrective action documentation tool.

THE NURSE AS A FIRST-TIME MANAGER OF A SMALL PATIENT GROUP

The RN responsible for direct care of a small group of patients is functioning as a first-line nurse manager. This nurse is responsible for linking each patient to the resources that the patient needs. This often involves supervising other licensed LPNs and UAP involved in direct patient care.

RELATING TO OTHER DISCIPLINES

Given the complexity of health care organizations in the United States, the successful interconnection among departments is a potential source of tremendous strength. The RN who understands the functions of the respiratory therapists, pharmacists, dieticians, social workers, case managers, and vendors for durable medical equipment will be able to efficiently incorporate their contributions in planning for effective patient care. In many settings, diagnosis-specific care plans or clinical practice guidelines articulate the anticipated relationships among disciplines. For example, a care plan for a patient admitted for a CVA may include consultation with physical therapy on day two and an evaluation for home care needs on day three. It is important for nurses to develop strong relationships with representatives of the many other disciplines whose practices interface with the nursing role.

DELEGATION TO TEAM MEMBERS

In the current health care environment, lengths of stay (LOS) are shorter despite increased patient acuity and complexity. The nurse who is responsible for a group of patients also needs to work with other nurses and licensed and unlicensed personnel to provide safe patient care. This usually involves delegating specific responsibilities to others. A nurse who delegates effectively assigns routine tasks to a coworker, freeing the RN for more-complex planning or care. As a starting point, an RN needs to refer to the Nurse Practice Act for the state the nurse is practicing in. This document limits or defines the responsibilities that may be delegated. For example, in some states, LPNs may draw blood but may not start IV lines. This can also vary from hospital to hospital. The nurse needs to follow all such policies in decisions about delegation.

The RN must also consider the skills and knowledge of coworkers in order to delegate well. This allows the nurse to give teammates the opportunity to work within their competencies. The RN needs to match the coworkers skills with the delegated task. The RN may ask the LPN what materials he or she usually uses for a particular wound dressing. At the same time, the RN needs to ensure that the LPN knows what must be reported back, for example, in this case, a saturated dressing. The RN must continue to evaluate the ongoing needs of the patient.

It is easy to fall into the trap of overdelegating or underdelegating, particularly for new nurses. Some nurses are hesitant to delegate activities to others because they are afraid their teammates will resent being asked to do a specific task. They worry they will be seen as lazy or lacking ability. Or they may hesitate to delegate out of a belief that they can do the task better or faster themselves.

Other nurses delegate more care than is appropriate or safe. Nurses who overdelegate may do so because they are poor time managers or because they personally lack the skill required. It may be that they failed to first assess their patients or are unfamiliar with their coworkers' competencies.

Performance feedback is a crucial element of delegation. It is important to openly recognize team members' contributions to safe patient care. In an instance in which the nurse is not satisfied with the outcome of a delegated task, it is equally important to discuss the assignment with the coworker individually. Perhaps the nurse's directions were unclear, or misunderstood, or failed to include an important time frame. Taking the time to provide feedback demonstrates the respect and value a nurse places on her teammates' contributions.

LEVELS OF AUTHORITY

Sometimes, when one delegates an assignment to a team member, that person questions the parameters of the assignment. If, for example, the RN in charge of a group of patients delegates a patient's ostomy teaching to another RN on the team, that RN may hear that assignment several ways. For example, the RN may think, "I need to do the ostomy appliance change while the patient's wife is here." Or, "I need to assess what the patient has learned already and report back to the RN." Or, finally, "I need

ALBANY MEDICAL CENTER
Corrective Action Notice

Employee's Name: _____   Job Title: _____

Division: ( ) Center   ( ) College   ( ) Hospital   Department: _____

PART I: CORRECTIVE ACTION HISTORY

Date of Corrective Action	Reason For Corrective Action	Level of Corrective Action Applied
1. / /	_____	_____
2. / /	_____	_____
3. / /	_____	_____
4. / /	_____	_____
5. / /	_____	_____
( )	Check here if no previous corrective action issued	

PART II: CURRENT OFFENSE REQUIRING CORRECTIVE ACTION

Date of Offense: _____/_____/_____

Level of Corrective Action Being Applied: ( ) Written Warning   ( ) Final Warning

Category of Offense: ( ) Job Performance   ( ) Absenteeism/Tardiness   ( ) Misconduct   ( ) Other

Description of Offense: _____
_____
_____
_____
_____

Expected Improvement And Plan For Correction: _____
_____
_____
_____

Suspension Without Pay (Pending Investigation)
Description of Incident: _____
_____

_____   _____/_____/_____   Follow-Up Date: _____/_____/_____
Manager's Signature   Date

The offense(s) described above is in violation of Albany Medical Center's policies governing the conduct and/or performance standards of it's employees. The reason for and level of Corrective Action being issued has been fully explained to me, and I understand that I must correct my job performance and/or conduct immediately. My job performance and/or conduct must remain at an acceptable level following improvement or further action up to and including discharge will be taken.

_____   _____/_____/_____
Employee's Signature   Date

Original Copy: Human Resources (Hospital Paid Staff) College Personnel Services (College Paid Staff)   Department Copy: Manager   Employee Copy
H-170

Figure 29-6 Corrective action notice documentation tool. (Courtesy of Albany Medical Center, Albany, NY.)

to develop a teaching plan with the patient and begin to implement it today."

These three possibilities demonstrate the importance of delegating clearly and specifically and defining the level of authority being delegated. Sharon Cox, a nursing leadership consultant, describes four possible levels of authority to be used when delegating a task to a coworker (1997):

1. Collect data, find out the facts, assess the situation, and report back to the team leader.
2. Collect data, and make a recommendation back to the team leader.
3. Assess the situation, make a recommendation, report back, and then implement that recommendation.
4. Assess the situation, and carry out the task as the coworker believes is appropriate.

An agreement as to the level of authority at the time the task is delegated prevents each party from making inaccurate assumptions about the other's accountability for the delegated assignment. See Chapter 16 for more discussion of delegation.

THE CHARGE ROLE

Many hospital-based nurses, especially those who work evening or night shifts, rapidly progress from being assigned responsibility for a small group of patients to being assigned to the charge role for the shift. Particularly on medical and surgical floors, the charge nurse continues to care for a group of patients but also may coordinate care for the rest of the unit. This nurse may be responsible for assigning the workload of the nursing staff for the shift.

First-time charge nurses often have high expectations for their own performance, and they can easily become stressed in the new role. It is helpful to recognize that the nursing process—assessing, planning, implementing, and evaluating care—requires organizational and priority-setting skills that directly apply to the charge nurse role. It is a matter of perceiving and delegating patient care needs from the perspective of the unit as a whole. The new charge nurse must let go of the need to be perfect. Instead, the nurse should concentrate on staying organized and focused on what is best for the patients. It is also important to recognize and utilize the available resources for problem solving, such as coworkers or the facility supervisor.

ARTICULATING EXPECTATIONS As a first-time charge nurse, it is important to build relationships with other staff members as well as coworkers from other disciplines. One way to develop these relationships is by sharing expectations. This may be as simple as sitting down over coffee and agreeing to certain behaviors, such as "We will maintain a patient focus, as evidenced by answering call lights quickly." Some performance expectations may be more generic, applying to relationships more than specific patient care items, but they still need

REAL WORLD INTERVIEW

remember my first job in nursing about forty years ago. It was as a staff nurse on a general medical-surgical unit. I had a wonderful preceptor, Ed Fuss, RN. He worked with me and helped me until gradually I could assume my full role as a staff nurse on the unit. It took a while. It was very stressful to care for the forty-two patients on that unit. After my orientation period, I would sometimes be the only RN, though I would have several licensed practical nurses and nurse aids working with me. I had to quickly learn appropriate delegation techniques.

Nursing has been a great career for me. I have worked as a nurse in Indiana, Illinois, New York, Oklahoma, and Wisconsin. Besides other nursing positions that I have held, I often work as a per diem agency nurse in various Emergency departments. I find I can move quickly into the culture of a new unit by being friendly, helping others on the unit, and keeping my nursing skills up to date. I notice that people in other professions often complain about being concerned that they will lose their job. In nursing, I have not had to worry about job layoffs. I always have been able to get an interesting nursing job doing something I like.

I have had nurse friends who have worked as nurse practitioners, nurse chaplains, traveling nurses, seminar teachers, missionary nurses, nurse lawyers, nurse managers, informatics nurses, nurses in a homeless shelter, nurses on a cruise boat, etc. There are all kinds of nursing opportunities. I also like stopping at the scene of an accident and knowing I can help. It has been my privilege to be a nurse. How many other professions can say they save lives for a living!

Patricia Kelly, RN, MSN
Chicago, Illinois

CASE STUDY 29-1

You are the charge nurse for the evening shift on a general surgical floor. A patient care associate (PCA) working on your shift brings you a complaint. He says that the nurse he is assigned to work with this evening is not doing her share. She is sitting at the desk visiting with the unit secretary while he answers all the call lights. She has also assigned him the task of setting up a traction bed, which he has done only once in orientation two months ago. As the charge nurse, how would you respond to the PCA? Would you talk to the nurse he is working with? What is the priority issue in this situation?

to be clearly spelled out. For example, "If you disagree with me, you will talk to me about it before you discuss our disagreement with others." These specific expectations help establish a level of trust and prevent the need for mind reading. They open the doorway for clear communication so that when a problem develops, it is easier to approach the individual involved.

STRATEGIES FOR PROFESSIONAL GROWTH

New nurses are more likely to stay in their positions if they are challenged and have opportunities for professional growth. Some health care facilities have a wealth of available educational opportunities. Others, particularly smaller organizations, may require the nurse looking for experiences to be more creative. The best place to start is with the experts on and around the nursing unit. Suppose you have developed an interest in learning more about cardiac arrhythmias. If your hospital offers an EKG interpretation course, great! Sign up! If not, there are lots of other ways to grow in this area. Talk to your nurse manager and educator about your interest. Ask them about classes, or ask them to refer you to experts in your geographic area. Speak to the cardiologist making rounds on your unit. Ask for the name of an interventional cardiologist so you can observe a cardiac catheterization. Ask to spend a day shadowing in a coronary care unit. Do not limit your search to nurses and practitioners. Often other health disciplines overlap with nursing's interests, and you may be able to tap into opportunities with another discipline.

Not all nurses have the motivation or time for a lot of formal professional growth activities. What is important is to stay challenged. Find a particular skill or interest in your position, and expand it. What do you like best of all the things you did today? Working with the patient's family? Teaching the new diabetic? Starting that IV? Whatever it is, look for opportunities to become your unit's expert at it.

CROSS TRAINING

Given today's shortage of nurses, there is increased floating and offering nurses cross-training to new areas. Cross-training is another opportunity for individual growth. Although some organizations have strict guidelines to limit the practice of floating nurses, other health care facilities expect nurses to routinely float to either a related unit or an area particularly in need of assistance.

It is important for nurses in their first job to be articulate about their competencies for a new patient population if they are asked to float. They need to be sure the manager assigning them is aware of their experience level. Nurses should not accept total responsibility for an area or population in which they have not achieved competency. It may be more appropriate to assign an inexperienced nurse to specific tasks to help on the unit rather than asking that nurse to take a typical patient assignment on an unfamiliar unit.

One way to minimize the stress of being asked to float to a different unit is to volunteer ahead of time to cross-train to the new area. This has many advantages. It allows the nurse the opportunity to experience working with different ages or types of patients. Besides learning new skills, it gives a nurse the chance to see how the other half lives. For example, a nurse who has worked only on a medical floor may regard accepting an admission from the Emergency Department (ED) as something to be worked into the shift, based on other patient care needs. After cross training to the ED, and seeing admitted patients waiting on stretchers in the hall, that nurse may have a new appreciation of the need to negotiate for timely acceptance of ED admissions to the floor.

Cross-training has some long-term benefits as well. If a new nurse is considering a career in a specialty, spending some time cross-training to that population can help

REAL WORLD INTERVIEW

Here are a few lessons I learned as a new graduate:

1. You will manage to get every single type of body fluid on you at one time or another (blood, trach gunk, fistula juice, stomach residual, stool, urine). Bring a pair of backup scrubs to work.
2. You learn from your mistakes. I was taking care of a patient on an insulin drip during the night shift. She was up all night long and her daughter didn't think too highly of the care she was getting. When the patient and her daughter finally fell asleep, I skipped her 3 A.M. Accucheck. Her 4 A.M. Accucheck was 27. Needless to say, I have never skipped an Accucheck since.
3. If a preceptor shows you something, don't say that they are doing it wrong and then pull out a policy book. Your preceptor will hate you for life.
4. Never pass up an opportunity to learn something, even if you think you have seen it before. Maybe someone will teach you a new and better way to do it.
5. You will think you are ready for your first really sick patient, but you are not. The senior staff will help you through it. I still replay my first really sick patient in my head and think back to all the things I wish I had done differently. Luckily, no one else dwells on it. I am my worst critic!
6. Find a person besides your preceptor whom you admire, maybe for their nursing skill, their personality, or their way of making everything look easy. Ask them if they will mentor you. It doesn't need to be a super-serious conversation. I made mine a joke and asked a nurse if she would be my Nighttime Sensei. She accepted and to this day she has my back when things get crazy.
7. Always do the little things. I was a patient care tech before I was a nurse. I always make sure my rooms are stocked, everything is put away, my patient is clean, the patient's meds are in the drawer, etc. Little things like this can really help out your next coworker. There is nothing worse than walking into a patient's room and it looks like a bomb went off.
8. Always help out your coworkers. I work in an ICU, and there is a real sense of teamwork. As a new graduate, I always felt like I never had enough time to do my work, but I always made time to help the other nurses turn their patients, do a bath, move them to a chair, etc. That stuff doesn't take that long and your coworkers really appreciate it. Plus, next time you need help with something, easy or not, they will be there for you.
9. I think my first month off of orientation, I cried in the shower at least once a week. Some of it was about the patients I took care of, some was about working with not nice people, some of it was just because I needed to cry. I always tried to keep my emotions out of my workplace. Some people are very emotional at work, and it makes others uncomfortable. I am not saying that you can never cry at work or with a patient's family, but if you are crying during every shift, your coworkers will start to think that you can't handle your job.
10. I live by the mottos, "never show fear" and "do it right." Always walk into the patient's room with confidence. If you are doing something for the first time, run through it with someone experienced before going into the patient's room. You are taking care of someone's mom, dad, or child, and they are trusting you with their lives. Don't give them a reason to lose that trust.

Erin Mahoney, BSN, RN
Loyola University Hospital
Maywood, Illinois

the nurse decide whether she wants to pursue that field. Cross-training also is beneficial to the nurse seeking a new position. When a nurse is applying for a new job, experience in more than one clinical area enhances a resume and makes the individual a stronger candidate.

Some health care organizations reward nurses who volunteer to cross-train so they can safely float to different areas. These rewards may be monetary. Other institutions offer nonmonetary incentives, such as reduced weekend or holiday commitments, as rewards for cross training or floating.

IDENTIFYING A MENTOR

Developing a mentoring relationship with a more experienced, successful nurse is another mechanism for professional growth. A mentor coaches a novice nurse and helps the novice develop skills and career direction. A mentor may introduce the younger nurse to professional networking opportunities. A good person to assist the new nurse in a workplace ethical dilemma may well be his mentor.

How does a new nurse find a mentor? First, the new nurse needs to communicate a willingness to learn and grow. A newer nurse usually needs to seek out a prospective mentor rather than wait to be approached by one. An ideal mentor is an experienced nurse who is willing to support and counsel other nurses when asked. This may lead to a formal structured relationship or a more informal role-modeling association.

Nurses who have been successful preceptors are often potential mentors because they are committed to helping another nurse learn and grow. Even though the preceptor role is more narrow and defined, the role can easily be expanded to a more informal mentoring relationship.

The Internet is a newer mentoring resource. Nurses can develop relationships through special-interest chat rooms or by e-mailing experts in other geographic areas. There are forums for questions and answers, often on specific patient populations, disease processes, or operational issues. Want to get some expert advice on a particular patient problem? Spend some time on the Internet.

DEVELOPING PROFESSIONAL GOALS

After a new nurse has mastered the skills for day-to-day nursing care, what is next? How does a nurse measure professional growth? For many nurses, the answer to these questions is a clinical ladder.

CLINICAL LADDER

A **clinical ladder** is a program established by some health care organizations to encourage nurses to earn promotions and gain recognition and increased pay by meeting specific requirements. Although the criteria may vary, most programs have three or four distinct levels. Some also

REAL WORLD INTERVIEW

There is a national nursing shortage, most acutely realized in nursing specialty areas such as critical care, operating room, and pediatrics. Staffing and scheduling practices directly affect nursing personnel costs, patient care outcomes, and recruitment and retention of nurses. At a Midwest university hospital, a specialty cluster-nursing program was implemented to respond to the nursing shortage. The specialty cluster-nursing program consisted of grouping several inpatient units and related specialty clinics with similar patient care requirements together. Nurses hired into the cardiac, oncology, pediatrics, and trauma clusters are offered a special fellowship orientation program.

Nurses working the cardiac cluster can work on the cardiac medical intensive care unit, cardiac medical step-down unit, cardiac surgery intensive care unit, and cardiac surgery step-down unit. Nurses working the medical cluster can work on pulmonary, geriatric, psychiatry, and general medicine inpatient units. Nurses working the neuroscience cluster can work on orthopedics, rehabilitation, and neurology inpatient units. Nurses working the oncology cluster can work on the pediatric oncology clinic, adult oncology unit, or the adult hematology/oncology clinic or adult surgical unit. Nurses working the pediatric cluster can work on the infant/toddler, adolescent, hematology, and pediatric intensive care inpatient units. Nurses working the surgical cluster can work on general surgery, plastics and otolaryngology, transplant, peripheral vascular, and security inpatient units. Finally, nurses working the trauma cluster can work on the trauma life support intensive care unit, Emergency Department, burn unit, and general surgery inpatient unit.

This program creates opportunities for nurses to develop expertise and specialty knowledge in patient populations that cross multiple units. Nurses skilled in the specialty cluster are preassigned to one or more settings within the cluster based on projected staffing requirements. Staffing adjustments are made for each scheduling period for patient acuity changes, changes in patient volume, extended leaves, and sick leaves. Scheduling specialty cluster staff prior to the beginning of a work schedule minimizes floating of unit-based staff on a shift-by-shift basis. The cluster program with the fellowship orientation has become an effective nurse retention strategy.

Patricia Dianne Padjen, RN, MBA, MS, EdD
Manager, EMS Program
Madison, Wisconsin

offer the nurse the opportunity to seek promotion in a specific track, within a clinical, educational, or managerial focus. Thus, it is possible for a new nurse to choose a clinical nursing track and move through the organization's promotional levels by meeting those requirements. For example, to be promoted from a new graduate level to a Level II RN, the nurse may be required to complete a specialty course such as Advanced Cardiac Life Support (ACLS) or EKG interpretation, join a unit-based or hospital-based committee, and finish the preceptor course. Besides offering opportunity for promotion, these programs offer an objective way to measure a nurse's achievements. Clinical ladders can be time-consuming to complete, yet they provide valuable information.

SPECIALTY CERTIFICATIONS

Many health care organizations encourage their staff to become certified. Nearly all nursing specialties now offer board certification exams to validate expert knowledge of that particular discipline. Emergency nurses may sit for the Certified Emergency Exam and the Advanced Cardiac Life Support Exam. Nurses who specialize in critical

CRITICAL THINKING 29-3

You have just begun interviewing for your first nursing job.

What type of nursing recognition programs would appeal to you? For you, would monetary or scheduling rewards be more of an incentive to cross-train on another unit? What are some measurable professional goals for your first year as an RN?

care may take the critical care certifying exam to earn their CCRN. Successfully passing a certification exam is another measure of professional growth and offers the benefit of national recognition of one's credentials.

KEY CONCEPTS

- When choosing a first nursing position, it is important to contemplate the differences in developmental opportunities between specialty and general medical-surgical units. Environmental, scheduling, and orientation options are also important considerations.

- Organizational orientation is both general and unit based. Orientation is a time for developing strong relationships with preceptors and members of other disciplines, as well as for mastering competencies needed for safe patient care.

- Nurses receive performance feedback both informally and as part of periodic evaluations. This input is valuable in developing personal goals.

- Health care organizations have mechanisms to recognize employee contributions. Many of these programs reward success, both monetarily and through recognition programs. Corrective action programs can be used to coach an employee who is having performance problems and to foster change in an employee who is failing to follow policies.

- Given the increasing complexity of health care today, it is crucial for the first-time nurse to develop strong relationships with team members and representatives of other health care disciplines. The new nurse needs to delegate appropriately and identify specific levels of authority with coworkers. Relationships with coworkers are enhanced when staff members mutually agree to performance expectations.

- Professional growth is important for job satisfaction. Organizational opportunities for growth include clinical ladders and developing mentoring relationships. Cross-training is another means to expand experiences and can be helpful in defining future career plans.

KEY TERMS

clinical ladder	self-scheduling
progressive discipline	360-degree feedback

REVIEW QUESTIONS

1. General orientation includes which of the following?
   A. Information all nurses new to a facility need
   B. Mastery of unit-specific processes
   C. Patient care for a specific diagnostic group of patients
   D. Patient care for a specific age group of patients

2. Which of the following is usually NOT necessary to do in your first job in nursing?
   A. Learning to be organized
   B. Developing a good attendance record
   C. Refining your assessment skills
   D. Completing written performance evaluations of the UAP that report to you

3. Preceptors who work with new nursing graduates should have all of the following characteristics EXCEPT
   A. be clinically experienced.
   B. enjoy teaching.
   C. a commitment to the preceptor role.
   D. the ability to float to specialty units.

4. The corrective action process usually contains all of the following EXCEPT
   A. a verbal warning.
   B. a written warning.
   C. a final warning.
   D. a transfer to another unit.

REVIEW ACTIVITIES

1. You will be graduating from your nursing program in three months. Identify several possible employment opportunities in your desired locale. Prepare examples of questions you will ask as part of choosing a position. What factors are most important to you in choosing a position?

2. You have been working as a new graduate for a year and have done well. Your nurse manager asks you to be the relief charge nurse on your unit for the 3 P.M. to 11 P.M. shift. What type of orientation will you need for this position? How can you work with a mentor to do well in this position?

3. You are interested in the concept of 360-degree feedback. Who could you ask to give you feedback on your clinical performance to achieve 360-degree feedback?

4. Review a recent nurse salary survey in a nursing journal. How do nursing salaries in your area compare?

EXPLORING THE WEB

- There are many Websites specific to nursing employment opportunities. Try some of these:
  www.rnwanted.com
  www.healthopps.com
  www.healthcareers-online.com
  www.nursingcenter.com
  www.healthjobsusa.com

- If you have a specialty area in mind, it is worth the time to explore the Web for more details. How will this help you as you prepare for interviews?

- Look up the Association of Pediatric/Hematology Oncology Nurses: *www.apon.org*

  Association of Rehabilitation Nurses:
  www.rehabnurse.org

  Association of Women's Health, Obstetric and Neonatal Nurses: *www.awhonn.org*

- If you are interested in trauma nursing, try *www.emergency.com*

REFERENCES

Baggs, J. G., & Ryan, S. A. (1990). ICU nurse-physician collaboration and nursing satisfaction. *Nursing Economic$, 8*(6), 386–392.

Brunt, B. A. (2005). Models, measurement, and strategies in developing critical thinking skills. *Journal of Continuing Education in Nursing, 36*(6), 255–262.

Cardillo, D. W. (2001). *Your first year as a nurse.* Roseville, CA: Prima.

Cox, S. H. (1997, November). *Motivation and morale: Coin of the realm.* Symposium conducted at Nursing Management Congress, Chicago, IL.

Kramer, M. (1974). *Reality shock: Why nurses leave nursing.* St. Louis, MO: Mosby.

Snodgrass, S. G. (2001, June 10). Wish you were a star? Become one! *Chicago Tribune,* D1.

Zerwekh, J., & Claborn, J. (2006). *Nursing Today: Transitions and Trends.* St Louis: Elsevier.

SUGGESTED READINGS

Albaugh, J. A. (2005). Resolving the nursing shortage: Nursing job satisfaction on the rise. *Urology Nursing, 25*(4), 293–284.

Amos, M. A., Hu, J., Herrick, C. A. (2005). The impact of team building on communication and job satisfaction of nursing staff. *Journal of Nursing Staff, Development, 21*(1), 10–18.

Andrews, D. R., & Dziegielewski, S. F. (2005). The nurse manager: Job satisfaction, the nursing shortage and retention. *Journal of Nursing Management, 13*(4), 286–295.

Hegney, D., Plank, A., & Parker, V. (2006). Extrinsic and intrinsic work values: Their impact on job satisfaction in nursing. *Journal of Nursing Management, 14*(4), 271–281.

Impollonia, M. (2004). How to impress nursing recruiters to get the job you want. *Imprint, 51*(1), 11–15.

Jarvi, M., & Uusitalo, T. (2004). Job rotation in nursing: A study of job rotation among nursing personnel from the literature and via a questionnaire. *Journal of Nursing Management, 12*(5), 337–347.

Makinen, A., Kivimaki, M., Elovainia, M., Virtanen, M., & Bond, S. (2003). Organization of nursing care as a determinant of job satisfaction among hospital nurses. *Journal of Nursing Management, 11*(5), 299–306.

Morris, K. (2004). I have been fired from my job. My employer says that I will be reported to the Board of Nursing and may face criminal charges. *Ohio Nurses Revue, 79*(1), 16.

Mrayyan, M. (2003). Nurse autonomy, nurse job satisfaction and client satisfaction with nursing care: Their place in nursing data sets. *Canadian Journal of Nursing Leadership, 16*(2), 74–82.

Murrells, T., Clinton, M., & Robinson, S. (2005). Job satisfaction in nursing: Validation of a new instrument for the UK. *Journal of Nursing Management, 13*(4), 296–311.

Tremayne, P., Moriarty, A., & Harrison, P. (2005). Starring role. Preparing for job interviews is often an ad hoc affair for nursing students. *Nursing Standards, 19*(27), 80.

Tzeng, H. M. (2004). Nurses' self-assessment of their nursing competencies, job demands and job performance in the Taiwan hospital system. *International Journal of Nursing Studies, 41*(5), 487–496.

Wu, L., & Norman, I. J. (2006). An investigation of job satisfaction, organizational commitment and role conflict and ambiguity in a sample of Chinese undergraduate nursing students. *Nursing Education Today, 26*(4), 304–314.

CHAPTER 30

Healthy Living: Balancing Personal and Professional Needs

Mary Elaine Koren, RN, PhD

TO NURSE

To Care

To Solace

To Touch

To Feel

To Hurt

To Need

To Heal others,

As well as ourselves

(Carol Battaglia, 1996).

OBJECTIVES

Upon completion of this chapter, the reader should be able to:

1. Generate a personal definition of health.
2. Apply the six concepts of physical, intellectual, emotional, professional, social, and spiritual health to your life.
3. Devise strategies to maintain physical, intellectual, emotional, professional, social, and spiritual health.
4. Summarize occupational health hazards that are present in the work setting.
5. Devise methods of personal financial planning.

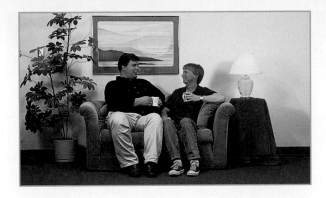

You get up early to work the day shift. On your drive to work, you grab a cup of coffee and a doughnut to sustain you through the morning. It is one of those busy days. The phone is ringing off the hook, patients are not stable, family members are demanding, practitioners are slow to answer your page, and the laboratory delivers misinformation. It is now noon, and there is no time for lunch. You run down to the vending machines for a Coke and peanut butter crackers to keep you going until the end of your shift. Five o'clock rolls around and you have worked two hours overtime and are exhausted. You are already late for your community meeting this evening. You race through a fast-food restaurant for a hamburger, fries, and a milkshake. When you finally arrive home late in the evening, you reward yourself with cookies and a bowl of ice cream and fall into bed. You have given so much throughout the day. There has been little time for yourself and for good nutrition.

What factors contributed to your busy day and poor eating habits in this scenario?

What recommendations would you have to decrease your stress and improve your nutrition in this scenario?

Can eating become a crutch for your daily stress?

How can you model the behaviors you teach your patients?

Nursing is a caring profession. Nurses spend their days helping others, many times at the expense of themselves. But who is there to care for the nurse at the end of the shift? If there is nothing left for them, they will not be able to give to their patients. Those that they care for also look to them to model healthy living. If they do not try to live by the standards set for their patients, they will lose a certain amount of credibility in their patients' eyes. How then can they balance the demands of work with their personal needs? The first step is to gather information. This chapter provides an overview of good health. Many strategies for healthy living are discussed based on six organizing concepts. This chapter also discusses financial planning and occupational health hazards for nurses.

DEFINITION OF HEALTH

Patients and nurses alike strive to maintain good health. But what does health mean? There are various ways of defining health. The *New Oxford Dictionary for Writers and Editors: The Essential A–Z Guide to the Written Word* (Ritter, Brown, & Stevenson, 2005) defines health as "the state of being free from illness or injury" (p. 779). Health as a concept has been in the literature since the inception of modern nursing. Florence Nightingale described health as "being well and using every power the individual possesses to the fullest extent" (Nightingale, 1969 [1860], p. 334). The World Health Organization (2006) describes **health** as a "state of complete physical, social, and mental well-being, and not merely the absence of disease or infirmity. Health is a resource for everyday life, not the object of living. It is a positive concept emphasizing social and personal resources as well as physical capabilities."

Pender, Murdaugh, and Parsons (2005) view health as multidimensional and consisting of biophysical, spiritual, environmental, and cultural aspects. Health changes over the course of a lifetime, and gender differences are often evident. Health can also be affected by the environment and culture we live in. Roy and Andrews (1999) define health as "a state or a process of being and becoming an integrated and whole person" (p. 31). Not only is health a complex concept, but it is also dynamic and in a constant state of change.

Health is holistic and multidimensional. All the parts of the whole must be in balance and work together to produce the end result of good health.

GOALS FOR HEALTHY PEOPLE 2010

In January 2000, more than 1,500 individuals, health professionals, and organizations convened in Washington, D.C. to discuss health promotion and disease prevention for the United States population (U.S. Department of Health and Human Services, 2001). The task was to outline specific goals that would enable Americans to maintain their health and avoid disease.

Healthy People 2010 has developed two overall goals for the nation: (1) to encourage those of all ages to increase their life expectancy as well as improve their overall quality of life and (2) to eliminate disparities among various pockets of the population. Ten leading health indicators will be used to measure the overall goals for the nation. Each of these leading indicators reflects a major health concern for the twenty-first century (Table 30-1).

TABLE 30-1	HEALTHY PEOPLE 2010 INDICATORS	
Physical activity	Responsible sexual behavior	Environmental quality
Overweight and obesity	Mental health	Immunization
Tobacco use	Injury and violence	Access to health care
Substance abuse		

Source: www.healthypeople.gov

CRITICAL THINKING 30-1

What does health mean? McWilliam, Spence Laschinger, and Weston (1999) interviewed twenty-three nursing and medical students and preceptors to obtain their definition of good health. Participants defined health in a broad sense as not only the absence of disease but also general overall well-being. A student in the study stated that "the way you live your life is going to play a role in how you practice" (p. 101). Maintaining good health is not only important to a nurse's overall well-being, but it will also affect the quality of care provided to patients. Only when you feel good are you able to deliver optimal patient care. Nurses also serve as role models for patients.

How then can nurses, when under tremendous stress on a daily basis, strive toward good health? As you think about your own health, how would you define health? What inhibits you from engaging in healthy behaviors?

AREAS OF HEALTH

Health is a complex and dynamic state of being. A healthy person must balance various aspects in life to achieve and maintain good health. When one area of life is affected, general health is also affected. There is overlap among each area, but for purposes of discussion in this chapter, health has been divided into the following six areas: physical health, intellectual health, emotional health, professional health, social health, and spiritual health (Figure 30-1).

Our bodies are dynamic and ever changing. Each area of health is constantly adjusting to outside stimuli and attempting to bring balance in life. For example, when someone is tired, fatigue can slow mental acuity. It is easy to become short tempered, which in turn can affect our relationships with others. By making a conscious decision to sleep longer, we can potentially influence not only our physical well-being but also our ability to think clearly, our emotional state, and how we relate to others. The remainder of this chapter will explore in more depth each of the various areas of health.

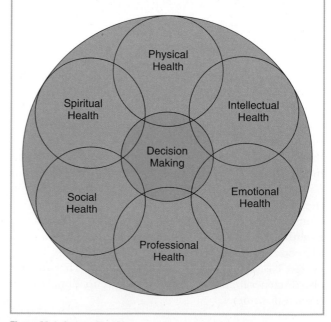

Figure 30-1 Areas of health.

PHYSICAL HEALTH

Physical health, the first area of health, encompasses nutrition as well as exercise coupled with a balanced amount of sleep. Physical health also includes health-preventive behaviors such as avoiding smoking and having annual Pap smears and other screening procedures that detect health problems early.

The first step in maintaining good physical health is to do an assessment. Table 30-2 provides a self-assessment of physical health. This tool is designed to assess trends only.

NUTRITION

Good nutrition is ingesting foods that provide a balanced diet. Maintaining good nutrition—one aspect of physical health—is often a difficult task. Finding the time and motivation to eat a nutritious diet in our fast-paced world is not easy. When we eat properly, we feel better and perform tasks at a higher level. The U.S. Department of Agriculture has age-specific and gender-specific recommendations for grains, vegetables, fruit, milk, and meat or beans at www.mypyramid.gov.

CALCULATION OF BODY MASS INDEX

A method for assessing body weight in relation to height is to calculate the body mass index (BMI). You can calculate this at www.nhlbisupport.com/bmi. The National Institute of Health (n.d.) has established the following guidelines for interpretation of the BMI:

- 18.5 to 24.9 is optimal health
- 25 to 29.9 is overweight
- 30 and above is obese
- Below 18.5 is considered underweight

BENEFITS OF EXERCISE

Following nutritional guidelines is not enough to maintain physical health. Daily exercise is another essential ingredient for healthy living. Exercise provides many benefits. It can improve cardiovascular function by lowering cholesterol and blood pressure and strengthening heart muscle. Exercise can boost the immune response to disease. Weight-bearing exercises are especially helpful for calcium uptake in bones. Exercise also improves flexibility and endurance and decreases fat deposition. Exercise can also make you feel better mentally. With exercise usually comes fewer depressive thoughts, less anxiety, an increase in self-confidence, and increased mental acuity (World Health Organization, 2006). The U.S. Surgeon General (U.S. Department of Health and Human Services, 2006b) recommends thirty minutes of physical exercise most days of the week. If the intent is to maintain weight and prevent further weight gain, about sixty minutes of daily exercise may be needed. You may also be interested in specific exercises for a particular sport.

TABLE 30-2 PHYSICAL HEALTH ASSESSMENT	Yes	No
1. I eat three balanced meals a day.	———	———
2. I exercise 30 minutes every day.	———	———
3. I enjoy exercising.	———	———
4. I exercise with a friend.	———	———
5. I rarely eat between meals.	———	———
6. I sleep 8 hours a night.	———	———
7. I wake up refreshed most mornings.	———	———
8. I sleep soundly without waking up during the night.	———	———
9. I don't smoke.	———	———
10. I implement recommended health screenings for my age category, such as mammogram, papsmear, dental cleaning and so on.	———	———
11. I avoid risky health behaviors, for example, drugs, tanning booths, unprotected sex, and so on.	———	———

PRACTICAL EXERCISE SUGGESTIONS

There are many different types of exercise from which to choose. Find one that you are passionate about and one that you truly enjoy. Finding friends who participate in the same activity can help you keep the commitment. When you decide, try to engage in the activity daily for thirty minutes at a time. Start slowly and gradually build the intensity and duration.

There are many ways to get exercise. You can set up an exercise program using DVDs or reference books. Following is a list of some suggestions:

- Walking
- Jogging
- Cycling
- Swimming
- Rowing
- Yoga and tai chi
- Golf and tennis
- Skiing
- Team sports, such as volleyball or basketball
- Dancing

If you are having trouble getting started, you can spend time at a health spa. There are many spas throughout the country, tailored to various budgets. Visit www.spafinder.com for other ideas.

SLEEP

Sleep is another aspect of physical health. It is not uncommon for nurses to sleep less than eight hours per night. Nurses who work nights may find it especially difficult to sleep for an uninterrupted block of time. Nurses who are constantly changing shifts are more susceptible to sleep deprivation. It is estimated that it can take from four to six weeks to change sleeping patterns. In spite of this, nurses may work multiple shifts within a week. Still other nurses work ten- and twelve-hour shifts and do not have a lot of time between shifts before they are back at work again. If it is necessary to swing to a different shift, it is best to rotate from days to evenings to nights. People generally adapt better if shift rotation is done clockwise. Practitioners, family members, and critically ill patients place heavy demands on nurses. Many nurses find it a challenge to leave thoughts of patients and the day's activities at work. This also contributes to insomnia.

CRITICAL THINKING 30-2

Keep a diary for one week of all that you eat, the type and amount of exercise you do, and how many hours of sleep you get each night. See Figure 30-2 for a sample activity diary. At the end of the week, assess to see how well you have taken care of yourself. Is this a typical week? Do you need to make any changes? Were there any surprises? You can also record for several weeks and compare the outcomes.

	Breakfast	Lunch	Dinner	Snacks	Exercise Type/ Duration	Hours of Sleep
Monday						
Tuesday						
Wednesday						
Thursday						
Friday						
Saturday						
Sunday						

Figure 30-2 Sample activity diary.

ASSESSMENT OF SLEEP DEPRIVATION

How do you know if you are sleep deprived? Assess your sleepiness index by answering eight simple questions using the Epworth Sleepiness Scale by visiting the following Website: http://provigil.com. Test your knowledge regarding sleep deprivation with the tools, quizzes, and sleep diary at the National Sleep Foundation Website, www.sleepfoundation.org. Click on Tools and Quizzes.

DELETERIOUS EFFECTS OF SLEEP DEPRIVATION

Current research indicates that there are many negative effects of sleep deprivation. Sleep-deprived individuals become petulant and find it difficult to remember or concentrate on the simplest tasks. Nurses who work more than 12 hours a day or commit to more than 60 hours per week are at the greatest risk of making errors that can impact patient safety (Institute of Medicine, 2004). Patient safety is the utmost concern. The drive home after work for a nurse can be equally as dangerous. For each extra shift worked during one month, there is a 9.1% increased risk of a motor vehicle accident during the commute home from work. Nurses who work rotating shifts are at the greatest risk of fatigue compared to those committed to one shift. Nurses who rotate to evenings or nights are almost twice as likely to nod off while driving home (Frank, 2005). A period of twenty-four hours of wakefulness is equivalent to a blood alcohol level of 0.10% (Dawson & Reid, 1997).

There is no magic formula to guarantee a good night's sleep, but the following suggestions may improve the quality of your sleep life:

- Make sleep a priority. Make a conscious decision to obtain adequate sleep every night.
- Do not use caffeine as a stimulant to stay awake or alcohol as a tool to fall asleep.
- Try drinking warm milk or decaffeinated tea at bedtime. Establish a routine before bed that is repeated nightly.
- Reserve your bed only for sleeping. Watching television or doing paperwork in bed can cause sleepiness early and interfere with sleep patterns.
- If thoughts of work prevent you from falling asleep, write your worries on a piece of paper. Leave your thoughts on paper and make a plan to deal with worries the next day while awake.

Other steps that nurses can take to prevent fatigue include the following:

- Use evidence-based fatigue guidelines.
- Take an uninterrupted 15-minute break every four hours.
- Join the safety committee at work.

- Rotate shift work clockwise, when possible, that is, days, evenings, nights.
- Build in a sanctioned short nap, especially on the night shift.
- Share a ride home or use public transportation. (Frank, 2005; Hughes & Rogers, 2004)

Adequate sleep, good nutrition, and proper exercise all go hand in hand. When you are tired, you may eat more to compensate for the lack of sleep. Overeating can lead to unnecessary weight gain. And the weight gain and fatigue can lead to a lack of exercise. Proper balance among the three is critical.

INTELLECTUAL HEALTH

Intellectual health is the second area of health and encompasses those activities that maintain intellectual curiosity. Intellectual health consists of the knowledge you accumulate and the ability to think. Intellectually healthy people are able to clearly process information and make sound decisions. They learn from experience, are flexible, and remain open to new ideas. For purposes of this chapter, the term *intellectual health* also includes personal financial planning.

The first step in maintaining intellectual health is assessment. Table 30-3 contains an assessment tool for intellectual health; this tool is designed to assess trends only.

INTELLECTUAL ACUITY

Just as it is important to find a type of exercise you are passionate about, so it is important to find some activity outside nursing that is of interest. The list is endless—antique shopping, reading, painting, sewing, photography, and so on. Develop a new hobby. Keep your mind sharp by staying abreast of developments within your interest area. Another way to maintain intellectual acuity is to establish and maintain a financial portfolio.

PERSONAL FINANCIAL PLANNING

The first step in personal financial planning is to identify your annual salary. The average nursing salary for RNs is $58,600. For nurses with five or less years, the mean annual income is $43,500 (Mee, 2005).

Next, begin to think about the percentage of your salary you want to save; most experts recommend 10% to 15%. There is no better time than now to invest in your future. Now is the time to begin saving for such things as a home, your children's education, and even retirement no matter what your age.

Note that a nurse who is making $50,000 annually will make $1,800,000 in a thirty-year working career. If this

TABLE 30-3	INTELLECTUAL HEALTH ASSESSMENT		
		Yes	**No**
1. I read at least one book a month.		_____	_____
2. I have a hobby I enjoy.		_____	_____
3. I belong to a club or organization.		_____	_____
4. I save 10% of my income in a 401K, 403b, or a Roth IRA savings plan for retirement.		_____	_____
5. I have invested in a mutual bond fund.		_____	_____
6. I have invested in a mutual stock fund.		_____	_____
7. I know how much money I have invested in Social Security.		_____	_____
8. I have a money market account.		_____	_____
9. I plan to buy a home soon.		_____	_____

nurse invests $200 per month at 12% interest for the 30 years, the nurse will have more than $1,000,000 in a retirement account at age sixty-five. Check the Web resources in this chapter for investing sites to review. Savings for retirement are three-pronged: (1) Social Security funds, (2) retirement funds, and (3) additional personal savings.

SOCIAL SECURITY

Social Security is automatically taken out of every paycheck by the federal government. The benefits from Social Security will not cover all retirement expenses especially with today's projected life span and inflation. You will need other retirement money. You should annually check the accuracy of your Social Security account by reviewing the information sent to you by the Social Security Administration.

RETIREMENT FUNDS

The most common retirement funds are the 401K or 403b plans. The primary difference between the two is that the 403b is a plan offered by a nonprofit organization, and the 401K is offered by a for-profit organization. For purposes of this discussion, the term 403b will be used.

Both the employee and employer contribute money to a 403b. This is a great way to save because many health care institutions will match the funds that you contribute. The maximum annual contribution by law is $10,500 or 20% of earned salary. After your money is put into the fund, it is tax sheltered, meaning you do not pay any taxes on the amount contributed until it is withdrawn. For example, if you earn $58,000 per year and contribute $5,800 to the 403b, you will be taxed on only $52,200 of income. If the money is withdrawn before you reach the age of $59^1/_2$, you will pay a 10% federal penalty. This is

an incentive to keep the money in the account until retirement; the plan should be considered a long-term investment.

Each retirement plan offers a number of investment options such as stock funds or bond funds. Some plans severely limit the number of investment options. To learn more about the risks and benefits of various funding options, consult *Morningstar* or *Consumer Reports*. (See Exploring the Web at the end of this chapter.)

INDIVIDUAL RETIREMENT ACCOUNT (IRA) Another type of retirement fund is the individual retirement account (IRA). This fund may or may not be tax deductible, depending upon your income level. There are two kinds of IRAs: the traditional IRA and the Roth. Funds placed in a Roth IRA account grow tax free and are tax free when withdrawn at retirement. Money from a Roth IRA can be withdrawn early, tax free, if used for the purchase of your first home (Table 30-4).

PERSONAL SAVINGS VEHICLES

After investing in retirement funds, you also have a few more options for investment. You can open a **money market account**. This is similar to a bank checking account, although it often requires a larger minimum amount of money to open the account. The interest rate is higher than that of a passbook savings account or a traditional bank checking account, and you have check-writing privileges. This is a place for money that you may need to quickly access.

You also have the option to invest in stock mutual funds, bond mutual funds, individual stocks, or individual bonds outside of your retirement account. You have the option of investing in individual stocks and bonds, but

TABLE 30-4	TIME VALUE OF MONEY

A nurse who invests $2,000 yearly at an 8% annual rate of return, beginning at age twenty will earn over $850,000 by age 65 versus a nurse who makes the same yearly investment but waits and begins at age 30. The latter nurse will earn only about $350,000 by age 65.

such an investment requires more research. You can start by reviewing Valueline at your local library (see "Exploring the Web" at the end of this chapter for Valueline). The key to successful investment is to diversify, meaning to spread your money around in many different types of investment options, stocks, bonds, mutual funds, and so on.

BUYING REAL ESTATE

Owning your own home is a smart investment (Silbiger, 2005). When purchasing a home, obtain as much information as possible. Research properties in the area you want to buy. Investigate the school system, tax base, typical list price, and average time of homes on the market. Drive by and examine the neighborhood. Is this where you would want to live? Next, plan how to finance the property. Work with a real estate agent.

HOW TO EDUCATE YOURSELF

There are many ways to learn more about investments. Try taking a course on personal finance at your junior college. You can also go to the Internet for advice (see "Exploring the Web" at the end of this chapter).

Another option is to hire a financial planner, however, this can become expensive. Check Fidelity for free advice at www.fidelity.com. The last suggestion is to read. Many of the books on the best-sellers list discuss personal finance. Suze Orman (1997) is an author that many find easy to understand and very relevant. Good financial magazines include *Money, Kiplinger's,* and *Consumer Reports;* read an article periodically, they become more interesting as you learn.

REAL WORLD INTERVIEW

Buying your first home is probably the smartest and biggest investment you will ever make. If you are currently renting, buying a home is a good start to a secure financial future. While renting has its pluses, that is, no long term commitment and no lawn care or maintenance, it does have its downfalls. For example, the rent you are paying every month goes into your landlord's pocket and does not benefit you in any way. When your lease is up and you move on, you have nothing to show for your hard-earned money.

Let us say that the rent you have been paying is $600 a month. For the same monthly payment, you could qualify for a $100,000 mortgage. Of course there will be other expenses such as utilities, maintenance, insurance, and taxes, but every penny you spend towards your mortgage will build financial security for you.

Once you are a homeowner, there are many advantages. You can write off all of your taxes and interest on April 15th. This can reduce the tax you owe or give you a bigger tax refund. Another advantage to owning your home is that year after year, your property will probably go up in value due to appreciation. When you decide to sell, your property value may have gone up several thousand dollars. This builds more financial security for you and makes it easier to buy a more expensive home. Today there are literally hundreds of programs to help you with home buying. Whether you have good credit, no credit, bankruptcy, or no down payment, you still may qualify to purchase a home. Make sure you always choose a reputable realtor who knows the market and has your best interest at hand. This will be the first step to gathering information that you can use to find your dream home.

Pamela Gwozdz, Realtor
Next Chicago Realty
Chicago, Illinois

EMOTIONAL HEALTH

Emotional health is the third area of health. Our emotions express how we are feeling about an event. Emotions can be intense, and each emotion evokes a strong response. Our challenge as human beings is to acknowledge the emotion and then respond appropriately. It is important to have balance between our thought processes and the emotion we are feeling; otherwise, disharmony occurs. Emotions are what make us human. Truly, emotions are one of our greatest gifts and add spice to our lives (Dossey, Keegan, & Guzzetta, 2005).

EMOTIONAL INTELLIGENCE

Emotional intelligence is the ability to recognize your own feelings and the feelings of those around you and manage your emotions in a positive manner. Emotional intelligence requires a mix of practice and skill. Emotional intelligence includes these five basic emotional and social competencies:

- *Self-awareness:* Knowing what you are feeling in the moment and using these preferences to guide your decision making, having a realistic assessment of your abilities, and a well-grounded sense of self-confidence.
- *Self-regulation:* Handling your emotions so that they facilitate rather than interfere with the task at hand, being conscientious and delaying gratification to pursue goals, and recovering well from emotional distress.
- *Motivation:* Using your deepest preferences to move and guide you toward your goals, to help you take initiative and strive to improve, and to persevere in the face of setbacks and frustrations.
- *Empathy:* Sensing what people are feeling, being able to take their perspective, and cultivating rapport and attunement with a broad diversity of people.
- *Social skills:* Handling emotion in relationships well and accurately reading social situations and networks, interacting smoothly; using appropriate skills to persuade and lead, and negotiate and settle disputes for cooperation and team work (Goleman, 1998).

Take a minute to assess your emotional health (Table 30-5). This tool is designed to assess trends only. The first step toward emotional health is acknowledgment of feelings.

ANGER

Anger is a common emotion that we all sometime or another feel. As a matter of fact, anger is pervasive in our society today. There is road rage, airplane rage, outraged customers, and rage at youth sporting events. The causes for the anger are numerous and may be due to rapid change in society, primarily the result of high technology; a lack of privacy, because we are accessible to work at all hours through cell phones, blackberries, and beepers; a sense of entitlement; a lack of family connection; and perhaps overcrowding.

There seems to be a spillover of anger into the nursing profession. Thomas (2003) has found numerous sources for nurses' anger: inadequate staffing and unreasonable

TABLE 30-5	**EMOTIONAL HEALTH ASSESSMENT**		
		Yes	**No**
1. I don't often get angry.		———	———
2. When I do get angry, I keep my anger under control.		———	———
3. I laugh every day.		———	———
4. My friends make me laugh.		———	———
5. I reward myself for something every day.		———	———
6. I am aware of my emotions and am confident in my decision making.		———	———
7. I can handle my emotions appropriately.		———	———
8. I am motivated to constantly improve.		———	———
9. I am empathetic to others.		———	———
10. I can handle social situations.		———	———

workload, mismanagement of patients, lack of administrative support, demeaning treatment by other health care providers, feeling like scapegoats for mistakes within the system, and feeling powerless to influence difficult situations.

WAYS TO COPE WITH ANGER

Thomas (2003) recommends numerous ways nurses can learn to cope with anger at work. Make a commitment to be supportive and honest with coworkers. Reach out to colleagues, and don't be afraid to disclose your honest opinion and utilize self-disclosure. Don't get caught up in workplace gossip. Discuss difficult situations with a confidant. Obtain skills in conflict resolution by taking classes in assertiveness training, bargaining, and negotiating. You may need to seek counseling if your anger is intense or sustained.

Sometimes anger and frustration are caused by sensory overload or overcommitment. It is important to have time for yourself. If nurses are to be effective caretakers, they first must care for themselves. Saying no, be it to a supervisor, friend, or family member, may at times be necessary. Learn to say no.

HUMOR

Laughter is the best medicine. Laughter has many benefits such as helping to boost the immune system, promoting relaxation, and decreasing blood pressure, heart rate, and respiratory rate (Holistic Online, 2006). But best of all, laughter is contagious and it is free. Laughter is a critical stress reliever (Figure 30-3).

WAYS TO MAKE YOU LAUGH

Set a goal for yourself—not to let a day go by without a hearty laugh. Surround yourself with people who can joke about life. Read a humorous book; watch a funny television program or movie. See how many people you can get to smile in a day. Treat others at work to a little laughter. It is a great way to engender trust and teamwork. You can also learn to appreciate the humor at work. Visit "Ivy Push," the acting name of Hob Osterlund MS, RN, CHTP, who has created DVDs of comical nursing situations. You can obtain more information about her shows at www.ivypush.com.

STRESS MANAGEMENT

Many things can be done to relieve the emotional stress of life. See Table 30-6 for a few suggestions.

If these suggestions do not help, there are other options. You can seek out professional counseling. And yes, sometimes nurses need a little extra help. You would be the first to call a counselor for a patient, so why not help yourself? There are also employee assistance programs that can help. Ask your human resource department at work.

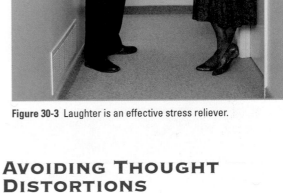

Figure 30-3 Laughter is an effective stress reliever.

AVOIDING THOUGHT DISTORTIONS

Research on thinking processes has shown that people make mistakes in the way they perceive information and think about the world around them. When people are depressed, their automatic thoughts are loaded with distorted thinking. If you can recognize this distorted thinking (Table 30-7), you can begin to turn life in a more positive direction.

PROFESSIONAL HEALTH

Professional health is the fourth element of health. You are professionally healthy when you are satisfied with your career choice and have continual opportunities for growth. A professionally healthy individual is goal directed and seeks every opportunity to obtain knowledge and new learning experiences. You can assess your professional health by using Table 30-8. This tool is designed to assess trends only.

WAYS TO MAINTAIN PROFESSIONAL HEALTH

There are numerous ways to continue to advance your career. Ask yourself where you want to be 5, 10, and 15 years from now. If you do not have an overall plan, work can become very monotonous.

TABLE 30-6	STRESS RELIEF SUGGESTIONS	
Meditate	Do relaxation exercises	Be polite to all
Think peaceful thoughts	Do something different for lunch	Take a walk
See things as others might	Give yourself a pat on the back	Read
Forgive your mistakes	Join a support group	Join a club
Do not procrastinate	Talk about your worries	Sing a song
Set realistic goals	Be affectionate	Forgive and forget
Do a good deed	View problems as a challenge	Listen to music
Vary your routine	Get/give a massage	Take a hot bath
Appreciate what you have	Say a prayer	Call an old friend
Focus on the positive	Expect to be successful	Let go of the need to be perfect

EVIDENCE FROM THE LITERATURE

Citation: Salmond, S., & Ropis, P. E. (2005). Job stress and general well-being: A comparative study of medical-surgical and home care nurses. *MedSurg Nursing, 14*(5), 301–309.

Discussion: The purpose of this research was to assess differences in job stress between medical-surgical nurses and home care nurses and determine if job stress influences general well-being. Using a comparative, descriptive design, a convenience sample of eighty-nine nurses from both medical-surgical and home health settings were surveyed. A subset of ten nurses, five from each setting, provided qualitative data gathered from in-depth interviews. Medical-surgical nurses scored significantly higher on the instrument that measures severity and frequency of job stress, and they indicated less professional support than their counterpart in the study. Those nurses who scored higher on job stress were significantly more likely to report negative mood states. Medical-surgical nurses and home care nurses both stated that excessive paperwork contributed the most to workplace stress. However, the two specialty area nurses differed in other major stressors in the workplace.

Implications for Practice: Data from nursing research can increase the awareness of what contributes to job stress. Increased awareness is the first step to alleviating the problem. This study indicates the need to support nurses in the work force by implementing more team development. Team enhancement can occur by ensuring the competency of all health care workers and promoting positive interpersonal relations with other team members. Older, experienced nurses can serve as mentors for younger nurses. Clinical nurse specialist or clinical experts can serve as resource persons for the staff. Every opportunity should be taken to build team spirit. The first step to change is acknowledging the problem of stress on the job.

It is important to seek out others within the health care field. Find a more experienced nurse you can relate to or who can act as a mentor. This nurse can provide guidance and support when problems arise. Network with other nurses and health care professionals. You can learn an enormous amount from others. Keep in touch with some of your favorite faculty members. They will enjoy hearing from you and can also offer useful advice. Join at least one professional organization. Attend as many workshops and professional meetings as possible. Many of these presentations may be paid for by your employer. After attending professional conferences, do

TABLE 30-7   THOUGHT DISTORTIONS

Thought Distortion	Example
All-or-nothing thinking: seeing things only in absolutes.	If I leave this area of nursing, no one will respect me.
Overgeneralization: interpreting every small setback as a never-ending pattern of defeat.	Everyone here is so smart; I'm a real loser.
Dwelling on negatives: ignoring multiple positive experiences.	I made a mistake. I'm not good enough to be a nurse.
Jumping to conclusions: assuming that others are reacting negatively without definite evidence.	I don't know why I study. Everyone thinks I'm going to fail this competency test anyway.
Pessimism: automatically predicting that things will turn out badly.	It's only a matter of time before everything falls apart for me.
Reasoning from feeling: thinking that if one feels bad, one must be bad.	My head hurts because I'm a bad person.
Obligations: living life around a succession of too many "shoulds," "shouldn'ts," "musts," "oughts," and "have-tos."	I should volunteer for that committee because my nursing director wants me to. It will impress my boss.

Source: Compiled with information from Frisch, N. C., & Frisch, L. E. (2006). *Psychiatric mental health nursing* (3rd ed.). Clifton Park, NY: Thomson Delmar.

TABLE 30-8   PROFESSIONAL HEALTH ASSESSMENT

	Yes	No
1. I have professional goals including certification and/or additional nursing education.	____	____
2. I have a mentor.	____	____
3. I have attended at least three educational workshops in the past year.	____	____
4. I subscribe to three nursing journals.	____	____
5. I belong to at least one professional organization.	____	____
6. I use appropriate personal protective equipment.	____	____
7. I never recap a needle.	____	____
8. I use good body mechanics when transferring patients.	____	____
9. I follow standards of care when handling gaseous waste, disinfectants, and chemotherapy.	____	____
10. I follow standards of care in dealing with radiation equipment and environmental hazards.	____	____
11. I don't abuse alcohol and/or drugs.	____	____
12. I protect myself from workplace violence.	____	____

not forget to apply for continuing education units (CEUs). You might want to return to school for an advanced degree. Refer to Table 30-6 for ways to deal with the stress of school, work, and family commitments.

Read as often as possible. If questions arise at work, come home and look up the information in your books or on the Internet, or go to the health care library. Subscribe to at least three professional journals related to your specialty area.

OCCUPATIONAL HAZARDS COMMON AMONG NURSES

An important aspect of professional health is avoidance of occupational hazards. The U.S. Department of Labor Statistics (2006) reports that health care and social assistance workers rank second highest in percentage of nonfatal workplace injuries reported in 2004, the latest statistics available (Figure 30-4).

The survey reports the number of new work-related illness cases that are recognized, diagnosed, and reported during the year. Some conditions, for example, long-term latent illnesses caused by exposure to carcinogens, often are difficult to relate to the workplace and are not adequately recognized and reported. These long-term latent illnesses are believed to be understated in the survey's illness measures. In contrast, the overwhelming majority of the reported new illnesses are easier to directly relate to workplace activity, for example, contact dermatitis, carpal tunnel syndrome, or back injuries.

There are numerous suggestions for safeguarding against various hazards in the workplace. For purposes of discussion, occupational hazards can be divided into four major categories: (1) infectious agents, (2) environmental agents, (3) physical agents, and (4) chemical agents. See Table 30-9.

INFECTIOUS AGENTS

Infectious agents can be transferred through direct contact with an infected patient or through exposure to infected body fluids. The major infectious agents for health care workers are HIV, herpes, tuberculosis, and hepatitis. A recent survey of fifty-eight hospitals found that 44% of the needlestick injuries were sustained by nurses compared to 15% by medical practitioners (IHCWSC, 2006). Nurses have the largest amount of direct patient contact and are at the greatest risk for exposure to blood-borne pathogens. The chance of a seroconversion, which occurs when a serological test for antibodies changes from a negative reading to a positive reading, varies according to the disease exposure. The estimated risk for infection for HIV after needle exposure is from 0.29% to 0.56%. The risk for hepatitis B ranges between 6% and 30% for nonimmunized personnel, whereas hepatitis C carries an estimated risk of 6% (Lee, Botteman, Xanthakos, & Nicklasson, 2005).

Although the majority of infectious agents are transmitted through blood, herpes simplex virus can be transmitted by direct contact with an infected lesion. Hepatitis A is transmitted primarily via diarrhea as a result of poor hygienic practices among health care workers. The overall incidence of tuberculosis (TB) is gradually increasing, and there are certain regional differences. For example, in 2004, the rate of cases per 100,000 population differed

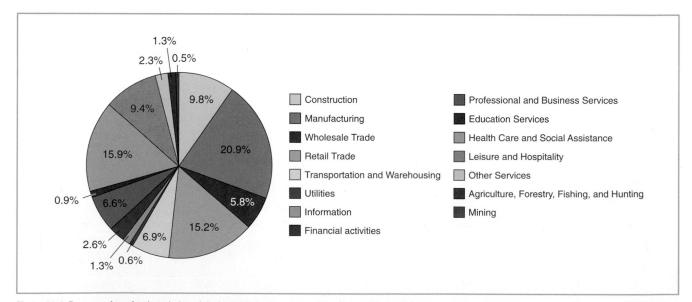

Figure 30-4 Percent of nonfatal workplace injuries by industry sector, 2004. (From *Injuries, illnesses, and fatalities* by U.S. Department of Labor Statistics, 2004. Retrieved April 30, 2007 from www.bls.gov/iif/oshsum.htm#04Summary%20Tables.)

TABLE 30-9	SAFEGUARDS FOR OCCUPATIONAL HAZARDS

Infectious Agents

- Do not recap needles.
- Use needle-free intravascular access devices.
- Place needle disposal containers near point of use of needles.
- Use personal protective equipment.
- Report all needle-stick injuries.
- Wash hands before and after each patient contact.

Physical Agents

- Follow standards of care for dealing with radiation/laser equipment.
- Assess work area for amount of noise.
- Eliminate excessive noise in the workplace.
- Implement good body mechanics.
- Follow ergonomic safety guidelines from OSHA. (Dept. of Government Affairs, 2006b)

Environmental Agents

- Develop a violence reduction plan.
- Rotate shifts clockwise—day to evening to night (Rogers, 1997).
- Assess for dangerous chemicals in your workplace.
- Determine whether OSHA standards are in place.
- Be aware of bio-terrorist alert plans.

Chemical Agents

- Utilize effective ventilation systems.
- Develop standards of care for handling hazardous agents.
- Protect pregnant nurses from handling chemotherapy during the first trimester.
- Use appropriate nonlatex barrier protections.
- Develop policies and procedures to ensure safety from latex allergies.

---

by states: 1.0 in Wyoming, 7.1 in New York, 8.3 in California, and 14.6 in the District of Columbia. The overall rate for TB in the United States in 2004 was 4.9 per 100,000 people, and in 2000, the rate was only 3.5 per 100,000 people (CDC, 2006).

ENVIRONMENTAL AGENTS

Another group of occupational hazards is environmental agents. These include all those agents within the hospital that may lead to injury. The most prevalent include violence, shift work, air quality, mold and fungus, and bioterrorism. Nurses are at risk for workplace violence. Employment in a health care facility is considered one of the most dangerous jobs in the United States. In a recent study, nearly half a million nurses per year reported being victims of some type of violence in the workplace (Department of Government Affairs, 2006a).

Poor air quality in the workplace is yet another environmental risk that may lead to symptoms such as shortness of breath, eye and nose irritation, headaches, contact dermatitis, joint pain, memory problems, and reproductive difficulties. Glutaraldehyde, a chemical used to disinfect many commonly used instruments, can emit

a hazardous gas. Lasers used in operating rooms can emit hazardous gaseous material in the form of either laser plume or chemical byproducts of laser smoke. It is essential that nurses be protected from the byproducts of lasers by high-efficiency smoke evacuators. Nurses need to be aware of and follow laser procedure safety guidelines (Anderson, 2004). Air quality can also be influenced by mold and fungus, which are often found in carpeting and in ceiling tiles. The presence of mold and fungus can lead to asthma and other respiratory problems. Most hospitals have some type of bio-terrorist alert plan. Nurses play an active role in dealing with any type of bio-terrorist disaster.

PHYSICAL AGENTS

Physical agents are another occupational hazard and include radiation, noise, and back strain. Radiation exposure is common among health care workers. Radiation is used for both diagnostic and treatment interventions. Persons exposed to excessive amounts of radiation are at risk for cancer. Nurses can protect themselves from the effects of radiation by following agency guidelines and wearing a dosimeter that measures the amount of

EVIDENCE FROM THE LITERATURE

Citation: Nelson, A., Fragala, G., & Menzel, N. (2003, February). Myths and facts about back injuries in nursing. *American Journal of Nursing, 103*(2), 32–36.

Discussion: Manual lifting and other patient-handling tasks are high-risk activities for both nurses and patients. The prevalence of work-related back injuries in nursing is among the highest of any profession internationally. Annual prevalence rates of nursing-related back pain range from 33.9% in New Zealand to 47% in the United States to 66.8% in the Netherlands. The year 2000 incidence rate for back injuries involving days away from work was 181.6 per 10,000 full-time workers in nursing homes and 90.1 for hospitals, compared with incidence rates of 98.4 for truck drivers, 70 for construction workers, 56.3 for miners, 47.1 for agricultural workers, and 43.2 for workers in manufacturing. The rising rate of obesity also increases the risk of injury to nurses and other health care workers who handle patients. Patients studied in a Veterans Administration hospital who required lifting ranged from 91 lbs. to 387 lbs. and averaged 169 lbs. The need to protect nurses from injury must direct efforts to the following in the future:

- Ergonomic assessment of patient care environments
- Engineering controls, such as new ceiling-mounted mechanical lifting devices designed to reduce manual patient handling
- Standardized protocol for assessing the handling and moving of patients
- Algorithms for deciding about the number of personnel and type of equipment needed to handle and move patients safely
- A new education model that includes hospital-unit peer leaders who would ensure that workers use equipment competently and who could help change nursing practice

Several misconceptions about how best to prevent musculoskeletal injuries when handling and moving patients are discussed in this article, which is the first of a two-part series.

Several emerging technologies and strategies that can improve nursing safety for both patients and nurses, based on engineering and administrative controls, are also discussed.

Implications for Practice: Attention to the facts should help nurses prevent back injuries. These back injuries have the potential to disrupt or end a nurse's career.

---

radiation exposure. Pregnant nurses working with radiation should declare their pregnancy to their employer as soon as possible (Duke University, 2006). Laser treatment carries the risk of eye and skin injury if the instruments are not handled properly. Noise is another physical hazard that can lead to hearing loss. Excessive noises that occur over a long period of time can lead to irritability and inability to concentrate. High levels of noise are deleterious for both nurses and patients. Special care units are especially noisy with alarms, ventilators, suction equipment, monitors, call lights, and so on. Lifting patients improperly is yet another risk factor for nurses. RNs rank sixth among all U.S. occupations for risk of incurring a muscular skeletal disorder that requires time off from work (Department of Government Affairs, 2006b). Be aware of institutional guidelines for ergonomics. Many new mechanical patient-lifting devices are now available that protect nurses from potential injury.

CHEMICAL AGENTS

Another occupational hazard is chemical agents such as anesthetic agents, antineoplastic drugs, disinfectants, latex gloves, hazardous agents, and drug and alcohol abuse. Questions still remain as to the negative effects of anesthesia on health care workers. Nurses working in the operating room should continue to protect themselves by ensuring proper ventilation and appropriate disposition of waste products (Allen, 2004).

Hazardous drugs are any medication that nurses may be exposed to either during preparation or administration of medication that poses a potential health risk. These drugs require special handling due to inherent toxicities (Polovich, 2004). Strict adherence to the agency guidelines are essential when handling these hazardous drugs.

Disinfectants are chemical agents that are of concern to nurses. Besides the gaseous effects of glutaraldehyde, which were discussed earlier, glutaraldehyde can also cause skin problems. Ethylene oxide, a chemical commonly used to sterilize surgical equipment, has been reported to have carcinogenic effects.

Latex glove exposure is another type of chemical concern for nurses. It has been reported that approximately 8% to 13% of health care workers are allergic to latex (AANA, 2006). Reactions to latex range from a simple contact dermatitis to a more systemic reaction to an anaphylactic crisis. Yet another concern for nurses is the potential for personal misuse of drugs and/or alcohol. The ANA estimates 6% to 8% of nurses may have a substance-abuse problem. This is similar to the national average for drug abuse. Nurses should be aware of the potential for addiction and abuse.

SOCIAL HEALTH

Social health is another significant area of health. The essence of social health is interacting with other people. Having the ability to relate to others is essential for life. Few can survive completely alone. We relate to people at various levels—some we know intimately, and others are mere acquaintances. These relationships occur within the immediate and extended family; at work; and within the local, national, and international community. These relationships give meaning to our lives. There are times when relationships cause distress and pain and other times when they bring great joy. We strive toward harmony in all relationships. It is human nature to seek out others and grow in relationships (Dossey et al., 2005). Take a minute to assess your status with relationships by taking the self-assessment in Table 30-10. This tool is designed to assess trends only.

CASE STUDY 30-1

You are a nurse admitting Mrs. Zakima, an 84-year-old female. You received the following report from the emergency room. Her vital signs are, BP 140/70, RR 30, HR 80. The patient has bilateral rales, 2+ pitting pedal edema, weighs 350 pounds, and her height is 5' 5". Mrs. Zakima is a transfer from a nursing home. She is being admitted for symptoms related to congestive heart failure. She has a past history of hypertension, diabetes, rheumatoid arthritis, dementia, and MRSA. Mrs. Zakima is being admitted to your unit. In preparing the room that she will be admitted to, what do you need to keep in mind with regards to noise, safety, and universal precautions?

What safety precautions would you put in place to protect yourself, that is, ergonomics, universal precautions, and so forth?

After reviewing her chart, you find she is taking the following medications: methotrexate, zestril, toprol, and lasix. What other precautions should you take with this patient?

TABLE 30-10   SOCIAL HEALTH ASSESSMENT

	Yes	No
1. I go out with my friends at least once a week.	_____	_____
2. I see my family at least twice a month.	_____	_____
3. I have one friend I can confide in.	_____	_____
4. I have a wide diversity of professional, family, neighborhood, and church friends.	_____	_____
5. I have other friends besides nurses.	_____	_____
6. I do volunteer work.	_____	_____

REAL WORLD INTERVIEW

I try to integrate my personal and professional life by organizing and prioritizing at the beginning of each day. Each night I outline with my family who needs to be where and how my husband and I will get the children to their various activities. In this way, I know my family will be taken care of during the day while I am at work. My family is my first priority. I view my social life in much the same manner. What needs to be accomplished today and how will I go about achieving this?

I organize my professional life every morning before I officially begin my day. I ask myself what are the issues that most need my attention today. Each Friday is "turnaround time." I assess the events of the week and determine all the good things that I did and those things that I could improve upon. I make sure I reward myself for the positives. I encourage all my managers to implement this weekly method of evaluation.

I have also developed a competency-based checklist for my managers. This is a tool that I use to continually assess and guide improvement of the managers. The tool outlines communication, leadership, decision making, interpersonal skills, just to name a few. I may begin by going over the assessment areas weekly and gradually taper the time needed to teach and assess the managers. Once the manager has mastered an area, there is no longer a need to use the tool. It is my goal for the managers to exhibit competency in all areas.

Another way that I try to keep balance in my life is to work hard and play hard. I make sure that I have fun on my weekends. It is important that I have humor in my life on a daily basis. My staff can laugh at me and I at them. This is healthy and a great stress reliever. Family and friends are very important to me. I try to incorporate family and friends into my daily life.

Corinne Haviley, RN, MS
Director of Medicine Nursing
Northwestern Memorial Hospital
Chicago, Illinois

IMPACT OF SOCIAL RELATIONSHIPS

The positive effects of social support on health outcomes have been documented in the literature (Breedlove, 2005). If these interactions are frequent, that only adds to good health. In other words, the more you see your friends, the healthier you become. The variety of those relationships may also keep you healthy. The greater the diversity of the relationships, such as professional, family, neighborhood, or church relationships, the more likely you are to remain healthy.

Try to interact with friends in person as often as possible. Cell phones and e-mail are helpful forms of communication, but nothing is more effective than face-to-face conversation. Be careful, though, to stay away from negative relationships and people who do not treat you well. Sometimes it is difficult to end a friendship, but if the relationship is destructive, it may be in your best interest to end it.

Another way to build relationships is through rituals. For example, celebrate Christmas with friends by seeing *The Nutcracker* or play tennis with a friend once a week.

But do not forget about your friends of the past. Phone a friend from the past or contact a family member you have argued with.

Finally, another way to establish friendships is through volunteerism. For example, join the American Red Cross as a disaster volunteer or pursue another activity that you find rewarding. It is also a good way to be aware of community issues.

SPIRITUAL HEALTH

Spiritual health is the last area of health. Spirituality is an elusive term that is difficult to define. It can be viewed as the essence of being, that which gives meaning and direction in life, and the principles of good living. It may also be your relationship with a higher being, other individuals, or your environment (Dossey et al., 2005). See Table 30-11.

There has been increased attention in the nursing profession regarding the spiritual needs of patients. However, little has been said about the spiritual needs of nurses themselves (McEwan, 2004). Nurses function in a fast-paced and stressful environment, which often leads

TABLE 30-11   SPIRITUAL HEALTH ASSESSMENT

	Yes	No
1. I pray or meditate every day.	____	____
2. I believe in a higher power.	____	____
3. I attend meetings at a place of worship regularly.	____	____
4. I spend time each day in quiet contemplation.	____	____
5. I read spiritual books.	____	____
6. I listen to spiritual audiotapes.	____	____
7. I am at peace.	____	____
8. I feel confident when confronted with new situations.	____	____
9. I maintain a daily journal.	____	____

to job dissatisfaction, burnout, and potentially suboptimal patient care. Some hospitals are addressing the spiritual well-being of nurses as a way to cope with these current demands by offering the RISEN (Re-Investing Spirituality and Ethics in our Network) program. The RISEN program helps nurses become more conscious and committed to their own spiritual growth in order to facilitate the healing process in others (Ollier, 2004).

RELIGION AND HEALTH

Koenig (1999), a leader in spirituality research, found that older adults who are religiously active (based on church attendance) are more physically fit and live longer than those who are less religious. In the past decade, there have been numerous studies documenting the positive effects of religiosity and spirituality on psychological and physical health (Berry, 2005). It appears that those who are more religious or spiritual have a greater chance of adjusting to life and maintaining good health. See the "Suggested Readings" for other resources on spirituality.

DECISION MAKING

Every day, we make decisions. Some days, we may decide to care for others and put their needs before our own. But still other days, we need to care for and nurture ourselves. The decision is always up to us. These decisions are often complicated and difficult to make. The goal of this chapter has been to provide you with some thoughts that will guide your decisions concerning your health.

CRITICAL THINKING 30-3

Take a minimum of ten minutes to sit and think about the day's activities. Make sure you are comfortable and will not be interrupted by any outside stimuli. Ask yourself what was good about the day and what might have been improved. What can you learn from today's events? If you choose the early morning as a time of reflection, you can also use this time to plan your day. It is a time for relaxation just for you. Try reading some inspirational passages (see the "Suggested Readings" section for some ideas). Or you might find soaking in the bathtub to be the best alternative. No matter how busy you become, do not forget to save time for yourself. The busier you become, the more important it is to take time to reflect and relax. Be good to you!

REAL WORLD INTERVIEW

I have learned a lot in the nine months that I have practiced nursing. I used to say yes to overtime each time when asked. I thought I needed the experience and that I owed it to the staff. I have since learned to say no. I have also learned that I need to take care of me. I used to come home and eat a lot and fall into bed. I gained weight and felt awful. Now I either go for a walk or to the health club after work. I volunteer at my church youth organization part-time whenever I can. I have also developed my own routine in delivering patient care. I am better organized and leave on time. I have gained more confidence in my clinical decisions. For example, I had a patient who I thought should not be extubated from the ventilator. I tried to voice my opinion to the resident on call but was overridden by the attending physician. The charge nurse was also supportive of keeping the patient intubated. As it turned out, the patient was extubated for a half-hour and then reintubated. I felt bad for the unnecessary procedure for the patient, but it did boost my confidence. I know now that in the future, I will be even more assertive with physicians concerning the welfare of my patients.

When I am scared in a clinical situation, I try not to let fear paralyze me. I try to think everything through logically. I have found that the better I understand what I am doing, the better nurse I become. I'm always trying to learn new things. I've been to about five seminars this year, and I subscribe to three nursing journals. I want to learn as much as I can.

Nayiri M. Birazian, RN
New Staff Nurse
Maywood, Illinois

CASE STUDY 30-2

You have been working for a home health agency for about one year now. One of your best friends at work, another nurse, asks your advice about how to maintain a healthier lifestyle. She states she is ten pounds overweight and does not really exercise much. She says she feels like all she does is work and come home and go to sleep. She says she does not have fun in life anymore. She states that college life is great compared to all the stress at work.

What advice would you give your friend about how to stay healthy? What would your first priority be in offering suggestions? What other major areas of consideration would you explore with your friend?

KEY CONCEPTS

- Nurses can care for themselves by maintaining a healthy lifestyle.

- Health is not just the absence of disease, but a balance among physical, intellectual, professional, social, and spiritual well-being.

- Health is multidimensional with areas that interact and overlap. If one dimension is altered, all other areas are impacted.

- Physical health includes good nutrition, proper exercise, and adequate sleep.

- It is important to strengthen your intellectual health and keep current in both personal and professional areas.

- An important piece of intellectual health is adequate financial planning. Now is the time to begin saving.

- Emotional health includes laughter and control of anger.

- Maintaining many different types of relationships helps keep you healthy.

- Spiritual well-being provides direction and meaning in life.

- To stay healthy, you must make a conscious decision to maintain each of the six areas of health: physical, intellectual, emotional, professional, social, and spiritual health. The choice is yours.

KEY TERMS

health
money market account
physical health

REVIEW QUESTIONS

1. You are trying to maintain a healthy diet. Which of the following would you include in your daily consumption? Mark all that are appropriate.
   _____ A. Peanut butter
   _____ B. Four glasses of fruit juice
   _____ C. Green leafy vegetables
   _____ D. White bread
   _____ E. Nuts
   _____ F. Whole milk
   _____ G. Yogurt

2. You have just calculated your BMI to be 28. How much exercise would be appropriate for you?
   A. 30 minutes three days a week
   B. 30 minutes every day
   C. 60 minutes three days a week
   D. 60 minutes daily

3. You work in the operating room, and notice that your hands have become very itchy and have small papules. What would be the most appropriate first action to take?
   A. Wear only nonlatex gloves in the future
   B. Ignore the situation
   C. Make a conscious effort to apply hand cream after washing your hands
   D. Apply a corticosteroid cream

4. The CNS for your unit has just passed you in the cafeteria. You are generally on very good terms with her. She does not acknowledge your presence. The most probable explanation for this is which of the following?
   A. You must have done something wrong with one of your patients yesterday.
   B. She has something else on her mind and didn't see you.
   C. She doesn't want to acknowledge you in front of other nursing leaders because you are only a staff nurse.
   D. She doesn't want to acknowledge you because you are one of the worst nurses on your unit.

REVIEW ACTIVITIES

1. Try doing a short relaxation exercise. Take a deep breath in and let it out. Take slow, deep breaths that originate from the diaphragm. Tighten the muscles in your right arm for thirty seconds and release. Your arm should feel totally limp and relaxed. Do the same with your left arm. Tighten the muscles in your right leg for thirty seconds and release. Repeat with the left leg. Pull in your stomach muscles for thirty seconds and release. Tighten the muscles in your buttocks and release. Continue to breathe in and out deeply. You can practice this brief exercise anytime or anywhere. If you are having a particularly hectic day, take a minute to do a relaxation exercise. You can vary the exercise by flexing any group of muscles you want.

2. Your best friend is getting married next month, and you are the maid of honor. You have been invited to a shower to be held out of town in honor of your friend this next weekend. You have already purchased a nonrefundable airline ticket to attend the shower. You work in a very small ICU. You have been working ten- and twelve-hour shifts and are near exhaustion. Your head nurse calls you two days before you are to leave for the shower and asks you to work the weekend. One of the staff has been involved in a serious car accident, and there is no one else to work. What would you do?

   If you work this weekend, you would disappoint your best friend and lose the money for your ticket. You are already exhausted, and you do not know how effective you would be at work. You know you need the break.

   If you do not work, you would be letting the rest of the staff down. They have been there for you, and now it is your turn to help them. You find it very hard to say no. You are a young nurse and you should "pay your dues." How could you relax when you know that you are needed elsewhere?

3. You are interviewing for your first job. You are attending the human resource session of orientation. Which investment benefits would you be most concerned about and why?

EXPLORING THE WEB

- Calculate your BMI and determine your life expectancy and health risks at
  www.healthstatus.com

- Try one of the following sites to retrieve information on dietary supplements, nutrition, and alternative medicine:
  www.mypyramid.gov
  www.nutritionsite.com

- Vanguard: *www.vanguard.com*
  Click on *Personal Investors* and then click on the *Planning & Education* tab, where you will find basic retirement planning information. Note especially the index funds.

- Note two Websites for retirement information: (*www.quicken.com*) and Charles Schwab (*www.schwab.com* and click on *Planning and Retirement*). Various investment firms also have retirement information at their Websites.

- Fidelity Investments: *www.fidelity.com*
  Click on *Retirement & Guidance* and follow the different retirement options.

- Valueline: *www.valueline.com*

- Morningstar: *www.morningstar.com*
  Click on *Retirement.*

- Consumer Reports: *www.online.consumerreports.org*

Resources for Violence Prevention

- The ANA's Workplace Violence: Can You Close the Door? Call (800) 274-4ANA
  www.nursingworld.org

- Guidelines for Preventing Workplace Violence for Healthcare and Social Service Workers. U.S. Department of Labor, OSHA 3148-1996, available online: *www.osha-slc.gov*

- Violence Potential Assessment Tool. Contact Victoria Carroll at (970) 416-6811.

Resources for Needle Sticks

General resource links:

- Safer Needle Devices: Protecting Health Care Workers: *www.osha-slc.gov*

- American Nurses Association: *www.nursingworld.org*

- Centers for Disease Control and Prevention: *www.cdc.gov*

Resources for Latex Allergy

- ANA's position paper on Latex Allergy: *www.nursingworld.org*
  or call (800) 274-4ANA

- OSHA *www.osha-slc.gov*

Resource for Back Strain

- Occupational Safety and Health Administration's ergonomics information: *www.osha-slc.gov*
  Call (202) 693-1999.

REFERENCES

Allen, G. (2004). Evidence for practice: Surgical team members' exposure to inhalational anesthetics. *Association of Operating Room Nurses Journal, 79*(1), 235.

American Association of Nurse Anesthetists. (2006). *AANA latex glove protocol.* Retrieved January 30, 2006, from http://www.aana.com/crna/prof/latex.asp

Andersen, K. (2004). Safe use of lasers in the operating room: What perioperative nurses should know. *AORN Journal, 79*(1), 171.

Berry, D. (2005). Methodological pitfalls in the study of religiosity and spirituality *Western Journal of Nursing Research, 27*(5), 628–647.

Breedlove, G . (2005). Perceptions of social support from pregnant and parenting teens using community-based doulas. *Journal of Perinatal Education, 14*(3),15–22.

Centers for Disease Control and Prevention. (2006). *Guidelines for preventing the transmission of Mycobacterium tuberculosis in health-care settings.* Retrieved January 20, 2006, from http://www.cdc.gov

Dawson, D., & Reid, K. (1997). Fatigue, alcohol and performance impairment. *Nature, 338*(6639), 235.

Department of Government Affairs. (2006a). *Health care worker safety.* Retrieved January 30, 2006, from http://www.anapoliticalpower.org

Department of Government Affairs. (2006b). *Safe patient handling and the OSHA ergonomics standard.* Retrieved January 30, 2006, from http://www.anapoliticalpower.org

Duke University Medical Center. (2006). *Radiation safety considerations for nurses at Duke.* Retrieved January 30, 2006, from http://www.safety.duke.edu/RadSafety/nurses/default.asp

Dossey, B. M., Keegan, L., & Guzzetta, C. E. (2005). Holistic nursing: A handbook for practice. Sudbury, MA: Jones and Bartlett Publishers.

Frank, M. B. (2005). Practicing under the influence of fatigue (PUIF): A wake-up call for patients and providers. *The National Association of Neonatal Nurses, 5*(2), 55–61.

Frisch, N. C., & Frisch, L. E. (2006). *Psychiatric mental health nursing* (3rd ed.). Clifton Park, NY: Thomson Delmar Learning.

Goleman, D. (1998). *Working with emotional intelligence.* Bantam Doubleday Dell Publishing Group.

Holistic Online. (2006). *Therapeutic benefits of laughter.* Retrieved January 28, 2006, from http://www.holistic-online.com/ Humor_Therapy/humor_therapy_benefits.htm

Hughes, R. G., & Rogers, A. E. (2004). First do no harm: Are you tired. *American Journal of Nursing, 104*(3), 36–38.

Institute of Medicine. (2004). Keeping patients safe: Transforming the work environment of nurses. Washington, DC: National Academies Press.

International Health Care Worker Safety Center (IHCWSC). (2006). Uniform needlestick and sharp injury report 58 hospital, 2001. University of Virginia. Retrieved January 28, 2006, from http://www.healthsystem.virginia.edu/internet/epinet/soi01.cfm

Koenig, H. G. (1999). The healing power of faith. *Annals of Long-Term Care, 7*(10), 381–384.

Lee, J. M., Botteman, M. F., Xanthakos, N., & Nicklasson, L. (2005). Needlestick injuries in the United States: Epidemiologic, economic and quality of life issues. *American Association of Occupational Health Nurses Journal, 53*(3), 117–134.

McEwan, W. (2004). Spirituality in nursing? What are the issues? *Orthopaedic Nursing, 23*(5), 321–326.

McWilliam, C. L., Spence Laschinger, H. K., & Weston, W. (1999). Health promotion amongst nurses and physicians: What is the human experience? *American Journal of Health Behavior, 23*(2), 95–103.

Mee, C. (2005). Nursing 2005 salary survey. *Nursing 2005, 35*(10), 321–326.

National Institute of Health. (n.d.). *Body mass index calculator.* Retrieved February 2, 2002, from http://www.nhlbi.nih.gov/guidelines/obesity/bmi_tbl.htm

Nelson, A., Fragala, G., & Menzel, N. (2003, February). Myths and facts about back injuries in nursing. *American Journal of Nursing, 103*(2), 32–36.

Nightingale, F. (1969). Notes on Nursing. New York: Dover. (Original work published 1860.)

Ollier, C. (2004). Body and spirit: Nurturing strategies help nurses cope with on the job stress. *COR Health, LLC, 4*(12), 5–8.

Pender, N. J., Murdaugh, C. L., & Parsons, M. A. (2005). *Health promotion in nursing Practice.* Upper Saddle River, NJ: Pearson Prentice Hall.

Polovich, M. (2004). Safe handling of hazardous drugs. *Online Journal of Issues in Nursing, 9*(3).

Ritter, R. M., Brown, L., & Stevenson, A. (Eds.). (2005). *New Oxford Dictionary for Writers and Editors: The Essential A-Z Guide to the Written Word.* Oxford University Press.

Rogers, B. (1997). Health hazards in nursing and health care: An overview. *American Journal of Infection Control, 25*(3), 248–261.

Roy, C., & Andrews, H. A. (1999). *The Roy Adaptation Model.* Stamford, CT: Appleton & Lange.

Salmond, S., & Ropis, P. E. (2005). Job stress and general well-being: A comparative study of medical-surgical and home care nurses. *MedSurg Nursing, 14*(5), 301–309.

Silbiger, S. (2005). *The 10-day MBA.* New York: Harper Collins.

Thomas, S. P. (2003). Anger: The mismanaged emotion. *Medsurg Nursing, 12*(2), 351–357.

U.S. Department of Agriculture. (2006). *My pyramid.* Retrieved January 5, 2006, from http://www.mypyramid.gov/downloads.miniposter.pdf

U.S. Department of Health and Human Services. (2001). *Healthy People 2010: Goals.* Retrieved January 2, 2002, from http://www.health.gov/healthypeople/LHI/lhiwhat.htm

U.S. Department of Health and Human Services (2006b). *Exercise and fitness.* Retrieved February 5, 2006, from http://www.hhs.gov/safety/index.shtml#exercise

U.S. Department of Labor Statistics. (2006). *Injuries and illnesses.* Retrieved January 12, 2006, from http://www.bls.gov/iif/oshsum.htm#04Summary%News%20Release

World Health Organization. (2006). *Benefits of physical activity.* Retrieved December 30, 2005, from http://www.who.int/moveforhealth/advocacy/information_sheets/benefits.en.index.html

SUGGESTED READINGS

Blocks, M. (2005). Practical solutions for safe handling. *Nursing 2005, 35*(10), 44–45.

Boston Women's Health Book Collective. (2005). *Our bodies ourselves.* New York: Simon & Schuster Incorporated.

Canfield, J., Hansen, M. V., Mitchell-Autio, N., & Thiemas, L. (2001). *Chicken soup for nurses' souls.* Deerfield Beach, FL: Health Communications, Inc.

Dunham, K. S. (2004). *How to survive and maybe even love nursing school.* Philadelphia: F. A. Davis Company.

Frankl, V. (1984). *Man's search for meaning.* New York: Simon & Schuster, Inc.

Gladwell, M. (2005). *Blink.* New York: Little Brown & Company.

Hunt, L. (2005). Sit-down comedy. Meet Ivy Push, nursing's funny girl. *American Journal of Nursing, 105*(7), 110–111.

Kingma, D. R., & Markova, D. (1993). *Random acts of kindness.* Berkeley, CA: Conari Press.

Remen, R. N. (1996). *Kitchen table wisdom.* New York: Wisdom Riverhead Books.

U.S. Department of Health and Human Services (2006a). Healthy People 2010: Goals. Retrieved January 22, 2006, from http://www.healthypeople.gov

Warren, R. (2002). *The purpose driven life.* Grand Rapids, MI: Zondervan.

Weil, A. (2004). *Natural health, natural medicine.* New York: Mifflin Company.

Wright, L. A. (2005). *Spirituality, suffering, and illness.* Philadelphia: F. A. Davis Company.

CHAPTER 31

NCLEX Preparation and Professionalism

Patricia Kelly, RN, MSN

For us who nurse, our nursing is a thing, which, unless in it we are making progress every year, every month, every week, take my word for it, we are going back (Florence Nightingale, 1872).

OBJECTIVES

Upon completion of this chapter, the reader should be able to:

1. Outline preparation for the NCLEX.
2. Relate factors associated with NCLEX RN performance.
3. Outline components of organizing a review to prepare for NCLEX.
4. Identify elements of a profession.
5. Analyze commitment to professional development.

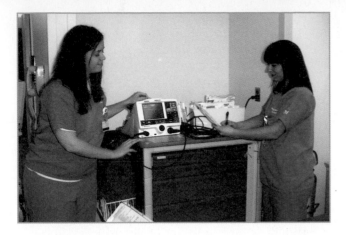

Anwar will be graduating from his nursing education program in two months. He plans to focus his current efforts on preparing to take the NCLEX-RN Licensure Examination. He knows that three areas of examination preparation are having the knowledge, being adept at testing, and controlling test anxiety.

How should he prepare for the examination?

Where should he focus?

How can he decrease his test anxiety?

A new graduate from an educational program that prepares RNs will take the **NCLEX**, the national nursing licensure examination prepared under the supervision of the National Council of State Boards of Nursing. NCLEX is taken after graduation and prior to

practice as an RN. It is wise to schedule the exam date soon after graduation. The examination is given across the United States at professional testing centers. Graduates submit their credentials to the state board of nursing in the state in which licensure is desired. After the state board accepts the graduate's credentials, the graduate can schedule the examination. This examination ensures a basic level of safe registered nursing practice to the public and is essential to working as a professional RN. The examination follows a test plan formulated on four categories of client needs that RNs commonly encounter. The concepts of the nursing process—caring, communication and documentation, and teaching/learning—are integrated throughout the four major categories of client needs (NCSBN, 2007). See Table 31-1. This chapter discusses preparation for NCLEX. It also discusses components of professionalism needed by RNs.

NCLEX EXAMINATION

Candidates receive between 75 and 265 questions on the NCLEX examination during the testing session. Of these questions, fifteen questions are being piloted to determine their psychometric value and validity for use in future NCLEX examinations. Students cannot determine whether they passed or failed the NCLEX examination from the number of questions they receive during

TABLE 31-1   NCLEX TEST PLAN

Client Needs Tested	Percent of Test Questions
Safe, effective care environment:	
Management of care	13–19%
Safety and infection control	8–14%
Physiologic integrity:	
Basic care and comfort	6–12%
Pharmacological and parenteral therapies	13–19%
Reduction of risk potential	13–19%
Physiological adaptation	11–17%
Psychosocial integrity:	6–12%
Health promotion and maintenance:	6–12%

Source: NCLEX Test Plan, 2007, www.ncsbn.org

their session. Candidates are allowed up to 6 hours to complete the NCLEX, which means that they could take the entire 6 hours to complete as few as seventy-five test items. However, because candidates do not know how many test items they will be required to answer, they should progress through the exam as though they will have to answer all 265 items. This means they should allow just over 1 minute per question. A 10-minute break is mandatory after 2 hours of testing. An optional 10-minute break may be taken after another 90 minutes of testing.

Each test question is presented to the student. If the student answers the question correctly, a slightly more difficult item will follow, and the level of difficulty will increase with each item until the candidate misses an item. If the student misses an item, a slightly less difficult item will follow, and the level of difficulty will decrease with each item until the student has answered an item correctly. This process continues until the student has achieved a definite passing or definite failing score. The least number of questions a student can take to complete the exam is seventy-five. Fifteen of these questions will be pilot questions, and they will not count toward the student's score. The other sixty questions will determine the student's score on the NCLEX.

HOW THE EXAMINATION IS CONSTRUCTED

The National Council of State Boards of Nursing (NCSBN) is the central organization for the independent member boards of nursing, which includes the fifty states, the District of Columbia, Guam, and the Virgin Islands. The member boards are divided into four regional areas, which supervise the selection of test item writers, representing educators and clinicians, whose names are suggested by the individual state boards of nursing. This provides for regional representation in the testing of nursing practice. All test items are validated in at least two approved nursing textbooks or references.

The National Council contracts with a professional testing service to supervise writing and validation of test items by the item writers. This professional service works closely with the Examination Committee of the National Council in the test-development process. The National Council and the state boards are responsible for the administration and security of the test. The exam is a computer examination known as CAT (Computerized Adaptive Testing). The exam is taken on a computer, utilizing state-of-the-art technology.

TEST QUESTION FORMATS AND SAMPLES

There are several formats for questions. Multiple-choice questions may be four-option, single-answer items or multiple-choice, multiple-option items that require more than one response. There may be fill-in-the-blank questions or questions that ask the test taker to identify an area on a picture or a graphic. The computer screen displays the question and the answer choices. There may also be examination questions that require responses to be placed in the correct order.

SAMPLE QUESTIONS

The various formats for test questions are illustrated here.

Test Question 1—Fill in the blanks

A man underwent an exploratory laparoscopy yesterday. He is on strict intake and output. Calculate his intake and output for an 8-hour period.

Intake	Output
IV-0.9% NS at 125 ml/hr	Foley urine output 850 ml
PO-1 ounce ice chips	NG tube-200 ml
NG irrigant-NS 15 ml Q 2 H	
Intake _____	Output _____

Test Answer 1

Intake = 1,090 ml; Output = 1,050 ml

125 ml/hr (125 ml × 8 hr) is 1,000 ml. 1 ounce of ice chips is 30 ml;

NG irrigant 15 ml q 2 hr (15 ml × 4) is 60 ml for a total of 1,090 ml.

Output is 850 ml urine and 200 ml of nasogastric drainage for a total of 1050 ml (Stein, 2005).

Test Question 2—Question that requires more than one response

The nurse is caring for a client who has a nasogastric tube attached to low wall suction. The suction is not working. Which of the following is the nurse likely to note when assessing the client? Select all that apply.

_____ Client vomits.

_____ Client has a distended abdomen.

_____ There is no nasogastric output in the past 2 hours.

_____ There are large amounts of nasogastric output.

Test Answer 2

"Client vomits" should be checked. The purpose of the nasogastric tube is to remove stomach contents. If it is not working, the client is likely to vomit.

"Client has a distended abdomen" should be checked. The purpose of the nasogastric tube is to remove stomach contents. If it is not working, the client is likely to have a distended abdomen.

"There is no nasogastric output in the past 2 hours" should be checked. The purpose of the nasogastric tube is to remove stomach contents. If it is not working, the client will have no output from the tube.

"There are large amounts of nasogastric output" should not be checked. The purpose of the nasogastric tube is to remove stomach contents. If it is not working, the client will have no output from the tube (Stein, 2005).

Test Question 3—Single-answer, multiple-choice questions

The following patients are on a medical-surgical nursing care unit:

359-1 Mr. A., 59, had an exploratory laparoscopy with permanent colostomy 2 days ago. He has an IV, PCA, indwelling urinary catheter, and nasogastric drainage to low wall suction. He is receiving IV push Decadron.

359-2 Mr. B., 86, suffered a cerebrovascular accident 1 week ago. He has a private sitter because he is confused. He has left-sided paralysis.

360-1 Mrs. C., 35, is a 23-hour admit for a myelogram. She is ready for discharge and needs her discharge teaching reinforced.

360-2 Miss D., 29, has severe asthma. She is experiencing some respiratory difficulty. She is on an aminophylline drip and IV steroids.

361-1 Mrs. E., 75, a newly diagnosed diabetic, requires reinforcement about insulin administration.

361-2 Mrs. F., 95, was admitted from a nursing home with dehydration and hypokalemia. She will be receiving KCl 10 mEq IV in 50 ml D5W × 3.

These clients will be assigned to one LPN and one RN. Which is the best assignment?

1. RN: 359-1, 359-2, 360-1;
   LPN: 360-2, 361-1, 361-2.
2. RN: 359-1, 360-2, 361-2
   LPN: 359-2, 360-1, 361-1.
3. RN: 360-2, 361-1, 361-2;
   LPN: 359-1, 359-2, 360-1.
4. RN: 360-1, 360-2, 361-1;
   LPN: 359-1, 359-2, 361-2 (Stein, 2005)

Test Answer 3

The RN should assume care for the patient in 359-1 because he is receiving recurring IV push medication and requires teaching about his colostomy; 360-2 because of the acute problems with asthma requiring very close respiratory assessment, IV aminophylline, and steroids; 361-2 as she will be receiving IV potassium and must be observed closely for signs and symptoms of fluid and electrolyte imbalances. The LPN should assume care for 359-2, 360-1, and 361-1. The LPN can teach the client going home from a myelogram using a standard teaching protocol and can reinforce postmyelogram diabetic teaching.

The LPN may not be able to give IV medications that the client in 360-2 requires depending on the state. The client in 361-2 is a newly diagnosed diabetic with teaching needs and is more appropriately assigned to the RN.

The LPN cannot give the IV push medication required by the client in 359-1.

Test Question 4—Fill in the blanks

Heparin is ordered to be given at 6 units/hr. The solution is 20,000 units/500 cc. How many units per hour will that deliver to the patient?

Test Answer 4

$$\frac{20{,}000 \text{ U.}}{500 \text{ cc}} = \frac{40 \text{ U.}}{1 \text{ cc}} = 40 \times 6 = 240 \text{ units per hour}$$

Test Question 5—Identify the height of the fundus at 22 weeks on this picture.

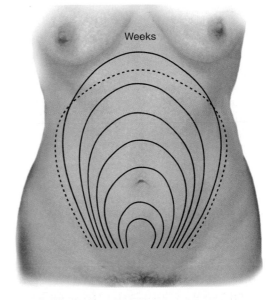

Test Answer 5—The fundus is located at this site at 22 weeks.

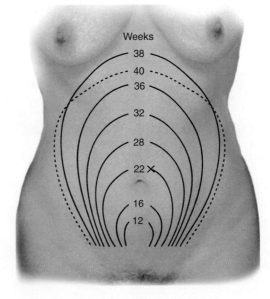

Test Question 6—Put in correct order

Put these steps in the correct order to insert a Foley catheter.

1. Check integrity of Foley balloon.
2. Attach drainage bag to bed.
3. Send urine specimen to laboratory.
4. Cleanse meatus.
5. Spread the labia.
6. Insert the foley.

Test Answer 6

1. Check integrity of Foley balloon.
5. Spread the labia.
4. Cleanse meatus.
6. Insert the Foley.
2. Attach drainage bag to bed.
3. Send urine specimen to laboratory.

ORIENTATION TO THE EXAMINATION

Each candidate is oriented to the computer before the examination starts. Because the exam is geared to the candidate's skill level, each candidate will have a unique computer adapted test (CAT). Each exam will include some experimental questions. The experimental questions are interspersed throughout the examination so the candidate will answer all questions with equal effort. The time period allowed for each candidate to complete the exam includes the exam instructions explaining how to use the mouse, the spacebar, and the Enter key, as well as samples representing each type of question in the exam and rest breaks.

The NCLEX-RN is scored by computer, and a pass/fail grade is reported. A criterion-referenced approach is used to set the passing score. This provides for the candidate's test performance to be compared with a consistent standard criteria. After administration of the CAT, candidates are notified of their success or failure by the board of nursing of the state in which they wrote the examination. Successful candidates are notified that they have passed. Unsuccessful candidates are provided with a diagnostic profile that describes their overall performance on a scale from low to high and their performance on the questions testing their abilities to meet client needs (Stein, 2005).

POSSIBLE PREDICTORS OF NCLEX SUCCESS

Several factors have been identified in research studies as being associated with performance on the NCLEX examination. Some of these factors are identified in Table 31-2.

NCLEX-RN REVIEW BOOKS AND COURSES

In preparing to take the NCLEX, the new graduate may find it useful to focus preparation in three areas: NCLEX knowledge review, NCLEX test question practice, and test anxiety control. Review books often include nursing content, sample test questions, or both. They frequently include computer software disks with test questions. The test questions may be arranged in the NCLEX book by clinical content area, or they may be presented in one or more comprehensive examinations covering all areas of the NCLEX. Listings of these review books are available at www.amazon.com. It is helpful to use several of these books and computer software when preparing for the NCLEX. Focus on NCLEX review books developed in the past three years.

Some resources for test anxiety reduction include a Tame Test Anxiety CD-ROM by Richard Driscoll, and two books: *Taking the Anxiety Out of Taking Tests* by Susan Johnson, and *Passing Exams Without Anxiety* by David Acres.

NCLEX review courses are also available. Brochures advertising these programs are often sent to schools and are available in many sites nationwide. The quality of these programs can vary, and students may want to ask former nursing graduates and faculty for recommendations. A review course is available at www.ncsbn.org.

TABLE 31-2	POSSIBLE PREDICTORS OF NCLEX SUCCESS
■ HESI Exit Exam	■ GPA in science and nursing theory courses
■ Verbal SAT score	■ Competency in American English language
■ ACT score	■ Reasonable family responsibilities or demands
■ High school rank and grade point average (GPA)	■ Absence of emotional distress
■ Undergraduate nursing program GPA	■ Critical thinking competency

EVIDENCE FROM THE LITERATURE

Citation: Wendt, A. (2003, Nov.–Dec.). The NCLEX-RN examination. *Nurse Educator, 28*(6), 276–280.

Discussion: Changes in the 2004 NCLEX-RN Test Plan and information about the alternate item formats for the NCLEX examination are discussed. Details about the new test plan and sample alternate items are identified. The 2000 NCLEX Test plan is contrasted with the 2004 Test Plan.

Implications for Practice: Nurses can use this information to prepare to take the NCLEX. Review knowledge and practice test questions in all areas of the test plan. Note that the latest exams include alternate style test questions. The percentage of questions in each area of the 2007 test plan is exactly the same as the 2004 test plan.

REAL WORLD INTERVIEW

My best advice to anyone preparing for the NCLEX is to take lots of practice tests. I answered close to 1,500 questions in preparation, and I feel it did me a world of good. I kept my nursing textbooks handy, and when I ran into something I didn't know, I looked it up.

Amanda Meadows, RN, BSN
Chicago, Illinois

EXIT EXAMINATIONS

Many nursing programs administer an examination to students at the completion of their nursing program. Two of these exams are the National League for Nursing (NLN) RN Pre-NCLEX Readiness test and the Health Educations System, Inc. (HESI) Exit Exam. New graduates will want to review their performance on any of these exams because these results will help identify their weaknesses and help focus their review sessions.

Students who examine their feedback from an Exit Exam have important information that can help them focus their review for the NCLEX. A strategy for examining this feedback and organizing this review is outlined in the following section.

ORGANIZING YOUR REVIEW

In preparing for NCLEX, identify your strengths and weaknesses. If you have taken an Exit Exam, note any content strength and weakness areas. Look carefully at the elements of the NCLEX test plan (refer to Table 31-1). Complete a self-needs analysis (Table 31-3), and establish a schedule that permits you to cover completely all the material to be learned. Note any nursing program course or clinical content areas in which you scored below a grade of B. Purchase one or more of the NCLEX review books. It is useful to review questions developed by different authors. Review content in the review books in any of your weak content areas. Take a comprehensive exam in the review book or on the computer software disk and analyze your performance. Try to answer as many questions correctly as you can. As you study, be sure to actually practice taking the examinations. Do not just jump ahead to the answer section until you have completed the examination. Completing the examination in this way may improve your examination performance.

Next, after you have completed the comprehensive examination, review the answers and rationales for any weak content areas and take another comprehensive exam. Repeat this process until you are doing well in all clinical content areas and in all areas of the NCLEX examination plan. Use methods of memory improvement that will work for you. Mnemonic devices, where a letter represents the first letter of each item in a sequence, are an effective means of recalling information as you study (Table 31-4).

Mental imagery is the technique of forming pictures in your mind to help you remember details of the sequence of events, such as the administration of an injection. Try practicing self-recitation to improve your study habits. Reciting to yourself the material being learned will promote retention of the information being studied. Concentrate on the information you identified in your self-needs analysis.

Do a general review of the common patient diseases, medications, diagnostic tests, and nursing procedures

TABLE 31-3   SELF NEEDS ANALYSIS

Anxiety level (circle)   1   2   3   4   5   6   7   8   9   10

Weak content areas identified on NCLEX Test Plan in Table 31-1, exit exam, or another comprehensive exam:

_____

_____

Nursing courses below B: _____

Predictors from Table 31-2 _____

_____

Weak content areas identified in any common patient conditions:

■ Mental Health, for example, schizophrenia, manic depressive, anxiety, personality disorders, eating disorders, abuse, and so on. _____

■ Women's Health, for example, antepartum care, intrapartum care, postpartum care, newborn care, and so on.

_____

■ Adult Health, for example, cancer, myocardial infarction, diabetes, pneumonia, HIV, hepatitis, cholecystectomy, lobectomy, nephrectomy, cardiac arrest, thyroidectomy, shock, appendectomy, and so on.

_____

■ Children's Health, for example, leukemia, cardiovascular surgery, fractures, cancer, tonsillectomy, asthma, wilm's tumor, cleft palate, and so on. _____

Weak content areas identified in any of the following areas:

■ Therapeutic Communication

■ Growth and development (developmental milestones and toys)

■ Management, delegation, and priority setting

■ Medications

■ Defense mechanisms

■ Immunizations

■ Diagnostic and laboratory tests

Organize Your Study

Your study schedule could look like the following:

Day 1:   Practice adult health test questions. Score the test, analyze your performance, and review test question rationales and content weaknesses. Practice deep breathing, relaxation exercises, and positive thinking, as needed.

Day 2:   Practice women's health test questions. Repeat above process.

Day 3:   Practice children's health test questions. Repeat above process.

Day 4:   Practice mental health test questions. Repeat above process.

Day 5:   Continue with content review and test question practice in all weak content areas. Practice deep breathing, relaxation exercises, and positive thinking. Continue this process until you are doing well in all areas.

TABLE 31-4	MNEMONIC DEVICE

It is "OK" to have your blood tested while on Anticoagulants. This is a memory device to assist you in remembering the antidote for Coumadin overdose, that is, the antidote for Oral Coumadin is Vitamin K (OK). Remembering this can help you eliminate the antidote for the other anticoagulant, Intravenous Heparin. Heparin's antidote is Protamine Sulfate.

in each major nursing content area, as well as defense mechanisms, communication tips, and growth and development.

Practice visualization and relaxation techniques as needed. Plan to use any or all of the following to control your anxiety level:

- Guided imagery, which requires using your imagination to create a relaxing sensory scene on which to concentrate
- Breathing exercises
- Relaxation exercises
- Relaxation audio tapes (Stein, 2005)

These strategies will assist you in conquering the three areas necessary for successful test taking—anxiety control, content review, and test question practice.

Organize the material so that you will be able to review all the need-to-know information within the allotted study time period. Your schedule should have allowed you to complete your review so you can close your books and do something relaxing on the night before the examination.

NUTRITION, SLEEP, AND WARDROBE

You will function best if you are well nourished. Plan to eat three well-balanced meals a day for at least three days prior to the examination. Be careful when choosing the food you consume within twenty-four hours of the examination. Avoid foods that will make you thirsty or cause intestinal distress. Minimize the potential of a full bladder midway through the examination by limiting the amount of fluids you drink and by allowing sufficient time at the test site to use the bathroom before entering the room.

Plan to allow sufficient time in your schedule the week before the examination to provide yourself with the minimum sleep you need to function effectively for at least three days prior to the examination. Plan your wardrobe ahead of time. Shoes and clothes that fit you comfortably will not distract your thought processes during the examination. Include a comfortable sweater. Your clothes for the test day should be ready to wear by the night before the examination. If you wear glasses or contact lenses, take along

CASE STUDY 31-1

Analyze your learning needs based on Table 31-3. Use Table 31-5 to identify your best time to practice NCLEX question and review content. Complete the schedule for the next week. When is your best time to study? Review the question of the week and note the NCLEX review course at the NCSBN site, www.learningext.com.

an extra pair of glasses. If you are taking medications on a regular basis, continue to do so during this period of time. Introduction of new medications should be avoided until after completion of the examination (Stein, 2005).

WHEN TO STUDY

Identify your personal best time. Are you a day person? Are you a night person? Study when you are fresh. Arrange to study one or more hours daily. Use Table 31-5 to organize your study.

Students who use this technique should increase their confidence in their ability to do well on the NCLEX.

SOME FINAL TIPS

Table 31-6 has some final tips on reviewing for NCLEX. Table 31-7 is a Medication Study Guide Excerpt to aid you in your NCLEX preparation. Use this guide as a starting point in your medication review for NCLEX.

PROFESSIONALISM

After you successfully pass your NCLEX-RN, you will join the profession of nursing. Experts in the social sciences are considered the authorities on what makes an occupation

TABLE 31-5 ORGANIZING YOUR NCLEX STUDY

	M	T	W	R	F	S	S
8–9							
9–10							
10–11							
11–12							
12–1							
1–2							
2–3							
3–4							
4–5							
5–6							
6–7							
7–8							
8–9							
9–10							

REAL WORLD INTERVIEW

A Dean that I know talks about the fact that she failed what was called in those days "the boards." She tells her students that it was the most traumatic event of her life (or at least one of the most traumatic events). When you have given it "your all" to complete a nursing curriculum, you want to be a successful NCLEX candidate. The HESI Exit Exam can help you achieve that goal. Look at your score printout and review any subject area that has a HESI score of less than 850. Remember, HESI scores are NOT percentage scores, but research data indicate that those who have HESI scores of 850 or above have a 94% probability of passing the NCLEX-RN (Nibert, Young, & Adamson, 2002).

Susan Morrison, PhD, RN
President, Health Education Systems, Inc. (HESI)
Houston, Texas

EVIDENCE FROM THE LITERATURE

Citation: Gordon, S., & Nelson, S. (2006). *Moving beyond the virtue script in nursing in the complexities of care.* Ithaca, NY: ILR Press.

Discussion: Author discusses the concept that images of hearts and angels and the emphasis on caring and health in nursing trivializes what is in fact highly skilled knowledge work that addresses the important role of nurses in care of the sick. The author states that hospital administrators, politicians, and the public won't expand the effort to decode nursing. Nurses must articulate a vivid picture of how nurses as a profession protect their patients. Nursing is facing a crisis because potential recruits don't understand that nurses prevent fatal complications and assess and monitor their patients using knowledge-based scientific care. An emphasis on caring devalues the nursing role, attracting the wrong recruits and driving practitioners from the role. Many nurses are tough-minded professionals who value their technical and practical expertise. They are often dismissed as uncaring. The author asks, isn't using technology and knowledge to prevent complications an act of caring?

Implications for Practice: Nurses must monitor nursing-sensitive indicators and demonstrate the lifesaving role nurses play with their patients using knowledge-based scientific practice.

TABLE 31-6 SELECTED NCLEX TIPS

- Remember Maslow. Physical needs are met first, for example, airway, breathing, circulation (ABCs) threats
  - □ Airway
    - Altered level of consciousness (LOC)
    - Unconscious
    - Foreign object in airway
  - □ Breathing
    - Asthma
    - Suicide threat
  - □ Circulation
    - Cardiac arrest
    - Shock
- Safety needs are met second, for example, safety and infection control threats
  - □ Confusion
  - □ Tuberculosis
  - □ Noninfectious patient away from infectious patient
- Psychological needs and teaching needs are met after physical and safety needs are met. Don't choose a test question answer that gives the patient psychological support or meets teaching needs until the patient's physical and safety needs have been met.
- Remember the nursing process—Assess your patient first, then plan, implement, and evaluate.
- Keep all your patients safe, for example, airway open, side rails up, IV access line in place on unstable patient; monitor vital signs, pulse oximeter, cardiac rhythm, urine output, as needed.
- Know delegation guidelines for RNs, LPNs, and UAPs. Observe the five rights of delegation, that is, the right task, the right circumstance, the right person, the right direction/communication, and the right supervision. See Chapter 16.
  - □ The RN assures quality care of all patients, especially complex patients. RNs delegate care of stable patients with predictable outcomes.
  - □ The RN uses patient care data such as vital signs, collected either by the nurse or others, to make clinical judgments. The RN continuously monitors and evaluates patient care and delegates care involving standard, unchanging procedures to LPNs and UAPs.

(Continues)

TABLE 31-6	**SELECTED NCLEX TIPS (CONTINUED)**

☐ The RN never delegates patient assessment, teaching, evaluation (ATE), or judgment.

☐ LPNs can perform medication administration (includes IV meds in some states), sterile dressings, Foley insertions, and so on.

☐ UAPs can perform basic care, for example, vital sign measurement, bathing, transferring, ambulating, communicating with patients, and stocking supplies.

☐ In some states, LPNs can insert IVs, pass nasogastric tubes, and so on, with documented competency.

☐ In some states, UAPs can perform venipuncture, do blood glucose tests, insert Foley catheters, and so on, with documented competency.

☐ When delegating care, don't mix the care of a patient with an infection with a patient who has decreased immunity, for example, a patient with HIV, diabetes, steroids, the very young, the very old, and so on.

■ In answering test questions, do the following:

☐ When choosing priorities, choose the first answer you would do if you were alone and could only do one thing at a time. Don't think that one RN will do one thing, and another RN will do another thing.

☐ Assume you have the practitioner's order for any possible choices. NCLEX is usually looking for the correct nursing action, not the medical action.

☐ Assume you have perfect staffing, plenty of time, and all the necessary equipment for any possible test question choices. Choose the answer that indicates the best nursing care possible.

☐ Assume you are able to give perfect care "by the book." Don't let your personal clinical experience direct you to choose a test answer that is less than high-quality care.

☐ Remember to care for the patient first and then check the equipment.

■ Know the most common adult, maternal-child, and psychological health care disorders. For each disorder, know the medications, laboratory and diagnostic tools, procedures, and treatments commonly used.

■ Know common medications (see Table 31-7).

■ Know common laboratory norms, for example, sodium, potassium, blood sugar, complete blood count, hematocrit, prothrombin time, partial thromboplastin time, international normalized ratio (INR), arterial blood gas (ABG), cardiac enzymes, digoxin level, dilantin level, lithium level, blood urea nitrogen (BUN), creatinine, and specific gravity of urine.

■ Know communication techniques—look for answers that give patients support and allow the patient to keep talking and verbalize their concerns and problems. Be their comforting nurse, not their therapist. Avoid advice.

■ Know common food choices included in special diets, for example, low sodium diet, diabetic diet, and so on.

■ Know the defense mechanisms.

■ Know growth and development, such as the developmental tasks for each childhood stage, toys for each childhood stage, and so on.

■ Know immunization schedules.

■ Prepare mentally with the following:

☐ Anxiety control and relaxation techniques

☐ Regular exercise

☐ Thinking positively and avoiding negative people.

☐ Avoiding thought distortions (see Chapter 30).

■ Remember—you graduated from an accredited nursing program. You can do it!

---

a profession. Although there is some variation in actual criteria, there is general agreement in several areas:

■ Professional status is achieved when an occupation involves a unique practice that carries individual responsibility and is based upon theoretical knowledge.

■ The privilege to practice is granted only after the individual has completed a standardized program of highly specialized education and has demon-strated an ability to meet the standards for practice.

■ The body of specialized knowledge is continually developed and evaluated through research.

■ The members are self organizing and collectively assume the responsibility of establishing standards for education in practice. They continually evaluate the quality of services provided to protect the individual members and the public.

TABLE 31-7   MEDICATION STUDY GUIDE EXCERPT—COMPLETE/ADD TO AS YOU STUDY

General Tips

1. Drowsiness and changes in vital signs are a side effect of many medications given for their analgesic, antiemetic, antiseizure, tranquilizer, sedative/hypnotic, antihistamine, or antianxiety effects.

2. Note that if drowsiness is a side effect listed in the following Table, consider the need to monitor airway, level of consciousness (LOC), blood pressure (BP), pulse (P), respirations (R), pulse oximetry, and cardiac monitor. Maintain side rails up and fall precautions; avoid driving.

3. Note that if the drug is a cardiac drug, consider the need to monitor LOC, cardiac monitor, BP, P, R, and pulse oximetry.

4. BP medication guidelines: Monitor BP and P. Consider need to monitor postural hypotension and maintain fall precautions; many of these meds also cause impotence.

Category	Word Prefix/Suffix	Examples	Nursing Implications
Analgesic		Morphine	Drowsiness
Analgesic and Antitussive		Codeine	Drowsiness Codeine may cause constipation
Antiemetics		Ondansetron (Zofran)	Drowsiness
Phenothiazines Antiemetic	zine	Promethazine (Phenergan) Hydroxyzine (Vistaril)	Drowsiness Phenergan, given Z-track IM
Anti anxiety Anti psychotic		Chlorpromazine (Thorazine) Prochlorperazine (Compazine) Fluphenazine (Prolixin)	Extrapyramidal (EPS) effects, Parkinsonism, akathisia (restless), dystonia (jerky movement and spasms, check airway), tardive dyskinesia (involuntary movements) Teach to report symptoms early
Sedative/Hypnotic		Zolpidem (Ambien) Zaleplon (Sonata) Eszopiclone (Lunesta) Haloperidol (Haldol)	Drowsiness
Benzodiazepines Tranquilizer Hypnotic Antianxiety Antiseizures Anesthetic	azepam	Diazepam (Valium) Clonazepam (Klonopin) Lorazepam (Ativan) Flurazepam (Dalmane) Midazolam (Versed)	Drowsiness Check for habituation; taper dose when discontinued Monitor bone marrow and liver and kidney function Versed used for short-term sedation; monitor patient closely Romazicon reverses sedative effect of benzodiazepines
Antihistamine Allergic responses		Benadryl (Dyphenhydramine)	Drowsiness

(Continues)

TABLE 31-7		MEDICATION STUDY GUIDE EXCERPT—COMPLETE/ADD TO AS YOU STUDY (CONTINUED)

Category	Word Prefix/Suffix	Examples	Nursing Implications
SSRI		Fluoxetine (Prozac)	Take two to four weeks to take effect
		Sertraline (Zoloft)	Don't use with MAO inhibitors
		Paroxetine (Paxil)	
Antipsychotic Lithium		Lithium	0.5–1.5 therapeutic drug level
			Monitor for toxicity (diarrhea, vomiting, drowsiness, muscle weakness, lack of coordination) to avoid coma, convulsions, and death
			Drowsiness
Anticonvulsant		(Phenytoin) Dilantin	Therapeutic drug level 10–20
			SE-gingival hyperplasia (enlarged gums)
			Flush IV Dilantin with saline only
Anticoagulant	parin	Heparin	Monitor bleeding, for example, stool, gums, urine, bruising, and so on
		Enoxaparin (Lovenox)	Check PTT
			Heparin given IV
			Antidote: protamine sulfate
Anticoagulant		Coumadin (Warfarin)	Monitor bleeding, for example, stool, gums, urine, bruising, and so on
			Check PTT and INR
			Given oral
			Antidote: Vitamin K
Angiotensin Converting Agent (ACE Inhibitor) Antihypertensive	pril	Lisinopril (Zestril)	BP med guidelines above
		Captopril (Capoten)	Monitor white blood cells (WBC)
		Benzapril (Lotensin)	
		Enalapril (Vasotec)	
		Quinapril (Acupril)	
Angiotensin Receptor Blocking Agents Antihypertensive	sartan	Losartan (Cozaar)	BP med guidelines above
		Telmisartan (Micardis)	
		Irbesartan (Avapro)	
		Valsartan (Diovan)	
Beta Blockers Antihypertensive	olol	Metoprolol (Lopressor)	BP med guidelines above
		Atenolol (Tenormin)	Monitor for bronchospasm, bradycardia
		Esmolol (Brevibloc)	Check blood urea nitrogen (BUN)

TABLE 31-7	MEDICATION STUDY GUIDE EXCERPT—COMPLETE/ADD TO AS YOU STUDY (CONTINUED)		

Category	Word Prefix/Suffix	Examples	Nursing Implications
Antihypertensive	pres	Clonidine (Catapres) Hydralazine (Apresoline)	BP med guidelines above
Calcium channel blockers Antihypertensive	pine	Nifedipine (Procardia) Amlodipine (Norvasc)	BP med guidelines above
Digoxin (Lanoxin)		Digoxin (Lanoxin)	Pulse—Hold if pulse below 60 for adult, below 70 in older child, and below 90 in infant and young child Monitor digoxin drug levels; Norm is 0.8–2.0 Check halos around lights, nausea, and vomiting Increased digoxin toxicity if patient is hypokalemic
Antiarrhythmic	caine	Lidocaine	Monitor toxicity CNS toxicity: (anxiety, restlessness, disorientation, blurred vision, nausea/vomiting, tremors/seizure, respiratory depression leading to cardiac arrest and cardiac effects, such as sinus bradycardia, arrhythmias, and hypotension)
Epinephrine		Epinephrine (Adrenalin)	Use for cardiac arrest, anaphylaxis Monitor BP and P
Antihyperlipidemic Lowers cholesterol	vastatin	Lovastatin (Mevacor) Atorvastatin (Lipitor) Pravastatin (Pravachol) Simvastatin (Zocor)	Check liver function test (LFT), blood urea nitrogen (BUN), creatinine, and cholesterol Check lens opacity
Bronchodilator		Albuterol	Monitor breath sounds, rapid pulse, and anxiety Often given per nebulizer
Diuretic		Lasix (Furosemide)	Monitor intake and output Check K
Diuretic		Aldactone (Spironolactone)	K-sparing diuretic Check K

(Continues)

TABLE 31-7	MEDICATION STUDY GUIDE EXCERPT—COMPLETE/ADD TO AS YOU STUDY (CONTINUED)

Category	Word Prefix/Suffix	Examples	Nursing Implications
Osmotic diuretic		Mannitol	Used for cerebral and eye edema
			Monitor urine output and electrolytes
Potassium		Potassium	Electrolyte
			Give slowly IV; use IV pump for infusions
			Potassium can kill if given quickly
			Be sure patient has adequate urine output before giving
Calcium	Cal	Calcium gluconate	Monitor calcium levels
CNS depressant given to preeclamptic patient to prevent seizures		Magnesium Sulfate	Hold dose and notify practitioner if toxicity occurs, for example, respirations below 12, urine output less than 100 cc in 4 hours, absent deep tendon reflexes, blood level greater than 8
May be used to stop preterm labor contractions			Therapeutic drug level 5–8 Antidote: Calcium gluconate
Insulin		Insulin	Many types, short acting, intermediate acting, long acting
Decreases blood sugar		Give common examples of each type—know peak time of each	Regular insulin is only type given IV
		Regular	Monitor blood sugar
		NPH	
		PZI	
		Lente	
Oral hypoglycemic	ide	Glyburide	Monitor blood sugar
Antiinfectives	mycin	Gentamycin (Garamycin)	Monitor for ototoxicity, seizures, blood dyscrasias, nephrotoxicity, rash, allergy
	cin	Streptomycin (Streptomycin)	Monitor peak and trough
		Tobramycin (Tobrex)	
		Amikacin (Amikin)	
		Vancomycin	
Anti-infective	Ceph	Cephalexin (Keflex)	Check allergy, LFT, renal function
Cephalosporin	Cef	Ceftriaxone (Rocephin)	
		Cefadroxil (Duricef)	
Antiviral	vir	Ritonavir (Norvir)	Monitor nausea and vomiting, tremors, confusion
Protease Inhibitors		Zidovudine (Retrovir)	LFT, creatinine
		Acyclovir (Zovirax)	
		Valacyclovir (Valtrex)	
		Ganciclovir (Cytovene)	

TABLE 31-7	MEDICATION STUDY GUIDE EXCERPT—COMPLETE/ADD TO AS YOU STUDY (CONTINUED)

Category	Word Prefix/Suffix	Examples	Nursing Implications
Chemotherapy drugs Wear gloves when handling Follow OSHA guidelines Highly toxic		Cytoxan Methotrexate Adriamylin Oncovin Taxol Hormonal Agents Hercaptia	Given in combination with other chemotherapy drugs Push fluids Monitor toxicity, for example, renal, liver, heart, bone marrow function—Monitor alopecia, stomatitis, nausea and vomiting, WBC, RBC, neutrophils, and so on.
Anti Tuberculosis (TB) Medication		Rifampin Isoniazid (INH) Ethambutal Pyrazinamide	Rifampin turns urine and bodily fluids orange, stains soft contacts, and reduces effectiveness of oral contraceptives Give medications in combination therapy to treat TB INH increases dilantin levels Prevent neuropathy by giving Pyrazinamide (Vitamin B6) with INH Monitor LFT and renal function Monitor vision with ethambutal May need to take meds one–two years
Steroids Antiinflammatory Many antiinflammatory uses for conditions such as CVA, Asthma, Arthritis, and so on	sone	Decadron (Dexamethasone) Prednisolone (Delta Cortef) Prednisone (Deltasone) Methylprednisolone (Solu-Cortef, Depo-Medrol)	Monitor "S's" sex, sad, stress, sight, sleep, susceptibility, sugar, sodium Decreases sex (hormones), stress (inflammatory response), sight (glaucoma and cataracts), and potassium Increases susceptibility (infection, ulcers), sugar (hyperglycemia), sad (mood), sodium (edema), and osteoporosis Wean off medication to avoid adrenal crisis and shock
Cox II Enzyme Blockers	cox	Celecoxib (Celebrex) Valdecoxib (Bextra)	Tinnitus/GI bleed Check platelets Check Renal function
Histamine 2 Antagonists H2 Antagonists Inhibit gastric acid secretion	tidine	Ranitidine (Zantac) Famotidine (Pepcid) Tagamet (Cimetidine)	Confusion/seizures Check BUN

(Continues)

TABLE 31-7		MEDICATION STUDY GUIDE EXCERPT—COMPLETE/ADD TO AS YOU STUDY (CONTINUED)	
Category	**Word Prefix/Suffix**	**Examples**	**Nursing Implications**
Proton Pump Inhibitors Suppress gastric acid secretion	prazole	Lansoprazole (Prevacid) Esomeprazole (Nexium) Rabeprazole (Aciphex) Pantoprazole (Protonix)	Gastro esophageal reflux disease (GERD), check LFT Rash, headache
Antidiarrheal		Lomotil	Decrease gastric motility
Miotic eye drops		Pilocarpine	Constrict the pupil—reduce intraocular pressures
Mydriatric eye drops		Atropine	Dilate the pupil
Ammonia detoxicant and Stimulant laxative		Lactulose	Decreases ammonia in encephalopathy associated with liver cirrhosis Monitor ammonia levels
Biologic response modifier		Epogen, Neupogen, Neumega	Use as needed, for example, use Epogen to treat anemia, Neupogen to treat neutrophilia, and Neumega to treat low platelets
Antacid		Mylanta, Riopan, Gelusil	Neutralize or reduce gastric acid
Uterine stimulant		Oxytocin (Pitocin)	Initiates/augments labor Given immediately post delivery of placenta to avoid trapped placenta Monitor fetal heart rate (FHR), BP, and pulse
Inhibit uterine contractions		Ritodrine (Yutopar)	Monitor for increased FHR
Rhogam		Rhogam	Blood product given to Rh negative mother if father is Rh positive Not given to mother with positive indirect Coombs; she is already sensitized to fetal cells and has developed antibodies Given to Rh negative women after miscarriage, abortion, trauma, or any procedure that increases risk of maternal-fetal blood exchange

Source: Unpublished manuscript, Patricia Kelly, RN, MSN, and Gabriel Hernandez, RPh.

There is a trend in recent years to call every occupation a profession. Have you heard of "professional baseball players" and "professional automobile mechanics"? There has been a tendency to confuse professionalism and profession. The term "professionalism" generally refers to an individual's commitment and dedication to the occupation. Professionalism often also refers to the attitude, appearance, and conduct of the individual. Whether an occupation is a profession requires more analysis. Figure 31-1 refers to some of the classic studies about the characteristics of a profession (Mitchell & Grippando, 1994). Figure 31-2 lists some of the various values, behaviors, and attributes that may be exhibited by a "professional" (Mitchell & Grippando, 1994).

Flexner, 1915

- Intellectual activities
- Activities based on knowledge
- Activities can be learned
- Activities must be practical
- Techniques are teachable
- A strong organization exists
- Altruism motivates the work

Pavalko, 1971

- Work based on systematic body of theory and abstract knowledge
- Work has social value
- Length of education required for specialization
- Service to public
- Autonomy
- Commitment to profession
- Group identity and subculture
- Existence of a code of ethics

Bixler and Bixler, 1959

- Specialized body of knowledge
- Growing body of knowledge
- New knowledge used to improve education and practice
- Autonomous practice
- Service above personal gain
- Compensation through freedom of action, continuing professional growth, and economic security

Public Law 93-360 on Collective Bargaining

- Predominantly intellectual work
- Varied work requirements
- Requires discretion and judgment
- Results cannot be standardized over time
- Requires advanced instruction and study

Figure 31-1 Characteristics of a profession. (Courtesy, Mitchell, G. M., and Grippando, P. R. (1994). *Nursing perspectives and issues.* Clifton Park, NY: Thomson Delmar Learning.)

Professional Values:

Caring	Freedom	Justice
Altruism	Esthetics	Truth
Equality	Human Dignity	Ethical
Nonjudgmental		

Professional Behaviors and Attributes:

Appearance	Stress Management
Time-Management Skills	Self-Evaluation
Self-Discipline	Initiative
Maintenance of Licensure/Certification	Motivation
Participation in Institutional/Community Activities	Creativity
Participation in Continuing Education	Effective Communication
Political Awareness	
Reading Professional Journals	
Participation in Nursing Research	

Figure 31-2 Characteristics of a professional. (Courtesy, Mitchell, G. M., and Grippando, P. R. (1994). *Nursing perspective and issues.* Clifton Park, NY: Thomson Delmar Learning.)

CRITICAL THINKING 31-1

Y ou may use a Website to contact your members of Congress. You may also contact them through the U.S. Capitol at (202) 224-3121. How could you use these contact sites to improve care for your patients or advocate for an important health care issue or the professional role of the nurse?

CASE STUDY 31-2

N ote the professional behaviors and attitudes characteristic of a professional shown previously in Figure 31-2. Which professional behaviors and attributes do you have? Make a one-year and a five-year plan in any areas you feel that you need to work on. Use Table 31-8. Review your list with a professional mentor.

TABLE 31-8 PLAN FOR PROFESSIONALISM

Behavior/Attribute	One-Year Goals	Five-Year-Goals
Appearance		
Time-management skills		
Self-discipline		
Licensure/certification		
Institutional/community activity participation		
Continuing education		
Political awareness		
Professional journals		
Nursing research participation		
Stress management		
Self-evaluation		
Initiative		
Motivation		
Creativity		
Communication		

THE FUTURE

As nursing goes forward into the future, the answer to whether nurses are professionals will continue to be developed by you, the nursing profession, and society as a whole (Table 31-9). Some of the answers depend on the development of nursing theory and the move to increase nursing academic credentials to a minimum of a baccalaureate degree. This degree is increasingly viewed as minimum professional preparation.

NURSE-SENSITIVE OUTCOMES

The existence of professional nursing benefits patients who develop lower rates of nurse-sensitive outcomes,

TABLE 31-9	**DEVELOPING A PROFESSIONAL STYLE**

1. Assess your current education and experience.

2. As you start your new nursing role, review the following on your unit:
   - Most common medical diagnoses
   - Most common nursing diagnoses
   - Most common medications and IV solutions
   - Most common diagnostic tests
   - Most common laboratory tests
   - Most common nursing and medical interventions and treatments

3. Set goals for any additional education and experience that you may need.

4. Review your own job description and the role and the job description of nursing and other health care and medical staff you work with.

5. Identify the names and contact information of all nursing, medical, and health care staff you work with.

6. Discuss delegation with your preceptor, and observe how the preceptor delegates to others.

7. Observe the impact of delegation on both the delegate and the person delegated to.

8. Remember the golden rule; do unto others as you would want them to do unto you.

9. Recognize that, under the law, the RN holds the responsibility and accountability for nursing care.

10. Practice assertiveness and work at being direct, open, and honest in your new role.

11. Exercise your power with kindness to all.

12. Hold others accountable for their responsibilities as spelled out in their job description.

13. Be open to performance improvement feedback about your personal delegation style.

14. Modify your communication approach to fit the needs of patients, staff, and yourself.

15. Take action to assure your patients receive high-quality, safe care.

CRITICAL THINKING 31-2

Go to the Website, www.sandiego.edu, and review some of the nursing theorists, for example, Nightingale, King, Orem, Parse, Roy, and others. How does nursing theory influence your practice of nursing as a professional? Pick one of the theories, and comment on how your practice of nursing may fit with the theory.

CRITICAL THINKING 31-3

Have you ever witnessed a "failure to rescue" or witnessed a nurse "rescuing" a patient? Would the patient have lived if the nurse was not present? Use Figure 31-2 to develop your own professional behavior and style. How will you rescue your patients?

EVIDENCE FROM THE LITERATURE

Citation: Wu, Y., Larrabee, J. H., & Putman, H. P. (2006, Jan.–Feb.). Caring behaviors inventory. *Nursing Research, 55*(1), 18–25.

Discussion: A short instrument for patient use is presented to measure the process of nurse caring. Elements of the patient instrument include patient assessment of the knowledge and skill, respectfulness, connectedness of the nurse, and so forth. Some of the areas presented to be assessed by the nurse include responding quickly to the patient's call; knowing how to give shots, IVs, and so on; attentively listening to the patient; and spending time with the patient. All twenty-four elements of the Caring Behaviors Inventory are presented.

Implications for Practice: Nurses interested in measuring the impact of their patient care can use this instrument to do so and improve their practice.

including lower death rates of patients from one of the following life-threatening complications: pneumonia, shock, cardiac arrest, urinary tract infection, gastrointestinal bleeding, sepsis, deep vein thrombosis, and "failure to rescue" (Needleman, Buerhaus, Mattke, Stewart, & Zelevinsky, 2002).

KEY CONCEPTS

- The NCLEX-RN Test Plan reviews patient needs in the following areas:
  safe, effective care environment; physiologic integrity; psychosocial integrity; and health promotion and maintenance.

- There are several new types of questions on NCLEX-RN.

- Multiple risk factors are associated with NCLEX-RN performance identified in Table 31-2.

- Nursing Exit Examinations are given by many schools of nursing.

- It is useful to have a plan to review any NCLEX-RN weaknesses.

- NCLEX-RN tips can help you prepare for the examination.

- A medication guide is useful to study for NCLEX.

- There are many characteristics of a profession.

- There are many characteristics of a professional.

- Nurses regularly take nursing action to prevent the incidence of nurse-sensitive outcomes in their patients.

KEY TERM

NCLEX

REVIEW QUESTIONS

1. The least number of questions a graduate nurse can take to complete the NCLEX is which of the following?
   A. 60
   B. 75
   C. 90
   D. 120

2. Which of the following client needs are tested in the NCLEX test plan? Choose all that apply.
   _____ A. Safe, effective care environment
   _____ B. Physiologic integrity
   _____ C. Psychosocial integrity
   _____ D. Health promotion and maintenance

3. Types of test questions that may appear on NCLEX include which of the following? Choose all that apply.
   _____ A. Single-option, multiple choice
   _____ B. Fill in the blank
   _____ C. True/False
   _____ D. Multiple-option, multiple-choice

REVIEW ACTIVITIES

1. Set up a group to study for NCLEX with several of your friends. Arrange to meet to discuss how your NCLEX review is going. Have each member of the group buy a NCLEX review book from a different publisher. Practice answering questions for one to two hours daily. Don't mark your answers in the review book. Share your review books with each other to increase your exposure to various authors' test questions.

2. Review Pavalko's characteristics of a profession in Figure 31-1. Is nursing a profession?

EXPLORING THE WEB

- Review NCLEX review books at *www.amazon.com* How many different books published in the past three years did you see on the topic of NCLEX Review?

- Go to *www.ncsbn.org* Note what you see there. Explore the site.

- Go to *www.learningext.com* Note: NCSBN's Review for the NCLEX is offered through this NCSBN learning extension. This self-paced, online review features NCLEX-style questions, interactive exercises, topic-specific course exams, and a diagnostic pretest that can help you develop a personal study plan. Visit this site every Monday to see its new NCLEX-RN test question samples.

REFERENCES

Gauwitz, D. (2007). *Complete Review for NCLEX-RN.* Clifton Park, NY: Thomson Delmar Learning.

Gordon, S., & Nelson, S. (2006). *Moving beyond the virtue script in nursing in the complexities of care.* Ithaca, NY: ILR Press.

Mitchell, G. M., & Grippando, P. R. (1994). *Nursing perspectives and issues.* Clifton Park, NY: Thomson Delmar Learning.

Needleman, J., Buerhaus, P., Mattke, S., Stewart, M., & Zelevinsky, K. (2002). Nurse-staffing levels and the quality of care in hospitals. *New England Journal of Medicine, 346*(22), 1715–1722.

Nibert, A., Young A., & Adamson, C. (2002). Predicting NCLEX success with the HESI Exit Exam: Fourth annual validity study. *Computers, Informatics, Nursing, 20*(6), 261–267.

Stein, A. M. (2005). *NCLEX-RN review* (5th ed.). Clifton Park, NY: Thomson Delmar Learning.

Wendt, A. (2003, Nov.–Dec.). The NCLEX-RN examination. *Nurse Educator, 29*(6), 276–280.

Wu, Y., Larrabee, J. H., & Putnam, H. P. (2006, Jan.–Feb.). Caring Behaviors Inventory. *Nursing Research, 55*(1), 18–25.

SUGGESTED READINGS

Aucoin, J. W., & Treas, L. (2005). Assumptions and realities of the NCLEX-RN. *Nursing Education Perspective, 26*(5), 268–271.

Baggs, J. G., Smith, P. L., & Ryan, S. A. (1990). ICU nurse-physician collaboration and nursing satisfaction. *Nursing Economics, 8*(6), 386–392.

Beeman, P. B., & Waterhouse, J. K. (2003). Post-graduation factors predicting NCLEX-RN success. *Nurse Educator, 28*(6), 257–260.

Candela, L., Michael, S. R., & Mitchell, S. (2003). Ethical debates. *Nurse Educator, 28*(1), 37–39.

Cathcart, E. B. (2003). Using the NCLEX-RN to argue for BSN preparation: Barking up the wrong tree. *Journal of Professional Nursing, 19*(3), 121–122.

Crow, C. S., Handley, M., Morrison, R. S., & Shelton, M. M. (2004). Requirements and interventions used by BSN programs to promote and predict NCLEX-RN success: A national study. *Journal of Professional Nursing, 20*(3), 174–186.

Cunningham, H., Stacciarini, J. M., & Towle, S. (2004). Strategies to promote success on the NCLEX-RN for students with English as a second language. *Nurse Educator, 29*(1), 15–19.

Daley, L. K., Kirkpatrick, B. L., Frazier, S. K., Chung, M. L., & Moser, D. K. (2003). Predictors of NCLEX-RN success in a baccalaureate nursing program as a foundation for remediation. *Journal of Nursing Education, 42*(9), 390–398.

DiBartolo, M. C., & Seldomridge, L. A. (2005). A review of intervention studies to promote NCLEX-RN success of baccalaureate students. *Nurse Educator, 30*(4), 166–171.

Downey, T. A. (2003). Predictive NCLEX success with the HESI exit examination: Fourth annual validity study. *Computer, Informatics, Nursing, 21*(6), 296–297; author reply 297–299.

Downey, T. A., & Nibert, A. T. (2003). Indicia: Letters to the editor and reply. *Computers, Informatics, Nursing, 21*(6), 296–299.

English, J. B., & Gordon, D. K. (2004). Successful student remediation following repeated failures on the HESI exam. *Nurse Educator, 29*(6), 266–268.

Frith, K. H., Sewell, J. P., & Clark, D. J. (2005). Best practices in NCLEX-RN readiness preparation for baccalaureate student success. *Computer, Informatics, Nursing, 23*(6), 322–329.

Giddens, J., & Gloeckner, G. W. (2005). The relationship of critical thinking to perform on the NCLEX-RN. *Journal of Nursing Education, 44*(2), 85–90.

Griffiths, M. J., Papastrat, K., Czekanski, K., & Hagan, K. (2004). The lived experience of NCLEX failure. *Journal of Nursing Education, 43*(7), 322–325.

Hanks, C., & Lauchner, K. (1999). Indicia: Letters to the editor. *Computers in Nursing, 17*(6), 241–246.

Hart, K. (2005, Nov.). What do men in nursing really think? *Nursing,* 46–48.

Higgins, B. (2005). Strategies for lowering attrition rates and raising NCLEX-RN pass rates. *Journal of Nursing Education, 44*(12), 541–547.

Kirkpatrick, J. M., Billings, D. M., Hodson-Carlton, K., Cummings, R. B., Dorner, J., Jeffries, et al. (2000). Computerized test development software. A comparative review updated. *Computers in Nursing, 18*(2), 72–86.

Lauchner, K., Newman, M., & Britt, R. (1999). Predicting licensure success with a computerized comprehensive nursing exam: The HESI Exit Exam. *Computers in Nursing, 17*(3), 120–125.

Lewis, C. (2005). *Predictive accuracy of the HESI Exit Exam on NCLEX-RN pass rates and effects of progression policies on nursing student Exit Exam scores.* Unpublished doctoral dissertation, Texas Woman's University, Denton, TX.

Major, D. A. (2005). OSCE's—seven years on the bandwagon: The progress of an objective structured clinical evaluation programme. *Nursing Education Today, 25*(6), 442–454.

Mayne, L., & Glascoff, M. (2002). Service learning: Preparing a healthcare workforce for the next century. *Nursing Educator, 27*(4), 191–194.

Miller, J. C. (2003). Twelve frequently asked questions about the NCLEX-RN. *Imprint, 50*(1), 73–75.

Miller, J. C. (2004). Tips on passing the NCLEX-RN. *Imprint, 51*(1), 61–62.

Miller, J. C. (2005). Tips on taking the NCLEX-RN. *Imprint, 52*(1), 28–32.

Morrison, S., & Free, K. W. (2001). Writing multiple-choice test items that promote and measure critical thinking. *Journal of Nursing Education, 40*(1), 17–24.

Morrison, S., Free, K. W., & Newman, M. (2002). Do progression and remediation policies improve NCLEX-RN pass rates? *Nurse Educator, 27*(2), 94–96.

Morrison, S. (2004). Test construction and analysis: Can I do it? In L. Caputi & L. Engelmann (Eds.), *Teaching Nursing: The art and science* (Vol. 1, pp. 366–387). Chicago: College of DuPage Press.

Morrison, S., Adamson, C., Nibert, A. T., & Hsia, S. (2004). HESI Exams: An overview of reliability and validity. *Computers, Informatics, Nursing, 22*(4), 220–226.

Morrison, S. (2005). Improving NCLEX-RN pass rates through internal and external curriculum evaluation. In M. Oermann & K. Heinrich (Eds.), *Annual review of nursing education: Strategies for teaching assessment and program planning* (Vol. 3, pp. 77–94). New York: Springer Publishing Co.

NCLEX practice questions. (2005). *Nursing, 35*(8), 68–70.

Newman, M., Britt, R., & Lauchner, K. (2000). Predictive accuracy of the HESI Exit Exam: A follow-up study. *Computers in Nursing, 18*(3), 132–136.

Nibert, A. (2003). New graduates: A precious critical care resource. *Critical Care Nurse, 23*(5), 47–50.

Nibert, A. (2005). Benchmarking for progression: Implications for students, faculty, and administrators. In L. Caputi (Ed.), *Teaching nursing: The art and science* (Vol. 3, pp. 314–335). Chicago: College of DuPage Press.

Nibert, A., & Young, A. (2001). A third study on predicting NCLEX success with the HESI Exit Exam. *Computers in Nursing, 19*(4), 172–178.

Nibert, A., Young, A., & Britt, R. (2003). The HESI Exit Exam: Progression benchmark and remediation guide. *Nurse Educator, 28*(3), 141–145.

Olshansky, E. (2004). In consideration of BSN-to-PhD programs. *Journal of Professional Nursing, 20*(1), 1–2.

O'Neill, T. R., Marks, C. M., & Reynolds, M. (2005). Reevaluating the NCLEX-RN passing standard. *Journal of Nursing Measures, 13*(2), 147–165.

Poorman, S. G., & Mastorovich, M. L. (2004). A clinical strategy to help students with leadership/management NCLEX questions. *Nurse Educator, 29*(4), 142–143.

Poster, E. C. (2004). Psychiatric nursing at risk: The new NCLEX-RN test plan. *Perspective Psychiatric Care, 40*(2), 43–44.

Reising, D. L. (2003). The relationship between computer testing during a nursing program and NCLEX performance. *Computers, Informatics, Nursing, 21*(6), 326–329.

Schwarz, K. A. (2005). Making the grade: Help staff pass the NCLEX-RN. *Nursing Management, 36*(3), 38–44.

Seldomridge, L. A., & Dibartolo, M. C. (2004). Can success and failure be predicted for baccalaureate graduates on the computerized NCLEX-RN? *Journal of Professional Nursing, 20*(6), 361–368.

Siktberg, L. L., & Dillard, N. L. (2001). Assisting at-risk students in preparing for NCLEX-RN. *Nurse Educator, 26*(3), 150–152.

Spector, N., & Sheets, V. (2004). NCLEX results to disclose or not disclose. *JONAS Health Law Ethics Regulations, 6*(2), 38–39.

Spurlock, D. R. Jr., & Hanks, C. (2004). Establishing progression policies with the HESI Exit Examination: A review of the evidence. *Journal of Nursing Education, 43*(12), 539–545.

Waterhouse, J. K., & Beeman, P. B. (2003). Predicting NCLEX-RN success: Can it be simplified? *Nursing Education Perspective, 24*(1), 35–39.

Wendt, A. (2003). Mapping geriatric nursing competencies to the 2001 NCLEX-RN test plan. *Nursing Outlook, 51*(4), 152–157.

Wissmann, J., Hauck, B., & Clawson, J. (2002). Assessing nurse graduate leadership outcomes: The "typical day" format. *Nurse Educator, 27*(1), 32–36.

Wood, R. M. (2005). Student computer competence and the NCLEX-RN examination: Strategies for success. *Computer, Informatics, Nursing, 23*(5), 241–243.

Yin, T., & Burger, C. (2003). Predictors of NCLEX-RN success of associate degree nursing graduates. *Nurse Educator, 28*(5), 232–236.

Young, J., Urden, L. D., Wellman, D. S., & Stoten, S. (2004). Management curriculum redesign: Integrating customer expectations for new leaders. *Nurse Educator, 29*(1), 41–44.

ABBREVIATIONS

AACN	American Association of Critical Care Nurses
AACN	American Association of Colleges of Nursing
AAHP	American Association of Health Plans
AAN	American Academy of Nursing
AANA	American Association of Nurse Anesthetists
AARP	American Association of Retired Persons
ACLS	Advanced Cardiac Life Support
ACNP	Acute Care Nurse Practitioner
ACS	American Cancer Society
ADA	American Dietetic Association
ADL	Activity of Daily Living
ADN	Associate Degree in Nursing
AHA	American Hospital Association
AHRQ	Agency for Healthcare Research and Quality
AIDS	Acquired Immune Deficiency Syndrome
AMA	American Medical Association
ANA	American Nurses Association
ANCC	American Nurses Credentialing Center
AONE	American Organization of Nurse Executives
APHA	American Public Health Association
AWHONN	Association of Women's Health, Obstetric, and Neonatal Nurses
BLS	Basic Life Support
BMI	Body Mass Index
BSN	Bachelor of Science in Nursing

BTIPA	Brooks' Theory of Intrapersonal Awareness
CAMH	Comprehensive Accreditation Manual for Hospitals
CARING	Capital Area Roundtable on Informatics in Nursing
CCQHC	Consumer Coalition for Quality Health Care
CCRN	Critical Care Registered Nurse
CCU	Coronary Care Unit
CDC	Centers for Disease Control and Prevention
CEO	Chief Executive Officer
CEU	Continuing Education Unit
CFO	Chief Financial Officer
CHF	Congestive Heart Failure
CINAHL	Cumulative Index to Nursing and Allied Health Literature
CIS	Clinical Information System
CMP	Comprehensive Metabolic Panel
CMS	Centers for Medicare and Medicaid Services
CN3	Clinical Nurse 3
CNA	Canadian Nurses Association
CNM	Certified Nurse Midwife
CNS	Clinical Nurse Specialist
CNS/NP	Clinical Nurse Specialist/Nurse Practitioner
CON	Certificate Of Need
COPC	Community-Oriented Primary Care

CPR	CardioPulmonary Resuscitation
CPR	Computerized Patient Record
CPRI	Computer-based Patient Record Institute
CQI	Continuous Quality Improvement
CRNA	Certified Registered Nurse Anesthetist
CU	Consumers Union
CVA	CerebroVascular Accident
DM	Disease Management
DRG	Diagnosis-Related Group
EBC	Evidence-Based Care
EBM	Evidence-Based Medicine
EBNP	Evidence-Based Nursing Practice
EBP	Evidence-Based Practice
EMTALA	Emergency Medical Treatment and Active Labor Act
ENIAC	Electronic Numerical Integrator and Computer
ERCP	Endoscopic Retrograde CholangioPancreatography
ERG	Existence-Relatedness-Growth Theory
ET Nurse	Enterostomal Therapy Nurse
FTE	Full-Time Equivalent
GI Lab	GastroIntestinal Laboratory
HCFA	Health Care Financing Administration
HIMSS	Health Information and Management Systems Society
HIPAA	Health Insurance Portability and Accountability Act
HIV	Human Immunodeficiency Virus
HMO	Health Maintenance Organization
IADL	Instrumental Activity of Daily Living
ICN	International Council of Nurses
ICU	Intensive Care Unit
IOM	Institute of Medicine
IRA	Individual Retirement Account
JBIEBNM	Joanna Briggs Institute for Evidence-Based Nursing & Midwifery
JC	Joint Commission
LOS	Length Of Stay
LPN/LVN	Licensed Practical Nurse/Licensed Vocational Nurse
MBNQA	Malcolm Baldridge National Quality Award
MBTI	Myers-Briggs Type Indicator
MDI	Metered-Dose Inhaler
MEDLARS	Medical Literature Analysis and Retrieval System
MeSH	Medical Subject Headings
MIS	Medical Information System
MRI	Medical Records Institute
MS-HUG	Microsoft Healthcare Users Group
MSN	Master's Degree in Nursing
NANDA	North American Nursing Diagnosis Association
NANN	National Association of Neonatal Nurses
NAP	Nursing Assistive Personnel
NAPNAP	National Association of Pediatric Nurses and Practitioners
NAPQ	Nosek-Androwich Profit: Quality Matrix
NCLEX	National Council of State Boards of Nursing Licensure Examination
NCQA	National Committee on Quality Assurance
NCSBN	National Council of State Boards of Nursing
NGC	National Guideline Clearinghouse
NHPPD	Nursing Hours Per Patient Day
NIH	National Institutes of Health
NLM	National Library of Medicine
NLN	National League for Nursing
NNP	Neonatal Nurse Practitioner
NP	Nurse Practitioner
NRP	Neonatal Resuscitation Program
NWIG-AMIA	Nursing Working Informatics Group of the American Medical Informatics Association
OB	Organizational Behavior
OR	Operating Room
OSHA	Occupational Safety and Health Administration
PALS	Pediatric Advanced Life Support
PC	Personal Computer
PCA	Patient Care Associate
PCS	Patient Classification System
PDCA	Plan Do Check Act
PDSA	Plan Do Study Act
PERT	Program Evaluation and Review Technique
P-F-A	Purpose-Focus-Approach
PHN	Public Health Nurse
PI	Performance Improvement
POD	PostOperative Day
POS	Point Of Service
POSDCORB	Planning, Organizing, Supervising, Directing, Coordinating, Reporting, and Budgeting

PPO	Preferred Provider Organization	**UAP**	Unlicensed Assistive Personnel
QI	Quality Improvement	**UC**	Ubiquitous Computing
RN	Registered Nurse	**URL**	Universal Resource Locator
RVU	Relative Value Unit	**USDHHS**	United States Department of Health and Human Services
SCHIP	State Children's Health Insurance Program	**UTI**	Urinary Tract Infection
SPAN	Staff Planning and Action Network	**VA**	Veterans Affairs
SWOT	Strengths, Weaknesses, Opportunities, Threats	**VAK**	Visual, Auditory, Kinesthetic
		VR	Virtual Reality
TB	Tuberculosis	**WHO**	World Health Organization
TEFRA	Tax Equity and Fiscal Responsibility Act	**WOC nurse**	Wound, Ostomy, Continence Nurse
TQI	Total Quality Improvement	**WWW**	World Wide Web

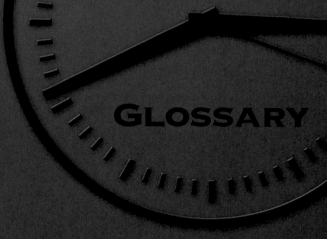

GLOSSARY

360-degree feedback System in which an individual is assessed by a variety of people to provide a broader perspective.

absenteeism The rate of employee absences from work.

accountability Being responsible and answerable for actions or inactions of self or others in the context of delegation.

accounting Activity that nurse managers engage in to record and report financial transactions and data.

acculturated Becoming like people in a new country by adopting their conditions, customs, and language.

activities of daily living Activities related to toileting, bathing, grooming, dressing, feeding, mobility, and verbal and written personal communication.

activity log Time-management technique to assist in determining how time is used by periodically recording activities.

administrative law Body of law created by administrative agencies in the form of rules, regulations, orders, and decisions to protect the rights of citizens.

administrative principles General principles of management that are relevant to any organization.

affective domain Learning domain centered on attitudes, or what the learner feels and believes.

assault Offer to or threat of touching another in an offensive manner without that person's permission.

assignment Distribution of work that each staff member is to accomplish on a given shift or work period.

authority Power and/or right to make decisions.

autocratic leadership Centralized decision-making style with the leader making decisions and using power to command and control others.

autonomy An individual's right to self-determination; individual liberty.

battery Touching of another person without that person's consent.

behavioral objective Statement of specific and measurable behavior that should result from the teaching session.

benchmark A quantitative or qualitative standard or point of reference used in measuring or judging quality or value.

benchmarking Continuous process of measuring products, service, and practices against the toughest competitors or those customers recognized as industry leaders (Camp, 1994).

beneficence The duty to do good to others and to maintain a balance between benefits and harms.

bioethics Ethics specific to health care; serves as a framework to guide behavior in ethical dilemmas.

bureaucratic organization Hierarchy with clear superior-subordinate communication and relations, based on positional authority, in which orders from the top are transmitted down through the organization via a clear chain of command.

capital budget Accounts for the purchase of major new or replacement equipment.

career planning Ongoing process that involves a personal and professional self-assessment, setting goals, searching for a job, preparing a cover letter and resume, and participating in an interview including follow-up.

change Making something different from what it was.

change agent One who is responsible for implementation of a change project.

civil law That body of law that governs how individuals relate to each other in everyday matters.

clinical ladder A promotional model that acknowledges that staff members have varying skill sets based on their education and experience. As such, depending on skills and experience, staff members may be rewarded differently and carry differing responsibilities for patient care and the governance and professional practice of the work unit.

clinical pathway Care management tool that outlines the expected clinical course and outcomes for a specific patient type.

cognitive domain Learning domain centered on knowledge, or what the learner knows.

communication An interactive process that occurs when a person (the sender) sends a verbal or nonverbal message to another person (the receiver) and receives feedback.

conflict Disagreement about something of importance to each person involved.

connection power Extent to which nurses are connected with others having power.

consensus All group members can live with and fully support the decision, regardless of whether they totally agree.

consideration Activities that focus on the employee and emphasize relating and getting along with people.

constitution A set of basic laws that specifies the powers of the various segments of the government and how these segments relate to each other.

construction budget Developed when renovation or new structures are planned.

contingency theory Style that acknowledges that other factors in the environment influence outcomes as much as leadership style and that leader effectiveness is contingent upon or depends upon something other than the leader's behavior.

contract law Rules that regulate certain transactions between individuals and/or legal entities such as businesses. Also governs transactions between businesses.

cost shifting Process of assigning financial charges from one cost center to another cost center.

cost center Departmental subsection or unit for tracking of financial data.

critical thinking Thinking about your thinking while you're thinking in order to make your thinking better.

culture A broad term that includes the beliefs, customs, and patterns of behavior and the institutions of a particular group of people.

cultural competence Providing culturally sensitive care through behaviors, attitudes, and policies that are congruent within health care.

dashboard Documentation tool providing a snapshot image of pertinent information and activity reflecting a point in time.

decision making Considering and selecting interventions from a repertoire of actions that facilitate the achievement of a desired outcome.

delegation Transferring to a competent individual the authority to perform a selected nursing task in a selected situation.

democratic leadership Style in which participation is encouraged and authority is delegated to others.

desired optimal outcomes Best possible objectives to be achieved given the resources at hand.

diagnostic-related groups Patient groupings established by the government for reimbursement purposes; these groupings are identified by patient diagnosis or condition, surgical procedure, age, comorbidity, or complications.

direct care Time spent providing hands-on care to patients.

direct patient care activities Patient care activities that include patient contact, such as bathing, providing medications, and so forth.

direct expenses Expenses that are directly associated with patient care (for example, medical and surgical supplies and drugs).

employee-centered leadership Style with a focus on the human needs of subordinates.

enabling objective Objective that identifies secondary behaviors that contribute to, or enable, achievement of terminal objectives.

episodic care unit Unit that sees patients for defined episodes of care; examples include dialysis or ambulatory care units.

ethical dilemma A conflict between two or more ethical principles for which there is no correct decision.

ethics The doctrine that the general welfare of society is the proper goal of an individual's actions rather than egoism; the branch of philosophy that concerns the distinction between right from wrong on the basis of a body of knowledge, not just on the basis of opinions.

ethnicity Identifies a person or group based on religious or national cultural group.

ethnocentrism Belief that one's own culture or ethnic group is better than all other groups.

evaluation Process of determining the success of teaching; it can measure the patient's learning and the teaching's effectiveness.

evidence-based care Recognized by nursing, medicine, health care institutions, and health policy makers as care based on state-of-the-art science reports. It is a process approach to collecting, reviewing, interpreting, critiquing, and evaluating research and other relevant literature for direct application to patient care.

evidence-based medicine (EBM) The conscientious, explicit, and judicious use of current best evidence in making decisions about the care of individual patients. The practice of evidence-based medicine means integrating individual clinical expertise with the best available external clinical evidence from systematic research.

evidence-based nursing practice Conscientious, explicit, and judicious use of theory-derived, research-based information in making decisions about care delivery to individuals or groups of individuals and in consideration of individual needs and preferences.

evidence-based practice Conscientious, explicit, and judicious use of current best evidence in making decisions about the care of individual patients.

expert power Power derived from the knowledge and skills nurses possess.

external forces Influences originating outside the organization, for example, the labor force and the economy.

false imprisonment Occurs when people are incorrectly led to believe they cannot leave a place.

fidelity The principle of promise keeping; the duty to keep one's promise or word.

fixed costs Expenses that are constant and are not related to productivity or volume.

focus groups Small groups of individuals selected because of a common characteristic (for example, a specific patient population, patients in day surgery, new diabetics, and so on) who are invited to meet in a group and respond to questions about a topic in which they are expected to have interest or expertise.

formal leadership When a person is in a position of authority or in a sanctioned role within an organization that connotes influence.

full-time equivalent Measure of the work commitment of an employee who works five days a week or forty hours per week for fifty-two weeks per year.

functional health status Ability to care for oneself and meet one's human needs.

functional nursing Care delivery model that divides the nursing work into functional roles that are then assigned to one of the team members.

gap The space between where the organization is and where it wants to be.

gap analysis An assessment of the differences between the expected magnet requirements and the organization's current performance on those requirements.

generation A group that shares birth years, age, location, and significant life events.

goal Specific aim or target that the unit wishes to attain within the time span of one year.

Good Samaritan laws Laws that have been enacted to protect the health care professional from legal liability for actions rendered in an emergency when the professional is giving service without pay.

grapevine An informal communication channel where information moves quickly and is often inaccurate.

Hawthorne effect   Term coined to reflect the findings of a research study that demonstrated that a change in employee behavior occurs as a result of being observed.

health   State of complete physical, social, and mental well-being, and not merely the absence of disease or infirmity.

health assets   Health-promoting attributes of individuals/families, communities, and systems.

health care systems disparities   Differences in health care system access and quality of care for different racial, ethnic, and socioeconomic population groups that persist across settings, clinical areas, age, gender, geography, health needs, and disabilities.

health determinants   Variables that include biological, psychosocial, environmental (physical and social), and health systems factors or etiologies that may cause changes in the health status of individuals, families, groups, populations, and communities. Health determinants may be assets (positive factors) or risks (negative factors).

health disparities   Differences in health risks and health status measures that reflect the poorer health status that is found disproportionately in certain population groups.

health literacy   Represents the cognitive and social skills that determine the motivation and ability of individuals to gain access to, understand, and use information in ways that promote and maintain good health.

health-related quality of life   Those aspects of life that are influenced either positively or negatively by one's health status and health risk factors.

health risk factors   Modifiable and nonmodifiable variables that increase or decrease the probability of illness or death; synonym is health determinants.

health status   Level of health of an individual, family, group, population, or community; the sum of existing health risk factors, level of wellness, existing diseases, functional health status, and quality of life.

high quality-of-work-life environments   A type of work environment in which the quality of the human experience in the workplace meets and surpasses employee expectations.

high-performance organizations   An organization that operates in a way that brings out the best in people and produces sustainable high performance over time.

indirect care   Time spent on activities that support patient care but are not done directly to the patient.

indirect expenses   Expenses that are referred to such items as utilities, such as gas, electric, and phones, that are not directly related to patient care.

indirect patient care activities   These are often necessary to support the patients and their environment, and only incidentally involve direct patient contact.

informal leader   Individual who demonstrates leadership outside the scope of a formal leadership role or as a member of a group, rather than as the head or leader of the group.

information power   Nurses who influence others with the information they provide to the group are using information power.

initiating structure   Style that involves an emphasis on the work to be done, a focus on the task and production.

innovation   Process of creating new services or products.

inpatient unit   Hospital unit that provides care to patients twenty-four hours a day, seven days a week.

instrumental activities of daily living   Activities related to food preparation and shopping; cleaning; laundry; home maintenance; verbal, written, and electronic communications; financial management; and transportation, as well as activities to meet social and support needs, manage health care needs, access community services and resources, and meet spiritual needs.

intellectual capital   An individual's knowledge, skills, and abilities that have value and portability in a knowledge economy.

interpersonal communication   Concerned with communication between individuals.

intrapersonal communication   Self-talk.

intuitive thinking   An innate feeling that nurses develop that helps them to act in certain situations.

job-centered leaders   Style that focuses on schedules, cost, and efficiency with less attention to developing work groups and high-performance goals.

job satisfaction   How organizational members feel about their job.

justice   The principle of fairness that is served when an individual is given that which he or she is due, owed, deserves, or can legitimately claim.

knowledge workers   Health care professionals who are well educated and technologically savvy and see themself as owning their intellectual capital.

laissez-faire leadership   Passive and permissive style in which the leader defers decision making.

leader-member relations   Feelings and attitudes of followers regarding acceptance, trust, and credibility of the leader.

leadership   Process of influence whereby the leader influences others toward goal achievement.

learner analysis   Process of identifying the learner's unique characteristics and needs.

learning domains   Taxonomies, or classifications, of learning.

learning organization   Learning organizations promote professional practice through the encouragement of personal mastery, an awareness of our mental models, and team learning.

learning style   Particular manner in which an individual responds to and processes learning.

legitimate power   Power derived from the position a nurse holds in a group; it indicates the nurse's degree of authority.

lesson plan   Document that provides the blueprint for the teaching session; it lists the objectives, topics, format, strategies, materials, and evaluation used in the teaching session.

living will   Document voluntarily signed by patients that specifies the type of care they desire if and when they are in a terminal state and cannot sign a consent form or convey this information verbally.

magnet hospitals   High-quality health care organizations that have met the rigorous nursing excellence requirements as determined by the American Nurses Credentialing Center (ANCC) and that are a supportive and collegial practice setting that incorporates principles of organizational behavior to achieve positive individual, group, and organizational outcomes.

maintenance or hygiene factors (Herzberg)   Elements such as salary, job security, working conditions, status, quality of supervision, and relationships with others that prevent job dissatisfaction.

malpractice   Professional's wrongful conduct in discharge of professional duties or failure to meet standards of care for the profession, which results in harm to another individual entrusted to the professional's care.

management   Process of coordinating actions and allocating resources to achieve organizational goals.

management process   Function of planning, organizing, coordinating, and controlling.

margin   Profit.

marginalization   Separation of a group away from the mainstream because of religious or cultural beliefs.

methodology   Structured, standardized approach for developing teaching.

mission   Call to live out something that matters or is meaningful; an organization's mission reflects the purpose and direction of the health care agency or a department within it.

mission statement   A formal expression of the purpose or reason for existence of the organization.

modular nursing   Care delivery model that is a kind of team nursing that divides a geographical space into modules of patients with each module having a team of staff led by an RN to care for them.

money market account   Similar to a bank checking account though it often requires a larger minimum amount of money to open the account and often has a higher interest rate for your money.

morality   Behavior in accordance with custom or tradition; usually reflects personal or religious beliefs.

motivation   Whatever influences our choices and creates direction, intensity, and persistence in our behavior.

motivation factors (Herzberg)   Elements such as achievement, recognition, responsibility, advancement, and the opportunity for development that all contribute to job satisfaction.

NCLEX   The national nursing licensure examination prepared under the supervision of the National Council of State Boards of Nursing.

negligence   Failure to provide the care a reasonable person would ordinarily provide in a similar situation.

nonmaleficence   The principle of doing no harm.

nonproductive hours   Paid time not devoted to patient care; includes benefit time such as vacation, sick time, and education time.

novice to expert model (by Benner) Provides a framework that when developed into a clinical or career promotion ladder, facilitates professional staff development by building on the skill sets and experience of each practitioner. Benner's model acknowledges that there are tasks, competencies, and outcomes that practitioners can be expected to have acquired based on five levels of experience: novice, advanced beginner, competent, proficient, and expert.

nursing-sensitive indicators Measures that reflect the outcome of nursing action.

nursing assistive personnel Unlicensed personnel to whom nursing tasks are delegated and who work in structured nursing organizations.

objective Measurable step that must be taken to reach a goal.

operational budget Account for the income and expenses associated with day-to-day activity within a department or organization.

open systems Entities that must interact with the environment to survive.

organizational change Planned change in an organization to generally improve efficiency.

organization A coordinated and deliberately structured social entity consisting of two or more individuals functioning on a relatively continuous basis to achieve a predetermined set of goals.

organizational behavior The study of human behavior in organizations.

organizational commitment How committed or loyal employees feel to the goals of the organization.

organizational effectiveness An organization's sustainable high performance in accomplishing its mission and objectives.

Pareto principle Principle, developed by Pareto, a 19th century economist, which states that 20% of focused effort results in 80% of outcome results, or conversely that 80% of unfocused effort results in 20% of results.

patient acuity Measure of nursing workload that is generated for each patient.

patient-centered care Care delivery model in which care and services are brought to the patient.

patient classification system (PCS) System for distinguishing among different patients based on their acuity, functional ability, or resource needs.

patient-focused care A model of differentiated nursing practice that emphasizes quality, cost, and value.

personal change Alteration made voluntarily for one's own reasons, usually for self-improvement.

philosophy Statement of beliefs based on core values and rational investigations of the truths and principles of knowledge, reality, and human conduct.

philosophy of an organization A value statement of the principles and beliefs that direct the organization's behavior.

physical health Encompasses nutrition and exercise coupled with a balanced amount of rest; health preventive behaviors such as avoiding smoking; and health screening behaviors that detect health problems early such as an annual Pap smear.

political voice An increase in the number of voices supporting or opposing an issue.

politics Process by which people use a variety of methods to achieve their goals.

population-based health care practice Development, provision, and evaluation of multidisciplinary health care services to population groups experiencing increased health risks or disparities, in partnership with health care consumers and the community in order to improve the health of the community and its diverse population groups.

population-based nursing practice Practice of nursing in which the focus of care is to improve the health status of vulnerable or at-risk population groups within the community by employing health promotion and disease prevention interventions across the health continuum.

position power Degree of formal authority and influence associated with the leader.

power Ability to create, get, and use resources to achieve one's goals.

power of attorney Legal document executed by an individual (principal) granting another person (agent) the right to perform certain activities in the principal's name.

practice guideline Descriptive tool or standardized specifications for care of the typical patient in the typical situation; these guidelines are developed by a formal process that incorporates the best scientific evidence of effectiveness and expert opinion. Synonyms or near synonyms include practice parameter, preferred practice pattern, algorithm, protocol, and clinical standard.

primary nursing   Care delivery model that clearly delineates the responsibility and accountability of the RN and places the RN as the primary provider of nursing care to patients.

problem solving   Active process which starts with a problem and ends with a solution.

process   Set of causes and conditions that repeatedly come together in a series of steps to transfer inputs into outcomes.

productivity   Quantity and quality of output an employee generates for an organization.

productive hours   Hours worked and available for patient care.

professional change   Alteration made in position or job such as obtaining education or credentials.

professional judgment   Intellectual (educated, informed) process that a nurse exercises in forming an opinion and reaching a clinical decision based upon an analysis of the available evidence.

profit   Determined by the relationship of income to expenses.

progressive discipline   System in which the manager and employee's mutual goal is to take steps to correct performance in order to bring it back to an acceptable level; it offers a stepwise process with opportunities for continued feedback and clarification of expectations.

protective factors   Patient strengths and resources that the patients can use to combat health threats that compromise core human functions.

psychomotor domain   Learning domain centered on skills, or what the learner does.

public law   General classification of law, consisting generally of constitutional, administrative, and criminal law. Public law defines a citizen's relationship with government.

quality assurance   Inspection approach to ensure that minimum standards of patient care quality are maintained in health care institutions.

quality improvement   Systematic process of organizationwide participation and partnership in planning and implementing continuous improvement methods to understand and meet or exceed customer needs and expectations.

quality of life   Level of satisfaction one has with the actual conditions of one's life, including satisfaction with socioeconomic status, education, occupation, home, family life, recreation, and the ability to enjoy life, freedom, and independence.

race   Geographical or global human population distinguished by genetic traits and physical characteristics such as skin color or facial features.

referent power   Power derived from how much others respect and like any individual, group, or organization.

reflective thinking   Watching or observing ourselves as we perform a task or make a decision about a certain situation.

resilience   The social and psychosocial capacity of individuals and groups to adapt, succeed, and persevere over time in the face of recurring threats to psychosocial and physiologic integrity.

resources   People, money, facilities, technology, and rights to properties, services, and technologies.

respect for others   Acknowledgement of the right of people to make their own decisions.

responsibility   Reliability, dependability, and the obligation to accomplish work when one accepts an assignment.

resume   Brief summary of your background, training, and experience as well as your qualifications for a position.

revenue   Income generated through a variety of means (for example, billable patient services, investments, and donations to the organization).

self-scheduling   Process in which staff on a unit collectively decide and implement the monthly work schedule.

sentinel event   Unexpected occurrence involving death or serious physical or psychological injury to a patient.

shared governance   Situation where nurses and managers work together to define their roles and expected outcomes, holding everyone accountable for their role and expected outcomes.

shift action plan Written plan based on a shift assessment that sets the priorities for the accomplishment of shift outcomes.

situational leadership A framework that maintains that there is no one best leadership style, but rather that effective leadership lies in matching the appropriate leadership style to the individual's or group's level of motivation and task-relevant readiness.

skill mix Percentage of RN staff compared to other direct care staff [LPNs and UAP].

sources of power Combination of conscious and unconscious factors that allow an individual to influence others to do as the individual wants.

spiritual distress A NANDA nursing diagnosis where an individual has an impaired ability to integrate meaning and purpose in life through the individual's connectedness with self, others, art, music, literature, nature, or a power greater than oneself.

staffing plan Plan that articulates how many and what kind of staff are needed, by shift and day, to staff a unit or department.

stakeholder Provider, employer, customer, patient, or payer who may have an interest in, and seek to influence, the decisions and actions of an organization.

stakeholders People or groups with an interest in the performance of the organization, for example, customers, competitors, suppliers, government, and regulatory agencies.

stakeholder assessment A systematic consideration of all potential stakeholders to ensure that the needs of each of these stakeholders are incorporated in the planning phase.

strategic plan The sum total or outcome of the processes by which an organization engages in environmental analysis, goal formulation, and strategy development with the purpose of organizational growth and renewal.

strategic planning A process that is designed to achieve goals in dynamic, competitive environments through the allocation of resources.

substitutes for leadership Variables that may influence or have an effect on followers to the same extent as the leader's behavior.

supervision Provision of guidance or direction, oversight evaluation, and followup by the licensed nurse for accomplishment of a nursing task delegated to UAP.

SWOT analysis A tool that is frequently used to conduct environmental assessments. SWOT stands for Strengths, Weaknesses, Opportunities, and Threats.

system Interdependent group of items, people, or processes with a common purpose.

task structure Involves the degree that work is defined, with specific procedures, explicit directions and goals.

taxonomy System that orders principles into a grouping or classification.

team Small number of people with complementary skills who are committed to a common purpose, performance goals, and approach for which they are mutually accountable.

team nursing Care delivery model that assigns staff to teams that then are responsible for a group of patients.

terminal objective Objective that identifies major behaviors that contribute to achievement of the overall session goal.

Theory X View that in bureaucratic organizations, employees prefer security, direction, and minimal responsibility; coercion, threats, or punishment are necessary because people do not like the work to be done.

Theory Y View that in the context of the right conditions, people enjoy their work, they can show self-control and discipline, are able to contribute creatively and are motivated by ties to the group, the organization, and the work itself; belief that people are intrinsically motivated by their work.

Theory Z View of collective decision making and a focus on long-term employment that involves slower promotions and less direct supervision.

time management Set of related common-sense skills that helps you use your time in the most effective and productive way possible.

tort A civil wrong for which a remedy may be obtained.

transformational leader Leader who is committed to a vision that empowers others.

turnover Number of employees who resigned divided by the total number of employees during the same time period.

values   Personal beliefs about the truth of ideals, standards, principles, objects, and behaviors that give meaning and direction to life.

variable costs   Costs that vary with volume and will increase or decrease depending on the number of patients.

variance   Difference between what was budgeted and the actual cost.

veracity   The obligation to tell the truth.

voting block   Group that represents the same political position or perspective.

whole systems shared governance   When the entire organization adopts an organizational structure based on the principles of partnership, equity, accountability, and ownership.

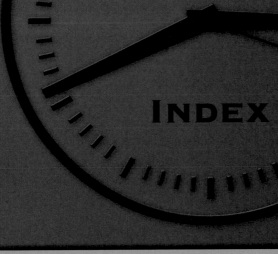

INDEX

H

M

S

T

U